a **LANGE** medical book

Basic and Clinical Pharmacology

Third Edition

Edited By

Bertram G. Katzung, MD, PhD

Professor of Pharmacology
Department of Pharmacology
University of California, San Francisco

**Appleton
&Lange**

Norwalk, Connecticut/Los Altos, California

Copyright © 1987 by Appleton & Lange
A Publishing Division of Prentice-Hall
Copyright © 1984, 1982 by Lange Medical Publications

Spanish Edition: Editorial El Manual Moderno. S.A. de C.V.,
Av. Sonora 206, Col. Hipodromo, 06100-Mexico, D.F.

87 88 89 90 / 10 9 8 7 6 5 4 3 2 1

Prentice-Hall of Australia, Pty. Ltd., Sydney
Prentice-Hall Canada, Inc.
Prentice-Hall Hispanoamericana, S.A., Mexico
Prentice-Hall of India Private Limited, New Delhi
Prentice-Hall International (UK) Limited, London
Prentice-Hall of Japan, Inc., Tokyo
Prentice-Hall of Southeast Asia (Pte.) Ltd., Singapore
Whitehall Books Ltd., Wellington, New Zealand
Editora Prentice-Hall do Brasil Ltda., Rio de Janeiro

Library of Congress Cataloging-in-Publication Data
Basic & clinical pharmacology.

"A Lange medical book."
Includes bibliographies and index.
1. Pharmacology. I. Katzung, Bertram G. II. Title.
Basic and clinical pharmacology. [DNLM: 1. Pharmacology.
QV 4 B3102]
RM300.B285   1987   615'.1   86-22352
ISBN 0-8385-0553-8

Cover: M. Chandler Martylewski

PRINTED IN THE UNITED STATES OF AMERICA

Table of Contents

Preface

This book is designed to serve as a complete textbook of pharmacology for students in the health sciences and for health practitioners. The guiding principle in its preparation has been that it should be both authoritative and readable. Each chapter provides current and concise coverage of both basic pharmacology and relevant aspects of clinical pharmacology.

Chapters are grouped to correspond to the organization of most survey courses: general principles; drugs acting on the autonomic nervous system, the cardiovascular system, and the kidneys; autacoids and respiratory drugs; central nervous system agents, including drugs of abuse; metabolic and endocrine agents; antimicrobial and antineoplastic chemotherapeutic agents; toxicology; and special topics. This organization allows students to learn the most general principles first, then apply these principles to the best-studied and -understood drug groups, and then go on to other groups in a logical fashion.

Within each chapter, the relationship between the basic pharmacology of the drugs and the pathophysiology of the diseases treated is made clear. The material is organized as follows: First the drug group is characterized on the basis of its major common features, including the receptors and the diseases involved. If a prototype drug for the group exists, it is described. Next, the chemistry and pharmacokinetics of the group are discussed. The presentation of the basic material is completed with a thorough discussion of the mechanism of action and major cellular and organ level effects of the group. The clinical applications of the group are then succinctly described. Too often, texts emphasize the basic pharmacology of drugs without placing them in clinical perspective, thus preventing students from relating their basic science knowledge to their clinical experience.

The third edition has been substantially revised and includes the following new features:

- A new chapter on *Principles of Toxicology*. This chapter covers the basic principles of toxicology and provides an up-to-date description of industrial and environmental toxicology.

- A new chapter on *Geriatric Pharmacology*. This chapter covers the special aspects of drug treatment of the elderly, including changes in drug disposition and drug responsiveness.

- Adoption of the international convention for naming autonomic receptors.

- In the chapter on prescription writing, a section on "unlabeled" uses of drugs that describes uses which are legitimate even though not approved by the FDA.

Finally, every chapter has been carefully updated and revised to ensure that it is the most current and useful source of information available on the topic.

Students and instructors may be interested in the accompanying study guide: *Pharmacology: A Review* (Lange, 1985). This book may be used as a syllabus for regular pharmacology courses or for independent preparation for examinations.

I am pleased to note that the Spanish language edition of *Basic & Clinical Pharmacology* has been well received and that translations into French, Indonesian, Italian, and Portuguese are under way. I also wish to acknowledge the continuing expert assistance of the staff at Lange Medical Publications, whose contributions are greatly appreciated.

Suggestions and comments about *Basic & Clinical Pharmacology* should be sent to me at the Department of Pharmacology, 1210-S, University of California, San Francisco, CA 94143.

Bertram G. Katzung, MD, PhD

San Francisco
October, 1986

The Authors

David F. Altman, MD
Associate Clinical Professor of Medicine, Department of Medicine, University of California, San Francisco.

Michael J. Aminoff, MD, FRCP
Professor of Neurology, Department of Neurology, University of California, San Francisco.

J. Desmond Baggot, MVM, MRCVS, PhD, DSc
Professor of Veterinary Pharmacology, School of Veterinary Medicine, and Chairman, Department of Veterinary Pharmacology and Toxicology, University of California, Davis, California.

Steven L. Barriere, PharmD
Specialist in Infectious Diseases, Department of Pharmaceutical Services; Adjunct Associate Professor of Medicine, Division of Infectious Diseases, University of California Medical Center, Los Angeles.

Charles E. Becker, MD
Professor of Medicine, Department of Medicine, University of California, San Francisco.

Leslie Z. Benet, PhD
Professor and Chairman, Department of Pharmacy, School of Pharmacy, University of California, San Francisco.

Neal L. Benowitz, MD
Associate Professor of Medicine and Clinical Pharmacology, Department of Medicine, University of California, San Francisco.

Barry A. Berkowitz, PhD
Vice President, Biological Sciences and Biopharmaceutical Research and Development, Smith Kline & French Laboratories, Philadelphia.

Daniel D. Bikle, MD, PhD
Assistant Professor of Medicine, Department of Medicine, and Co-Director, Special Diagnostic and Treatment Unit, University of California, San Francisco, and Veterans Administration Medical Center, San Francisco.

Henry R. Bourne, MD
Professor of Pharmacology and Medicine, Departments of Pharmacology and Medicine, and Chairman, Department of Pharmacology, University of California, San Francisco.

Homer A. Boushey
Associate Professor of Medicine, Department of Medicine, University of California, San Francisco.

Alan Burkhalter, PhD
Professor of Pharmacology, Department of Pharmacology, University of California, San Francisco.

Neal Castagnoli, Jr., PhD
Professor of Chemistry and Pharmaceutical Chemistry, Department of Pharmaceutical Chemistry, University of California, San Francisco.

Kanu Chatterjee, MB, FRCP
Lucie Stern Professor of Cardiology, Professor of Medicine, Cardiology Division, Department of Medicine, University of California, San Francisco.

Martin S. Cohen, MD
Director of Pediatrics, Scenic General Hospital, Modesto, California.

Maria Almira Correia, PhD
Associate Professor of Pharmacology, Department of Pharmacology, University of California, San Francisco.

Betty J. Dong, PharmD
Associate Clinical Professor of Pharmacy, Division of Clinical Pharmacy, University of California, San Francisco.

Oscar L. Frick, MD, PhD
Professor of Pediatrics, Department of Pediatrics, University of California, San Francisco.

Alan Goldfien, MD
Professor of Medicine, Departments of Medicine, Obstetrics, Gynecology, and Reproductive Sciences, and Cardiovascular Research Institute, University of California, San Francisco.

Robert S. Goldsmith, MD, DTM&H
Professor of Tropical Medicine and Epidemiology, Department of Epidemiology and International Health, University of California, San Francisco.

Marc E. Goldyne, MD, PhD
Associate Professor in Residence, Dermatology and Medicine, Department of Dermatology and Medicine, University of California, San Francisco, and Assistant Chief, Department of Dermatology, Veterans Administration Medical Center, San Francisco.

Francis S. Greenspan, MD
Clinical Professor of Medicine and Radiology, Department of Medicine, and Chief, Thyroid Clinic, University of California, San Francisco.

Philip D. Hansten, PharmD
Professor of Clinical Pharmacy, Department of Pharmacy, Washington State University College of Pharmacy, Pullman, Washington.

Brian B. Hoffman, MD
Assistant Professor of Medicine and Pharmacology, Stanford University School of Medicine, Stanford, California, and Veterans Administration Medical Center, Palo Alto, California.

Nicholas H.G. Holford, MB, ChB, MSc, MRCP (UK), FRACP
Senior Lecturer, Departments of Pharmacology and Clinical Pharmacology, University of Auckland Medical School, Auckland, New Zealand.

Leo E. Hollister, MD
Professor of Medicine and Psychiatry, Stanford University School of Medicine, and Senior Medical Investigator, Veterans Administration Hospital, Palo Alto, California.

Michael J. Holtzman, MD
Cardiovascular Research Institute and Department of Medicine, University of California, San Francisco.

Luc M. Hondeghem, MD, PhD
Associate Professor of Pharmacology, Department of Pharmacology, University of California, San Francisco.

Ernest Jawetz, MD, PhD
Professor of Microbiology and Medicine Emeritus, Department of Microbiology, University of California, San Francisco.

John P. Kane, MD, PhD
Professor of Medicine, Department of Medicine, University of California, San Francisco.

John H. Karam, MD
Professor of Medicine in Residence, Metabolic Research Unit, University of California, San Francisco.

Bertram G. Katzung, MD, PhD
Professor of Pharmacology, Department of Pharmacology, University of California, San Francisco.

Mary Anne Koda-Kimble, PharmD
Clinical Professor of Pharmacy, Division of Clinical Pharmacy, School of Pharmacy, University of California, San Francisco.

David C. Klonoff, MD
Clinical Instructor in Medicine, Department of Medicine, University of California, San Francisco.

Nancy M. Lee, PhD
Adjunct Associate Professor, Department of Pharmacology, University of California, San Francisco.

Paul W. Lofholm, PharmD
Associate Clinical Professor of Pharmacy, School of Pharmacy, University of California, San Francisco.

Lisa A. Lybecker, PharmD
Adjunct Assistant Professor, Department of Family and Community Medicine, and Assistant Professor of Clinical Pharmacy, Department of Pharmacy Practice, University of Utah, Salt Lake City.

Howard I. Maibach, MD
Professor of Dermatology, Department of Dermatology, University of California, San Francisco.

Mary J. Malloy, MD
Clinical Professor of Pediatrics and Medicine, Departments of Pediatrics and Medicine, University of California, San Francisco.

Jay W. Mason, MD
Professor of Internal Medicine, and Chief, Division of Cardiology, University of Utah College of Medicine, Salt Lake City.

Ronald D. Miller, MD
Professor and Chairman of Anesthesia and Professor of Pharmacology, Department of Anesthesia, University of California, San Francisco.

John Mills, MD
Associate Professor of Medicine, Microbiology, and Clinical Pharmacy, University of California, San Francisco, and Chief, Infectious Disease Unit, San Francisco General Hospital, San Francisco.

Roger A. Nicoll, MD
Professor of Pharmacology and Physiology, Department of Pharmacology, University of California, San Francisco.

Kent R. Olson, MD
Director, San Francisco Bay Area Regional Poison Center, San Francisco General Hospital, Attending Emergency Physician, Eden Hospital, Castro Valley, California, and Assistant Chief, Emergency Medicine, Highland Hospital, Oakland, California.

Robert A. O'Reilly, MD
Chairman, Department of Medicine, Santa Clara Valley Medical Center, Professor of Medicine, Stanford University School of Medicine, and Clinical Professor of Medicine, Department of Medicine, University of California, San Francisco.

William W. Parmley, MD
Professor of Medicine, Department of Medicine, Cardiology Division, University of California, San Francisco, and Chief of Cardiology, H. C. Moffitt Hospital, San Francisco.

William H. Pitlick, PhD
Deputy Director, Convulsive, Developmental, and Neuromuscular Disorders Program, National Institutes of Health, Bethesda, Maryland.

Gabriel L. Plaa, PhD
Professor de Pharmacologie, Département de Pharmacologie, Faculté de Médecine, Université de Montréal, Montréal.

Roger J. Porter, MD
Chief, Medical Neurology Branch, National Institutes of Health, Bethesda, Maryland, Clinical Professor of Neurology and Adjunct Professor of Pharmacology, Uniformed Services University of the Health Sciences, Bethesda, Maryland, and Consultant-Lecturer in Neurology, National Naval Medical Center, Bethesda, Maryland.

Ian A. Reid, PhD
Professor of Physiology, Department of Physiology, University of California, San Francisco.

Curt A. Ries, MD
Clinical Professor of Medicine and Hematology-Oncology, Department of Medicine, University of California, San Francisco.

James M. Roberts, MD
Professor of Obstetrics and Gynecology and Reproductive Sciences, Department of Obstetrics and Gynecology, and Senior Staff, Cardiovascular Research Institute, University of California, San Francisco.

Dirk B. Robertson, MD
Assistant Professor of Dermatology, Department of Dermatology, Emory University School of Medicine, Atlanta.

Sydney E. Salmon, MD
Professor of Medicine (Hematology-Oncology), Department of Internal Medicine, and Director, Arizona Cancer Center, University of Arizona College of Medicine, Tucson.

Daniel V. Santi, MD, PhD
Professor of Biochemistry and Pharmaceutical Chemistry, Department of Biochemistry and Biophysics and Pharmaceutical Chemistry, University of California, San Francisco.

Alan C. Sartorelli, PhD
Professor, Department of Pharmacology, and Director, Comprehensive Cancer Center, Yale University School of Medicine, New Haven, Connecticut.

Martin A. Shearn, MD
Clinical Professor of Medicine, Department of Medicine, University of California, San Francisco.

Anthony Trevor, PhD
Professor of Pharmacology and Toxicology, Department of Pharmacology, University of California, San Francisco.

Ching Chung Wang, PhD
Professor of Pharmaceutical Chemistry, Department of Pharmaceutical Chemistry, University of California, San Francisco.

David G. Warnock, MD
Associate Professor of Medicine and Pharmacology in Residence, Departments of Medicine and Pharmacology, University of California, San Francisco, and Chief, Nephrology Section, Veterans Administration Medical Center, San Francisco.

August M. Watanabe, MD
Professor of Medicine and Pharmacology, and Chairman, Department of Medicine, Indiana University School of Medicine, Indianapolis.

E. Leong Way, PhD
Professor of Pharmacology and Toxicology, Department of Pharmacology, University of California, San Francisco.

Walter L. Way, MD
Professor of Anesthesia and Pharmacology, Department of Anesthesia, University of California, San Francisco.

Introduction

Bertram G. Katzung, MD, PhD

Pharmacology can be broadly defined as the science dealing with interactions between living systems and molecules, especially chemicals introduced from outside the system. This definition thus includes **medical pharmacology**—the science of materials used to prevent, diagnose, and treat disease—as well as the important role played by chemicals in the environment that *cause* disease and the use of certain chemicals as molecular probes for the study of normal biochemistry and physiology. **Toxicology** is that branch of pharmacology that deals with the undesirable effects of chemicals in biologic systems.

What is or is not a **drug** can be broadly or narrowly defined. For our purposes, a drug will be any small molecule that, when introduced into the body, alters the body's function by interactions at the molecular level. There is clearly some overlap with endocrinology in this definition. This is as it should be, since hormones are properly considered drugs whether introduced from outside the body ("exogenous") in any amount or released internally in increased amounts by administration of a stimulant agent. Poisons are drugs whether administered with criminal or suicidal intent or encountered inadvertently in the environment.

Drugs vary in molecular size. Molecules as small as carbon monoxide and lithium ion and as large as thrombolytic enzymes fall within the above functional definition. However, the great majority of drugs fall into the molecular weight range of 100–1000. There is a reason for this: As noted below, a drug is often introduced for practical reasons into a part of the body remote from the target tissue. To be absorbed and distributed to the target organ, the drug molecule must be capable of diffusion (or transport by carrier mechanisms). With some exceptions, molecules within the narrow range of MW 100–1000 are capable of convenient administration and efficient absorption and distribution.

Drugs also vary in their chemical nature. On the one hand, there are highly reactive alkylating agents such as mechlorethamine; on the other, "inert" anesthetic gases such as xenon. The various classes of organic compounds—carbohydrates, proteins, and lipids—are all represented. Many drugs are weak acids or weak bases. This fact has important implications for the way they are handled by the body, since the pH differences between different compartments of the body may alter the degree of ionization of such compounds (see below).

Drug-Body Interactions

The interactions between a drug and the biologic system are conveniently divided into 2 classes: **pharmacodynamic** interactions, the effects of the drug on the body; and **pharmacokinetic** interactions, the way in which the body handles the drug. The quantitative aspects of pharmacodynamics—the drug receptor concept and dose-response relationships—are discussed in Chapter 2. The principles of pharmacokinetics—absorption, distribution, metabolism, and excretion—are presented in Chapter 3. Some of the introductory concepts used in discussing these interactions are presented in this chapter.

Drug Permeation

As noted above, movements of drug molecules—into the body from the site of administration (absorption), between different parts of the body (distribution), and out of the body (excretion)—are important characteristics of any useful therapeutic agent. Because the body is protected from the outside world and is itself internally compartmentalized by membrane barriers to the free movement of water and solute, permeation of drug molecules across membranes plays a role in all 3 of these processes.

There are 4 major mechanisms by which drugs move across barriers.

A. Aqueous Diffusion: This is a pathway of limited capacity across most barriers, eg, the epithelial lining of the surfaces of the body, such as the cornea, gut, and bladder. Because these cells are connected by tight junctions, only molecules small enough (less than MW 100–150, eg, Li^+, methanol) to pass through very small aqueous pores permeate these barriers by the aqueous route. In contrast, most capillaries have very large pores between cells that allow molecules as large as MW 20,000–30,000 to pass. The capillaries of most of the brain lack these pores, but they are found in a few areas of the central nervous system: the pituitary gland, the pineal gland, the median eminence, the area postrema, and the choroid plexus.

B. Lipid Diffusion: Movement across cell membranes by solution in the lipids of the membrane, with passive transfer across the lipid driven by a concentration gradient, is one of the most important mechanisms of drug permeation. Obviously, a high degree of lipid solubility relative to aqueous solubility (often quantitated as the octanol/water or olive oil/water partition coefficient) will favor this mode of permeation. However, since drugs must first be in aqueous solution to gain access to the lipid membrane, too low a level of water solubility is undesirable.

A great many drugs are weak acids or weak bases. Such molecules are relatively *more water-soluble when ionized (polar) and more lipid-soluble when un-ionized*. The pH of the environment will determine the degree of ionization of weak acids and bases according to the Henderson-Hasselbalch equation ("protonated" = combined with a proton, H^+):

$$\log \left(\frac{\text{Protonated form}}{\text{Unprotonated form}} \right) = pK_a - pH \quad \ldots (1)$$

For weak acids, eg, phenobarbital,

$$HA \rightleftharpoons H^+ + A^- \qquad \ldots (2)$$

The pK_a of phenobarbital is 7.4 (Table 1–1). Therefore, if phenobarbital is being excreted in an acid urine, more of the drug will be protonated (un-ionized) and readily reabsorbable by permeation across the lipid membranes of renal tubular cells. In an alkaline urine, more of the drug will be dissociated (ionized), poorly soluble in lipid, and more rapidly excreted. The magnitude of this effect can be estimated by applying the Henderson-Hasselbalch equation (equation 1):

For pH 6.4:

$$\log \left(\frac{HA}{A^-} \right) = 7.4 - 6.4 = 1$$

antilog $(1) = 10$

Therefore, the ratio of readily reabsorbed (protonated) to poorly reabsorbed (dissociated) phenobarbital is 10 when the urine pH is 6.4.

For pH 8.0:

$$\log \left(\frac{HA}{A^-} \right) = 7.4 - 8.0 = -0.6$$

antilog $(-0.6) = 0.25$

Therefore, in alkaline urine, most of the phenobarbital is dissociated (charged) and therefore readily excreted. In treating a patient who has taken an overdose of phenobarbital, alkalinizing the urine is one method of hastening elimination of the drug.

For weak bases, eg, pyrimethamine, an antimalaria drug:

$$H^+ + RNH_2 \rightleftharpoons RN^+H_3 \qquad \ldots (3)$$

and, as before,

$$\log \left(\frac{\text{Protonated form}}{\text{Unprotonated form}} \right) = pK_a - pH \quad \ldots (1)$$

The pK_a of pyrimethamine is 7.0 (Table 1–1). Therefore, at pH 8.0, the ratio of the protonated to the unprotonated form is 0.1; at pH 7.0, the ratio is 1; and at pH 6 it is 10. However, the protonated form of a base is the ionized, poorly lipid-soluble form. Thus, in contrast to phenobarbital, more of the pyrimethamine is in the more lipid-soluble form in alkaline environments than in acid ones.

Most weak bases used in pharmacology are substituted amines. Because the nitrogen atom can form bonds with one, 2, 3, or 4 carbon atoms, we can speak of primary, secondary, tertiary, and quaternary amines. Pyrimethamine is a primary amine, since only one of the nitrogen bonds is to a carbon atom. Secondary and tertiary amines can also acquire a proton and become charged, as in the example given above. Quaternary amines, on the other hand, are permanently charged, since the carbon-nitrogen bond is not subject to change by physiologic pH alterations.

The degree of ionization of weak electrolytes is not the only factor that influences its lipid solubility, but it is especially important in those body compartments in which the pH may change. For instance, the gastric pH may vary between 1.5 and 7 and the pH of the urine between 5.5 and 8. For drugs that have moderately high lipid solubility in the un-ionized form (and that therefore permeate very readily), changes of pH of this magnitude can have considerable clinical significance. For example, phenobarbital is cleared 7 times more rapidly into alkaline urine than into acid urine. Mecamylamine, an antihypertensive drug and a weak base, is cleared almost 80 times more rapidly into acidic than into alkaline urine.

In contrast, the clearance of some weak acids and bases is not significantly influenced by urine pH. An example is penicillin, which is very water-soluble in both ionized and un-ionized forms and is, therefore, cleared very rapidly regardless of urine pH.

C. Via Special Carriers (Facilitated Diffusion): A few classes of drugs are transported by special carriers in the membranes of cells. Such carriers include those for amino acids in the "blood-brain barrier" and those for weak acids in the proximal convoluted tubule of the kidney.

D. Pinocytosis (Receptor-Mediated Endocytosis): Drugs of exceptionally large size (over MW 1000) enter cells primarily by pinocytosis—the process of engulfing extracellular material within membrane vesicles. This is of importance for some drugs, most of them polypeptides.

Factors Influencing Permeation

For most mechanisms of permeation, the rate of drug transfer is a function of the surface area available for transfer and, in the case of a passive process, of the concentration gradient driving it. Thus, transfer across the lipid barrier of organs with very large surface areas (lung, small intestine) is usually much faster than across small areas (stomach). The concentration gradient depends upon processes on both sides of the membrane. In a typical example of drug absorption from a

Table 1–1. Ionization constants of some common drugs.

Drug	pK$_a$*	Drug	pK$_a$*	Drug	pK$_a$*
Weak acids		**Weak bases (cont'd)**		**Weak bases (cont'd)**	
Acetaminophen	9.5	Amiloride	8.7	Methadone	8.4
Acetazolamide	7.2	Amphetamine	9.8	Methamphetamine	10.0
Ampicillin	2.5	Atropine	9.7	Methyldopa	10.6
Aspirin	3.5	Bupivacaine	8.1	Methysergide	6.6
Chlorothiazide	6.8, 9.4†	Chlordiazepoxide	4.6	Metoprolol	9.8
Chlorpropamide	5.0	Chloroquine	10.8, 8.4†	Morphine	7.9
Cromolyn	2.0	Chlorpheniramine	9.2	Nicotine	7.9, 3.1†
Ethacrynic acid	3.5	Chlorpromazine	9.3	Norepinephrine	8.6
Furosemide	3.9	Clonidine	8.3	Pentazocine	9.7
Ibuprofen	4.4, 5.2†	Cocaine	8.5	Phenylephrine	9.8
Levodopa	2.3	Codeine	8.2	Physostigmine	7.9, 1.8†
Methotrexate	4.8	Cyclizine	8.2	Pilocarpine	6.9, 1.4†
Methyldopa	2.2, 9.2†	Desipramine	10.2	Pindolol	8.8
Penicillamine	1.8	Diazepam	3.3	Procainamide	9.2
Pentobarbital	8.1	Dihydrocodeine	8.8	Procaine	9.0
Phenobarbital	7.4	Diphenhydramine	9.0	Promazine	9.4
Phenytoin	8.3	Diphenoxylate	7.1	Promethazine	9.1
Propylthiouracil	8.3	Ephedrine	9.6	Propranolol	9.4
Salicylic acid	3.0	Epinephrine	8.7	Pseudoephedrine	9.8
Sulfadiazine	6.5	Ergotamine	6.3	Pyrimethamine	7.0
Sulfapyridine	8.4	Fluphenazine	8.0, 3.9†	Quinidine	8.5, 4.4†
Theophylline	8.8†	Guanethidine	11.4, 8.3†	Scopolamine	8.1
Tolbutamide	5.3	Hydralazine	7.1	Strychnine	8.0, 2.3†
Warfarin	5.0	Imipramine	9.5	Terbutaline	10.1
Weak bases		Isoproterenol	8.6	Thioridazine	9.5
Albuterol (salbutamol)	9.3	Kanamycin	7.2	Tolazoline	10.6
Allopurinol	9.4, 12.3†	Lidocaine	7.9		
Alprenolol	9.6	Metaraminol	8.6		

*The pK$_a$ is that pH at which the concentrations of the ionized and un-ionized forms are equal.
†More than one ionizable group.

site of subcutaneous administration, the amount of drug administered will determine the concentration on one side (the gradient source). The rate of removal of drug will determine the concentration on the other side (the gradient sink). Thus, a high blood flow will rapidly replace blood in which drug has dissolved with blood containing no drug, thereby maintaining a high concentration gradient. Vasodilator substances are typically absorbed very rapidly because they increase blood flow, whereas vasoconstrictor drugs are absorbed more slowly because they decrease flow.

Absorption of Drug Into the Body

Use of a drug almost always involves transfer of the agent into the bloodstream. Exceptions include topical application for local effect on the skin or mucous membranes and oral administration of drugs that act from within the intestinal lumen such as antacids and some laxatives. However, even when the site of therapeutic action is in one of these locations, absorption into the bloodstream may occur and may have undesirable effects.

In addition to the factors described above that affect drug permeation, absorption into the blood is significantly influenced by the **route of administration.** In addition to the intravenous route, which bypasses the absorption process, the important routes of administration are oral, inhalational, topical, transdermal,

subcutaneous, intramuscular, and buccal (sublingual). Less commonly, the intra-arterial, intrathecal, and rectal routes may be used.

The **oral route** is most commonly used because of its convenience and, for most drugs, efficiency of absorption. The large surface area of the gastrointestinal tract, the mixing of its contents, and the differences in pH at different levels favor effective absorption of drugs given in this way. However, the acid and enzymes secreted by the patient and the biochemical activity of the resident microbiologic flora also have the capacity to destroy some drugs before they are absorbed. Some penicillins are ineffective when given orally because they are rapidly inactivated by gastric acid. Polypeptide hormones such as insulin are hydrolyzed in the intestine and therefore must be given **parenterally** (by a nongastrointestinal route).

Because the gut is lined by epithelium with tight junctions, absorption of most drugs is by lipid diffusion. Thus, the basic rules of lipid permeation described above apply.

The **inhalational route** of administration, in addition to its obvious role in the use of gaseous anesthetics and other therapeutic gases, can be used for pharmacologic agents that vaporize readily, eg, amyl nitrite, and for drugs that can be dispersed in an aerosol of fine aqueous droplets, eg, certain ergot derivatives. Because of the very large surface area of the alveolar membrane and the high blood flow through the lungs, therapeutic gases of suitable solubility characteristics are rapidly absorbed from the lungs.

The airway itself is an important target of drugs used in asthma; the use of aerosols for delivery to the bronchi constitutes a type of topical adminstration.

The **topical route** includes application, for local effect, to the skin, the eye, the nose and throat, and the vaginal surface. (Drugs are occasionally used topically in the rectum for their anti-inflammatory effect. More often, the rectal route is used as an alternative to oral adminstration, for systemic effects.) The **transdermal route** utilizes application of drugs to the skin for systemic effects. Prolonged blood levels of some drugs can be achieved by this method because they are slowly absorbed. The skin constitutes a multilayered lipid barrier with special pharmacokinetic features as discussed in Chapter 65. The basic principles of lipid permeation apply to the skin and to the other body surfaces mentioned above.

The **buccal route** is an important one for drugs that must be self-administered but are too rapidly inactivated by the liver to be useful after ingestion. Some drugs are so rapidly metabolized by the liver that when absorbed from the stomach and small intestine into the portal circulation they are more than 90% inactivated before reaching the systemic circulation. Blood flow through the buccal mucosa is high, and venous drainage is into systemic veins, not the portal circulation. Therefore, drugs such as nitroglycerin are effective in much lower dosage when placed under the tongue than when swallowed.

When drugs must be given by **injection,** several options are available. The **intravenous route** is the most direct and bypasses the absorption barriers. It is also the most hazardous, because a very high concentration of drug is delivered to the target organs very rapidly. Drugs in aqueous solution injected **intramuscularly** are often absorbed fairly rapidly. "Depot" injections of drug dissolved in oil can be used to provide a slowly absorbed reservoir of drug. Some formulations provide significant levels of drug for weeks after a single injection. Some drugs cannot be given by this route because they cause pain and tissue damage at the site of injection. **Subcutaneously** injected drugs are usually more slowly absorbed. Irritating substances are particularly painful when given by this route, and large volumes are not feasible unless they contain hyaluronidase, an enzyme that facilitates the spread of the injected solution through the tissue.

Special routes of adminstration are also available or under development for producing high local concentrations of toxic agents and for long-term therapy of chronic conditions. To achieve a high local concentration of a chemotherapeutic or antibacterial drug, **intra-arterial** or **intrathecal** injections can be given for acute or intermittent treatment. If continuous therapy is required, reservoirs of drug together with the necessary intra-arterial or intrathecal catheter can be surgically implanted near the target organ. These techniques permit the use of much higher concentrations of drug in the target tissue than can be tolerated by the rest of the body. Long-term therapy with drugs that must normally be injected, eg, insulin, can also be carried out with implantable reservoirs. Such reservoirs may be equipped with radiofrequency-controlled pumps to permit regulation of the rate of infusion. However, at the present time, such devices appear to offer little or no advantage over traditional intermittent injection techniques.

Distribution of Drug Within the Body

Once a drug has been absorbed into the blood, it may be distributed to different physical compartments of the body (Table 1–2). If avidly bound to plasma proteins, it may remain in the vascular compartment until eliminated. Small water-soluble molecules may be freely distributed in the total body water. Drugs that are highly lipid-soluble (eg, DDT) are ultimately distributed to fat. Drugs that are not tightly bound to cells or proteins within the blood leave the vascular compartment, at a rate and to an extent governed by the permeability principles outlined above. Certain ions, especially the heavy metals and fluoride, are slowly sequestered in bone (Table 1–2).

Such compartments of the body, since they constitute actual physical entities, may be considered *real* volumes of potential distribution. However, many drugs are not simply dissolved in these volumes but bind to cell surfaces and intercellular macromolecules. If the volume in which a drug is dissolved is computed by dividing the total amount of drug present by the measured concentration, the *apparent* volume of distribution is obtained. Because some drugs are almost 100% bound by tissue structures, leaving only a small amount in solution, the apparent volume of distribution may be extremely large—much larger than the total volume of the body (Chapter 3, Part I). Although the apparent volume of distribution is obviously an abstract rather than a real entity, it is nevertheless more useful than the real volume of distribution for purposes of pharmacokinetic calculation.

The most important of the factors that determine drug distribution are protein binding, blood flow, membrane permeation, and tissue solubility.

Table 1–2. Physical volumes (in L/kg) of examples of body compartments into which drugs may be distributed.

Compartment and Volume	Examples
Total body water (0.6 L/kg*)	Small water-soluble molecules: eg, ethanol.
Extracellular water (0.2 L/kg)	Larger water-soluble molecules: eg, mannitol.
Blood (0.08 L/kg); plasma (0.04 L/kg)	Strongly plasma protein–bound molecules and very large molecules: eg, heparin.
Fat (0.2–0.35 L/kg)	Highly lipid-soluble molecules: eg, DDT.
Bone (0.07 L/kg)	Certain ions: eg, lead, fluoride.

*An average figure. Total body water in a young lean male might be 0.7 L/kg; in an obese woman, 0.5 L/kg.

In the blood, drugs may bind to albumin and several other serum proteins. The degree to which this occurs is usually measured as the percentage of total drug in the blood that is not dialyzable, ie, bound to large molecules (Table 3–1). Binding sites on these molecules are sometimes referred to as **inert binding sites** to differentiate them from **receptor binding sites,** since binding to albumin brings about no specific pharmacologic response, whereas (by definition) binding to the drug receptor alters the function of the cell that contains the receptor site. Binding to nonreceptor proteins also takes place outside the vascular compartment and may account for a significant fraction of the total drug in the body.

Drug molecules bound to inert binding sites are not available for diffusion or interaction with receptors. They are, however, in equilibrium with free drug, so that alterations in the concentration of free drug will result in changes in the amount (but not the percentage) bound.

Nonreceptor protein binding sites are not very specific—eg, many weak acids with different pharmacologic effects bind to the same or closely related plasma protein sites. Therefore, different drugs may compete for the same binding sites. This can have important consequences if a high percentage of a potent drug ("A") is bound, since the binding sites must be loaded to achieve a therapeutic concentration of free drug in the plasma. Addition of a second drug ("B") that competes for the same inert binding site (but not the receptor site) may cause a marked increase in the concentration of free "A" and thus precipitate toxicity. This and other types of pharmacokinetic drug interaction are described in Appendix I.

Blood flow determines how rapidly drug molecules are delivered to a given tissue and how effectively the concentration gradient between blood and tissue is maintained. Therefore, drugs equilibrate rapidly between the blood and organs with a high blood flow (Table 1–3). If the drug is very soluble or bound in the cells of these organs—eg, lipid-soluble drugs in the brain—then a very high concentration may be achieved at the steady state. Conversely, if an organ is sufficiently massive, eg, skeletal muscle, large amounts of drug may be distributed to it without ever reaching a very high concentration.

Table 1–3. Blood flow to some important tissues of the body (based on a 70-kg human).

Tissue	Mass (kg)	Blood Flow (mL/min)	Flow (Percent of Cardiac Output)
Brain	1.4	750	13.9
Heart	0.3	250	4.7
Liver	2.9	1500	27.8
Kidneys	0.3	1260	23.3
Skeletal muscle	34.4	840	15.6
Skin	4.0	462	8.6
Placenta and fetus (term)	3.8	500	9
Whole body	70	5400	100

Elimination of Drugs From the Body & Termination of Drug Effect

Termination of drug effect is sometimes dependent upon excretion from the body. More commonly, termination of effect is the result of **biotransformation** to inactive products that are then excreted. A few drugs are given in a pharmacologically inactive ("prodrug") form and metabolized into another form that is pharmacologically active. Therefore, drug excretion and drug metabolism must be considered separately, as in Chapter 3.

The major organs for drug excretion are the kidneys, the liver, the gastrointestinal tract, and the lungs. Other minor routes of drug excretion are sweat and milk.

A. Kidneys: Drugs may be excreted by the kidneys by 2 processes, glomerular filtration and tubular secretion, and reabsorbed usually by passive diffusion. Glomerular filtration is a passive, nonsaturable process that removes molecules up to the size of small proteins. Therefore, drugs that are effectively bound to plasma protein are poorly filtered; and conversely, drugs that are not bound are cleared from the blood at a rate approximately equal to creatinine clearance (Chapter 3, Part I). Some drugs are actively secreted by special mechanisms located in the mid segment of the proximal convoluted tubule. Drugs that are weak acids, including many diuretic drugs, are secreted in this manner and may compete with endogenous acids such as uric acid for the carrier. Active secretion is a saturable process.

Once in the tubular urine, the drug is exposed to the lipid membrane of the nephron; highly lipid-soluble molecules will be rapidly reabsorbed; more water-soluble ones are likely to be excreted. Metabolism of many drugs results in a less lipid-soluble product (Chapter 3, Part II); such metabolites are less likely than the parent drug to be reabsorbed from the tubular lumen.

B. Liver: The liver is the most important organ for drug metabolism. Bile may contain higher concentrations of metabolites than of the parent molecule, especially if the metabolite is sufficiently polar to be reabsorbed poorly from bile. A few drugs appear to be actively secreted into the bile, eg, certain cardiac glycosides, antibiotics, and quaternary ammonium cholinergic blocking agents.

Drugs and their metabolites that are secreted into bile are carried by the biliary ducts and the common duct to the duodenum. Some drug may then be absorbed from the lumen of the intestine and appear again unchanged in the blood. This recycling of drug is termed **enterohepatic circulation.**

C. Gastrointestinal Tract: The walls of the stomach and intestines constitute large lipid membranes across which drugs can be transferred from blood to lumen. This passive diffusion is occasionally of importance when a weakly basic drug is present in very high concentration in the blood, eg, after self-administration of a large dose of morphine. Any morphine that diffuses into the acidic environment of the

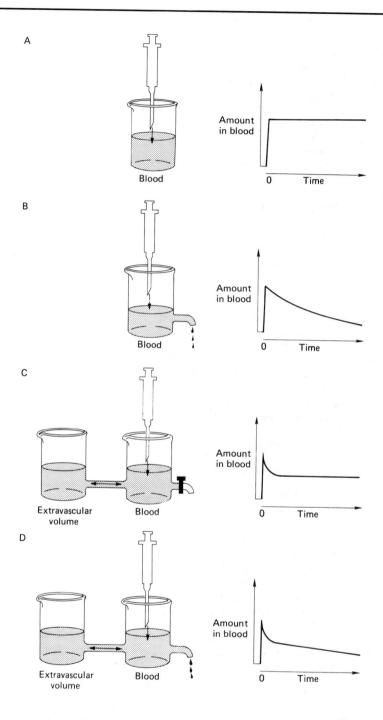

Figure 1–1. Models of drug distribution and elimination. The effect of adding drug to the blood by rapid intravenous injection is represented by expelling a known amount of the agent into a beaker. The time course of the amount of drug in the beaker is shown in the graphs at the right. In the first example *(A)*, there is no movement of drug out of the beaker, so the graph shows only a steep rise to maximum followed by a plateau. In the second example *(B)*, a route of elimination is present, and the graph shows a slow decay after a sharp rise to a maximum. Because the level of material in the beaker falls, the "pressure" driving the elimination process also falls, and the slope of the curve decreases, approaching the steady state asymptotically. This is an exponential decay curve. In the third model *(C)*, drug placed in the first compartment (blood) equilibrates rapidly with the second compartment (extravascular volume) and the amount of drug in "blood" declines logarithmically to a new steady state. The fourth model *(D)* illustrates a more realistic combination of elimination mechanism and extravascular equilibration. The resulting graph shows an early distribution phase followed by the slower elimination phase. These curves can be linearized by plotting the logarithm of the amount of drug against time.

stomach would be almost 100% ionized (pK$_a$ 7.9, pH 1.5–2.5) and poorly reabsorbed. Such trapped drug could then be removed by lavage. (If the morphine were not removed from the stomach, it would pass into the more alkaline environment of the intestine and be promptly reabsorbed.)

D. Lungs: The lungs are the most important route of excretion of gaseous anesthetics but a relatively unimportant route for most other drugs.

E. Minor Routes: Inconsequential amounts of drugs are excreted by the sweat and salivary glands. Similarly, the amount of drug excreted in milk is usually a small fraction of the total excreted. However, for the nursing infant, the drug in the milk may constitute a significant dose (Chapter 63).

History of a Single Administration of a Drug

As will be emphasized in Chapters 2 and 3, the most important factor determining the intensity of pharmacologic response is the concentration of drug at the receptor sites in the target tissue. It would be desirable to monitor this concentration to guide the adjustment of dosage, interpretation of treatment failure, etc, but direct tissue measurements are not often feasible in clinical practice. Therefore, blood (or plasma)

concentrations are usually measured when pharmacokinetic studies are done.

The pharmacokinetic history of a drug dose, determined by repeatedly measuring its blood concentration after a single administration, provides useful information for developing a concept or "model" about how the body handles the drug. In their simplest form, such models can be thought of as systems of compartments into which the drug is placed at the time of administration or into which it diffuses. Fig 1–1 illustrates these concepts. For many drugs, the history of concentration in the blood is fairly well predicted by a 2-compartment model like that shown in Fig 1–1D. An example of 2-compartment behavior by a real drug is shown in Fig 1–2. Many other drugs exhibit more complex curves when analyzed in this way. A few drugs display simpler kinetic behavior. For example, a drug that is retained within the vascular compartment does not manifest a distribution phase. If such a drug were to enter the body and be neither metabolized nor excreted, it might produce the graph shown in Fig 1–1A.

Drug Groups

The proper use of a drug requires an understanding of its pharmacokinetic properties and its pharmacody-

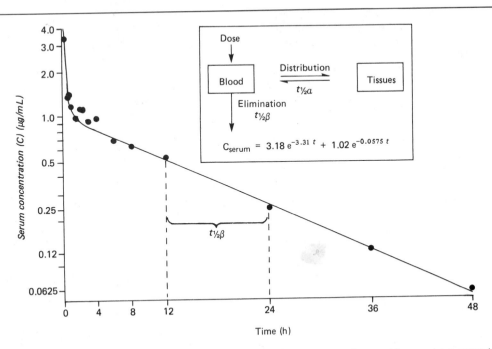

Figure 1–2. Serum concentration–time curve after administration of 25 mg of chlordiazepoxide as an intravenous bolus to a 75-kg man. The experimental data are plotted on a semilogarithmic scale as filled circles. If the drug is assumed to follow 2-compartment kinetics (inset), the initial curvilinear portion of the data represents the distribution phase, with drug moving into the tissues. The linear portion of the curve represents drug elimination. The equation shown in the inset was fitted to the data and generated the smooth curve passing through the data points. The **elimination half-life** ($t_{1/2\beta}$) can be extracted in 2 ways: graphically, by measuring the time between any 2 points that differ by 2-fold plasma concentration; and numerically, from the exponent of the second term of the equation, ie, $t_{1/2\beta} = 0.693 \div 0.0575 = 12$ hours. (t = time.) See Chapter 3, Part I for additional details. (Modified and reproduced, with permission, from Greenblatt DJ, Koch-Weser J: Drug therapy: Clinical pharmacokinetics. *N Engl J Med* 1975;**293**:702.)

namic interactions. To learn each pertinent fact about each of the many hundreds of drugs mentioned in this book is impractical, and fortunately, unnecessary. Therapeutic agents fall naturally into about 50 or 60 groupings on the basis of similarities in therapeutic effects or mechanisms of action. Thus, if the major pharmacodynamic and pharmacokinetic features of a prototype drug are learned, the characteristics of many of the other agents in the same drug group can often be inferred.

Information Sources

The references at the end of each chapter in this book were selected to provide information specific to those chapters. Three textbooks (listed alphabetically below) provide more general discussions and references:

Bowman WC, Rand MJ: *Textbook of Pharmacology,* 2nd ed. Blackwell Scientific, 1980. [A large textbook with a chemical and comparative pharmacology orientation.]

Gilman AG et al (editors): *Goodman and Gilman's The Pharmacological Basis of Therapeutics,* 7th ed. Macmillan, 1985. [A large textbook with a medical orientation.]

Goldstein A, Aronow L, Kalman SM: *Principles of Drug Action,* 2nd ed. Wiley, 1974. [A specialized text emphasizing general principles: receptor concepts, dose-response principles, pharmacokinetics, biochemical toxicology.]

Specific questions relating to basic or clinical research are best answered by searching the general pharmacology journals and the clinical specialty serials. Two periodicals can be recommended as especially useful sources of current information about drugs: *The New England Journal of Medicine,* which publishes much original drug-related research as well as frequent reviews of topics in pharmacology; and *The Medical Letter on Drugs and Therapeutics,* which publishes critical reviews of new and old therapies, mostly pharmacologic.

Other sources of information pertinent to the USA should be mentioned: the "package insert," a summary of information the manufacturer is required to place in the prescription sales package; *Physicians' Desk Reference (PDR),* which is basically a compendium of package inserts published annually with supplements; *Facts and Comparisons,* a more complete loose-leaf drug information service with monthly updates; the *USP DI* (Vol 1, *Drug Information for the Health Care Provider*), a concise and impartial annual publication; and *AMA Drug Evaluations,* now in its fifth edition. The package insert consists of a brief description of the chemical and physical characteristics of the drug product, a description of its pharmacology, and lists of approved indications, contraindications, warnings, precautions, and adverse reactions. Information on the recommended dosage and the effects of overdosage are also provided. While this brochure contains much practical information, it is also used as a device to shift liability for untoward drug reactions from the manufacturer onto the practitioner. Therefore, the manufacturer typically lists every toxic effect ever reported, no matter how rare. A disadvantage of *PDR* is that it is industry-oriented rather than professionally oriented. Only those drugs are described that their manufacturers want to pay to have included. The *USP DI,* Vol 1, provides more complete information about more drugs.

The following addresses are provided for the convenience of readers wishing to obtain any of the publications mentioned above:

AMA Drug Evaluations
535 N. Dearborn Street
Chicago, IL 60610

Facts and Comparisons
J. B. Lippincott Co.
111 West Port Plaza, Suite 423
St. Louis, MO 63146

The Medical Letter on Drugs and Therapeutics
56 Harrison Street
New Rochelle, NY 10801

The New England Journal of Medicine
10 Shattuck Street
Boston, MA 02115

Physicians' Desk Reference
Box 2017
Mahopac, NY 10541

United States Pharmacopoeia Dispensing Information
12601 Twinbrook Parkway
Rockville, MD 20852

REFERENCES

Bowman WC, Rand MJ: Pages 40.1–40.28 in: *Textbook of Pharmacology,* 2nd ed. Blackwell Scientific, 1980.

Seeman P, Sellars EM, Roschlau WHE: Pages 1–89 in: *Principles of Medical Pharmacology,* 3rd ed. Univ of Toronto Press, 1980.

Drug Receptors & Pharmacodynamics

2

Henry R. Bourne, MD, & James M. Roberts, MD

The therapeutic and toxic effects of drugs result from their interactions with molecules in the patient. In most instances, drugs act by associating with specific macromolecules in ways that alter their biochemical or biophysical activity. This idea, now almost a century old, is embodied in the terms **receptive substances** and **receptor:** the component of a cell or organism that interacts with a drug and initiates the chain of biochemical events leading to the drug's observed effects.

Initially, the existence of receptors was inferred from observations of the chemical and physiologic specificity of drug effects. Thus, Ehrlich noted that certain synthetic organic agents had characteristic antiparasitic effects while other agents did not, although their chemical structures differed only slightly. Langley noted that curare did not prevent electrical stimulation of muscle contraction but did block contraction triggered by nicotine. From these simple beginnings, receptors have now become the central focus of investigation of drug effects and their mechanisms of action (pharmacodynamics). The receptor concept, extended to endocrinology, immunology, and molecular biology, has proved essential for explaining many complexities of biologic regulation. Drug receptors are now being isolated and characterized as macromolecules, thus opening the way to precise understanding of the molecular basis of drug action.

In addition to its usefulness for explaining biology, the receptor concept has immensely important practical consequences for the development of drugs and for making therapeutic decisions in clinical practice. These consequences—explained more fully in later sections of this chapter—form the basis for understanding the actions and clinical uses of drugs described in every chapter of this book. They may be briefly summarized as follows:

(1) **Receptors largely determine the quantitative relations between dose or concentration of drug and pharmacologic effects.** The receptor's affinity for binding a drug determines the concentration of drug required to form a significant number of drug-receptor complexes, and the total number of receptors often limits the maximal effect a drug may produce.

(2) **Receptors are responsible for selectivity of drug action.** The molecular size, shape, and electrical charge of a drug determine whether—and with what avidity—it will bind to a particular receptor among the vast array of chemically different binding sites available in a cell, animal, or patient. Accordingly, changes in the chemical structure of a drug can dramatically increase or decrease a new drug's affinities for different classes of receptors, with resulting alterations in therapeutic and toxic effects.

(3) **Receptors mediate the actions of pharmacologic antagonists.** Many drugs and endogenous chemical signals, such as hormones, regulate the function of receptor macromolecules as **agonists;** ie, they change the function of a macromolecule as a more or less direct result of binding to it. Pure pharmacologic **antagonists,** however, bind to receptors without directly altering the receptors' function. Thus, the effect of a pure antagonist on a cell or in a patient depends entirely upon its preventing the binding and blocking the biologic actions of agonist molecules. Some of the most useful drugs in clinical medicine are pharmacologic antagonists.

MACROMOLECULAR NATURE OF DRUG RECEPTORS

It is still true that the chemical structures and even the existence of receptors for most clinically useful drugs can only be inferred from the chemical structures of the drugs themselves. By noting which chemical groups are required for specific pharmacologic effects of chemical congeners of a drug, pharmacologists imagine the complementary shape and distribution of electrical charge of the receptor site. In recent years, however, investigators have begun to characterize drug receptors in biochemical terms. Most of these receptors turn out to be proteins, presumably because the polypeptide structure provides the necessary diversity and specificity of shape and charge.

The best-characterized drug receptors are **regulatory proteins,** which mediate the actions of endogenous chemical signals such as neurotransmitters, autacoids, and hormones. This class of receptors mediates effects of many of the most useful therapeutic agents, which either mimic actions of endogenous agonists or, acting as antagonists, prevent responses to endogenous chemical signals. Although the physiologist or endocrinologist may think of these regulatory proteins as the only class of receptors, virtually any kind of protein molecule may serve as a receptor for a drug. Other classes of proteins that have been clearly identified as drug receptors include **enzymes,** which may be inhibited (or, less commonly, activated) by binding a drug (eg, dihydrofolate reductase, the receptor for the antineoplastic drug methotrexate); **transport proteins** (eg, Na^+,K^+-ATPase, the membrane receptor for cardioactive digitalis glycosides); and **structural proteins** (eg, tubulin, the receptor for colchicine, an anti-inflammatory agent).

Of the membrane-bound proteins that serve as receptors for neurohormones and drugs, the nicotinic acetylcholine receptor is the best-characterized (see Chapter 6). This receptor is a pentamer composed of 5 peptide subunits with molecular weights ranging from 40,000 to 65,000. All 5 peptides span the membrane's lipid bilayer, but only one or 2 peptides bind acetylcholine, the neurotransmitter. The binding of acetylcholine triggers opening of a transmembrane channel through which sodium ions penetrate from the extracellular fluid into the cell, an event that initiates an excitatory postsynaptic potential in the nerve or muscle cells that are targets for nicotinic stimulation. Thus, the nicotinic receptor, a single oligomeric protein molecule, performs 2 distinct functions as a receptor: (1) specific recognition of a drug or regulatory ligand (binding of acetylcholine), and (2) initiation of a biochemical event (opening of the sodium channel) that leads to the characteristic response of the cell (an excitatory postsynaptic potential).

RELATION BETWEEN DRUG CONCENTRATION & RESPONSE

The relation between dose of a drug and the clinically observed response may be quite complex. In carefully controlled in vitro systems, however, the relation between concentration of a drug and its effect is often simple and can be described with mathematical precision. We will analyze this simple, idealized relation first because it underlies virtually all of the more complex relations between dose and effect that occur when drugs are given to patients.

Concentration-Effect Curves & Receptor Binding of Agonists

Even in intact animals or patients, responses to low doses of a drug usually increase in direct proportion to dose. As doses increase, however, the incremental response diminishes; finally, doses may be reached at which no further increase in response can be achieved. In idealized or in vitro systems, the relation between drug concentration and effect is described by a hyperbolic curve (Fig 2–1A), according to the following equation:

$$E = \frac{E_{max} \; C}{C + K_{act}}$$

where E is the effect observed at concentration C, E_{max} is the maximal response that can be produced by the drug, and K_{act} is the concentration of drug that produces half-maximal effect. This K_{act} concentration is often called the EC50 (concentration for 50% of maximal effect).

The resemblance of this hyperbolic relation to the mass action law that predicts association between 2 molecules of a given affinity suggested that drug agonists act by binding to ("occupying") a distinct class of biologic molecules with a characteristic affinity for the drug—the receptor. With the advent of radioactive receptor ligands, including both agonists and antagonists, this occupancy assumption has been amply confirmed for a number of drug-receptor systems. In these systems, the relation between drug bound to receptors (B) and the concentration of free (unbound) drug (C) depicted in Fig 2–1B is described by an analogous equation:

$$B = \frac{B_{max} \; C}{C + K_D}$$

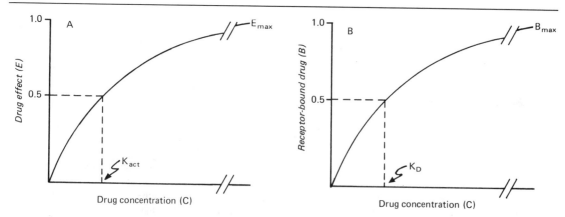

Figure 2–1. Relations between drug concentration and drug effect **(A)** or receptor-bound drug **(B)**. The drug concentrations at which effect or receptor occupancy are half-maximal are denoted K_{act} and K_D, respectively.

in which B_{max} indicates the concentration of bound drug at infinitely high concentrations of free drug, and K_D (the equilibrium dissociation constant) indicates the concentration of free drug at which half-maximal binding is observed. The value of B_{max} indicates the total number of receptors in the cell or tissue available for binding the drug, while the K_D characterizes the receptor's affinity for binding the drug in a reciprocal fashion: If the K_D concentration is low, binding affinity is high, and vice versa.

Note also that the K_{act} and K_D may be identical but need not be so, as discussed below.

Graphic representation of dose-response data is frequently improved by plotting the drug effect (ordinate) against the *logarithm* of the dose or concentration (abscissa). The effect of this purely mathematical maneuver is to transform the hyperbolic curve of Fig 2–1 into a sigmoid curve with a linear midportion (for example, Fig 2–8). This linearization makes easier the comparison of different dose-response curves, as indicated below.

Competitive & Irreversible Antagonists

Receptor antagonists act by binding to the receptor but do not activate it. The effects of these antagonists result from preventing agonists (other drugs or endogenous regulatory molecules) from binding to and activating receptors. Such antagonists are divided into 2 classes depending on whether or not they reversibly compete with agonists for binding to receptors. The 2 classes of receptor antagonism produce quite different concentration-effect and concentration-binding curves in vitro and exhibit important practical differences in therapy of disease.

In the presence of a fixed concentration of agonist, increasing concentrations of a **competitive antagonist** progressively inhibit the agonist response; high antagonist concentrations prevent response completely (Fig 2–2). The concentration of a competitive antagonist that inhibits 50% of the response observed with a fixed concentration of agonist is called the IC50. Note, however, that the IC50 of an antagonist is different for every concentration of agonist used. This is because the inhibition is competitive, so that high enough concentrations of agonist can overcome the effect of any fixed concentration of antagonist. (The converse is also true.) As a result, in the presence of a fixed concentration of competitive antagonist, an agonist concentration-effect curve (Fig 2–3A) has the same E_{max} as does the curve seen in the absence of antagonist; however, concentrations of agonist required for producing any given level of effect are increased, and the curve is shifted to the right.

The concentration (C′) of an agonist required to produce a given effect in the presence of a fixed concentration [I] of a competitive antagonist is greater than the agonist concentration (C) required to produce the same effect in the absence of the antagonist. The

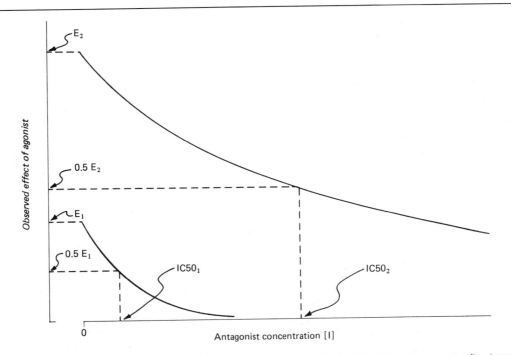

Figure 2–2. Increasing concentrations of a competitive antagonist progressively diminish the response to a fixed concentration of agonist. The IC50 concentration of antagonist is greater if the concentration of agonist is greater (upper versus lower curve).

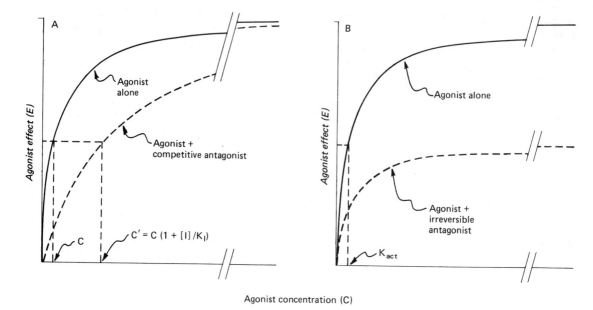

Figure 2–3. Changes in agonist dose-effect curves produced by a competitive antagonist *(A)* or by an irreversible antagonist *(B)*. In the presence of a competitive antagonist, higher concentrations of agonist are required to produce a given effect; thus, the agonist concentration (C′) required for a given effect in the presence of concentration [I] of an antagonist is the product of the concentration (C) required to produce the same effect in the absence of the antagonist times (1 + [I]/K_I). High agonist concentrations can overcome inhibition by a competitive antagonist. This is not the case with an irreversible antagonist, which reduces the maximal effect the agonist can achieve, although it may not change the K_{act}.

ratio of these 2 agonist concentrations (the "dose ratio") is related to the dissociation constant (K_I) of the antagonist by the Schild equation:

$$\frac{C'}{C} = 1 + \frac{[I]}{K_I}$$

Pharmacologists often use this relation to determine the K_I of a competitive antagonist. Even without knowledge of the relationship between agonist occupancy of the receptor and response, the K_I can be determined simply and accurately. A concentration response curve is obtained in the presence and absence of a fixed concentration of competitive antagonist; comparison of the agonist concentrations required to produce identical degrees of pharmacologic effect in the 2 situations reveals the K_I. If C′ is twice C, for example, then [I] = K_I.*

For the clinician, this mathematical relationship has 2 important therapeutic implications:

(1) The degree of inhibition produced by a competitive antagonist depends upon the concentration of unbound antagonist. Thus, the extent and duration of action of such a drug will depend upon its concentration in plasma and will be critically influenced by the rate of its metabolic clearance or excretion. Different patients receiving a fixed dose of propranolol, for example, exhibit a wide range of plasma concentrations,

owing to differences in clearance of the drug. As a result, the effects of a fixed dose of this competitive antagonist of norepinephrine may vary widely in patients, and the dose must be adjusted accordingly.

(2) The equation defines another important source of variability in clinical response to a competitive antagonist, ie, the concentration of agonist that is competing for binding to receptors. Here also propranolol provides a useful example: When this competitive β-adrenoceptor antagonist is administered in doses sufficient to block the effect of basal levels of the neurotransmitter norepinephrine, resting heart rate is decreased. However, the increase in release of norepinephrine and epinephrine that occurs with exercise, postural changes, or emotional stress may suffice to overcome competitive antagonism by propranolol and increase heart rate. Consequently, the physician who devises a dosage regimen for a competitive antagonist must always consider possible changes in endogenous agonist concentration that could influence therapeutic response.

Some receptor antagonists bind to the receptor in an **irreversible** or nearly irreversible fashion. The antagonist's affinity for the receptor may be so high that for practical purposes, the receptor is unavailable for binding of agonist. Other antagonists in this class produce irreversible effects because after binding to the receptor they form covalent bonds to the receptor. After occupancy of a substantial proportion of receptors by such an antagonist, the number of remaining unoccupied receptors may be so low that high concentrations of agonist cannot overcome the antagonism, and

---

*K_I values derived from such experiments agree with those determined by direct measurements of binding of radiolabeled competitive antagonists to receptors.

a maximal agonist response cannot be obtained (Fig 2–3B). A lower dose of an irreversible antagonist, however, may leave enough receptors unoccupied to allow achievement of maximum response to antagonist, although a higher agonist concentration will be required (see Receptor-Effector "Coupling" and Spare Receptors, below).

Therapeutically, irreversible antagonists present distinctive advantages and disadvantages. Once the noncompetitive antagonist has occupied the receptor, it need not be present in unbound form to inhibit agonist responses. Consequently, the duration of action of such an irreversible antagonist is relatively independent of its own rate of clearance and more dependent upon the rate of turnover of receptor molecules.

Phenoxybenzamine, an irreversible α-adrenoceptor antagonist, is used to reduce the increased blood pressure caused by catecholamines released from pheochromocytoma, a tumor of the adrenal medulla. If administration of phenoxybenzamine lowers blood pressure, blockade will be maintained even when the tumor episodically releases very large amounts of catecholamine. In this case, the ability to prevent responses to varying and high concentrations of agonist is a therapeutic advantage. If overdose occurs, however, a real problem may arise. If the α-adrenoceptor blockade cannot be overcome, excess effects of the drug must be antagonized "physiologically," eg, by using a pressor agent that does not act via alpha receptors.

Partial Agonists

Based on the maximal pharmacologic response that occurs when all receptors are occupied, agonists can be divided into 2 classes: **Partial agonists** produce a lower maximal response, at full receptor occupancy, than do **full agonists** (Fig 2–4A). As compared to full agonists, partial agonists produce concentration-effect curves that resemble the curves observed with full agonists in the presence of a noncompetitive antagonist that irreversibly blocks receptor sites (compare Figs 2–4A and 2–3B). Nonetheless, radioligand-binding experiments have demonstrated that partial agonists may occupy all receptor sites (Fig 2–4B) at concentrations that will fail to produce a maximal response comparable to that seen with full agonists (Fig 2–4A). In addition, the failure of partial agonists to produce a "full" maximal response is not due to decreased affinity for binding to receptors. Such drugs compete, frequently with high affinity, for the full complement of receptors. Indeed, the partial agonists' ability to occupy the total receptor population is indicated by the fact that partial agonists competitively inhibit the responses produced by full agonists.

The precise molecular mechanism that accounts for blunted maximal responses to partial agonists is not known. It is simplest to imagine that the partial agonist produces an effect on receptors that is intermediate between the effect produced by a full agonist and that produced by a competitive antagonist. The full agonist changes receptor conformation in a way that initiates subsequent pharmacologic effects of receptor occupancy, while the "pure" competitive antagonist produces no such change in receptor conformation; in this view, the partial agonist changes receptor conformation, but not to the extent necessary to result in full efficacy of the occupied receptor.

To express this idea, pharmacologists refer to the **efficacy** of a drug as a way of indicating the relation between occupancy of receptor sites and the pharmacologic response. A drug may have zero efficacy (ie, may be a pure antagonist) or any degree of efficacy greater than zero. Partial agonists can be viewed as drugs with such low efficacy that even occupancy of the full complement of receptors does not result in the maximal response that can be elicited by other ("full") agonists, which have higher efficacy. The reader will

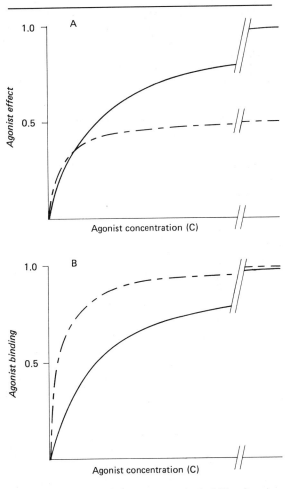

Figure 2–4. Comparison of a full agonist (solid lines) and a partial agonist (broken lines) with respect to effect **(A)** or receptor binding **(B)** at different agonist concentrations. In this example, the receptor has a higher affinity for the partial agonist than for the full agonist, so that a higher concentration of the latter is required for half-maximal binding. At high concentrations, however, the partial agonist produces a smaller maximal response than does the full agonist.

see that many drugs used as competitive antagonists are in fact weak partial agonists.

Receptor-Effector "Coupling" & Spare Receptors

Whatever its actual nature, the conformational change that occurs when a receptor is occupied by an agonist is only one of several steps necessary for expression of a full pharmacologic response. The transduction process between occupancy of receptors and drug response is often termed "coupling." The efficiency of receptor-effector coupling is determined by the ionic environment and by specific cellular components ("coupling factors," some of which have been biochemically identified for the actions of certain drugs), in addition to the receptor itself. Thus, agonist-receptor interactions presumably result in full or "tight" coupling of full agonists to response, in less tight coupling of partial agonists, and in "uncoupling" of pure antagonists. However, it is possible for even full agonists to become "uncoupled" from responses as the result of changes in coupling processes that take place distal to the receptor.

High efficiency of receptor-effector coupling may also be interpreted as the result of **spare receptors.** Receptors are said to be "spare" for a given pharmacologic response when the maximal response can be elicited by an agonist at a concentration that does not result in occupancy of the full complement of available receptors. Experimentally, spare receptors may be demonstrated by using noncompetitive (irreversible) antagonists to prevent binding of agonist to a proportion of available receptors and showing that high concentrations of agonist can still produce an undiminished maximal response (Fig 2–5). Thus, a maximal inotropic response of heart muscle to β-agonist amines can be elicited even under conditions where up to 90% of the beta receptors are occupied by a quasi-irreversible antagonist. Accordingly, myocardium is said to contain a large proportion of spare receptors.

Note, however, that spare receptors are not qualitatively different from nonspare ones. They are not "hidden" or unavailable, and they can be coupled to response. Fig 2–6 depicts one way of explaining how maximal response can occur without full occupancy of receptors. This will happen if the concentration or amount of a cellular component other than the receptor limits the coupling of receptor occupancy to response.

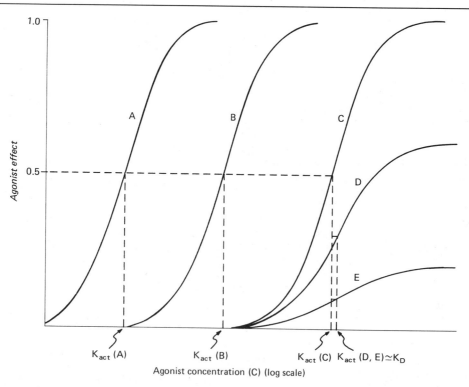

Figure 2–5. Experimental demonstration of spare receptors, using different concentrations of an irreversible antagonist. Curve *A* shows agonist response in the absence of antagonist. After treatment with a low concentration of antagonist (curve *B*), the curve is shifted to the right; maximal responsiveness is preserved, however, because the remaining available receptors are still in excess of the number required. In curve *C,* produced after treatment with a larger concentration of antagonist, the available receptors are no longer "spare"; instead, they are just sufficient to mediate an undiminished maximal response. Still higher concentrations of antagonist (curves *D* and *E*) reduce the number of available receptors to the point that maximal response is diminished. The apparent K_{act} of the agonist in curves *D* and *E* may approximate the K_D that characterizes the binding affinity of the agonist for the receptor.

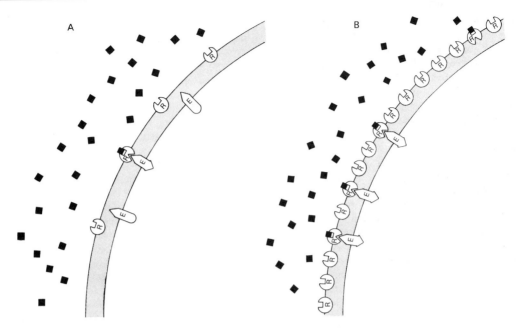

Figure 2–6. Spare receptors increase sensitivity to drug. In membrane **A (left),** the free concentration of agonist (■) is one-third the K_D concentration; this is sufficient to bind 25% of the 4 receptors (R) present, resulting in the formation of one agonist-receptor complex. [**Note:** Before going on, verify for yourself that free agonist at a concentration (C) one-third the K_D will occupy one-fourth of the total receptors. Remember that $B/B_{max} = C/(C + K_D)$.] Agonist occupancy of this one receptor changes its conformation so that it binds to and activates an effector molecule (E), resulting in a response. Because one of 3 effectors is stimulated by agonist-receptor complex, the response is 33% of maximum. In membrane **B (right),** the receptor concentration has been increased to 16, but the K_D for binding of agonist to receptors remains unchanged. As a result, the same free concentration of drug (one-third K_D) occupies 25% of the receptors. Now, however, this is *four* activated receptors, which results in activation of all 3 effectors and produces 100% response. Note that membrane **B** has one receptor that is occupied by drug but has no available effector molecule. This receptor is "spare," as are all the unoccupied receptors that could bind agonist at higher free agonist concentrations.

The spare receptor concept should help explain how the sensitivity of a cell or tissue to a particular concentration of agonist may depend not only on the affinity of the receptor for binding an agonist (characterized by the K_D) but also on the total concentration of receptors. Sensitivity may be expressed in terms of K_{act} or EC50, the concentration of agonist that results in half-maximal response. The K_D of the agonist-receptor interaction determines what fraction (B/B_{max}) of total receptors will be occupied at a given free concentration (C) of agonist, regardless of the receptor concentration:

$$\frac{B}{B_{max}} = \frac{C}{C + K_D}$$

If a tissue with 90% spare receptors has a receptor concentration of 100 per cell and if response is linearly related to occupancy, it will require the occupancy of 10 receptors (10%) for maximal response, and half-maximal response will be at an agonist concentration (K_{act}) that results in occupancy of 5% or 5 receptors per cell. K_{act} will be considerably lower than K_D. If receptor concentration is doubled to 200 per cell, it will still only require the occupancy of 10 receptors per cell for maximal response and 5 receptors per cell for half-

maximal response. This is now, however, 5 per 200, or only 2.5% of total receptors. Since the affinity of the receptor has not changed, a lower concentration of agonist will be sufficient to occupy 2.5% rather than 5% of receptors, and K_{act} will be decreased. Thus, it is possible to change the sensitivity of tissues with spare receptors by changing the receptor concentration. (Note, in passing, that changing the number of receptors does not usually change the free concentration of drug achieved by administering a given dose. This is because the concentration of receptors in a tissue is usually very small relative to effective concentrations of drugs.)

An important biologic consequence of spare receptors is that they allow agonists with low affinity for receptors to produce full responses at low concentrations, to the extent that K_{act} is lower than K_D. This is important because ligands with low affinity (high K_D) dissociate rapidly from receptors, allowing rapid termination of biologic responses. High binding affinity (low K_D), on the other hand, would result in slow dissociation of agonist from receptor and correspondingly slower reversal of a biologic response.

Other Mechanisms of Drug Antagonism

Not all of the mechanisms of antagonism involve interactions of drugs or endogenous ligands at a single type of receptor. Indeed, **chemical antagonists** need not involve a receptor at all. Thus, one drug may antagonize the actions of a second drug by binding to and inactivating the second drug. For example, protamine, a protein that is positively charged at physiologic pH, is used clinically to counteract the effects of heparin, an anticoagulant that is negatively charged; in this case, one drug antagonizes the other simply by binding it and making it unavailable for interactions with proteins involved in formation of a blood clot.

The clinician often uses drugs that take advantage of **physiologic antagonism** between endogenous regulatory pathways. Many physiologic functions are controlled by opposing regulatory pathways. For example, several catabolic actions of the glucocorticoid hormones lead to increased blood sugar, an effect that is physiologically opposed by insulin. Although glucocorticoids and insulin act on quite distinct receptor-effector systems, the clinician must sometimes administer insulin to oppose the hyperglycemic effects of glucocorticoid hormones, whether the latter are elevated by endogenous synthesis (eg, an inoperable tumor of the adrenal cortex) or as a result of glucocorticoid therapy.

In general, use of a drug as a physiologic antagonist produces effects that are less specific and less easy to control than are the effects of a receptor-specific antagonist. Thus, for example, to treat bradycardia caused by increased vagal tone associated with the acute pain of myocardial infarction, the physician could use isoproterenol, a β-adrenoceptor agonist that increases heart rate by mimicking sympathetic stimulation of the heart. However, use of this physiologic antagonist would be less rational—and potentially more dangerous—than would use of a receptor-specific antagonist such as atropine (a competitive antagonist at the muscarinic receptors through which vagal stimuli slow heart rate).

CLASSIFICATION OF RECEPTORS

As we have seen, the existence of a specific drug receptor is usually inferred from studying the **structure-activity relationship** of a group of structurally similar congeners of the drug that mimic or antagonize its effects. Thus, if a series of related agonists exhibits identical relative potencies in producing 2 distinct effects, it is likely that the 2 effects are mediated by similar or identical receptor molecules. In addition, if the same molecular species of receptor mediates both effects, a competitive antagonist will inhibit both responses with the same K_I; a second competitive antagonist will inhibit both responses with its own characteristic K_I. Thus, studies of the relation between structure and activity of a series of agonists and antagonists can identify a species of receptor that mediates a set of pharmacologic responses.

Exactly the same experimental procedure can show that observed effects of a drug are mediated by different species of receptors. In this case, effects mediated by different receptors may exhibit different orders of potency among agonists, and different K_I values for each competitive antagonist.

Evidence that a particular drug acts via 2 or more distinct receptors usually presents an important therapeutic opportunity, because it suggests the possibility of developing new drugs that will exhibit enhanced selectivity for one receptor over the other. Such opportunities have been extensively exploited with the receptors for histamine, acetylcholine, and norepinephrine. Thus, for example, β-adrenoceptor antagonists can block cardioacceleration produced by norepinephrine without preventing catecholamine regulation of arteriolar constriction, which is mediated by α-adrenoceptors. Similarly, α-adrenoceptor agonists can induce vasoconstriction without stimulating beta receptors in the heart (see Chapter 8). Clinical uses of receptor-selective drugs are described in many chapters of this book (see Chapter 6 for acetylcholine receptors; Chapter 15 for histamine receptors). In each case, the endogenous autacoid or neurotransmitter produces multiple effects in the intact patient, and it is therapeutically advantageous to stimulate or block one set of effects without substantially affecting others. This principle is illustrated in Fig 2–7.

RELATION BETWEEN DRUG DOSE & CLINICAL RESPONSE

We have dealt with receptors as molecules and shown how receptors can quantitatively account for the relation between dose or concentration of a drug and pharmacologic responses, at least in an idealized system. When faced with a patient who needs treatment, the physician must make a choice among a variety of possible drugs and devise a dosage regimen that is likely to produce maximal benefit and minimal toxicity. Because the patient is never an idealized system, the physician will not have precise information about the physicochemical nature of the receptors involved, the number of receptors, or their affinity for drugs. Nonetheless, in order to make rational therapeutic decisions, the physician must understand how drug-receptor interactions underlie the relations between dose and response in nonideal patients, the nature and causes of variation in pharmacologic responsiveness, and the clinical implications of selectivity of drug action.

Dose & Response in Patients

A. Graded Dose-Response Relations: To choose among drugs and to determine appropriate doses of a drug, the physician must know the relative **pharmacologic potency** and **maximal efficacy** of the drugs in relation to the desired therapeutic effect. These 2 important terms, often confusing to students and clinicians, can be explained by reference to Fig 2–8, which depicts graded dose-response curves that relate log dose of 4 different drugs to the magnitude of a particular therapeutic effect, eg, lowering of blood

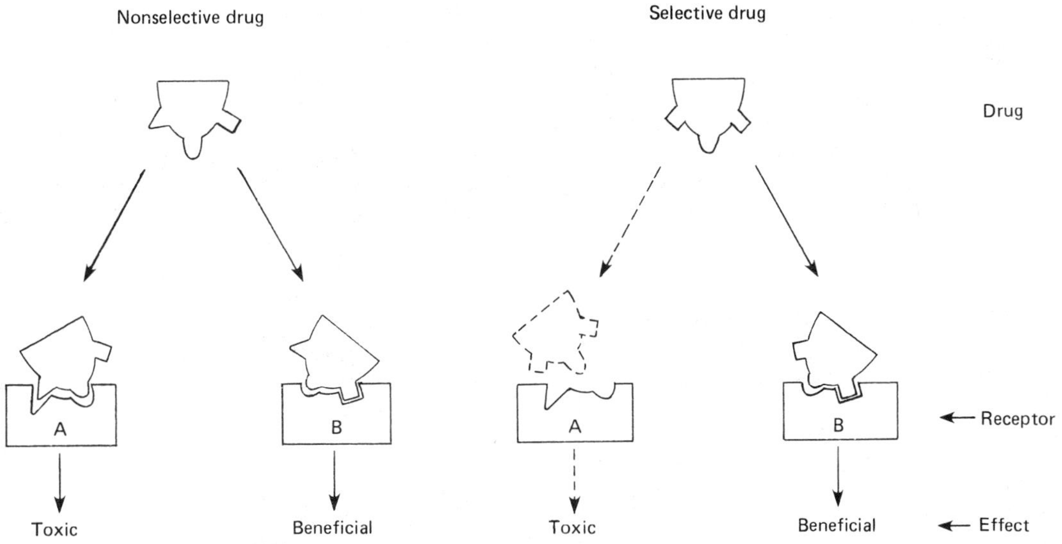

Nonselective drug

Selective drug

Drug

← Receptor

Toxic Beneficial Toxic Beneficial ← Effect

Figure 2–7. Receptor selectivity. Receptors A and B mediate toxic (unwanted) or beneficial (therapeutic) effects, respectively. A nonselective drug binds equally well to both types of receptor, while a selective drug binds with higher affinity to receptor B than to receptor A.

pressure in a hypertensive patient or increasing urinary excretion of sodium in a patient with congestive heart failure.

1. Potency–Drugs A and B are said to be more potent than drug C because of their relative positions along the **dose axis** of Fig 2–8. Potency thus refers to the dose or concentration of a drug required to produce a given effect (or degree of effect). Accordingly, drug B is more potent than drug A with respect to the lower part of the response range (eg, for a response 25% of maximal); this is because drug B produces this degree of response at a lower concentration than does drug A. If one is considering a greater degree of effect (eg, 90% of maximum response), then drug A is more potent than drug B—indeed, drug B, a partial agonist, has zero potency in the higher range of responses, because its maximal efficacy is less than that of drug A (see below).

Potency of a drug depends in part on the affinity (K_D) of receptors for binding the drug and in part on the efficiency with which drug-receptor interaction is coupled to response. Both affinity and coupling efficiency contribute to the K_{act} or EC50 of a particular drug-response relation in vitro, as described above. When a drug is administered to a patient, its potency also depends upon its ability to reach the relevant receptors. Thus, a drug's potency may depend upon its route of administration, absorption, distribution through the body, and clearance from the blood or from its site of action.

While the potency of a drug clearly is important for determining the dose to be used, there is no reason to consider the relative potencies of 2 drugs in deciding which one to administer to a patient. (Low potency would only be important if the drug had to be administered in inconveniently large amounts.)

For therapeutic purposes, the potency of a drug should be stated in dosage units, usually in terms of a particular therapeutic end point (eg, 50 mg for mild sedation, 1 μg/kg/min for an increase in heart rate of 25 beats/min). Relative potency, the ratio of equieffective doses (0.2, 10, etc), may be used in comparing one drug with another.

2. Maximal efficacy–This parameter reflects the limit of the dose-response relation on the **response axis.** Drugs A, C, and D in Fig 2–8 have equal maximal efficacy, while all have greater maximal efficacy than does drug B. The maximal efficacy (sometimes referred to simply as **efficacy**) of a drug is obviously crucial for making clinical decisions. It may be determined by the drug's mode of interactions with recep-

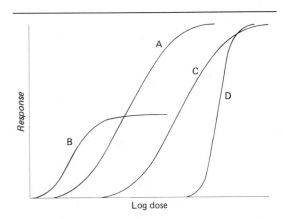

Figure 2–8. Graded dose-response curves for 4 drugs, illustrating different pharmacologic potencies and different maximal efficacies.

tors (as with partial agonists, described above)* or by characteristics of the receptor-effector system involved. Thus, diuretics that act on one portion of the nephron may produce much greater excretion of fluid and electrolytes than diuretics that act elsewhere. In addition, the efficacy of a drug for achieving a therapeutic end point (eg, increased cardiac contractility) may be limited by the drug's propensity to cause a toxic effect (eg, fatal cardiac arrhythmia) even if the drug could otherwise produce a greater therapeutic effect.

B. Shape of Dose-Response Curves: While the responses depicted in curves A, B, and C of Fig 2–8 approximate the shape of a simple Michaelis-Menten relation (transformed to a logarithmic plot), some clinical responses do not. Extremely steep dose-response curves (eg, curve D) may have important clinical consequences if the upper portion of the curve represents an undesirable extent of response (eg, coma caused by a sedative-hypnotic). Steep dose-response curves in patients could result from cooperative interactions of several different actions of a drug (eg, effects on brain, heart, and peripheral vessels, all contributing to lowering of blood pressure). Such steep dose-response curves could also be produced by a receptor-effector system in which most receptors must be occupied before any effect is seen or by unusual pharmacokinetic properties of a drug that create a threshold dose below which little or no drug can reach the receptors responsible for its action (see Chapter 3).

C. Quantal Dose-Effect Curves: Despite their usefulness for characterizing the actions of drugs, graded dose-response curves of the sort described above have certain limitations in their application to clinical decision making. For example, such curves may be impossible to construct if the pharmacologic response is an either/or (quantal) event, such as prevention of convulsions, arrhythmia, or death. Furthermore, the clinical relevance of a quantitative dose-response relationship in a single patient, no matter how precisely defined, may be limited in application to other patients, owing to the great potential variability among patients in severity of disease and responsiveness to drugs.

Some of these difficulties may be avoided by determining the dose of drug required to produce a specified magnitude of effect in a large number of individual patients or experimental animals and plotting the cumulative frequency distribution of responders versus the log dose (Fig 2–9). The specified quantal effect may

*Note that "maximal efficacy," used in a therapeutic context, does not have exactly the meaning the term implies in the more specialized context of drug-receptor interactions, described earlier in this chapter. In an idealized in vitro system, efficacy refers to the relative maximal efficacy of agonists and partial agonists that act via the same receptor. In therapeutics, efficacy refers to the extent or degree of an effect that can be achieved in the intact patient. Thus, therapeutic efficacy may be affected by the characteristics of a particular drug-receptor interaction, but it also depends upon a host of other factors, noted in the text.

be chosen on the basis of clinical relevance (eg, relief of headache) or for preservation of safety of experimental subjects (eg, using low doses of a cardiac stimulant and specifying an increase in heart rate of 20 beats/min as the quantal effect), or it may be an inherently quantal event (eg, death of an experimental animal). For most drugs, the doses required to produce a specified quantal effect in individuals are lognormally distributed; ie, a frequency distribution of such responses plotted against the log of the dose produces a gaussian normal curve of variation (Fig 2–9). When these responses are summated, the resulting cumulative frequency distribution constitutes a quantal dose-effect curve (or dose-percent curve) of the proportion or percentage of individuals who exhibit the effect plotted as a function of log dose (Fig 2–9).

The quantal dose-effect curve is often characterized by stating the **median effective dose** (ED50), the dose at which 50% of individuals exhibit the specified quantal effect. Similarly, the dose required to produce a particular toxic effect in 50% of animals is called the **median toxic dose** (TD50). If the toxic effect is death of the animal, a **median lethal dose** (LD50) may be experimentally defined. Such values provide a convenient way of comparing the potencies of drugs in experimental and clinical settings: Thus, if the ED50s of 2 drugs for producing a specified quantal effect are 5 and 500 mg, respectively, then the first drug can be said to be 100 times more potent than the second for that particular effect. Similarly, one can obtain a valuable index of the selectivity of a drug's action by comparing its ED50s for 2 different quantal effects in a population (eg, cough suppression versus sedation for opiate drugs; increase in heart rate versus increased vasoconstriction for sympathomimetic amines; anti-inflammatory effects versus sodium retention for corticosteroids; etc).

Quantal dose-effect curves may also be used to generate information regarding the margin of safety to be expected from a particular drug used to produce a specified effect. One measure, which relates the dose of a drug required to produce a desired effect to that which produces an undesired effect, is the **therapeutic index.** In animal studies, the therapeutic index is usually defined as the ratio of the TD50 to the ED50 for some therapeutically relevant effect. The clinical usefulness of a drug usually relates to a much more conservative definition of therapeutic index and critically depends upon the severity of the disease under treatment. Thus, for the treatment of headache the physician might require a very large therapeutic index, defined as the ratio of the dose required to cause serious toxicity in a very small percentage of subjects (TD0.001) to the dose required to ameliorate headache in a very large proportion of subjects (ED99). For treatment of a lethal disease, such as Hodgkin's lymphoma, an acceptable therapeutic index might be defined less stringently.

Finally, note that the quantal dose-effect curve and the graded dose-response curve summarize somewhat different sets of information, although both appear

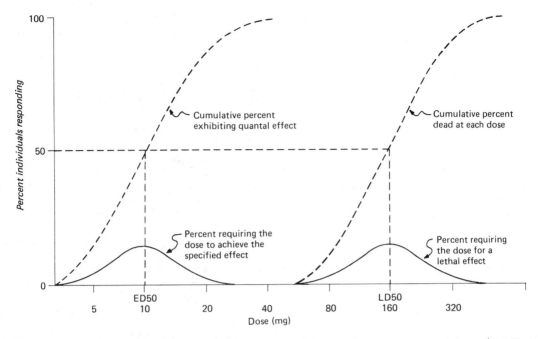

Figure 2–9. Quantal dose-effect curves. Solid curves indicate the frequency distribution of doses of drug required to produce a specified effect; ie, the curves show the percentage of animals that required a particular dose to exhibit the effect. Dashed lines indicate the cumulative frequency distribution of responses, which are lognormally distributed.

sigmoid in shape on a semilogarithmic plot (compare Figs 2–8 and 2–9). Critical information required for making rational therapeutic decisions can be obtained from each type of curve: Both curves provide information regarding the **potency** and **selectivity** of drugs; the graded dose-response curve indicates the **maximal efficacy** of a drug; and the quantal dose-effect curve indicates the potential **variability** of responsiveness among individuals.

Variation in Drug Responsiveness

Individuals may vary considerably in their responsiveness to a drug; indeed, a single individual may respond differently to the same drug at different times during the course of treatment. Occasionally, individuals exhibit an unusual or **idiosyncratic** drug response, one that is infrequently observed in most patients. These idiosyncratic responses are usually caused by genetic differences in metabolism of the drug or by immunologic mechanisms, including allergic reactions.

Quantitative variations in drug response are in general more common and more clinically important: An individual patient is **hyporeactive** or **hyperreactive** to a drug in that the intensity of effect of a given dose of drug is diminished or increased in comparison to the effect seen in most individuals. (*Note:* The term **hypersensitivity** usually refers to allergic or other immunologic responses to drugs.) With some drugs, the intensity of response to a given dose may change during the course of therapy; in these cases, responsiveness usually decreases as a consequence of continued drug administration, producing a state of relative **tol-**

erance to the drug's effects. When responsiveness diminishes rapidly after administration of a drug, the response is said to be subject to **tachyphylaxis.**

The general clinical implications of individual variability in drug responsiveness are clear: The physician must be prepared to change either the dose of drug or the choice of drug, depending upon the response observed in the patient. Even before administering the first dose of a drug, the physician should consider factors that may help in predicting the direction and extent of possible variation in responsiveness. These include the propensity of a particular drug to produce tolerance or tachyphylaxis as well as the effects of age, sex, body size, disease state, and simultaneous administration of other drugs.

Four general mechanisms may contribute to variation in drug responsiveness among patients or within an individual patient at different times. The classification described below is necessarily artificial in that most variation in clinical responsiveness is caused by more than one mechanism. Nonetheless, the classification may be useful because certain mechanisms of variation are best dealt with according to different therapeutic strategies:

A. Alteration in Concentration of Drug That Reaches the Receptor: Patients may differ in the rate of absorption of a drug, in distributing it through body compartments, or in clearing the drug from the blood (see Chapter 3). Any of these pharmacokinetic differences may alter the concentration of drug that reaches relevant receptors and thus alter clinical response. These differences can often be predicted on the basis of age, weight, sex, disease state, or liver and kidney function of the patient, and such predictions may be used to guide quantitative decisions regarding an initial dosing regimen. Repeated measurements of drug concentrations in blood during the course of treatment are often helpful in dealing with the variability of clinical response caused by pharmacokinetic differences among individuals.

B. Variation in Concentration of an Endogenous Receptor Ligand: This mechanism contributes greatly to variability in responses to pharmacologic antagonists. Thus, propranolol, a β-adrenoceptor antagonist, will markedly slow the heart rate of a patient whose endogenous catecholamines are elevated (as in heart failure or pheochromocytoma) but will not affect the resting heart rate of a well-trained marathon runner. A partial agonist may exhibit even more dramatically different responses: Saralasin, a weak partial agonist at angiotensin II receptors, lowers blood pressure in patients with hypertension caused by increased angiotensin II production and raises blood pressure in patients who produce low amounts of angiotensin.

In assessing clinical response to antagonist drugs, the physician must always make a judgment about the probable stimulation of receptors by endogenous agonists. Thus, unsatisfactory response to a dose of a competitive antagonist might be due to greatly elevated endogenous agonist, and a larger dose of antagonist would be appropriate. Alternatively, the unsatisfactory response might be due to low rates of stimulation by agonist; this would suggest that the diagnosis is wrong and that a different mode of therapy, rather than more drug, is indicated.

C. Alterations in Number or Function of Receptors: Experimental studies have documented changes in drug responsiveness caused by increases or decreases in the number of receptor sites or by alterations in the efficiency of coupling of receptors to distal effector mechanisms. Although such changes have not been rigorously documented in human beings, it is likely that they account for much of the individual variability in response to some drugs, particularly those that act at receptors for hormones, biogenic amines, and neurotransmitters. In some cases, the change in receptor number is caused by other hormones; for example, thyroid hormones increase both the number of beta receptors in rat heart muscle and the cardiac sensitivity to catecholamines. Similar changes probably contribute to the tachycardia of thyrotoxicosis in patients and may account for the usefulness of propranolol, a β-adrenoceptor antagonist, in ameliorating symptoms of this disease.

In other cases, the agonist ligand itself induces a decrease in the number ("down regulation") or coupling efficiency of its receptors. Receptor-specific desensitization mechanisms presumably act physiologically to allow cells to adapt to changes in rates of stimulation by hormones and neurotransmitters in their environment. These mechanisms may contribute to tachyphylaxis or tolerance to the effects of some drugs, particularly the biogenic amines and their con-

geners. Recent investigations suggest, in addition, that similar adaptive mechanisms may be responsible for so-called "overshoot" phenomena that follow withdrawal of certain drugs (propranolol, opiates, some antihypertensive agents, etc). Thus, for example, an antagonist may actually raise the number of receptors in a cell by preventing down regulation caused by endogenous agonist; when the antagonist is withdrawn, the elevated receptor number allows an exaggerated response to physiologic concentrations of agonist.

Therapeutic strategies required to deal with receptor-specific changes in drug responsiveness vary according to the clinical situation. In some cases, the dose of an agonist must be increased to achieve a continuing satisfactory response, while in other cases different or additional drugs should be administered. Cessation of treatment with certain drugs should be gradual and carefully monitored.

D. Changes in Components of Response Distal to Receptor: Although a drug initiates its actions by binding to receptors, the response observed in a patient depends on the functional integrity of biochemical processes in the responding cell and physiologic regulation by interacting organ systems. Clinically, changes in these postreceptor processes represent the largest and most important class of mechanisms that cause variation in responsiveness to drug therapy.

Before initiating therapy with a drug, the physician should be aware of patient characteristics that may limit the clinical response. These characteristics include the age, sex, and general health of the patient and—most importantly—the severity and pathophysiologic mechanism of the disease. Once treatment is begun, the most important potential cause of failure to achieve a satisfactory response is that the diagnosis is wrong or physiologically incomplete. Thus, congestive heart failure will not respond satisfactorily to agents that increase myocardial contractility if the underlying pathologic mechanism is unrecognized stenosis of the mitral valve rather than myocardial insufficiency. Conversely, drug therapy will always be most successful when it is accurately directed at the pathophysiologic mechanism responsible for the disease.

When the diagnosis is correct and the drug is appropriate, treatment may still not produce an optimal result. An unsatisfactory therapeutic response can often be traced to compensatory mechanisms in the patient that respond to and oppose the beneficial effects of the drug. Compensatory increases in sympathetic nervous tone and fluid retention by the kidney, for example, can contribute to tolerance to antihypertensive effects of a vasodilator drug. In such cases, additional drugs may be required to achieve a useful therapeutic response.

Clinical Selectivity: Beneficial Versus Toxic Effects of Drugs

Although we classify drugs according to their principal actions, it is clear that *no drug causes only a single, specific effect.* Why is this so? It is exceedingly unlikely that any kind of drug molecule will bind to only a single molecular species of receptor, if only because the number of potential receptors in a patient is astronomically large. (Consider that the human genome codes for approximately 10^4 different peptide gene products and that the chemical complexity of each of these peptides is sufficient to provide many different potential binding sites.) Even if the chemical structure of a drug allowed it to bind to only one kind of receptor, the biochemical processes controlled by such receptors would take place in multiple cell types and would be coupled to many other biochemical functions; as a result, the patient and the physician would probably perceive more than one drug effect.

Accordingly, drugs are only *selective*—rather than specific—in their actions, because they bind to one or a few types of receptor more tightly than to others, and because these receptors control discrete processes that result in distinct effects. As we have seen, selectivity can be measured by comparing binding affinities of a drug to different receptors or by comparing ED50s for different effects of a drug in vivo. In drug development and in clinical medicine, selectivity is usually considered by separating effects into 2 categories: **beneficial** or **therapeutic effects** versus **toxic effects.** Pharmaceutical advertisements and physicians occasionally use the term **side effect,** implying that the effect in question is insignificant or occurs via a pathway that is to one side of the principal action of the drug; such implications are frequently erroneous.

It is important to recognize that the designation of a particular drug effect as either therapeutic or toxic is a value judgment and not a statement about the pharmacologic mechanism underlying the effect. As a value judgment, such a designation depends on the clinical context in which the drug is used.

It is only because of their selectivity that drugs are useful in clinical medicine. Thus, it is important, both in the management of patients and in the development and evaluation of new drugs, to analyze ways in which beneficial and toxic effects of drugs may be related, in order to increase selectivity and usefulness of drug therapy. Fig 2–10 depicts 3 possible relations between the therapeutic and toxic effects of a drug based on analysis of the receptor-effector mechanisms involved.

A. Beneficial and Toxic Effects Mediated by the Same Receptor-Effector Mechanism: Much of the serious drug toxicity in clinical practice represents a **direct pharmacologic extension** of the therapeutic actions of the drug. In some of these cases (bleeding caused by anticoagulant therapy; hypoglycemic coma due to insulin), toxicity may be avoided by judicious management of the dose of drug administered, guided by careful monitoring of effect (measurements of blood coagulation or serum glucose) and aided by ancillary measures (avoiding tissue trauma that may lead to hemorrhage; regulation of carbohydrate intake). In still other cases, the toxicity may be avoided by not administering the drug at all, if the therapeutic indication is weak or if other therapy is

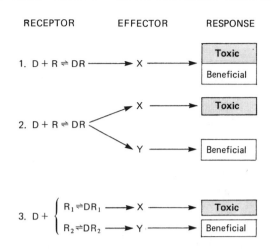

Figure 2–10. Possible relations between the therapeutic and toxic effects of a drug, based on different receptor-effector mechanisms. Therapeutic implications of these different relations are discussed in the text.

available (eg, sedative-hypnotics ordinarily should not be used to treat patients whose complaints of insomnia are due to underlying mental depression).

In certain situations, a drug is clearly necessary and beneficial but produces unacceptable toxicity when given in doses that produce optimal benefit. In such situations, it may be necessary to add another drug to the treatment regimen. For example, guanethidine (Chapter 10) lowers blood pressure in essential hypertension by inhibiting cardiovascular stimulation by sympathetic nerves; as an inevitable consequence, patients will suffer from symptoms of postural hypotension if the dose of drug is large enough. (Note that postural hypotension has been called a "side effect" of guanethidine, although in fact it is a direct effect, closely related to the drug's principal therapeutic action.) Appropriate management of such a problem takes advantage of the fact that blood pressure is regulated by changes in blood volume and tone of arterial smooth muscle in addition to the sympathetic nerves. Thus, concomitant administration of diuretics and vasodilators may allow the dose of guanethidine to be lowered, with relief of postural hypotension and continued control of blood pressure.

B. Beneficial and Toxic Effects Mediated by Identical Receptors But in Different Tissues or by Different Effector Pathways: Examples of drugs in this category include digitalis glycosides, which may be used to augment cardiac contractility but also produce cardiac arrhythmias, gastrointestinal effects, and changes in vision (all probably mediated by inhibition of Na^+, K^+-ATPase in cell membranes); methotrexate, used to treat leukemia and other neoplastic diseases, which also kills normal cells in bone marrow and gastrointestinal mucosa (all mediated by inhibition of the enzyme dihydrofolate reductase); and congeners of glucocorticoid hormones, used to treat asthma or inflammatory disorders, which also can produce protein catabolism, psychosis, and other toxicities (all thought to be mediated by similar or identical glucocorticoid receptors). In addition to these and other well-documented examples, it is likely that "side effects" of many drugs are mediated by receptors identical to those which produce the recognized beneficial effect.

Three therapeutic strategies are used to avoid or mitigate this sort of toxicity. *First,* the drug should always be administered at the lowest dose that produces acceptable benefit, recognizing that complete abolition of signs or symptoms of the disease may not be achieved. *Second* (as described above for guanethidine), adjunctive drugs that act through different receptor mechanisms and produce different toxicities may allow lowering the dose of the first drug, thus limiting its toxicity (eg, use of other immunosuppressive agents added to glucocorticoids in treating inflammatory disorders). *Third,* selectivity of the drug's actions may be increased by manipulating the concentrations of drug available to receptors in different parts of the body. Such "anatomic" selectivity may be achieved, for example, by aerosol administration of a glucocorticoid to bronchi or by selective arterial infusion of an antimetabolite into an organ containing tumor cells.

C. Beneficial and Toxic Effects Mediated by Different Types of Receptors: Therapeutic advantages resulting from new chemical entities with improved receptor selectivity were mentioned earlier in this chapter and are described in detail in later chapters. Such drugs include the α- and β-adrenoceptor agonists and antagonists, the H_1 and H_2 antihistamines, nicotinic and muscarinic blocking agents, and receptor-selective steroid hormones. All of these receptors are grouped in functional families, each responsive to a small class of endogenous agonists. The receptors—and their associated therapeutic uses—were discovered by analyzing effects of the physiologic chemical signals—catecholamines, histamine, acetylcholine, and corticosteroids.

A number of other drugs were discovered in a similar way, although they may not act at receptors for known hormones or neurotransmitters. These drugs were discovered by exploiting toxic or side effects of other agents, observed in a different clinical context. Examples include quinidine, the sulfonylureas, thiazide diuretics, tricyclic antidepressants, monoamine oxidase inhibitors, and phenothiazine antipsychotics among many others.

It is likely that some of these drugs will eventually be shown to act via receptors for endogenous agonists, as was recently established for morphine, a potent analgesic agent. Morphine has been shown to act on receptors physiologically stimulated by the opioid peptides. Pharmacologists are now beginning to subclassify the opioid receptors, in a fashion reminiscent of earlier studies of autonomic receptors.

Thus, the propensity of drugs to bind to different classes of receptor sites is not only a potentially vexing problem in treating patients—it also presents a continuing challenge to pharmacology and an opportunity for developing new and more useful drugs.

REFERENCES

Ariens EJ: Intrinsic activity: Partial agonists and partial antagonists. *J Cardiovasc Pharmacol* 1983;**5**:S8.

Baxter JD, Funder JW: Hormone receptors. *N Engl J Med* 1979; **301**:1149.

Goldstein A, Aronow L, Kalman SM: *Principles of Drug Action: The Basis of Pharmacology,* 2nd ed. Wiley, 1974.

Iversen LL, Iversen SD, Snyder SH (editors): *Handbook of Psychopharmacology.* Vol 2: *Principles of Receptor Research.* Plenum Press, 1975.

Kaplan SA: Cell receptors. *Am J Dis Child* 1984;**138**:1140.

Lefkowitz RJ, Caron MG, Stiles GL: Mechanisms of membrane-receptor regulation: Biochemical, physiological, and clinical insights derived from studies of the adrenergic receptors. *N Engl J Med* 1984;**310**:1570.

Roberts JM: The transfer of information into cells. *Obstet Gynecol Annu* 1985;**14**:1.

Williams LT, Lefkowitz RJ: *Receptor Binding Studies in Adrenergic Pharmacology.* Raven Press, 1978.

Pharmacokinetics: I. Absorption, Distribution, & Excretion

3

Leslie Z. Benet, PhD

When a clinician prescribes a drug and the patient takes it, their main concern is with the effect on the patient's disease. However, as illustrated in Fig 3–1, several processes are going forward from the time a dose is administered until the appearance of any therapeutic effect. These pharmacokinetic processes, defined in Chapter 1, determine how rapidly and in what concentration and for how long the drug will appear at the target organ. The 3 steps shown at the top of Fig 3–1—**input, distribution,** and **loss**—are the major pharmacokinetic variables. In most cases, input will consist of absorption from the most convenient site that meets the requirements for speed and completeness of absorption. For most drugs, oral administration is appropriate, and measurable concentrations of the drug in the blood result. The pattern of the concentration-time curve in the blood is a function of the input, distribution, and loss factors. In this chapter, we will examine the quantitative aspects of these relationships.

A fundamental hypothesis of pharmacokinetics is that a relationship exists between a pharmacologic or toxic effect of a drug and the concentration of the drug in a readily accessible site of the body (eg, blood). This hypothesis has been documented for many drugs (Table 3–1), although for some drugs no clear relationship has been found between pharmacologic effect and plasma or blood concentrations. In most cases, the concentration of drug in the general circulation will be related to its concentration at the site of action. The drug will then elicit a number of pharmacologic effects at the site of action. These pharmacologic effects may include toxic effects in addition to the desired clinical effect. The clinician then must balance the toxic potential of a particular dose of a drug with its efficacy to determine the utility of that agent in that clinical situation (Fig 3–1). Pharmacokinetics plays its role in the dose efficacy scheme by providing the quantitative relationship between drug efficacy and drug dose, with the aid of measurements of drug concentrations in various biologic fluids. The importance of pharmacokinetics in patient care rests upon the improvement in drug efficacy and reduction in toxicity that can be attained when the measurement of drug levels in the general circulation is added to traditional methods of predicting the dose of the drug. Knowledge of the relationship between efficacy and drug concentration measurements allows the clinician to take into account the various pathologic and physiologic features of a particular patient that make him or her different from the normal individual in responding to a dose of the drug.

PHARMACOKINETIC VARIABLES

Several pathologic and physiologic processes dictate dosage adjustment in individual patients (eg, heart failure, renal failure). They do so by modifying specific pharmacokinetic parameters. The 2 basic variables are **clearance,** the measure of the ability of the body to eliminate the drug, and **volume of distribution,** the measure of the apparent space in the body available to contain the drug.

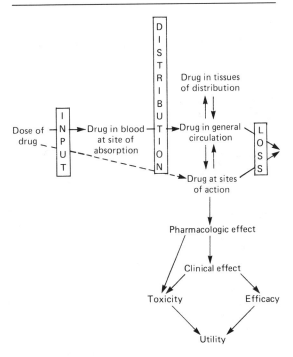

Figure 3–1. A schematic representation of the dose-effect relationships of a drug. (Modified and reproduced, with permission, from Benet LZ: Effect of route of administration and distribution on drug action. *J Pharmacokinet Biopharm* 1978;**6:**559.)

Table 3–1. Pharmacokinetic and pharmacodynamic parameters for selected drugs.*

Drug	Oral Availability (percent)	Urinary Excretion (percent)	Bound in Plasma (percent)	Clearance (mL/min)†	Volume of Distribution (L)†	Half-Life (hours)	Effective‡ Concentrations	Toxic‡ Concentrations
Acetaminophen	88 ± 15	3 ± 1	0–15	350 ± 100	67 ± 8	2.0 ± 0.4	10–20 µg/mL	>300 µg/mL
Acyclovir	15–30	67 ± 15	15 ± 4	330 ± 80	50 ± 17	2.4 ± 0.7		
Amikacin		98	4	91 ± 42	19 ± 4	2.3 ± 0.4		
Amoxicillin	93 ± 10	52 ± 15	18	370 ± 90	29 ± 13	1.0 ± 0.1		
Amphotericin B		3	>90	30 ± 6	280 ± 28	15 ± 2 days		
Ampicillin	62 ± 17	82 ± 10	18 ± 2	270 ± 50	20 ± 5	1.3 ± 0.2		
Aspirin§	68 ± 3	1.4 ± 1.2	49	650 ± 80	11 ± 2	0.25 ± 0.3	See Salicylic acid.	
Atenolol	56 ± 30	85	<5	97	39 ± 20	6.3 ± 1.8	1 µg/mL	
Captopril	65	50	30	890 ± 210	49 ± 6	1.9 ± 0.5	50 ng/mL	
Carbamazepine§	>70	<1	74 ± 3	89 ± 37	98 ± 26	15 ± 5	6.5 ± 3 µg/mL	>9 µg/mL
Cephalexin	90 ± 9	91 ± 18	14 ± 3	300 ± 80	18 ± 2	0.90 ± 0.18		
Cephalothin		52	71 ± 3	470 ± 120	18 ± 8	0.57 ± 0.32		
Chloramphenicol	75–90	5 ± 1	53 ± 5	170 ± 14	66 ± 4	2.7 ± 0.8		
Chlordiazepoxide§	100	<1	96.5 ± 1.8	38 ± 34	21 ± 2	10 ± 3	>0.7 µg/mL	
Chloroquine	89 ± 16	55 ± 14	61 ± 9	750 ± 120	13,000 ± 4,600	8.9 ± 3.1 days		0.25 µg/mL
Chlorpropamide	>90	20 ± 18	87	2.1 ± 0.4	6.8 ± 0.8	33 ± 6		
Cimetidine	62 ± 6	62 ± 20	19	540 ± 130	70 ± 14	1.9 ± 0.3	0.8 µg/mL	
Clonidine	100	62 ± 11		210 ± 84	150 ± 30	8.5 ± 2	0.5–1.5 ng/mL	
Cyclosporine	34 ± 11	<1	96	650 ± 70	250 ± 190	16 ± 8	100–400 ng/mL	>400 ng/mL
Diazepam§	100	<1	98.7 ± 0.2	27 ± 4	77 ± 20	43 ± 13	>600 ng/mL	
Digitoxin	>90	32 ± 15	97 ± 1	3.9 ± 1.3	38 ± 10	6.7 ± 1.7 days	>10 ng/mL	>35 ng/mL
Digoxin	70 ± 13	60 ± 11	25 ± 5	130 ± 67	640 ± 200	39 ± 13	>0.8 ng/mL	>2 ng/mL
Diltiazem§	44 ± 10	<4	78 ± 3	810 ± 130	370 ± 120	3.2 ± 1.3		
Disopyramide	83 ± 11	55 ± 6	30–70	84 ± 28	41 ± 11	6.0 ± 1.0	3 ± 1 µg/mL	>8 µg/mL
Erythromycin	35 ± 25	12 ± 7	84 ± 3	640 ± 290	55 ± 31	1.6 ± 0.7		
Ethambutol	77 ± 8	79 ± 3	20–30	600 ± 60	110 ± 14	3.1 ± 0.4		>10 µg/mL
Furosemide	61 ± 17	66 ± 7	98.8 ± 0.2	140 ± 30	7.7 ± 1.4	1.5 ± 0.1		25 µg/mL
Gentamicin		>90	<10	90 ± 25	18 ± 6	2–3		
Hydralazine	20–60	1–15	87	3900 ± 900	105 ± 70	1.0 ± 0.3	100 ng/mL	
Imipramine§	27 ± 8	0–2	94.8 ± 0.5	1050 ± 280	1600 ± 600	18 ± 7	100–300 ng/mL	>1 µg/mL
Indomethacin	98	15 ± 8	90	140 ± 30	18 ± 5	2.4 ± 0.4	0.3–3 µg/mL	>6 µg/mL
Labetalol	20 ± 5	<5	50	1500 ± 630	700 ± 140	5.2 ± 1.3	0.13 µg/mL	
Lidocaine	35 ± 11	2 ± 1	70 ± 5	640 ± 170	77 ± 28	1.8 ± 0.4	1.5–6 µg/mL	>6 µg/mL
Lithium	100	95 ± 15	0	25 ± 8	55 ± 24	22 ± 8	0.6–1.2 meq/L	>2 meq/L
Meperidine	52 ± 3	1–25	58 ± 9	1200 ± 350	310 ± 60	3.2 ± 0.8	0.4–0.7 µg/mL	
Methotrexate	65	85 ± 11	58 ± 7	110 ± 20	67 ± 14	7.2 ± 2.1		10 µg/mL
Metoprolol	38 ± 14	10 ± 3	13	1050 ± 210	290 ± 50	3.2 ± 0.2	25 ng/mL	
Metronidazole§	99 ± 8	<10	10	90 ± 20	77 ± 28	8.5 ± 2.9	3–6 µg/mL	
Morphine	20–33	6–10	35 ± 2	1100 ± 140	230 ± 60	3.0 ± 1.2	65 ng/mL	
Moxalactam		76 ± 12	50	120 ± 30	19 ± 6	2.1 ± 0.7		
Nifedipine	45 ± 28	~0	98	720 ± 360	84 ± 35	3.4 ± 1.2		
Nortriptyline	51 ± 5	2 ± 1	92 ± 2	500 ± 130	1300 ± 300	31 ± 13	50–140 ng/mL	>500 ng/mL
Phenobarbital	100 ± 11	24 ± 5	51 ± 3	4.3 ± 0.9	38 ± 2	4.1 ± 0.8 days	10–25 µg/mL	>30 µg/mL

Table 3–1 (cont'd). Pharmacokinetic and pharmacodynamic parameters for selected drugs.*

Drug	Oral Availability (percent)	Urinary Excretion (percent)	Bound in Plasma (percent)	Clearance (mL/min)[†]	Volume of Distribution (L)[†]	Half-Life (hours)	Effective[‡] Concentrations	Toxic[‡] Concentrations
Phenytoin	98 ± 7	2	89 ± 23	Dose-dependent	45 ± 3	Dose-dependent	>10 μg/mL	>20 μg/mL
Prazosin	57 ± 10	<1	95 ± 1	210 ± 20	42 ± 9	2.9 ± 0.8		
Procainamide[§]	83 ± 16	67 ± 8	16 ± 5	350–840	130 ± 20	3.0 ± 0.6	3–14 μg/mL	>14 μg/mL
Propranolol[§]	36 ± 10	<1	93 ± 1	840 ± 210	270 ± 40	3.9 ± 0.4	20 ng/mL	
Pyridostigmine	14 ± 3	80–90		600 ± 120	77 ± 21	1.9 ± 0.2	50–100 ng/mL	
Quinidine	80 ± 15	18 ± 5	90 ± 3	330 ± 130	190 ± 80	6.2 ± 1.8	2–6 μg/mL	>8 μg/mL
Ranitidine	52 ± 11	69 ± 6	15 ± 3	730 ± 80	130 ± 20	6.2 ± 1.8	2–6 μg/mL	>6 μg/mL
Salicylic acid	100	2–30	Dose-dependent	Dose-dependent	12 ± 2	Dose-dependent	150–300 μg/mL	
Sulfamethoxazole	100	15–30	62 ± 5	22 ± 3	15 ± 1.4	10 ± 5		
Sulfisoxazole	96 ± 14	49 ± 8	91 ± 1	23 ± 3.5	10.5 ± 1.4	6.6 ± 0.7		
Terbutaline	15 ± 6	57 ± 14	25	210 ± 35	98 ± 28	16 ± 3	3 ng/mL	
Tetracycline	77	58 ± 8	65 ± 3	120 ± 20	105 ± 6	11 ± 1.5		
Theophylline	96 ± 8	13	56 ± 4	48 ± 21	35 ± 11	8.1 ± 2.4	10–20 μg/mL	>20 μg/mL
Tobramycin		90	<10	77	18 ± 6	2.2 ± 0.1		
Tocainide	89 ± 5	38 ± 7	10 ± 15	180 ± 35	210 ± 15	14 ± 2	6–15 μg/mL	
Tolbutamide	93 ± 10	0	96 ± 1	21 ± 3	11 ± 2	5.9 ± 1.4	80–240 μg/mL	
Trimethoprim	100	80–90	35–40	150 ± 40	130 ± 15	11 ± 1.4		
Tubocurarine		63 ± 35	50 ± 8	160 ± 50	21 ± 8	2.0 ± 1.1	0.6 ± 0.2 μg/mL	
Valproic acid	100 ± 10	<5	93 ± 1	7.7 ± 1.4	9.1 ± 2.8	14 ± 3	55–100 μg/mL	>150 μg/mL
Vancomycin		>90	55 ± 3	76 ± 5	27 ± 4	5.6 ± 1.8		
Verapamil	19 ± 12	<3	90 ± 2	830 ± 350	280 ± 60	4.8 ± 2.4	100 ng/mL	
Warfarin	100	0	99	3.2 ± 1.7	7.7 ± 0.7	37 ± 15	2.2 ± 0.4 μg/mL	

*The values in this table represent the parameters determined when the drug is administered to healthy normal volunteers or to patients who are generally free from disease except for the condition for which the drug is being prescribed. The values presented here are adapted, with permission, from Benet LZ, Sheiner LB: Design and optimization of dosage regimens: Pharmacokinetic data. Pages 1663–1733 in: *Goodman and Gilman's The Pharmacological Basis of Therapeutics,* 7th ed. Gilman AG et al (editors). Macmillan, 1985. This source must be consulted for the effects of disease states on the pertinent pharmacokinetic parameters.

†For a standard 70-kg person.

‡No pharmacodynamic values are given for antibiotics since these vary depending upon the infecting organism.

§One or more metabolites are active.

Volume of Distribution

As briefly introduced in Chapter 1, volume of distribution (V_d) relates the amount of drug in the body to the concentration of drug (C) in blood or plasma:

$$V_d = \text{Amount of drug in body} \div C \quad \ldots (1)$$

Volume of distribution is defined in terms of blood or plasma concentrations, depending upon the fluid measured, and reflects the apparent space available in both the general circulation and the tissues of distribution in Fig 3–1. The plasma volume of a normal 70-kg man is 3 L, blood volume about 5.5 L, extracellular fluid outside plasma 12 L, and total body water about 42 L. However, many drugs exhibit volumes of distribution, according to equation (1), far in excess of these known body fluid volumes. For example, when

500 μg of digoxin is in the body of a healthy young 70-kg male, a plasma concentration of about 0.78 ng/mL will result. Dividing the amount of drug in the body by the plasma concentration yields a volume of distribution for digoxin of 645 L—about 9 times the total body volume of a 70-kg man. This serves to emphasize that volume of distribution does not represent a real volume but must be considered as the size of the pool of body fluids that would be required if the drug were distributed equally throughout all portions of the body. In fact, digoxin, which is relatively hydrophobic, is distributed into muscle and adipose tissue, leaving a very small amount of drug in the plasma. Volume of distribution can change as a function of several variables, including the patient's age, sex, and disease. For example, the same 500 μg of digoxin in a middle-aged patient with congestive heart failure might yield a con-

centration of 1 ng/mL, corresponding to a 500-L volume of distribution.

Depending on the pK_a of the drug, the degree of plasma protein binding, the partition coefficient of the drug in the fatty tissues, and the degree of binding to other tissues within the body, volume of distribution may vary widely. For example, plasma volumes of distribution ranging from 7 to 13,000 L/70 kg are represented in Table 3–1. The antimalarial quinacrine has been reported to exhibit an apparent volume of distribution approaching 50,000 L. For a drug extensively bound to plasma proteins but not to tissue proteins, most of the drug in the body will be retained in the blood, and the volume of distribution will have a lower limit of approximately 7 L, as exemplified by chlorpropamide, furosemide, and warfarin in Table 3–1. In contrast, drugs such as imipramine, nortriptyline, and propranolol have high volumes of distribution even though over 90% of the drug in the blood is bound to plasma proteins. These drugs are even more extensively bound to tissue protein than to plasma protein. If plasma protein binding is more sensitive to pathologic changes than tissue binding, we might expect to see a linear relation between V_d and the unbound fraction in plasma, as has been shown for propranolol in patients with liver disease.

Clearance

Drug clearance principles are similar to the clearance concepts of renal physiology, in which creatinine or urea clearance is defined as the rate of elimination of the compound in the urine relative to the plasma drug concentration (UV ÷ P). At the simplest level, clearance of a drug is the rate of elimination by all routes relative to the concentration of drug in any biologic fluid:

$$Cl = \text{Rate of elimination} \div C \qquad \ldots (2)$$

Clearance (Cl) is usually defined as blood clearance (Cl_b), plasma clearance (Cl_p), or clearance based on unbound or free drug concentration (Cl_u), depending on the concentration measured for the right side of equation (2) $(C_b, C_p, \text{ or } C_u)$.

In Table 3–1, the plasma clearance of amikacin is reported as 91 mL/min, with 98% of the drug excreted in the urine unchanged. In other words, the kidney is able to remove this drug from approximately 89 mL of plasma per minute. Since clearance is usually constant in a stable patient, the rate of elimination of amikacin will depend on the concentration of drug in the plasma as required by equation (2). Propranolol is cleared at a rate of 840 mL/min, almost exclusively by nonrenal routes, especially the liver. In this case, the liver is able to remove this drug from 840 mL of plasma per minute. For the drugs listed in Table 3–1, one of the highest plasma clearances is that for imipramine, 1050 mL/min, a value 50% greater than the plasma flow to the liver, the dominant organ of elimination for this drug. However, since this drug distributes readily into red blood cells $(C_{rbc} \div C_p \sim 2.7)$, the amount of

drug delivered to the excretory organ is considerably higher than plasma flow indicates. The clearance measured in terms of blood concentration is in the physiologic range of blood flow measurements. Thus, like volume of distribution, *plasma* clearance may assume proportions that are not "physiologic." A drug that is concentrated in the red blood cells (eg, mecamylamine) can manifest a plasma clearance of tens of liters per minute. However, if blood concentration is used to define clearance, the maximum clearance possible is equal to the sum of blood flows to the various organs of elimination. For a drug eliminated solely by the liver, blood clearance is therefore limited by the flow of blood to that organ, approximately 1500 mL/min (Table 1–3). It is important to note the additive character of clearance. Elimination of drug from the body may involve processes occurring in the kidney, the lung, the liver, and other organs. Dividing the rate of elimination at each organ by the concentration of drug presented to it (eg, plasma concentration) yields the respective clearance at that organ. Added together, these separate clearances equal total systemic clearance:

$$\frac{\text{Rate of elimination}_{\text{kidney}}}{C_p} = Cl_{\text{renal}} \qquad \ldots (3a)$$

$$\frac{\text{Rate of elimination}_{\text{liver}}}{C_p} = Cl_{\text{liver}} \qquad \ldots (3b)$$

$$\frac{\text{Rate of elimination}_{\text{other}}}{C_p} = Cl_{\text{other}} \qquad \ldots (3c)$$

$$Cl_{\text{renal}} + Cl_{\text{liver}} + Cl_{\text{other}} = Cl_{\text{systemic}} \qquad \ldots (3d)$$

The example provided in equations (3a–d) indicates that the drug is eliminated by liver, kidney, and other tissues and that these routes of elimination account for all of the pathways by which the drug leaves the body. "Other" tissues of elimination could include the lungs, salivary glands, sweat glands, partition into the gut, and additional sites of metabolism, eg, hydrolysis in blood or muscle.

The 2 major sites of drug elimination are the kidneys and the liver. Clearance of unchanged drug in the urine represents renal clearance. Within the liver, drug elimination occurs via biotransformation of parent drug to one or more metabolites, or excretion of unchanged drug into the bile or both. The pathways of biotransformation are discussed in part II of this chapter. For most drugs, clearance is constant over the plasma or blood concentration range encountered in clinical settings, ie, elimination is not saturable, and the rate of drug elimination is directly proportionate to concentration (equation [2]). For drugs that exhibit saturable or dose-dependent elimination (eg, phenytoin, salicylic acid), clearance will vary depending on the concentration of drug that is achieved (Table 3–1). Dosage adjustments with such drugs are more complex than those for drugs with nonsaturable elimination and are discussed in Chapter 67.

A further definition of clearance is useful in understanding the effects of physiologic and pathologic variables on drug elimination, particularly with respect to a specific organ. The rate of elimination of a drug by a single organ can be defined in terms of the blood flow entering and exiting from the organ and the concentration of drug in the blood. The rate of presentation of drug to the organ is the product of blood flow and entering drug concentration ($Q \times C_i$), while the rate of exit of drug from the organ is the product of blood flow and exiting drug concentration ($Q \times C_o$). The difference between these rates at steady state is the rate of drug elimination:

$$\text{Rate of elimination} = Q \times C_i - Q \times C_o \quad \dots (4)$$

Dividing equation (4) by concentration of drug entering the organ of elimination (C_i), an expression for organ clearance of drug is obtained:

$$Cl_{organ} = \frac{Q \times C_i - Q \times C_o}{C_i} \quad \dots (5a)$$

$$= Q \times \frac{C_i - C_o}{C_i} = Q \times ER \quad \dots (5b)$$

As shown in equation (5b), the expression $(C_i - C_o) \div C_i$ can be referred to as the extraction ratio (ER) of the drug.

The concepts developed in equations (5a) and (5b) are illustrated in Fig 3–2, where the loss of drug from the body via the hepatic route is separated from the other loss processes. Consider a drug that is efficiently removed from the blood by hepatic processes. The concentration of drug in the blood leaving the liver will be small; the extraction ratio will approach unity; and clearance of the blood will be limited by hepatic blood flow. Drugs highly extracted by the liver (eg, hydralazine, imipramine, lidocaine, meperidine, morphine, nortriptyline, propranolol, verapamil; Table 3–1) are restricted in their rate of elimination not by intrahepatic processes but by the rate at which they can be transported in the blood to hepatic sites of elimination. The availability of drugs that are highly extracted by the liver is sensitive to small changes in the hepatic extraction ratio. For a drug that is completely absorbed from the gastrointestinal tract and enters the liver without biotransformation, the systemic availability of the drug (F) is diminished by the extent of hepatic extraction:

$$F = 1 - ER \quad \dots (6)$$

Small changes in ER for a highly extracted drug can result in dramatic changes in availability, as will be discussed in the following section.

Clearance is probably the most important pharmacokinetic term to be considered in defining a rational

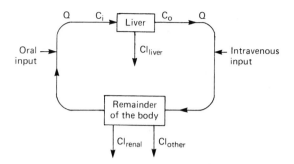

Figure 3–2. The clearance of drug by the liver is separated from the remaining systemic clearance to illustrate the effects of blood flow (Q) and extraction ratio [$(C_i - C_o) \div C_i$] on organ clearance and to illustrate that following oral drug dosing some of the absorbed drug may not be available to the remainder of the body owing to hepatic elimination during the "first pass" through the liver.

drug dosage regimen. In most cases, the clinician would like to maintain steady-state drug concentrations within a known therapeutic range (Table 3–1). Steady state will be achieved when the dosing rate (rate of active drug entering the systemic circulation) equals the rate of drug elimination. Therefore,

$$\text{Dosing rate} = Cl \times C_{ss} \quad \dots (7)$$

Thus, if the desired steady-state concentration (plasma or blood) is known, the clearance value in that patient will dictate the dosing rate.

Two additional pharmacokinetic variables, half-life and bioavailability, must be considered when designing appropriate drug dosage regimens.

Half-Life

Half-life ($t_{1/2}$) is an expression of the relationship between volume and clearance. For the simplest case (and the most useful in designing drug dosage regimens), the body may be considered as a single compartment (as illustrated in Fig 1–1B) of a size equal to the volume of distribution (V_d). However, the organs of elimination can only clear drug from the blood or plasma in direct contact with the organ. Thus, the time course of drug in the body will depend on both the volume of distribution and the clearance:

$$t_{1/2} = 0.693 \ V_d \div Cl \quad \dots (8)$$

Half-life is a useful kinetic parameter in that it indicates the time required to attain steady state or to decay from steady-state conditions after a change (ie, starting or stopping) in a particular rate of drug administration (the dosing regimen). However, as an indicator of either drug elimination or distribution, it has little value. Early studies of drug pharmacokinetics in diseased subjects were compromised by reliance on drug half-life as the sole measure of alterations in drug disposition. Disease states can affect both of the physiologically related parameters, volume of distribution and clearance; thus, the derived parameter, $t_{1/2}$, will not necessarily reflect the expected change in drug elimination.

Bioavailability

Bioavailability is defined as the fraction of unchanged drug reaching the systemic circulation following administration by any route. For an intravenous dose of the drug, bioavailability is equal to unity. For a drug administered orally, bioavailability may be less than unity for several reasons. The drug may be incompletely absorbed. It may be metabolized in the gut, the gut wall, the portal blood, or the liver prior to entry into the systemic circulation. It may undergo enterohepatic cycling with incomplete reabsorption following elimination into the bile. Biotransformation of some drugs in the liver following oral administration is an important factor in the pharmacokinetic profile, as discussed below. Data on bioavailability following oral drug administration are set forth in Table 3–1 as percentages of dose available to the systemic circulation.

Absorption, Bioavailability, & Routes of Administration

In addition to the definition given above, bioavailability is often used to indicate the *rate* at which an administered dose reaches the general circulation. The difference between the 2 definitions of bioavailability—ie, the extent and the rate of availability—is illustrated in Fig 3–3. This figure depicts the concentration-time curve for a hypothetical drug prepared in 3 different dosage formulations. Dosage forms A and B are designed so that the drug is absorbed into the blood at the same rate but twice as fast as in dosage form C. The times at which drug concentrations reach a peak are identical for dosage forms A and B and occur earlier than the peak time for dosage form C. In general, the relative order of peak times following the administration of different dosage forms of the drug thus corresponds to the rates of availability of the drug from the various dosage forms. The extent of availability may be measured by using either drug concentration in the blood or drug amounts in the urine. The area under the blood concentration–time curve (area under the curve, AUC) for a drug is a common measure of the extent of availability. In Fig 3–3, the areas under curves A and C are identical and twice as great as the area under curve B. For most drugs, drug clearance is linear (a constant function of concentration), and the relative areas under the curve or the total amounts of unchanged drug excreted in the urine quantitatively describe the relative availability of the drug from the different dosage forms. However, even in nonlinear cases, where clearance is dose-dependent, the relative areas under the curve will yield a measurement of the rank order of availability from different dosage forms or from different sites of administration.

Since there is usually a minimum effective concentration (mec) of drug in the blood (Fig 3–3) that is necessary to elicit a clinical effect (note Effective Concentrations in Table 3–1), both the rate and the extent of input or availability can affect the clinical efficacy of a drug. In many cases, the duration of pharmacologic

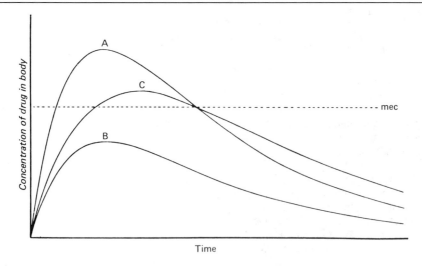

Figure 3–3. Blood concentration-time curves illustrating how changes in the rate and extent of drug availability can influence both the duration of action and the efficacy of a dose of a drug. The dotted line indicates the minimum effective concentration (mec) of the drug in the body. *Case A:* Drug is absorbed and is available rapidly and completely. This product will produce a prompt and prolonged response. *Case B:* Drug is absorbed at the same rate as in case A but is only half as available. There will be no clinical response, since the mec is not reached. *Case C:* Drug is absorbed at half the rate shown in cases A and B but is 100% available. The formulation produces a delayed and less prolonged response when compared to case A. (Modified and reproduced, with permission, from Benet LZ: Input factors as determinants of drug activity: Route, dose, dosage regimen, and the drug delivery system. Chap 2, pp 9–23, in: *Principles and Techniques of Human Research and Therapeutics*. McMahon FG Jr [editor]. Futura, 1974.)

effect is a function of the length of time the blood concentration curve is above the minimum effective concentration, and the intensity of the effect is usually a function of the height of the blood level curve above the minimum effective concentration.

Thus, for the 3 different dosage forms depicted in Fig 3–3, there would be significant differences in the levels of clinical effectiveness. Dosage form B would require twice the dose to attain blood levels equivalent to those of dosage form A. Table 3–1 contains only measures of the extent of availability following oral dosing. No measures of the rate of availability are provided, since the fractional *extent* (F) is more useful than the *rate* of availability to estimate the amount of drug in the body. Differences in rate of availability may become important for drugs given as a single dose, such as a hypnotic used to induce sleep. In this case, drug from dosage form A would reach its minimum effective concentration earlier than from dosage form C; concentrations from A would also reach a higher level and remain above the minimum effective concentration for a longer period. In a multiple dosing regimen, dosage forms A and C would yield the same average blood level concentrations, although dosage form A would show somewhat greater maximum and lower minimum concentrations.

Extraction Ratio & the First-Pass Effect

For most drugs, disposition or loss from the biologic system is independent of input, where disposition is defined as what happens to the active drug after it reaches a site in the circulation where drug concentration measurements can be made. Although disposition processes may be independent of input, the inverse is not necessarily true, since disposition can markedly affect the extent of availability. Drug absorbed from the stomach and the intestine must pass through the liver before reaching a site in the circulation that can be sampled for measurement (Fig 3–2). Thus, if a drug is metabolized in the liver or excreted in bile, some of the active drug absorbed from the gastrointestinal tract will be inactivated by hepatic processes before the drug can reach the general circulation and be distributed to its sites of action. If the metabolizing or biliary excreting capacity of the liver is great, the effect on the extent of availability will be substantial (first-pass effect). As stated in equation (6), the systemic availability of a drug metabolized in the liver will be decreased by the hepatic extraction ratio when the drug is given orally (ie, $F = 1 - ER$ for a drug completely absorbed and eliminated only by hepatic processes). Thus, if the hepatic clearance for a drug is large ($ER = Cl_{liver} \div Q_{liver}$), the extent of availability for this drug will be low when it is given by a route that yields first-pass metabolic effects. This decrease in availability is a function of the physiologic site from which absorption takes place, and no amount of dosage form modification can improve the fractional availability. Of course, therapeutic blood levels may still be reached by this route of administration if

larger doses are given. However, in this case, the levels of the drug metabolites will be increased significantly over those that would occur following intravenous administration, especially if the drug has a large volume of distribution. Therefore, the toxicity potential and elimination kinetics of the metabolites must be thoroughly understood before a decision to administer a large oral dose is made.

Drugs with high extraction ratios will show marked intersubject variability in bioavailability because of variations in hepatic function or blood flow or both. Consider a drug with an extraction ratio of 0.95 that falls to 0.90 as a result of hepatic impairment. In this instance, the bioavailability of the drug will double, from 0.05 to 0.10. These relationships can explain the marked variability in plasma or blood drug concentrations that occurs among individuals given similar doses of a highly extracted drug. Small variations in hepatic extraction between individuals will result in large differences in availability and plasma drug concentrations. These considerations are also pertinent for hepatic disease states accompanied by significant intrahepatic or extrahepatic circulatory shunting and in the presence of surgically created anastomoses between the portal system and the systemic venous circulation. For drugs that are highly extracted by the liver, shunting of blood past hepatic sites of elimination will result in substantial increases in drug availability, whereas for drugs that are poorly extracted by the liver (for which the difference in equations [4] and [5] between entering and exiting drug concentration is small), shunting of blood past the liver will cause little change in drug availability. Drugs in Table 3–1 that are poorly extracted by the liver are chlordiazepoxide, chlorpropamide, diazepam, digitoxin, phenytoin, theophylline, tolbutamide, and warfarin.

The first-pass effect can be avoided to a great extent by use of sublingual tablets and to some extent by use of rectal suppositories. The capillaries in the lower and mid sections of the rectum drain into the inferior and middle hemorrhoidal veins, which in turn drain into the inferior vena cava, thus bypassing the liver. However, suppositories tend to move upward in the rectum into a region where veins that lead to the liver, such as the superior hemorrhoidal, predominate. In addition, there are extensive anastomoses between the superior and middle hemorrhoidal veins; thus, only about 50% of a rectal dose can be assumed to bypass the liver. The lungs represent a good temporary clearing site for a number of drugs, especially basic compounds, as a result of partition into lipid tissues. The lungs also provide a filtering function for particulate matter that may be given by intravenous injection. The lung may serve as a site of first-pass loss by excretion and possible metabolism for drugs administered by nongastrointestinal ("parenteral") routes.

THE USE OF PHARMACOKINETICS IN DESIGNING A DOSAGE REGIMEN

The "dosage" of a drug represents a decision about 4 variables: (1) the amount of drug to be administered at one time; (2) the route of administration; (3) the interval between doses; and (4) the period of time over which drug administration is to be continued. The choice of the route of administration and the implications of this choice upon the extent and rate of drug availability were discussed in the previous section. Most patterns of administration fall into 2 classes, both of which may be described using pharmacokinetic principles: (1) continuous input by intravenous infusion (or any route that delivers drug at a constant rate), and (2) a series of intermittent drug doses, usually of equal size and given at approximately equally spaced intervals.

Maintenance Dose

In most clinical situations, drugs are administered in such a way as to maintain a steady state of drug in the body. Thus, calculation of the appropriate maintenance dose is a primary goal. To maintain the chosen steady state, all that is needed is to adjust dosage so that the rate of drug input (dosing rate) equals the rate of drug loss, ie, rate in = rate out. This relation was previously defined at steady state in equation (7):

$$\text{Dosing rate} = \text{Cl} \times \text{C}_{ss} \qquad \ldots (7)$$

Dosing rate is also defined as the product of the extent of availability (F) and the dose divided by the dosing interval. Thus, if the clinician can specify the desired plasma drug concentration and knows the clearance and availability for that drug in a particular patient, the appropriate dosing rate can be calculated.

Example: A steady-state plasma theophylline concentration of 15 μg/mL is desired to relieve acute bronchial asthma in a patient. If the patient is a nonsmoker and otherwise normal except for the asthmatic condition, we may use the mean clearance given in Table 3–1, ie, 48 mL/min/70 kg. Since the drug will be given as an intravenous infusion, F = 1.

$$\text{Dosing rate} = \text{Cl}_p \times \text{C}_{p,ss}$$

$$= \frac{48 \text{ mL}}{\text{min}/70 \text{ kg}} \times 15 \text{ } \mu\text{g/mL}$$

$$= 720 \text{ } \mu\text{g/min}/70 \text{ kg}$$

Therefore, in this patient, the proper infusion rate would be 0.72 mg/min, or 43.2 mg/h/70 kg. The drug might also be given as a series of bolus intravenous doses every 2 or 4 hours, for example. If the acute asthmatic attack is relieved, the clinician might then want to maintain this plasma level using oral theophylline at intervals of 8, 12, or even 24 hours. When a series of multiple doses is given, the concen-

tration term in equation (7) becomes the average of plasma concentrations over the dosing interval, $\text{C}_{p_{avg}}$ (Fig 3–4).

$$\frac{\text{F} \times \text{Dose}}{\text{Dosing interval}} = \text{Cl}_p \times \text{C}_{p_{avg}}$$

$$\text{Dose} = (43.2 \text{ mg/h}/70 \text{ kg}) \times (\text{Dosing interval})$$

$$\simeq 85 \text{ mg every 2 hours, or 340 mg every}$$
$$8 \text{ hours, or 1020 mg every 24 hours}$$

Note that the steady-state plasma level upon continuous infusion or the average plasma level following multiple dosing depends only on the primary disposition parameter, clearance. The values for volume of distribution and half-life are not needed to determine the average plasma concentration for a given dosing rate or for the reverse, determining the dosing rate for a desired plasma steady-state concentration.

Although the above equations are most useful in estimating the average drug concentrations, Fig 3–4 shows that at different dosing intervals the plasma level time curves will have different maximum and minimum values even though the average level will always be 15 μg/mL. If the clinician chose to infuse theophylline at a continuous rate of 720 μg/min, the level of 15 μg/mL would be maintained continuously. However, with intermittent dosing, eg, at intervals of 2, 8, or 24 hours, the maximum and minimum levels would differ. A simplified way of calculating these maximum ($\text{C}_{p,ss_{max}}$) and minimum ($\text{C}_{p,ss_{min}}$) values is given in equations (9) and (10):

$$\text{C}_{p,ss_{max}} = \frac{\text{F} \times \text{Dose} \div \text{V}_d}{\text{Fraction lost in a dosing interval}}$$

$$= \frac{1020 \text{ mg}/35 \text{ L}}{0.88} = 33.1 \text{ } \mu\text{g/mL} \qquad \ldots (9)$$

$$\text{C}_{p,ss_{min}} = \text{C}_{p,ss_{max}} \times \frac{\text{Fraction remaining}}{\text{after dosing interval}}$$

$$= (33.1 \text{ } \mu\text{g/mL})(0.12) = 4 \text{ } \mu\text{g/mL} \qquad \ldots (10)$$

The calculations in equations (9) and (10) were made assuming oral doses of 1020 mg per 24 hours of a drug with a half-life of 8 hours and an oral availability of about 1 (Table 3–1) and a patient with a V_d of 35 L. The denominator of equation (9), the fraction lost in a dosing interval, may be easily calculated when one knows the half-life. For example, a 24-hour dosing interval was chosen for theophylline; assuming a half-life of 8 hours, 50% of the dose would be lost in the first 8 hours, 75% in 16 hours, and 88% in 24 hours. Therefore, only 12% would remain at the end of the 24-hour dosing interval. Thus, with this dosing regimen, a maximum level of 33.1 and a minimum level of 4 μg/mL would be achieved. This would not be a good dosing scheme, since potentially toxic levels (>20

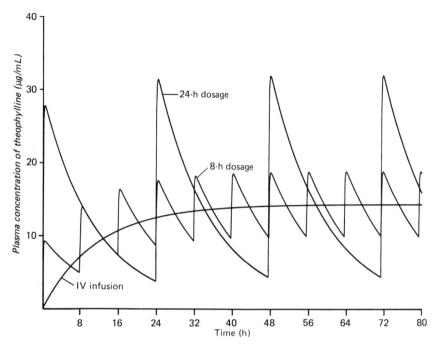

Figure 3–4. Relationship between frequency of dosing and maximum and minimum plasma concentrations when a steady-state theophylline plasma level of 15 μg/mL is desired. The smoothly rising line shows the plasma concentration achieved with an intravenous infusion of 43.2 mg/h. The doses for 8-hourly administration are 340 mg; for 24-hourly administration, 1020 mg. In each of the 3 cases, the mean steady-state plasma concentration is 15 μg/mL.

μg/mL) would be maintained for over 5 hours, and levels below the minimum effective concentration (10 μg/mL) would be expected over 10 hours during each 24-hour dosing interval. A better choice would be 340 mg every 8 hours, where the fraction lost in a dosing interval would be 0.5, and maximum and minimum levels at steady state would be 19.4 and 9.7 μg/mL, respectively. However, in both cases, the average drug concentration would still be 15 μg/mL. In the above example, the fraction of drug eliminated from the body was derived from the simple relationship that states that 50% of the amount *remaining* to be eliminated is eliminated in each successive half-life. Thus, it takes 5 half-lives after cessation of therapy for a drug to be almost entirely (97%) eliminated from the body. It is interesting to note that this same relationship also applies to drug accumulation within the body toward a plateau that occurs with multiple dosing and constant rates of intravenous infusion (Fig 3–4).

In contrast to estimates of dosage rates and average steady-state levels, which may be determined independently of any pharmacokinetic model, using only clearance (equation [7]), the determination of maximum and minimum steady-state levels requires pharmacokinetic model assumptions. Equations (9) and (10) assume that the drug follows a one-compartment body model (Fig 1–1B) and that the absorption rate is much faster than the elimination rate. For the calculation of estimated maximum and minimum concentrations in a clinical situation, these assumptions are reasonable.

Loading Dose

When the time to reach steady state is appreciable, as it is for drugs with long half-lives, it may be desirable to administer a loading dose that promptly raises the concentration of drug in plasma to the projected steady-state value. In theory, only the amount of the loading dose need be computed, not the rate of its administration; to a first approximation, this is so. The amount of drug required to achieve a given steady-state concentration in the *plasma* is the amount that must be in the *body* when the desired steady state is reached. (For intermittent dosage schemes, the amount is that at the average concentration.) The volume of distribution (V_d) is the proportionality factor that relates the total amount of drug in the body to the concentration in the plasma (C_p); if a loading dose is to achieve the desired steady-state concentration, then:

$$\text{Loading dose} = \text{Amount in the body at steady state}$$

$$= C_{p,ss} \times V_d \qquad \ldots (11)$$

For the theophylline example above, the loading dose would be 525 mg (15 μg/mL × 35 L). For most drugs, the loading dose can be given as a single dose by the chosen route of administration. Up to this point, we have ignored the fact that some drugs follow complicated multicompartment pharmacokinetics, eg, the distribution process of Fig 3–1, illustrated by the 2-compartment model in Fig 1–2. This is justified in the great majority of cases where pharmacokinetics is used as a tool in developing drug dosage regimens and in elucidating or predicting the effects of physiologic or pathologic changes in the patient. However, in some cases the distribution phase may not be ignored, particularly in connection with the calculation of loading doses. If the rate of absorption is rapid relative to distribution (this is always true for intravenous bolus administration), the concentration of drug in plasma that results from an appropriate loading dose can initially be considerably higher than desired. Severe toxicity may occur, albeit transiently. This may be particularly important, for example, in the administration of antiarrhythmic drugs, where an almost immediate toxic response is obtained when plasma concentrations exceed a particular level. Thus, while the estimation of the amount of a loading dose may be quite correct, the rate of administration can sometimes be crucial in preventing excessive drug concentrations, and slow administration of an intravenous drug (over minutes rather than seconds) is almost always wise. For intravenous doses of theophylline, initial injections should be given over a 20-minute period to avoid the possibility of high plasma levels during the distribution phase.

THE EFFECT OF DISEASE ON PHARMACOKINETIC PROCESSES

Disease states may modify all of the variables listed in Table 3–1. The ability to predict or understand how pathologic conditions may modify drug kinetics requires an understanding of the interrelationship between the variables. Clearance is the most important parameter in the design of drug dosage regimens. As shown in equation (5), clearance of an eliminating organ may be defined in terms of blood flow to the organ and the extraction ratio. The concepts embodied in equations (2), (5), and (7) are statements that can be derived from consideration of mass balance of a drug across an eliminating organ at steady state. No model is required to derive these equations. However, simple expressions for clearance, blood flow, and extraction cannot account for the full complexity of hepatic or renal drug elimination. For example, these equations do not account for drug binding to blood and tissue components, nor do they permit an estimation of the intrinsic ability of the liver or kidney to eliminate a drug in the absence of limitations imposed by blood flow. To extend the relationship of equation (5) to include expressions for protein binding and intrinsic clearance, it is necessary to formulate a model to describe organ elimination of drugs. The simplest model relating the extraction ratio to physiologic parameters is the so-called venous equilibration or well-stirred model. This approach assumes that the unbound drug concentration leaving the organ is equal to the unbound concentration inside the organ and that the intrinsic ability to metabolize or clear drug (Cl_{int}) is equal to the rate of elimination divided by the unbound concentration in

the organ. The clearance (with respect to blood concentration) for the eliminating organ then becomes

$$Cl = Q \times \frac{fu \times Cl_{int}}{Q + fu \times Cl_{int}} \qquad \ldots (12)$$

where fu is the unbound fraction of drug in blood and Q is the blood flow.

Equation (12) demonstrates that when the capability of the eliminating organ to metabolize the drug is large in comparison to the rate of drug presentation to the organ (fu $\times Cl_{int} >> Q$), the clearance will approximate the organ blood flow:

$$Cl \simeq Q \qquad \ldots (13)$$

ie, drug elimination is limited by blood flow rate, and the compound is called a high-extraction-ratio drug. On the other hand, when the metabolic capability is small in comparison to the rate of drug presentation ($Q >> fu \times Cl_{int}$), the clearance will be proportionate to the unbound fraction of drug in blood and the intrinsic clearance, ie,

$$Cl \simeq fu \times Cl_{int} \qquad \ldots (14)$$

The drug is then called a low-extraction-ratio drug. When the capability for elimination is of the same order of magnitude as the blood flow, clearance is dependent upon the blood flow as well as on the intrinsic clearance and plasma protein binding (equation [12]). Equation (12) clarifies a number of important experimental results. For example, enzyme induction or hepatic disease may change the rate of imipramine metabolism in an isolated hepatic microsomal enzyme system, but no change in clearance is found in the whole animal with similar hepatic changes. This is explained by the fact that imipramine is a high-extraction-ratio drug and clearance is limited by blood flow rate (equation [13]), so that changes in Cl_{int} due to enzyme induction or liver disease have no effect on clearance. Also, although imipramine is highly protein-bound (Table 3–1), changes in protein binding due to disease or competitive binding should have no effect on clearance even though volume of distribution is changed. In the latter case, a change in volume of distribution with no change in clearance will result in a change in half-life (equation [8]), although the elimination mechanisms have not been altered.

The differences between clearance and half-life are important in defining the underlying mechanisms for the effect of a disease state on drug disposition. For example, the half-life of diazepam increases with age (Fig 3–5). One explanation for this change is that the ability of the liver to metabolize this drug decreases as a function of age. However, when clearance is plotted against age for 20 normal individuals (Fig 3–6), it is apparent that there is no correlation with age. The increasing half-lives illustrated in Fig 3–5 actually result from changes in the volume of distribution with age;

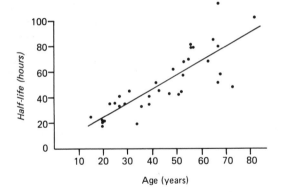

Figure 3–5. Correlation of diazepam half-life and age. (Modified and reproduced, with permission, from Klotz U et al: The effects of age and liver disease on the disposition and elimination of diazepam in adult man. *J Clin Invest* 1975;**55**:347. Copyright © 1975 by The American Society for Clinical Investigation.)

the metabolic processes responsible for eliminating the drug are fairly constant.

In many reports hepatic disease has been shown to reduce drug clearance and prolong half-life. However, for many other drugs known to be eliminated by hepatic processes, no changes in clearance or half-life have been noted with hepatic disease. This reflects the fact that hepatic disease does not always affect the hepatic intrinsic clearance. This may be due to the multiplicity of liver metabolizing enzymes available to degrade drugs and other exogenous compounds (see Chapter 3, Part II). At present, there is no reliable marker of hepatic drug-metabolizing function that can be used to predict changes in liver clearance in a manner analogous to the changes in drug renal clearance

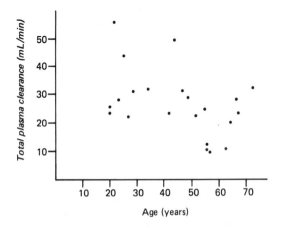

Figure 3–6. Relationship of plasma clearance of diazepam with age. (Modified and reproduced, with permission, from Klotz U et al: The effects of age and liver disease on the disposition and elimination of diazepam in adult man. *J Clin Invest* 1975;**55**:347. Copyright © 1975 by The American Society for Clinical Investigation.)

that can be predicted as a function of creatinine clearance (see below).

Generally, hepatic impairment would be expected to reduce clearance and prolong half-life or to cause no change in drug elimination. However, there is some evidence that hepatic disease can also increase clearance and shorten half-life. For example, the clearance of tolbutamide may increase and its half-life decrease with no change in volume of distribution in individuals with acute viral hepatitis during the acute phase of illness in comparison to the recovery period. Tolbutamide is a low-extraction-ratio drug, and its hepatic clearance may be described by equation (14). The explanation for the observations appears to be an increase in the unbound fraction of drug in plasma (fu) in the absence of a change in Cl_{int}. The half-life is changed, since total clearance is changed without a change in volume of distribution. For many drugs, volume of distribution would be expected to increase as the free fraction of drug in plasma increases. However, the volume of distribution for tolbutamide is quite small (11 L/70 kg from Table 3–1), and the majority of the distribution space is related to blood volume, which is independent of fu.

Pharmacokinetic changes in renal disease may also be explained in terms of clearance concepts. However, since the net renal excretion of a drug is determined by filtration, active secretion, and reabsorption, the treatment of renal clearance is more complicated than that described above. Renal clearance can be described by the following equation:

$$Cl_{renal} = (Cl_{RF} + Cl_{RS}) \times (1 - FR) \quad \ldots (15)$$

where Cl_{RF} is renal filtration clearance, Cl_{RS} is renal secretion clearance, and FR is the fraction of drug filtered and secreted that is reabsorbed. The rate of filtration depends upon the volume of fluid that is filtered in the glomerulus and the unbound concentration of drug in plasma, because proteins and drugs bound to proteins are not filtered. The volume filtered is usually estimated from inulin or creatinine clearance. The renal filtration can usually be expressed as

$$Cl_{RF} = fu \times Cl_{cr} \quad \ldots (16)$$

where Cl_{cr} is the creatinine clearance.

The secretion of drug in the kidney will depend on the relative binding of drug to the active transport carriers in relation to the binding to plasma proteins, the degree of saturation of these carriers, transfer of the drug across the tubular membrane, and the rate of delivery of the drug to the secretory site. With a model that combines these factors, the influence of changes in protein binding, blood flow, and number of functioning nephrons may be predicted and explained in a manner analogous to the examples given above for hepatic elimination.

ADJUSTMENT OF THE DOSAGE REGIMEN FOR THE INDIVIDUAL PATIENT

Attainment of an appropriate maintenance dosage regimen often requires adjustment for that patient. It is reasonable to assume that the usual recommended dose of a drug has been determined from appropriate experience with many "typical" cases. If a particular patient being treated is not expected to differ from the "typical" one with respect to *sensitivity* to the drug, one may adjust the usual maintenance dosage regimen on the basis of the patient's clearance of the drug. This requires computation or measurement of clearance for the patient (and bioavailability, if it will differ from usual) by the methods described below, and use of the following equation:

$$\text{Dosing rate}_{\text{patient}} = \text{Dosing rate}_{\text{typical}} \times \frac{Cl_{\text{patient}}}{Cl_{\text{normal}}}$$

$$\dots (17)$$

At the corrected dosing rate, the patient's mean steady-state concentration of drug will be identical to that achieved in the presumably successful treatment of a "typical" patient.

When an intermittent regimen is adjusted for an individual patient, one may choose to alter the dose given per dosing interval, the dosing interval, or both. As a rule, adjustment of the amount of each dose, not the interval, is preferred. Adjustments of dosage are usually made to compensate for smaller-than-usual clearances. If the amount of each dose is reduced to compensate for reduced clearance, then fluctuations about the mean steady-state concentration will be smaller. For most drugs, a more constant concentration-time profile is not only acceptable but desirable.

Estimates of clearance must often be adjusted when patients have alterations in renal function. The quantities required for this adjustment are the fraction of normal renal function remaining and the fraction of drug usually excreted unchanged in the urine. The latter parameter appears in Table 3–1; the former can be estimated as the ratio of the patient's creatinine clearance to a normal creatinine clearance (100–120 mL/min/70 kg). If creatinine clearance has not been measured, it may be estimated from measurements of the concentration of creatinine in serum, using one of several different equations and nomograms (see Chapter 67).

Example: Renal clearance of digoxin in a patient with depressed renal function (Cl_{cr} = 30 mL/min/70 kg) may be estimated as follows (see values in Table 3–1):

$$Cl_{\text{renal, normal}} = Cl \times \text{Fraction excreted unchanged}$$

$$= (130 \text{ mL/min/70 kg}) \times (0.60)$$

$$= 78 \text{ mL/min/70 kg} \qquad \dots (18)$$

$$Cl_{\text{renal, patient}} = \frac{Cl_{\text{cr, patient}}}{Cl_{\text{cr, normal}}} \times Cl_{\text{renal, normal}}$$

$$= \frac{30}{120} \times 78 \text{ mL/min/70 kg}$$

$$= 20 \text{ mL/min/70 kg} \qquad \dots (19)$$

$$Cl_{\text{patient}} = Cl_{\text{renal}} + Cl_{\text{nonrenal}}$$

$$= 20 + 52 = 72 \text{ mL/min/70 kg} \dots (3d)$$

Nonrenal clearance in equation (3d) was estimated as the difference between total and renal clearance in the normal person, which is assumed not to change in the patient with renal impairment. The oral dosing rate in a normal patient could be calculated using equation (7), assuming that an average plasma level of 1.2 ng/mL was desired and F = 0.70 (see Table 3–1). This would result in a dosing rate of 223 ng/min, or 0.32 mg/d for a 70-kg patient with normal renal function. Substituting this usual dosing rate into equation (17) along with the normal clearance (130 mL/min/70 kg; Table 3–1) and the calculated patient clearance of 72 mL/min from equation (3d), and assuming no change in F, yields a patient dosing rate of 0.18 mg/d. The above calculations provide a first estimate of the dosing rate. As described in greater detail in Chapter 67, drug level monitoring for drugs such as digoxin will allow the clinician to adjust the dose more accurately in a case like this one.

REFERENCES

Benet LZ, Massoud N, Gambertoglio JG (editors): *The Pharmacokinetic Basis of Drug Treatment*. Raven Press, 1984.

Benet LZ, Sheiner LB: Design and optimization of dosage regimens: Pharmacokinetic data. Pages 1663–1733 in: *Goodman and Gilman's The Pharmacological Basis of Therapeutics*, 7th ed. Gilman AG et al (editors). Macmillan, 1985.

Benet LZ, Sheiner LB: Pharmacokinetics: The dynamics of drug absorption, distribution, and elimination. Pages 3–34 in:

Goodman and Gilman's The Pharmacological Basis of Therapeutics, 7th ed. Gilman AG et al (editors). Macmillan, 1985.

Bennett WM et al: Drug prescribing in renal failure: Dosing guidelines for adults. *Am J Kidney Dis* 1983;**3**:155.

Evans WE, Schentag JJ, Jusko WJ (editors): *Applied Pharmacokinetics: Principles of Therapeutic Drug Monitoring*. Applied Therapeutics, 1980.

Klotz U et al: The effects of age and liver disease on the disposition and elimination of diazepam in adult man. *J Clin*

Invest 1975;**55**:347.

Oie S, Benet LZ: Altered drug disposition in disease states. Chap 29, pp 277–287, in: *Annual Reports in Medicinal Chemistry*. Vol 15. Hess HJ (editor). Academic Press, 1980.

Rowland M, Benet LZ, Graham GG: Clearance concepts in pharmacokinetics. *J Pharmacokinet Biopharm* 1973;**1**:123.

Sheiner LB, Rosenberg BG, Marathe VV: Estimation of population characteristics of pharmacokinetic parameters from routine clinical data. *J Pharmacokinet Biopharm* 1977;**5**:445.

Wagner JG: *Fundamentals of Clinical Pharmacokinetics*. Drug Intelligence, 1975.

Wilkinson GR, Shand DG: A physiologic approach to hepatic drug clearance. *Clin Pharmacol Ther* 1975;**18**:377.

Williams RL, Benet LZ: Drug pharmacokinetics in cardiac and hepatic disease. *Annu Rev Pharmacol Toxicol* 1980;**20**:389.

Williams RL et al: Influence of acute viral hepatitis on disposition and plasma binding of tolbutamide. *Clin Pharmacol Ther* 1977;**21**:301.

Pharmacokinetics: II. Drug Biotransformation

Maria Almira Correia, PhD, & Neal Castagnoli, Jr., PhD

Humans are daily exposed to a wide variety of foreign compounds called **xenobiotics**—substances absorbed across the lungs or skin or, more commonly, ingested either unintentionally as compounds present in food and drink or deliberately as drugs for therapeutic or "recreational" purposes. Exposure to environmental xenobiotics may be inadvertent and accidental and may even be inescapable. Some xenobiotics are innocuous, but many can provoke biologic responses both pharmacologic and toxic in nature that are discussed in Chapters 60–62. These biologic responses often depend on conversion of the absorbed substance into an active metabolite. The discussion that follows is applicable to xenobiotics in general as well as to drugs and to some extent to endogenous compounds.

WHY IS DRUG BIOTRANSFORMATION NECESSARY?

Renal excretion plays a pivotal role in terminating the biologic activity of a few drugs, particularly those that have small molecular volumes or possess polar characteristics such as functional groups fully ionized at physiologic pH. Most drugs do not possess such physicochemical properties. Pharmacologically active organic molecules tend to be lipophilic and remain unionized or only partially ionized at physiologic pH. They are often strongly bound to plasma proteins. Such substances are not readily filtered at the glomerulus. The lipophilic nature of renal tubular membranes also facilitates the reabsorption of hydrophobic compounds following their glomerular filtration. Consequently, most drugs would have a prolonged duration of action if termination of their action depended solely on renal excretion. An alternative process that may lead to the termination or alteration of biologic activity is metabolism. In general, lipophilic xenobiotics are transformed to more polar and hence more readily excretable products. The role metabolism may play in the inactivation of lipid-soluble drugs can be quite dramatic. For example, lipophilic barbiturates such as thiopental and phenobarbital would have half-lives greater than 100 years if it were not for their metabolic conversion to more water-soluble compounds.

Metabolic products are often less active than the parent drug and may even be inactive. However, some biotransformation products have enhanced activity or toxic properties, including mutagenicity, teratogenicity, and carcinogenicity. This observation undermines the once popular theory that drug-biotransforming enzymes evolved as a biochemical defense mechanism for the detoxification of environmental xenobiotics. It is noteworthy that the synthesis of endogenous substrates such as steroid hormones, cholesterol, and bile acids involves many enzyme-catalyzed pathways associated with the metabolism of xenobiotics. The same is true of the formation and excretion of endogenous metabolic products such as bilirubin, the end catabolite of heme. Finally, drug-metabolizing enzymes have been exploited through the design of pharmacologically inactive pro-drugs that are converted in vivo to pharmacologically active molecules.

THE ROLE OF BIOTRANSFORMATION IN DRUG DISPOSITION

Most metabolic biotransformations occur at some point between absorption of the drug into the general circulation and its renal elimination. A few transformations occur in the intestinal lumen or intestinal wall. In general, all of these reactions can be assigned to one of 2 major categories, called phase I and phase II reactions (Fig 3–7).

Phase I reactions usually convert the parent drug to a more polar metabolite by introducing or unmasking a functional group ($-OH$, $-NH_2$, $-SH$). Often these metabolites are inactive, although in some instances activity is only modified.

If phase I metabolites are sufficiently polar, they may be readily excreted. However, many phase I products are not eliminated rapidly and undergo a subsequent reaction in which an endogenous substrate such as glucuronic acid, sulfuric acid, acetic acid, or an amino acid combines with the newly established functional group to form a highly polar conjugate. Such conjugation or synthetic reactions are the hallmarks of phase II metabolism. A great variety of drugs undergo these sequential biotransformation reactions, although in some instances the parent drug may already possess a functional group that may form a conjugate directly. For example, the hydrazide moiety of isoniazid is known to form an N-acetyl conjugate—in a phase II reaction—that is a substrate for a phase I

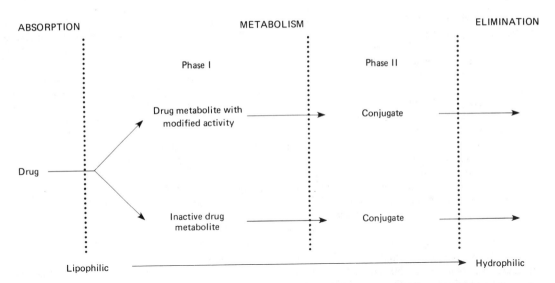

Figure 3–7. Phase I and phase II reactions in drug biodisposition. Phase II reactions may also precede phase I reactions.

type reaction, namely, hydrolysis to isonicotinic acid (Fig 3–8). Thus, phase II reactions may actually precede phase I reactions.

WHERE DO DRUG BIOTRANSFORMATIONS OCCUR?

Although every tissue has some ability to metabolize drugs, the liver is the principal organ of drug metabolism. Other tissues that display considerable activity include the gastrointestinal tract, the lungs, the skin, and the kidneys. Following oral administration, many drugs (eg, isoproterenol, meperidine, pentazocine, morphine) are absorbed intact from the small intestine and transported first via the portal system to the liver, where they undergo extensive metabolism.

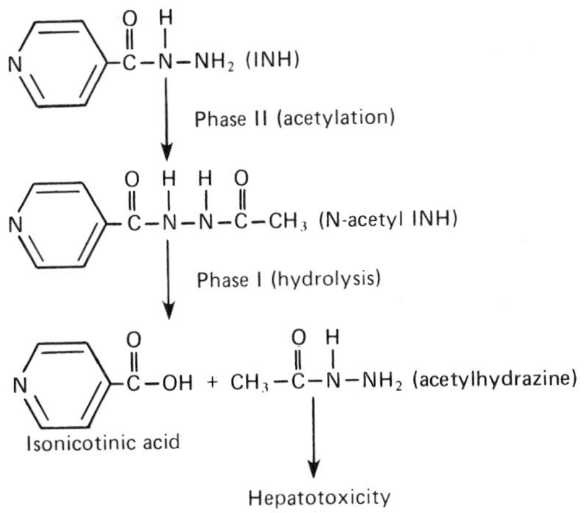

This process has been called a **first-pass effect.** Some orally administered drugs (eg, clonazepam, chlorpromazine) are more extensively metabolized in the intestine than in the liver. Thus, intestinal metabolism may contribute to the overall first-pass effect. First-pass effects may so greatly limit the bioavailability of orally administered drugs that alternative routes of administration must be employed to achieve therapeutically effective blood levels. The lower gut harbors intestinal microorganisms that are capable of many biotransformation reactions. In addition, drugs may be metabolized by gastric acid (eg, penicillin), digestive enzymes (eg, polypeptides such as insulin), or by enzymes in the wall of the intestine (eg, sympathomimetic catecholamines).

Although drug biotransformation in vivo can occur by spontaneous, noncatalyzed chemical reactions, the vast majority are catalyzed by specific cellular enzymes. At the subcellular level, these enzymes may be located in the endoplasmic reticulum, mitochondria, cytosol, lysosomes, or even the nuclear envelope or plasma membrane.

MICROSOMAL MIXED FUNCTION OXIDASE SYSTEM

Many drug-metabolizing enzymes are located in the lipophilic membranes of the endoplasmic reticulum of the liver and other tissues. When these lamellar membranes are isolated by homogenization and fractionation of the cell, they re-form into vesicles called **microsomes.** Microsomes retain most of the morphologic and functional characteristics of the intact membranes, including the rough and smooth surface features of the rough (ribosome-studded) and smooth (no ribosomes) endoplasmic reticulum. Whereas the rough microsomes tend to be dedicated to protein synthesis, the smooth microsomes are relatively rich in

Figure 3–8. Phase II activation of isoniazid (INH) to a hepatotoxic metabolite.

enzymes responsible for oxidative drug metabolism. In particular, they contain the important class of enzymes known as the mixed function oxidases (MFO), or monooxygenases. The activity of this enzyme system requires both a reducing agent (NADPH) and molecular oxygen; in a typical reaction, one molecule of oxygen is consumed (reduced) per substrate molecule, with one oxygen atom appearing in the product and the other in the form of water.

In this oxidation-reduction process, 2 microsomal enzymes play a key role. The first of these is a flavoprotein, NADPH-cytochrome P-450 reductase. One mol of this enzyme (molecular weight $\sim$ 80,000) contains 1 mol each of flavin mononucleotide (FMN) and flavin adenine dinucleotide (FAD). Because cytochrome c can serve as an electron acceptor, the enzyme is often referred to as NADPH–cytochrome c reductase. The second microsomal enzyme is a hemoprotein called cytochrome P-450 and serves as the terminal oxidase. The name cytochrome P-450 is derived from the spectral properties of this hemoprotein. In its reduced (ferrous) form, it binds carbon monoxide to give a ferrocarbonyl adduct that absorbs maximally in the visible region of the electromagnetic spectrum at 450 nm. As with other naturally occurring heme-containing proteins, the iron present in this molecule is complexed with protoporphyrin IX. Over half of the heme synthesized in the liver is committed to hepatic cytochrome P-450 formation. The relative abundance of cytochrome P-450, as compared to that of the reductase in the liver, contributes to making cytochrome P-450 heme reduction the rate-limiting step in hepatic drug oxidations.

Microsomal drug oxidations require cytochrome P-450, cytochrome P-450 reductase, NADPH, and molecular oxygen. A simplified scheme of the oxidative cycle is presented in Fig 3–9. Briefly, oxidized (Fe^{3+}) cytochrome P-450 combines with a drug substrate to form a binary complex (step ①). NADPH donates an electron to the flavoprotein reductase, which in turn reduces the oxidized cytochrome P-450–drug complex (step ②). A second electron is introduced from NADPH via the same flavoprotein reductase, which serves to reduce molecular oxygen and to form

an "activated oxygen"–cytochrome P-450–substrate complex (step ③). This complex in turn transfers "activated" oxygen to the drug substrate to form the oxidized product (step ④).

The potent oxidizing properties of this activated oxygen permit oxidation of a large number of substrates. Substrate specificity is very low for this enzyme complex. High solubility in lipids is the only common structural feature of the wide variety of structurally unrelated drugs and chemicals that serve as substrates in this system (Table 3–2).

Enzyme Induction

An interesting feature of some of these chemically dissimilar drug substrates is their ability, on repeated administration, to "induce" cytochrome P-450 by enhancing the rate of its synthesis or reducing its rate of degradation. Induction results in an acceleration of metabolism and usually in a decrease in the pharmacologic action of the inducer and also of coadministered drugs. However, in the case of drugs metabolically transformed to reactive intermediates, enzyme induction may exacerbate drug-mediated tissue toxicity.

Various substrates appear to induce forms of cytochrome P-450 having different molecular weights and exhibiting different substrate specificities and immunochemical and spectral characteristics. The 2 isozymes that have been most extensively studied are (1) cytochrome P-450b, or LM_2 (for liver microsomal form 2), which is induced by treatment with phenobarbital; and (2) cytochrome P-448 (cytochrome P_1-450, or P-450c, or LM_4), which is induced by polycyclic aromatic hydrocarbons, of which 3-methylcholanthrene is a prototype. Environmental pollutants are capable of inducing cytochrome P-450. For example, exposure to benzo(a)pyrene, present in tobacco smoke, charcoal-broiled meat, and other organic pyrolysis products, is known to induce cytochrome P-448 and to alter the rates of drug metabolism in both experimental animals and in humans. Other environmental chemicals known to induce specific cytochrome P-450 isozymes include the polychlorinated biphenyls (PCBs), which are used widely in industry as insulating materials and plasticizers, and 2,3,7,8-

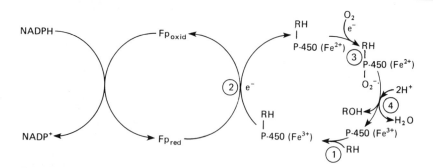

Figure 3–9. Cytochrome P-450 cycle in drug oxidations. (RH = parent drug; ROH = oxidized metabolite; Fp = flavoprotein; e⁻ = electron.)

Table 3–2. Phase I reactions.

Reaction Class	Structural Change	Drug Substrates
Oxidations Cytochrome P-450–dependent oxidations: Aromatic hydroxylations		Acetanilide, propranolol, phenobarbital, phenytoin, phenylbutazone, amphetamine, warfarin, 17α-ethinyl estradiol, naphthalene, benzpyrene.
Aliphatic hydroxylations	$RCH_2CH_3 \rightarrow RCH_2CH_2OH$ $RCH_2CH_3 \rightarrow RCHCH_3$ $\quad\quad\quad\quad\quad\;\; OH$	Amobarbital, pentobarbital, secobarbital, chlorpropamide, ibuprofen, meprobamate, glutethimide, phenylbutazone, digitoxin.
Epoxidation	$\quad\quad\quad\quad H\;\;O\;\;H$ $RCH{=}CHR \rightarrow R{-}C{-}C{-}R$	Aldrin.
Oxidative dealkylation N-Dealkylation	$RNHCH_3 \rightarrow RNH_2 + CH_2O$	Morphine, ethylmorphine, benzphetamine, aminopyrine, caffeine, theophylline.
O-Dealkylation	$ROCH_3 \rightarrow ROH + CH_2O$	Codeine, p-nitroanisole.
S-Dealkylation	$RSCH_3 \rightarrow RSH + CH_2O$	6-Methylthiopurine, methitural.
N-Oxidation Primary amines	$RNH_2 \rightarrow RNHOH$	Aniline, chlorphentermine.
Secondary amines	R_1 $\quad\;\; NH \rightarrow \quad\;\; N{-}OH$ R_2	2-Acetylaminofluorene, acetaminophen.
Tertiary amines	R_1 $R_2{-}N \rightarrow R_2{-}N \rightarrow O$ R_3	Nicotine, methaqualone.
S-Oxidation	R_1 $\quad\;\; S \rightarrow \quad\;\; S{=}O$ R_2	Thioridazine, cimetidine, chlorpromazine.
Deamination	$\quad\quad\quad\quad\;\; OH$ $RCHCH_3 \rightarrow R{-}C{-}CH_3 \rightarrow R{-}CCH_3 + NH_3$ $\;\;\, NH_2 \quad\quad\quad NH_2 \quad\quad\quad\;\; O$	Amphetamine, diazepam.
Desulfuration	R_1 $\quad\;\; C{=}S \rightarrow \quad\;\; C{=}O$ R_2	Thiopental.
	R_1 $\quad\;\; P{=}S \rightarrow \quad\;\; P{=}O$ R_2	Parathion.
Dechlorination	$CCl_4 \rightarrow [CCl_3^{\cdot}] \rightarrow CHCl_3$	Carbon tetrachloride.
Cytochrome P-450–independent oxidations:		
Amine oxidases	$RCH_2NH_2 \rightarrow RCHO + N_2$	Phenylethylamine, epinephrine.
Dehydrogenations	$RCH_2OH \rightarrow RCHO$	Ethanol, chloral hydrate.
Reductions Azo reductions	$RN{=}NR_1 \rightarrow RNH{-}NHR_1 \rightarrow RNH_2 + R_1NH_2$	Prontosil, tartrazine.
Nitro reductions	$RNO_2 \rightarrow RNO \rightarrow RNHOH \rightarrow RNH_2$	Nitrobenzene, chloramphenicol, clorazepam, dantrolene.
Carbonyl reductions	$RCR' \rightarrow RCHR'$ $\;\; \| \quad\quad\quad\;\; \|$ $\;\; O \quad\quad\quad\;\; OH$	Metyrapone, methadone, naloxone.
Hydrolyses Esters	$R_1COOR_2 \rightarrow R_1COOH + R_2OH$	Procaine, succinylcholine, aspirin, clofibrate, methylphenidate.
Amides	$RCONHR_1 \rightarrow RCOOH + R_1NH_2$	Procainamide, lidocaine, indomethacin.

tetrachlorodibenzo-*p*-dioxon (dioxin, TCDD), a trace by-product of the chemical synthesis of the defoliant 2,4,5-trichlorophenol.

Enzyme Inhibition

Other drug substrates may inhibit cytochrome P-450 enzyme activity. A well-known inhibitor is proadifen (SK&F 525-A). This compound binds avidly to the cytochrome molecule and thereby competitively inhibits the metabolism of potential substrates. Cimetidine is a popular therapeutic agent that has been found to impair the in vivo metabolism of other drugs (Table 3–5) by the same mechanism. Some substrates irreversibly inhibit cytochrome P-450 via covalent interaction of a metabolically generated reactive intermediate that may react with either the apoprotein or the heme moiety of the cytochrome. A growing list of such inhibitors includes the steroids ethinyl estradiol, norethindrone, and spironolactone; the anesthetic agent fluroxene; the barbiturates secobarbital and allobarbital; the analgesic sedatives allylisopropylacetylurea, diethylpentenamide, and ethchlorvynol; the solvent carbon disulfide; and propylthiouracil.

PHASE II REACTIONS

Parent drugs or their phase I metabolites that contain suitable chemical groups often undergo coupling or conjugation reactions with an endogenous substance to yield drug conjugates (Table 3–3). In general, conjugates are polar molecules that are readily excreted and often inactive. Conjugate formation involves high-energy intermediates and specific transfer enzymes. Such enzymes (transferases) may be located in microsomes or in the cytosol. They catalyze the coupling of an activated endogenous substance (such as the uridine 5'-diphosphate [UDP] derivative of glu-

curonic acid) with a drug (or endogenous compound), or of an activated drug (such as the S-CoA derivative of benzoic acid) with an endogenous substrate. Because the endogenous substrates originate in the diet, nutrition plays a critical role in the regulation of drug conjugations.

Drug conjugations were once believed to represent terminal inactivation events and as such have been viewed as "true detoxification" reactions. However, this concept must be modified, since it is now known that certain conjugation reactions (O-sulfation of N-hydroxyacetylaminofluorene and N-acetylation of isoniazid) may lead to the formation of reactive species responsible for the hepatotoxicity of the drug.

CLINICAL RELEVANCE OF DRUG METABOLISM

The dose and the frequency of administration required to achieve effective therapeutic blood and tissue levels vary in different patients because of individual differences in drug distribution and rates of drug metabolism and elimination. These differences are determined by genetic factors and nongenetic variables such as age, sex, liver size, liver function, circadian rhythm, body temperature, and nutritional and environmental factors such as concomitant exposure to inducers or inhibitors of drug metabolism. The discussion that follows will summarize the most important variables relating to drug metabolism that are of clinical relevance.

Individual Differences

Individual differences in metabolic rate depend on the nature of the drug itself. Thus, within the same population, steady-state plasma levels may reflect a 30-fold variation in the metabolism of one drug and

Table 3–3. Phase II reactions.

Type of Conjugation	Endogenous Reactant	Transferase (Location)	Types of Substrates	Examples
Glucuronidation	UDP glucuronic acid.	UDP-glucuronyl transferase (microsomes).	Phenols, alcohols, carboxylic acids, hydroxylamines, sulfonamides.	Nitrophenol, morphine, acetaminophen, diazepam, N-hydroxydapsone, sulfathiazole, meprobamate, digitoxin, digoxin.
Acetylation	Acetyl-CoA.	N-Acetyl transferase (cytosol).	Amines.	Sulfonamides, isoniazid, clonazepam, dapsone, mescaline.
Glutathione conjugation	Glutathione.	GSH-S-transferase (cytosol, microsomes).	Epoxides, arene oxides, nitro groups, hydroxylamines.	Ethacrynic acid, bromobenzene.
Glycine conjugation	Glycine.	Acyl-CoA glycine transferase (mitochondria).	Acyl-CoA derivatives of carboxylic acids.	Salicylic acid, benzoic acid, nicotinic acid, cinnamic acid, cholic acid, deoxycholic acid.
Sulfate conjugation	Phosphoadenosyl phosphosulfate.	Sulfotransferase (cytosol).	Phenols, alcohols, aromatic amines.	Estrone, aniline, phenol, 3-hydroxycoumarin, acetaminophen, methyldopa.
Methylation	S-Adenosylmethionine.	Transmethylases (cytosol).	Catecholamines, phenols, amines, histamine.	Dopamine, epinephrine, pyridine, histamine, thiouracil.

only a 2-fold variation in the metabolism of another. Genetic factors that influence enzyme levels account for some of these differences. Succinylcholine, for example, is metabolized only half as rapidly in persons with genetically determined defects in pseudocholinesterase as in normals. Analogous pharmacogenetic differences are seen in the acetylation of isoniazid and the hydroxylation of warfarin. Similarly, genetically determined defects in the oxidative metabolism of debrisoquine, phenacetin, guanoxan, sparteine, and phenformin have been recently reported. The defects are apparently transmitted as autosomal recessive traits and may be expressed at any one of the multiple metabolic transformations that a chemical might undergo in vivo. Environmental factors also contribute to individual variations in drug metabolism. Cigarette smokers metabolize some drugs more rapidly than nonsmokers because of enzyme induction (see p 38). Industrial workers exposed to some pesticides metabolize certain drugs more rapidly than nonexposed individuals. Such differences make it difficult to determine effective and safe doses of drugs that have narrow therapeutic indices.

Age & Sex

Increased susceptibility to the pharmacologic or toxic activity of drugs has been reported in very young and old patients as compared to young adults. Although this may reflect differences in absorption, distribution, and elimination, differences in drug metabolism cannot be ruled out—a possibility supported by studies in other mammalian species indicating that drugs are metabolized at reduced rates during the prepubertal period and senescence. Slower metabolism could be due to reduced activity of metabolic enzymes or reduced availability of essential endogenous cofactors. Similar trends have been observed in humans, but incontrovertible evidence is yet to be obtained.

Sex-dependent variations in drug metabolism have been well documented in rats but not in other rodents. Young adult male rats metabolize drugs much faster than mature female rats or prepubertal male rats. These differences in drug metabolism have been clearly associated with androgenic hormones. A few clinical reports suggest that similar sex-dependent differences in drug metabolism also exist in humans for benzodiazepines, estrogens, and salicylates.

Drug-Drug Interactions During Metabolism

Many substrates, by virtue of their relatively high lipophilicity, are retained not only at the active site of the enzyme but remain nonspecifically bound to the lipid membrane of the endoplasmic reticulum. In this state, they may induce microsomal enzymes; depending on the residual drug levels at the active site, they also may competitively inhibit metabolism of a simultaneously administered drug. Such drugs include various sedative-hypnotics, tranquilizers, anticonvulsants, and insecticides (see Table 3–4 and Appendix I). Patients who routinely ingest barbiturates, other sedative-hypnotics, or tranquilizers may require con-

Table 3–4. Partial list of drugs that enhance drug metabolism in humans.

Inducer	Drug Whose Metabolism Is Enhanced
Chlorcyclizine	Steroid hormones
Ethchlorvynol	Warfarin
Glutethimide	Antipyrine, glutethimide, warfarin
Griseofulvin	Warfarin
Phenobarbital and other barbiturates*	Barbiturates, chloramphenicol, chlorpromazine, cortisol, coumarin anticoagulants, desmethylimipramine, digitoxin, doxorubicin, estradiol, phenylbutazone, phenytoin, quinine, testosterone
Phenylbutazone	Aminopyrine, cortisol, digitoxin
Phenytoin	Cortisol, dexamethasone, digitoxin, theophylline
Rifampin	Coumarin anticoagulants, digitoxin, glucocorticoids, methadone, metoprolol, oral contraceptives, prednisone, propranolol, quinidine

* Secobarbital is an exception. See Table 3–5 and text.

siderably higher doses of warfarin or dicumarol, when being treated with these oral anticoagulants, to maintain a prolonged prothrombin time. On the other hand, discontinuation of the sedative may result in reduced metabolism of the anticoagulant and bleeding—a toxic effect of the enhanced plasma levels of the anticoagulant. Similar interactions have been observed in individuals receiving various combination drug regimens such as tranquilizers or sedatives with contraceptive agents, sedatives with anticonvulsant drugs, and even alcohol with hypoglycemic drugs (tolbutamide).

It must also be noted that an inducer may enhance not only the metabolism of other drugs but also its own metabolism. Thus, continued use of a drug may result in one form of tolerance—progressively reduced effectiveness due to enhancement of its own metabolism.

Conversely, simultaneous administration of 2 or more drugs may result in impaired elimination of the more slowly metabolized drug and prolongation or potentiation of its pharmacologic effects (Table 3–5). Both competitive substrate inhibition and irreversible substrate-mediated enzyme inactivation may augment plasma drug levels and lead to toxic effects from drugs with narrow therapeutic indices. For example, it has been shown that dicumarol inhibits the metabolism of the anticonvulsant phenytoin and leads to the expression of side effects such as ataxia and drowsiness. Similarly, allopurinol both prolongs the duration and enhances the chemotherapeutic action of mercaptopurine by competitive inhibition of xanthine oxidase. Consequently, to avoid bone marrow toxicity, the dose of mercaptopurine is usually reduced in patients receiving allopurinol. Cimetidine, a drug used in the treatment of peptic ulcer, has been shown to potentiate the pharmacologic actions of anticoagulants and seda-

Table 3–5. Partial list of drugs that inhibit drug metabolism in humans.

Inhibitor	Drug Whose Metabolism Is Inhibited
Allopurinol, chloramphenicol, isoniazid	Antipyrine, dicumarol, probenecid, tolbutamide
Cimetidine	Chlordiazepoxide, diazepam, warfarin
Dicumarol	Phenytoin
Diethylpentenamide	Diethylpentenamide
Disulfiram	Antipyrine, ethanol, phenytoin, warfarin
Ethanol	Chlordiazepoxide (?), diazepam (?), methanol
Nortriptyline	Antipyrine
Oral contraceptives	Antipyrine
Phenylbutazone	Phenytoin, tolbutamide
Secobarbital	Secobarbital

tives. The metabolism of chlordiazepoxide has been shown to be inhibited by 63% after a single dose of cimetidine; such effects are reversed within 48 hours after withdrawal of cimetidine. For such interactions to occur, drug metabolism must follow zero-order kinetics (see Chapter 3, Part I). Elimination of most drugs proceeds, however, by exponential (first-order) kinetics, thus greatly reducing the probability of such metabolically dependent interactions.

Impairment of metabolism may also result if a simultaneously administered drug irreversibly inactivates a common metabolizing enzyme, as is the case with secobarbital or novonal (diethylpentenamide) overdoses. These compounds, in the course of their metabolism by cytochrome P-450, inactivate the enzyme and result in impairment of their own metabolism and that of other cosubstrates.

Interactions Between Drugs & Endogenous Compounds

Various drugs require conjugation with endogenous substrates such as glutathione, glucuronic acid, and sulfuric acid for their inactivation. Consequently, different drugs may compete for the same endogenous substrates, and the faster-reacting drug may effectively deplete endogenous substrate levels and impair the metabolism of the slower-reacting drug. If the latter has a steep dose-response curve or a narrow margin of safety, potentiation of its pharmacologic and toxic effects may result.

Diseases Affecting Drug Metabolism

Acute or chronic diseases that affect liver architecture or function markedly affect hepatic metabolism of some drugs. Such conditions include fat accumulation, alcoholic hepatitis, active or inactive alcoholic cirrhosis, hemochromatosis, chronic active hepatitis, biliary cirrhosis, and acute viral or drug hepatitis. Depending on their severity, these conditions impair hepatic drug-metabolizing enzymes, particularly microsomal oxidases, and thereby markedly affect drug

elimination. For example, the half-lives of chlordiazepoxide and diazepam in patients with liver cirrhosis or acute viral hepatitis are greatly increased, with a corresponding prolongation of their effects. Consequently, these drugs may cause coma in patients with liver disease when given in ordinary doses.

Liver cancer has been reported to impair hepatic drug metabolism in humans. For example, aminopyrine metabolism is slower in patients with malignant hepatic tumors than in normal controls. These patients also exhibit markedly diminished aminopyrine clearance rates. Studies of liver biopsy specimens from patients with hepatocellular carcinoma also indicate impaired ability to oxidatively metabolize drugs in vitro. This is associated with a correspondingly reduced cytochrome P-450 content.

Cardiac disease, by limiting blood flow to the liver, may impair disposition of those drugs whose metabolism is flow-limited (Table 3–6). These drugs are so readily metabolized by the liver that hepatic clearance is essentially equal to liver blood flow. Pulmonary disease may affect drug metabolism as indicated by the impaired hydrolysis of procainamide and procaine in patients with chronic respiratory insufficiency and the increased half-life of antipyrine in patients with lung cancer. Impairment of enzyme activity or defective formation of enzymes associated with heavy metal poisoning or porphyria also results in reduction of hepatic drug metabolism. For example, lead poisoning has been shown to increase the half-life of antipyrine in humans.

Although the effects of endocrine dysfunction on drug metabolism have been well explored in experimental animal models, corresponding data for humans with endocrine disorders are scanty. Thyroid dysfunction has been associated with altered metabolism of some drugs and of some endogenous compounds as well. Hypothyroidism increases the half-life of antipyrine, digoxin, methimazole, and practolol, whereas hyperthyroidism has the opposite effect. A few clinical studies in diabetic patients indicate no apparent impairment of drug metabolism, as reflected by the half-lives of antipyrine, tolbutamide, and phenylbutazone. In contrast, the metabolism of several drugs is impaired in male rats treated with diabetogenic agents such as alloxan or streptozocin. These alterations are abolished by administration of insulin, which has no direct influence on hepatic drug-metabolizing enzymes. Malfunctions of the pituitary, adrenal cortex, and gonads markedly impair hepatic drug metabolism

Table 3–6. Rapidly metabolized drugs whose hepatic clearance is blood flow–limited.

Alprenolol	Lidocaine
Amitriptyline	Meperidine
Clomethiazole	Morphine
Desipramine	Pentazocine
Imipramine	Propoxyphene
Isoniazid	Propranolol
Labetalol	Verapamil

in rats. On the basis of these findings, it may be supposed that such disorders could significantly affect drug metabolism in humans. However, until sufficient evidence is obtained from clinical studies in patients, such extrapolations must be considered tentative.

METABOLISM OF DRUGS TO TOXIC PRODUCTS

It is becoming increasingly evident that metabolism of drugs and other foreign chemicals may not always be an innocuous biochemical event leading to detoxification and elimination of the compound. Indeed, several compounds have been shown to be metabolically transformed to reactive intermediates that are toxic to various organs. Such toxic reactions may not be apparent at low levels of exposure to parent compounds when alternative detoxification mechanisms are not yet overwhelmed or compromised and the availability of endogenous detoxifying cosubstrates (glutathione, glucuronic acid, sulfate) is not limited. However, when these resources are exhausted, the toxic pathway may prevail resulting in overt organ toxicity or carcinogenesis. The number of specific examples of such drug-induced toxicity is expanding rapidly. An example is acetaminophen (paracetamol)–induced hepatotoxicity (Fig 3–10). This analgesic antipyretic drug is quite safe in therapeutic doses (1.2 g/d). It normally undergoes glucuronidation and sulfation to the corresponding conjugates, which together comprise 95% of the total excreted metabolites. The alternative cytochrome P-450–dependent glutathione (GSH) conjugation pathway accounts for the remaining 5%. When acetaminophen intake far exceeds therapeutic doses, the glucuronidation and sulfation pathways are saturated, and the cytochrome P-450–dependent pathway becomes increasingly important. Little or no hepatotoxicity results as long as glutathione is available for conjugation. However, with time, hepatic glutathione is depleted faster than it can be regenerated, and accumulation of a reactive and toxic metabolite occurs. In

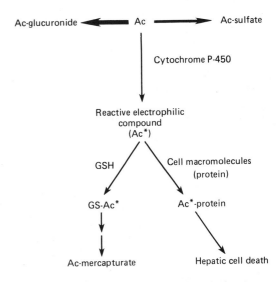

Figure 3–10. Metabolism of acetaminophen (Ac) to hepatotoxic metabolites. (GSH = glutathione; GS = glutathione moiety; Ac* = reactive intermediate.)

the absence of intracellular nucleophiles such as glutathione, this reactive metabolite (thought to be an N-hydroxylated product or an N-acetylbenzoiminoquinone) reacts with nucleophilic groups present on cellular macromolecules such as protein, resulting in hepatotoxicity (Fig 3–10).

The chemical and toxicologic characterization of the electrophilic nature of the reactive acetaminophen metabolite has led to the development of effective antidotes—cysteamine and acetylcysteine (Mucomyst). Administration of acetylcysteine (the safer of the 2) within 24 hours following acetaminophen overdosage has been shown to protect victims from fulminant hepatotoxicity and death.

Similar mechanistic interpretations can be invoked to explain the nephrotoxicity of phenacetin and the hepatotoxicity of aflatoxin and of benzo(a)pyrene, a pyrolytic product of organic matter present in cigarette tar and smoke and in smoked foods.

REFERENCES

Desmond PV et al: Cimetidine impairs elimination of chlordiazepoxide (Librium) in man. *Ann Intern Med* 1980;**93**:266.

Hodgson E, Guthrie FE (editors): *Introduction to Biochemical Toxicology*. Elsevier/North Holland, 1980.

Jenner P, Testa B (editors): *Concepts in Drug Metabolism*. Part B of: *Drugs and the Pharmaceutical Science Series*. Vol 10. Marcel Dekker, 1981.

La Du BN, Mandel G, Way EL (editors): *Fundamentals of Drug Metabolism and Drug Disposition*. Williams & Wilkins, 1971.

Minchin RF, Boyd MR: Localization of metabolic activation and deactivation systems in the lung: Significance to the pulmonary toxicity of xenobiotics. *Annu Rev Pharmacol Toxicol* 1983;**23**:217.

Ortiz de Montellano PR, Correia MA: Suicidal destruction of cytochrome P-450 during oxidative drug metabolism. *Annu Rev Pharmacol Toxicol* 1983;**23**:481.

Testa B, Jenner P (editors): *Drug Metabolism: Chemical and Biological Aspects*. Marcel Dekker, 1976.

4

Basic & Clinical Evaluation of New Drugs

Bertram G. Katzung, MD, PhD, & Barry Berkowitz, PhD

During the past 50 years, the introduction of hundreds of new drugs in many previously unknown drug groups—as well as major improvements in traditional drug groups—has converted the management of many diseases that were once nontreatable, life-threatening, or fatal into routine treatment exercises. One cause of this remarkable change is a radical improvement in the means of developing and testing new drugs. This process has been greatly accelerated by new technology and by economic and governmental stimuli; in most countries, the testing of drugs is now regulated by legislation and closely monitored by departments of government. This chapter summarizes the process by which new therapeutic agents are researched and developed. While the examples used reflect the process in the USA, the pathway generally is the same worldwide.

Enormous costs, ranging from $70 to $100 million, are involved in the development of a single new drug. These costs are incurred in the labor invested in rejected molecules—5000–10,000 new molecules are generated for each successful new drug introduced—and in the cost of detailed basic and clinical studies and promotion of the ultimate candidate molecule. For example, the development of ethambutol, an antituberculosis agent, involved the testing of several thousand molecules to find the lead compound; ethambutol itself was one of 600 analogs subsequently synthesized. For this and other reasons, most new drugs are developed in the industrial laboratories of pharmaceutical companies. The fact that substantial economic rewards can be had if a new drug proves successful provides a major stimulus for continued effort by the companies.

DRUG DISCOVERY

Most new drug candidates are identified through one of 3 approaches: chemical modification of a known molecule, screening of natural products or previously discovered chemical entities for biologic activity, or rational drug design based on an understanding of biologic mechanisms. The development of

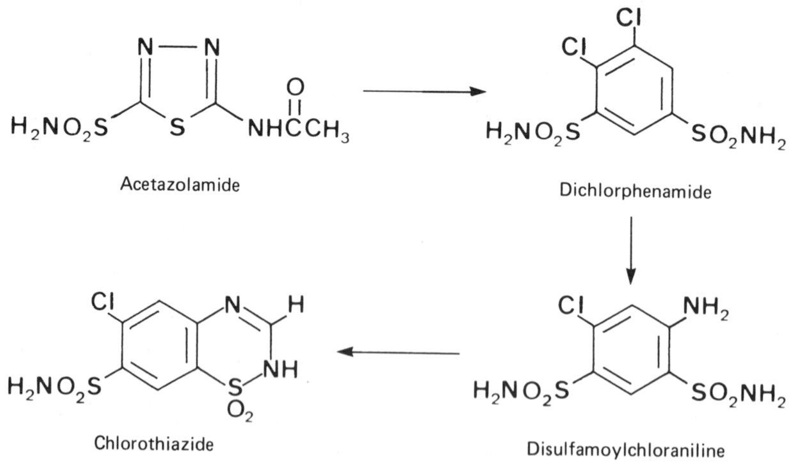

Figure 4–1. Development of chlorothiazide from the carbonic anhydrase inhibitors. The arrows indicate historical steps, not chemical reactions. Acetazolamide was one of the first effective carbonic anhydrase inhibitors. Dichlorphenamide was subsequently synthesized and was found to cause an increased ratio of sodium chloride to sodium bicarbonate in the urine, a desirable effect, when it produced a diuresis. Disulfamoylchloraniline was less potent than dichlorphenamide, but when cyclized by acylation it yielded chlorothiazide, the first member of the thiazide drug group.

thiazide diuretics from the much less useful carbonic anhydrase inhibitors (Chapter 14) is an example of the first approach (Fig 4–1). The discovery of streptomycin, a product of soil-dwelling microorganisms, illustrates the second approach. Knowledge of different types of histamine receptors was the cornerstone of the synthesis of H_2 histamine antagonists and the development of cimetidine. Regardless of the source of the molecule, a critical pathway of pharmacologic testing and characterization is followed—screening. A variety of biologic assays at the molecular, cellular, organ, and whole animal levels are used to define the activity and selectivity of the drug. The type and number of initial screening tests depend on the pharmacologic goal. Anti-infective drugs will be tested first against a variety of infectious organisms; hypoglycemic drugs are tested first for their ability to lower blood sugar; etc. However, the molecule is usually studied for a broad array of actions. This has the advantage of demonstrating unsuspected effects and occasionally discloses a previously unsuspected therapeutic action.

Some of the more detailed studies performed during drug discovery testing are listed in Table 4–1 and define the **pharmacologic profile** of the drug. For example, a broad range of tests would be performed on a drug designed to act as an antagonist at vascular alpha-adrenoceptors for the treatment of hypertension. At the molecular level, the compound would be screened for receptor binding affinity to cell membranes containing alpha receptors. Selectivity for other receptors and receptor subtypes would be determined. Since binding sites on enzymes frequently resemble cell receptor sites, the activity on appropriate enzymes would be determined. Early studies would be done on the enzymes of drug metabolism such as liver cytochrome P-450 to determine whether the molecule of interest is likely to be a substrate or inhibitor of these enzymes in therapeutic concentrations.

Effects on cell function would be studied to determine evidence of the efficacy of the compound. Evidence for whether the drug is an agonist or antagonist would be obtained. Isolated tissues would be utilized to further determine the pharmacologic activity and selectivity of the compound. Comparisons with other muscle preparations and with reference compounds would be undertaken. At each step in this pathway, the compound would have to meet specific performance criteria to be carried further.

Whole animals would be used for studies of the drug on organ systems and disease models. Cardiovascular and renal function studies would be first carried out in normal animals. For this antihypertensive drug, animals with hypertension would then be treated to characterize the compound. Evidence of oral and parenteral efficacy and duration of action would be collected. If the agent possessed useful activity, it would be further studied for possible side effects on other major organ systems, including respiratory, gastrointestinal, endocrine, and central nervous systems.

These studies might suggest the need for further chemical modification to achieve more desirable pharmacokinetic or pharmacodynamic properties. For example, oral administration studies might show that the drug was poorly absorbed or rapidly metabolized in the liver; modification to improve bioavailability might be indicated. If the drug is to be administered chronically, an assessment of tolerance development would be made. For drugs related to those known to cause physical dependency, abuse potential would also be studied. An explanation of pharmacologic mechanism would be sought.

The result of this procedure (which may have to be repeated several times to produce a promising molecule) is a **lead compound,** ie, a leading candidate for a successful new drug. A patent application may be filed for novel compounds that are efficacious or for previously known chemical entities that may have new therapeutic utility.

Advances in molecular biology and biotechnology have brought new approaches and new problems to the drug discovery and development process. The production and use of polypeptides and proteins as drugs were limited previously by their structural complexity. Because they could not be easily synthesized, supply was limited to minute amounts extracted from animal and cadaver tissues. Now we can identify, isolate, and sequence the genes that code for many of these molecules. Insertion of the genes in bacteria, yeasts, or mammalian cells makes it possible to synthesize, isolate, and purify large amounts of the desired protein or peptide. Human insulin, human growth hormone, interferon, hepatitis vaccine, and tissue plasminogen activator are currently available for use or in clinical trials and are the first drugs to be produced by these biotechnology approaches.

PRECLINICAL SAFETY & TOXICITY TESTING

Candidate drugs that survive the initial screening and profiling procedures must be carefully evaluated for potential risk before clinical testing is begun. Depending on the proposed use of the drug, preclinical toxicity testing includes most or all of the procedures shown in Table 4–2. While no chemical can be certified as completely "safe" (*free* of risk), since every chemical is toxic at some level of dosage, it is possible to estimate the risk associated with exposure to the chemical under specified conditions.

The major kinds of information needed from the preclinical toxicity study are (1) acute toxicity—effects of large single doses up to the lethal level; (2) subacute and chronic toxicity—effects of multiple doses, which are especially important if the drug is intended for chronic use in humans; (3) effects on reproductive functions, including teratogenicity; (4) carcinogenicity; (5) mutagenicity; and (6) investigative toxicology. In addition to the studies shown in Table 4–2, several quantitative estimates are desirable.

Table 4–1. Pharmacologic profile tests.

Experimental Method or Target Organ	Species/Tissue	Route of Administration	Measurement
Molecular			
Receptor binding (example: α-adrenoceptors)	Cell membrane fractions from organs or cultured cells	In vitro	Receptor affinity and selectivity.
Enzyme activity (examples: tyrosine hydroxylase, dopamine-β-hydroxylase, monoamine oxidase)	Sympathetic nerves/adrenal glands; purified enzymes	In vitro	Enzyme inhibition and selectivity.
Cytochrome P-450	Liver	In vitro	Enzyme inhibition; effects on drug metabolism.
Cellular			
Cell function	Cultured cells	In vitro	Evidence for receptor activity—agonism or antagonism (example: effects on cyclic nucleotides).
Isolated tissue	Blood vessels: arteries/veins, heart, lung, ileum (rat or guinea pig)	In vitro	Effects on vascular contraction and relaxation; selectivity for vascular receptors; effects on other smooth muscles.
Systems/disease models			
Blood pressure	Dog, cat (anesthetized)	Parenteral	Systolic-diastolic changes.
	Rat, hypertensive (conscious)	Oral	Antihypertensive effects.
Cardiac effects	Dog (conscious)	Oral	Electrocardiography.
	Dog (anesthetized)	Parenteral	Inotropic, chronotropic effects, cardiac output, total peripheral resistance.
Peripheral autonomic nervous system	Dog (anesthetized)	Parenteral	Effects on response to known drugs and electrical stimulation of central and peripheral autonomic nerves.
Respiratory effects	Dog, guinea pig	Parenteral	Effects on respiratory rate/amplitude, bronchial tone.
Diuretic activity	Dog	Oral, parenteral	Natriuresis, kaliuresis, water diuresis, renal blood flow, glomerular filtration rate.
Gastrointestinal effects	Rat	Oral	Gastrointestinal motility/secretions.
Circulating hormones, cholesterol, blood sugar	Rat/dog	Parenteral, oral	Serum concentration.
Blood coagulation	Rabbit	Oral	Coagulation time, clot retraction, prothrombin time.
Central nervous system	Mouse, rat	Parenteral, oral	Degree of sedation, muscle relaxation, locomotor activity, stimulation.

These include the "no-effect" dose, the maximum dose at which the specified toxic effect is not seen; the minimum lethal dose, the smallest dose that is observed to kill any animal; and, if necessary, the median lethal dose (LD50), the dose that kills approximately 50% of the animals (see Chapter 2). Historically the latter value (LD50) was calculated with a high degree of precision and was used to compare toxicities of compounds relative to their therapeutic doses. It is now realized that a high degree of precision may not be necessary to compare toxicity (Malmfors and Teiling reference). Therefore, the median lethal dose is now an approximate value estimated from the smallest number of animals possible. These doses are used to calculate the initial dose to be tried in humans, usually taken as 1/100–1/10 of the no-effect dose.

It is important to recognize the limitations of pre-

Table 4–2. Safety tests.

	Approach	Comment
Acute toxicity	Acute dose that is lethal in approximately 50% of animals. Determine maximum tolerated dose. Usually 2 species, 2 routes, single dose.	Compare with therapeutic dose.
Subacute toxicity	Three doses, 2 species. Up to 6 months may be necessary prior to clinical trial. The longer the duration of expected clinical use, the longer the subacute test.	Clinical chemistry, physiologic signs, autopsy studies, hematology, histology, electron microscopy studies. Identify target organs of toxicity.
Chronic toxicity	One to 2 years. Required when drug is intended to be used in humans for prolonged periods. Usually run concurrently with clinical trial.	Goals of subacute and chronic tests are to show which organs are susceptible to drug toxicity. Tests as noted above for subacute.
Effect on reproductive performance	Effects on animal mating behavior, reproduction, parturition, progeny, birth defects.	Examines fertility, teratology, perinatal and postnatal effects, lactation.
Carcinogenic potential	Two years, 2 species. Required when drug is intended to be used in humans for prolonged periods.	Hematology, histology, autopsy studies.
Mutagenic potential	Effects on genetic stability of bacteria (Ames test) or mammalian cells in culture; dominant lethal test in mice.	Increasing interest in this problem.
Investigative toxicology	Determine sequence and mechanisms of toxic action. Develop new methods for assessing toxicity.	May allow rational and earlier design of safer drugs.

clinical testing, especially if one is to be directly involved in the clinical study of a new drug. These include the following:

(1) Toxicity testing is time-consuming and expensive. The total cost of preclinical pharmacology and toxicology studies was estimated to be $41 million per successful drug in 1979. Two to 5 years may be required to collect and analyze data.

(2) Large numbers of animals must be used to obtain preclinical data. This is a proper cause of ethical concern for scientists, and progress is being made toward reducing the numbers required while still obtaining valid data (see Malmfors and Teiling and Zbinden and Flury-Reversi references). Unfortunately, some segments of the public are attempting to suppress all animal testing in the erroneous belief that such testing is obsolete or unnecessary and that all essential data can be obtained from cell cultures or computer models.

(3) Extrapolation of toxicity data from animals to humans is not completely reliable (see Dixon reference). For any given compound, the total toxicity data from all species have a very high predictive value for its toxicity in humans. However, the problems noted above place limitations on the amount of information it is practical to obtain.

(4) For statistical reasons, rare adverse effects are unlikely to be detected, just as in clinical trials (see below).

EVALUATION IN HUMANS

Federal law in the USA requires that the study of new drugs in humans be conducted in accordance with certain stringent requirements. Scientifically valid results are not guaranteed simply by conforming to government regulations, however, and the design and execution of a good clinical trial requires the efforts of a clinician-scientist or clinical pharmacologist, a statistician, and frequently other professionals as well. The need for careful design and execution is based upon 3 major factors inherent in the study of any therapeutic measures—pharmacologic or nonpharmacologic—in humans:

(1) **The variable natural history of most diseases:** Most diseases tend to wax and wane in severity; some disappear spontaneously with time; even malignant neoplasms may undergo spontaneous remissions. A good experimental design must take into account the natural history of the disease under study by evaluating a large enough population of subjects over a sufficiently long period of time. Additional protection against errors of interpretation caused by fluctuations in severity of the manifestations of disease is provided by utilizing a **cross-over design,** which consists of alternating periods of administration of test drug, placebo preparation, and standard drug control, if any, in each subject. These sequences are systematically varied, so that different subsets of patients receive each of the possible sequences of treatment. An example of such a design is shown in Table 4–3.

(2) **The presence of other diseases and risk factors:** Known or unknown diseases and risk factors

Table 4–3. Typical cross-over design for comparing a mythical new analgesic, "Novent," with placebo and a known active drug, aspirin, in the management of chronic pain. Each therapeutic period lasts 7 days.

Patient Group	Medication Given		
	Week 1	Week 2	Week 3
I	Aspirin	Placebo	"Novent"
II	Placebo	"Novent"	Aspirin
III	"Novent"	Aspirin	Placebo

(including life-styles of subjects) may influence the results of a clinical study. For example, some diseases alter the pharmacokinetics of drugs (Chapter 3). Concentrations of a blood component being monitored as a measure of the effect of the new agent may be influenced by other diseases or other drugs. Attempts to avoid this hazard usually involve the cross-over technique (when feasible) and proper selection and assignment of patients to each of the study groups. This requires that careful medical and pharmacologic histories (including use of recreational drugs) be obtained and that statistically valid methods of randomization be used in assigning subjects to particular study groups.

(3) **Subject and observer bias:** Most patients tend to respond in a positive way to any therapeutic intervention by interested, caring, and enthusiastic medical personnel. The manifestation of this phenomenon in the subject is the **placebo response** (Latin "I shall please") and may involve objective physiologic and biochemical changes as well as changes in subjective complaints associated with the disease. It is usually quantitated by administration of an inert material, with exactly the same physical appearance, odor, consistency, etc, as the active dosage form. The magnitude of the response varies considerably from patient to patient. However, the incidence of the placebo response is fairly constant, being observed in 20–40% of patients in almost all studies. Placebo "toxicity" also occurs but usually involves subjective effects: stomach upset, insomnia, sedation, etc.

Observer bias includes the unconscious as well as any conscious tendency of people evaluating the response of subjects to find an anticipated result.

Subject bias effects can be quantitated—and discounted from the response measured during active therapy—by the **single-blind design.** This involves use of a placebo or dummy medication, as described above, which is administered to the same subjects in a cross-over design, if possible, or to a separate control group of subjects. Observer bias can be taken into account by disguising the identity of the medication being used—placebo or active form—from both the subjects and the personnel evaluating the subjects' responses (**double-blind design**). In this design, a third party holds the code identifying each medication packet, and the code is not broken until all of the clinical data have been collected.

The Food & Drug Administration

The Food and Drug Administration (FDA) is the administrative body that oversees the drug evaluation process in the United States and grants approval to market new drug products. The authority of the FDA to regulate drug marketing derives from several pieces of legislation (Table 4–4). If a drug has not been shown through adequately controlled testing to be safe and effective for a specific use, it cannot be marketed in interstate commerce for this use.

Of course it is impossible, as noted above, to certify that a drug is absolutely safe, ie, free of all risk. It is possible, however, to identify most of the hazards likely to be associated with use of the drug and to place some statistical limits on frequency of occurrence of such events in the population under study. As a result, an operational and pragmatic definition of "safety" can usually be reached that is based upon the nature and incidence of drug-associated hazards as compared to the hazard of nontherapy of the target disease.

Table 4–4. Major legislation pertaining to drugs in the USA.

Law	Purpose and Effect
Pure Food & Drug Act of 1906	Prohibited mislabeling and adulteration of drugs.
Opium Exclusion Act of 1909	Prohibited importation of opium.
Amendment (1912) to the Pure Food & Drug Act	Prohibited advertising claims if they were both false and fraudulent.
Harrison Narcotics Act of 1914	Established regulations for the use of opium, opiates, and cocaine (marihuana added in 1937).
Food, Drug, & Cosmetic Act of 1938	Required that new drugs be **safe** as well as pure (but did not require proof of efficacy).
Durham-Humphrey Act of 1952	Vested in the FDA the power to determine which products could be sold without prescription.
Kefauver-Harris Amendment (1962) to the Food, Drug, & Cosmetic Act	Required proof of **efficacy** as well as safety for new drugs and for drugs released since 1938; established guidelines for reporting of information about adverse reactions, clinical testing, and advertising of new drugs.
Comprehensive Drug Abuse Prevention & Control Act (1970)	Outlined strict controls on the manufacture, distribution, and prescribing of habit-forming drugs; established programs to prevent and treat drug addiction.
Drug Price Competition & Patent Restoration Act of 1984	Abbreviated new drug applications for generic drugs. Requires bioequivalence data. Patent life extended by amount of time drug was delayed by FDA review process. Cannot exceed 5 extra years or extend to more than 14 years post-NDA approval.

THE IND & NDA

Once a drug is judged ready to be studied in humans, a Notice of Claimed Investigational Exemption for a New Drug (IND) must be filed with the FDA. The IND includes (1) information on composition and source of the drug, (2) manufacturing information, (3) all data from animal studies, (4) clinical plans and protocols, and (5) names and credentials of physicians who will conduct the trials.

It often requires 4–6 years of clinical testing to accumulate all required data and to fulfill regulatory requirements. Testing is begun after sufficient acute and subacute animal toxicity studies have been completed. Chronic safety testing in animals is usually done concurrently with clinical trials. In each of the 3 formal phases of clinical trials, volunteers or patients must be informed of the investigational status of the drug as well as possible risks and must be allowed to decline or to consent to participate and receive the drug. These regulations are based on the principles set forth in the "Declaration of Helsinki" (see Editor's Page reference). In addition to the approval of the sponsoring organization and the FDA, an interdisciplinary "institutional review board" at the facility where the clinical drug trial will be conducted critically reviews the request for testing in humans.

In phase 1, the effects of the drug as a function of dosage are established in a small number of healthy volunteers. Phase 1 trials are done to determine whether humans and animals show significantly different responses to the drug and to establish the probable limits of the clinical dosage range. These trials are nonblind, ie, both the investigators and the subjects know what is being given. Many predictable toxicities are detected in this phase (Table 4–5, Clinical Pharmacology Phase). Pharmacokinetic measurements of absorption, half-life, and metabolism are often done in phase 1. Such studies are usually performed in clinical research centers by specially trained clinical pharmacologists.

In phase 2, the drug is studied for the first time in patients with the target disease to determine safety and efficacy. A small number of patients (10–150) are studied in great detail. A single-blind design is often used, with an inert placebo medication and an older active drug (positive control) in addition to the investigational agent. Phase 2 trials also are usually done in special clinical centers. A broader range of toxicities may be detected in this phase (Table 4–5, Controlled Evaluation Phase).

In phase 3, the drug is evaluated in much larger numbers of patients, sometimes thousands. Using information gathered in phases 1 and 2, trials are designed to minimize errors caused by placebo effects, variable courses of the disease, etc. Therefore, double-blind and cross-over techniques (like that of Table 4–3) are frequently employed. Phase 3 trials are usually in clinical settings similar to those anticipated for the ultimate use of the drug. Phase 3 studies are difficult to design and execute and are usually very ex-

Table 4–5. Drug-related toxic manifestations in humans. Order of clinical evaluation.*

1. **Clinical Pharmacology Phase**
   (1) Related to *desired* pharmacologic, biochemical, or endocrine effects. Exaggerated effect at recommended dose.
   (2) Related to *desired* pharmacologic, biochemical, or endocrine effects. Drug acting on wrong target organ.
   (3) Related to *undesired* pharmacologic, biochemical, or endocrine effects.
   (4) Related to tissue irritation and damage on direct contact (topical and parenteral agents only).
2. **Controlled Evaluation Phase**
   (1) Related to *desired or undesired* pharmacologic, biochemical, or endocrine effects, requiring preexisting disease.
   (2) Related to *desired or undesired* pharmacologic, biochemical, or endocrine effects, requiring contributing iatrogenic and other exogenous factors.
   (3) Related to interference with absorption of nutrients.
   (4) Related to interference with natural defense mechanisms.
   (5) Related to tissue storage or precipitation of drugs or metabolites.
   (6) Toxic effects on the fetus.
   (7) Related to sensitization and allergic reactions.
3. **Broad Trial Phase**
   (1) Related to sensitization and allergic reactions that may require contributing exogenous factors.
   (2) Related to idiosyncrasy (unknown mechanisms).

*Modified and reproduced, with permission, from Abrams WB, Bagdon RE, Zbinden G: Techniques of animal and clinical toxicology. Page 61 in: *Animal and Clinical Pharmacologic Techniques in Drug Evaluation*. Nodine JH, Siegler PE (editors). Copyright © 1964 by Year Book Medical Publishers, Inc., Chicago.

pensive, because of the large numbers of patients involved and the masses of data that must be collected and analyzed. The investigators are usually specialists in the disease being treated. Certain toxic effects, especially those caused by sensitization, may first become apparent in phase 3 (Table 4–5, Broad Trial Phase).

If phase 3 results are positive, application will be made for permission to market the new agent. The process of applying for marketing approval requires submission of a New Drug Application (NDA) to the FDA. The application contains, often in hundreds of volumes, full reports of all preclinical and clinical data pertaining to the drug under review. A decision on approval by the FDA may take 3 years or longer. In cases where an urgent need is perceived (eg, cancer chemotherapy), the process of preclinical and clinical testing and FDA review may be considerably abbreviated.

Once approval to market a drug has been obtained, phase 4 begins. This constitutes an attempt to monitor the safety of the new drug under actual conditions of use in large numbers of patients. Initial release of the agent may be limited to selected medical centers, which agree to report all unexpected effects to the FDA and the manufacturer. Spontaneous reporting by physicians of adverse drug effects to the company and FDA also occurs. Final release of a drug for general prescription use should be accompanied by a vigilant postmarketing surveillance program. The importance of careful and complete reporting of toxicity after marketing approval by the FDA can be appreciated by noting that many important drug-induced effects have an incidence of 1:10,000 or less. Table 4–6 shows the sample size required to detect a drug-induced increase of events that occur with different frequencies in the untreated population (and some examples of such events). Because of the small numbers of subjects in phases 1–3, such low-incidence drug effects will not generally be detected before phase 4, no matter how carefully the studies are executed. Phase 4 has no fixed duration.

The time from the filing of a patent application to approval for marketing of a new drug may be 5 years or more. Since the lifetime of a patent is 17 years in the USA, the owner of the patent (usually a pharmaceutical company) has exclusive rights for marketing the product for only a limited time. Because the review process with the FDA can be lengthy, the time during which a drug is under review can be added to the patent life. However, the length of extension (up to 5 years) cannot extend the total life of the patent to more than 14 years post-NDA approval. After expiration of the patent, any company may produce and market the drug without paying license fees to the original patent owner. However, a trademark—the proprietary name given by the company to its version of the drug—may be legally protected indefinitely. Therefore, pharmaceutical companies are strongly motivated to give their new drugs easily remembered trade names. For example, "Librium" is the trade name for the sedative-hypnotic drug whose generic name is "chlordiazepoxide." For the same reason, the company's advertising material will emphasize the trade name. In 1978, almost 80% of prescriptions specified the drug by trade name. (See section on generic prescribing in Chapter 69.)

ADVERSE REACTIONS TO DRUGS

Severe adverse reactions to marketed drugs are uncommon, although less dangerous toxic effects, as noted in the subsequent chapters of this book, are frequent for some drug groups. Life-threatening reactions probably occur in less than 2% of patients admitted to medical wards (see *Br Med J* editorial reference). The mechanisms of the various toxicities listed in Table 4–5 can be conveniently grouped into 2 categories: type A ("augmented"), which are manifestations of excessive pharmacologic effect and therefore predictable; and type B ("bizarre"), which are manifestations of immunologic or unknown mechanisms (see Rawlins reference). Type A reactions are usually discovered by pharmacologists and toxicologists before a drug reaches phase 3 trials. Type B reactions may not be recognized until a drug has been on the market for many years and are therefore usually discovered by clinicians. It is therefore important that practitioners be aware of the various types of allergic reactions to drugs. These include IgE-mediated reactions such as anaphylaxis, urticaria, and angioedema; IgG- or IgM-mediated reactions of the lupus erythematosus type; IgG-mediated responses of the serum sickness type, which involve vasculitis; and cell-mediated allergies involved in contact dermatitis. They are discussed in Chapter 59.

EVALUATING A CLINICAL DRUG EVALUATION

The periodical literature is the chief source of clinical information about new drugs, especially those very recently released for general use. Such information may include new indications or major new toxicities and contraindications. Therefore, health practitioners should be familiar with the sources of such information (noted in Chapter 1) and should be prepared to evaluate it. Certain general principles can be applied to such evaluations and are discussed in detail in the Riegelman and Smith references listed below. These principles are conveniently stated in the form of questions every reader should ask while examining the paper.

(1) Were appropriate ethical and procedural safeguards available to the patients? Adherence to standards such as those laid down in the Declaration of Helsinki is enforced by the NIH for federally supported clinical research, by institutional review boards, and by responsible medical journals publishing the results of such studies.

(2) What were the objectives of the study? Are the

Table 4–6. Study size as a function of effect frequency.*

Number of exposed people required to detect a 2-fold increase in incidence of a rare effect with a 20% probability of missing a real effect and a 5% probability of concluding that an effect exists when one does not. One nonexposed control is required per exposed subject. If the drug increases the risk more than 2-fold, the number of subjects required is decreased.

Frequency of Effect in Nonexposed Controls	Example	Number of Exposed Subjects Required
1/100	Any congenital cardiac defect†	1800
1/1000	Facial clefts‡	18,000
1/10,000	Tricuspid atresia§	180,000
1/100,000	Myocardial infarction**	1,800,000

* Modified and reproduced, with permission, from Finkle W: Sample size requirements for detection of drug-induced disease. Report of Joint Commission on Prescription Drug Use, Appendix V, 1980.
†Frequency of all forms of congenital cardiac malformations is about one in 111 live births.
‡Frequency of facial cleft malformations is about one in 700 live births.
§Frequency of tricuspid value atresia is about one in 8500 live births.
** Frequency of myocardial infarction in women nonsmokers 30–39 years of age is about 4 in 100,000.

goals clearly defined and stated? A poorly defined goal such as "to study the effects of minoxidil" (an antihypertensive drug) is much less likely to lead to useful results than a clearly defined objective such as "to measure the effect of minoxidil on renal function in severely hypertensive males above age 45."

(3) Were the experimental methods appropriate to the study goals? Does the author state the accuracy and precision (reproducibility) of the methods? Are the methods sensitive enough so that small but biologically important changes could be detected?

(4) How were the patients selected? Were there enough? Are they representative of the population most likely to receive the drug or the population in which the reader would like to use the drug? If the project was a long-term or outpatient study, were any patients lost to follow-up? How was this accounted for? Were placebo and positive control treatments included? How were patients assigned to the various groups? Was a cross-over design feasible and was one used? Were patients receiving any other therapy during the trial? How was this controlled or accounted for? Were appropriate statistical tests applied?

(5) Do the data, even if sound, justify the conclusions? Does the drug offer significant advantages of efficacy or safety over existing agents or is it merely new? Extrapolation from the study population to other groups must be very carefully scrutinized.

A well-written report of a good clinical study usually provides explicit answers to all of the above questions. Lack of clear answers to these questions justifies skepticism about the investigation.

REFERENCES

Adverse drug reactions. (Editorial.) *Br Med J* 1981;**282:**1819.

Beyer KH: *Discovery, Development, and Delivery of New Drugs*. SP Medical & Scientific Books, 1978.

Bezold C: *The Future of Pharmaceuticals: The Changing Environment for New Drugs*. Wiley, 1981.

Dixon RL (editor): Extrapolation of laboratory toxicity data to man: Factors influencing the dose-toxic response relationship. (Symposium.) *Fed Proc* 1980;**39:**53.

Editor's Page: Code of ethics of the World Medical Association: Declaration of Helsinki. *Clin Res* 1966;**14:**193.

Glantz SA: *Primer of Biostatistics*. McGraw-Hill, 1981.

Jick H: Drugs: Remarkably nontoxic. *N Engl J Med* 1974;**291:** 824.

Malmfors T, Teiling A: LD50: Its value for the pharmaceutical industry in safety evaluation of drugs. *Acta Pharmacol Toxicol* 1983;**52(Suppl 2):**229.

Rawlins MD: Clinical pharmacology: Adverse reactions to drugs. *Br Med J* 1981;**282:**974.

Riegelman RK: *Studying a Study and Testing a Test: How to Read the Medical Literature*. Little, Brown, 1981.

Schwartzman D: *Innovation in the Pharmaceutical Industry*. Johns Hopkins Univ Press, 1976.

Silverman M, Lee PR: *Pills, Profit, and Politics*. Univ of California Press, 1974.

Sloan D et al: Drug evaluation after marketing. *Ann Intern Med* 1979;**90:**257.

Smith W: Drug choice in disease. Chapter 1 in: *Clinical Pharmacology: Basic Principles in Therapeutics*, 2nd ed. Melmon KL, Morrelli HF (editors). Macmillan, 1978.

Venning GR: Identification of adverse reactions to new drugs. (5 parts.) *Br Med J* 1983;**286:**199, 289, 365, 458, 544.

Zbinden G, Flury-Reversi M: Significance of LD50-test for the toxicological evaluation of chemical substance. *Arch Toxicol* 1981;**47:**77.

5

Introduction to Autonomic Pharmacology

Bertram G. Katzung, MD, PhD

The nervous system and the endocrine system are the major means by which body functions are controlled and integrated. They have several properties in common, including high-level integration in the brain, ability to influence processes in distant regions of the body, and extensive use of negative feedback. The major difference between the nervous and endocrine systems is in the mode of transmission of information. In the case of the endocrine system, transmission is largely chemical, via blood-borne hormones (see Chapter 35). The nervous system, on the other hand, relies primarily on rapid electrical transmission of information over nerve fibers. However, between nerve cells—and between nerve cells and their effector cells—signals are usually carried by chemical rather than electrical impulses. This chemical transmission takes place through the release of small amounts of transmitter or "neuromediator" substances from the nerve terminals into the region of the synapse. The chemical transmitter crosses the synaptic cleft by diffusion and activates (or inhibits) the postsynaptic cell by binding to a specialized receptor molecule.

Within the nervous system, one can discern 2 major functional subdivisions. The **autonomic division** is largely independent in that its activities are not under direct conscious control. It is concerned primarily with visceral functions—cardiac output, blood flow to various organs, digestion, elimination, etc—necessary for life. The other major division of the nervous system, the **somatic division,** is largely nonautomatic and is concerned with consciously controlled functions such as locomotion as well as respiration and posture. Autonomic pharmacology is the study of those drugs that affect the autonomic nervous system itself or autonomic receptors on the effector cells controlled by the autonomic nervous system (cardiac muscle, smooth muscle, and glands). To understand the selectivity and actions of these drugs, it is necessary to understand the autonomic nervous system at the anatomic, biochemical, and physiologic levels.

ANATOMY OF THE AUTONOMIC NERVOUS SYSTEM
(See Fig 5–1.)

The autonomic nervous system lends itself to division on anatomic grounds into 2 major portions: the

sympathetic (thoracolumbar) division and the **parasympathetic (craniosacral)** division. Both divisions originate in nuclei within the central nervous system and give off preganglionic fibers that exit from the brain stem or spinal cord. The sympathetic division contains discrete motor ganglia lying principally in 2 chains on either side of the spinal column; the parasympathetic division consists largely of groups of motor ganglia distributed diffusely in the walls of the organs innervated. The 2 divisions are further differentiated by the fact that their preganglionic efferent fibers originate in different portions of the central nervous system. The parasympathetic preganglionic fibers leave the central nervous system via cranial nerves (especially the third, seventh, ninth, and tenth) and the third and fourth sacral spinal roots. The sympathetic preganglionic axons leave the central nervous system via the thoracic and lumbar roots. In addition to these clearly defined peripheral motor portions of the autonomic nervous system, there are large numbers of afferent—sensory—fibers that impinge on important integrating centers in the hypothalamus and medulla to evoke the motor activity carried to the effector cells by the efferent fibers described above.

It is important to remember that the terms sympathetic and parasympathetic are anatomic ones and do not depend on the type of transmitter chemical released from the nerve endings nor on the kind of effect—excitatory or inhibitory—evoked by nerve activity.

NEUROTRANSMITTER CHEMISTRY OF THE AUTONOMIC NERVOUS SYSTEM

A different classification of autonomic nerve cells can be based on the transmitter molecules released from their terminal boutons and varicosities. A large number of peripheral autonomic nervous system fibers synthesize and release acetylcholine; they are **cholinergic** fibers—ie, they act by releasing acetylcholine. These include all preganglionic efferent autonomic fibers and the somatic (nonautonomic) motor fibers to skeletal muscle as well. Thus, almost all efferent fibers leaving the central nervous system are cholinergic. In addition, all parasympathetic postganglionic and a few sympathetic postganglionic fibers are cholinergic. In contrast, most postganglionic sympathetic

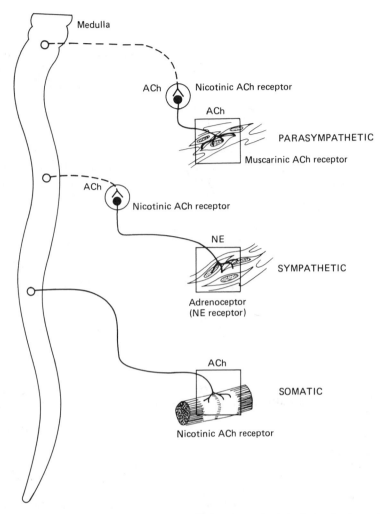

Figure 5–1. Schematic diagram comparing some anatomic and pharmacologic features of autonomic and somatic motor nerves. Because most parasympathetic ganglia are in or near the wall of the innervated organ, parasympathetic preganglionic nerves are long and postganglionic ones are short. Conversely, sympathetic ganglia are near the spinal cord; therefore, preganglionic fibers are short and postganglionic fibers long. Only the primary transmitter substances are shown: ACh = acetylcholine; NE = norepinephrine.

fibers release norepinephrine (noradrenaline); they are **noradrenergic** (often called simply "adrenergic") fibers—ie, they act by releasing norepinephrine. These chemical characteristics are presented schematically in Fig 5–1. A few sympathetic fibers release acetylcholine (see below). There is considerable evidence that dopamine is released by some peripheral sympathetic fibers. Adrenal medullary cells, which are embryologically analogous to postganglionic sympathetic neurons, release a mixture of epinephrine and norepinephrine.

The terminals of cholinergic neurons contain large numbers of small membrane-bound vesicles concentrated near the synaptic portion of the cell membrane. These clear vesicles contain acetylcholine in high concentration and certain other molecules (eg, peptides) that may act as cotransmitters. Most of the acetylcholine is synthesized in the cytoplasm from choline and acetyl-CoA through the catalytic action of the enzyme choline acetyltransferase (Fig 5–2). Acetyl-CoA is synthesized in mitochondria, which are present in large numbers in the nerve ending. Choline is transported by a membrane carrier mechanism from the extracellular fluid into the neuron terminal. Synthesis is thus a rather simple process and is capable of supporting a very high rate of synaptic release. Vesicular storage of acetylcholine is accomplished by the packaging of "quanta" of acetylcholine molecules (usually 1000–50,000 molecules per quantum) in membranes cycled in from the neuronal surface. Release of transmitter occurs when an action potential reaches the terminal and triggers sufficient influx of calcium ions to "destabilize" the storage vesicles. Fusion of the vesicular membranes with the terminal membrane occurs, with exocytotic expulsion of several hundred quanta of acetylcholine molecules and cotransmitter into the

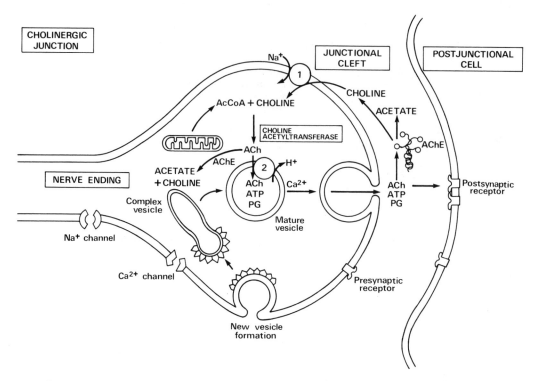

Figure 5–2. Schematic illustration of a generalized cholinergic junction (not to scale). Two cellular structures, the cholinergic nerve terminal (left) and the postjunctional cell (right), are separated by the junctional (synaptic) cleft. Choline is transported into the nerve terminal by carrier (1) that cotransports sodium ion, using the sodium gradient for energy. This transport can be inhibited by hemicholinium. Inside the nerve terminal, choline combines with activated acetate (AcCoA), in a reaction catalyzed by choline acetyltransferase, to form acetylcholine (ACh). Formation of storage vesicles is initiated by the deposition of clathrin molecules on the inner surface of the terminal membrane (shown as the fencelike structure on the new vesicle). Upon being pinched off from the surface, a "complex vesicle" is formed that eventually gives rise to a mature storage vesicle. ACh is transported into the storage vesicle by the action of a carrier (2) that utilizes the outward flux of protons as its source of energy. ATP and proteoglycan (PG) are also stored in the vesicle. Release of transmitter occurs when an action potential, carried down the axon by the action of voltage-sensitive sodium channels, invades the nerve terminals. Voltage-sensitive calcium channels in the terminal membrane are opened, allowing an influx of calcium. The increase in intracellular calcium causes fusion of vesicles with the surface membrane, resulting in exocytotic expulsion of ACh, ATP, and proteoglycan into the junctional cleft. This step is blocked by botulin. ACh reaching prejunctional and postjunctional receptors modifies the function of the corresponding cell. (*Note:* Some cholinergic junctions appear to lack prejunctional receptors.) ACh also diffuses into contact with the enzyme acetylcholinesterase (AChE), a polymeric enzyme that splits ACh into choline and acetate. At some cholinergic junctions, a polypeptide cotransmitter, vasoactive intestinal polypeptide (VIP), is released along with ACh into the junctional cleft.

synaptic cleft. The physiologic role of the cotransmitter is not known.

After release from the presynaptic terminal, acetylcholine molecules may bind to and activate an acetylcholine receptor (**cholinoceptor**). Eventually (and usually very rapidly), all of the acetylcholine released will diffuse within range of an **acetylcholinesterase** molecule. Acetylcholinesterase (AChE) very efficiently splits acetylcholine into choline and acetate, neither of which has significant potency, and thereby terminates the action of the transmitter (Fig 5–2). Most cholinergic synapses are richly supplied with acetylcholinesterase; the half-life of acetylcholine in the synapse is therefore very short. In addition, acetylcholinesterase is found in other tissues, eg, red blood cells. (Another cholinesterase with a lower specificity for acetylcholine, butyrocholinesterase [pseudocholinesterase], is found in blood plasma, liver, glia, and many other tissues.)

Adrenergic neurons also store their transmitter substances in membrane-bound vesicles (Fig 5–3), but the synthesis of the catecholamine transmitters is more complex than that of acetylcholine, as indicated in Fig 5–4. In the adrenal medulla and certain areas of the brain, norepinephrine is further converted to epinephrine. In noradrenergic neurons, a portion of the norepinephrine is apparently not stored in vesicles but exists in a protected form in the neuronal cytoplasm; this secondary pool is not released by nerve action potentials but may be expelled by the action of certain indirect-acting sympathomimetic drugs such as tyramine. Several important transport mechanisms in the noradrenergic nerve terminal are potential sites of drug action. One of these, located in the terminal cell

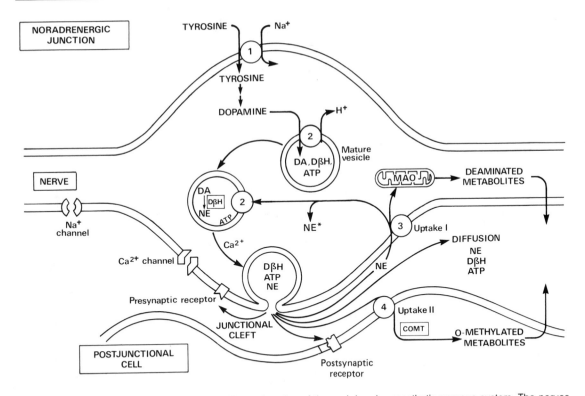

Figure 5–3. Schematic diagram of the neuroeffector junction of the peripheral sympathetic nervous system. The nerves terminate in complex networks with varicosities or enlargements that form synaptic junctions with effector cells. Some of the processes occurring in the noradrenergic varicosity are analogous to those in cholinergic terminals, eg, new vesicle formation in the varicosity. Tyrosine is transported into the noradrenergic varicosity by a carrier (1) that is linked to sodium uptake. Tyrosine is hydroxylated to dopa and then decarboxylated to form dopamine (DA) in the cytoplasm. Dopamine is transported into the vesicle by a carrier mechanism (2) that can be blocked by reserpine. The same carrier transports norepinephrine (NE) and several other amines into these granules. Dopamine is converted to norepinephrine through the catalytic action of dopamine-β-hydroxylase (DβH). ATP is also present in high concentration in the vesicle. Release of transmitter occurs when an action potential is conducted to the varicosity by the action of voltage-sensitive sodium channels. Depolarization of the varicosity membrane opens voltage-sensitive calcium channels and results in an increase in intracellular calcium. The elevated calcium facilitates exocytotic fusion of vesicles with the surface membrane and expulsion of norepinephrine, ATP, and some of the dopamine-β-hydroxylase. Release is blocked by drugs such as guanethidine and bretylium. Norepinephrine reaching either pre- or postsynaptic receptors modifies the function of the corresponding cells. Norepinephrine also diffuses out of the cleft, or it may be transported into the cytoplasm of the varicosity (uptake I [3], blocked by cocaine, tricyclic antidepressants) or into the postjunctional cell (uptake II [4]). The nonvesicular norepinephrine, shown schematically as NE*, can be released by tyramine and a variety of the other indirectly acting adrenergic agonists.

membrane, actively transports norepinephrine and similar molecules into the cell cytoplasm (Fig 5–3, carrier 3). It can be inhibited by such agents as cocaine and the tricyclic antidepressants. A second high-affinity carrier for catecholamines is located in the wall of the storage vesicle itself and can be inhibited by a different class of drugs, the reserpine alkaloids (Fig 5–3, carrier 2).

Release of the vesicular content from noradrenergic nerve endings is believed to be similar to the calcium-dependent process described above for cholinergic terminals. In addition to the primary transmitter (norepinephrine), ATP, dopamine-β-hydroxylase, and certain polypeptides are also released into the synaptic cleft. It is not known whether any of these cotransmitters play a significant role in adrenergic transmission.

Norepinephrine and epinephrine can be metabolized by several enzymes, as shown in Fig 5–5. Because of the high activity of monoamine oxidase in the mitochondria of the nerve terminal, there is a significant turnover of norepinephrine even in the resting terminal. Since the metabolic products are excreted in the urine, an estimate of catecholamine turnover can be obtained from laboratory analysis of total metabolites (sometimes referred to as "total VMA and metanephrines") in a 24-hour urine sample. However, metabolism is not the primary mechanism for termination of action of norepinephrine physiologically released from noradrenergic nerves. Termination of noradrenergic transmission results from several processes including simple diffusion away from the receptor site (with ultimate metabolism in the plasma or liver) and reuptake into the nerve terminal (**uptake**

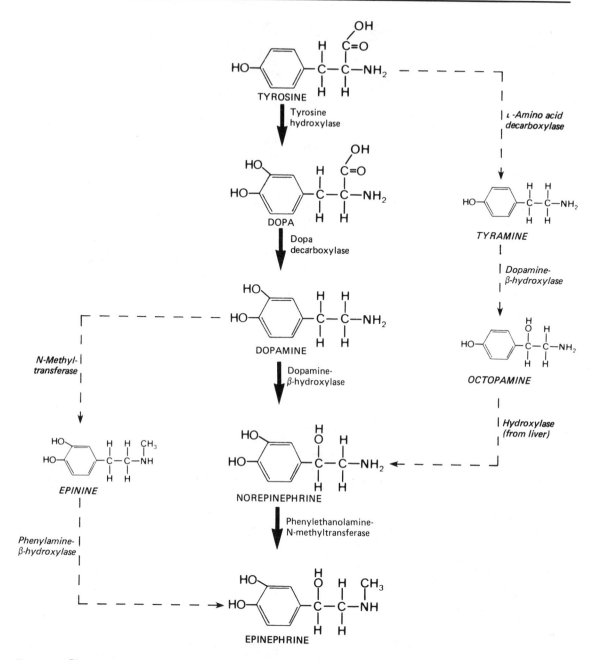

Figure 5–4. Biosynthesis of catecholamines. The alternative pathways shown by the dashed arrows have not been found to be of physiologic significance in humans. However, tyramine and octopamine may accumulate in patients treated with monoamine oxidase inhibitors. (Reproduced, with permission, from Greenspan FS, Forsham PH: *Basic & Clinical Endocrinology*, 2nd ed. Lange, 1986.)

I) or into perisynaptic glia or smooth muscle cells (**uptake II**) (Fig 5–3).

AUTONOMIC RECEPTORS

Less is known about the biochemical nature of autonomic receptors than of transmitters, but this field is one of the most active research areas in pharmacology.

Historically, indirect structure-activity analyses, with careful comparisons of the potency of series of autonomic analogs, led to the definition of different autonomic receptor subtypes (Table 5–1). The acetylcholine receptor subtypes were named after the alkaloids originally used in their identification: muscarine and nicotine. These nouns are readily converted into adjectives—thus, muscarinic and nicotinic receptors. In the case of receptors associated with noradrenergic

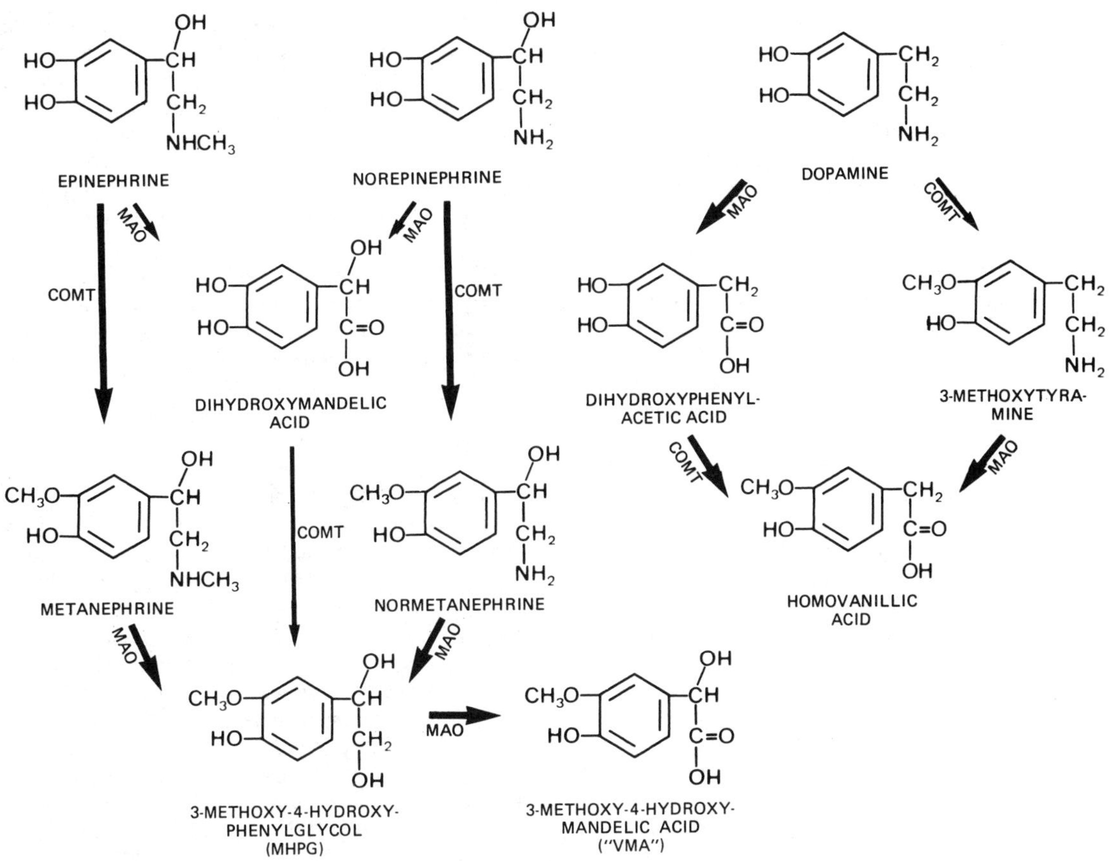

Figure 5–5. Metabolism of catecholamines by catechol-O-methyltransferase (COMT) and monoamine oxidase (MAO). (Modified and reproduced, with permission, from Greenspan FS, Forsham PH: *Basic & Clinical Endocrinology,* 2nd ed. Lange, 1986.)

Table 5–1. Autonomic receptor types.

Name	Typical Locations
Cholinoceptors Muscarinic	Parasympathetic effector cells: smooth muscle, cardiac muscle, exocrine glands; brain.
Nicotinic	Autonomic ganglia, skeletal muscle neuromuscular end-plate, spinal cord.
Adrenoceptors Alpha$_1$	Postsynaptic effector cells, especially smooth muscle.
Alpha$_2$	Presynaptic adrenergic nerve terminals, platelets, lipocytes, smooth muscle.
Beta$_1$	Postsynaptic effector cells, especially heart; lipocytes, brain, presynaptic noradrenergic nerve terminals.
Beta$_2$	Postsynaptic effector cells, especially smooth muscle.
Dopamine	Brain and postsynaptic effectors, especially vascular smooth muscle of the splanchnic and renal vascular beds. Presynaptic receptors on nerve terminals, especially in the heart, vessels, and gastrointestinal system.

nerves, the coining of simple adjectives from the names of the agonists (noradrenaline, phenylephrine, isoproterenol, etc) was not practicable. Therefore, the term **adrenoceptor** is widely used to describe receptors that respond to catecholamines, especially norepinephrine. By analogy, the term **cholinoceptor** denotes receptors that respond to acetylcholine. In North America, receptors were colloquially named after the nerves that usually innervate them—thus, **adrenergic** (or noradrenergic) **receptors** and **cholinergic receptors.** These terms are still used in some quarters, including older textbooks. Development of selective blocking drugs has led to the naming of subclasses within these major types, eg, within the adrenergic class, α_1 and α_2 receptors differ in both agonist and antagonist selectivity. Specific examples of such selective drugs are given in the chapters that follow. More recently, much progress has been made in isolating and purifying receptor proteins. Detailed characterization of the peptide sequences of these proteins and their 3-dimensional conformations should lead to the development of even more specific agonists and antagonists.

FUNCTIONAL ORGANIZATION OF AUTONOMIC ACTIVITY

A basic understanding of the interactions of autonomic components with each other and with their effector organs is essential for an appreciation of the actions of autonomic drugs, especially because of their significant "reflex" effects.

Central Integration

At the highest level—midbrain and medulla—the 2 divisions of the autonomic nervous system and the endocrine system are integrated with each other and with information from higher central nervous system centers. These interactions are such that early investigators called the parasympathetic system a **trophotropic** one (ie, leading to growth) and the sympathetic system an **ergotropic** one (ie, leading to energy expenditure) that was activated for "fight or flight." While such terms offer little insight into the mechanisms involved, they do provide simple descriptions applicable to many of the actions of the systems (Table 5–2). For example, slowing of the heart and stimulation of digestive activity are typical energy-conserving trophotropic actions of the parasympathetic system. In contrast, cardiac stimulation, increased blood sugar, and cutaneous vasoconstriction are responses produced by sympathetic discharge that are suited to fighting or surviving attack.

At a more subtle level of interactions in the brain stem, medulla, and spinal cord, there are important cooperative interactions between the parasympathetic and sympathetic systems. For some organs, sensory fibers in the parasympathetic system exert reflex control over motor outflow in the sympathetic system. Thus, the sensory baroreceptor fibers in the glossopharyngeal nerve have a major influence on sympathetic outflow from the vasomotor center. This example is developed in greater detail below. Similarly, parasympathetic sensory fibers in the wall of the urinary bladder significantly influence sympathetic inhibitory outflow to that organ.

Cardiovascular Reflexes

The reflexes that control or are controlled by autonomic nerve activity are particularly important in understanding cardiovascular responses to autonomic drugs. As indicated in Fig 5–6, the primary controlled variable in cardiovascular function is **mean arterial pressure.** Changes in any variable contributing to mean arterial pressure (eg, peripheral vascular resistance) will evoke homeostatic secondary responses that tend to compensate for the directly evoked change. The **homeostatic response** may sometimes be sufficient to prevent any change in mean arterial pressure. A slow infusion of norepinephrine provides a useful example. This agent produces direct effects on both vascular and cardiac muscle. It is a powerful vasoconstrictor and, by increasing peripheral vascular resistance, tends to increase mean arterial pressure. In the absence of reflexes, its effect on the heart is also

stimulatory—ie, it increases heart rate and contractile force. However, in a subject with intact reflexes, the negative feedback baroreceptor response to increased mean arterial pressure causes decreased sympathetic outflow to the heart and a powerful increase in parasympathetic (vagus nerve) discharge at the cardiac pacemaker. As a result, the *net* effect of ordinary pressor doses of norepinephrine is to produce a marked increase in peripheral vascular resistance, a moderate increase in mean arterial pressure, and a consistent *slowing* of heart rate. Bradycardia is thus a reflex or compensatory response elicited by this agent and is *the exact opposite of the drug's direct action;* yet it is completely predictable if the integration of cardiovascular function by the autonomic nervous system is understood.

Presynaptic Regulation

The principle of negative feedback control is also found at the presynaptic level of autonomic function. While not yet as completely understood as the baroreceptor reflex, an important presynaptic feedback inhibitory control mechanism has been shown to exist in noradrenergic fibers. An α_2 receptor located on the presynaptic nerve terminals is activated by norepinephrine and similar molecules; activation diminishes further release of norepinephrine from the nerve ending. Conversely, a presynaptic beta receptor may facilitate the release of norepinephrine. Selective activation of α_2 receptors by a drug might be expected to reduce sympathetic effects by attenuating endogenous norepinephrine release. Certain antihypertension drugs may act in this way (clonidine, α-methylnorepinephrine). Inhibitory control of transmitter release is not limited to inhibition by the transmitter itself. Evidence also strongly implicates prostaglandins and polypeptides in the regulation of norepinephrine release. Presynaptic regulation by a variety of endogenous chemicals probably occurs in all nerve fibers.

Postsynaptic Regulation

Postsynaptic regulation can be considered from 2 perspectives: modulation by the prior history of activity (which may up- or down-regulate receptor number; see Chapter 2) and modulation by other temporally associated events. The first mechanism has been well documented in several autonomic receptor-effector systems. The second mechanism usually involves modulation of each primary transmitter-receptor event by simultaneous events evoked by the same or other transmitters acting on different receptors.

Ganglionic transmission is a good example of this hierarchy. The postganglionic cells are activated (depolarized) as a result of binding of an appropriate ligand (acetylcholine or nicotine) to a nicotinic acetylcholine receptor. The primary spike response (fast excitatory postsynaptic potential; EPSP) evoked by this event is often followed by a small and slowly developing but relatively long-lasting hyperpolarizing afterpotential—an inhibitory postsynaptic potential (IPSP). This in turn is followed by a small, slow exci-

Table 5–2. Direct effects of autonomic nerve activity on some organ systems.

Organ	Effect of			
	Sympathetic		Parasympathetic	
	Action*	Receptor†	Action	Receptor†
Eye				
Iris				
Radial muscle	Contracts	α	. . .	. . .
Circular muscle	. . .	. . .	Contracts	M
Ciliary muscle	[Relaxes]	β	Contracts	M
Heart				
Sinoatrial node	Accelerates	β_1	Decelerates	M
Ectopic pacemakers	Accelerates	β_1	. . .	. . .
Contractility	Increases	β_1	Decreases (atria)	M
Vascular smooth muscle				
Skin, splanchnic vessels	Contracts	α	. . .	M‡
Skeletal muscle vessels	Relaxes	β_2	. . .	. . .
	[Contracts]	α	. . .	. . .
	Relaxes	M§	. . .	. . .
Bronchiolar smooth muscle	Relaxes	β_2	Contracts	M
Gastrointestinal tract				
Smooth muscle				
Walls	Relaxes	β_2	Contracts	M
Sphincters	Contracts	α	Relaxes	M
Secretion	. . .	. . .	Increases	M
Myenteric plexus	Inhibits	α	. . .	. . .
Genitourinary smooth muscle				
Bladder wall	Relaxes	β_2	Contracts	M
Sphincter	Contracts	α	Relaxes	M
Uterus, pregnant	Relaxes	β_2	. . .	. . .
	Contracts	α	. . .	. . .
Penis, seminal vesicles	Ejaculation	α	Erection	M
Skin				
Pilomotor smooth muscle	Contracts	α	. . .	. . .
Sweat glands				
Thermoregulatory	Increases	M	. . .	. . .
Apocrine (stress)	Increases	α	. . .	. . .
Metabolic functions				
Liver	Gluconeogenesis	α/β_2**	. . .	. . .
Liver	Glycogenolysis	α/β_2	. . .	. . .
Fat cells	Lipolysis	α_2, β_1††	. . .	. . .

*Less important actions are in brackets.

†Specific receptor type: α = alpha, β = beta, M = muscarinic.

‡Most blood vessels have uninnervated muscarinic receptors.

§Vascular smooth muscle in skeletal muscle has sympathetic cholinergic dilator fibers.

**Depends on species.

††Alpha$_2$ inhibits; β_1 stimulates.

Table 5–3. Steps in autonomic transmission: Effects of drugs.

Process	Drug Example	Site	Action
Action potential propagation	Local anesthetics, tetrodotoxin,[1] saxitoxin.[2]	Nerve axons.	Block sodium channels; block conduction.
Transmitter synthesis	Hemicholinium.	Cholinergic nerve terminals: membrane.	Blocks uptake of choline and slows synthesis.
	α-Methyltyrosine (metyrosine).	Adrenergic nerve terminals and adrenal medulla: cytoplasm.	Blocks synthesis.
Transmitter storage	Carbachol.	Cholinergic terminals: vesicles.	Promotes release.
	Reserpine.	Adrenergic terminals: vesicles.	Promotes depletion.
Transmitter release	Many.[3]	Nerve terminal membrane receptors.	Modulate release.
	Mg^{2+}, Ca^{2+} influx inhibitors.	Nerve terminal membrane Ca^{2+} channels.	Reduce transmitter release.
	Botulinus toxin.	Cholinergic vesicles.	Prevents release.
	Latrotoxin.[4]	Cholinergic and adrenergic vesicles.	Causes explosive release.
	Tyramine, amphetamine.	Adrenergic nerve terminals.	Promote transmitter release.
Transmitter uptake after release	Cocaine, tricyclic antidepressants.	Adrenergic nerve terminals.	Inhibit uptake; increase transmitter effect on postsynaptic receptors.
	6-Hydroxydopamine.	Adrenergic nerve terminals.	Destroys the terminals.
Receptor activation/ blockade	Norepinephrine.	Receptors at adrenergic junctions.	Binds α receptors; causes contraction.
	Phentolamine.	Receptors at adrenergic junctions.	Binds α receptors; prevents activation.
	Isoproterenol.	Receptors at adrenergic junctions.	Binds β receptors; activates adenylate cyclase.
	Propranolol.	Receptors at adrenergic junctions.	Binds β receptors; prevents activation.
	Nicotine.	Receptors, cholinergic junctions (autonomic ganglia, neuromuscular end-plates).	Binds nicotinic receptors; opens ion channel in postsynaptic membrane.
	Tubocurarine.	Neuromuscular end-plates.	Prevents activation.
	Bethanechol.	Receptors, parasympathetic effector cells (smooth muscle, cardiac muscle, glands).	Binds muscarinic receptors; releases inositol trisphosphate and activates guanylate cyclase.
	Atropine.	Receptors, parasympathetic effector cells.	Binds muscarinic receptors; prevents activation.
Enzymatic inactivation of transmitter	Neostigmine.	Cholinergic synapses (acetylcholinesterase).	Inhibits enzyme; prolongs and intensifies transmitter action.
	Tranylcypromine.	Adrenergic nerve terminals (monoamine oxidase).	Inhibits enzyme; increases stored transmitter pool.

[1]Toxin of puffer fish, California newt.
[2]Toxin of *Gonyaulax* (red tide organism).
[3]Norepinephrine, dopamine, acetylcholine, angiotensin II, various prostaglandins, etc.
[4]Black widow spider venom.

tatory postsynaptic potential. These slow potentials serve to modulate the responsiveness of the postsynaptic cell to subsequent primary excitatory presynaptic nerve activity. (See Chapter 19 for further examples.)

PHARMACOLOGIC MODIFICATION OF AUTONOMIC FUNCTION

Because the transmission of information involves different mechanisms in different segments of the autonomic nervous system, some drugs produce highly specific effects while others are nonselective in their actions. A summary of the steps in transmission of impulses, from the central nervous system to the autonomic effector cells, is presented in Table 5–3. Drugs such as local anesthetics are very nonselective in their action, since they act on a process that is common to all neurons. On the other hand, drugs that act on the biochemical processes involved in transmitter synthesis and storage are more selective, since the biochemistry of adrenergic transmission is very different from that of cholinergic transmission. Activation or blockade of effector cell receptors offers the maximum

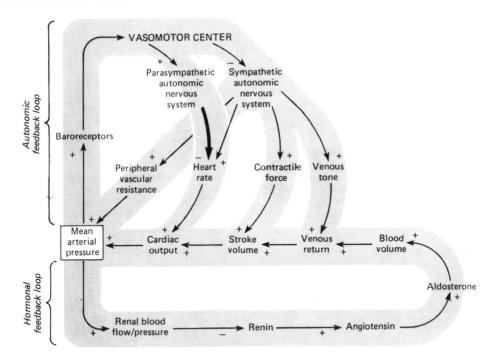

Figure 5–6. Autonomic and hormonal control of cardiovascular function. Note that at least 2 feedback loops are present, the autonomic nervous system loop and the hormonal loop. In addition, each major loop has several components. Thus, the sympathetic autonomic nervous system directly influences the 4 major variables, peripheral vascular resistance, heart rate, force, and venous tone. The vagus directly influences heart rate. Angiotensin II directly increases peripheral vascular resistance (not shown), and the sympathetic autonomic nervous system probably directly increases renin secretion (not shown). The plus and minus signs on the arrows indicate the direction of change in the variables pointed to when activity of the preceding variable is increased. For example, an increase in mean arterial pressure causes an *increase* in renal blood flow; an increase in renal blood flow causes a *decrease* in renin release; an increase in plasma renin causes an *increase* in angiotensin production, etc.

flexibility and selectivity of effect: adrenoceptors are easily distinguished from cholinoceptors. Furthermore, several subgroups can be selectively activated or blocked within each major type.

The next 4 chapters provide the information needed to take advantage of this useful diversity of autonomic processes.

REFERENCES

Andersson K-E, Sjögren C: Aspects on the physiology and pharmacology of the bladder and urethra. *Prog Neurobiol* 1982;**19**:71.

Berridge MJ: Inositol trisphosphate and diacylglycerol as second messengers. *Biochem J* 1984;**220**:345.

Burnstock G: Neurotransmitters and trophic factors in the autonomic nervous system. *J Physiol (Lond)* 1981;**313**:1.

Central integration of cardiovascular control. Central cardiovascular control: A distributed neural network. (Symposium.) Manning JW (chairman). *Fed Proc* 1980;**39**:2485.

Complexities of transmission in autonomic ganglia. (Symposium.) Volle RL (chairman). *Fed Proc* 1980;**39**:2980.

Dixon WR, Mosimann WF, Weiner N: The role of presynaptic feedback mechanisms in regulation of norepinephrine release by nerve stimulation. *J Pharmacol Exp Ther* 1979;**209**:196.

Furchgott RF: Role of endothelium in responses of vascular smooth muscle to drugs. *Annu Rev Pharmacol Toxicol* 1984;**24**:175.

Glick G, Braunwald E: Relative roles of the sympathetic and

parasympathetic nervous systems in the reflex control of heart rate. *Circ Res* 1965;**16**:363.

Gootman PM: Development of the autonomic nervous system. (Symposium.) *Fed Proc* 1983;**42**:1619.

Guyton AC et al: Relative importance of venous and arterial resistances in controlling venous return and cardiac output. *Am J Physiol* 1959;**196**:1008.

Hakanson R, Sundler F: The design of the neuroendocrine system: A unifying concept and its consequences. *Trends Pharmacol Sci* 1983;**4**:41.

Higgins CB, Vatner SF, Braunwald E: Parasympathetic control of the heart. *Pharmacol Rev* 1973;**25**:119.

Hokfelt T et al: Peptidergic neurones. *Nature* 1980;**284**:515.

Jan YN, Jan LY: Coexistence and corelease of cholinergic and peptidergic transmitters in frog sympathetic ganglia. *Fed Proc* 1983;**42**:2929.

Katzung BG: Myocardial toxicity as a result of altered membrane channel function. Pages 135–179 in: *Cardiovascular Toxicology*. Van Stee EW (editor). Raven, 1982.

Knoth J, Zallakian M, Njus D: Mechanism of proton-linked monoamine transport in chromaffin granule ghosts. *Fed Proc* 1982;**41**:2742.

Kohli JD, Glock D, Goldberg LI: Differential antagonism of postsynaptic (DA$_1$) and presynaptic (DA$_2$) peripheral dopamine receptors by substituted benzamides. Pages 97–108 in: *The Benzamides: Pharmacology, Neurobiology, and Clinical Aspects.* Rotrosen J, Stanley M (editors). Raven, 1982.

Langer SZ: Presynaptic regulation of the release of catecholamine. *Pharmacol Rev* 1980;**32**:337.

Langer SZ, Hicks PE: Alpha-adrenoreceptor subtypes in blood vessels: Physiology and pharmacology. *J Cardiovasc Pharmacol* 1984;**6**:S547.

Lentz TL: Cellular membrane reutilization and synaptic vesicle recycling. *Trends Neurosci* 1983;**6**:48.

Miyamoto MD: The actions of cholinergic drugs on motor nerve terminals. *Pharmacol Rev* 1977;**29**:221.

Motulsky HJ, Insel PA: Adrenergic receptors in man: Direct identification, physiologic regulation, and clinical alteration. *N Engl J Med* 1982;**307**:18.

Neff NH, Karoum F, Hadjiconstantinon M: Dopamine-containing small intensely fluorescent cells and sympathetic ganglion function. *Fed Proc* 1983;**42**:3009.

Parsons SM et al: Transport in the cholinergic synaptic vesicle. *Fed Proc* 1982;**41**:2765.

Pumplin DW, Reese TS: Action of brown widow spider venom and botulinum toxin on the frog neuromuscular junction examined with the freeze-fracture technique. *J Physiol (Lond)* 1977;**273**:443.

Ruffolo RR Jr: Peripheral alpha-adrenergic receptors: Introduction. (Symposium.) *Fed Proc* 1984;**43**:2908.

Simpson LL: The origin, structure, and pharmacological activity of botulinum toxin. *Pharmacol Rev* 1981;**33**:155.

Starke K: Presynaptic receptors. *Annu Rev Pharmacol Toxicol* 1981;**21**:7.

Timmermans PBMWM, van Zwieten PA: α_2 Adrenoceptors: Classification, localization, mechanisms, and targets for drugs. *J Med Chem* 1982;**25**:1389.

Volle RL: Complexities of transmission in autonomic ganglia. (Symposium.) *Fed Proc* 1980;**39**:2980.

Watanabe AM et al: Cardiac autonomic receptors: Recent concepts from radiolabeled ligand-binding studies. *Circ Res* 1982;**50**:161.

Willems JL et al: Neuronal dopamine receptors on autonomic ganglia and sympathetic nerves and dopamine receptors in the gastrointestinal system. *Pharmacol Rev* 1985;**37**:165.

Acetylcholine Receptor Stimulants

6

August M. Watanabe, MD

The acetylcholine receptor stimulants comprise a large group of drugs that mimic acetylcholine. The effects of acetylcholine cover a broad spectrum, depending upon the receptor type—muscarinic or nicotinic—that is activated. There is a correspondingly wide spectrum of potential actions for other molecules ("cholinomimetics") that activate acetylcholine receptors. Thus, one important basis for classification of these agents is their *spectrum* of action; another is their *mechanism* of action, since some cholinomimetic drugs directly bind to (and activate) cholinoceptors while a second important group acts indirectly by inhibiting the hydrolysis of endogenous acetylcholine (Fig 6–1).

SPECTRUM OF ACTION OF CHOLINOMIMETIC DRUGS

In some of the first studies of the parasympathetic nervous system, Sir Henry Dale found that the alkaloid **muscarine** mimicked the effects of parasympathetic nerve discharge, ie, the effects were **parasympathomimetic.** Direct application of muscarine to ganglia and to autonomic effector tissues (smooth muscle, heart, exocrine glands) showed that the parasympathomimetic action of the alkaloid was mediated only by receptors at the effector cells, not those in the ganglia. Therefore, by convention, the effects of acetylcholine itself and of other cholinomimetic drugs at autonomic neuroeffector junctions are referred to as parasympathomimetic effects, mediated by muscarinic receptors.

In contrast, the alkaloid **nicotine** was found to stimulate autonomic ganglia and skeletal muscle neuromuscular junctions but to have little effect on autonomic effector cells when applied in low concentrations. The ganglion and skeletal muscle receptors were therefore labeled nicotinic. When it was later demonstrated that acetylcholine is the physiologic transmitter substance at both muscarinic and nicotinic receptors, it was recognized that both receptors are subtypes of cholinoceptors.

Muscarinic receptors are located on plasma membranes of cells of organs innervated by parasympathetic nerves as well as on some tissues that are not innervated by parasympathetic nerves (Table 5–1). Nicotinic receptors are located on plasma membranes of parasympathetic and sympathetic postganglionic cells in autonomic ganglia and also on membranes of muscles innervated by somatic motor fibers (Fig 5–1). Because of the multiple sites of action of acetylcholine and the fact that it has both excitatory and inhibitory effects, unselective cholinoceptor stimulants can produce very diffuse and marked alterations in organ system function. Fortunately, drugs are available that have a degree of selectivity, so desired effects can be achieved while avoiding or minimizing undesired side

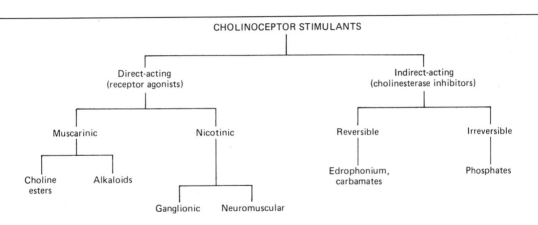

Figure 6–1. The major classes of acetylcholine receptor stimulants.

effects. This selectivity of action is based on several factors. Thus, some drugs stimulate muscarinic receptors selectively, whereas others selectively activate nicotinic receptors. Some agents stimulate nicotinic receptors in ganglia preferentially, whereas others act preferentially on nicotinic receptors at neuromuscular junctions. Organ selectivity can also be achieved by utilizing appropriate routes of administration ("pharmacokinetic selectivity"). For example, muscarinic stimulants can be administered topically to the external surface of the eye to modify ocular function while minimizing systemic effects.

MODE OF ACTION OF CHOLINOMIMETIC DRUGS

The cholinoceptor stimulant drugs can be divided into 2 major categories on the basis of their mode of action: direct and indirect (Fig 6–1). The direct-acting agents directly bind to and activate the muscarinic or nicotinic receptors. The indirect-acting agents produce their primary effects by inhibiting the action of acetylcholinesterase, which hydrolyses acetylcholine to choline and acetic acid (Fig 5–2). By inhibiting acetylcholinesterase, the indirect-acting drugs increase the concentration of endogenous acetylcholine in the synaptic clefts and neuroeffector junctions, and the excess acetylcholine in turn stimulates cholinoceptors to evoke increased responses.

Some cholinesterase inhibitors, even in low concentration, also inhibit butyrocholinesterase (pseudocholinesterase), and most inhibit this enzyme when they are present in high concentrations. However, since this enzyme is not important in the physiologic termination of action of synaptic acetylcholine, inhibition of its action plays little role in the action of indirect-acting cholinoceptor stimulants. Some cholinesterase inhibitors also have a modest direct action as well; this is especially true of some quaternary carbamates, eg, neostigmine, which activate neuromuscular nicotinic cholinoceptors.

Metoclopramide is a new drug that has some effects which appear cholinomimetic. Experimental data suggest that this compound can augment acetylcholine release from postganglionic cholinergic nerve terminals. The actions of metoclopramide are reduced or abolished by atropine. The mechanism by which metoclopramide augments acetylcholine release from cholinergic nerve terminals is unknown. In addition, studies with isolated tissues suggest that metoclopramide has other effects, including dopamine antagonism. Metoclopramide does not inhibit cholinesterase. Because its mechanism of action is not yet defined and because its use is largely restricted to gastrointestinal indications, it is discussed in Chapter 66.

I. BASIC PHARMACOLOGY OF THE DIRECT-ACTING CHOLINOCEPTOR STIMULANTS

The direct-acting cholinomimetic drugs can be divided on the basis of chemical structure into esters of choline (including acetylcholine) and alkaloids (such as muscarine and nicotine). A few of these drugs have a high degree of specificity for the muscarinic or for the nicotinic receptor. Many have effects on both receptors; acetylcholine is typical.

Chemistry & Pharmacokinetics
A. Structure: Four important esters of choline that have been studied extensively are shown in Fig 6–2. Because they contain the quaternary ammonium group, they are permanently charged and relatively insoluble in lipids. Many naturally occurring and synthetic cholinomimetic drugs that are not choline

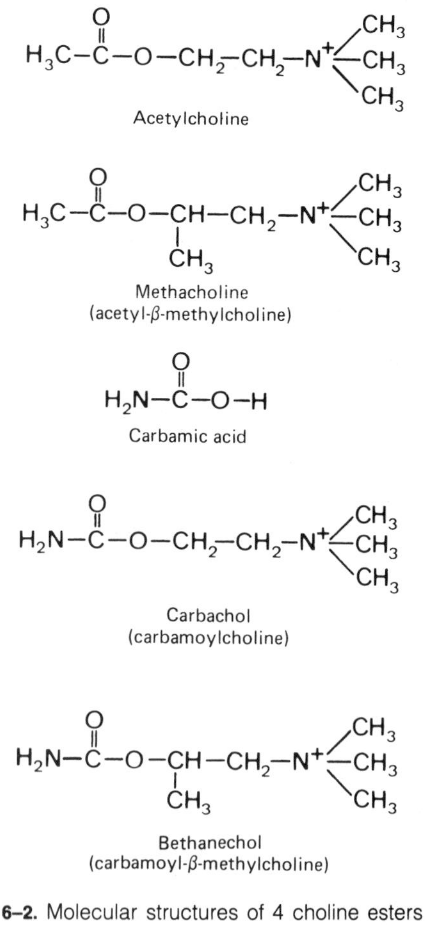

Figure 6–2. Molecular structures of 4 choline esters and carbamic acid. Acetylcholine and methacholine are acetic acid esters of choline and β-methylcholine, respectively. Carbachol and bethanechol are carbamic acid esters of the same alcohols.

esters have been identified; a few of these are shown in Fig 6–3.

B. Absorption, Distribution, and Metabolism: The choline esters all have similar absorption and distribution characteristics, dominated by their low lipid solubility; they are poorly absorbed and poorly distributed into the central nervous system. Although they are all hydrolyzed in the gastrointestinal tract (and less active by the oral route), they differ markedly in their susceptibility to hydrolysis by cholinesterase in the body. Acetylcholine is very rapidly hydrolyzed, as described in Chapter 5; large amounts must be infused intravenously to achieve levels high enough to produce detectable effects. A large intravenous bolus injection has a brief effect, typically 5–20 seconds, whereas intramuscular and subcutaneous injections produce only local effects. Methacholine is at least 3 times more resistant to hydrolysis and produces systemic effects even when given subcutaneously. The carbamic acid esters, carbachol and bethanechol, are completely resistant to hydrolysis by cholinesterase and have correspondingly longer durations of action. Presence of the β-methyl group (methacholine, bethanechol) reduces the potency of these drugs at the nicotinic receptor (Table 6–1).

The tertiary cholinomimetic alkaloids (pilocarpine, nicotine, lobeline; Fig 6–3) are well absorbed from most sites of administration. Nicotine, a liquid, is

Table 6–1. Properties of choline esters.

Choline Ester	Susceptibility to Cholinesterase	Muscarinic Action	Nicotinic Action
Acetylcholine chloride	+ + + +	+ + +	+ + +
Methacholine chloride	+	+ + + +	+
Carbachol chloride	None	+ +	+ + +
Bethanechol chloride	None	+ +	None

sufficiently lipid-soluble to be absorbed across the skin. Muscarine, a quaternary amine, is less completely absorbed from the gastrointestinal tract than the tertiary amines but is nevertheless toxic when ingested, eg, in mushrooms. Excretion of these amines is chiefly by the kidneys. Clearance of tertiary amines can be accelerated by acidification of the urine. Oxotremorine is an extremely potent synthetic muscarinic agonist that has been used as a research tool. It is well distributed into the central nervous system. Lobeline is a plant derivative with lower potency than nicotine but with a similar spectrum of action. Dimethylphenylpiperazinium (DMPP) is a potent synthetic nicotinic stimulant with little access to the central nervous system.

Pharmacodynamics

A. Mechanism of Action: Activation of the

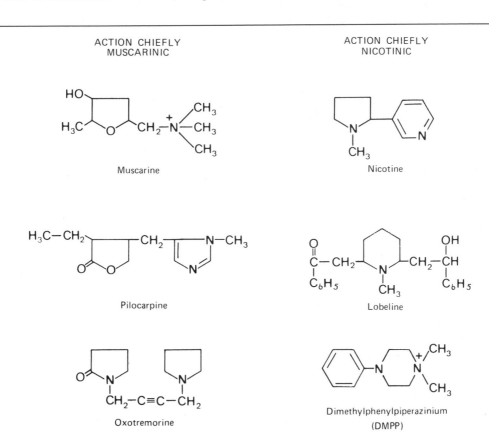

ACTION CHIEFLY
MUSCARINIC

Muscarine

Pilocarpine

Oxotremorine

ACTION CHIEFLY
NICOTINIC

Nicotine

Lobeline

Dimethylphenylpiperazinium
(DMPP)

Figure 6–3. Structures of some cholinomimetic alkaloids and synthetic analogs.

parasympathetic nervous system modifies organ function by 2 major mechanisms. First, acetylcholine released from parasympathetic nerves can activate muscarinic receptors on effector organs to alter organ function directly. Second, acetylcholine released from parasympathetic nerves can interact with muscarinic receptors on sympathetic nerve terminals to inhibit the release of norepinephrine. By this mechanism, the parasympathetic system indirectly alters organ function by modulating the effects of the sympathetic nervous system.

The subcellular or biochemical mechanism by which muscarinic stimulants alter cellular function continues to be investigated. Several cellular events occur when muscarinic receptors are activated, one or more of which might serve as "second messengers" for muscarinic activation. Muscarinic agonists can increase cellular concentrations of cGMP. The role of cGMP in cellular regulation has not, however, been established. The activation of muscarinic receptors also increases potassium flux across cell membranes. However, it is not yet known whether alterations in potassium channels are directly coupled to muscarinic receptors or if one or more intervening "messengers" are involved in mediating the change in ion flux. Muscarinic agonists also accelerate the turnover of inositol phospholipids in membranes of cells that possess muscarinic receptors (see Berridge reference, Chapter 5). What role this effect has in mediating muscarinic actions remains to be established. Finally, it has been shown that muscarinic receptors are coupled to adenylate cyclase in an inhibitory manner. Activation of muscarinic receptors in these tissues results in inhibition of adenylate cyclase activity. Moreover, muscarinic agonists can attenuate the activation of adenylate cyclase and modulate the increase in cAMP levels induced by hormones such as catecholamines. These muscarinic effects on cAMP generation are paralleled by attenuation of the physiologic response of the organ to stimulatory hormones.

The mechanism of nicotinic receptor activation has been studied in great detail, taking advantage of 3 factors: The receptor is present in extremely high concentration in the membranes of the electric organs of electric fish; α-bungarotoxin, a component of certain snake venoms, is tightly bound to the receptors and readily labeled as a marker for isolation procedures; and activation of the receptor results in easily measured electrical and ionic changes in the cells involved. The nicotinic receptor appears to be a pentamer of 4 types of glycoprotein subunits (one monomer occurs twice) with a total molecular weight of about 250,000. It has one or 2 receptor sites that, when activated by a nicotinic agonist, cause a conformational change in the protein that allows sodium and potassium ions to diffuse rapidly down their concentration gradients. Thus, the primary effect of nicotinic receptor activation is depolarization of the nerve cell or neuromuscular end-plate bearing the receptor.

If activation of the nicotinic receptor is prolonged, effector response is abolished; ie, the postganglionic neuron stops firing and the skeletal muscle cell relaxes. Furthermore, the continued presence of the nicotinic agonist prevents recovery of the postjunctional membrane. In this way, a state of "depolarizing blockade" is induced that is refractory to reversal by other agonists.

B. Organ System Effects: Most of the direct organ system effects of muscarinic cholinoceptor stimulants are readily predicted from a knowledge of the effects of parasympathetic nerve stimulation (Table 5–2) and the distribution of muscarinic receptors. Effects of a typical agent such as acetylcholine are listed in Table 6–2. The effects of nicotinic agonists are similarly predictable from a knowledge of the physiology of the autonomic ganglia and skeletal muscle motor end-plate.

1. Eye–Muscarinic agonists instilled into the conjunctival sac cause contraction of the smooth muscle of the iris sphincter (miosis) and of the ciliary muscle (accommodation). As a result, the iris is pulled away from the angle of the anterior chamber, and the trabecular meshwork at the base of the ciliary muscle is

Table 6–2. Effects of direct-acting cholinoceptor stimulants. Only the direct effects are indicated; homeostatic responses to these direct actions may be important (see text).

Organ	Response
Eye	
Sphincter muscle of iris	Contraction (miosis).
Ciliary muscle	Contraction for near vision.
Heart	
Sinoatrial node	Decrease in rate (negative chronotropy).
Atria	Decrease in contractile strength (negative inotropy). Decrease in refractory period.
Atrioventricular node	Decrease in conduction velocity (negative dromotropy).
Ventricles	Small decrease in contractile strength.
Blood vessels	
Arteries	Dilatation.
Veins	Dilatation.
Lung	
Bronchial muscle	Contraction (bronchoconstriction).
Bronchial glands	Stimulation.
Gastrointestinal tract	
Motility	Increase.
Sphincters	Relaxation.
Secretion	Stimulation.
Urinary bladder	
Detrusor	Contraction.
Trigone and sphincter	Relaxation.
Glands	
Sweat, salivary, lacrimal, nasopharyngeal	Secretion.

opened up. Both effects facilitate the outflow of aqueous humor into the canal of Schlemm, which drains the anterior chamber.

2. Cardiovascular system–The primary cardiovascular effects of muscarinic agonists are reduction in peripheral vascular resistance and changes in heart rate. The direct effects shown in Table 6–2 are modified by important homeostatic reflexes, as described in Chapter 5 and depicted in Fig 5–6. Intravenous infusions of minimal effective doses of acetylcholine in humans (eg, 20–50 μg/min) cause vasodilatation, resulting in a reduction in blood pressure, often accompanied by a reflex increase in heart rate. Larger doses of acetylcholine produce bradycardia and decreased conduction velocity through the atrioventricular node in addition to the hypotensive effect.

The direct cardiac actions of muscarinic stimulants include an important increase in membrane potassium permeability in atrial muscle cells and probably in the cells of the sinoatrial and atrioventricular nodes as well. In addition, cholinoceptor stimulants decrease the slow inward calcium current in atrial and nodal cells of at least some species. Both of these actions could contribute to the observed slowing of pacemaker rate and the hyperpolarization and decreased contractility of atrial cells. As noted above, the direct slowing of sinoatrial rate and atrioventricular conduction that is produced by muscarinic agonists is often opposed by reflex sympathetic discharge, elicited by the decrease in blood pressure. The resultant interaction between sympathetic and parasympathetic effects is complex because of the previously described muscarinic modulation of sympathetic influences that occurs by inhibition of norepinephrine release and by postjunctional cellular effects. Therefore, the net effect on heart rate depends on local concentrations of the agonist in the heart and in the vessels and on the level of reflex responsiveness. Parasympathetic innervation of the ventricles is much less than that of the atria. Also, activation of muscarinic receptors in ventricles results in much less physiologic effect than that seen following activation of these receptors in atria. However, the effects of muscarinic activation on ventricular function are enhanced by the muscarinic modulation of sympathetic effects as described above.

The precise mechanism by which muscarinic stimulants bring about vascular smooth muscle relaxation is poorly understood. Preparations of isolated strips of vascular smooth muscle prepared in the traditional way are usually *contracted* by acetylcholine and its congeners even though the same vessels can be shown to dilate in intact animals. A possible explanation for this paradox has become available through the observation that isolated vascular strips relax like their counterparts in the intact animal if care is taken to avoid damaging or removing the intima of the vessel. This and other evidence suggest that the effect of muscarinic vasodilators may be to facilitate production of an endogenous vasodilator substance or to inhibit the production of a vasoconstrictor by the intima of the vessels (see Furchgott reference).

The cardiovascular effects of all of the choline esters are similar to those of acetylcholine, the main difference being in their potency and duration of action. Because of the resistance of methacholine, carbachol, and bethanechol to acetylcholinesterase, lower doses given intravenously are sufficient to produce effects similar to those of acetylcholine, and the duration of action of these synthetic choline esters is longer. The cardiovascular effects of most of the cholinomimetic natural alkaloids and synthetic analogs are also generally similar to those of acetylcholine. Pilocarpine is an exception. When given intravenously, it often produces hypertension after a brief initial hypotensive response. The longer-lasting hypertensive effect can be traced to ganglionic discharge caused by activation of slow excitatory postsynaptic potentials (Chapter 5). This effect, like the hypotensive effect, can be blocked by atropine, an antimuscarinic drug.

3. Respiratory system–The smooth muscle of the bronchial tree is contracted by muscarinic stimulants. In addition, the glands of the tracheobronchial mucosa are stimulated to secrete. This combination of effects can occasionally cause symptoms, especially in individuals with asthma.

4. Gastrointestinal tract–Administration of muscarinic agonists, like stimulation of the parasympathetic nervous system, causes an increase in secretory and motor activity of the gut. The salivary and gastric glands are strongly stimulated; the pancreas and small intestinal glands less so. Peristaltic activity is increased throughout the gut, and most sphincters are relaxed. Stimulation of contraction in this organ system has been shown to involve depolarization of the smooth muscle cell membrane and increased calcium influx.

5. Genitourinary tract–Muscarinic agonists stimulate the detrusor muscle and relax the trigone and sphincter muscles of the bladder, thus promoting voiding. The human uterus is not notably sensitive to muscarinic agonists.

6. Miscellaneous secretory glands–Muscarinic agonists stimulate the secretory activity of sweat, lacrimal, and nasopharyngeal glands.

7. Central nervous system–The central nervous system contains both muscarinic and nicotinic receptors, the brain being relatively richer in muscarinic sites and the spinal cord containing a preponderance of nicotinic sites. The physiologic role of these receptors is discussed in Chapter 19. In spite of the smaller ratio of nicotinic:muscarinic receptors in the brain, nicotine and lobeline (Fig 6–3) have important effects on the brain stem and cortex. The mild alerting action of nicotine absorbed from inhaled tobacco smoke is the best-known of these effects. In larger concentrations, nicotine induces tremor, emesis, and stimulation of the respiratory center. At still higher levels, nicotine causes convulsions, which may terminate in fatal coma. The lethal effects on the central nervous system and the fact that nicotine is readily absorbed form the basis for the use of nicotine as an insecticide. Dimethylphenylpiperazinium (DMPP), a synthetic nicotinic stimulant (Fig 6–3), is relatively free of these central effects because it does not cross the blood-brain barrier.

8. Peripheral nervous system–The autonomic **ganglia** are important sites of nicotinic synaptic action. All of the nicotinic agents shown in Fig 6–3 are capable of causing marked activation of the nicotinic receptors, resulting in firing of action potentials in the postganglionic neurons. The action is the same on both parasympathetic and sympathetic ganglia. The initial response therefore often resembles simultaneous discharge of both parasympathetic and sympathetic nervous systems. In the case of the cardiovascular system, the effects of nicotine are chiefly sympathomimetic. Dramatic hypertension is produced by parenteral injection of nicotine; sympathetic tachycardia may alternate with a vagally mediated bradycardia. In the gastrointestinal and urinary tracts, the effects are largely parasympathomimetic: nausea, vomiting, diarrhea, and voiding of urine are commonly observed.

A second class of nicotinic sites consists of **chemoreceptors** on sensory nerve endings—especially certain chemosensitive nerve endings in the coronary arteries and the carotid and aortic bodies. Activation of these endings elicits complex medullary responses, including respiratory stimulation and vagal discharge.

9. Neuromuscular junction–The nicotinic receptors on the neuromuscular end-plate apparatus are similar but not identical to the receptors in the autonomic ganglia. Both types respond to acetylcholine and nicotine. (However, as discussed in Chapter 7, they differ in their structural requirements for nicotinic blocking drugs.) When applied directly (by iontophoresis or by intra-arterial injection), an immediate depolarization of the end-plate results, caused by an increase in permeability to sodium ions. Depending on the synchronization of depolarization of end-plates throughout the muscle, the contractile response will vary from disorganized fasciculations of independent motor units to a strong contraction of the entire muscle. Depolarizing nicotinic agents that are not rapidly hydrolyzed (like nicotine itself) cause rapid development of depolarization blockade, discussed further in Chapter 7. In the case of skeletal muscle, this block is manifested as flaccid paralysis.

II. BASIC PHARMACOLOGY OF THE INDIRECT-ACTING CHOLINOCEPTOR STIMULANTS

The actions of acetylcholine released from autonomic and somatic motor nerves are terminated by enzymatic destruction of the molecule. Hydrolysis is accomplished by the action of acetylcholinesterase, a protein with a molecular weight of about 320,000, which is present in high concentrations in cholinergic synapses. The indirect-acting cholinomimetics have their primary effect at the active site of this enzyme, although some also have direct actions at nicotinic receptors. By far the most important use of these chemicals is as insecticides; a few have therapeutic applications. The chief differences between members of the group are chemical and pharmacokinetic—their pharmacodynamic properties are almost identical.

Chemistry & Pharmacokinetics

A. Structure: The commonly used cholinesterase inhibitors fall into 3 chemical groups: (1) simple alcohols bearing a quaternary ammonium group, eg, edrophonium; (2) carbamic acid esters of alcohols bearing quaternary or tertiary ammonium groups (carbamates, eg, neostigmine); and (3) organic derivatives of phosphoric acid (organophosphates, eg, isoflurophate). Examples of the first 2 groups are shown in Fig 6–4. Edrophonium, neostigmine, and ambenonium are synthetic quaternary ammonium agents used in medicine. Physostigmine (eserine) is a naturally occurring tertiary amine of greater lipid solubility that is also used in therapeutics. Carbaryl (carbaril) is typical of a large group of carbamate insecticides designed for very high lipid solubility, so that absorption into the insect and distribution to the central nervous system is very rapid.

A few of the estimated 50,000 organophosphates are shown in Fig 6–5. Many of the organophosphates (echothiophate is an exception) are highly lipid-soluble liquids. Isoflurophate (diisopropylfluorophosphate, DFP) was one of the first organophosphates synthesized and is one of the best-studied. It is no longer available for clinical use but has been superseded by better agents. Soman is an extremely potent "nerve gas." Echothiophate, a thiocholine derivative, is of clinical interest because it retains the very long duration of action of other organophosphates but is more stable in aqueous solution. Parathion and malathion are thiophosphate insecticides that are inactive as such; they are converted to the phosphate derivatives in animals and plants. They are somewhat more stable than compounds like isoflurophate and soman, making them more suitable for use as insecticides.

B. Absorption, Metabolism, and Distribution: Absorption of the quaternary carbamates from the conjunctiva, skin, and lungs is predictably poor, since their permanent charge renders them relatively insoluble in lipids. Similarly, much larger doses are required for oral administration than for parenteral injection. Distribution into the central nervous system is negligible. Physostigmine, in contrast, is well absorbed from all sites and can be used topically in the eye (Table 6–3). It is distributed into the central nervous system and is more toxic. However, even nonpolar carbamates used as insecticides are poorly absorbed across the skin—the ratio of dermal:oral lethal doses for this group is much higher than the ratios for the organophosphate pesticides. The carbamates are relatively stable in aqueous solution but can be metabo-

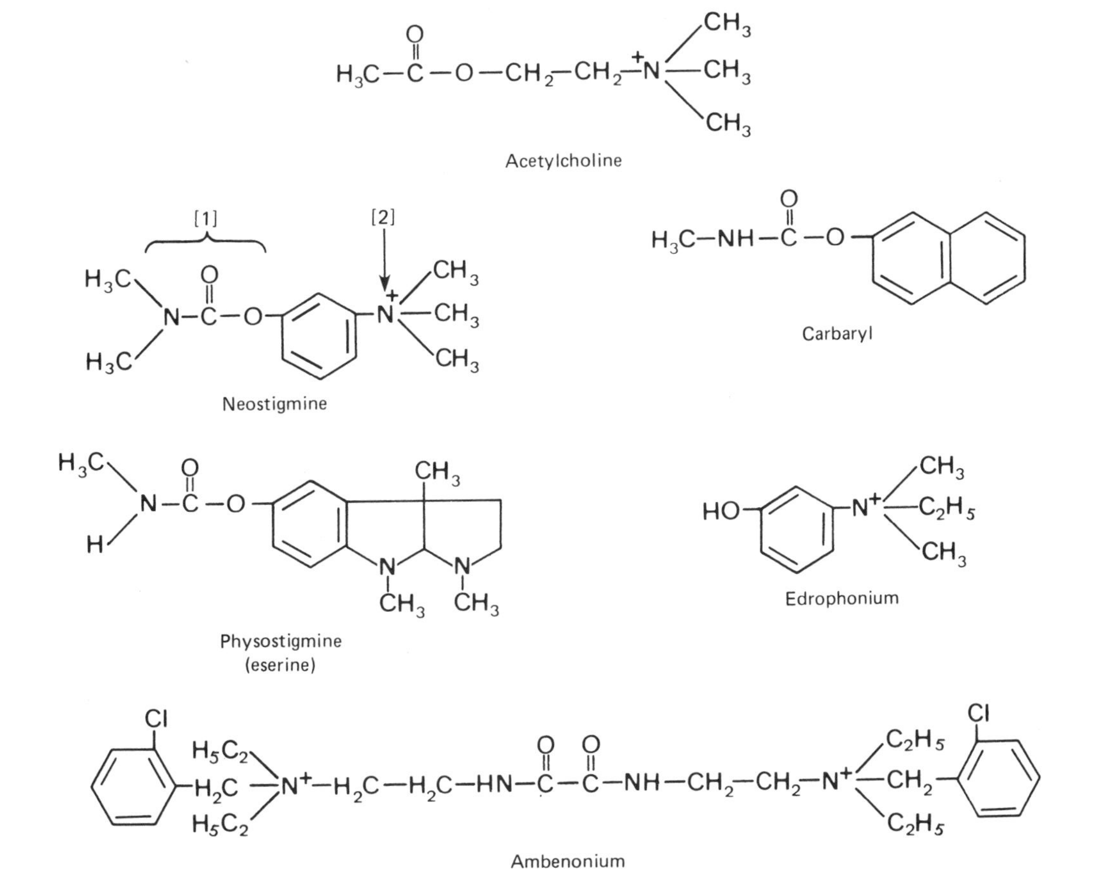

Figure 6–4. Cholinesterase inhibitors. Neostigmine exemplifies the typical compound that is an ester of carbamic acid ([1]) and a phenol bearing a quaternary ammonium group ([2]). Physostigmine, a naturally occurring carbamate, is a tertiary amine. Acetylcholine is shown in the same orientation (acid left, alcohol right) for reference. Edrophonium and ambenonium are not esters but bind to the active site of the enzyme.

lized by nonspecific esterases in the body, as well as by cholinesterase. However, the half-life of their effect is determined by the stability of the inhibitor-enzyme complex (see Mechanism of Action, below), not by metabolism or excretion.

The organophosphate cholinesterase inhibitors (except for echothiophate) are well absorbed from the skin, lung, gut, and conjunctiva—thereby making them dangerous to humans and highly effective as insecticides. They are relatively less stable than the carbamates when dissolved in water and thus have a limited half-life in the environment (as compared to the other major class of insecticides, the halogenated hydrocarbons, eg, DDT). Echothiophate is highly polar and more stable than most other organophosphates. It can be made up in aqueous solution for ophthalmic use and retains its activity for weeks.

The thiophosphate insecticides (parathion, malathion, and related compounds) are very lipid-soluble and are rapidly absorbed by all routes. They must be activated in the body by conversion to the oxygen analogs (Fig 6–5), a process that occurs rapidly in both insects and vertebrates. Malathion and certain other

Table 6–3. Uses and duration of action of cholinesterase inhibitors used in therapeutics.

	Uses	Approximate Duration of Action
Alcohols		
Edrophonium (Tensilon)	Myasthenia gravis, ileus, arrhythmias	5–15 minutes
Carbamates and related agents		
Neostigmine (Prostigmin, etc)	Myasthenia gravis, ileus	½–2 hours
Pyridostigmine (Mestinon, etc)	Myasthenia gravis	3–6 hours
Physostigmine	Glaucoma	½–2 hours
Ambenonium (Mytelase)	Myasthenia gravis	4–8 hours
Demecarium (Humorsol)	Glaucoma	4–6 hours
Organophosphates		
Echothiophate (Phospholine, etc)	Glaucoma	100 hours

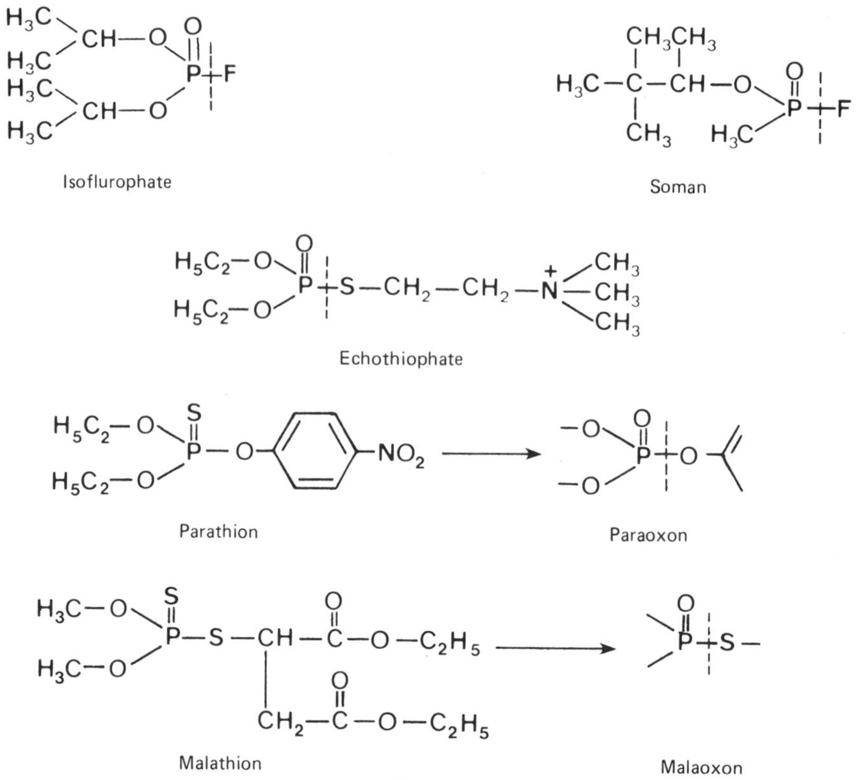

Figure 6–5. Structures of some organophosphate cholinesterase inhibitors. The dashed lines indicate the bond that is hydrolyzed in binding to the enzyme.

organophosphate insecticides are also rapidly metabolized by other pathways to inactive products in birds and mammals, but not in insects; these agents are therefore considered safe enough for sale to the general public. Unfortunately, fish are not able to detoxify malathion, and significant die-offs have occurred from the heavy use of this agent on and near waterways. Parathion is not detoxified effectively in vertebrates; thus, it is considerably more dangerous to humans and livestock and is not available for general public use.

All of the organophosphates except echothiophate are fully distributed to all parts of the body, including the central nervous system. Poisoning with these agents therefore includes an important component of central nervous system toxicity.

Pharmacodynamics

A. Mechanism of Action: Acetylcholinesterase is an extremely active enzyme. In the initial step, acetylcholine binds to the enzyme active site and is hydrolyzed, yielding free choline and the *acetylated* enzyme. In the second step, the covalent acetylenzyme bond is split, with the addition of water. The entire process takes place in approximately 150 microseconds.

All of the cholinesterase inhibitors exert their effects by inhibiting acetylcholinesterase and thereby increasing the concentration of endogenous acetylcholine in the vicinity of cholinoceptors. However, the

molecular details of their interaction with the enzyme vary according to the 3 chemical subgroups mentioned above.

The first group, of which edrophonium is the major example, consists of quaternary alcohols. These agents bind reversibly (by means of electrostatic forces) to the active site, thus preventing access by acetylcholine. The enzyme-inhibitor complex does not involve a covalent bond and is correspondingly short-lived (on the order of 2–10 minutes). The second group consists of carbamate esters, eg, neostigmine and physostigmine. These agents undergo a 2-step hydrolysis sequence analogous to that described for acetylcholine. However, the covalent bond of the *carbamylated* enzyme is considerably more resistant to the second (hydration) process, and this step is correspondingly prolonged (on the order of 30 minutes to 6 hours). The third group consists of the organophosphates. These agents also undergo initial binding and hydrolysis by the enzyme, resulting in a *phosphorylated* active site. The covalent phosphorus-enzyme bond is extremely stable and hydrolyzes in water at a very slow rate (hundreds of hours). After the initial binding-hydrolysis step, the phosphorylated enzyme complex may undergo a process called **aging**. This process apparently involves the breaking of one of the oxygen-phosphorus bonds of the inhibitor and results in further strengthening of the phosphorus-enzyme bond. The rate of aging varies with the particular organophosphate compound. If given before aging has occurred, strong nucleophiles like pralidoxime are able to split the phosphorus-enzyme bond and can be used as "cholinesterase regenerator" drugs for organophosphate insecticide poisoning (Chapter 7). Once aging has occurred, the enzyme-inhibitor complex cannot be split, even with oxime compounds.

Because of the marked differences in duration of action, the organophosphate inhibitors are sometimes referred to as "irreversible" cholinesterase inhibitors, relegating edrophonium and the carbamates to the category of "reversible" inhibitors. In fact, the molecular mechanisms of action of the 3 groups do not support this simplistic description, but the terms are frequently used.

B. Organ System Effects: The most prominent pharmacologic effects of cholinesterase inhibitors are on the cardiovascular and gastrointestinal systems, the eye, and the skeletal muscle neuromuscular junction. Because the primary action is to potentiate the action of endogenous acetylcholine, the effects are similar (but not always identical) to the effects of the direct-acting cholinomimetic agonists.

1. Central nervous system–In low concentrations, the lipid-soluble cholinesterase inhibitors cause diffuse activation of the EEG and a subjective alerting response. In higher concentrations, they cause generalized convulsions, which may be followed by coma and respiratory arrest.

2. Eye, respiratory tract, gastrointestinal tract, urinary tract–The effects of the cholinesterase inhibitors on these organ systems, all of which are well innervated by the parasympathetic nervous system, are qualitatively quite similar to the effects of the direct-acting cholinomimetics.

3. Cardiovascular system–The cholinesterase inhibitors can increase activation in both sympathetic and parasympathetic ganglia supplying the heart and at the acetylcholine receptors on neuroeffector cells (cardiac and vascular smooth muscles) that receive cholinergic innervation.

In the heart, the effects on the parasympathetic limb predominate. Thus, administration of cholinesterase inhibitors such as edrophonium, physostigmine, or neostigmine leads to effects on the heart that mimic the effects of vagal nerve activation. Heart rate decreases, conduction velocity through the atrioventricular junction diminishes, atrial contractility decreases, and cardiac output falls. The fall in cardiac output is contributed to by the bradycardia, decreased atrial contractility, and some reduction in ventricular contractility. The latter effect occurs as a result of prejunctional modulation of sympathetic activity (inhibition of norepinephrine release) as well as inhibition of postjunctional cellular sympathetic effects. When administered to patients who have undergone cardiac transplantation (which causes degeneration of the nerve endings in the transplanted heart), the same drugs have no effect. These results indicate that the effects of these drugs are dependent on endogenous acetylcholine released from vagal nerve endings.

The effects of cholinesterase inhibitors on vascular smooth muscle and on blood pressure are less marked than the effects of direct-acting muscarinic agonists. This is because indirect-acting drugs can modify the tone of only those vessels that are innervated by cholinergic nerves and because the net effects on vascular tone may represent activation of both the parasympathetic and sympathetic nervous systems. Since few vascular beds receive cholinergic innervation (Chapter 5), the cholinomimetic effect is minimal. Furthermore, although activation of cholinergic nerves (at ganglia and neuroeffector junctions) would tend to lower vascular resistance and blood pressure, activation of sympathetic ganglia would tend to oppose these hypotensive effects.

The *net* cardiovascular effects of moderate doses of cholinesterase inhibitors therefore consist of modest bradycardia, a fall in cardiac output, and no change or a modest fall in blood pressure. Large (toxic) doses of these drugs cause more marked bradycardia and hypotension.

4. Neuromuscular junction–The cholinesterase inhibitors have important therapeutic and toxic effects at the skeletal muscle neuromuscular junction. Low (therapeutic) concentrations moderately prolong and intensify the actions of physiologically released acetylcholine. This results in increased strength of contraction, especially in muscles weakened by curarelike neuromuscular blocking agents or by myasthenia gravis. At higher concentrations, the accumulation of acetylcholine may result in fibrillation of muscle fibers. Antidromic firing of the motor neuron may also occur, resulting in fasciculations that involve an entire motor unit. With marked inhibition of acetylcholinesterase, membrane depolarization becomes sustained and neuromuscular blockade may ensue.

Some quaternary carbamate cholinesterase inhibitors, eg, neostigmine, have an additional *direct* nicotinic agonist effect at the neuromuscular junction. This may contribute to the effectiveness of these agents in the therapy of myasthenia.

III. CLINICAL PHARMACOLOGY OF THE CHOLINOCEPTOR STIMULANTS

The major therapeutic uses of the cholinoceptor stimulants are for diseases of the eye (glaucoma, accommodative esotropia), the gastrointestinal and urinary tracts (postoperative atony, neurogenic bladder), the neuromuscular junction (myasthenia gravis, curare-induced neuromuscular paralysis), and the heart (certain atrial arrhythmias). Cholinesterase inhibitors are occasionally used in the treatment of atropine overdosage.

Clinical Uses
A. The Eye: Glaucoma is a disease characterized

by increased intraocular pressure. There are 2 types of acquired glaucoma: primary, which can be subdivided into angle-closure and open-angle types; and secondary, eg, caused by surgical procedures. Muscarinic stimulants and cholinesterase inhibitors can reduce intraocular pressure by facilitating outflow of aqueous humor and possibly also by diminishing the rate of its secretion. Of the direct agonists, methacholine, carbachol, and pilocarpine have been used for treatment of glaucoma. Among the cholinesterase inhibitors, physostigmine, demecarium, echothiophate, and isoflurophate have been extensively studied.

Acute angle-closure glaucoma is a medical emergency that is usually treated initially with drugs but frequently requires surgery for permanent correction. Initial therapy often consists of a combination of a direct muscarinic agonist and a cholinesterase inhibitor (eg, pilocarpine plus physostigmine). Once the intraocular pressure is controlled and the danger of loss of vision is diminished, the patient can be prepared for corrective surgery (iridectomy). Open-angle glaucoma and some cases of secondary glaucoma are chronic diseases that are not amenable to surgical correction. Consequently, therapy is based on long-term pharmacologic management that relies heavily on the use of cholinoceptor-stimulating drugs as well as epinephrine, the beta-adrenoceptor–blocking drugs, and acetazolamide. Of the cholinomimetics, the ones in current favor include pilocarpine (as drops, or a long-acting plastic film reservoir of drug [Ocusert] placed in the conjunctival sac) and physostigmine (drops). Longer-acting agents (demecarium, echothiophate) are reserved for cases in which control of the intraocular pressure cannot be achieved with other agents.

Accommodative esotropia (strabismus caused by hypermetropic accommodative error) in young children is sometimes diagnosed and treated with cholinomimetic agonists. Dosage is similar to or higher than that used for glaucoma.

B. Gastrointestinal and Urinary Tracts: In clinical disorders that involve depression of smooth muscle activity *without obstruction*, cholinomimetic agonists with direct or indirect muscarinic effects may be helpful. These disorders include postoperative ileus (atony or paralysis of the stomach or bowel following surgical manipulation) and congenital megacolon. Urinary retention may occur postoperatively or postpartum or may be secondary to spinal cord injury or disease (neurogenic bladder). Cholinomimetic agonists are also sometimes used to increase the tone of the lower esophageal sphincter in patients with reflux esophagitis. Of the choline esters, bethanechol is the most widely used for these disorders. For gastrointestinal problems, it is usually administered orally in a dose of 10–25 mg 3–4 times daily. In patients with urinary retention, bethanechol can be given subcutaneously in a dose of 5 mg and repeated in 30 minutes if necessary. Of the cholinesterase inhibitors, neostigmine is the most widely used for these applications. For paralytic ileus or atony of the urinary bladder,

neostigmine can be given subcutaneously in a dose of 0.5–1 mg. If patients are able to take the drug by mouth, neostigmine can be given orally in a dose of 15 mg. In all of these clinical situations, the clinician must be certain that there is no mechanical obstruction to outflow prior to using the cholinomimetic. Otherwise, the drug may exacerbate the problem and may even cause perforation as a result of increased pressure.

C. Neuromuscular Junction: Myasthenia gravis is a disease of the skeletal muscle neuromuscular junctions. An autoimmune process causes production of antibodies that decrease the number of functional nicotinic receptors on the postjunctional end-plate. The characteristic symptoms of weakness and fatigability that remit with rest and worsen with exercise may affect any skeletal muscle but most often involve the small muscles of the hand, head, neck, and extremities. Frequent findings are ptosis, diplopia, difficulty in speaking and swallowing, and extremity weakness. Severe disease may affect all the muscles, including those necessary for respiration. The disease resembles the neuromuscular paralysis produced by d-tubocurarine and similar nondepolarizing neuromuscular blocking drugs (Chapter 25). Patients with myasthenia are exquisitely sensitive to the action of curariform drugs and other drugs that interfere with neuromuscular transmission, eg, aminoglycoside antibiotics.

Cholinesterase inhibitors—but not direct-acting acetylcholine receptor agonists—are extremely valuable in the therapy of myasthenia. (Some patients also respond to immunosuppressant therapy such as adrenocorticosteroids and cyclophosphamide.)

Edrophonium is frequently used as a diagnostic test for myasthenia. Two milligrams are injected intravenously after obtaining baseline measurements of muscle strength. If no reaction occurs after 45 seconds, an additional 8 mg may be injected. Some clinicians divide the 8-mg dose into 2 doses of 3 and 5 mg given at 45-second intervals. If the patient has myasthenia gravis, an improvement in muscle strength that lasts about 5 minutes will usually be observed.

Edrophonium is also used to assess the adequacy of treatment with the longer-acting cholinesterase inhibitors in patients with documented myasthenia gravis. If excessive amounts of cholinesterase inhibitor have been used, patients may become paradoxically weak because of nicotinic depolarizing blockade of the motor end-plate. These patients may also exhibit symptoms of excessive stimulation of muscarinic receptors (abdominal cramps, diarrhea, increased salivation, excessive bronchial secretions, miosis, bradycardia). Small doses of edrophonium (1–2 mg intravenously) will produce no relief or even worsen weakness if the patient is receiving excessive cholinesterase inhibitor therapy. On the other hand, if the patient improves with edrophonium, an increase in cholinesterase inhibitor dosage may be indicated. Clinical situations in which severe myasthenia (myasthenic crisis) must be distinguished from excessive drug therapy (cholinergic crisis) usually occur in very ill myasthenic patients and must be managed in hospital with adequate emergency and support systems (eg, mechanical ventilators) available.

Chronic long-term therapy of myasthenia gravis is usually accomplished with neostigmine, pyridostigmine, or ambenonium. The doses are titrated to optimum levels based on changes in muscle strength. These agents are relatively short-acting and therefore require frequent dosing (every 2–4 hours for neostigmine and every 3–6 hours for pyridostigmine and ambenonium; Table 6–3). Sustained-release preparations are available but should be used only at night and if needed. Longer-acting cholinesterase inhibitors such as the organophosphate agents are not used, because the dose requirement in this disease changes too rapidly to permit smooth control with long-acting drugs.

If muscarinic side effects are prominent, they can be controlled by the administration of antimuscarinic drugs such as atropine. Frequently, tolerance to the muscarinic effects of the cholinesterase inhibitors develops, so atropine treatment is not required.

Neuromuscular blockade is frequently produced as an adjunct to surgical anesthesia, using nondepolarizing neuromuscular relaxants such as curare, pancuronium, and newer agents (Chapter 25). Following the surgical procedure, it is usually desirable to reverse this pharmacologic paralysis promptly. This can be easily accomplished with cholinesterase inhibitors; neostigmine and edrophonium are the drugs of choice. They are given intravenously or intramuscularly for prompt effect.

D. Heart: The short-acting cholinesterase inhibitor edrophonium has been used for treatment of supraventricular tachyarrhythmias, particularly paroxysmal supraventricular tachycardia. By potentiating the effects of endogenous acetylcholine released at the atrioventricular junction, atrioventricular conduction velocity is diminished, the number of supraventricular impulses conducted into the ventricles may be reduced, and an excessive ventricular rate may be slowed. Edrophonium may also convert the abnormal supraventricular tachyarrhythmia into normal sinus rhythm. Edrophonium usually is given intravenously in a dose of 5–10 mg (0.15 mg/kg) administered over 30 seconds. Carotid sinus massage may be performed after giving the drug if the ventricular rate has not slowed.

E. Antimuscarinic Drug Intoxication: Atropine intoxication is potentially lethal in children (Chapter 7) and may cause prolonged severe behavioral disturbances in adults. The tricyclic antidepressants, when taken in overdosage (often with suicidal intent), also cause severe muscarinic blockade (Chapter 28). Because the muscarinic receptor blockade produced by all these agents is competitive in nature, it can be overcome by increasing the amount of endogenous acetylcholine present at the neuroeffector junctions. Physostigmine has been used for this application, because it enters the central nervous system

and reverses the central as well as the peripheral signs of muscarinic blockade. Physostigmine salicylate is given in intravenous boluses of 0.5–2 mg repeated at 5- to 10-minute intervals until an effect is noted. However, as explained in the next chapter, such therapy is used only in patients with dangerous elevation of body temperature or very rapid supraventricular tachycardia.

Toxicity

The toxic potential of the cholinoceptor stimulants varies markedly depending on the absorption of the drug, its access to the central nervous system, and its metabolism.

A. Direct-Acting Muscarinic Stimulants: Drugs such as pilocarpine and the choline esters cause predictable signs of muscarinic excess when given in overdosage. These effects include nausea, vomiting, diarrhea, salivation, sweating, cutaneous vasodilatation, and bronchial constriction. The effects are all blocked competitively by atropine and its congeners.

Certain mushrooms, especially those of the genus *Inocybe*, contain muscarinic alkaloids. Ingestion of these mushrooms causes typical signs of muscarinic excess within 15–30 minutes. Treatment is with atropine, 1–2 mg parenterally. (*Amanita muscaria*, the first source of muscarine, contains very low concentrations of the alkaloid.)

B. Direct-Acting Nicotinic Stimulants: Nicotine itself is the only common cause of this type of poisoning. The acute toxicity of the alkaloid is well-defined but much less important than the chronic effects associated with smoking. In addition to its occurrence in tobacco, nicotine is also used in a number of insecticides.

1. Acute toxicity—The fatal dose of nicotine is approximately 40 mg, or 1 drop of the pure liquid. This is the amount of nicotine in 2 regular cigarettes. Fortunately, most of the nicotine in cigarettes is destroyed by burning or escapes via the "side-stream" smoke. Ingestion of nicotine insecticides and of tobacco by infants and children is usually followed by vomiting, limiting the amount of the alkaloid absorbed.

The toxic effects of a large dose of nicotine are simple extensions of the effects described previously. The most dangerous are (1) central stimulant actions, which cause convulsions and may progress to coma and respiratory arrest; (2) skeletal muscle end-plate depolarization, which may lead to depolarization blockade and respiratory paralysis; and (3) hypertension and cardiac arrhythmias.

Treatment of acute nicotine poisoning is largely symptom-directed. Muscarinic excess resulting from parasympathetic ganglion stimulation can be controlled with atropine. Central stimulation is usually treated with parenteral anticonvulsants such as diazepam. Neuromuscular blockade is not responsive to pharmacologic treatment and may require mechanical respiration.

Fortunately, nicotine is metabolized and excreted relatively rapidly. Patients who survive the first 4 hours usually recover completely if hypoxia and brain damage have not occurred.

2. Chronic nicotine toxicity–The health costs of tobacco smoking to the smoker and its socioeconomic costs to the general public are still incompletely understood. However, the 1979 Surgeon General's Report on Health Promotion and Disease Prevention stated that "cigarette smoking is clearly the largest single preventable cause of illness and premature death in the United States." This statement was underscored by the 1983 and 1985 reports of the US Department of Health and Human Services, which estimated that up to 30% of the 565,000 coronary heart disease deaths and 30% of the 416,000 cancer deaths in the USA each year were attributable to smoking. Unfortunately, the fact that the most important of the tobacco-associated diseases are delayed in onset reduces the health incentive to stop smoking. Furthermore, the fact that society— through private or national health insurance programs—subsidizes the extraordinary cost of tobacco-associated diseases reduces the personal financial incentive to control smoking in addicted users.

It is not known to what extent nicotine *per se* contributes to the well-documented adverse effects of chronic tobacco use. It appears highly probable that nicotine contributes to the elevated risk of vascular disease and sudden coronary death associated with smoking. It is also probable that nicotine contributes to the high incidence of ulcer recurrences in smokers with peptic disease.

C. Cholinesterase Inhibitors: The acute toxic effects of the cholinesterase inhibitors, like those of the direct-acting agents, are direct extensions of their pharmacologic actions. The major source of such intoxications is pesticide use in agriculture and in the home. Approximately 100 organophosphate and 20 carbamate cholinesterase inhibitors are available in pesticides and veterinary vermifuges used in the USA.

Acute intoxication must be recognized and treated promptly in patients with heavy exposure. The dominant initial signs are those of muscarinic excess: miosis, salivation, sweating, bronchial constriction, vomiting, and diarrhea. Central nervous system involvement usually follows rapidly, accompanied by peripheral nicotinic effects, especially depolarizing neuromuscular blockade. Therapy always includes (1) maintenance of vital signs—respiration in particular may be impaired; (2) decontamination to prevent further absorption—this may require removal of all clothing and washing of the skin in cases of exposure to dusts and sprays; and (3) atropine parenterally in large doses, given as often as required to control signs of muscarinic excess (Chapter 7). Therapy often also includes treatment with pralidoxime as described in Chapter 7.

Chronic exposure to certain organophosphate compounds, including some organophosphate cholinesterase inhibitors, causes neuropathy associated with demyelination of axons. Triorthocresylphosphate, an additive in lubricating oils, is the prototype agent of this class. The effects are not caused by cholinesterase inhibition.

REFERENCES

Brown JH, Wetzel GT, Dunlap J: Activation and blockade of cardiac muscarinic receptors by endogenous acetylcholine and cholinesterase inhibitors. *J Pharmacol Exp Ther* 1982; **223:**20.

Burnstock G: Neurotransmitters and trophic factors in the autonomic nervous system. *J Physiol (Lond)* 1981;**313:**1.

Cady B: Cost of smoking. (Letter.) *N Engl J Med* 1983; **308:**1105.

Drachman DH: Myasthenia gravis. (2 parts.) *N Engl J Med* 1978;**298:**136, 186.

Fielding JE: Smoking: Health effects and control. (2 parts.) *N Engl J Med* 1985;**313:**491, 555.

Finkbeiner AE, Bissada NK, Welch LT: Uropharmacology: Choline esters and other parasympathomimetic drugs. *Urology* 1977;**10:**83.

Furchgott RF et al: Endothelial cells as mediators of vasodilation of arteries. *J Cardiovasc Pharmacol* 1984;**6:**S336.

Granacher RP, Baldessarini RJ: Physostigmine: Its use in acute anticholinergic syndrome with antidepressant and antiparkinson drugs. *Arch Gen Psychiatr* 1975;**32:**375.

Havener WH: Pages 261–417 in: *Ocular Pharmacology*, 5th ed. Mosby, 1983.

Hobbiger F: Pharmacology of anticholinesterase drugs. Pages 487–581 in: *Neuromuscular Junction*. Vol 42. Zaimis E (editor). *Handbuch der Experimentellen Pharmakologie*. Springer-Verlag, 1976.

Levy MN, Martin PJ: Neural control of the heart. Pages 581–620 in: *Handbook of Physiology: The Cardiovascular System I*. American Physiological Society, 1979.

Molitor H: A comparative study of the effects of five choline compounds used in therapeutics: Acetylcholine chloride, acetyl-beta-methylcholine chloride, carbaminoyl choline, ethyl ether beta-methylcholine chloride, carbaminoyl beta-methylcholine chloride. *J Pharmacol Exper Ther* 1936; **58:**337.

Parasympathetic neuroeffector mechanisms in the heart. (Symposium.) *Fed Proc* 1984;**43:**2597.

Raftery MA et al: Acetylcholine receptor: Complex of homologous subunits. *Science* 1980;**208:**1454.

Richelson E, El-Fakahamy E: The molecular basis of neurotransmission at the muscarinic receptor. *Biochem Pharmacol* 1981;**30:**2887.

Root WS, Hoffman FG (editors): Pages 97–322 in: *Physiological Pharmacology*. Vol 3. Academic Press, 1967.

Smoking and cardiovascular disease. *MMWR* 1984;**32:**677.

Watanabe AM et al: Cardiac autonomic receptors: Recent concepts from radiolabeled ligand-binding studies. *Circ Res* 1982;**50:**161.

Watanabe AM et al: Muscarinic cholinergic receptor modulation of beta-adrenergic receptor affinity for catecholamines. *J Biol Chem* 1978;**253:**4833.

Wieland T: Poisonous principles of mushrooms of the genus *Amanita*. *Science* 1968;**159:**946.

Acetylcholine Receptor Antagonists

7

Bertram G. Katzung, MD, PhD

Just as cholinoceptor agonists are divided into muscarinic and nicotinic subgroups on the basis of their specific receptor affinities, so the antagonists acting on these receptors fall into 2 major families: the **antimuscarinic** and **antinicotinic** agents. Muscarinic receptors are apparently very similar throughout the body; only limited selectivity for different muscarinic receptors has been achieved through modification of chemical structure. Nicotinic receptors, on the other hand, are readily divided on the basis of differential blockade by 2 subgroups: ganglion-blocking and neuromuscular blocking agents.

This chapter presents the general pharmacology of the muscarinic receptor–blocking drugs and some aspects of the ganglion-blocking nicotinic antagonists. The neuromuscular nicotinic antagonists are discussed in Chapter 25.

I. BASIC PHARMACOLOGY OF THE MUSCARINIC RECEPTOR–BLOCKING DRUGS

Because the effects of parasympathetic autonomic discharge can be blocked by muscarinic antagonists, they are often called parasympatholytic drugs. However, they do not "lyse" parasympathetic nerves, and they have some effects that are not predictable from block of the parasympathetic nervous system. For these reasons, the term "antimuscarinic" is preferable.

Naturally occurring compounds with antimuscarinic effects have been known and used for millenia as medicines, poisons, and cosmetics. The prototype of these drugs is **atropine.** Many similar plant alkaloids are known, and hundreds of synthetic antimuscarinic compounds have been prepared.

Chemistry & Pharmacokinetics

A. Source and Chemistry: Atropine and its naturally occurring congeners are tertiary ammonium alkaloid esters of tropic acid (Fig 7–1).

Atropine (hyoscyamine) is found in the plant *Atropa belladonna*, or deadly nightshade, and in *Datura stramonium*, also known as jimsonweed (Jamestown) or thorn apple. **Scopolamine** (hyoscine) occurs in *Hyoscyamus niger*, or henbane. Scopolamine is the

$l(-)$ stereoisomer and is obtained as such from the plant. Naturally occurring atropine is $l(-)$-hyoscyamine, but the compound readily racemizes, so the commercial material is racemic d,l-hyoscyamine. The $l(-)$ isomers of both alkaloids are at least 100 times more potent than the $d(+)$ isomers.

Semisynthetic tertiary ammonium analogs are produced by esterifying a natural base, eg, tropine, the base in atropine, with different acids. Thus, homatropine is the mandelic acid ester of tropine. A variety of fully synthetic molecules have antimuscarinic effects; the tertiary members of these classes (Fig 7–2) are often used for their effects in the eye or the central nervous system. Many antihistaminic (Chapter 15), antipsychotic (Chapter 27), and antidepressant (Chapter 28) drugs have similar structures and, predictably, significant antimuscarinic effects.

Quaternary ammonium antimuscarinic agents have been developed to reduce central nervous system effects. These drugs include both semisynthetic and synthetic molecules (Fig 7–2).

B. Absorption: The natural alkaloids and most tertiary antimuscarinic drugs are well absorbed from the gut and across the conjunctival membrane. When applied in a suitable vehicle, some, eg, scopolamine, are even absorbed across the skin (transdermal route). In contrast, only 10–30% of a dose of a quaternary antimuscarinic drug is absorbed after oral administration, reflecting the decreased lipid solubility of the charged molecule.

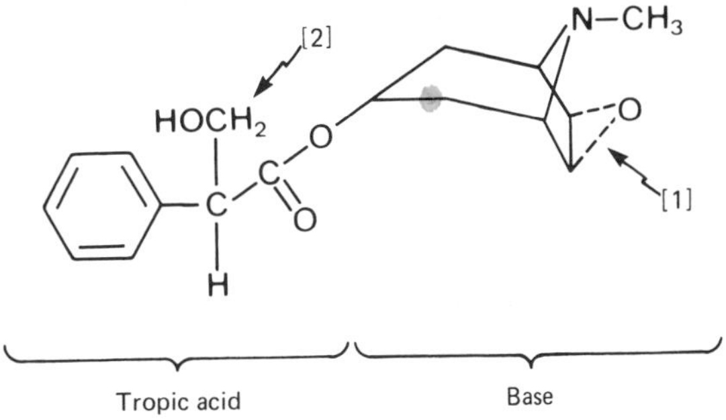

Figure 7–1. The structure of atropine (oxygen at [1] is missing) or scopolamine (oxygen present). In homatropine, the hydroxymethyl at [2] is replaced by a hydroxyl group, and the oxygen at [1] is absent.

Quaternary amines for gastrointestinal applications (peptic disease, hypermotility):

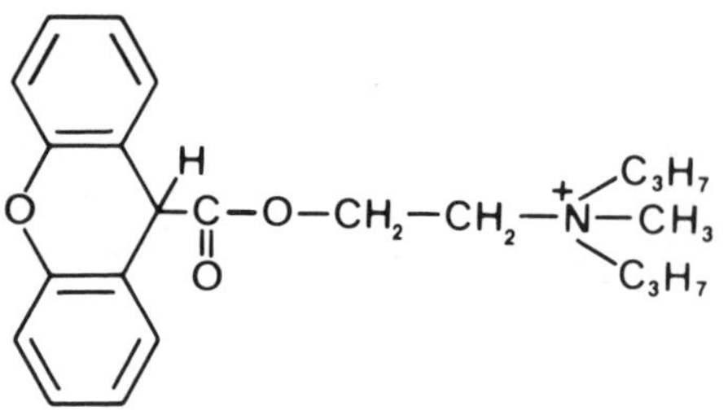

Propantheline

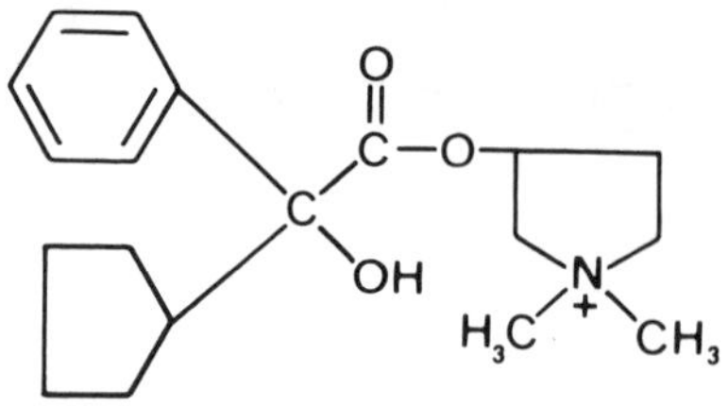

Glycopyrrolate

Quaternary amine for use in asthma:

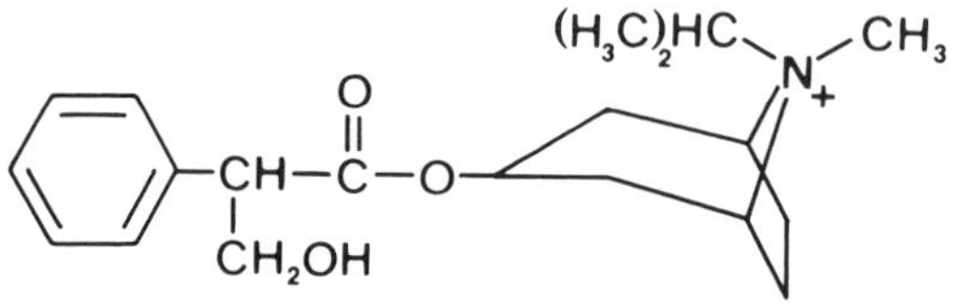

Ipratropium

Tertiary amines for peripheral applications:

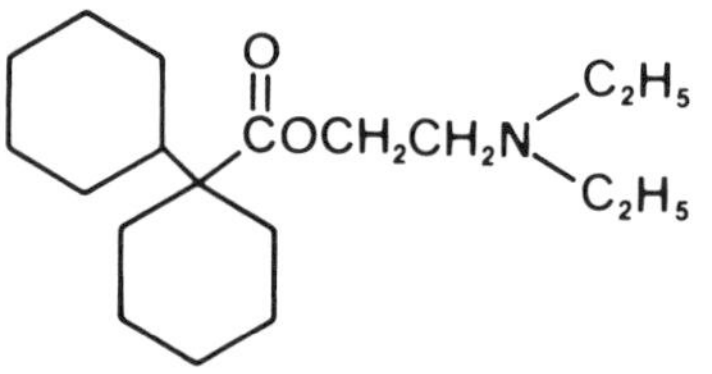

Dicyclomine
(peptic disease, hypermotility)

Tropicamide
(mydriatric, cycloplegic)

Tertiary amine for Parkinson's disease:

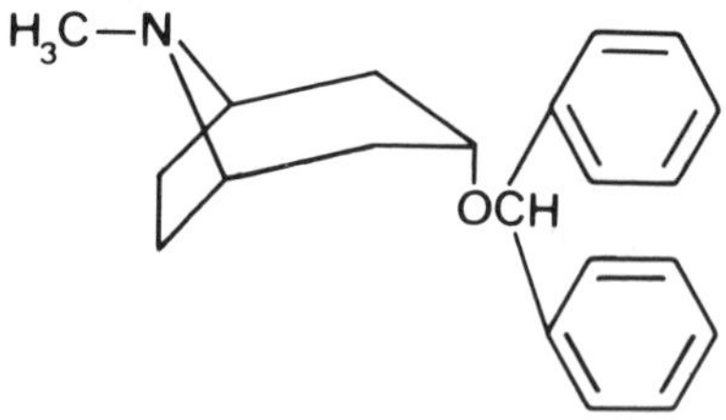

Benztropine

Figure 7–2. Structures of some semisynthetic and synthetic antimuscarinic drugs.

C. Distribution: Atropine and the other tertiary agents are widely distributed after absorption. Significant levels are achieved in the central nervous system within 30 minutes to 1 hour and may limit the dose tolerated when the drug is taken for its peripheral effects. The quaternary derivatives are very poorly taken up by the brain and therefore are relatively free of these central nervous system side effects.

D. Metabolism and Excretion: Atropine disappears rapidly from the blood after administration. About 80% of the dose is excreted in the urine, with a half-life of 2 hours. Most of the rest appears in the urine with a half-life of 13–38 hours. About a third of the dose is excreted unchanged, with some free tropine base and some glucuronide metabolites accounting for a portion of the remainder. The effect of the drug on parasympathetic function declines rapidly in all organs except the eye. Effects on the iris and ciliary muscle persist for 48–72 hours.

Certain species, notably rabbits, have a specific enzyme—atropine esterase—that confers almost complete protection against the toxic effects of atropine by rapidly metabolizing the drug.

Pharmacodynamics

A. Mechanism of Action: Atropine causes reversible blockade of the actions of acetylcholine at muscarinic receptors—ie, blockade by a small dose of atropine can be overcome by a larger concentration of acetylcholine or equivalent muscarinic agonist. This suggests competition for a common binding site. The interaction may not be so simple, however, since in vitro studies suggest that in some tissues there may be 3 separate sites (or 3 different states) for agonist binding but only one for antagonists. Furthermore, antagonist binding appears to involve a 2-step sequence from an initial rapidly reversible antagonist-receptor complex to a more slowly reversible complex. In any case, the result of binding to the muscarinic receptor is to prevent the actions described in Chapter 6 such as the synthesis of cGMP that are brought about by acetylcholine and other muscarinic agonists.

The effectiveness of antimuscarinic drugs varies with the tissue under study and with the source of agonist. The tissues most sensitive to atropine are the salivary, bronchial, and sweat glands. Secretion of acid by the gastric parietal cells is the least sensitive. Smooth muscle autonomic effectors and the heart are intermediate in responsiveness. In most tissues, antimuscarinic agents are much more effective in blocking exogenously administered cholinoceptor agonists than endogenously released acetylcholine.

Atropine is highly selective in its action. Its potency at nicotinic receptors is much lower than at muscarinic receptors; in clinical use, actions at nonmuscarinic receptors are generally undetectable. Most synthetic antimuscarinic drugs are considerably less specific. The overlap of side effects of the antihistamine and antidepressant drugs has been mentioned. Furthermore, quaternary antimuscarinic drugs have more antinicotinic effects than atropine and can produce some of the symptoms of ganglionic blockade.

B. Organ System Effects:

1. Central nervous system—In the doses usually used clinically, atropine has mild stimulant effects on medullary centers, especially the vagal nucleus, and a slower, longer-lasting sedative effect. The central vagal stimulant effect is frequently sufficient to cause bradycardia, which is later supplanted by tachycardia as the drug's antimuscarinic effects at the sinoatrial node become manifest. Scopolamine has more marked sedative effects, producing drowsiness when given in recommended dosages and amnesia in sensitive individuals. In toxic doses, atropine and scopolamine cause excitement, agitation, hallucinations, and coma.

The tremor of Parkinson's disease is reduced by centrally acting antimuscarinic drugs, and atropine—in the form of belladonna extract—was one of the first drugs used in the therapy of this disease. As discussed in Chapter 26, parkinsonian tremor and rigidity seem to result from an excess of cholinergic activity and a deficiency of dopaminergic activity in the basal ganglia-striatal system. Thus, the combination of an antimuscarinic agent with a dopaminelike drug (levodopa) may provide a more effective therapeutic approach than either drug alone.

Vestibular disturbances, especially motion sickness, appear to involve muscarinic cholinergic transmission. Scopolamine is often effective in preventing or reversing these disturbances.

2. Eye—The pupillary constrictor muscle is dependent on muscarinic-cholinoceptor activation. This activation is effectively blocked by topical atropine and other tertiary antimuscarinic drugs and results in unopposed sympathetic dilator activity and **mydriasis**. Dilated pupils were apparently considered cosmetically desirable during the Renaissance and account for the name belladonna (Italian, "beautiful lady") applied to the plant and its active extract.

The second most important ocular effect of atropine is paralysis of the ciliary muscle, or **cycloplegia**. The result of cycloplegia is loss of the ability to accommodate; the fully atropinized eye cannot focus for near vision.

Both mydriasis and cycloplegia are therapeutically useful in ophthalmology. They are also potentially hazardous, since acute glaucoma may be precipitated in patients with a narrow anterior chamber (Chapter 6).

A third (less important) ocular effect of antimuscarinic drugs is reduction of lacrimal secretion. Patients occasionally complain of dry or "sandy" eyes when receiving large doses of antimuscarinic drugs.

3. Cardiovascular system—The atria of the heart are heavily innervated by parasympathetic (vagal) nerve fibers, and the sinoatrial node is therefore sensitive to muscarinic receptor blockade. The effect in the isolated, innervated, and spontaneously beating heart is a clear blockade of vagal slowing and a relative tachycardia. In patients, tachycardia is seen consistently when moderate to high therapeutic doses are given. However, as noted above, lower doses cause central vagal *stimulation* and may result in initial bradycardia before the effects of peripheral vagal block become manifest. The same mechanisms operate in the control of atrioventricular node function; in the presence of high vagal tone, administration of atropine can significantly reduce the PR interval of the ECG. Muscarinic effects on atrial muscle are similarly blocked, but except in atrial flutter and fibrillation these effects are of no clinical significance. The ventricles, because of a lower degree of control by muscarinic mechanisms, are less affected by antimuscarinic drugs at therapeutic levels. In toxic concentrations, the drugs can cause intraventricular conduction block by an unknown mechanism.

The blood vessels receive little or no direct innervation from the parasympathetic nervous system. However, as noted in Chapter 5, sympathetic cholinergic nerves cause vasodilatation in the skeletal muscle vascular bed. This vasodilatation can be blocked by atropine. Furthermore, almost all vessels contain muscarinic receptors that mediate vasodilatation (Chapter 6). These receptors respond to circulating direct-acting muscarinic agonists, and they are readily blocked by antimuscarinic drugs. At toxic doses, and in a few patients at normal doses, antimuscarinic agents cause cutaneous vasodilatation, especially in the blush area. The mechanism is unknown.

The net cardiovascular effects of atropine in patients with normal hemodynamics are not dramatic: tachycardia may occur, but there is little effect on blood pressure. However, the effects of administered direct-acting muscarinic stimulants (Chapter 6) are easily prevented.

4. Respiratory system–Both smooth muscle and secretory glands of the airway receive vagal innervation and contain muscarinic receptors. Even in normal individuals, some bronchodilatation and reduction of secretion can be measured after administration of atropine. The effect is much more dramatic in patients with airway disease, although the antimuscarinic drugs are not as useful as the beta-adrenoceptor stimulants in the treatment of asthma (Chapter 18). Nevertheless, the antimuscarinic agents are valuable in some patients with asthma. In addition, they are frequently used prior to administration of inhalant anesthetics to reduce the accumulation of secretions in the trachea and the possibility of laryngospasm.

5. Gastrointestinal tract–Blockade of muscarinic receptors has dramatic effects on motility and some of the secretory functions of the gut. However, since local hormones and noncholinergic neurons also modulate gastrointestinal function, even complete muscarinic block cannot totally abolish activity in this organ system. As in other tissues, exogenously administered muscarinic stimulants are more effectively blocked than the effects of parasympathetic (vagal) nerve activity.

The effects of antimuscarinic blockade on salivary secretion are marked; dry mouth is a frequent symptom in patients taking antimuscarinic drugs for Parkinson's disease or peptic ulcer. Gastric secretion is blocked less effectively: the volume and amount of acid, pepsin, and mucin are all reduced, but large doses of atropine may be required. Basal secretion is blocked more effectively than that stimulated by food, nicotine, or alcohol (Chapter 66). Pancreatic and intestinal secretion is little affected by atropine; these processes are primarily under hormonal rather than vagal control.

Motility of gastrointestinal smooth muscle is more broadly affected than is secretory activity in the gut. In general, the walls of the viscera are relaxed, and both tone and propulsive movements are diminished. Therefore, gastric emptying time is prolonged, and intestinal transit time is lengthened. Diarrhea due to overdose with parasympathomimetic agents is readily

eliminated, and even that caused by nonautonomic agents can usually be temporarily controlled. However, intestinal "paralysis" induced by antimuscarinic drugs is temporary; local mechanisms will usually reestablish at least some peristalsis after 1–3 days of antimuscarinic drug therapy.

Several of the synthetic antimuscarinic agents are said to have "spasmolytic" activity in excess of their antimuscarinic effects. This is the result of selection of agents, through screening tests in isolated tissue, that relax the gut in the absence as well as the presence of cholinoceptor stimulants.

6. Genitourinary tract–Smooth muscle of the ureters and bladder wall is relaxed by the antimuscarinic action of atropine and its analogs. This action is useful in the treatment of spasm induced by mild inflammatory conditions, but it also poses a hazard of precipitating urinary retention in elderly men, who may have prostatic hypertrophy (see Clinical Pharmacology). The antimuscarinic drugs have no significant effect on the uterus.

7. Sweat glands–Thermoregulatory sweating is suppressed by atropine. The muscarinic receptors on eccrine sweat glands are innervated by sympathetic cholinergic fibers and are readily accessible to antimuscarinic drugs. In adults, body temperature is elevated by this effect only if large doses are administered, but in infants and children even ordinary doses may cause "atropine fever."

II. CLINICAL PHARMACOLOGY OF THE ANTIMUSCARINIC DRUGS

Therapeutic Applications
A. Central Nervous System Disorders:
1. Parkinson's disease–As described in Chapter 26, the treatment of Parkinson's disease is often an exercise in polypharmacy, since no single agent is fully effective over the (usually prolonged) course of the disease. Most of the large number of antimuscarinic drugs promoted for this application (Table 26–1) were developed before levodopa became available. Their use is accompanied by all of the adverse effects described below, but the drugs remain useful in the attempt to control the disease in many patients.

2. Motion sickness–Certain vestibular disorders respond to antimuscarinic drugs (and to antihistaminic agents with antimuscarinic effects). Scopolamine is one of the oldest remedies for seasickness and is still as effective as any more recently introduced agent. It can be given by injection as well as by mouth. A newer dosage form, the transdermal patch, results in significant blood levels over 24–48 hours. Unfortunately, useful doses usually cause significant sedation and dry mouth.

B. Ophthalmologic Disorders: Accurate measurement of refractive error in uncooperative patients, eg, young children, requires ciliary paralysis. In addition, ophthalmoscopic examination of the retina is greatly facilitated by mydriasis. Therefore, antimuscarinic agents, administered topically as eye drops or in ointment form, are extremely helpful in doing a complete examination. For adults and older children, the shorter-acting drugs are preferred (Table 7–1). For younger children, the greater efficacy of atropine is sometimes necessary, but the possibility of antimuscarinic poisoning is correspondingly increased. Loss of drug from the conjunctival sac via the nasolacrimal duct into the nasopharynx is diminished by the use of atropine ointment.

Antimuscarinic drugs should never be used for mydriasis unless cycloplegia or prolonged action is required. Alpha-adrenoceptor stimulant drugs, eg, phenylephrine, produce a short-lasting mydriasis that is usually sufficient for funduscopic examination (Chapter 8).

A second ophthalmologic use is to prevent synechia formation in uveitis and iritis. The longer-acting preparations, especially homatropine, are valuable for this indication.

C. Gastrointestinal Disorders: A major application of the antimuscarinic drugs is in the treatment of peptic ulcer and hypermotility of the gut. This subject is discussed in some detail in Chapter 66. The quaternary semisynthetic and synthetic agents (Table 7–2) are favored for this purpose, since central nervous system side effects are diminished. Unfortunately, large doses are required to effectively reduce gastric acid secretion, which means that patients with peptic ulcer will have dry mouth, blurred vision, and urinary hesitancy when these drugs are used as the principal treatment. Fortunately, when combined with H_2 histamine receptor antagonists, much lower doses can be useful and side effects correspondingly diminished.

In the treatment of common traveler's diarrhea and other mild or self-limited conditions of hypermotility, the antimuscarinic agents, especially in combination with an opioid antidiarrheal drug, are extremely useful. The classic combination of atropine with diphenoxylate, a nonanalgesic congener of meperidine, is

Table 7–1. Antimuscarinic drugs used in ophthalmology.

Drug	Preparation	Duration of Mydriasis (days)	Duration of Cycloplegia (days)
Atropine	Drops, ointment, 0.5%, 1%, 2%, and 3%	7–10	7–12
Scopolamine	Drops, ointment, 0.2%, 0.25%, and 0.3%	3–7	3–7
Homatropine	Drops, 1%, 2%, and 5%	1–3	1–3
Cyclopentolate (Cyclogyl)	Drops, 0.5%, 1%, and 2%	1	¼–1
Tropicamide (Mydriacyl)	Drops, 0.5% and 1%	¼	¼

Table 7–2. Antimuscarinic drugs used in gastrointestinal and genitourinary conditions.

Drug	Usual Dose (mg)
Quaternary amines	
Anisotropine (Valpin 50)	50
Clidinium (Quarzan)	2.5
Glycopyrrolate (Glycobarb, Robinul)	1
Hexocyclium (Tral)	25
Isopropamide (Darbid)	5
Mepenzolate (Cantil)	25
Methantheline (Banthine)	50
Methscopolamine (Pamine)	2.5
Oxyphenonium (Antrenyl)	5
Propantheline (Pro-Banthine)	15
Tertiary amines	
Atropine	0.4
Dicyclomine (Bentyl, etc)	10–20
Oxyphencyclimine (Daricon)	10
Scopolamine	0.4
Tridihexethyl (Pathilon)	25

available under many names in both tablet and liquid form.

D. Cardiovascular Disorders: Marked vagal discharge sometimes accompanies the pain of myocardial infarction and may result in sufficient depression of sinoatrial or atrioventricular node function to impair cardiac output. Rare individuals without other detectable cardiac disease have hyperactive carotid sinus reflexes and may experience faintness or even syncope as a result of vagal discharge in response to pressure on the neck, eg, from a tight collar. Such individuals may benefit from the judicious use of atropine or a related antimuscarinic agent.

E. Respiratory Disorders: The use of atropine became part of routine preoperative medication when anesthetics such as ether were used, because these irritant anesthetics caused a marked increase in bronchial secretion and were associated with frequent episodes of laryngospasm. These hazardous effects were prevented by preanesthetic injection of atropine or scopolamine. The latter drug also produced significant amnesia for the events associated with surgery and obstetric delivery, a side effect that was considered desirable. On the other hand, urinary retention and intestinal hypomotility following surgery could be significantly exacerbated by the use of the antimuscarinic drug.

With the advent of effective and nonirritant inhalational anesthetics such as halothane and enflurane, it would seem that the major reason for the routine use of antimuscarinic drugs as preanesthetic medication has been eliminated.

Inhalation of smoke from burning leaves of *Datura stramonium* has been used for centuries as a remedy for bronchial asthma. "Asthmador" cigarettes containing *D stramonium* were available without prescription for this application until recently. As described in Chapter 18, the hyperactive neural bronchoconstrictor reflex present in most individuals with asthma is mediated by the vagus, acting on muscarinic receptors on bronchial smooth muscle cells. **Ipratropium** (Fig 7–2), a synthetic analog of atropine, is being studied as an inhalational drug for use in asthma. The aerosol route of administration provides the obvious advantages of maximal concentration at the bronchial target tissue with reduced systemic effects. This application is discussed in greater detail in Chapter 18.

F. Cholinergic Poisoning: Severe cholinergic excess is an important medical emergency, especially in rural communities where the use of cholinesterase inhibitor insecticides is common, and in cultures where wild mushrooms are eaten.

As noted in Chapter 6, both the nicotinic and the muscarinic effects of the cholinesterase inhibitor insecticides can be life-threatening. To reverse the muscarinic effects, a tertiary (not quaternary) amine drug must be used (preferably atropine), since the central nervous system effects as well as the peripheral effects of the organophosphate insecticides must be treated. Large doses of atropine may be needed to combat the muscarinic effects of agents like parathion: 1–2 mg of atropine sulfate may be given intravenously every 5–15 minutes until signs of effect (dry mouth, reversal of miosis) appear. The drug may have to be repeated many times, since the acute effects of the anticholinesterase agent may last for 24–48 hours.

A second class of compounds, capable of regenerating active enzyme from the organophosphorus-cholinesterase complex, is also available for the treatment of organophosphorus insecticide poisoning. These **oxime** agents include pralidoxime (PAM), diacetylmonoxime (DAM), and obidoxime.

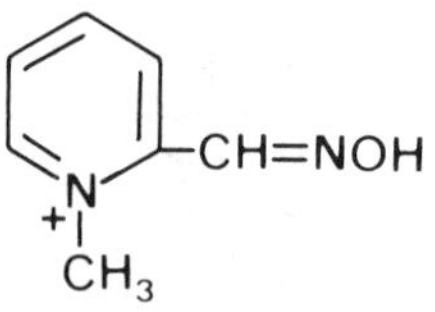

Pralidoxime

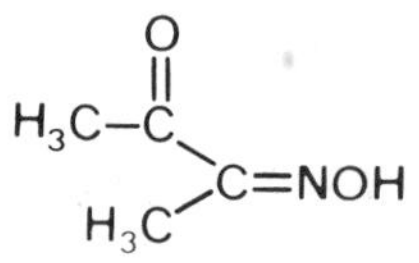

Diacetylmonoxime

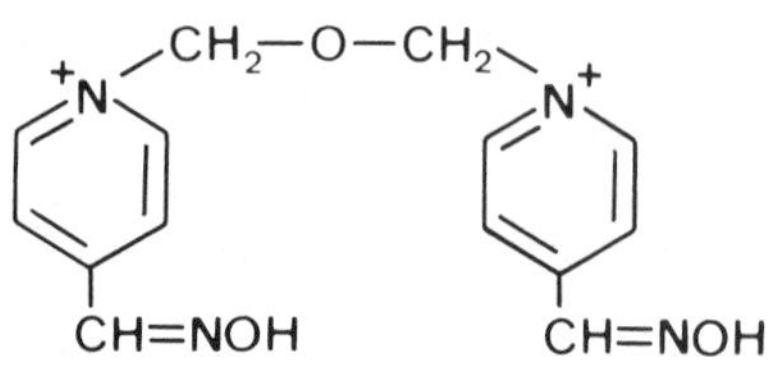

Obidoxime

The oxime group (=NOH) has a very high affinity for the phosphorus atom, and these drugs are able to hydrolyze the phosphorylated enzyme if the complex has not "aged" (Chapter 6). Obidoxime is the most potent of these oximes. Pralidoxime is the most extensively studied of the 3 agents shown above and the only one available for clinical use in the USA. It is most effective in regenerating the cholinesterase associated with skeletal muscle neuromuscular junctions. Because of its positive charge, it does not enter the central nervous system and is ineffective in reversing the central effects of organophosphate poisoning. Diacetylmonoxime, on the other hand, does cross the blood-brain barrier and, in experimental animals, can regenerate some of the central nervous system cholinesterase. The effect of the oximes on cholinesterase carbamylated by the carbamate cholinesterase inhibitors is controversial.

Pralidoxime is administered by intravenous infusion, 1–2 g given over 15–30 minutes. In high doses, pralidoxime can induce neuromuscular weakness and other side effects. Further details of treatment of anticholinesterase toxicity are given in Chapter 62.

Mushroom poisoning has traditionally been divided into rapid-onset and delayed-onset types. The rapid-onset type is usually apparent within 15–30 minutes following ingestion of the mushrooms. It is often characterized entirely by signs of muscarinic excess: nausea, vomiting, diarrhea, vasodilatation, reflex tachycardia (occasionally bradycardia), sweating, salivation, and sometimes bronchoconstriction. Although *Amanita muscaria* contains muscarine (the alkaloid was named after the mushroom), numerous other alkaloids, including *antimuscarinic* agents, are found in this fungus. In fact, ingestion of *A muscaria* may produce signs of atropine poisoning, not muscarine excess. Other mushrooms, especially those of the *Inocybe* genus, cause rapid-onset poisoning of the muscarinic excess type. Parenteral atropine, 1–2 mg, is effective treatment in such intoxications.

Delayed-onset mushroom poisoning, usually caused by *Amanita phalloides*, manifests its first symptoms 6–12 hours after ingestion. Although the initial symptoms usually include nausea and vomiting, the mechanism involves hepatic and renal cellular injury. Atropine is of no value in this form of mushroom poisoning (see Chapter 62).

G. Other Applications: Atropine and quaternary antimuscarinic drugs have been used in the treatment of urinary urgency caused by minor inflammatory bladder disorders. This approach does provide some symptomatic relief, although it is no substitute for specific antimicrobial therapy if cystitis is caused by infection. The antimuscarinic agents have also been used in urolithiasis to relieve the ureteral smooth muscle spasm caused by passage of the stone. However, their usefulness in this condition is debatable.

Hyperhidrosis is sometimes reduced by the antimuscarinic agents. However, relief is incomplete at best.

Adverse Effects

Because of the broad range of antimuscarinic effects, treatment with atropine or its congeners directed at one organ system almost always induces undesirable effects in other organ systems. Thus, mydriasis and cycloplegia are "adverse" effects when an antimuscarinic agent is being used to reduce gastrointestinal secretion or motility, even though they are "therapeutic" effects when the drug is used in ophthalmology.

At higher concentrations, atropine causes block of all parasympathetic functions; these are predictable from the organ system effects described above. However, even in gram quantities, atropine is a remarkably safe drug *in adults*. Atropine poisoning has occurred as a result of attempted suicide, but recent cases are more apt to be due to attempts to induce hallucinations. Poisoned individuals manifest dry mouth, mydriasis, tachycardia, hot and flushed skin, agitation, and delirium for as long as a week. Body temperature is frequently elevated.

Unfortunately, children are much more sensitive to the hyperthermic effects of atropine. Although accidental administration of over 400 mg has been followed by recovery, deaths have followed doses as small as 2 mg. Therefore, atropine should be considered a highly dangerous drug when overdose occurs in infants or children.

The pharmacologic treatment of overdose with atropine and its tertiary congeners in both children and adults is reserved for patients with severe drug-induced supraventricular tachycardia or marked elevation of body temperature and consists of giving **physostigmine** (Chapter 6). This tertiary cholinesterase inhibitor reverses muscarinic blockade in the central nervous system as well as the periphery. Given *slowly* intravenously (1–4 mg in adults; 0.5–1 mg in children), physostigmine is relatively safe and effective. Severe hyperthermia in children should also be treated with cooling blankets (not aspirin). Seizures may be treated with intravenous diazepam.

Poisoning caused by high doses of the quaternary antimuscarinic drugs is associated with all of the peripheral signs of parasympathetic blockade but few or none of the central nervous system effects of atropine. These more polar drugs may cause significant ganglionic blockade, however, with marked orthostatic hypotension (see below). Treatment of the antimuscarinic effects, if required, can be carried out with a quaternary cholinesterase inhibitor such as neostigmine. Reversal of hypotension may require the administration of a sympathomimetic drug such as phenylephrine or methoxamine.

Contraindications

Contraindications to the use of antimuscarinic drugs are relative, not absolute. Obvious muscarinic excess, especially that caused by cholinesterase inhibitors, can always be treated with atropine.

Antimuscarinic drugs are contraindicated in patients with glaucoma, especially angle-closure glaucoma. Even systemic use of moderate doses may precipitate angle closure (and acute glaucoma) in patients with shallow anterior chambers.

In elderly men, atropine should always be used with caution, and probably never in those with a history of prostatic hypertrophy.

Because the antimuscarinic drugs slow gastric emptying, they may increase symptoms in patients with *gastric* ulcer. If a stomach ulcer is to be treated pharmacologically, antacids and H_2 histamine antagonists are preferred (see Chapter 66).

III. BASIC & CLINICAL PHARMACOLOGY OF THE GANGLION-BLOCKING DRUGS

These agents block the action of acetylcholine and similar agonists at the nicotinic receptors of both parasympathetic and sympathetic autonomic ganglia. Some members of the group also (or perhaps exclusively) block the ionic channel that is gated by the nicotinic cholinoceptor. Because of their ability to block all autonomic outflow, the ganglion-blocking drugs are still important and useful in pharmacologic and physiologic research. However, their lack of selectivity confers such a broad range of undesirable side effects that they have been almost abandoned for clinical use. Their major remaining therapeutic application is for blood pressure control.

Chemistry & Pharmacokinetics

All of the ganglion-blocking drugs of interest are synthetic amines. The first to be recognized as having this action was **tetraethylammonium (TEA)**. Because of the very short duration of action of TEA, **hexamethonium ("C6")** was developed and was soon introduced into clinical medicine as the first effective drug for management of hypertension. As shown in Fig 7–3, there is an obvious relationship between the structures of the normal agonist acetylcholine and the nicotinic antagonists tetraethylammonium and hexamethonium. It is interesting that decamethonium, the "C10" analog of hexamethonium, is an effective neuromuscular depolarizing blocking agent.

Because the quaternary ammonium compounds are poorly and erratically absorbed after oral administration, **mecamylamine**, a secondary ammonium compound, was developed to improve the degree and extent of absorption from the gastrointestinal tract. **Trimethaphan**, a short-acting ganglion blocker, is inactive by the oral route and is given by intravenous infusion (Chapter 10).

Pharmacodynamics

A. Mechanism of Action: As noted above, the nicotinic receptors of the ganglia, like those of the skeletal muscle neuromuscular junction, are subject to both depolarizing and nondepolarizing blockade. Nicotine itself, carbamylcholine, and even acetylcholine (if given with a cholinesterase inhibitor) can produce depolarizing ganglion block.

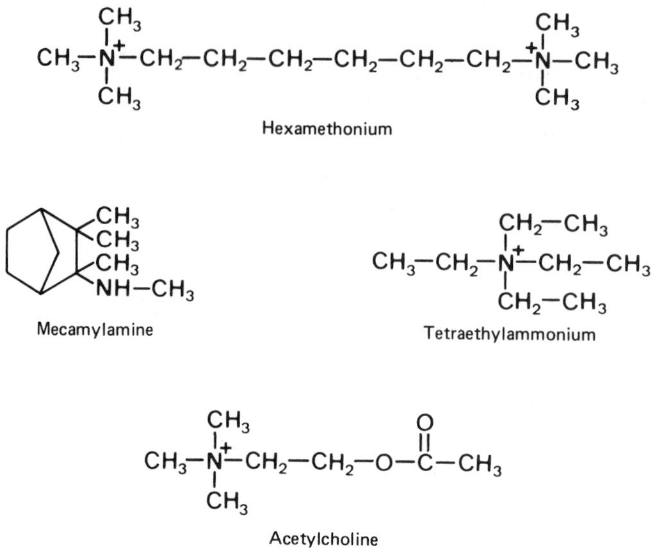

Figure 7–3. Some ganglion-blocking drugs. Acetylcholine is shown for reference. The structure of trimethaphan is shown in Fig 10–4.

All of the drugs presently used as ganglion blockers are generally classified as nondepolarizing competitive antagonists. Evidence from recent studies suggests that hexamethonium actually produces most of its block by occupying sites in or on the ion channel that is controlled by the acetylcholine receptor, not by occupying the cholinoceptor itself. In contrast, trimethaphan appears to block the nicotinic receptor, not the channel. According to older studies, block can be at least partially overcome by increasing the concentration of normal agonists, eg, acetylcholine.

As noted in Chapter 5, other receptors on the postganglionic cell modulate the ganglionic transmission event. However, their effects are not sufficient to overcome large doses of the hexamethonium-trimethaphan group.

B. Organ System Effects:

1. Central nervous system–The quaternary ammonium agents and trimethaphan are devoid of central effects because they do not cross the blood-brain barrier. Mecamylamine readily enters the central nervous system. Sedation, tremor, choreiform movements, and mental aberrations have all been reported as effects of the latter drug.

2. Eye–Because the ciliary muscle receives significant innervation only from the parasympathetic nervous system, the ganglion-blocking drugs cause a predictable cycloplegia with loss of accommodation. The effect on the pupil is not so easily predicted, since the iris receives both sympathetic innervation (mediating pupillary dilation) and parasympathetic innervation (mediating pupillary constriction). Because parasympathetic tone is usually dominant, ganglionic blockade usually causes moderate dilatation of the pupil.

3. Cardiovascular system–The blood vessels receive chiefly vasoconstrictor fibers from the sympathetic nervous system; therefore, ganglion blockade causes a very important decrease in arteriolar and venomotor tone. The blood pressure may drop precipitously, because both peripheral vascular resistance and venous return are decreased (see Fig 5–6). Hypotension is especially marked in the upright position (orthostatic hypotension), because postural reflexes that normally prevent venous pooling are blocked.

Cardiac effects include diminished contractility and, because the sinoatrial node is usually dominated by the parasympathetic nervous system, a moderate tachycardia.

4. Gastrointestinal tract–Secretion is reduced, although not enough to effectively treat peptic disease. Motility is profoundly inhibited, and constipation may be marked.

5. Other systems–Genitourinary smooth muscle is partially dependent on autonomic innervation for normal function. Ganglion blockade therefore causes hesitancy in urination and may precipitate urinary retention in men with prostatic hypertrophy. Sexual function is impaired in that both erection and ejaculation may be prevented by moderate doses.

Thermoregulatory sweating is blocked by the ganglion-blocking drugs. However, hyperthermia is not a problem except in very warm environments, because cutaneous vasodilatation is usually sufficient to maintain a normal body temperature.

6. Response to autonomic drugs–Because the effector cell receptors (muscarinic, alpha, and beta) are not blocked, patients receiving ganglion-blocking drugs are fully responsive to autonomic drugs acting on the effector cell receptors. In fact, responses may be exaggerated, because homeostatic reflexes, which normally moderate autonomic responses, are absent.

Clinical Applications & Toxicity

Because of the availability of more selective autonomic blocking agents, the applications of the ganglion blockers are limited to the lowering of blood pressure. The great efficacy of trimethaphan, when aided by the orthostatic hypotensive effect of venous pooling, is valuable in the treatment of hypertensive emergencies as described in Chapter 10. Controlled hypotension can be of value in neurosurgery to reduce bleeding in the operative field. The short, controllable effect of trimethaphan lends itself to this application as well. Trimethaphan has also been used in acute pulmonary edema to reduce pulmonary vascular pressure.

The toxicity of the ganglion-blocking drugs is limited to the autonomic effects already described. For most patients, these effects are intolerable except for acute use.

REFERENCES

Antimuscarinic Drugs

Becker CE et al: Diagnosis and treatment of *Amanita phalloides*-type mushroom poisoning. *West J Med* 1976; **125**:100.

Birdsall NJM, Burgen SAV, Hulme EC: The binding of agonists to brain muscarinic receptors. *Mol Pharmacol* 1978;**14**:723.

Bowers J, Forbes J, Freston J: Effect of nighttime anisatropine methylbromide (AMB) on duodenal ulcer healing: A controlled trial. *Gastroenterology* 1977;**72**:1032.

Crowell EB, Ketchum JS: The treatment of scopolamine-induced delirium with physostigmine. *Clin Pharmacol Ther* 1967;**8**:409.

Duvoisin RC: Cholinergic-anticholinergic antagonism in parkinsonism. *Arch Neurol* 1967;**17**:124.

Epstein SE, Redwood DR, Smith ER: Atropine and acute myocardial infarction. *Circulation* 1972;**45**:1273.

Feldman M et al: Effect of low-dose propantheline on food-stimulated gastric acid secretion. *N Engl J Med* 1977; **297**:1427.

Fordtran JS: Placebos, antacids and cimetidine for duodenal ulcer. *N Engl J Med* 1978;**298**:1081.

Glick G, Braunwald E: Relative roles of the sympathetic and parasympathetic nervous systems in the reflex control of heart rate. *Circ Res* 1965;**16**:363.

Gowdy JM: Stramonium intoxication: Review of symptomatology in 212 cases. *JAMA* 1972;**221**:585.

Greenblatt DJ, Shader RI: Anticholinergics. *N Engl J Med* 1973;**288**:1215.

Kalser SC, McLain PL: Atropine metabolism in man. *Clin Pharmacol Ther* 1970;**11**:214.

Petrie, GR, Palmer KNV: Comparison of aerosol ipratropium bromide and salbutamol in chronic bronchitis and asthma. *Br Med J* 1975;**1**:430.

Richelson E, El-Fakahany E: The molecular basis of neurotransmission at the muscarinic receptor. *Biochem Pharmacol* 1981;**30**:2887.

Rumack BH: Anticholinergic poisoning: Treatment with physostigmine. *Pediatrics* 1973;**52**:449.

Shader RI, Greenblatt DJ: Belladonna alkaloids and synthetic anticholinergics: Uses and toxicity. Pages 103–147 in: *Psychiatric Complications of Medical Drugs*. Shader RI (editor). Raven Press, 1972.

Yamamura HI, Snyder SH: Muscarinic cholinergic receptor binding in the longitudinal muscle of the guinea pig ileum with (^{3}H) quinuclidinyl benzilate. *Mol Pharmacol* 1974; **10**:861.

Ganglion-Blocking Drugs

Mason DFJ: Ganglion-blocking drugs. Pages 363–387 in: *Physiological Pharmacology: A Comprehensive Treatise.* Vol 3. Root WS, Hoffman FG (editors). Academic Press, 1967.

Rang HP: The action of ganglionic blocking drugs on the synaptic responses of rat submandibular ganglion cells. *Br J Pharmacol* 1982;**75**:151.

Salem MR: Therapeutic uses of ganglionic blocking drugs. *Int Anesthesiol Clin* 1978;**16**:171.

Stone CA et al: Ganglionic blocking properties of 3-methylaminoisocamphane hydrochloride (mecamylamine): A secondary amine. *J Pharmacol Exp Ther* 1956;**117**:169.

Volle RL: Ganglionic transmission. *Am Rev Pharmacol* 1969;**9**:135.

Wang HH, Tim LMP, Katz RL: A comparison of the cardiovascular effects of sodium nitroprusside and trimethaphan. *Anesthesiology* 1977;**46**:40.

8

Adrenoceptor-Activating Drugs

Brian B. Hoffman, MD

The sympathetic nervous system is an important regulator of the activities of organs such as the heart and peripheral vasculature (see Chapter 5), especially in responses to stress. The ultimate effects of sympathetic stimulation are mediated by release of norepinephrine from nerve terminals that serve to activate the adrenoceptors on postsynaptic sites. Also, in response to stress, the adrenal medulla releases epinephrine, which is transported in the blood to target tissues. Drugs that partially or completely mimic the actions of epinephrine or norepinephrine—**sympathomimetics**—would be expected to have a wide range of effects. An understanding of the pharmacology of these agents is thus a logical extension of what we know about the physiologic role of the catecholamines. Some of these drugs act directly on adrenoceptors; others act indirectly, their actions dependent on the release of endogenous catecholamines. Both types of sympathomimetics ultimately cause activation of adrenoceptors, leading to some of the characteristic effects of catecholamines.

I. BASIC PHARMACOLOGY OF ADRENOCEPTOR-ACTIVATING DRUGS

Identification of Adrenoceptors

The effort to understand the molecular mechanisms by which catecholamines act has a long and rich history. A great conceptual debt is owed to the work of Langley and Ehrlich 75–100 years ago putting forth the hypothesis that drugs have their effects by interacting with specific "receptive" substances. Ahlquist, in 1948, rationalized a large body of observations by his conjecture that catecholamines acted via 2 principal receptors. He termed these receptors alpha and beta. Alpha receptors are those which exhibit the potency series epinephrine $\geq$ norepinephrine $>>$ isoproterenol. Beta receptors have the potency series isoproterenol $>$ epinephrine $\geq$ norepinephrine. Ahlquist's hypothesis was dramatically confirmed by the development of drugs that specifically antagonize alpha or beta receptors (see Chapter 9). Subsequently, it was found that there are at least 2 subtypes of beta receptors, designated β_1 and β_2. Beta$_1$ and β_2 receptors are operationally defined by their affinities for epinephrine and norepinephrine: β_1 receptors have approximately

equal affinity for epinephrine and norepinephrine, whereas β_2 receptors have a higher affinity for epinephrine than for norepinephrine.

More recently, it has been recognized that there are also at least 2 subgroups of alpha receptors (α_1 and α_2). The subtypes of alpha receptors are defined by their affinities for alpha receptor–blocking drugs such as prazosin (see Chapters 9 and 10).

Examples of sympathomimetic agonists that are relatively selective for these receptor subgroups are listed in Table 8–1 along with some nonselective agents. **Selectivity** means that a drug may preferentially activate one subgroup of receptors at concentrations too low to activate another subgroup. For example, norepinephrine preferentially activates β_1 receptors as compared to β_2 receptors. However, selectivity is not usually absolute, and at higher concentrations related classes of receptor may also be occupied by the drug. As a result, the "numeric" subclassification of adrenergic receptors is clinically important only for drugs that have relatively marked selectivity.

Molecular Mechanisms of Sympathomimetic Action

A. Alpha Receptors: The mechanisms involved in the activation of alpha receptors by catecholamines are not well understood. In addition to the method of identification by agonist potency series described above, α-adrenoceptors have been identified in a variety of tissues by measuring the binding of radiolabeled compounds that are considered to have a high affinity for these receptors, eg, dihydroergocryptine, prazosin, and yohimbine. These radioligands have been utilized to measure the number of receptors in tissues and to determine the affinity (by displacement of the radio-

Table 8–1. Relative selectivity of adrenoceptor agonists.

	Receptor
Alpha-agonists	
Phenylephrine, methoxamine	α_1-selective
Epinephrine, norepinephrine	$\alpha_1 \sim \alpha_2$
Clonidine, α-methylnorepinephrine	α_2-selective
Beta-agonists	
Norepinephrine, dobutamine, prenalterol	β_1-selective
Isoproterenol, epinephrine	$\beta_1 \sim \beta_2$
Fenoterol, albuterol, terbutaline, metaproterenol	β_2-selective

labeled ligand) of other drugs that interact with the receptors. Such studies have been used to define the α_1 and α_2 selectivity of the agents listed in Table 8–1.

The most commonly observed effect of α_1-receptor activation is a rise in cytosolic calcium concentration. This effect does not appear to involve a change in adenylate cyclase activity or cAMP concentration in cells, except perhaps in certain regions of the brain. The mechanism by which this increase in calcium occurs is unclear. In certain smooth muscle cells, α_1-receptor activation leads to an influx of calcium across the membrane, probably through the opening of "receptor-operated" calcium channels (Fig 11–4). Alpha$_1$-receptor activation in many cells leads to the breakdown of polyphosphoinositides into inositol trisphosphate and diacylglycerol. Inositol trisphosphate may be directly involved in the release of sequestered calcium into the cytoplasm. Diacylglycerol activates a recently discovered protein kinase, termed C kinase. The physiologic significance of C kinase is not yet clear; however, in some cells it promotes cell division. The increased concentration of calcium leads to the activation of distinct calcium-dependent protein kinases (Fig 11–4). These calcium-dependent enzymes are distinct from cAMP-dependent protein kinases.

Certain α_2 receptors inhibit adenylate cyclase activity and bring about a fall in intracellular cAMP levels. While this effect has been well documented, it is not clear whether this action is the exclusive or major expression of α_2-receptor activation. Thus, α_2-receptor agonists cause a fall in platelet cAMP levels and cause platelet aggregation, but it is not clear that aggregation is the result of the decrease in cAMP. Alpha$_2$ inhibition of adenylate cyclase is brought about through the mediation of an inhibitory regulatory protein ("N_i") that couples the α_2 receptor to the cyclase (Fig 8–1). This inhibitory coupling protein has some features in common with the stimulatory coupling protein (see below).

B. Beta Receptors: Like alpha receptors, beta receptors can be identified and their ligands characterized by means of radiolabeled compounds that have a high and selective affinity for them. Derivatives of the beta-antagonists have been particularly useful in this application and have made possible the isolation and purification of the receptor protein.

The mechanism of action of beta-agonists has been studied in considerable detail. Activation of both β_1 and β_2 receptors results in activation of adenylate cyclase and increased conversion of ATP to cAMP. Activation of the cyclase enzyme is mediated by a stimulatory guanine nucleotide–dependent coupling protein analogous to the inhibitory "N" protein identified with certain α_2 receptors (Fig 8–1). Indeed, there are now known to be structural homologies as well as differences between N_s and N_i. cAMP is the major "second messenger" of beta-receptor activation. For example, in the liver of many species, beta-receptor activation increases cAMP synthesis, which leads to a cascade of events culminating in the activation of glycogen phosphorylase (Fig 8–2). Additional details are given in Chapter 35. In the heart, beta-receptor activation increases the influx of calcium across the cell membrane and its sequestration inside the cell. Beta-receptor activation also promotes the relaxation of smooth muscle. While the mechanism is uncertain, it may involve the phosphorylation of myosin light chain kinase (Fig 11–4).

Chemistry & Pharmacokinetics

Beta-phenylethylamine may be considered the parent compound from which sympathomimetic drugs are derived (Fig 8–3). This compound consists of a benzene ring with an ethylamine side chain. Substitutions

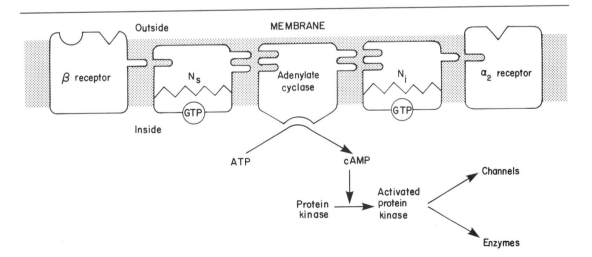

Figure 8–1. Hypothetical arrangement of β and α_2 receptors and the coupling proteins that regulate adenylate cyclase activity. The GTP-dependent coupling "N" proteins are subscripted "s" (stimulatory) or "i" (inhibitory) on the basis of their observed effects on cAMP production. cAMP facilitates the activation of a group of protein kinases, enzymes that phosphorylate and thereby modulate a variety of cell components, 2 of which are listed.

Catecholamine + Beta receptor $\xrightarrow{\text{Activates}}$ Adenylate cyclase $\longrightarrow$ cAMP $\xrightarrow{\text{Activates}}$

Protein kinase $\xrightarrow{\text{Activates}}$ Phosphorylase kinase $\xrightarrow{\text{Activates}}$ Glycogen phosphorylase

Figure 8–2. Activation of liver glycogen phosphorylase by cAMP. Interaction of a catecholamine or related sympathomimetic drug with beta receptors in liver leads to enhanced cAMP synthesis. The cAMP binds to a subunit of protein kinase. Consequently, protein kinase activates phosphorylase kinase, which in turn activates glycogen phosphorylase.

may be made (1) on the terminal amino group, (2) on the benzene ring, and (3) on the α or β carbons. Substitution by $-OH$ groups at the 3 and 4 positions yields sympathomimetic drugs collectively known as **catecholamines**. The effects of modification of β-phenylethylamine are to change the affinity of the drugs for alpha and beta receptors as well as to influence the intrinsic ability to activate the receptors. Sympathomimetic drugs may activate both alpha and beta receptors; however, the relative alpha-receptor versus beta-receptor activity spans the range from almost pure alpha activity (methoxamine) to almost pure beta activity (isoproterenol).

A. Substitution on the Amino Group: Increasing the size of alkyl substituents tends to increase beta-receptor activity. For example, methyl substitution on norepinephrine, yielding epinephrine, enhances activity at β_2 receptors. Beta activity is further enhanced with isopropyl substitution (isoproterenol). Beta$_2$-selective agonists generally require a large amino substituent group. The larger the substituent on the amino group, the lower the activity at alpha receptors; eg, isoproterenol is very weak at alpha receptors.

B. Substitution on the Benzene Ring: Maximal alpha and beta activity is found with catechola-

mines (drugs having $-OH$ groups at the 3 and 4 positions). The absence of one or the other of these groups, particularly the hydroxyl at C3, without other substitutions on the ring may dramatically reduce the potency of the drugs. For example, phenylephrine (Fig 8–4) is much less potent than epinephrine; indeed, beta activity is almost negligible except at high concentrations. However, catecholamines are subject to inactivation by catechol-O-methyltransferase (COMT), an enzyme found in gut and liver (Chapter 5). Therefore, absence of one or both $-OH$ groups on the phenyl ring increases the bioavailability after oral administration and prolongs the duration of action. Furthermore, absence of ring $-OH$ groups increases the distribution of the molecule into the central nervous system. For example, ephedrine (Fig 8–4) is orally active, has a prolonged duration of action, and produces central nervous system effects not observed with the catecholamines.

C. Substitution on the Alpha Carbon: Substitutions at this site block oxidation by monoamine oxidase (MAO) and prolong the action of such drugs, particularly for noncatecholamines. Ephedrine and amphetamine are examples of α-substituted compounds (Fig 8–4). Alpha-methyl compounds are also

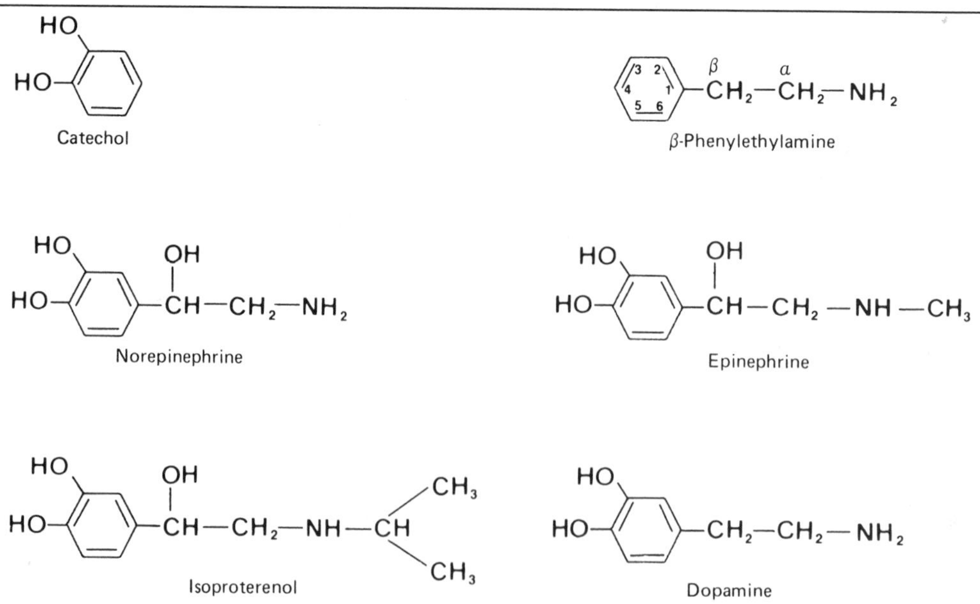

Figure 8–3. Phenylethylamine and some important catecholamines. These compounds are derivatives of β-phenylethylamine. Catechol is shown for reference.

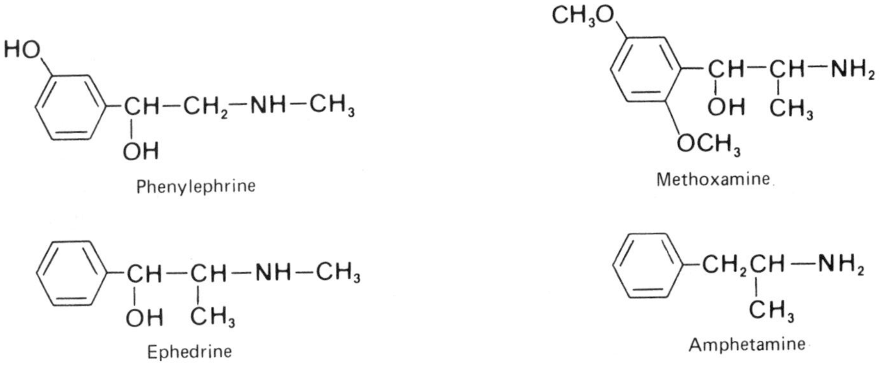

Figure 8–4. Some examples of noncatecholamine sympathomimetic drugs.

called phenylisopropylamines. In addition to their resistance to oxidation by MAO, phenylisopropylamines have an enhanced ability to displace catecholamines from storage sites in noradrenergic nerves. Therefore, at least a portion of their activity is dependent upon the presence of normal norepinephrine stores in the body; they are *indirectly* acting sympathomimetics.

ORGAN SYSTEM EFFECTS OF SYMPATHOMIMETIC DRUGS

General outlines of the cellular actions of sympathomimetics are presented in Tables 5–2 and 8–2. The net effect of a given drug in the intact organism depends on its relative receptor affinity (alpha or beta), intrinsic activity, and the compensatory reflexes evoked by its direct actions.

Cardiovascular System

A. Blood Vessels: Vascular smooth muscle tone

is regulated by adrenoceptors; consequently, catecholamines are important in controlling peripheral vascular resistance and venous capacitance. Alpha receptors increase arterial resistance, whereas β_2 receptors promote smooth muscle relaxation. There are major differences in receptor types in the various vascular beds. The skin vessels have predominantly alpha receptors and constrict in the presence of catecholamines, as do the splanchnic vessels. Vessels in skeletal muscle may constrict or relax, depending on whether alpha or beta receptors are activated. Thus, the overall effects of a sympathomimetic drug on blood vessels depend on the relative activities at alpha and beta receptors and the anatomic sites of the vessels affected (Table 8–3).

B. Heart: Direct effects on the heart are determined largely by β_1 receptors, although β_2 and to a lesser extent α receptors have also been implicated. Beta-receptor activation results in increased calcium

Table 8–2. Distribution of adrenoceptor subtypes.

Type	Tissue	Actions
Alpha₁	Most vascular smooth muscle.	Contraction.
	Pupillary dilator muscle.	Contraction (dilates pupil).
	Pilomotor smooth muscle.	Erects hair.
	Rat liver.	Glycogenolysis.
Alpha₂	Postsynaptic CNS adrenoceptors.	Probably multiple.
	Platelets.	Aggregation.
	Adrenergic and cholinergic nerve terminals.	Inhibition of transmitter release.
	Some vascular smooth muscle.	Contraction.
	Fat cells.	Inhibition of lipolysis.
Beta₁	Heart, fat cells, CNS.	Activates adenylate cyclase.
Beta₂	Respiratory, uterine, and vascular smooth muscle.	Activates adenylate cyclase.

Table 8–3. Cardiovascular response to sympathomimetic amines.*

	Phenyl-ephrine	Epi-nephrine	Isopro-terenol
Vascular resistance (tone)			
Cutaneous, mucous membranes (α)	↑ ↑	↑ ↑	0
Skeletal muscle (β_2, α)	↑	↓	↓ ↓
Renal (α)	↑	↑	↓
Splanchnic (α)	↑ ↑	↓ or ↑↑	↓
Total peripheral resistance	↑ ↑ ↑	↓ or ↑↑	↓ ↓
Venous tone	↑	↑	↓
Cardiac			
Contractility (β_1)	0 or ↑	↑ ↑ ↑	↑ ↑ ↑
Heart rate (predominantly β_1)	↓ ↓ (vagal reflex)	↑ or ↓	↑ ↑ ↑
Stroke volume	0, ↓, ↑	↑	↑
Cardiac output	↓	↑	↑ ↑
Blood pressure			
Mean	↑ ↑	↑	↓
Diastolic	↑ ↑	↓ or ↑↑	↓ ↓
Systolic	↑ ↑	↑ ↑	0 or ↓
Pulse pressure	0	↑ ↑	↑ ↑

*(↑ = increase; ↓ = decrease; 0 = no change.)
†Small doses decrease, large doses increase.

influx in cardiac cells. This has both electrical (Fig 8–5) and mechanical consequences. Pacemaker activity, both normal (sinoatrial node) and abnormal (eg, Purkinje fibers), is increased (positive chronotropic effect). Conduction velocity in the atrioventricular node is increased, and the refractory period is decreased. Intrinsic contractility is increased (positive inotropic effect), and relaxation is accelerated. As a result, the twitch response of isolated cardiac muscle is increased in tension but abbreviated in duration. In the intact heart, intraventricular pressure rises and falls more rapidly, and ejection time is decreased. These direct effects are easily demonstrated in the absence of reflexes evoked by changes in blood pressure, eg, in isolated myocardial preparations and in patients with ganglionic blockade. In the presence of normal reflex activity, the direct effects on heart rate may be dominated by a reflex response to blood pressure changes.

C. Blood Pressure: The effects of sympathomimetic drugs on blood pressure can be explained on the basis of their effects on the heart, the peripheral vascular resistance, and the venous return (Fig 5–6; Table 8–3). A relatively pure alpha-agonist such as phenylephrine increases peripheral resistance and venous tone (Fig 8–6). The enhanced arterial constriction may lead to a marked rise in blood pressure. In the presence of normal cardiovascular reflexes, the rise in blood pressure elicits a baroreceptor-mediated increase in vagal tone with slowing of heart rate. However, cardiac output may not diminish in proportion to this reduction in rate, since increased venous return may increase stroke volume; furthermore, direct alpha-adrenoceptor stimulation of the heart may have a modest positive inotropic action. While these are the expected effects of pure alpha-agonists in normal subjects, their use in hypotensive patients probably would not lead to these brisk reflex responses.

The blood pressure response to a pure beta-adreno-

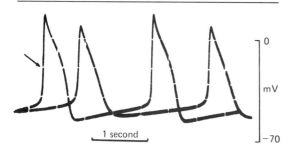

Figure 8–5. Effect of epinephrine on the transmembrane potential of a pacemaker cell in the frog heart. The arrowed trace was recorded after the addition of epinephrine. Note the increased slope of diastolic depolarization and decreased interval between action potentials. This pacemaker acceleration is typical of β_1-stimulant drugs. (Modified and reproduced, with permission, from Brown H, Giles W, Noble S: Membrane currents underlying rhythmic activity in frog sinus venosus. In: *The Sinus Node: Structure, Function, and Clinical Relevance.* Bonke FIM [editor]. Martinus Nijhoff, 1978.)

ceptor agonist is quite different. Stimulation of beta receptors in the heart increases cardiac output. A relatively pure beta-agonist such as isoproteronol also decreases peripheral resistance by dilating certain vascular beds. The net effect is to maintain or slightly increase systolic pressure while permitting a fall in diastolic pressure owing to enhanced diastolic runoff. The actions of drugs with both alpha and beta effects (eg, epinephrine and norepinephrine) are discussed below.

Eye

The radial pupillary dilator muscle of the iris contains alpha receptors; activation by drugs such as phenylephrine causes mydriasis. Alpha and beta stimulants also have important effects on intraocular pressure via poorly understood mechanisms. These effects are important in the treatment of glaucoma. Beta stimulants relax the ciliary muscle to an insignificant degree, causing a minor decrease in accommodation.

Respiratory Tract

Bronchial smooth muscle contains β_2 receptors that cause relaxation. Activation of these receptors thus results in bronchodilation (Table 8–2 and Chapter 18). The blood vessels of the upper respiratory tract mucosa contain α receptors; the decongestant action of alpha stimulants is clinically useful (see part II of this chapter).

Gastrointestinal Tract

Relaxation of gastrointestinal smooth muscle can be brought about by both α- and β-stimulant agents. Beta receptors appear to be located directly on the smooth muscle cells and mediate relaxation via hyperpolarization and decreased spike activity in these cells. Alpha stimulants are thought to decrease muscle activity *indirectly* by acting presynaptically to reduce the release of acetylcholine and possibly other stimulants.

Genitourinary Tract

The human uterus contains α and β_2 receptors. The fact that the beta receptors mediate relaxation can be clinically useful in pregnancy (see part II). The bladder base and urethral sphincter contain α receptors that mediate contraction and therefore promote continence. The β_2 receptors of the bladder wall mediate relaxation. Ejaculation is dependent upon normal α-receptor activity.

Exocrine Glands

The salivary glands contain adrenoceptors that regulate the secretion of amylase and water. However, certain sympathomimetic drugs—eg, clonidine, an α_2-selective agonist used in the treatment of hypertension—produce symptoms of dry mouth. The mechanism of this effect is uncertain; it is likely that central nervous system effects are responsible, although other (peripheral) effects may contribute.

The apocrine sweat glands, located on the palms of the hands and a few other areas, respond to alpha stim-

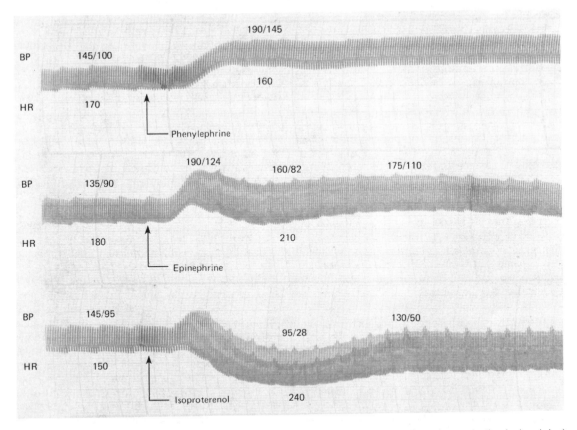

Figure 8–6. Effects of an alpha-selective (phenylephrine), beta-selective (isoproterenol), and nonselective (epinephrine) sympathomimetic, given as an intravenous bolus injection to a dog. (BP = blood pressure; HR = heart rate.) Reflexes are blunted but not eliminated in this anesthetized animal.

ulants with increased sweat production. These are the nonthermoregulatory glands usually associated with psychologic stress. (The diffusely distributed, thermoregulatory eccrine sweat glands are regulated by acetylcholine receptors.)

Metabolic Effects

Sympathomimetic drugs have important effects on intermediary metabolism. Activation of β_1-adrenoceptors in fat cells leads to increased lipolysis. Human lipocytes also contain α_2 receptors that inhibit lipolysis by decreasing intracellular cAMP. Sympathomimetic drugs enhance glycogenolysis in the liver, which leads to increased glucose release into the circulation. In the human liver, the effects of catecholamines are probably mediated by beta receptors, although alpha receptors may also play a role. Catecholamines in high concentrations may also cause metabolic acidosis. Activation of β_2-adrenoceptors by endogenous epinephrine or by sympathomimetic drugs promotes the uptake of potassium into cells, leading to a fall in extracellular potassium. This may lead to a fall in the plasma potassium concentration during stress or protect against a rise in plasma potassium during exercise.

Effects on Endocrine Function

Catecholamines are important endogenous regulators of hormone secretion from a number of glands. Insulin secretion is stimulated by beta receptors and inhibited by α_2 receptors. Similarly, renin secretion is stimulated by β and inhibited by α_2 receptors; indeed, beta-receptor antagonist drugs may lower plasma renin at least in part by this mechanism. Adrenoceptors also modulate the secretion of parathormone, calcitonin, thyroxine, and gastrin; however, the physiologic significance of these control mechanisms is unclear.

SPECIFIC SYMPATHOMIMETIC DRUGS

Catecholamines

Epinephrine (adrenaline) is a very potent vasopressor; the mechanism responsible for the rise in systolic blood pressure that occurs after epinephrine release or administration relates to its positive inotropic and chronotropic actions on the heart (predominantly β_1 receptors) and the vasoconstriction induced in many vascular beds (α receptors). Epinephrine also activates β_2 receptors in certain vessels, leading to their dilatation. Consequently, total peripheral resistance may actually fall, explaining the fall in diastolic pressure that is sometimes seen with epinephrine injection (Fig 8–6).

Norepinephrine (levarterenol, noradrenaline) and epinephrine have similar effects on β_1 receptors in the heart; however, norepinephrine is comparatively less potent at α receptors. More importantly, norepinephrine has relatively little effect on β_2 receptors. Consequently, norepinephrine increases peripheral resistance and both diastolic and systolic blood pressure. Compensatory vagal reflexes tend to overcome the direct positive chronotropic effects of norepinephrine; however, the positive inotropic effects are maintained.

Isoproterenol (isoprenaline) is an extremely potent beta-receptor agonist, having little effect on alpha receptors. The drug has positive chronotropic and inotropic actions; because isoproterenol activates beta receptors almost exclusively, it is a potent vasodilator. These actions lead to a marked increase in cardiac output associated with a fall in diastolic and mean arterial pressure and a lesser decrease or a slight increase in systolic pressure (Table 8–3; Fig 8–6).

Dopamine, the immediate metabolic precursor of norepinephrine, activates β_1 receptors in the heart. At low doses it has relatively little effect on peripheral resistance. However, at higher rates of infusion, it activates vascular alpha receptors, leading to vasoconstriction. Thus, high concentrations may mimic the actions of epinephrine. More importantly, it dilates renal and splanchnic resistance vessels by activating **dopamine receptors** that are not blocked by α- or β-blocking drugs. Similar dopamine receptors are found in the central nervous system and autonomic ganglia. The effect on renal blood flow may be clinically useful.

Dobutamine is a relatively β_1-selective synthetic catecholamine; it is discussed below.

Other Sympathomimetics

These agents are of interest because of pharmacokinetic features (oral activity, distribution to the central nervous system) or because of relative selectivity for specific receptor subclasses.

Phenylephrine has been described above as an example of a relatively pure α-agonist (Table 8–3; Fig 8–6). It acts directly on the receptors. Because it is not a catechol derivative (Fig 8–4), it is not inactivated by COMT and has a much longer duration of action than the catecholamines. It is an effective mydriatic and decongestant and can be used to raise the blood pressure.

Methoxamine. The pharmacologic actions of methoxamine are similar to those of phenylephrine, since it is predominantly a direct-acting alpha-receptor agonist. It may cause prolonged increase in blood pressure due to vasoconstriction; it also causes a vagally mediated bradycardia. Methoxamine is available for parenteral use; clinical applications are rare and limited to hypotensive states.

Ephedrine occurs in various plants and has been used in China for over 2000 years; it was introduced into Western medicine approximately 60 years ago as the first orally active sympathomimetic drug. Because it is a noncatechol phenylisopropylamine (Fig 8–4), it has high bioavailability and a long duration of action. As is the case with many other phenylisopropylamines, a significant fraction of the drug is excreted unchanged in the urine. Since its pK_a is greater than 9, its excretion can be accelerated by acidification of the urine.

Ephedrine acts primarily through the release of stored catecholamines; in addition, it has some direct actions on adrenoceptors. It is nonselective and mimics epinephrine in its spectrum of effects. Because it gains access to the central nervous system, it causes a mild amphetaminelike stimulation that is not seen with the catecholamines.

Clinically, ephedrine is utilized when a prolonged duration of effect is desired, particularly after oral administration. The main applications are in asthma, as a nasal decongestant, and as a pressor agent.

Xylometazoline and oxymetazoline. Xylometazoline and oxymetazoline are direct-acting alpha-agonists. These drugs have been used as nasal decongestants because of their ability to promote vasoconstriction in the nasal mucosa. When taken in large doses, oxymetazoline may cause hypotension, presumably because of a central clonidinelike effect.

Amphetamines. Amphetamine is a phenylisopropylamine (Fig 8–4) that is important because of its use and misuse as a central nervous system stimulant (see Chapter 30). Its pharmacokinetics are similar to those of ephedrine, but amphetamine enters the central nervous system even more readily and has a much more marked stimulant effect on mood and alertness and a depressant effect on appetite. Its peripheral actions are mediated primarily through the release of catecholamines. **Methamphetamine** (N-methylamphetamine) is very similar to amphetamine with an even higher ratio of central to peripheral actions. **Phenmetrazine** (see Fig 30–1) is a variant phenylisopropylamine with amphetaminelike effects. It has been promoted as an anorexiant and is also a popular drug of abuse. **Methylphenidate** is an amphetamine variant with major pharmacologic effects and abuse potential similar to those of amphetamine.

Hydroxyamphetamine (4-hydroxyamphetamine) enters the central nervous system very poorly but has peripheral effects by virtue of its ability to release stored catecholamines. Its highly specialized application illustrates how knowledge of a drug's basic mechanism of action can be applied to clinical problems. Horner's syndrome is a condition resulting from interruption of the sympathetic nerves to the face, including the eye, in which it causes miosis. The syndrome can be caused by either preganglionic or postganglionic lesions. Because a postganglionic lesion leads to degeneration of the adrenergic nerve endings and loss of stored catecholamines in the iris, the abnormally constricted pupil in such a case will not dilate in response to an indirect-acting sympathomimetic (hydroxyamphetamine), but it does respond to phenylephrine, which acts directly on the alpha receptors. In contrast, a patient with a preganglionic lesion will show a normal response to both drugs, since the postganglionic fibers remain intact.

Receptor-Selective Sympathomimetic Drugs

Alpha$_2$-selective agonists are used in the treatment of hypertension. Clonidine and methyldopa are discussed in Chapter 10. Guanfacine and guanabenz have similar modes of action.

Beta-selective agonists have become important because of the separation of β_1 and β_2 effects that has been achieved. Although this separation is incomplete, it is sufficient to reduce side effects in several clinical applications.

Beta$_1$-selective agents include dobutamine and a partial agonist, prenalterol (Fig 8–7). Because they are less effective in activating vasodilator β_2 receptors, they may increase cardiac output with less reflex tachycardia than occurs with nonselective β-agonists such as isoproterenol. Some of the important pharmacologic effects of dobutamine are critically dependent on the use of a racemic mixture. It is likely that one of the stereoisomers of dobutamine has alpha-receptor activity; this action tends to reduce vasodilatation and may also contribute to the positive inotropic action caused by the isomer with predominantly beta-receptor activity. These agents are currently under study for the treatment of congestive heart failure and cardiogenic shock. A major limitation with these drugs, as with other direct-acting sympathomimetic agents, is that tolerance to their effects may develop with prolonged use.

Beta$_2$-selective agents have achieved an important place in the treatment of asthma and are discussed in Chapter 18. An additional application is as uterine relaxants in premature labor (ritodrine; see part II). Some examples of drugs currently in use are shown in Figs 8–7 and 18–4; many more are available or under investigation.

Special Sympathomimetics

Cocaine is a local anesthetic with a sympathomimetic action that results from inhibition of transmitter reuptake at noradrenergic synapses (Chapter 5). It readily enters the central nervous system and produces an intense response that has made it a very heavily abused drug (Chapter 30).

Tyramine (Fig 5–4) is a normal by-product of tyrosine metabolism in the body and is also found in high concentrations in fermented foods such as cheese, beer, and wine. It is readily metabolized by MAO and is normally inactive if ingested. If administered parenterally, it has an indirect sympathomimetic action caused by the release of stored catecholamines. Thus, its spectrum of action is similar to that of norepinephrine. In patients treated with MAO inhibitors, which are used as antidepressants (see Chapter 28), tyramine may reach the systemic circulation and can be converted to octopamine (Fig 5–4), a false transmitter that is stored in sympathetic nerve endings (Chapter 10).

II. CLINICAL PHARMACOLOGY OF ADRENOCEPTOR-ACTIVATING DRUGS

The rationale for the use of sympathomimetic drugs in therapy rests on a knowledge of the physiologic effects of catecholamines on tissues. Selection of a particular sympathomimetic drug from the host of

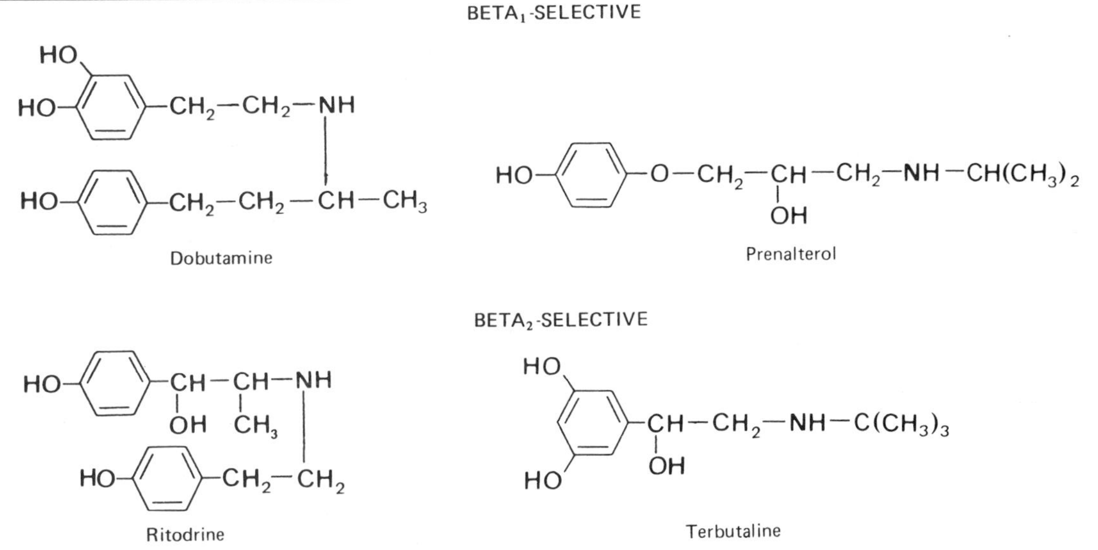

Figure 8–7. Examples of β_1- and β_2-selective agonists.

compounds available depends upon such factors as whether activation of α, β_1, or β_2 receptors is desired; the duration of action desired; and the preferred route of administration. Sympathomimetic drugs are very potent and can have profound effects on a variety of organ systems, particularly the heart and peripheral circulation. When these agents are used parenterally, great caution is indicated. In most cases, rather than using fixed doses of the drugs, careful monitoring of pharmacologic response is required to determine the appropriate rate of infusion. Generally, it is desirable to use the minimum dose required to achieve the desired response. The adverse effects of these drugs are generally understandable in terms of their known physiologic effects.

Cardiovascular Applications

A. Conditions in Which Blood Flow or Pressure Is to Be Enhanced: **Hypotension** may occur in a variety of settings such as volume contraction, cardiac arrhythmias, adverse reactions to medications such as antihypertensive drugs, and infection. If cerebral, renal, and cardiac perfusion is maintained, hypotension itself does not usually require vigorous direct treatment. Rather, placing the patient in the recumbent position and ensuring adequate fluids—while the primary problem is determined and treated—is usually the correct course of action. The use of sympathomimetic drugs merely to elevate a blood pressure that is not an immediate threat to the patient may increase morbidity (see p 93). Sympathomimetic drugs may be utilized in a hypotensive emergency to preserve cerebral and coronary blood flow. Such situations might arise in severe hemorrhage, spinal cord injury, or overdose of antihypertensive or central nervous system depressant medications. The treatment is usually of short duration while indicated fluids or blood are being administered. Direct-acting alpha-agonists such as norepinephrine, phenylephrine, or methoxamine can be utilized in this setting if vasoconstriction is desired.

Shock is a complex acute cardiovascular syndrome that results in a critical reduction in perfusion of vital tissues and a wide range of systemic effects. Shock is usually associated with hypotension, an altered mental state, oliguria, and metabolic acidosis. If untreated, shock usually progresses to a refractory deteriorating state and death. The 3 major mechanisms responsible for shock are hypovolemia, cardiac insufficiency, and altered vascular resistance. Volume replacement and treatment of the underlying disease are the mainstays of the treatment of shock. While sympathomimetic drugs have been utilized in virtually all forms of shock, their efficacy is unclear. In most forms of shock, vasoconstriction mediated by the sympathetic nervous system is already intense. Indeed, efforts aimed at reducing rather than increasing peripheral resistance may be more fruitful. A decision to use vasoconstrictors or vasodilators is best made on the basis of information about the underlying cause, which may require invasive monitoring.

Cardiogenic shock, usually due to massive myocardial infarction, has a poor prognosis. Mechanical perfusion and emergency cardiac surgery have been utilized in some settings. Optimal fluid replacement requires monitoring of pulmonary capillary wedge pressure. Positive inotropic agents such as dopamine or dobutamine may have a role in this situation. In low to moderate doses, these drugs may increase cardiac output and, compared with norepinephrine, cause relatively little peripheral vasoconstriction. Isoproterenol increases heart rate and work more than either dopamine or dobutamine.

Unfortunately, the patient with shock may not respond to general therapeutic maneuvers; the temptation is then great to use vasoconstrictors to maintain adequate blood pressure. While coronary perfusion may be improved, this gain may be offset by increased myocardial oxygen demands as well as more severe vasoconstriction in blood vessels to the abdominal viscera. Therefore, the goal of therapy in shock should be to optimize tissue perfusion, not blood pressure.

B. Conditions in Which Blood Flow Is to Be Reduced: Reduction of regional blood flow is desirable for achieving hemostasis in surgery, for reducing diffusion of local anesthetics away from the site of administration, and for reducing mucous membrane congestion. In each instance, alpha-receptor activation is desired, and the choice of agent depends upon the maximal efficacy required, the desired duration of action, and the route of administration.

Effective pharmacologic hemostasis, often required in facial, oropharyngeal, and nasopharyngeal surgery, requires drugs of high efficacy that can be administered by local application in high concentrations. Epinephrine is usually applied topically in nasal packs (epistaxis) or in a gingival string (gingivectomy). **Cocaine** is still sometimes used for nasopharyngeal surgery, because it combines a hemostatic effect with local anesthesia.

Combining alpha-agonists with local anesthetics greatly prolongs the duration of infiltration nerve block; the total dose (and the probability of toxicity) can therefore be reduced. **Epinephrine,** 1:200,000, is the favored agent for this application.

Mucous membrane decongestants reduce the discomfort of hay fever and, to a lesser extent, the common cold. Unfortunately, rebound hyperemia may follow the use of these agents, and repeated topical use of high concentrations may result in ischemic changes in the mucous membrane. Favored short-acting topical agents include phenylephrine and phenylpropanolamine in nasal sprays and ophthalmic drops. A longer duration of action, at the cost of much lower local concentrations and greater cardiac and central nervous system effects, can be achieved by the oral administration of agents such as ephedrine or one of its isomers, pseudoephedrine. Long-acting topical decongestants include xylometazoline and oxymetazoline. All of these mucous membrane decongestants are available as over-the-counter products (Chapter 68).

C. Cardiac Applications: Episodes of **parox-**

ysmal atrial tachycardia may be treated with alpha receptor–activating drugs such as phenylephrine or methoxamine. These drugs cause marked vasoconstriction, leading to a rise in blood pressure; the rise in blood pressure promotes a reflex vagal discharge that may convert the arrhythmia to sinus rhythm. The drugs should be given by slow intravenous infusion; caution must be utilized to prevent a dangerous rise in systolic blood pressure to greater than about 160 mm Hg. While these drugs are often effective in terminating this rhythm disturbance in patients who are hypotensive, generally safer alternatives may exist, such as the use of verapamil, edrophonium, or electrical cardioversion.

Catecholamines such as isoproterenol and epinephrine have also been utilized in the temporary emergency management of **complete heart block** and **cardiac arrest.** However, electronic pacemakers are both safer and more effective in heart block and should be inserted as soon as possible if there is any indication of continued high-degree block.

Congestive heart failure may respond to the positive inotropic effects of drugs such as dobutamine and prenalterol. Good results have also been reported following the use of β_2-selective agents used to reduce afterload by decreasing vascular resistance. These applications are discussed in Chapter 12. The development of tolerance or desensitization is a major limitation to the use of catecholamines in congestive heart failure.

Respiratory Applications

One of the most important uses of sympathomimetic drugs is in the therapy of bronchial asthma. This use is discussed in Chapter 18.

Anaphylaxis

Anaphylactic shock and related acute hypersensitivity reactions affect both the respiratory and the cardiovascular systems. The syndrome of bronchospasm, mucous membrane congestion, angioedema, and cardiovascular collapse usually responds rapidly to subcutaneous administration of **epinephrine,** 0.3–0.5 mg (0.3–0.5 mL of 1:1000 epinephrine solution). This drug is the agent of choice because of its great efficacy at α, β_1, and β_2 receptors; stimulation of all of these is helpful in reversing the pathophysiologic process. Glucocorticoids and antihistamines may occasionally be useful as secondary therapy in anaphylaxis; however, epinephrine is the initial treatment.

Ophthalmic Applications

Phenylephrine is an effective mydriatic agent frequently used to facilitate examination of the retina. It is also a useful decongestant for minor allergic hyperemia of the conjunctival membranes. The diagnostic use of hydroxyamphetamine has been described above.

Glaucoma responds to a variety of sympathomimetic and sympathoplegic drugs. **Epinephrine** and beta-blocking agents are among the most important therapies. Topical epinephrine (1–2% solution) low-ers intraocular pressure apparently both by decreasing aqueous humor formation and by increasing aqueous outflow. The efficacy of epinephrine may be related in part to desensitization of beta-adrenoceptor–mediated responses.

Genitourinary Applications

As noted above, β_2-selective agents relax the pregnant uterus. **Ritodrine, terbutaline,** and similar drugs have been used to suppress premature labor. In spite of some β_1 effects (tachycardia, arrhythmias), they are superior to ethanol and can be used chronically if the initial response is favorable.

Central Nervous System Applications

The amphetaminelike sympathomimetics have a mood-elevating (euphoriant) effect; this effect is the basis for the widespread abuse of this subgroup. The amphetamines also have an alerting, sleep-deferring action that is manifested by improved attention to repetitive tasks and by acceleration and desynchronization of the EEG. A therapeutic application of this effect is in the treatment of narcolepsy. The anorexiant effect of these agents is easily demonstrated in experimental animals. In obese humans, although an encouraging initial response may be observed, it is generally agreed that no long-term improvement in weight control can be achieved with amphetamines alone. A final application of the CNS-active sympathomimetics is in the **hyperkinetic syndrome** of children, a poorly defined and overdiagnosed behavioral syndrome consisting of short attention span, hyperkinetic physical behavior, and learning problems. Some patients with this syndrome respond well to low doses of the amphetaminelike drugs.

TOXICITY OF SYMPATHOMIMETIC DRUGS

The adverse effects of adrenoceptor agonists are primarily extensions of their receptor effects in the cardiovascular and central nervous systems.

Adverse cardiovascular effects seen with pressor agents include marked elevations in blood pressure, which may cause cerebral hemorrhage. Increased cardiac work may precipitate severe angina or myocardial infarction. Beta-stimulant drugs frequently cause tachycardia and, more significantly, may provoke serious ventricular arrhythmias. Sympathomimetic drugs may lead to myocardial damage, particularly after prolonged infusion. Special caution is indicated in elderly patients or those with hypertension or coronary artery disease. If an adverse effect requires urgent reversal, then a specific adrenoceptor antagonist should be used (see Chapter 9). For example, extravasation into subcutaneous tissues of norepinephrine being given by the intravenous route may lead to marked ischemia that can be reversed by alpha-adrenoceptor antagonists.

Central nervous system toxicity is rarely observed

with catecholamines or drugs such as phenylephrine. Phenylisopropylamines commonly cause restlessness, tremor, insomnia, and anxiety. In very high doses, a paranoid state may be induced. Therapy is discussed in Chapter 30.

REFERENCES

Barach EM et al: Epinephrine for treatment of anaphylactic shock. *JAMA* 1984;**251**:2118.

Caritis SN: Treatment of preterm labour: A review of the therapeutic options. *Drugs* 1983;**26**:243.

Colucci WS et al: Decreased lymphocyte beta-adrenergic–receptor density in patients with heart failure and tolerance to the beta-adrenergic agonist pirbuterol. *N Engl J Med* 1981; **305**:185.

Day MD: *Autonomic Pharmacology.* Churchill Livingstone, 1979.

Exton JH: Role of calcium and phosphoinositides in the actions of certain hormones and neurotransmitters. *J Clin Invest* 1985;**75**:1753.

Feely J, De Vane PJ, Maclean D: Beta-blockers and sympathomimetics. *Br Med J* 1983;**286**:1043.

Gilman AG: G proteins and dual control of adenylate cyclase. *Cell* 1984;**36**:577.

Goldberg LI: Dopamine: Clinical uses of an endogenous catecholamine. *N Engl J Med* 1974;**291**:707.

Himms-Hagen J: Sympathetic regulation of metabolism. *Pharmacol Rev* 1967;**19**:367.

Hoffman BB, Lefkowitz RJ: Adrenergic receptors in the heart. *Annu Rev Physiol* 1982;**44**:475.

Hoffman BB, Lefkowitz RJ: Alpha-adrenergic receptor subtypes. *N Engl J Med* 1980;**302**:1390.

Langer SZ: Presynaptic receptors and modulation of neurotransmission: Pharmacologic implications and therapeutic relevance. *Trends Neurosci* 1980;**3**:110.

Lefkowitz RJ, Stadel JM, Caron MG: Adenylate cyclase–coupled beta adrenergic receptors: Structure and mechanisms of activation and desensitization. *Annu Rev Biochem* 1983; **52**:159.

Leier CV, Unverferth DV: Dobutamine. *Ann Intern Med* 1983; **99**:490.

Motulsky HJ, Insel PA: Adrenergic receptors in man: Direct identifications and clinical alterations. *N Engl J Med* 1982; **307**:18.

Nelson HS: Beta adrenergic agonists. *Chest* 1982;**82**:33S.

Svedmyr W: Fenoterol: A beta₂-adrenergic agonist for use in asthma. *Pharmacotherapy* 1985;**5**:109.

Tarazi RC: Sympathomimetic agents in the treatment of shock. *Ann Intern Med* 1974;**81**:364.

Wurtman RJ: Catecholamines. (3 parts.) *N Engl J Med* 1965; **273**:637, 693, 746.

Adrenoceptor-Blocking Drugs

9

Brian B. Hoffman, MD

Since catecholamines play a role in a variety of important physiologic responses, drugs that antagonize adrenoceptors have obvious pharmacologic applications. The classification of adrenoceptors into alpha and beta types has been discussed in Chapter 8. The present chapter deals with drugs whose major effect is to antagonize the action of catecholamines by occupying either alpha or beta receptors, thus preventing their activation by the catecholamines.

In general, alpha receptor–blocking drugs have been very useful in the experimental exploration of autonomic nervous system function; surprisingly, they have thus far had only limited clinical application. Even though these drugs effectively block the vasoconstricting effect of catecholamines, their use in hypertension—with the exception of prazosin and labetalol—has been of little consequence. The place of alpha-receptor antagonists in the treatment of peripheral vascular disease is uncertain. In contrast, the beta receptor–blocking drugs have been found useful in a wide variety of clinical conditions.

I. BASIC PHARMACOLOGY OF THE ALPHA RECEPTOR–BLOCKING DRUGS

Alpha-receptor antagonists may be classified into 2 general categories: reversible and irreversible. Reversible antagonists may dissociate from the alpha receptor; irreversible drugs do not. Phentolamine and tolazoline are examples of reversible antagonists (Fig 9–1). Prazosin and labetalol, drugs used primarily for their antihypertensive effects, as well as several ergot derivatives (Chapter 15), are also reversible α-adrenoceptor blockers. Phenoxybenzamine, an agent related to the nitrogen mustards, forms a reactive ethyleneimonium intermediate (Fig 9–1) that covalently binds to the alpha-receptor site, resulting in irreversible blockade. Fig 9–2 illustrates the effects of a reversible drug in comparison with those of an irreversible agent.

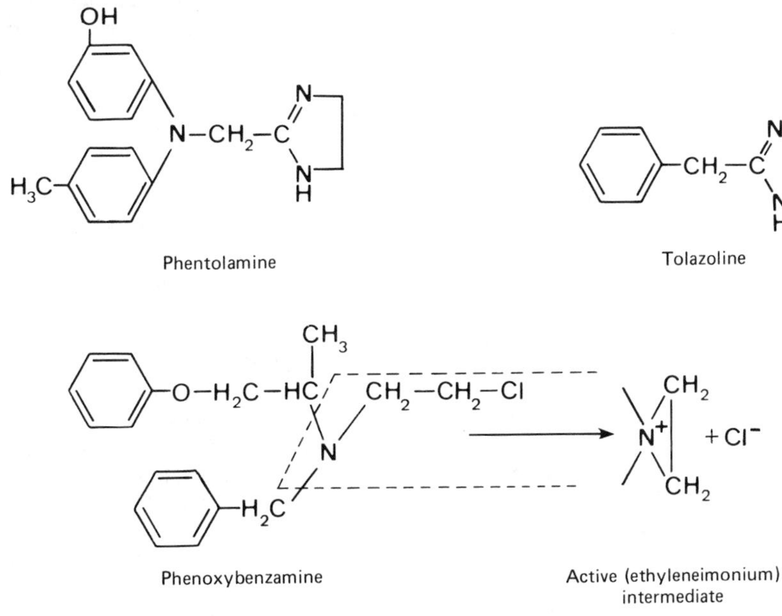

Figure 9–1. Structure of several alpha receptor–blocking drugs.

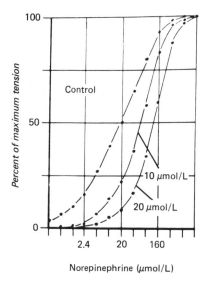
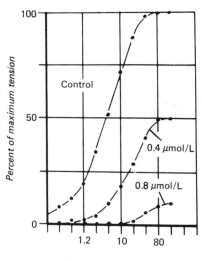

Figure 9–2. Dose-response curves to norepinephrine in the presence of 2 different α-adrenoceptor–blocking drugs. The tension produced in isolated strips of cat spleen, a tissue rich in alpha receptors, was measured in response to graded doses of norepinephrine. *Left:* Tolazoline, a reversible blocker, shifted the curve to the right without decreasing the maximum response when present at concentrations of 10 and 20 μmol/L. *Right:* Dibenamine, an analog of phenoxybenzamine and irreversible in its action, reduced the maximum response attainable at both concentrations tested. (Modified and reproduced, with permission, from Bickerton RK: The response of isolated strips of cat spleen to sympathomimetic drugs and their antagonists. *J Pharmacol Exp Ther* 1963;**142**:99.)

Pharmacologic Effects

A. Cardiovascular Effects: Because arteriolar and venous tone are determined to a large extent by alpha receptors on vascular smooth muscle, alpha receptor–blocking drugs cause a lowering of peripheral vascular resistance and blood pressure (Fig 9–3). They can prevent the pressor effects of usual doses of alpha-agonists; indeed, in the case of agonists with both α and β_2 effects (eg, epinephrine), they convert a pressor to a depressor response (Fig 9–3). This change in response is called **epinephrine reversal.** By inhibiting adrenergic-mediated venoconstriction, alpha blockers may cause postural hypotension and reflex tachycardia. Tachycardia may be more marked with agents that block α_2 presynaptic receptors in the heart (Table 9–1), since the augmented release of norepinephrine

will further stimulate beta receptors in the heart. Chronic use of alpha-antagonists may result in a compensatory increase in blood volume.

B. Other Effects: Minor effects that signal the blockade of alpha receptors in other tissues include reduced pupillary dilator tone, decreased adrenergic sweating, and nasal stuffiness. However, individual agents may have additional non–alpha-blocking effects that are far more important (see below).

SPECIFIC AGENTS

Phentolamine, an imidazoline derivative, is a potent competitive antagonist of alpha receptors. Phentolamine causes a reduction in peripheral resistance, through both alpha-receptor blockade and an additional nonadrenergic action on vascular smooth muscle. The cardiac stimulation induced by phentolamine may be in part reflex; however, a component of this stimulation is not dependent on baroreceptor activity. Alpha$_2$-receptor blockade may be involved. Phentolamine is about equally potent at α_1 and α_2 receptors. Phentolamine also inhibits responses to serotonin. Phentolamine is an agonist at muscarinic and H$_1$ and H$_2$ histamine receptors.

Phentolamine is poorly absorbed after oral administration. The principal adverse effects are related to cardiac stimulation, which may cause severe tachycardia, arrhythmias, and angina. Gastrointestinal stimu-

Table 9–1. Relative selectivity of antagonists for adrenoceptors.

	Receptor
Alpha-antagonists	
Prazosin, phenoxybenzamine	α_1-selective*
Phentolamine	$\alpha_1 = \alpha_2$
Yohimbine, tolazoline	α_2-selective*
Beta-antagonists	
Metoprolol, acebutolol, alprenolol, atenolol	β_1-selective*
Propranolol, timolol, nadolol, pindolol	$\beta_1 = \beta_2$
Butoxamine	β_2-selective*

*Selective means a *relatively higher* affinity for this receptor.

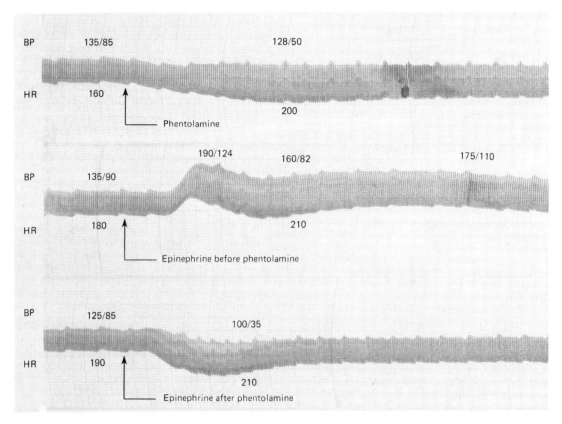

Figure 9–3. *Top:* Effects of phentolamine, an alpha receptor–blocking drug, on blood pressure in an anesthetized dog. Epinephrine "reversal" is demonstrated by tracings showing the response to epinephrine before *(middle)* and after *(bottom)* phentolamine. All drugs given intravenously. (BP = blood pressure; HR = heart rate.)

lation may cause diarrhea and increased gastric acid production.

Tolazoline is similar to phentolamine. It is somewhat less potent, but better absorbed from the gastrointestinal tract. It is rapidly excreted in the urine. Tolazoline has limited clinical applications in peripheral vasospastic disease and in the treatment of pulmonary hypertension in newborn infants with respiratory distress syndrome.

Ergot derivatives—eg, ergotamine, dihydroergotamine—cause reversible alpha-receptor blockade. However, most of the clinically significant effects of these drugs are the result of other actions (Chapter 15).

Phenoxybenzamine, because it binds covalently to alpha receptors, causes irreversible blockade of long duration (14–48 hours). It is somewhat selective for α_1 receptors, but less so than prazosin. The drug inhibits reuptake of released norepinephrine by presynaptic adrenergic nerve terminals. Phenoxybenzamine blocks histamine (H_1), acetylcholine, and serotonin receptors as well as alpha receptors.

The pharmacologic actions of phenoxybenzamine are primarily related to antagonism of alpha receptor–mediated events. Most importantly, phenoxybenzamine blocks adrenergic vasoconstriction. While phe-

noxybenzamine causes relatively little fall in blood pressure in supine individuals, it will reduce blood pressure when sympathetic tone is high, eg, as a result of upright posture or because of reduced blood volume. Cardiac output may be increased because of reflex effects and because of presynaptic effects on cardiac sympathetic nerves.

Phenoxybenzamine is absorbed after oral administration, though bioavailability is low. It may be used intravenously but not by other parenteral routes, because it is too irritating. The drug is usually given orally, starting with low doses of 10–20 mg/d and progressively increasing the dose until the desired effect is achieved. Less than 100 mg/d is usually sufficient to achieve adequate alpha-receptor blockade.

The adverse effects of phenoxybenzamine derive from its alpha receptor–blocking action; the most important are postural hypotension and tachycardia. Nasal stuffiness and inhibition of ejaculation also occur. Since phenoxybenzamine enters the central nervous system, it may cause less specific effects, including fatigue, sedation, and nausea. Since phenoxybenzamine is an alkylating agent, it may have other adverse effects that have not yet been characterized.

Prazosin is effective in the management of hypertension (Chapter 10). It was originally thought to be a direct-acting vasodilator, but it is now clear that the major pharmacologic action of prazosin is that of an extremely potent alpha-receptor antagonist. It is highly selective for α_1 receptors, having relatively low affinity for α_2 receptors. This may partially explain the relative absence of tachycardia seen with prazosin compared to phentolamine and phenoxybenzamine. Prazosin leads to relaxation of both arterial and venous smooth muscle.

Prazosin is extensively metabolized in humans; because of metabolic degradation by the liver, only about 50% of the drug is available after oral administration. The half-life is normally about 3 hours.

OTHER ALPHA-ADRENOCEPTOR ANTAGONISTS

Other alpha blockers include **yohimbine** (α_2-selective) and **trimazosin** (similar to prazosin but less potent). While yohimbine does not have an established clinical role, theoretically it could be useful in autonomic insufficiency by promoting neurotransmitter release by presynaptic blockade of α_2 receptors. Yohimbine may improve symptoms in some patients with painful diabetic neuropathies. It has been alleged that yohimbine improves or enhances sexual function; however, convincing evidence for this putative effect in humans is not yet available. Neuroleptic drugs such as chlorpromazine and haloperidol are potent alpha-receptor antagonists. While not used clinically to block alpha receptors, this action may contribute to the adverse effects of these drugs (eg, hypotension).

II. CLINICAL PHARMACOLOGY OF THE ALPHA RECEPTOR–BLOCKING DRUGS

Pheochromocytoma

The major clinical use of both phenoxybenzamine and phentolamine is in the management of pheochromocytoma. Pheochromocytoma is a tumor usually found in the adrenal medulla that releases a mixture of epinephrine and norepinephrine. Patients have many signs of catecholamine excess, including hypertension, tachycardia, and arrhythmias.

The diagnosis of pheochromocytoma is usually made on the basis of chemical assay of circulating catecholamines and urinary excretion of catecholamine metabolites, especially 3-hydroxy-4-methoxymandelic acid, metanephrine, and normetanephrine. Infusion of phentolamine has been advocated as a diagnostic test in patients suspected of harboring a pheochromocytoma, since patients with this tumor often manifest a greater-than-average drop in blood pressure in response to alpha-blocking drugs. However, measurement of circulating catecholamines and of urinary catecholamines and their metabolites is a more reliable and safer diagnostic approach. Provocative testing for pheochromocytoma by infusion of drugs such as histamine may cause dangerous blood pressure elevation if performed improperly. Unavoidable release of stored catecholamines sometimes occurs during operative manipulation of pheochromocytoma; the resulting hypertension may be controlled with phentolamine or nitroprusside.

Alpha-receptor antagonists are also useful in the preoperative management of patients with pheochromocytoma. Administration of phenoxybenzamine in the preoperative period will prevent precipitation of acute hypertensive episodes during studies undertaken to localize the tumor and will tend to reverse chronic changes resulting from excessive catecholamine secretion such as plasma volume contraction, if present. Furthermore, the patient's operative course may be simplified. Oral doses of 10–20 mg/d may be increased at intervals of several days until hypertension is controlled. Some physicians prefer to treat pheochromocytoma patients with phenoxybenzamine for many weeks before surgery, whereas others operate sooner. Beta-blocking drugs may be required after alpha-receptor blockade has been instituted to reverse the cardiac effects of excessive catecholamines. Beta-antagonists should not be employed prior to establishing effective alpha-receptor blockade, since unopposed beta-receptor blockade could theoretically cause blood pressure elevation from increased vasoconstriction. Phenoxybenzamine may be very useful in the chronic treatment of patients with inoperable or metastatic pheochromocytoma.

Pheochromocytoma is rarely treated with **metyrosine,** the α-methyl analog of tyrosine (α-**methyltyrosine**). This agent, in oral doses of 1–4 g/d, interferes with the synthesis of dopamine (Fig 5–4) and thereby decreases the amounts of norepinephrine and epinephrine secreted by the tumor. Metyrosine has no alpha-blocking effects but may act synergistically with phenoxybenzamine in the treatment of pheochromocytoma.

Hypertensive Emergencies

The alpha-adrenoceptor–blocking drugs have limited application in the management of hypertensive emergencies. They are most useful when increased blood pressure reflects excess circulating levels of alpha-agonist agents. Phentolamine can be used to control blood pressure in this circumstance, which may result from pheochromocytoma, overdosage of sympathomimetic drugs, or clonidine withdrawal. However, other drugs are generally preferable (Chapter 10).

Peripheral Vascular Disease

Although many alpha receptor–blocking drugs have been tried for treatment of peripheral vascular occlusive disease, there is no evidence that the effects are significant when morphologic changes limit flow in the vessels. Occasionally, individuals with Raynaud's syndrome and other conditions involving excessive reversible vasospasm in the peripheral circulation do receive significant benefit from phentolamine, tolazoline, or phenoxybenzamine.

Local Vasoconstrictor Excess

Phentolamine is also useful to reverse the intense local vasoconstriction caused by inadvertent infiltration of alpha-agonists into subcutaneous tissue during intravenous administration. The alpha-antagonist is administered by local infiltration into the ischemic tissue.

Urinary Obstruction

While the primary therapy for prostatic hypertrophy is surgery, alpha-receptor blockade with phenoxybenzamine has been found to be helpful in selected patients with urinary obstruction who are poor operative risks. The mechanism of action presumably involves partial relief of obstruction due to smooth muscle contraction in the enlarged prostate or in the bladder base. In addition, phenoxybenzamine may be useful in relieving bladder neck hypertonus in patients with spinal cord injury.

I. BASIC PHARMACOLOGY OF THE BETA RECEPTOR-BLOCKING DRUGS

Drugs in this category share the common feature of antagonizing the effects of catecholamines at β-adrenoceptors. Beta-blocking drugs occupy beta-receptors and competitively reduce receptor occupancy by catecholamines and other beta-agonists. (A few members of this group, used only for experimental purposes, bind irreversibly to beta receptors.) Most beta-blocking drugs in clinical use are pure antagonists; ie, the occupancy of a beta receptor by such a drug causes no activation of the receptor. However, certain beta receptor–blocking drugs cause partial activation of the receptor, albeit less than the full agonists epinephrine and norepinephrine. Another major difference among the many beta receptor–blocking drugs relates to their relative affinities at β_1 and β_2 receptors. Some of these antagonists have a higher affinity for β_1 than for β_2 receptors, and this selectivity for β_1 receptors may have important clinical implications. Other major differences among beta-antagonists relate to their pharmacokinetic characteristics and nonspecific membrane-stabilizing effects.

Chemically, the beta-receptor antagonist drugs (Fig 9–4) resemble isoproterenol (Fig 8–3), a potent beta-receptor agonist.

Pharmacokinetic Properties of the Beta-Receptor Antagonists

A. Absorption: Most of the drugs in this class are well absorbed after oral administration; peak con-

centrations occur 1–3 hours after ingestion. Sustained-release preparations of some of the drugs are available.

B. Bioavailability: Propranolol undergoes extensive hepatic ("first-pass") metabolism; its bioavailability is relatively low (Table 9–2). The proportion of drug reaching the systemic circulation increases as the dose is increased, suggesting that hepatic extraction mechanisms may become saturated. A major consequence of the low bioavailability of propranolol is that intravenous injection of the drug leads to much higher drug concentrations than are achieved after oral administration of the same dose. There is great individual variability in the plasma concentrations achieved after oral propranolol. Bioavailability is limited to varying degrees for all of the beta-antagonists except pindolol (Table 9–2).

C. Distribution and Clearance: The beta-antagonists are rapidly distributed and have large volumes of distribution. Propranolol crosses the blood-brain barrier. Most beta-antagonists are rapidly eliminated, with half-lives in the range of 2–5 hours. Propranolol and metoprolol are extensively metabolized in the liver, with little unchanged drug appearing in the urine. Pindolol and atenolol are less completely metabolized. Nadolol is excreted unchanged in the urine and has the longest half-life of any available beta blocker (up to 24 hours). Nadolol's half-life is prolonged in renal failure. The elimination of drugs such as propranolol may be prolonged in the presence of liver disease, diminished hepatic blood flow, or hepatic enzyme inhibition. It is notable that the clinical effects of these drugs are often prolonged well beyond the time predicted from half-life data.

Pharmacodynamics of the Beta-Receptor Antagonist Drugs

Most of the effects of these drugs are related to occupancy and blockade of beta receptors. However, some actions may be related to other effects, including partial agonist activity at beta receptors and local anesthetic action.

A. Effects on the Cardiovascular System: Beta-blocking drugs *lower* blood pressure. This effect

Table 9–2. Properties of several beta receptor–blocking drugs.

	Selectivity	Partial Agonist Activity	Local Anesthetic Activity	Elimination Half-Life (hours)	Approximate Bioavailability (percent)
Acebutolol	β_1	Yes	Yes	3–4	50
Atenolol	β_1	No	No	6–9	40
Labetalol	None	No	Yes	5	30
Metoprolol	β_1	No	Yes	3–4	50
Nadolol	None	No	No	14–24	33
Pindolol	None	Yes	Yes	3–4	90
Propranolol	None	No	Yes	3.5–6	30*
Timolol	None	No	No	4–5	50

*Bioavailability is dose-dependent.

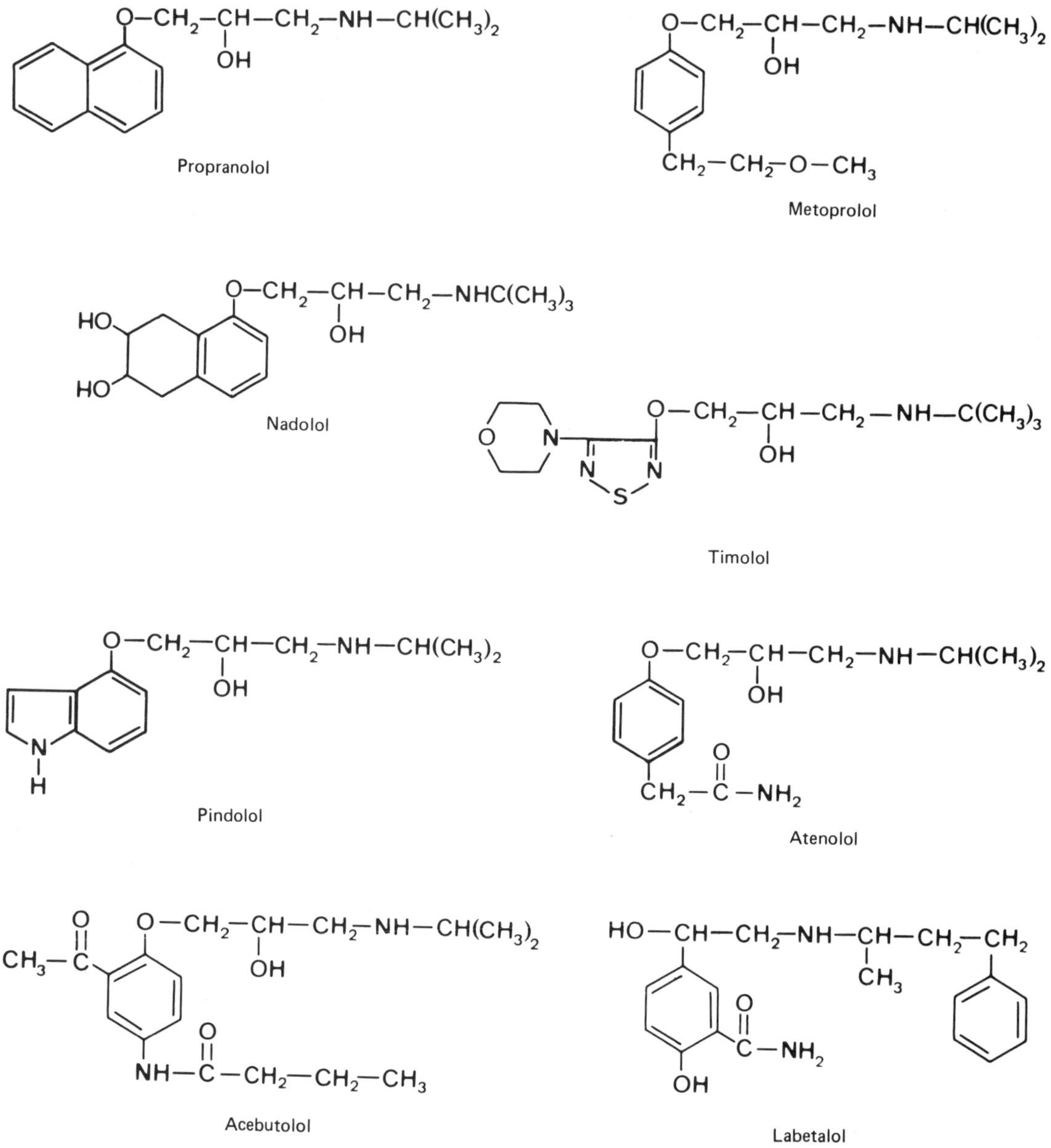

Figure 9–4. Structures of some beta-receptor antagonists.

is the result of several factors, some of them not fully understood. These factors include effects on the heart and blood vessels, the renin-angiotensin system, and possibly the central nervous system. Beta-adrenoceptor–blocking drugs are of major clinical importance in the treatment of hypertension (Chapter 10).

Beta-receptor antagonists have prominent effects on the heart (Fig 9–5). The negative inotropic and chronotropic effects are predictable from the role of adrenoceptors in regulating these functions. Slowed atrioventricular conduction with increased PR interval on the ECG is a related result of adrenoceptor blockade in the atrioventricular node. These effects may be clinically valuable in some patients but are potentially

hazardous in others. In the vascular system, beta-receptor blockade opposes β_2-mediated vasodilatation. This may result initially in a rise in peripheral resistance from unopposed alpha receptor–mediated effects. Beta-blocking drugs antagonize the release of renin caused by the sympathetic nervous system. As noted in Chapter 10, the relation between the effects on renin release and those on blood pressure is still being debated.

B. Effects on the Respiratory Tract: Blockade of the β_2 receptors in bronchial smooth muscle may lead to an increase in airway resistance, particularly in patients with asthma. Beta$_1$-receptor–selective antagonists such as metoprolol or atenolol may have some

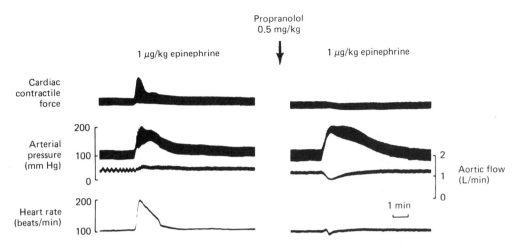

Figure 9–5. The effect in an anesthetized dog of the injection of epinephrine before and after propranolol. In the presence of a beta receptor–blocking agent, epinephrine no longer augments the force of contraction (measured by a strain gauge attached to the ventricular wall) nor increases cardiac rate. Blood pressure is still elevated by epinephrine because vasoconstriction is not blocked. (Reproduced, with permission, from Shanks RG: The pharmacology of beta sympathetic blockade. *Am J Cardiol* 1966;**18:**312.)

advantage over nonselective beta-antagonists when blockade of β_1 receptors in the heart is desired and β_2-receptor blockade is undesirable. However, no currently available β_1-selective antagonist is sufficiently specific to *completely* spare interactions with β_2-adrenoceptors.

C. Effects on the Eye: Several beta-blocking agents reduce intraocular pressure, especially in glaucomatous eyes. The mechanism of this action is poorly understood. Because of interspecies differences and differences in technique, many of the experimental data cannot be explained on the basis of a single mechanism of action. The mechanism usually reported is decreased aqueous humor production, but increased outflow has also been described.

D. Metabolic and Endocrine Effects: Beta-antagonists such as propranolol inhibit sympathetic nervous system stimulation of lipolysis. The effects on carbohydrate metabolism are less clear, although glycogenolysis in the liver is at least partially inhibited after beta blockade. However, glucagon is the primary counterregulatory hormone employed to combat hypoglycemia. It is unclear to what extent beta-antagonists impair recovery from hypoglycemia, although caution is advised about their use in insulin-dependent diabetics. This may be particularly important in diabetics with inadequate glucagon reserve or in pancreatectomized patients.

E. Effects Not Related to Beta Blockade: Partial beta-agonist activity was significant in the first beta-blocking drug synthesized, dichloroisoproterenol. It has been suggested that retention of some intrinsic sympathomimetic activity is desirable to prevent untoward effects such as precipitation of asthma. Pindolol and acebutolol are partial agonists (Table 9–2). It is not yet clear to what extent partial agonism is clinically valuable. However, these drugs may be useful

in patients who develop symptomatic bradycardia with pure beta-adrenoceptor antagonists.

Local anesthetic action, also known as "membrane-stabilizing" action, is a prominent effect of several beta blockers (Table 9–2). This action is the result of typical local anesthetic blockade of sodium channels and can be demonstrated in neurons, heart muscle, and skeletal muscle membrane. However, it is unlikely that these effects are important after systemic administration, since the concentration usually achieved by that route is too low for the anesthetic effects to be very evident.

SPECIFIC AGENTS
(See Table 9–2.)

Propranolol is the prototype beta-blocking drug. The spectrum of its actions shown in Table 9–2 is most remarkable for the degree of local anesthetic effect. In fact, propranolol is as potent as procaine in blocking nerve action potentials. It is also remarkable for its low and dose-dependent bioavailability, the result of extensive first-pass metabolism in the liver. A "long-acting" form of propranolol has recently become available; prolonged absorption of the drug may occur over a 24-hour period.

Metoprolol, altenolol, and acebutolol are representatives of the β_1-selective group of drugs. These agents may be safer in patients who experience bronchoconstrictive responses to propranolol.

Nadolol is unusual because of its very long duration of action; its spectrum of action is similar to that of timolol.

Timolol is a nonselective agent with no local anesthetic activity. It has excellent ocular hypotensive effects.

Pindolol and acebutolol are of interest because they have partial beta-agonist activity. They are effective in the major cardiovascular applications of the beta-blocking group (hypertension and angina).

Selective β_2-blocking drugs have not been actively sought because there is no obvious clinical application for them. An agent reported to possess some selectivity for β_2 receptors is butoxamine.

Labetalol is a reversible adrenoceptor antagonist with affinity for both alpha and beta receptors. Its affinity for alpha receptors is less than that of phentolamine, but labetalol is α_1-selective. Its nonselective beta-blocking potency is somewhat less than that of propranolol. Hypotension induced by this agent is accompanied by less tachycardia than occurs with phentolamine and similar alpha blockers.

Esmolol is a new ultra–short-acting investigational beta-adrenoceptor antagonist. It is a cardioselective compound with a duration of action in the range of 15–20 minutes after intravenous infusion, possibly because of rapid metabolism. Its major application thus far has been in the management of cardiac arrhythmias. To what extent such a compound will reduce the risk of beta-adrenoceptor antagonist therapy in critically ill patients remains to be determined.

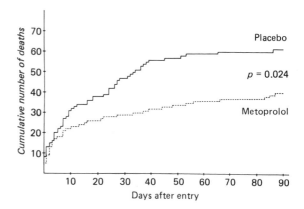

Figure 9–6. Cumulative number of deaths in 1395 patients with suspected acute myocardial infarction. Metoprolol was given to 698 patients and placebo to 697, starting as soon as possible after arrival in the hospital and continuing for 3 months. The difference between groups was highly significant, and after 90 days all patients were placed on metoprolol therapy. (Modified and reproduced, with permission, from Hjalmarson A et al: The Göteborg metoprolol trial: Effects on mortality and morbidity in acute myocardial infarction. *Circulation* 1983;67[Suppl 1]:I–26.)

II. CLINICAL PHARMACOLOGY OF THE BETA RECEPTOR–BLOCKING DRUGS

Hypertension

Many of the beta-adrenoceptor–blocking drugs have proved to be effective and well tolerated in hypertension. While many hypertensive patients will respond to a beta blocker used alone, the drug is most often used with either a diuretic or vasodilator. In spite of the short half-life of many beta-antagonists, these drugs may be administered once or twice daily and still have an adequate therapeutic effect. Labetalol, a competitive alpha- and beta-antagonist, is effective in hypertension, although its ultimate role is yet to be determined. Use of these agents is discussed in detail in Chapter 10.

Ischemic Heart Disease

Beta-adrenoceptor blockers reduce the frequency of anginal episodes and improve exercise tolerance in many patients with angina (Chapter 11). These actions relate to the blockade of cardiac beta receptors, resulting in decreased cardiac work and reduction in oxygen demand. Recent large-scale prospective studies indicate that the long-term use of timolol, propranolol, or metoprolol in patients who have had acute myocardial infarction may prolong survival (see Fig 9–6). Studies in experimental animals suggest that use of beta-receptor antagonists during the acute phase of a myocardial infarction may limit infarct size. However, their

use during the acute phase of myocardial infarction in patients is not usually undertaken.

Cardiac Arrhythmias

Beta-antagonists are effective in the treatment of both supraventricular and ventricular arrhythmias (Chapter 13). In cases of sinus tachycardia and supraventricular ectopic beats, the underlying disease should be treated rather than merely using a beta-antagonist. By increasing the atrioventricular nodal refractory period, beta-antagonists will slow ventricular response rates in atrial flutter and fibrillation. These drugs can also reduce ventricular ectopic beats, particularly if the ectopic activity has been precipitated by catecholamines.

Other Cardiovascular Disorders

Beta-receptor antagonists have been found to increase stroke volume in some patients with obstructive cardiomyopathy. This beneficial effect is thought to result from the slowing of ventricular ejection and decreased outflow resistance. Beta-antagonists are useful in dissecting aortic aneurysm to decrease the rate of development of systolic pressure. Recent experimental evidence suggests that—paradoxically—beta-antagonists may be effective in treating congestive heart failure in certain highly selected patients.

Glaucoma

Systemic administration of beta-blocking drugs was found serendipitously to reduce intraocular pressure in patients with glaucoma. Subsequently, it was found that topical administration also reduces intraocular pressure. Timolol has been favored for local use in the eye, because it lacks local anesthetic properties and is a pure antagonist. The mechanism by which timolol reduces intraocular pressure is unclear, but it may relate to decreased production of aqueous humor. Timolol appears to have an efficacy comparable to that of epinephrine or pilocarpine in open-angle glaucoma. While the maximal daily dose applied locally (1 mg) is small compared with the systemic doses commonly used in the treatment of hypertension or angina (10–60 mg), sufficient timolol may be absorbed from the eye to cause serious adverse effects on the heart and airways in susceptible individuals.

Betaxolol and levobunolol are newer beta-receptor antagonists that have recently been approved for the treatment of glaucoma. To what extent they may have fewer systemic side effects remains to be determined.

Hyperthyroidism

Excessive adrenergic activity is an important aspect of the pathophysiology of hyperthyroidism (Chapter 37), especially in relation to the heart. The beta-antagonists have salutary effects in this condition. The beneficial effects presumably relate to blockade of adrenoceptors and inhibition of peripheral conversion of thyroxine to triiodothyronine. The latter action may vary from one beta-antagonist to another. Propranolol is particularly efficacious in thyroid storm; it has been used cautiously in patients with this condition to control supraventricular tachycardias that often precipitate congestive heart failure.

Neurologic Diseases

Several studies suggest a beneficial effect of propranolol in reducing the frequency and intensity of migraine headache. The mechanism is not known. Since sympathetic activity may enhance certain tremors, it is not surprising that beta-antagonists have been found to reduce a variety of tremors. The somatic manifestations of anxiety may respond dramatically to low doses of propranolol, particularly when taken prophylactically. Propranolol is also of benefit in treating alcohol withdrawal.

Schizophrenia and the central nervous system manifestations of acute porphyria have also been reported to be alleviated by propranolol. However, most of the evidence for these effects is anecdotal.

CHOICE OF A BETA-BLOCKING DRUG

Propranolol is the standard against which all newer beta-antagonists promoted for systemic use should be measured. In many years of very wide use, it has proved to be a safe and effective drug for many indications. It is not clear that any of the newer beta-receptor blockers are superior to propranolol except in patients with reactive airways, who may be better managed with the β_1-selective agents metoprolol and atenolol. However, since the selectivity demonstrated by these drugs is far from complete, the risk of worsening airway obstruction is still significant. Since it is possible that some actions of a "beta-receptor antagonist" may

relate to some other effect of the drug, these drugs should not be considered interchangeable for all applications. For example, only beta-antagonists known to be effective in hyperthyroidism or in prophylactic therapy after myocardial infarction should be used for those indications. It is possible that the beneficial effects of one drug in these settings might not be shared by another drug in the same class. The possible advantages and disadvantages of beta blockers that are partial agonists have not been clearly defined in clinical settings.

CLINICAL TOXICITY OF THE BETA-RECEPTOR ANTAGONIST DRUGS

A variety of minor toxic effects have been reported for propranolol. Rash, fever, and other manifestations of drug allergy are rare. Central nervous system effects include sedation, sleep disturbances, and depression. It has been claimed that beta-receptor antagonist drugs with low lipid solubility will have a lower incidence of central nervous system side effects compared to compounds with higher lipid solubility. Further studies designed to compare the central nervous system adverse effects of various drugs are required before specific recommendations can be made, although it seems reasonable to try nadolol or atenolol in a patient who experiences unpleasant central nervous system side effects with other beta blockers. Experience with the newer members of this group is too limited to permit comparison of the incidence of toxic effects.

The major adverse effects of beta-receptor antagonist drugs relate to the predictable pharmacologic consequences of beta blockade. Beta$_2$-receptor blockade associated with the use of nonselective agents commonly causes worsening of preexisting asthma and other forms of airway obstruction without having these consequences in normal individuals. Indeed, relatively trivial asthma may become severe after beta blockade. While β_1-selective drugs may have less effect on airways than nonselective beta-antagonists, they must be used very cautiously, if at all, in patients with reactive airways.

Beta-receptor blockade depresses myocardial contractility and excitability. In patients with abnormal myocardial function, cardiac output may be dependent on sympathetic drive. If this stimulus is removed by beta blockade, cardiac decompensation may ensue. Great caution must be exercised in using beta-receptor antagonists in patients with myocardial infarction or compensated congestive heart failure. While an adverse cardiac effect of a beta-antagonist may be overcome directly with isoproterenol or with glucagon (glucagon stimulates the heart via glucagon receptors that are not blocked by beta-antagonists), neither of these methods is without hazard. A very small dose of a beta-antagonist (eg, 10 mg of propranolol) may provoke severe cardiac failure in a susceptible individual.

A much-studied but still unanswered question relates to possible hazards of abruptly discontinuing beta-antagonist therapy after chronic use. Evidence suggests that patients with ischemic heart disease may be at increased risk if beta blockade is suddenly interrupted. The mechanism of this effect is uncertain but might involve "up regulation" of the number of beta receptors. Until better evidence is available regarding the magnitude of the risk, prudence dictates the gradual tapering rather than abrupt cessation of dosage when these drugs are discontinued.

Similarly, the true incidence of hypoglycemic episodes provoked or exacerbated by beta-blocking agents is unknown. Nevertheless, it would be inadvisable to use beta-antagonists in insulin-dependent diabetics, particularly those with inadequate glucagon reserve, if reasonable alternatives are available.

Beta blockade may mask clinical signs of developing hyperthyroidism. With the increasing number of patients taking these medications for prolonged periods, this issue may become of more concern.

REFERENCES

Aellig W: Clinical pharmacologic investigations of the partial agonist activity of beta-adrenoceptor antagonists. *Hosp Formul* 1985;**20**:475.

Berthelsen S, Pettinger WA: A functional basis for classification of alpha adrenergic receptors. *Life Sci* 1977;**21**:595.

Beta-Blocker Heart Attack Trial Research Group: A randomized trial of propranolol in patients with acute myocardial infarction. 1. Mortality results. *JAMA* 1982;**247**:1707.

Byrd RC et al: Safety and efficacy of esmolol (ASL-8052: an ultra–short-acting beta-adrenergic blocking agent) for control of ventricular rate in supraventricular tachycardias. *J Am Coll Cardiol* 1984;**3**:394.

Cambridge D, Davey MJ, Massingham R: The pharmacology of antihypertensive drugs with special reference to vasodilators, alpha-adrenergic blocking agents and prazosin. *Med J Aust* 1977;**2(Suppl 1)**:2.

Feely J, Maclean D: New drugs: Beta-blockers and sympathomimetics. (Letter.) *Br Med J* 1983;**286**:1972.

Feely J, Peden N: Use of β-adrenoceptor blocking drugs in hyperthyroidism. *Drugs* 1984;**27**:425.

Frishman WH: *Clinical Pharmacology of the Beta-Adrenoceptor Blocking Drugs*, 2nd ed. Appleton-Century-Crofts, 1984.

Gerber JG, Nies AS: Beta-adrenergic blocking drugs. *Annu Rev Med* 1985;**36**:145.

Hjalmarson A et al: The Göteborg metoprolol trial: Effects on mortality and morbidity in acute myocardial infarction. *Circulation* 1983;**67(Suppl 1)**:I-26.

Hoffman BB, Lefkowitz RJ: Alpha-adrenergic receptor subtypes. *N Engl J Med* 1980;**302**:1390.

Langer SZ: Presynaptic receptors and modulation of neurotransmission: Pharmacological implications and therapeutic relevance. *Trends Neurosci* 1980;**3**:110.

Minneman KP, Pittman RN, Molinoff PB: β-Adrenergic receptor subtypes: Properties, distribution, and regulation. *Annu Rev Neurosci* 1981;**4**:419.

Nickerson M: The pharmacology of adrenergic blockade. *Pharmacol Rev* 1949;**1**:27.

Norwegian Multicenter Study Group: Timolol-induced reduction in mortality and reinfarction in patients surviving acute myocardial infarction. *N Engl J Med* 1981;**304**:801.

Potter DE, Rowland JM: Adrenergic drugs and intraocular pressure. *Gen Pharmacol* 1981;**12**:1.

Shand D: Clinical pharmacology of the beta-blocking drugs: Implications for the postinfarction patient. *Circulation* 1983;**67(Suppl 1)**:I-2.

Zaroshinski J et al: Ultra–short-acting beta blockers: A proposal for the treatment of the critically ill patient. *Life Sci* 1982;**31**:899.

Antihypertensive Agents

10

Neal L. Benowitz, MD, & Henry R. Bourne, MD

By some estimates, the arterial blood pressure of 15% of American adults is elevated to a degree that requires medical treatment. Sustained arterial hypertension damages blood vessels in kidney, heart, and brain and leads to an increased incidence of renal failure, coronary disease, and stroke. Effective pharmacologic lowering of blood pressure has been shown to prevent damage to blood vessels and to substantially reduce morbidity and mortality rates. Many effective drugs are available. Knowledge of their antihypertensive mechanisms and sites of action allows accurate prediction of efficacy and toxicity. As a result, rational use of these agents, alone or in combination, can lower blood pressure with minimal risk of toxicity in most patients.

HYPERTENSION & REGULATION OF BLOOD PRESSURE

Diagnosis

The diagnosis of hypertension is based on repeated, reproducible measurements of elevated blood pressure. The diagnosis serves primarily as a prediction of consequences for the patient; it seldom includes a statement about the cause of hypertension.

Epidemiologic studies indicate that the risks of damage to kidney, heart, and brain are directly related to the extent of blood pressure elevation. Even mild hypertension (diastolic blood pressure $\geq$ 90 mm Hg) in young or middle-aged adults increases the risk of eventual end organ damage. The risks—and therefore the urgency of instituting therapy—increase in proportion to the magnitude of blood pressure elevation. The risk of end organ damage at any level of blood pressure or age is greater in black people and relatively less in premenopausal women than in men. Other positive risk factors include a family history of cardiovascular disease, smoking, hyperlipidemia, diabetes, and manifestations of end organ damage at the time of diagnosis.

It should be noted that the diagnosis of hypertension depends on measurement of blood pressure and not upon symptoms reported by the patient. In fact, hypertension is usually asymptomatic until overt end organ damage is imminent or has already occurred.

Etiology of Hypertension

A specific cause of hypertension can be established in perhaps no more than 10% of patients. It is important to consider specific causes in each case, however, because some of them are amenable to definitive surgical treatment: renal artery constriction, coarctation of the aorta, pheochromocytoma, Cushing's disease, and primary hyperaldosteronism.

Patients in whom no specific cause of hypertension can be found are said to have **essential hypertension.*** In most cases, elevated blood pressure is associated with an overall increase in resistance to flow of blood through arterioles, while cardiac output is usually normal. Meticulous investigation of autonomic nervous system function, baroreceptor reflexes, the renin-angiotensin-aldosterone system, and the kidney has failed to identify a primary abnormality as the cause of increased peripheral vascular resistance in essential hypertension.

Elevated blood pressure is usually caused by a combination of several abnormalities (multifactorial). Epidemiologic evidence points to genetic inheritance, psychologic stress, and environmental and dietary factors (increased salt and perhaps decreased calcium intake) as perhaps contributing to the development of hypertension. Increase in blood pressure with aging does not occur in populations with low daily sodium intake. Patients with labile hypertension appear more likely than normal controls to have blood pressure elevations after salt loading.

Normal Regulation of Blood Pressure

According to the hydraulic equation, arterial blood pressure (BP) is directly proportionate to the product of the rate of blood flow (cardiac output, CO) and the resistance to passage of blood through precapillary arterioles (peripheral vascular resistance, PVR):

$$BP = CO \times PVR$$

Physiologically, in both normal and hypertensive individuals, blood pressure is maintained by moment-to-moment regulation of cardiac output and peripheral vascular resistance, exerted at 3 anatomic sites (Fig 10–1): arterioles, postcapillary venules (capacitance vessels), and heart. A fourth anatomic control site, the kidney, contributes to maintenance of blood pressure by regulating the volume of intravascular fluid. Baro-

---

*The adjective originally was intended to convey the now abandoned idea that blood pressure elevation was *essential* for adequate perfusion of diseased tissues. The term now serves as a reminder that we know "essentially" very little about the cause of this kind of hypertension.

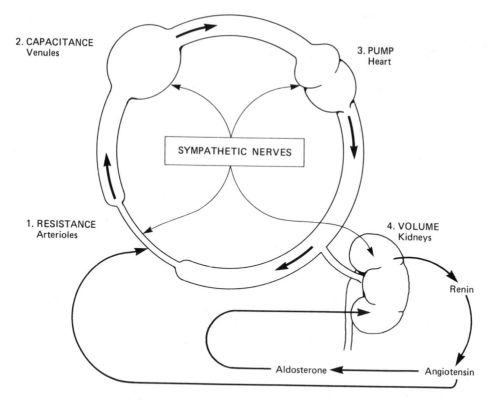

Figure 10–1. Anatomic sites of blood pressure control.

reflexes, mediated by sympathetic nerves, act in combination with humoral mechanisms, including the renin-angiotensin-aldosterone system, to coordinate function at these 4 control sites and to maintain normal blood pressure.

Blood pressure in an untreated hypertensive patient is controlled by the same mechanisms that are operative in normotensive subjects. Regulation of blood pressure in hypertensives differs from normal in that the baroreceptors and the renal blood volume–pressure control systems appear to be "set" at a higher level of blood pressure. All antihypertensive drugs act by interfering with these normal mechanisms, which are reviewed below.

A. Postural Baroreflex: (Fig 10–2.) Baroreflexes are responsible for rapid, moment-to-moment adjustments in blood pressure, such as in transition from a reclining to an upright posture. Central sympathetic neurons arising from the vasomotor area of the medulla are tonically active. Carotid baroreceptors are stimulated by the stretch of the vessel walls brought about by the internal pressure (blood pressure). Baroreceptor activation inhibits central sympathetic discharge. Conversely, reduction in stretch results in a reduction in baroreceptor firing. Thus, in the case of a transition to upright posture, baroreceptors sense the reduction in pressure that results from pooling of blood in the veins below the level of the heart as reduced wall stretch, and sympathetic discharge is disinhibited. The reflex acts through sympathetic nerve

endings to increase peripheral vascular resistance (constriction of arterioles) and cardiac output (direct stimulation of the heart and constriction of capacitance vessels, which increases venous return to the heart), thereby restoring normal blood pressure. The same baroreflex acts in response to any event that lowers arterial pressure, including a primary reduction in peripheral vascular resistance (eg, caused by a vasodilating agent) or a reduction in intravascular volume (eg, due to hemorrhage or to loss of salt and water via the kidney).

B. Renal Response to Decreased Blood Pressure: Via control of blood volume, the kidney is primarily responsible for long-term blood pressure control. A reduction in renal perfusion pressure causes intrarenal redistribution of blood flow and increased reabsorption of salt and water. In addition, decreased pressure in renal arterioles as well as sympathetic neural activity (via β-adrenoceptors) stimulates production of renin, which increases production of angiotensin II (see Fig 10–1 and Chapter 16). Angiotensin II causes (1) direct constriction of resistance vessels and (2) stimulation of aldosterone synthesis in the adrenal cortex, which increases renal sodium absorption and intravascular blood volume.

Therapeutic Implications

Because antihypertensive therapy is not usually directed at a specific cause, it necessarily depends upon interfering with normal physiologic mechanisms that

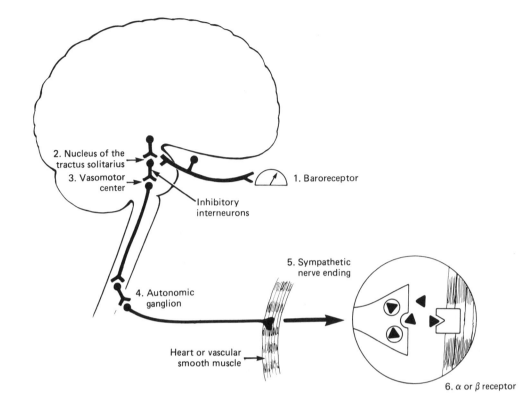

Figure 10–2. Baroreceptor reflex arc.

regulate blood pressure. The risk of toxicity from treatment is high, because hypertension is treated, in effect, by creating another disease.

Antihypertensive therapy is administered to an asymptomatic patient, for whom it provides no direct relief from discomfort; instead, the benefit of lowering blood pressure lies in preventing disease and death at some future time. The natural human tendency to weigh present inconvenience and discomfort more heavily than future benefit means that a major problem—perhaps *the* major problem—in antihypertensive therapy is that of providing consistent, effective drug therapy over many years ("patient compliance").

It is essential to balance the risks of toxicity from drug treatment against the risks of not treating, which are proportionate to the extent of blood pressure elevation before treatment and vary according to the characteristics of individual patients. Accordingly, no single mode of treatment will be suitable for more than a small proportion of hypertensive patients.

I. BASIC PHARMACOLOGY OF ANTIHYPERTENSIVE AGENTS

All antihypertensive agents act at one or more of the 4 anatomic control sites depicted in Fig 10–1 and produce their effects by interfering with normal mech-

anisms of blood pressure regulation. A useful classification of these agents categorizes them according to the principal regulatory site or mechanism on which they act (Table 10–1). Because of their common mechanisms of action, drugs within each category tend to produce a similar spectrum of toxicities. The categories include the following:

(1) Diuretics, which lower blood pressure by depleting the body of sodium and reducing blood volume.

(2) Sympatholytic agents, which lower blood pressure by reducing peripheral vascular resistance, inhibiting cardiac function, and increasing venous pooling in capacitance vessels. (The latter 2 effects reduce cardiac output.) These agents are further subdivided according to their putative sites of action in the sympathetic reflex arc (see below).

(3) Direct vasodilators, which reduce pressure by relaxing vascular smooth muscle, thus dilating resistance vessels and—to varying degrees—increasing capacitance as well.

(4) Agents that block production or action of angiotensin and thereby reduce peripheral vascular resistance and (potentially) blood volume.

Hypertension is often treated by a combination of 2 or more drugs, each acting by a different mechanism. The rationale for polypharmacy is that each of the drugs acts on one of a set of interacting, mutually compensatory regulatory mechanisms for maintaining blood pressure. Thus, partial impairment of one regu-

Table 10–1. Classification of antihypertensive agents.

Diuretics
  Low maximal efficacy
    Indapamide (Lozol)
    Phthalimidines
    Thiazides
  High maximal efficacy
    Bumetanide (Bumex)
    Ethacrynic acid (Edecrin)
    Furosemide (Lasix)
  Potassium-sparing
    Amiloride (Midamor)
    Spironolactone (Aldactone)
    Triamterene (Dyrenium)

Sympatholytic agents
  Act on central nervous system
    Clonidine (Catapres)
    Guanabenz (Wytensin)
    Methyldopa (Aldomet)
  Act on autonomic ganglia
    Trimethaphan (Arfonad)
  Act on postganglionic sympathetic neuron
    Guanadrel (Hylorel)
    Guanethidine (Ismelin)
    Monoamine oxidase inhibitors
    Reserpine
  Receptor blockers
    α-Adrenoceptors
      Phenoxybenzamine (Dibenzyline)
      Phentolamine (Regitine)
      Prazosin (Minipress)
    β-Adrenoceptors
      Atenolol (Tenormin)
      Labetalol (Normodyne, Trandate)
      Metoprolol (Lopressor)
      Nadolol (Corgard)
      Pindolol (Visken)
      Propranolol (Inderal)
      Timolol (Blocadren)

Vasodilators
  Diazoxide (Hyperstat)
  Diltiazem (Cardizem)
  Hydralazine (Apresoline)
  Minoxidil (Loniten)
  Nifedipine (Adalat, Procardia)
  Nitroprusside (Nipride)
  Verapamil (Calan, Isoptin)

Inhibitors of renin-angiotensin system
  Captopril (Capoten)
  Enalapril (Vasotec)
  Saralasin (Sarenin)

latory mechanism increases the antihypertensive effect of impairing regulation by another mechanism. Similarly, a drug that interferes with one regulatory mechanism may be limited in its effectiveness by the normal compensatory response of a second mechanism. Finally, in some circumstances, a normal compensatory response accounts for the toxicity of an antihypertensive agent, and the toxic effect can be prevented by administering a second type of drug.

Thus, when hypertension does not respond ade-quately to a regimen of one or 2 drugs, a second or third drug from a different class is usually added.

DRUGS THAT ALTER SODIUM & WATER BALANCE

Dietary sodium restriction has been known for many years to decrease blood pressure in hypertensive patients. With the advent of diuretics, sodium restriction was thought to be less important. Recently, there has been renewed interest in dietary control of blood pressure as a relatively nontoxic therapeutic and even preventive measure. Several studies have shown that even modest dietary sodium restriction lowers blood pressure (although to varying extents) in many hypertensive individuals.

Mechanisms of Action & Hemodynamic Effects of Diuretics

Diuretics lower blood pressure primarily by depleting body sodium stores. The vasodilatation observed when intravenous diuretics are administered in the treatment of acute pulmonary edema is of doubtful antihypertensive usefulness over the long term. Initially, diuretics reduce blood pressure by reducing blood volume and cardiac output; peripheral vascular resistance may increase. After 6–8 weeks, cardiac output returns to normal while peripheral vascular resistance declines. Sodium is believed to contribute to vascular resistance by increasing vessel stiffness and neural reactivity, possibly related to increased sodium-calcium exchange with a resultant increase in intracellular calcium. These effects are reversed by diuretics or sodium restriction.

Indapamide is a nonthiazide sulfonamide diuretic with both diuretic and vasodilator activity. As a consequence of vasodilatation, cardiac output remains unchanged or increases slightly.

Diuretics are effective in lowering blood pressure by 10–15 mm Hg in most patients, and diuretics alone often provide adequate treatment for mild or moderate essential hypertension. In more severe hypertension, diuretics are used in combination with sympatholytic and vasodilator drugs to control the tendency toward sodium retention caused by these agents. Vascular responsiveness—ie, the ability to either constrict or dilate—is diminished by sympatholytic and vasodilator drugs, so that the vasculature behaves like a pipe with a constant diameter. As a consequence, blood pressure becomes exquisitely sensitive to blood volume. Thus, in severe hypertension, when multiple drugs are used, blood pressure may be well controlled when blood volume is 95% of normal but much too high when blood volume is 105% of normal.

Selection of Diuretics

The sites of action within the kidney and the pharmacokinetics of various diuretic drugs are discussed in

Chapter 14. Thiazide diuretics are appropriate for most patients with mild or moderate hypertension and normal renal and cardiac function. More powerful diuretics (eg, those acting on the loop of Henle) are necessary in severe hypertension, when multiple drugs with sodium-retaining properties are used; in renal insufficiency, when glomerular filtration rate is less than 30 or 40 mL/min; and in cardiac failure or cirrhosis, where sodium retention is marked.

Potassium-sparing diuretics are useful both to avoid excessive potassium depletion, particularly in patients taking digitalis, and to enhance the natriuretic effects of other diuretics.

Dosing Considerations

Although the pharmacokinetics and pharmacodynamics of the various diuretics differ, their common therapeutic end point in treating hypertension is daily natriuresis. However, it must be recognized that in steady-state conditions (as in long-term management of hypertension), daily sodium excretion is equal to dietary sodium intake. Diuretics are necessary to oppose the tendency toward sodium retention in a relatively sodium-depleted patient. Although thiazide diuretics are more natriuretic at higher doses (up to 100–200 mg of hydrochlorothiazide), when used as a single agent, lower doses (25–50 mg) exert as much antihypertensive effect as do higher doses. Thus, a threshold amount of body sodium depletion may be necessary for antihypertensive efficacy. In contrast to thiazides, the dose-response range for loop diuretics is many times greater than the usual therapeutic dose.

Toxicity of Diuretics

In the treatment of hypertension, the most common adverse effect of diuretics (except for potassium-sparing diuretics) is potassium depletion. Although mild degrees of hypokalemia are tolerated well by many patients, hypokalemia may be hazardous in persons taking digitalis, those who have chronic arrhythmias, or those with acute myocardial infarction. Potassium loss is coupled to reabsorption of sodium, and restriction of dietary sodium intake will therefore minimize potassium loss. Diuretics may also impair glucose tolerance and increase serum lipid concentrations. The possibility of increased risk of coronary artery disease associated with the metabolic effects of diuretics is currently under study.

DRUGS THAT ALTER SYMPATHETIC NERVOUS SYSTEM FUNCTION

In patients with moderate to severe hypertension, most effective drug regimens include an agent that inhibits function of the sympathetic nervous system. Drugs in this group are classified according to the site at which they impair the sympathetic reflex arc (Fig 10–2). This neuroanatomic classification explains prominent differences in cardiovascular effects of drugs and allows the clinician to predict interactions of these drugs with one another and with other drugs.

Most importantly, the subclasses of drugs exhibit different patterns of potential toxicity. Drugs that lower blood pressure by actions on the central nervous system tend to cause sedation and mental depression and may produce disturbances of sleep, including nightmares. Drugs that act by inhibiting transmission through autonomic ganglia produce toxicity from inhibition of parasympathetic regulation, in addition to profound sympathetic blockade. Drugs that act chiefly by reducing release of norepinephrine from sympathetic nerve endings cause effects that are similar to those of surgical sympathectomy, including inhibition of ejaculation, and hypotension that is increased by exercise and upright posture. Drugs that block postsynaptic adrenoceptors produce a more selective spectrum of effects depending on the class of receptor to which they bind.

A few of the drugs to be discussed appear to act at more than one anatomic site, although each (probably) works by a single biochemical mechanism. No clinically useful drug acts primarily on baroreceptors. The **veratrum alkaloids** lower blood pressure by increasing sensitivity of baroreceptors, but they are of only academic interest because they produce erratic therapeutic effects and cause unacceptable toxicity in patients.

Finally, we should note that *all* of the agents that lower blood pressure by altering sympathetic function can elicit compensatory effects through mechanisms that are not dependent on adrenergic nerves. Thus, the antihypertensive effect of any of these agents used alone may be limited by retention of sodium and expansion of blood volume. For these reasons, sympatholytic antihypertensive drugs are most effective when used concomitantly with a diuretic.

CENTRALLY ACTING SYMPATHOLYTIC DRUGS

Mechanism & Sites of Action

Methyldopa and clonidine reduce sympathetic outflow from vasopressor centers in the brain stem but allow these centers to retain their sensitivity to baroreceptor control. Accordingly, the antihypertensive and toxic actions of these drugs are generally less dependent on posture than are the effects of drugs such as guanethidine that act directly on peripheral sympathetic neurons.

Methyldopa (L-α-methyl-3,4-dihydroxyphenylalanine) is an analog of L-dopa and is converted to α-methylnorepinephrine; this pathway, illustrated in Fig 10–3, directly parallels the synthesis of norepinephrine from dopa (see Chapter 5). Alpha-methylnorepinephrine is stored in adrenergic nerve granules, where it stoichiometrically replaces norepinephrine, and is released by nerve stimulation to interact with postsynaptic adrenoceptors. However, this replacement of norepinephrine by a false transmitter in peripheral neurons is *not* responsible for methyldopa's antihypertensive effect, because the α-methylnorepinephrine released is an effective agonist at the α-adrenoceptors that mediate peripheral sympathetic constriction of arterioles and venules. Direct electrical stimulation of sympathetic nerves in methyldopa-treated animals produces sympathetic responses similar to those observed in untreated animals.

Indeed, methyldopa's antihypertensive action appears to be due to stimulation of central α-adrenoceptors by α-methylnorepinephrine or α-methyldopamine, based on the following evidence: (1) Much lower doses of methyldopa are required to lower blood pressure in animals when the drug is administered centrally by cerebral intraventricular injection rather than intravenously. (2) Alpha-receptor antagonists, administered centrally, block the antihypertensive effect of methyldopa, whether the latter is given centrally or intravenously. (3) Potent inhibitors of dopa decarboxylase, administered centrally, block methyldopa's antihypertensive effect, thus showing that metabolism of the parent drug is necessary for its action.

The antihypertensive action of **clonidine,** a 2-imidazoline derivative (Fig 10–4), was discovered in the course of testing the drug for use as a topically applied nasal decongestant. After intravenous injection, clonidine produces a brief rise in blood pressure followed by more prolonged hypotension. The pressor response is due to direct stimulation of α-adrenoceptors in arterioles. The drug is classified as a partial agonist at alpha receptors because it also inhibits pressor effects of other α-agonists.

Considerable evidence indicates that the hypotensive effect of clonidine is exerted at α-adrenoceptors in the medulla of the brain. In animals, the hypotensive effect of clonidine is prevented by central administration of α-antagonists. Clonidine reduces sympathetic and increases parasympathetic tone, resulting in blood pressure lowering and bradycardia. These observations suggest that clonidine sensitizes brain stem pressor centers to inhibition by baroreflexes.

Thus, studies of clonidine and methyldopa suggest that normal regulation of blood pressure involves central adrenergic neurons that modulate baroreceptor reflexes. Both drugs bind more tightly to α_2- than to α_1-adrenoceptors. Alpha$_2$ receptors are located presynaptically on membranes of peripheral vascular sympathetic neurons, where they inhibit norepinephrine release (see Chapter 5). It is possible that clonidine and α-methylnorepinephrine act in the brain to reduce norepinephrine release onto relevant receptor sites.

Guanabenz is a newly marketed centrally active antihypertensive drug that shares the central α-adrenoceptor–stimulating effects of clonidine.

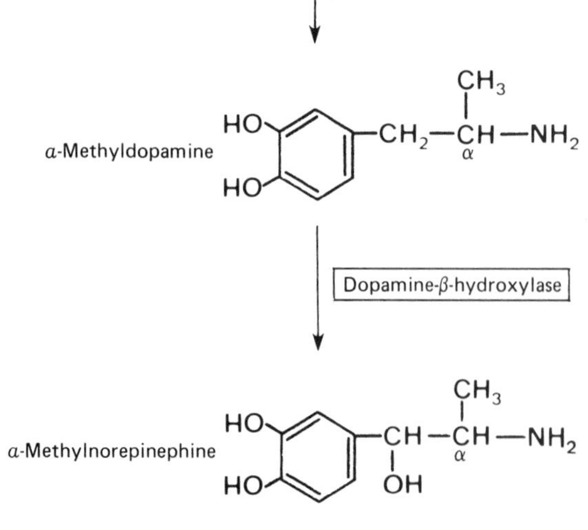

METHYLDOPA

Methyldopa is useful in the treatment of mild to moderately severe hypertension. It lowers blood pressure chiefly by reducing peripheral vascular resistance; there is little change in heart rate or cardiac output in most patients.

Most cardiovascular reflexes remain intact after administration of methyldopa, and blood pressure reduction is not markedly dependent upon maintenance of upright posture. Postural (orthostatic) hypotension sometimes occurs, particularly in volume-depleted patients. One potential advantage of methyldopa is that it causes reduction in renal vascular resistance, perhaps owing to reduced efficacy of α-methylnorepinephrine as a vasoconstrictor in renal arterioles.

Pharmacokinetics & Dosage

Owing to extensive first-pass metabolism (primarily O-sulfate conjugation by the gastrointestinal mucosa), the bioavailability of methyldopa is low, averaging 25%, and varies among individuals. About two-thirds of the drug that reaches plasma is cleared by renal excretion, with a terminal elimination half-life of 2 hours. Impaired renal function results in reduced drug clearance. Although there are no studies in this regard, some clinicians report greater efficacy and toxicity and recommend using lower doses in patients with renal failure.

An oral dose of methyldopa produces its maximal antihypertensive effect in 4–6 hours, and the effect can persist for up to 24 hours. Because the effect depends upon accumulation of a metabolite, α-methyl-

Figure 10–3. Metabolic activation of methyldopa.

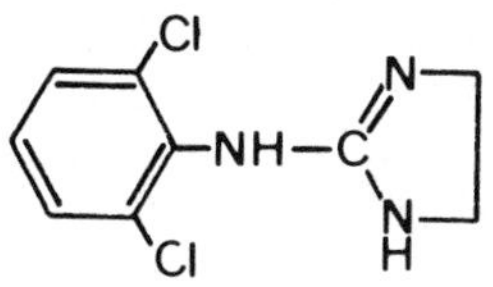

Clonidine

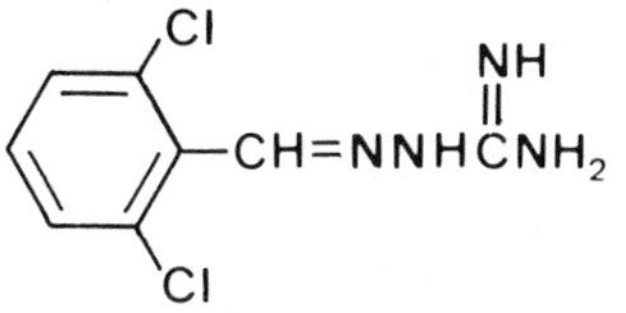

Guanabenz

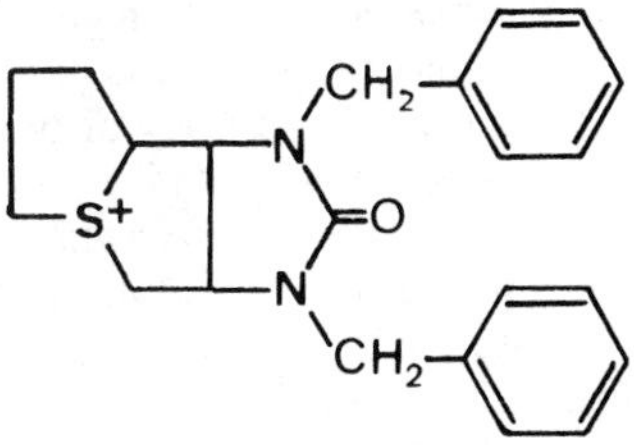

Trimethaphan

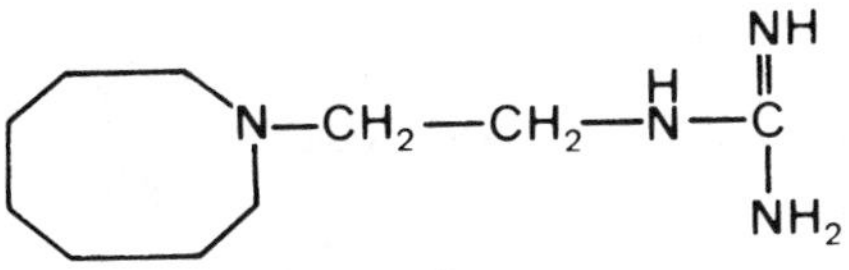

Guanethidine

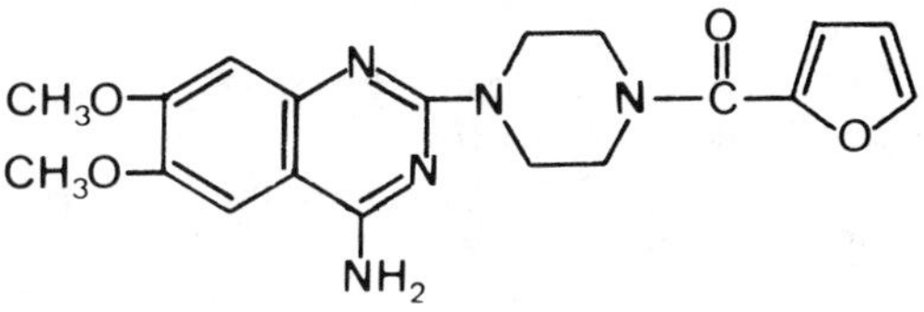

Prazosin

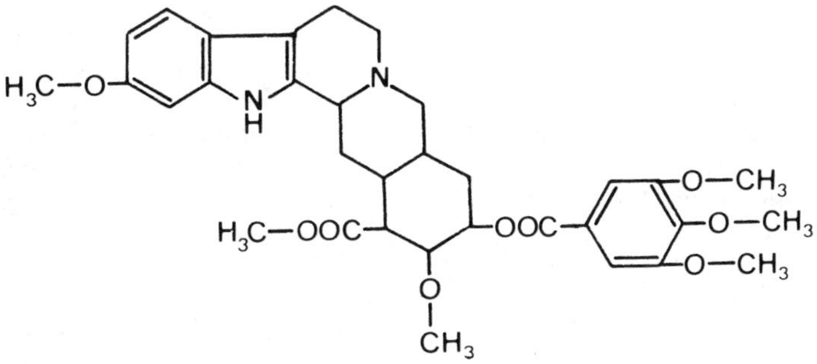

Reserpine

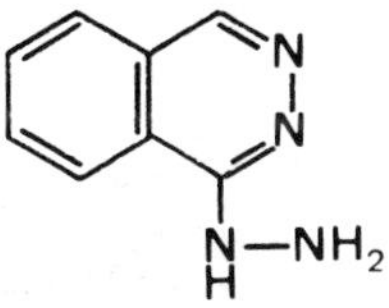

Hydralazine

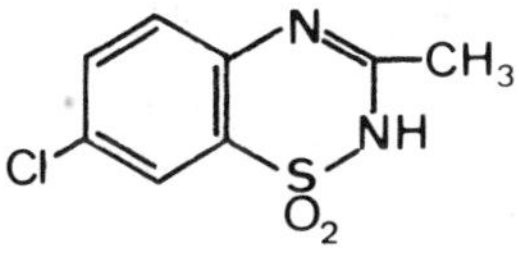

Diazoxide

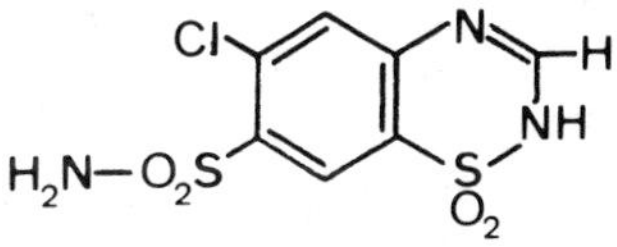

Chlorothiazide

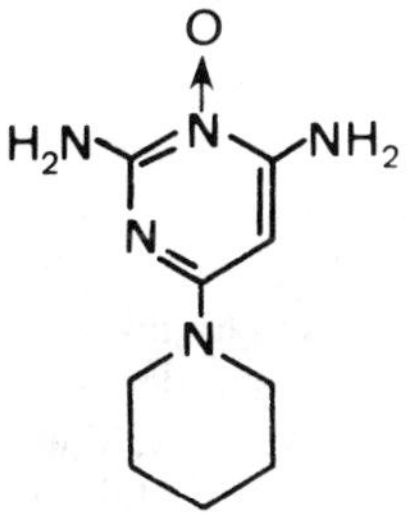

Minoxidil

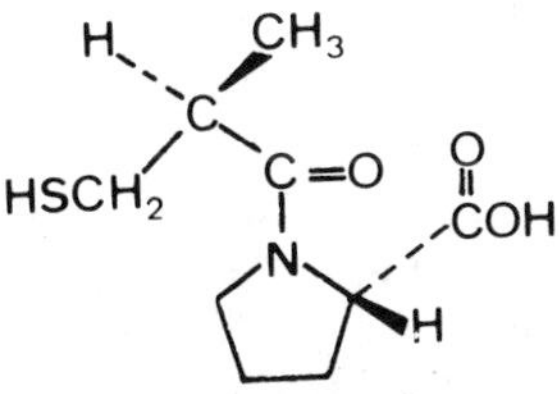

Captopril

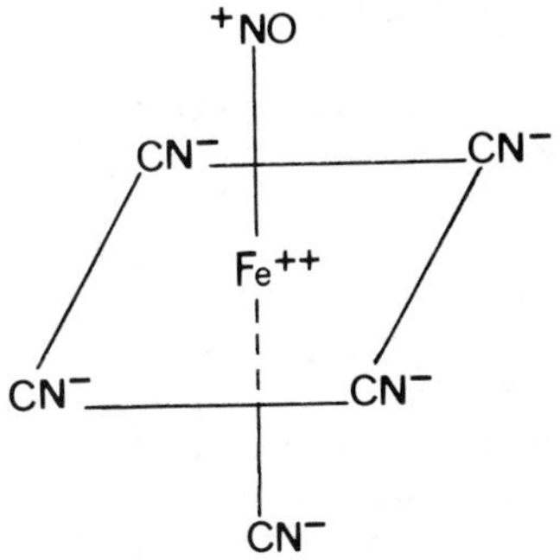

Nitroprusside

Figure 10–4. Chemical structures of antihypertensive drugs.

norepinephrine, the action persists long after the parent drug has disappeared from the circulation.

The maximal efficacy of methyldopa in lowering blood pressure is limited. In most patients, a dose of 2 g or less will produce maximal reduction in hypertension; if this result is not satisfactory, higher doses will usually not result in greater effects. The usual therapeutic dose is about 1–2 g/d orally in divided doses. In many patients, once-daily therapy is effective.

Toxicity

Most of the undesirable effects of methyldopa are referable to the central nervous sytem. Of these, the most frequent is overt sedation, particularly at the onset of treatment. With long-term therapy, patients may complain of persistent mental lassitude and impaired mental concentration. Nightmares, mental depression, vertigo, and extrapyramidal signs may occur but are relatively infrequent. Lactation, associated with increased prolactin secretion, can occur in either men or women treated with methyldopa. This toxicity is probably mediated by actions on dopaminergic mechanisms in the hypothalamus.

Other important adverse effects of methyldopa are development of a positive Coombs test, which sometimes makes cross-matching blood for transfusion difficult and rarely is associated with hemolytic anemia, as well as hepatitis and drug fever.

CLONIDINE

Hemodynamic studies indicate that blood pressure lowering by clonidine results from reduction of cardiac output due to decreased heart rate and relaxation of capacitance vessels, with no consistent change in peripheral vascular resistance.

Reduction in arterial blood pressure by clonidine is accompanied by decreased renal vascular resistance and maintenance of renal blood flow. As with methyldopa, clonidine reduces blood pressure in the supine position and only rarely causes postural hypotension. Pressor effects of clonidine are not observed after ingestion of therapeutic doses of clonidine, but severe hypertension can complicate overdosage.

Pharmacokinetics & Dosage

In healthy individuals, the bioavailability of clonidine averages 75% and the half-life is 8–12 hours. About half of the drug is eliminated unchanged in the urine, suggesting that lower than usual doses may be effective in patients with renal insufficiency.

Because of its relatively short half-life and the fact that its antihypertensive effect is directly related to blood concentration, clonidine must be given twice a day to maintain smooth blood pressure control. Therapeutic doses are commonly between 0.2 and 1.2 mg/d. However, as is not the case with methldopa, the dose-response curve of clonidine is such that increasing

doses are more effective (but also more toxic). The maximal recommended dose is 1.2 mg/d.

A transdermal preparation of clonidine that reduces blood pressure for 7 days after a single application has recently been marketed. This preparation appears to produce less sedation than clonidine tablets but is commonly associated with local skin reactions.

Toxicity

Dry mouth and sedation are frequent and may be severe. Both effects are centrally mediated and dose-dependent and coincide temporally with the drug's antihypertensive effect.

The drug should not be given to patients who are at risk of mental depression and should be withdrawn if depression occurs during therapy. Concomitant treatment with tricyclic antidepressants may block the antihypertensive effect of clonidine. The interaction is believed to be due to α-adrenoceptor–blocking actions of the tricyclics.

Withdrawal of clonidine after protracted use, particularly with high doses (greater than 1 mg/d), can result in life-threatening hypertensive crisis mediated by increased sympathetic nervous activity. Patients exhibit nervousness, tachycardia, headache, and sweating after omitting one or 2 doses of the drug. Although the incidence of severe hypertensive crisis is unknown, it is high enough to require that all patients who take clonidine be carefully warned of the possibility. If the drug must be stopped, this should be done gradually while other antihypertensive agents are being substituted. Treatment of the hypertensive crisis consists of reinstitution of clonidine therapy or administration of α- and β-adrenoceptor–blocking agents.

GANGLIONIC BLOCKING AGENTS

Historically, drugs that block stimulation of postganglionic autonomic neurons by acetycholine were among the first agents used in the treatment of hypertension. Most such drugs are no longer available clinically because of intolerable toxicities related to their primary action (see Chapter 5). Only cne drug in this class (trimethaphan) is still used to treat hypertension.

TRIMETHAPHAN

Trimethaphan camsylate (Fig 10–4) is administered intravenously to take advantage of its rapid action in treating hypertensive crisis and to induce controlled hypotension for neurosurgery. The dependence of ganglionic blockade on blood level of the drug allows precise titration of blood pressure while other drugs are taking effect.

The antihypertensive effect of trimethaphan is to a large extent dependent upon pooling of blood in capacitance vessels. Patients must be tilted head up (usually with blocks under the head of the bed) for effective blood pressure lowering. Conversely, excessive hypotension can be rapidly treated by reverse tilting.

ADRENERGIC NEURON BLOCKING AGENTS

These drugs lower blood pressure by preventing normal physiologic release of norepinephrine from postganglionic sympathetic neurons (see Chapter 5).

GUANETHIDINE

In high enough doses, guanethidine can produce profound sympathoplegia. The resulting high maximal efficacy of this agent made it the mainstay of outpatient therapy of severe hypertension in the 1960s. For the same reason, guanethidine can produce all of the toxicities expected from "pharmacologic sympathectomy," including marked postural hypotension, diarrhea, and impaired ejaculation.

The structure of guanethidine includes a highly basic nitrogen (Fig 10–4) that prevents its entry into the central nervous system. As a result, this drug has none of the central effects seen with many of the other antihypertensive agents described in this chapter.

Guanadrel is a guanethidinelike drug that has recently been released in the USA. **Bethanidine** and **debrisoquin,** antihypertensive agents not yet released for clinical use in the USA, are also similar in chemical structure and mechanism of antihypertensive action to guanethidine. **Bretylium,** an antiarrhythmic drug described in Chapter 13, is also structurally similar to guanethidine.

Mechanism & Sites of Action

Guanethidine inhibits the release of norepinephrine that occurs when a neuronal action potential reaches sympathetic nerve endings (Fig 10–5). This effect is probably responsible for most of the sympathoplegia that occurs in patients. Guanethidine is transported across the sympathetic nerve membrane by the same mechanism that transports norepinephrine itself, and uptake is essential for the drug's action. Once guanethidine has entered the nerve, it is concentrated in transmitter vesicles, where it replaces norepinephrine. Subsequently, the drug causes a gradual depletion of norepinephrine stores in the nerve ending.

Inhibition of norepinephrine release is probably related to guanethidine's local anesthetic properties. Although the drug does not impair axonal conduction in sympathetic fibers, local blockade of membrane electrical activity may occur in nerve endings, because the nerve endings specifically take up and concentrate the drug.

Because neuronal uptake is necessary for the hypotensive activity of guanethidine, drugs that block the catecholamine uptake process (see Chapter 5) block the uptake and subsequent effects of guanethidine. These include cocaine, tricyclic antidepressants, phenothiazines, phenoxybenzamine, and certain sympathomimetic amines.

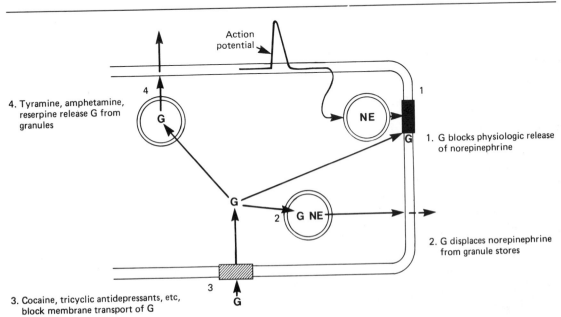

4. Tyramine, amphetamine, reserpine release G from granules

1. G blocks physiologic release of norepinephrine

2. G displaces norepinephrine from granule stores

3. Cocaine, tricyclic antidepressants, etc, block membrane transport of G

Figure 10–5. Guanethidine actions and drug interactions involving the adrenergic neuron. (G = guanethidine; NE = norepinephrine.)

When guanethidine first enters the neuron, norepinephrine is released. With usual doses, the amount of norepinephrine released is too small to have any significant effect; after rapid intravenous administration, however, sudden norepinephrine release can cause hypertension.

Guanethidine increases sensitivity to the hypertensive effects of exogenously administered sympathomimetic amines. This results from inhibition of neuronal uptake of such amines and, after long-term therapy with guanethidine, supersensitivity of effector smooth muscle cells, in a fashion analogous to the process that follows surgical sympathectomy (see Chapter 5).

The hypotensive action of guanethidine early in the course of therapy is associated with reduced cardiac output, due to bradycardia and relaxation of capacitance vessels, without consistent change in peripheral vascular resistance. With chronic therapy, cardiac output may return to normal, owing in part to blood volume expansion, while peripheral vascular resistance decreases. Blood flow to splanchnic and renal beds is decreased relative to flow to heart, muscle, and brain. Renal hemodynamic effects may explain in part the marked tendency toward sodium and water retention during guanethidine therapy.

Pharmacokinetics & Dosage

The bioavailability of guanethidine is variable (3–50%). It is 50% cleared by the kidney. Retention of drug in nerve endings and uptake into other sites account for the very large volume of distribution and long half-life (5 days) of guanethidine. Thus, with constant daily dosing, the onset of sympathoplegia is gradual (maximal effect in 1–2 weeks), and sympathoplegia persists for a comparable period after cessation of therapy.

The daily dose required for a satisfactory hypotensive response varies greatly among individual patients. For this reason, therapy is usually initiated at a low dose, eg, 10 mg/d. As patients require 1–2 weeks for the hypotensive effect of a given daily dosage level to reach maximum, the dose should not ordinarily be increased at intervals shorter than 2 weeks. Because of the drug's long duration of action, maintenance doses need not be taken more than once a day.

Toxicity

Therapeutic use of guanethidine is often associated with symptomatic postural hypotension and hypotension following exercise, particularly when the drug is given in high doses. However, when it is used in lower doses (25–50 mg/d) for mild to moderate hypertension, orthostatic hypotension is not a significant problem. Injudicious treatment (excessive doses or too rapid escalation in dosage) may produce dangerously decreased blood flow to heart and brain or even overt shock. Guanethidine-induced sympathoplegia in men may be associated with delayed or retrograde ejaculation. Guanethidine commonly causes diarrhea, which results from increased gastrointestinal motility due to

parasympathetic predominance in controlling the activity of intestinal smooth muscle.

Interactions with other drugs may complicate guanethidine therapy. Sympathomimetic agents at doses available in over-the-counter cold preparations can produce hypertension in patients taking guanethidine. Similarly, guanethidine can produce hypertensive crisis by releasing catecholamines in patients with pheochromocytoma. When tricyclic antidepressants are administered to patients taking guanethidine, the antihypertensive effect is attenuated, and severe hypertension may follow. A physician who is ignorant of this interaction may raise the dose of guanethidine; if the tricyclic antidepressant is then stopped, the patient may suffer severe hypotension or cardiovascular collapse from the unopposed action of guanethidine.

RESERPINE

Reserpine (Fig 10–4), an alkaloid extracted from the roots of an Indian plant, *Rauwolfia serpentina,* was one of the first effective drugs used on a large scale in the treatment of hypertension. At present, it is considered an effective and relatively safe drug for treating mild to moderate hypertension.

Mechanism & Sites of Action

Reserpine blocks the ability of adrenergic transmitter vesicles to take up and store biogenic amines, probably by interfering with an uptake mechanism that depends on Mg^{2+} and ATP (Fig 5–3). This effect occurs throughout the body, resulting in depletion of norepinephrine, dopamine, and serotonin in both central and peripheral neurons. Chromaffin granules of the adrenal medulla are also depleted of catecholamines, although to a lesser extent than are neurons elsewhere. Reserpine's effects on adrenergic vesicles appear irreversible; trace amounts of the drug remain bound to vesicular membranes for many days. Although sufficiently high doses of reserpine in animals can reduce catecholamine stores to zero, lower doses cause inhibition of neurotransmission that is roughly proportionate to the degree of amine depletion. Depletion of peripheral amines probably accounts for much of the beneficial antihypertensive effect, but a central component cannot be ruled out. The effects of low but clinically effective doses resemble those of centrally acting agents (eg, methyldopa) in that sympathetic reflexes remain largely intact, blood pressure is reduced in supine as well as in standing patients, and postural hypotension is mild. Reserpine readily enters the brain, and depletion of cerebral amine stores causes sedation, mental depression, and parkinsonism symptoms.

At lower doses used for treatment of mild hypertension, reserpine lowers blood pressure by a combination of decreased cardiac output and decreased peripheral vascular resistance.

Pharmacokinetics & Dosage

Absorption, clearance, and metabolism have not been well-defined. The drug disappears rapidly from the circulation, but its effects persist much longer, owing to irreversible inactivation of catecholamine storage granules, as described above.

The usual daily dose is less than 1 mg (typically, 0.25 mg), administered orally as a single dose. Although reserpine is available in injectable form, parenteral administration is rarely indicated.

Toxicity

At the low doses usually administered, reserpine produces little postural hypotension. Most of the unwanted effects of reserpine result from actions on the brain or gastrointestinal tract.

High doses of reserpine characteristically produce sedation, lassitude, nightmares, and severe mental depression; occasionally, these occur even in patients receiving low doses (0.25 mg/d). Much less frequently, ordinary doses of reserpine produce extrapyramidal effects resembling Parkinson's disease, probably as a result of dopamine depletion in the corpus striatum. Although these central effects are uncommon, it should be stressed that they may occur at any time, even after months of uneventful treatment. Patients with a history of mental depression should not receive reserpine, and the drug should be stopped if depression appears.

Reserpine rather often produces mild diarrhea and gastrointestinal cramps and increases gastric acid secretion. The drug should probably not be given to patients with a history of peptic ulcer.

PARGYLINE

Although pargyline and other inhibitors of monoamine oxidase have no place in the modern treatment of hypertension, their interesting mechanisms of action and their toxicity deserve mention. Pargyline is thought to lower blood pressure by increasing the concentration of an ineffective false transmitter in peripheral adrenergic nerve endings. Pargyline inhibits monoamine oxidase in gastrointestinal mucosa and thus allows unimpeded access of dietary tyramine to the systemic circulation. Tyramine is taken up into nerve endings and converted to octopamine (Fig 5–4), which partially replaces norepinephrine in catecholamine storage granules. Because octopamine is ineffective as a pressor agonist at postsynaptic alpha receptors, sympathoplegia results.

Depletion of endogenous norepinephrine is not complete enough, however, to prevent the severe toxicity that may result when pargyline-treated patients ingest the large quantities of tyramine found in certain wines and cheeses. In this situation, high concentrations of tyramine reach the nerve endings and release norepinephrine in large amounts onto sympathetic nerve endings, producing a hypertensive crisis. Pargyline is considered too dangerous for use in the treatment of hypertension because of the possibility of such hypertensive crises and because of its propensity to interact adversely with other drugs, including reserpine and opiates.

ADRENOCEPTOR ANTAGONISTS

The pharmacology of drugs that antagonize catecholamines at α- and β-adrenoceptors is presented in Chapter 9. Here we will concentrate on 2 drugs, propranolol and prazosin, primarily in relation to their use in treatment of hypertension. Other adrenoceptor antagonists will be considered only briefly.

PROPRANOLOL

Propranolol, a β-adrenoceptor–blocking agent, is very useful for lowering blood pressure in mild to moderate hypertension. In severe hypertension, propranolol is especially useful in preventing the reflex tachycardia that often results from treatment with direct vasodilators.

Mechanism & Sites of Action

Propranolol antagonizes catecholamines at both β_1- and β_2-adrenoceptors. Both its efficacy in treating hypertension as well as most of its toxic effects result from beta blockade. When propranolol is first administered to a hypertensive patient, blood pressure decreases primarily as a result of a decrease in cardiac output associated with bradycardia. With continued treatment, however, cardiac output returns toward normal while blood pressure remains low, owing to decreased peripheral vascular resistance.

Beta blockade in both brain and kidney has been proposed as contributing to the antihypertensive effect observed with β-receptor blockers. The brain appears unlikely to be the primary site of propranolol's action, because some beta blockers that do not readily cross the blood-brain barrier (eg, nadolol, described below) are nonetheless effective antihypertensive agents.

Propranolol inhibits the stimulation of renin production by catecholamines (mediated by β_2 receptors) in animals and humans. It is likely that part of propranolol's effect is due to depression of the renin-angiotensin-aldosterone system, described above. Nonetheless, propranolol reduces blood pressure in hypertensive patients with normal or even low renin activity. In addition, beta blockers relatively selective for β_1 receptors (such as metoprolol) are as effective in lowering blood pressure as is propranolol. Thus, depression of renin secretion cannot in itself account for propranolol's usefulness in treating hypertension.

We are left with the idea that with chronic propranolol therapy, a long-term readjustment to the initial reduction in cardiac output leads to sustained reduction in peripheral vascular resistance and therefore blood pressure.

In mild to moderate hypertension, propranolol produces a significant reduction in blood pressure without prominent postural hypotension.

Pharmacokinetics & Dosage

As described in Chapter 9, effective oral doses of propranolol are 10-fold (or more) greater than effective intravenous doses, owing to first-pass hepatic inactivation. The prominent first-pass effect partially accounts for the variability in doses required for clinically useful effects. The half-life is 3–6 hours.

Treatment of hypertension is usually started with 80 mg/d in divided doses. Effective antihypertensive doses range from 80 to 480 mg/d. Resting bradycardia and a reduction in the heart rate during exercise are indicators of propranolol's beta-blocking effect. Measures of these responses may be used as guides in regulating dosage. Propranolol can be administered once or twice daily.

Toxicity

The principal toxicities of propranolol result from blockade of cardiac, vascular, or bronchial beta receptors and are described in more detail in Chapter 9. The most important of these predictable extensions of the beta-blocking action occur in patients with reduced myocardial reserve, asthma, peripheral vascular insufficiency, and diabetes.

When propranolol is discontinued after prolonged regular use, some patients experience an abstinence syndrome, including nervousness, tachycardia, increased intensity of angina, or increase of blood pressure. Myocardial infarction has been reported in a few patients. Although the incidence of these complications is probably low, propranolol should not be discontinued abruptly. The withdrawal syndrome may involve "up regulation" or supersensitivity of β-adrenoceptors (see Chapter 2).

Propranolol also produces a low incidence of effects not clearly attributable to beta blockade, including diarrhea, constipation, nausea, and vomiting. Not infrequently, patients receiving propranolol complain of central nervous system effects reminiscent of those caused by methyldopa and clonidine, including nightmares, lassitude, mental depression, and insomnia.

Finally, propranolol may increase plasma triglycerides and decrease HDL-cholesterol, which theoretically could contribute to atherogenesis.

OTHER BETA-ADRENOCEPTOR–BLOCKING AGENTS

Of the large number of beta blockers tested, most have been shown to be effective in lowering blood pressure. The pharmacologic properties of 5 of these agents differ from those of propranolol in ways that may confer therapeutic benefit in certain clinical situations.

1. METOPROLOL

Metoprolol is approximately equipotent to propranolol in inhibiting stimulation of β_1-adrenoceptors such as those in the heart but 50- to 100-fold less potent than propranolol in blocking β_2 receptors. Although metoprolol is in other respects very similar to propranolol, its relative cardioselectivity may be advantageous in treating hypertensive patients who also suffer from asthma, diabetes, or peripheral vascular disease. Studies of small numbers of asthmatic patients have shown that metoprolol causes less bronchial constriction than propranolol at doses that produce equal inhibition of β_1-adrenoceptor responses. The cardioselectivity is not complete, however, and asthmatic symptoms have been exacerbated by metoprolol. Usual antihypertensive doses of metoprolol range from 100 to 450 mg/d.

2. NADOLOL & ATENOLOL

Nadolol, a nonselective beta-receptor antagonist, and atenolol, a β_1-selective blocker, are not appreciably metabolized and are excreted to a considerable extent in the urine. Both can be administered once daily, owing to relatively long half-lives in plasma. Nadolol is usually begun at a dosage of 40 mg/d; atenolol, at a dosage of 50 mg/d. Increases in dosage to obtain a satisfactory therapeutic effect should take place no oftener than every 4 or 5 days. Patients with reduced renal function should receive correspondingly reduced doses. It is claimed that atenolol produces fewer central nervous system–related effects than other more lipid-soluble beta-antagonists.

3. PINDOLOL

Pindolol is a beta blocker with intrinsic beta-adrenoceptor agonist activity. It lowers blood pressure by decreasing vascular resistance without decreasing cardiac output or heart rate. This may be particularly beneficial for patients with cardiac failure, bradyarrhythmias, or peripheral vascular disease. Usual daily doses range from 10 to 60 mg.

4. LABETALOL

Labetalol blocks both beta- and alpha-adrenoceptors. Beta blockade, which is nonselective, is predominant, with a 3:1 ratio of beta:alpha antagonism after oral dosing. Blood pressure is lowered by reduction of systemic vascular resistance without significant alteration in heart rate or cardiac output. Because of its combined alpha- and beta-blocking activity, labetalol is useful in treating the hypertension of pheochromocytoma and hypertensive emergencies. Oral daily doses of labetalol range from 200 to 2400 mg/d. Labetalol is given as repeated intravenous bolus injections of 20–80 mg to treat hypertensive emergencies.

PRAZOSIN

Mechanism & Sites of Action

Prazosin (Fig 10–4) produces most of its antihypertensive effect by blocking α_1 receptors in arterioles and venules. Although this agent is clearly effective in treating hypertension, its clinical advantages and disadvantages in comparison with older antihypertensive agents are not yet well-defined.

Prazosin's selectivity for α_1 receptors is well established and may explain why this agent produces less reflex tachycardia than do nonselective alpha-antagonists such as phentolamine. This receptor selectivity allows norepinephrine to exert unopposed negative feedback (mediated by presynaptic α_2 receptors) on its own release (see Chapter 5); in contrast, phentolamine blocks both pre- and postsynaptic alpha receptors, with the result that reflex stimulation of sympathetic neurons produces greater release of transmitter onto beta receptors and correspondingly greater cardio-acceleration.

Prazosin reduces arterial pressure by dilating both resistance and capacitance vessels. As expected, blood pressure is reduced more in the upright than in the supine position. Retention of salt and fluid occurs when prazosin is administered without a diuretic. The drug is clearly more effective when used in combination with other agents, such as propranolol and a diuretic, than when used alone.

Pharmacokinetics & Dosage

Prazosin is well absorbed but undergoes substantial first-pass metabolism in the liver. It is eliminated almost entirely by metabolism, with a plasma half-life of 3–4 hours, although the half-life of the antihypertensive effect is longer. Plasma concentrations are increased in patients with congestive heart failure, owing primarily to reduced first-pass metabolism.

Treatment with prazosin should be initiated with a low dose (1 mg 3 times daily) to prevent postural hypotension and syncope. Doses may be increased to 20 or 30 mg/d. Although long-term prazosin treatment causes relatively little postural hypotension, a number of patients develop bradycardia and a precipitous drop in standing blood pressure shortly after the first dose is absorbed. For this reason, the first dose should be administered at bedtime. While the mechanism of this first-dose phenomenon is not clear, it occurs more commonly in patients who are salt- and volume-depleted.

Aside from the first-dose phenomenon, the reported toxicities of prazosin are relatively infrequent and mild. These include dizziness, palpitations, headache, and lassitude. Some patients develop a positive test for antinuclear factor in serum while on prazosin therapy, but this has not been associated with rheumatic symptoms. Unlike diuretics and beta blockers, prazosin does not alter plasma lipid concentrations.

OTHER ALPHA-ADRENOCEPTOR–BLOCKING AGENTS

Phentolamine and **phenoxybenzamine** are useful in diagnosis and treatment of pheochromocytoma and in other clinical situations associated with exaggerated release of catecholamines (eg, phentolamine may be combined with propranolol to treat the clonidine withdrawal syndrome, described above). Their pharmacology is described in Chapter 9.

VASODILATORS

Mechanism & Sites of Action

Within this class of drugs are the oral vasodilators, hydralazine and minoxidil, which are used for long-term outpatient therapy of hypertension; the parenteral vasodilators, nitroprusside and diazoxide, which are used to treat hypertensive emergencies; and the calcium channel blockers, which are used in both circumstances.

All vasodilators relax smooth muscle of arterioles, thereby decreasing systemic vascular resistance. Sodium nitroprusside also relaxes veins. Decreased arterial resistance and decreased mean arterial blood pressure elicit compensatory responses, mediated by baroreceptors and the sympathetic nervous system (Fig 10–6), as well as renin, angiotensin, and aldosterone. These compensating responses counteract the hypotensive effect of the vasodilator. Because sympathetic reflexes are intact, vasodilator therapy does not cause orthostatic hypotension or sexual dysfunction.

Vasodilators work best in combination with other antihypertensive drugs that oppose the compensatory cardiovascular responses (Fig 10–6). Sympatholytic drugs are useful in blocking increases in heart rate, myocardial contractility, and plasma renin levels. Propranolol is particularly useful because cardiac sympathetic effects can be totally blocked without producing orthostatic hypotension. Diuretics are useful in preventing fluid retention and plasma volume expansion.

HYDRALAZINE

Hydralazine, a hydrazine derivative (Fig 10–4), dilates arterioles but not veins. It has been available for many years, although it was initially thought not to be particularly effective because tachyphylaxis to hypertensive effects developed rapidly. In recent years, the benefits of combination therapy have been better appreciated, and hydralazine has had a resurgence in use.

Pharmacokinetics, Metabolism, & Dosage

Hydralazine is well absorbed and rapidly metabolized by the liver during the first pass, so that bioavailability is low (averaging 25%) and variable

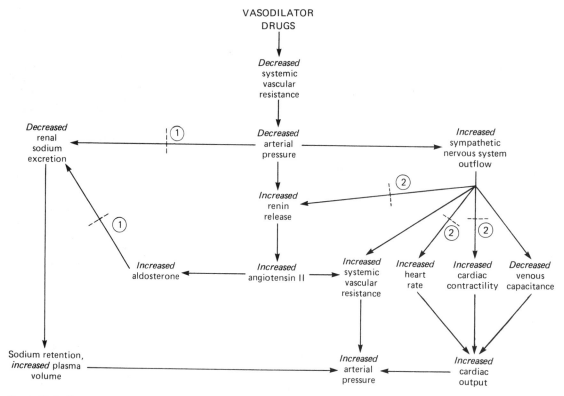

Figure 10–6. Compensatory responses to vasodilators; basis for combination therapy with beta blockers and diuretics. ① Effect blocked by diuretics. ② Effect blocked by beta blockers.

among individuals. It is metabolized in part by acetylation at a rate that appears to be bimodally distributed in the population. As a consequence, rapid acetylators have greater first-pass metabolism, lower bioavailability, and less antihypertensive benefit from a given dose than do slow acetylators. The half-life of hydralazine ranges from 2 to 4 hours, but vascular effects appear to persist longer than do blood concentrations—an observation that is consistent with experimental evidence of avid binding to vascular tissue.

Usual doses range from 40 to 200 mg/d. The higher dose was selected as the dose at which there is a small possibility of developing the lupus erythematosus–like syndrome described in the next section. However, higher doses result in greater vasodilatation and may be used if necessary. Dosing twice or 3 times daily provides smooth control of blood pressure.

Toxicity

The most common side effects of hydralazine are headache, nausea, anorexia, palpitations, sweating, and flushing. In patients with ischemic heart disease, reflex tachycardia and sympathetic stimulation may provoke angina or ischemic arrhythmias. With doses of 400 mg/d or more, there is a 10–20% incidence—chiefly in persons who slowly acetylate the drug—of a syndrome characterized by arthralgia, myalgia, skin rashes, and fever that resembles lupus erythematosus. The syndrome is not associated with renal damage and

is reversed by discontinuation of hydralazine. Peripheral neuropathy and drug fever are other serious but uncommon adverse effects.

MINOXIDIL

Minoxidil (Fig 10–4) is a very efficacious orally active vasodilator recently released for use in the USA. Like hydralazine, it dilates arterioles but not veins. Because of its greater potential antihypertensive effect, minoxidil should replace hydralazine when maximal doses of the latter are not effective or in patients with renal failure and severe hypertension, who do not respond well to hydralazine.

Pharmacokinetics, Metabolism, & Dosage

Minoxidil is well absorbed from the gastrointestinal tract and is metabolized, primarily by glucuronide conjugation, in the liver. Minoxidil is not protein-bound. Its half-life averages 4 hours, but its hypotensive effect after a single dose may persist for over 24 hours, probably as a result of avid binding to vascular smooth muscle.

Minoxidil is available only as an oral preparation. Generally, patients are started on 5 or 10 mg/d in 2 doses, and the daily dose is then gradually increased to 40 mg/d. Higher doses—up to 80 mg/d—have been used in treating severe hypertension.

Even more than with hydralazine, the use of minoxidil is associated with reflex sympathetic stimulation and sodium and fluid retention. Minoxidil must be used in combination with a beta blocker and a loop diuretic.

Toxicity

Tachycardia, palpitations, angina, and edema are observed when doses of beta blockers and diuretics are inadequate. Headache, sweating, and hypertrichosis, which is particularly bothersome in women, are relatively common. Minoxidil illustrates how one person's toxicity may become another person's therapy. Topical minoxidil is currently being evaluated as a stimulant to hair growth for correction of baldness.

SODIUM NITROPRUSSIDE

Sodium nitroprusside is a powerful parenterally administered vasodilator that is used in treating hypertensive emergencies as well as severe cardiac failure. Nitroprusside dilates both arterial and venous vessels, resulting in reduced peripheral vascular resistance and venous return.

In the absence of cardiac failure, blood pressure decreases, owing to decreased vascular resistance, while cardiac output does not change or decreases slightly. In patients with cardiac failure and low cardiac output, output increases owing to afterload reduction. Heart rate typically increases, but less than is observed with other vasodilators.

Pharmacokinetics, Metabolism, & Dosage

Nitroprusside (Fig 10–4) is a complex of iron, cyanide groups, and a nitroso moiety. It is rapidly metabolized by uptake into red blood cells, where cyanide is liberated. Cyanide in turn is metabolized by the mitochondrial enzyme rhodanase, in the presence of a sulfur donor, to thiocyanate. Thiocyanate is distributed in extracellular fluid and slowly eliminated by the kidney.

Nitroprusside rapidly lowers blood pressure, and its effects disappear soon after discontinuation. The infusion rate is increased until blood pressure is controlled or until an administration rate likely to result in toxicity is achieved. Sodium nitroprusside in aqueous solution is sensitive to light and must therefore be made up fresh before each administration and covered with opaque foil. Infusion solutions should be changed after several hours. Doses typically begin at 0.5 μg/kg/min and may be increased up to 10 μg/kg/min as necessary to control blood pressure. Because of its efficacy and rapid onset of effect, the drug should be administered by infusion pump and arterial blood pressure continuously monitored via intra-arterial recording.

Toxicity

The most serious toxicity is related to accumulation of cyanide: metabolic acidosis, arrhythmias, excessive hypotension, and death have resulted. In a few cases, toxicity after relatively low doses of nitroprusside suggested a defect in cyanide metabolism. Administration of sodium thiosulfate as a sulfur donor facilitates metabolism of cyanide. Hydroxocobalamin combines with cyanide to form the nontoxic cyanocobalamin. Both have been advocated for prophylaxis or treatment of cyanide poisoning during nitroprusside infusion. Thiocyanate may accumulate over the course of prolonged administration, usually a week or more, particularly in patients with renal insufficiency who do not excrete thiocyanate at a normal rate. Thiocyanate toxicity is manifested as weakness, disorientation, psychosis, muscle spasms, and convulsions, and the diagnosis is confirmed by finding serum concentrations greater than 10 mg/dL. Rarely, delayed hypothyroidism occurs, owing to thiocyanate inhibition of iodide uptake by the thyroid. Methemoglobinemia during infusion of nitroprusside has also been reported.

DIAZOXIDE

Diazoxide is an effective and relatively long-acting parenterally administered arteriolar dilator that is used to treat hypertensive emergencies. Injection of diazoxide results in a sudden fall in systemic vascular resistance and mean arterial blood pressure associated with substantial tachycardia and increase in cardiac output.

Pharmacokinetics & Dosage

Diazoxide (Fig 10–4) is similar chemically to the thiazide diuretics but has no diuretic activity. It is bound extensively to serum albumin and to vascular tissue. Diazoxide is both metabolized and excreted unchanged; its metabolic pathways are not well characterized. Its half-life is approximately 24 hours, but the relationship between blood concentration and hypotensive action is not well established. The blood pressure–lowering effect after a rapid injection is established within 5 minutes and lasts for 4–12 hours. It was initially thought that rapid injection was mandatory to saturate plasma protein binding so that free drug could reach vascular tissue, but this idea is no longer generally accepted. Blood pressure is in fact lowered by constant infusion, although the extent of lowering for a given total dose is greater after rapid administration.

When diazoxide was first marketed, a dose of 300 mg by rapid injection was recommended. It appears, however, that excessive hypotension can be avoided by beginning with smaller doses (75–100 mg). If necessary, doses of 150 mg may be repeated every 5 minutes until blood pressure is lowered satisfactorily. Nearly all patients respond to a maximum of 3 or 4 doses. Because of reduced protein binding, hypotension occurs after smaller doses in persons with chronic renal failure, and smaller doses should be administered to these patients. The hypotensive effects of diazoxide are also greater if patients are pretreated with beta blockers to prevent the reflex tachycardia and associated increase in cardiac output.

Toxicity

The most significant toxicity from diazoxide has been excessive hypotension, resulting from the recommendation to use a fixed dose of 300 mg in all patients. Such hypotension has resulted in stroke and myocardial infarction. The reflex sympathetic response can also provoke angina, electrocardiographic evidence of ischemia, and cardiac failure in patients with ischemic heart disease, and diazoxide should be avoided in this situation.

Diazoxide inhibits insulin release from the pancreas and is used to treat hypoglycemia secondary to insulinoma. Occasionally, hyperglycemia complicates diazoxide use, particularly in persons with renal insufficiency.

In contrast to the thiazide diuretics, diazoxide causes renal salt and water *retention*. However, because the drug is used for short periods only, this is rarely a problem.

CALCIUM CHANNEL BLOCKERS

Although primarily used thus far as antiarrhythmic and antianginal agents, calcium channel blockers also dilate peripheral arterioles and reduce blood pressure. The mechanism of action is inhibition of calcium influx in arterial smooth muscle.

Verapamil, nifedipine, and **diltiazem** are equally effective in lowering blood pressure, although none are yet approved for this use in the USA. Hemodynamic differences among calcium channel blockers may influence the choice of a particular agent. Nifedipine is the most selective as a vasodilator and has the least cardiac effect. Reflex sympathetic activation with slight tachycardia maintains or increases cardiac output in most patients. Verapamil has the greatest effect on the heart and may decrease heart rate and cardiac output. Diltiazem has intermediate actions. The pharmacology of these drugs is discussed in more detail in Chapter 11. Doses of calcium channel blockers used in treating hypertension are similar to those used in treating angina or coronary spasm. Nifedipine, sublingually or chewed in 10- to 20-mg doses, has gained recent popularity in emergency treatment of severe hypertension.

INHIBITORS OF ANGIOTENSIN

Although the causative roles of renin, angiotensin, and aldosterone in essential hypertension are still controversial, there do appear to be differences in the activity of this system among individuals. When controlled for daily sodium intake (assessed as 24-hour urinary sodium excretion) and serum potassium concentration, approximately 20% of patients with essential hypertension have inappropriately low and 20% have inappropriately high plasma renin activity. Blood pressure of patients with high-renin hypertension responds better to β-adrenoceptor blockers, which lower plasma renin activity, and to angiotensin inhibitors—supporting a role for excess renin and angiotensin in this population.

Mechanism & Sites of Action

Renin release from the kidney cortex is stimulated by reduced renal arterial pressure, sympathetic neural stimulation, and reduced sodium delivery or increased sodium concentration at the distal renal tubule. Renin acts upon renin substrate, an α_2-globulin, to split off the inactive decapeptide angiotensin I. Angiotensin I is then converted, primarily in the lung, to the arterial vasoconstrictor octapeptide angiotensin II, which is in turn converted in the adrenal gland to angiotensin III (Fig 10–7). Angiotensin II has vasoconstrictor and sodium-retaining activity. Angiotensin II and III both stimulate aldosterone release. Angiotensin may contribute to maintaining high vascular resistance in hypertensive states associated with high plasma renin activity, such as renal arterial stenosis, some types of intrinsic renal disease, and malignant hypertension, as well as in essential hypertension after treatment with sodium restriction, diuretics, or vasodilators. Three compounds that inhibit the action of angiotensin have been extensively evaluated in humans.

SARALASIN

Saralasin (1-sar-8-ala-angiotensin II) is an analog and competitive inhibitor of angiotensin II. Saralasin blocks the pressor and aldosterone-releasing effects of infused angiotensin II and lowers blood pressure in high-renin states such as renal artery stenosis. Saralasin also has weak agonist activity, however, so that rapid injection or administration to persons without high circulating angiotensin II may increase rather than decrease blood pressure. This drug has proved to be a valuable research tool in determining the role of angiotensin II in hypertension.

CONVERTING ENZYME INHIBITORS

Captopril (Fig 10–4) inhibits the converting enzyme peptidyl dipeptidase that hydrolyzes angiotensin I to angiotensin II and (under the name plasma kininase) inactivates bradykinin, a potent vasodilator. Unlike saralasin, captopril has no pressor activity. Thus, the hypotensive activity of captopril may result from an inhibitory action on the renin-angiotensin system and a stimulating action on the kallikrein-kinin system (Fig 10–7).

Enalapril (Fig 16–2) is a pro-drug that is converted by deesterification to a converting enzyme inhibitor, enalaprilat, with effects similar to those of captopril.

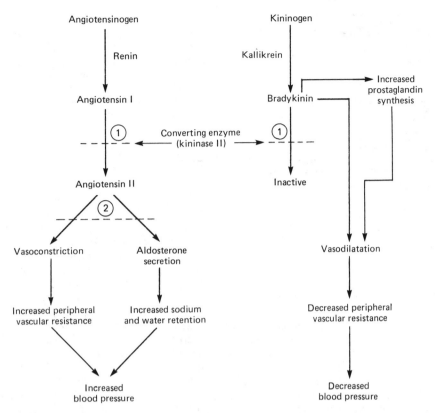

Figure 10–7. Sites of action of captopril and saralasin. ① Site of captopril blockade. ② Site of saralasin blockade.

Angiotensin II inhibitors lower blood pressure principally by decreasing peripheral vascular resistance. Cardiac output and heart rate are not significantly changed. Unlike direct vasodilators, these agents do not result in reflex sympathetic activation and can be used safely in persons with ischemic heart disease.

Although converting enzyme inhibitors are most effective in conditions associated with high plasma renin activity, there is no good correlation among subjects between plasma renin activity and hypotensive response. Accordingly, renin profiling is unnecessary.

Pharmacokinetics & Dosage

Captopril is rapidly absorbed, with a bioavailability of about 70% after fasting; bioavailability is decreased by 30–40% if the drug is taken with food. It is metabolized chiefly to disulfide conjugates with other sulfhydryl-containing molecules. Less than half of an oral dose of captopril is excreted unchanged in the urine. Captopril is distributed to most body tissues, with the notable exception of the central nervous system. Although the half-life is not clearly established, most captopril is eliminated from the body within 6 hours.

Captopril is initially administered in doses of 25 mg 2 or 3 times each day, taken 1–2 hours before meals. Maximal blood pressure response is seen 2–4 hours after the dose. At 1- to 2-week intervals, doses can be increased until blood pressure is controlled. Doses of 50–150 mg/d are effective for most patients. Because captopril is partly eliminated by the kidney, less frequent dosing has been recommended for patients with renal insufficiency, but data to support this suggestion are lacking.

Typical doses of enalapril are 10–20 mg twice daily. Peak concentrations of enalaprilat occur 3–4 hours after dosing with enalapril. The half-life of enalaprilat is about 11 hours.

Toxicity

Toxicity from captopril is uncommon but may be serious, including bone marrow suppression and proteinuria. Neutropenia or pancytopenia usually occurs in the first month of therapy and resolves after the drug is discontinued, although fatal cases have been reported. Proteinuria is associated with minimal changes in kidney basal membranes and is reversible after stopping captopril in most, but not all, cases. Serious toxicity has occurred primarily when captopril was given in high doses to patients with collagen vascular disease or renal insufficiency. It has been recommended that blood counts and urinalyses be performed frequently (every 2 weeks) in the first few months of treatment. Minor toxic effects seen more typically include altered sense of taste, allergic skin rashes, and drug fever, which may occur in as many as 10% of patients. The incidence of these side effects may be lower with enalapril.

II. CLINICAL PHARMACOLOGY OF ANTIHYPERTENSIVE AGENTS

Hypertension presents a unique problem in therapeutics. It is usually a lifelong disease that causes few symptoms until the advanced stages. For effective treatment, medicines that are expensive and often produce adverse effects must be consumed daily. Thus, the physician must establish with certainty that hypertension is persistent and requires treatment and must exclude secondary causes of hypertension that might be treated by definitive surgical procedures. Persistence of hypertension, particularly in persons with mild elevation of blood pressure, should be established by finding an elevated blood pressure on at least 3 different office visits. Ambulatory blood pressure monitoring may be the best predictor of risk and therefore of need for therapy in mild hypertension.

Once the presence of hypertension is established, the question of whether or not to treat and which drugs to use must be considered. The level of blood pressure, the age and sex of the patient, the severity of organ damage (if any) due to high blood pressure, and the presence of cardiovascular risk factors must all be considered. For example, an obese, apparently healthy middle-aged woman with mild hypertension and no cardiovascular risk factors might be treated with dietary caloric and sodium restriction and observation every 6 months. A young adult black man with mild hypertension but a strong family history of hypertension and coronary heart disease who has hyperlipidemia and is a heavy cigarette smoker should be treated more vigorously.

Opinion differs about the level of mild hypertension at which pharmacologic therapy should be initiated. Of concern in making the decision to treat mild hypertension is the possibility that the usual first-line drugs such as diuretics and propranolol may, by adversely affecting serum lipid profiles or impairing glucose tolerance, add to the risk of coronary heart disease, possibly offsetting the benefit of blood pressure reduction.

Once the decision is made to treat, a therapeutic regimen must be developed and the patient must be educated about the nature of hypertension and the importance of treatment. Selection of drugs is dictated by the level of blood pressure and the presence and severity of end organ damage. Severe high blood pressure with life-threatening complications requires more rapid treatment with more potent drugs. Most patients with essential hypertension, however, have had elevated blood pressure for months or years, and therapy is best initiated in a gradual fashion.

Successful treatment of hypertension requires that dietary instructions be followed and medications be taken as directed. Education about the natural history of hypertension and the importance of treatment as well as potential side effects of drugs is essential. Fol-

low-up visits should be frequent enough to convince the patient that the physician thinks the illness is serious. With each follow-up visit, the importance of treatment should be reinforced and questions—particularly concerning dosing or side effects of medication—encouraged. Other factors that may improve compliance are simplifying dosing regimens and having the patient monitor blood pressure at home.

OUTPATIENT THERAPY OF HYPERTENSION

A general approach to outpatient management of hypertension has been presented by the Joint National Committee on Detection, Evaluation, and Treatment of High Blood Pressure. It consists of a number of sequential steps, combining drugs with different sites of action to maximize lowering of blood pressure while minimizing toxicity. A modified version of the stepped-care approach is shown in Fig 10–8.

The initial step in treating hypertension may be nonpharmacologic. As discussed previously, sodium restriction may be effective treatment for as many as half of patients with mild hypertension. The average American diet contains about 200 meq of sodium per day. A reasonable dietary goal in treating hypertension is 70–100 meq of sodium per day, which can be achieved by not salting food during or after cooking and by avoiding processed foods that contain large amounts of sodium. Compliance with sodium restriction can be assessed by measuring 24-hour urinary excretion of sodium, which approximates sodium intake, before and after dietary instruction.

Weight reduction even without sodium restriction has been shown to normalize blood pressure in up to 75% of overweight patients with mild to moderate hypertension. Regular exercise has been shown in some but not all studies to lower blood pressure in hypertensive patients.

For most patients, diuretics are the first drug group used. Thiazide diuretics, combined with sodium restriction, are effective in normalizing blood pressure in most patients with mild hypertension and many with moderate hypertension. Loop diuretics are necessary in the presence of renal insufficiency with reduced glomerular filtration rate. Spironolactone may be used

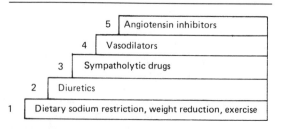

Figure 10–8. Stepped-care approach to treatment of hypertension.

in the presence of hyperaldosteronism due to tumor, cardiac failure, or cirrhosis. At least 1 month should be allowed to evaluate the maximal antihypertensive effect of a particular diuretic.

Sympatholytic drugs are the next step, although propranolol is also widely used as a first-step drug, particularly in younger persons with labile or high-renin essential hypertension or those unable to tolerate diuretics. All sympatholytic drugs are effective. Selection of a particular agent should be determined by anticipated side effects, convenience of use, cost, and physician preference. Propranolol is often chosen for physically active patients, because sedation is minimal and there is no orthostatic hypotension and less sexual dysfunction compared with other sympatholytic drugs. Centrally acting sympatholytics such as methyldopa and clonidine are more sedating—an effect that may be advantageous in the treatment of anxious patients. Because of its wide dose-response range, clonidine may be more effective than beta blockers in treating severe hypertension. Long-acting sympatholytic drugs such as reserpine and guanethidine are especially convenient, because they require only once-daily dosing and are less expensive than other sympatholytic agents. However, in larger doses required to treat more severe hypertension, reserpine causes excessive sedation and guanethidine causes orthostatic hypotension, diarrhea, and sexual dysfunction. Prazosin is effective in mild to moderate hypertension and is useful in patients who cannot tolerate beta blockers (because of asthma, for example) or the sedating effects of centrally active drugs. In more severe hypertension, prazosin can be combined successfully with beta blockers.

Vasodilators are added as the third drug class. Hydralazine has usually been started first, and if maximal doses are reached without adequate control of blood pressure, minoxidil is substituted. Doses of diuretics or beta blockers (or both) may have to be increased or, if other sympatholytic drugs are being used, beta blockers are added to control the tendency toward sodium retention and reflex sympathetic stimulation due to vasodilators. Constant body weight and a heart rate of 80 or less are useful end points in adjusting doses of diuretics and beta blockers, respectively.

There is no consensus about the next step to be taken if hypertension is still uncontrolled. Some authorities advise guanethidine, but this drug's unwanted effects may be incapacitating in severe hypertension, when large doses are required. Converting enzyme inhibitors or calcium channel blockers are probably better choices. They act by different mechanisms, may be additive or synergistic with actions of other drugs, and are usually well tolerated. Recently there has been movement toward use of these drugs as third-step (or even first- or second-step) drugs.

Assessment of blood pressure during office visits should include measurement of recumbent, sitting, and standing blood pressures. If a drug such as guanethidine that produces orthostatic hypotension is used, postexercise blood pressure should be measured as well. An attempt should be made to normalize blood pressure (mean blood pressure 100 mm Hg or less) in the posture or activity level that is customary for the patient. The extent of orthostatic hypotension and inhibition of reflex or exercise tachycardia are useful indicators of the effectiveness of or compliance with sympatholytic therapy. In addition to noncompliance with medication, causes of failure to respond to drug therapy include excessive sodium intake and inadequate diuretic therapy with excessive blood volume (this can be measured directly), and drugs such as antidepressants and over-the-counter sympathomimetics that can interfere with actions of some antihypertensive drugs or directly raise blood pressure.

MANAGEMENT OF HYPERTENSIVE EMERGENCIES

Despite the large number of patients with chronic hypertension, hypertensive emergencies are relatively rare. Marked or sudden elevation of blood pressure may be a serious threat to life, however, and prompt reduction of blood pressure is indicated. Most commonly, hypertensive emergencies occur in patients whose hypertension is severe and poorly controlled and in those who suddenly discontinue antihypertensive medications.

Clinical Presentation & Pathophysiology

Hypertensive emergencies include hypertension associated with vascular damage (termed malignant hypertension) and hypertension associated with hemodynamic complications such as cardiac failure, stroke, or dissecting aneurysm. The underlying pathologic process in malignant hypertension is a progressive arteriopathy with inflammation and necrosis of arterioles. Vascular lesions occur in the kidney, which releases renin, which in turn stimulates production of angiotension and aldosterone, which further increases blood pressure.

Hypertensive encephalopathy is a classic feature of malignant hypertension. Its clinical presentation consists of severe headache, mental confusion, and apprehension. Blurred vision, nausea and vomiting, and focal neurologic deficits are common. If untreated, the syndrome may progress to convulsions, stupor, coma, and even death over a period of 12–48 hours.

Treatment of Hypertensive Emergencies

The general management of hypertensive emergencies requires monitoring the patient in an intensive care unit with continuous recording of arterial blood pressure. Rapid treatment is essential. Fluid intake and output must be monitored carefully and body weight measured daily as an indicator of total body fluid volume during the course of therapy. The first medication to be administered is usually a diuretic. Because it is likely that the patient will have compromised renal function, a drug that works in the presence of renal insufficiency, such as furosemide, should be selected. An appreciable diuresis should occur within 30 minutes and enhance the antihypertensive effects of other medications.

Dialysis may be a necessary alternative to the loop diuretics, particularly in patients with oliguric renal failure. Dialysis can remove excess fluid, correct electrolyte disturbances, and control symptoms of uremia. Uremic symptoms may be confusing in evaluating patients with hypertensive encephalopathy.

Parenteral antihypertensive medications are used to lower blood pressure rapidly; as soon as reasonable blood pressure control is achieved, oral antihypertensive therapy should be substituted, because this allows smoother long-term management of hypertension. The drugs most commonly used to treat hypertensive emergencies are the vasodilators sodium nitroprusside and diazoxide. Other parenteral drugs that may be effective include labetalol, trimethaphan, hydralazine, reserpine, and methyldopa. Nonparenteral therapy with sublingual or chewed nifedipine—or oral captopril, prazosin, or clonidine—has recently been shown to be useful in the therapy of severe hypertension.

REFERENCES

Becker CE, Benowitz NL: Hypertensive emergencies. *Med Clin North Am* 1979;**63**:127.

Bertel O et al: Nifedipine in hypertensive emergencies. *Br Med J* 1983;**286**:19.

Chaffman M et al: Indapamide: A review of its pharmacodynamic properties and therapeutic efficacy in hypertension. *Drugs* 1984;**28**:189.

Cohn JN, Burke LP: Nitroprusside. *Ann Intern Med* 1979; **91**:752.

Colucci WS: Alpha-adrenergic receptor blockade with prazosin. *Ann Intern Med* 1982;**97**:67.

Edwards CRW, Padfield PL: Angiotensin-converting enzyme inhibitors: Past, present, and bright future. *Lancet* 1985;**1**:30.

Frishman WH: Pindolol: A new beta-adrenoceptor antagonist with partial agonist activity. *N Engl J Med* 1983;**308**:940.

Frohlich ED: Methyldopa: Mechanisms and treatment 25 years later. *Arch Intern Med* 1980;**140**:954.

Gifford RW Jr, Tarazi RC: Resistant hypertension: Diagnosis and management. *Ann Intern Med* 1978;**88**:661.

Graham RM, Pettinger WA: Prazosin. *N Engl J Med* 1979; **300**:232.

Helgeland A: Treatment of mild hypertension: A five year controlled drug trial. The Oslo study. *Am J Med* 1980;**69**:725.

Holland OB, Kaplan NM: Propranolol in the treatment of hypertension. *N Engl J Med* 1976;**294**:930.

Hypertension Detection and Follow-Up Program Cooperative Group: The effect of treatment on mortality in "mild" hypertension. *N Engl J Med* 1982;**307**:976.

Hypertension Detection and Follow-Up Program Cooperative Group: Five-year findings of the Hypertension Detection and Follow-Up Program. 1. Reduction in mortality of persons with high blood pressure, including mild hypertension. *JAMA* 1979;**242**:2562.

Joint National Committee on Detection, Evaluation, and Treatment of High Blood Pressure: Report of the Joint National Committee on Detection, Evaluation, and Treatment of High Blood Pressure: A cooperative study. *JAMA* 1977;**237**:255.

Joint National Committee on Detection, Evaluation, and Treatment of High Blood Pressure: The 1980 Report of the Joint National Committee on Detection, Evaluation, and Treatment of High Blood Pressure. *Arch Intern Med* 1980;**140**:1280.

Joint National Committee on Detection, Evaluation, and Treatment of High Blood Pressure: The 1984 Report of the Joint National Committee on Detection, Evaluation, and Treatment of High Blood Pressure. *Arch Intern Med* 1984;**144**:1045.

Kaplan NM: New approaches to the therapy of mild hypertension. *Am J Cardiol* 1983;**51**:621.

Koch-Weser J: Diazoxide. *N Engl J Med* 1976;**294**:1271.

Koch-Weser J: Drug therapy: Hydralazine. *N Engl J Med* 1976; **295**:320.

Koch-Weser J: Drug therapy: Metoprolol. *N Engl J Med* 1979; **301**:698.

Langford HG et al: Dietary therapy slows the return of hypertension after stopping prolonged medication. *JAMA* 1985; **253**:657.

Ledingham JGG: Management of hypertensive crises. *Hypertension* 1983;**5(Suppl III)**:114.

Leren P et al: Effect of propranolol and prazosin on blood lipids: The Oslo study. *Lancet* 1980;**2**:4.

Linas SL, Nies AS: Minoxidil. *Ann Intern Med* 1981;**94**:61.

Lowenstein J: Clonidine. *Ann Intern Med* 1980;**92**:74.

MacGregor GA: Dietary sodium and potassium intake and blood pressure. *Lancet* 1983;**1**:750.

Massie BM et al: Calcium channel blockers as antihypertensive agents. *Am J Med* 1984;**77(Suppl)**:135.

McCarron DA et al: Assessment of nutritional correlates of blood pressure. *Ann Intern Med* 1983;**93(Part 2)**:715.

McCarron DA et al: Blood pressure and nutrient intake in the United States. *Science* 1984;**224**:1392.

Michelson EL: Labetalol: An alpha- and beta-adrenoceptor blocking drug. *Ann Intern Med* 1983;**99**:553.

Multiple Risk Factor Intervention Trial Research Group: Multiple risk factor intervention trial. *JAMA* 1982;**248**:1465.

Murphy MB et al: Glucose intolerance in hypertensive patients treated with diuretics: A fourteen-year follow-up. *Lancet* 1982;**2**:1293.

Pickering TG et al: What is the role of ambulatory blood pressure monitoring in the management of hypertensive patients? *Hypertension* 1985;**7**:171.

Reisin E et al: Effect of weight loss without salt restriction on the reduction of blood pressure in overweight hypertensive patients. *N Engl J Med* 1978;**298**:1.

Report by the Management Committee: The Australian therapeutic trial in mild hypertension. *Lancet* 1980;**1**:1261.

Riley LJ Jr, Vlasses PH, Ferguson RK: Clinical pharmacology and therapeutic applications of the new oral converting enzyme inhibitor, enalapril. *Am Heart J* 1985;**109**:1085.

Smith WB et al: Antihypertensive effectiveness of intravenous labetalol in accelerated hypertension. *Hypertension* 1983; **5**:579.

Veterans Administration Cooperative Study Group on Antihypertensive Agents: Effects of treatment on morbidity in hypertension. 1. Results in patients with diastolic blood pressure averaging 115 through 129 mm Hg. *JAMA* 1967;**202**:1028.

Veterans Administration Cooperative Study Group on Antihypertensive Agents: Effects of treatment on morbidity in hypertension. 2. Results in patients with diastolic blood pressure averaging 90 through 114 mm Hg. *JAMA* 1970;**213**:1143.

Vidt DG, Bravo EL, Fouad FM: Captopril. *N Engl J Med* 1982;**306**:214.

Woosley RL, Nies AS: Guanethidine. *N Engl J Med* 1976; **295**:1053.

Vasodilators & the Treatment of Angina Pectoris

11

Bertram G. Katzung, MD, PhD, & Kanu Chatterjee, MB, FRCP

Vasodilator drugs are used in several conditions involving tissue ischemia, but the most important one is angina pectoris. Angina is caused by the accumulation of metabolites in striated muscle; angina pectoris is the strangling chest pain that occurs when coronary blood flow is inadequate to supply the oxygen required by the heart.

Ischemic heart disease is the most common serious health problem in many Western societies. By far the most frequent cause is atheromatous obstruction of the large coronary vessels. However, transient spasm of localized portions of these vessels can also cause significant myocardial ischemia and pain (variant or angiospastic angina).

The primary cause of angina pectoris is an imbalance between the oxygen requirement of the heart and the oxygen supplied to it via the coronary vessels. In classic angina, the imbalance occurs when the myocardial oxygen requirement increases, as during exercise. Classic angina is therefore "angina of effort." In variant angina, oxygen delivery decreases as a result of reversible coronary vasospasm. The primary objective of treatment in both forms of angina is to improve coronary blood flow. A secondary objective is reduction of the myocardial oxygen requirement. Both measures are used in clinical practice. Traditional treatment achieves the second goal through the use of organic nitrates—potent vasodilators—and several other classes of drugs. It is important to realize that the vasodilators useful in angina of effort do not act by dilating the obstructed coronary vessels but by dilating normal peripheral vessels and thus decreasing the work of the heart. Therefore, the term "coronary vasodilator" should be avoided. Furthermore, careful study of newer agents has shown that not all vasodilators are effective in angina and, conversely, that some agents useful in angina (eg, propranolol) are not vasodilators.

This chapter is divided into 2 sections. The first describes the basic pharmacology of 2 important classes of vasodilators: the nitrates and the calcium influx inhibitors. The second section describes the management of angina pectoris using these 2 classes of drugs and the β-adrenoceptor–blocking agents.

History

Angina pectoris was first described as a distinct clinical entity by William Heberden in the latter half of the 18th century. In the second half of the 19th century, it was found that amyl nitrite could provide transient relief. However, it was not until the introduction of nitroglycerin in 1879 that effective relief of acute episodes of angina became possible. Subsequently, many other vasodilators were introduced for the treatment of angina. However, when careful double-blind clinical trials were done, most of these agents were found to be no better than placebo. In fact, several of the classic studies of the placebo effect were carried out in patients with angina. With the introduction of β-adrenoceptor–blocking drugs, useful prophylactic therapy of angina became possible. More recently, the calcium influx blockers have been shown to be useful for prevention of anginal attacks, especially in variant angina.

I. BASIC PHARMACOLOGY OF VASODILATORS

NITRATES & NITRITES

Chemistry

These agents are simple nitric and nitrous acid esters of polyalcohols (Fig 11–1). They vary from extremely volatile liquids (amyl nitrite) through moderately volatile liquids (nitroglycerin) to solids (isosorbide dinitrate). Nitroglycerin may be considered the prototype of the group. Although it is used in the manufacture of dynamite, the formulations of nitroglycerin used in medicine are not explosive. The conventional sublingual tablet form of nitroglycerin may lose potency when stored as a result of volatilization and adsorption to plastic surfaces. Therefore, it should be kept in tightly closed glass containers. It is not sensitive to light.

Structure-activity studies indicate that all therapeutically active agents in this group are capable of releasing nitrite ion in vascular smooth muscle target tissues. Unfortunately, they all also appear to be capable of inducing cross-tolerance when given in large doses. Therefore, pharmacokinetic factors govern the choice of agent and mode of therapy when using the nitrates.

Pharmacokinetics

The use of organic nitrates is strongly influenced by

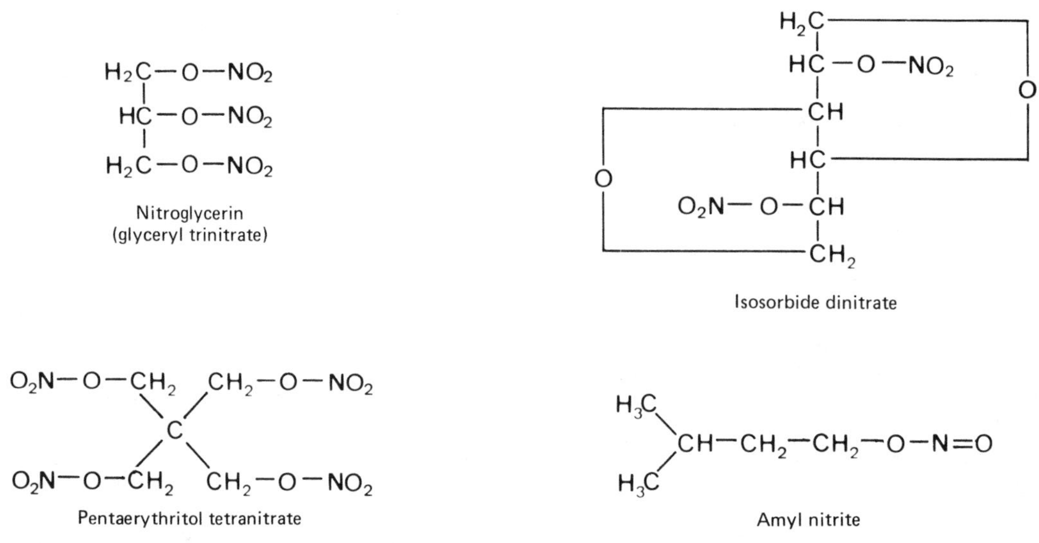

Figure 11–1. Chemical structures of 3 nitrates and amyl nitrite.

the existence of a high-capacity hepatic organic nitrate reductase that inactivates the drug. Therefore, bioavailability of all orally administered organic nitrates is very low (typically less than 10%). Consequently, the sublingual route is preferred for achieving a therapeutic blood level rapidly. Nitroglycerin and isosorbide dinitrate are both absorbed efficiently by this route and reach therapeutic blood levels within a few minutes. However, the total dose administered by this route must be limited to avoid excessive effects; therefore, the total duration of effect is brief, typically 15–30 minutes. When much longer duration of action is needed, oral preparations are available that contain an amount of drug sufficient to result in sustained systemic blood levels of drug or active metabolites. Other routes of administration available for nitroglycerin include transdermal absorption when applied to the skin as an ointment and buccal absorption from slow-release buccal preparations; these are described below.

Amyl nitrite and related nitrites are highly volatile liquids. Amyl nitrite is available in fragile glass ampules packaged in a protective cloth covering. The ampule can be crushed with the fingers, resulting in rapid release of inhalable vapors through the cloth covering. The inhalation route provides for very rapid absorption and, like the sublingual route, avoids the hepatic first-pass effect.

Once absorbed, the unchanged nitrate compounds have half-lives of only 2–8 minutes. The denitrated metabolites have much longer half-lives (1–3 hours). Of the nitroglycerin metabolites (2 dinitroglycerins and 2 mononitro forms), the dinitro derivatives have significant vasodilator efficacy; they probably provide most of the therapeutic effect of orally administered nitroglycerin. The 5-mononitrate metabolite of isosorbide dinitrate is an active metabolite of the latter drug

and is available for clinical use in the United Kingdom as isosorbide mononitrate (Elantan).

Excretion, primarily in the form of glucuronide derivatives of the denitrated metabolites, is largely by way of the kidney.

Pharmacodynamics

Nitroglycerin and its analogs are unusually selective drugs: in therapeutic doses, their action is almost exclusively on smooth muscle cells.

A. Mechanism of Action: Nitroglycerin is probably denitrated in the smooth muscle cell. The resulting nitric oxide (NO) is thought to react with a specific receptor. The latter appears to include sulfhydryl (−SH) groups, since tolerance to nitrite involves a decrease in tissue sulfhydryl groups, and tolerance can be reversed with dithiothreitol, a sulfhydryl-regenerating agent. Little is known of the steps linking receptor binding of nitric oxide and relaxation of smooth muscle. Some evidence suggests that an increase in cGMP is the first link. Other studies implicate the production of prostaglandin E or prostacyclin (PGI_2) as an important intermediate step. There is no evidence that autonomic receptors are involved in the primary nitrate response (although autonomic *reflex* responses are evoked when hypotensive doses are given).

B. Organ System Effects: Nitroglycerin relaxes all types of smooth muscle irrespective of the cause of the preexisting muscle tone (Fig 11–2). It has practically no direct effect on cardiac or skeletal muscle, and the reasons for this selectivity are unknown.

1. Vascular smooth muscle–All segments of the vascular system from large arteries through large veins relax in response to nitroglycerin (Fig 11–2). However, arterioles and precapillary sphincters are dilated less than other portions of the vascular tree, at least partly because of reflex responses. The primary

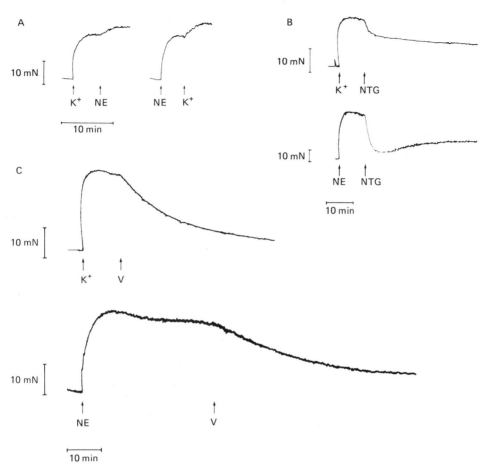

Figure 11–2. Effects of vasodilators on contractions of human vein segments studied in vitro. Panel **A** shows contractions induced by 2 vasoconstrictor agents, norepinephrine (NE) and potassium (K^+). Panel **B** shows the relaxation induced by nitroglycerin (NTG), 4 μmol/L. The relaxation is prompt. Panel **C** shows the relaxation induced by verapamil (V), 2.2 μmol/L. The relaxation is slower but more sustained. (Modified and reproduced, with permission, from Mikkelsen E, Andersson K-E, Bengtsson B: Effects of verapamil and nitroglycerin on contractile responses to potassium and noradrenaline in isolated human peripheral veins. *Acta Pharmacol Toxicol* 1978;**42**:14.)

direct result of an effective blood concentration is marked relaxation of the large veins with increased venous capacitance and decreased ventricular preload. Pulmonary vascular pressures and heart size are significantly reduced. In the absence of heart failure, cardiac output is reduced. Because venous capacitance is increased, orthostatic hypotension may be marked, and syncope can result. Dilatation of some large arteries may be significant: Temporal artery pulsations and a throbbing headache associated with meningeal artery pulsations are frequent side effects of nitroglycerin and amyl nitrite. In the presence of heart failure, preload is usually abnormally high; the nitrates and other vasodilators may have a beneficial effect on cardiac output in this condition (see Chapter 12).

The indirect effects of nitroglycerin consist of those reflexes evoked by baroreceptors responding to decreased arterial pressure (Fig 5–6). The primary mechanism of this reflex is sympathetic discharge; this consistently results in tachycardia and increased car-

diac contractility. In the case of very rapidly acting agents (eg, inhaled amyl nitrite), arterial dilatation may be so marked as to cause a reflex venoconstriction.

In the isolated coronary-perfused heart (Langendorf preparation) and in normal subjects without coronary disease, nitroglycerin can induce a significant, if transient, increase in total coronary blood flow. In contrast, there is no evidence that total coronary flow is increased in patients with angina due to atherosclerotic obstructive coronary artery disease. While some studies suggest that *redistribution* of coronary flow from normal to ischemic regions may play a role, most evidence suggests that relief of angina by nitroglycerin is the result of decreased myocardial oxygen requirement secondary to decreased preload and arterial pressure (see Clinical Pharmacology, below).

2. Other smooth muscle organs–Relaxation of smooth muscle of the bronchi, gastrointestinal tract (including biliary system), and genitourinary tract has been demonstrated experimentally. Because of their brief duration, these actions of the nitrates are rarely of any clinical value. During recent years, the use of amyl nitrite and isobutyl nitrite as recreational (sex-enhancing) drugs has become popular with some segments of the population. Isobutyl nitrite is not licensed or advertised as a drug but is sold over the counter under such names as Rush, Bolt, Locker Room, and Dr. Bananas.

3. Other effects–Nitrite ion reacts with hemoglobin (which contains ferrous iron) to produce **methemoglobin** (which contains ferric iron). Because methemoglobin has a very low affinity for oxygen, large doses of nitrites can result in pseudocyanosis, tissue hypoxia, and death. The plasma level of nitrite resulting from even large doses of organic and inorganic nitrates is too low to cause significant methemoglobinemia in adults. However, sodium nitrite is used as a curing agent for meats. In nursing infants, the intestinal flora is capable of converting significant amounts of inorganic nitrate, eg, from well water, to nitrite ion. Thus, inadvertent exposure to large amounts of nitrite ion can produce serious toxicity. One therapeutic application of this otherwise toxic effect of nitrite has been discovered. **Cyanide poisoning** results from complexing of cytochrome iron by the CN^- ion. Methemoglobin iron has a very high affinity for CN^-; thus, administration of sodium nitrite ($NaNO_2$) soon after cyanide exposure will regenerate active cytochrome. The cyanmethemoglobin produced can be further detoxified by the intravenous administration of sodium thiosulfate ($Na_2S_2O_3$); this results in formation of thiocyanate ion (SCN^-), a less toxic ion that is readily excreted. Methemoglobinemia, if excessive, can be treated by giving methylene blue intravenously.

Toxicity & Tachyphylaxis

The major acute toxicity of organic nitrates is a direct extension of therapeutic vasodilatation: orthostatic hypotension, tachycardia, and throbbing headache. With continuous exposure to nitrates, isolated smooth muscle may develop complete tachyphylaxis (tolerance), and the intact human becomes at least partially tolerant. Continuous exposure to high levels of nitrates can occur in the chemical industry, especially where explosives are manufactured. When contamination of the workplace with volatile organic nitrate compounds is severe, workers find that upon starting their work week (Monday), they suffer headache and transient dizziness. After a day or so, these symptoms disappear owing to the development of tolerance. Over the weekend, when exposure to the chemicals is reduced, tolerance disappears, so symptoms recur each Monday. A more serious hazard of industrial exposure is the development of dependence. This may affect workers after months or years of exposure and manifests itself as variant angina occurring after 1–2 days away from the source of nitrates, eg, on Sunday of a normal work week. In the most seriously affected individuals, coronary vasospasm may cause myocar-

dial infarction. There is no evidence that physical dependence develops as a result of the therapeutic use of nitrates for angina, even in large doses.

Nitrosamines are small molecules with the structure $R_2–N–NO$ formed from the combination of nitrates and nitrites with amines. Some nitrosamines are powerful carcinogens in animals, apparently through conversion to very reactive derivatives. While there is no direct proof that these agents cause cancer in humans, there is a strong epidemiologic correlation between the incidence of esophageal and gastric carcinoma and the nitrate content of food in different cultures. Nitrosamines are also found in tobacco and in cigarette smoke. There is no evidence that the small doses of nitrates used in the treatment of angina result in significant body levels of nitrosamines.

Mechanisms of Clinical Effect

The beneficial and deleterious effects of nitrate-induced vasodilatation are summarized in Table 11–1.

A. Nitrate Effects in Angina of Effort: Decreased venous return to the heart and the resulting reduction of intracardiac volume are the principal hemodynamic effects. Arterial pressure decreases. Decreased intraventricular pressure and left ventricular volume are associated with decreased wall tension (Laplace relation) and resulting decreased myocardial oxygen requirement. In rare instances, a paradoxic increase in myocardial oxygen demand may occur as a result of excessive reflex tachycardia and increased contractility.

Intracoronary or intravenous nitrate administration consistently increases the caliber of the epicardial coronary arteries. Coronary arteriolar resistance tends to decrease, though to a lesser extent. However, nitrates administered by the usual systemic routes consistently *decrease* overall coronary blood flow and myocardial oxygen consumption. Intracoronary injection of small doses of nitroglycerin, which increases

Table 11–1. Beneficial and deleterious effects of nitrates in the treatment of angina.

	Result
Potential beneficial effects	
Decreased ventricular volume	Decreased myocardial oxygen requirement.
Decreased arterial pressure	
Decreased ejection time	
Vasodilation of epicardial coronary arteries	Relief of coronary artery spasm.
Increased collateral flow	Improved perfusion to ischemic myocardium.
Decreased left ventricular diastolic pressure	Improved subendocardial perfusion.
Potential deleterious effects	
Reflex tachycardia	Increased myocardial oxygen requirement.
Reflex increase in contractility	
Decreased diastolic perfusion time due to tachycardia	Decreased myocardial perfusion.

total coronary blood flow but does not produce systemic hemodynamic effects, does not relieve angina. Yet systemic administration of nitroglycerin, which decreases arterial pressure and left ventricular volume, does relieve angina despite decreased coronary blood flow. These findings indicate that the relief of effort angina with nitrates is due primarily to decreased myocardial oxygen demand and not increased coronary blood flow.

B. Nitrate Effects in Variant Angina: In patients with variant angina, relaxation of smooth muscles of the epicardial coronary arteries, together with relief of coronary artery spasm, is the principal mechanism by which nitrates exert their beneficial effects. Although intracoronary nitroglycerin injection appears to be the most effective method for relieving coronary artery spasm, this method of administration has little relevance in the clinical management of patients.

C. Nitrate Effects in Unstable Angina: Nitrates are also useful in the treatment of unstable angina, but the precise mechanism for their beneficial effects is not clear. Because both increased coronary vascular tone and increased myocardial oxygen demand can precipitate rest angina in these patients, nitrates may exert their beneficial effects both by dilating the epicardial coronary arteries and simultaneously reducing myocardial oxygen demand.

Clinical Use of Nitrates

Some of the forms of nitroglycerin and its congeners are listed in Table 11–2. Because of its rapid onset of action (1–3 minutes), sublingual nitroglycerin is the most frequently used agent for the immediate treatment of angina. Because its duration of action is short (not exceeding 20–30 minutes), it is not a suitable agent for maintenance therapy. The onset of action of intravenous nitroglycerin is also rapid (minutes), but its hemodynamic effects are quickly reversed with discontinuation of its infusion. Its clinical application, therefore, is restricted to the treatment of severe, recurrent rest angina. Slowly absorbed preparations of nitroglycerin include a buccal form, an oral preparation, and several transdermal forms. These formulations are claimed to provide effective blood concentrations for long periods.

The hemodynamic effects of sublingual or chewable isosorbide dinitrate, pentaerythritol tetranitrate, and erythrityl tetranitrate are similar to those of nitroglycerin. The recommended dosage schedules for commonly used long-acting nitrate preparations, along with their duration of action, are listed in Table 11–2. Although transdermal administration may provide blood levels of nitroglycerin for 24 hours or longer, the hemodynamic effects usually do not persist for more than 6–8 hours. The clinical efficacy of slow-release forms of nitroglycerin in maintenance therapy of angina remains unestablished.

Clinical Toxicity

The most common untoward effects of nitrate ther-

Table 11–2. Nitrate and nitrite drugs used in the treatment of angina.

Drug	Dose	Duration of Action
"Short-acting"		
Nitroglycerin, sublingual	0.15–1.2 mg	10–30 minutes
Isosorbide, sublingual	2.5–5 mg	10–60 minutes
Amyl nitrite, inhalant	0.18–0.3 mL	3–5 minutes
"Long-acting"		
Nitroglycerin, oral sustained-action	6.5–13 mg per 6–8 hours	6–8 hours
Nitroglycerin, 2% ointment	1/2–2 inches per 4 hours	3–6 hours
Nitroglycerin, slow-release buccal	1–2 mg per 4 hours	3–6 hours
Nitroglycerin, slow-release transcutaneous	10–25 mg per 24 hours	24 hours or longer
Isosorbide dinitrate, sublingual	2.5–10 mg per 2 hours	1 1/2–2 hours
Isosorbide dinitrate, oral	10–60 mg per 4–6 hours	4–6 hours
Isosorbide dinitrate, chewable	5–10 mg per 2–4 hours	2–3 hours
Pentaerythritol tetranitrate	40 mg per 6–8 hours	6–8 hours
Erythrityl tetranitrate	10–40 mg per 6–8 hours	6–8 hours

apy are throbbing headache, which tends to decrease in intensity with continued therapy, and postural dizziness, weakness, or even frank syncope. Occasionally, excessive tachycardia occurs in response to hypotension, and angina may be worsened. Glaucoma, once thought to be a contraindication, does not worsen, and nitrates can be used safely in the presence of increased intraocular pressure. Nitrates, however, are contraindicated if intracranial pressure is elevated.

MOLSIDOMINE

Molsidomine is a new vasodilator of novel structure. It is not yet approved for use in the USA.

Molsidomine

Molsidomine is active when administered by the oral route and has a duration of action that may exceed 2 hours. The drug appears to have less effect on coronary arterial resistance than the nitrates, but it is an effective venodilator. Cardiac output and cardiac oxy-

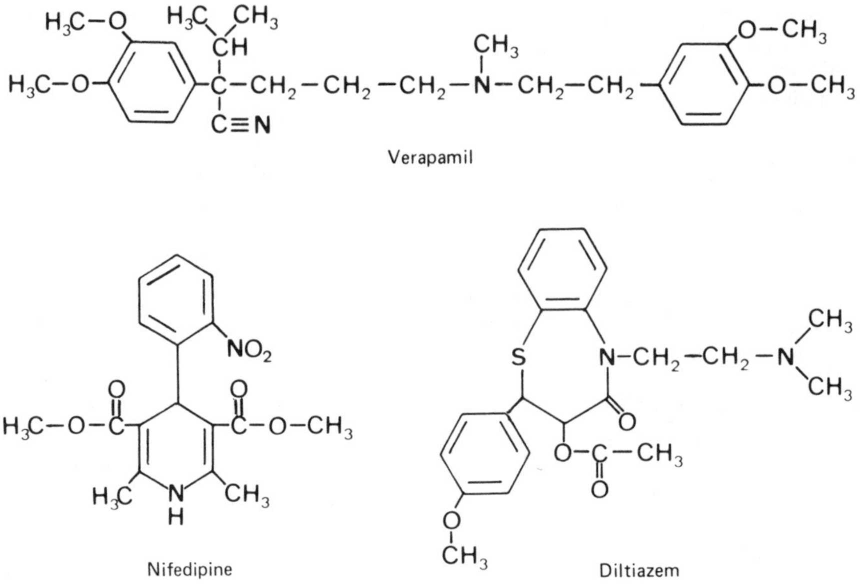

Figure 11–3. Chemical structures of several calcium influx–blocking drugs.

gen requirements are reduced as a result of decreased preload.

Like nitroglycerin and other nitrates, it improves exercise tolerance in patients with angina of effort. Unlike the nitrates, molsidomine may not cause sympathetic reflex tachycardia or increased cardiac contractility. Preliminary double-blind studies indicate that this new drug can reduce exercise-induced anginal pain and the intake of nitroglycerin by preventing the onset of angina. However, clinical experience with molsidomine is not yet sufficient to determine its potential advantages and disadvantages in the management of angina.

CALCIUM INFLUX–BLOCKING DRUGS

Chemistry

Verapamil, the first clinically useful member of this group, was the result of attempts to synthesize more active analogs of papaverine, a vasodilator alkaloid found in the opium poppy. Since then, dozens of agents of widely varying structure have been found to have the same fundamental pharmacologic action. A few of the clinically important agents are shown in Fig 11–3. Two older compounds, prenylamine and perhexiline, are still available in many countries (not the USA) but appear to have significant disadvantages in comparison with the agents shown. A large number of newer agents are under investigation. In spite of the diverse structures represented in this group, the drug receptor is stereoselective: the R (+) isomer of verapamil has much lower potency than the S (−) isomer.

Pharmacokinetics

The calcium influx blockers are orally active agents that readily bind to plasma protein (80–90%). First-pass hepatic metabolism is extensive for verapamil and diltiazem. Elimination half-lives are 3–6 hours, with nifedipine and verapamil being excreted primarily in the urine and diltiazem in the feces. All 3 compounds are extensively metabolized (Table 11–3).

Table 11–3. Pharmacokinetics of some calcium influx–blocking drugs.

Drug	Absorption	Onset of Action	Plasma Half-Life	Disposition
Verapamil	> 90% after oral administration.	< 1½ min after intravenous, 30 min after oral administration.	6 hours	About 90% bound to plasma protein; 85% first-pass hepatic elimination after oral administration. About 70% eliminated by kidney; 15% by gastrointestinal tract.
Nifedipine	> 90% after oral or sublingual administration.	< 1 min after intravenous, < 3 min after sublingual, < 20 min after oral administration.	4 hours	About 90% bound to plasma protein; metabolized to an acid lactate. Drug and metabolites excreted 80% in urine.
Diltiazem	70–90% after oral administration.	< 3 min after intravenous, > 30 min after oral administration.	3–4 hours	Little bound to plasma protein but extensively deactylated. Drug and metabolites excreted in feces.

Pharmacodynamics

A. Mechanism of Action: Calcium influx blockers bind to membrane structures responsible for the "slow inward current"—structures thought to be channels much like the sodium channels of nerve but relatively selective for calcium. Tissues that require calcium influx for normal activity are therefore susceptible to block by these agents (Fig 11–4).

Calcium channel blockade by these drugs resembles sodium channel blockade by local anesthetics. The drugs act from the inner side of the membrane and bind more effectively to channels in depolarized membranes. The block is partially reversible by elevating the concentration of calcium, although the levels of calcium required are not easily attainable. Partial reversal of block can also be obtained by the use of drugs that increase the transmembrane flux of calcium, such as sympathomimetics.

B. Organ System Effects:

1. Smooth muscle–Most types of smooth muscle are dependent on transmembrane calcium influx for normal resting tone and contractile responses. These cells are relaxed by the calcium influx inhibitors. Vascular smooth muscle appears to be the most sensitive (Fig 11–2), but similar relaxation can be shown for bronchiolar, gastrointestinal, and uterine smooth muscle. In the vascular system, arterioles appear to be more sensitive than veins; orthostatic hypotension is not a common side effect. Blood pressure can be reduced, especially with nifedipine. The reduction in peripheral vascular resistance is one mechanism by which these agents may benefit the patient with angina of effort. Reduction of coronary arterial tone has been demonstrated in patients with variant angina.

2. Cardiac muscle–Cardiac muscle is highly dependent upon calcium influx for normal function. Impulse generation in the sinoatrial node and conduction in the atrioventricular node may be reduced or blocked by all of the calcium influx inhibitors. Excitation-contraction coupling in all cardiac cells requires calcium influx, so these drugs reduce cardiac contractility and cardiac output in a dose-dependent fashion. This reduction in mechanical function is another mechanism by which the calcium influx inhibitors may reduce the oxygen requirement in patients with angina.

An additional benefit of calcium influx inhibition has been demonstrated in experimental myocardial infarction. Because ischemia causes membrane depolarization, calcium influx in ischemic cells is increased. Elevated intracellular calcium accelerates the activity of several ATP-consuming enzymes, which further depletes already marginal cellular energy stores, making the heart even more susceptible to ischemic damage. Protection by the calcium influx blockers against these damaging effects of calcium has been demonstrated by a reduction in the incidence of arrhythmias and in the ultimate size of developing infarctions in experimental animals.

Important differences between the available calcium influx inhibitors arise from the details of their interactions with cardiac ion channels and differences in their relative smooth muscle versus cardiac effects. Cardiac sodium channels are blocked by verapamil but

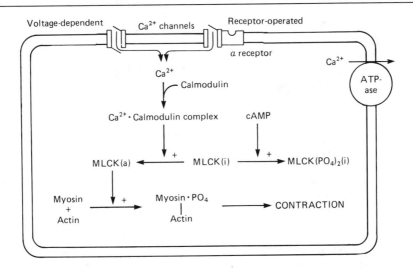

Figure 11–4. Schematic diagram of a vascular smooth muscle cell and some aspects of smooth muscle contraction. Calcium ion enters the cell through voltage-dependent or receptor-operated channels. Such receptors may include α-adrenoceptors. The Ca^{2+} ion forms a complex with the small protein calmodulin, and this complex activates an inactive (i) form of the enzyme myosin light chain kinase (MLCK). Activated myosin light chain kinase (MLCK[a]), in turn, activates the myosin ATPase sites that interact with actin and generate tension and shortening. The calcium influx blockers act primarily on the voltage-sensitive calcium channels. Calmodulin also facilitates removal of Ca^{2+} from the cell by a Ca-ATPase pump. cAMP has several interactions with this process: It facilitates the inactivation of myosin light chain kinase; it may inhibit formation of the Ca^{2+} • calmodulin complex; and it probably facilitates Ca^{2+} extrusion by Ca-ATPase in the cell membrane. These effects would all cause relaxation.

less effectively than are calcium channels. Sodium channel block is less marked with diltiazem and nifedipine. Verapamil and diltiazem interact kinetically with the calcium channel receptor in a different manner than nifedipine; they therefore block tachycardias in calcium-dependent cells, eg, the atrioventricular node, more selectively than does nifedipine. (See Chapter 13 for additional details.) On the other hand, nifedipine appears to block smooth muscle calcium channels at concentrations below those required for significant cardiac effects; it is therefore less depressant on the heart than verapamil or diltiazem.

3. Skeletal muscle–Skeletal muscle is not depressed by the calcium influx inhibitors because it utilizes intracellular pools of calcium to support excitation-contraction coupling and does not require transmembrane calcium influx.

4. Other effects–Calcium influx inhibitors interfere with stimulus-secretion coupling in glands and nerve endings. The effect has been demonstrated experimentally in measurements of the secretion of pituitary and pancreatic polypeptide hormones and release of transmitters from synaptosomes prepared from brain tissue. Verapamil has been shown to inhibit insulin release in humans, but the dosages required are greater than those used in management of angina.

Preliminary evidence suggests that the calcium influx inhibitors may also interfere with platelet aggregation in vitro and the development of atheromatous lesions in rabbits fed a high-fat diet. These effects have not yet been reproduced in human studies.

In addition to angina pectoris, calcium influx inhibitors have been used in the therapy of hypertension, hypertrophic cardiomyopathy, cardiac arrhythmias, migraine headache, Raynaud's syndrome, cerebrovascular accidents, and premature labor.

Toxicity

The most important toxic effects reported for the calcium influx blockers are direct extensions of their therapeutic action. Excessive inhibition of calcium influx can cause serious cardiac depression, including cardiac arrest, bradycardia, atrioventricular block, and congestive heart failure. These effects have been rare in clinical use. Patients receiving β-adrenoceptor–blocking drugs are more sensitive to the cardiodepressant effects of calcium influx inhibitors. Minor toxicity (not requiring discontinuation of therapy) includes flushing, edema, dizziness, nausea, and constipation.

Mechanisms of Clinical Effects

As mentioned previously, calcium influx inhibitors decrease myocardial contractile force, which in turn reduces myocardial oxygen requirements. Inhibition of calcium entry into arterial smooth muscle is associated with decreased arteriolar tone and systemic vascular resistance, resulting in decreased arterial and intraventricular pressure. Some of these drugs (eg, verapamil) also block alpha-adrenoceptors, which may contribute to peripheral vasodilatation. Thus, left

ventricular wall stress declines, which also reduces the myocardial oxygen requirements. Decreased heart rate with the use of some calcium influx–blocking agents (verapamil and diltiazem) causes a further decrease in myocardial oxygen demand. Calcium influx–blocking agents also relieve and prevent focal coronary artery spasm—the primary mechanism of variant angina. Use of these agents has thus emerged as the most effective treatment for this form of angina pectoris. As noted above, the calcium influx–blocking agents differ in their clinical cardiovascular effects. Sinoatrial and atrioventricular nodal tissues, which are mainly composed of "slow response" cells, are affected markedly by verapamil, moderately by diltiazem, and much less by nifedipine. Thus, verapamil and diltiazem decrease atrioventricular nodal conduction and are effective in the management of supraventricular reentry tachycardia and in decreasing ventricular responses in atrial fibrillation or flutter. Nifedipine does not affect atrioventricular conduction. Nonspecific sympathetic antagonism is most marked with diltiazem and much less with verapamil. Nifedipine does not appear to have this effect. Thus, significant reflex tachycardia in response to hypotension occurs most frequently with nifedipine and less so with verapamil. These differences in pharmacologic effects should be considered in selecting calcium influx–blocking agents in the management of angina.

Calcium influx–blocking agents are effective in the long-term management of chronic stable angina. A number of studies have demonstrated an increase in exercise duration and a significant delay in the onset of effort angina (Fig 11–5). The comparative efficacy of calcium influx–blocking drugs, beta-blocking agents, and nitrates has not been established; preliminary studies suggest that there is little difference between these agents. However, calcium blockers, beta blockers, and nitrates have all been shown to be more effective than placebo in reducing daily attacks of angina and in prolonging exercise tolerance. The combination of a beta blocker and a calcium antagonist appears to be more effective than either drug alone in improving exercise duration and tolerance.

Nifedipine, verapamil, and diltiazem are considerably more effective than the beta-adrenoceptor–blocking drugs in relieving and preventing ischemic episodes in patients with variant angina. In approximately 70% of patients, angina attacks are completely abolished; in another 20%, marked reduction of frequency of anginal episodes is observed. Prevention of coronary artery spasm (in the presence or absence of fixed arteriosclerotic coronary artery lesions) is the principal mechanism for this beneficial response.

In patients with unstable angina with recurrent ischemic episodes at rest, the addition of nifedipine to beta blocker and nitrate therapy can decrease the frequency of rest angina, the incidence of myocardial infarction, and the necessity for emergency myocardial revascularization.

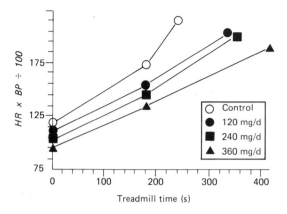

Figure 11–5. Effects of diltiazem on the "double product" in a group of 20 patients with angina of effort. In a double-blind study using a standard protocol, patients were tested on a treadmill during treatment with placebo and 3 doses of the drug. Heart rate (HR) and systolic blood pressure (BP) were recorded at 180 seconds of exercise (midpoints of lines) and at the time of onset of anginal symptoms (rightmost points). Note that the drug treatment decreased the double product at all times during exercise and prolonged the time to appearance of symptoms. (Data from Lindenberg BS et al: Efficacy and safety of incremental doses of diltiazem for the treatment of angina. *J Am Coll Cardiol* 1983;2:1129. Used with permission of the American College of Cardiology.)

Clinical Use of Calcium Influx–Blocking Drugs

The choice of a particular calcium influx–blocking agent should be made with knowledge of its specific potential adverse effects as well as of its pharmacologic properties. A combination of verapamil or diltiazem with beta blockers may produce atrioventricular block. Nifedipine does not decrease atrioventricular conduction and therefore can be used more safely in the presence of atrioventricular conduction abnormalities. Combined beta blocker and verapamil therapy may cause depression of ventricular function. In the presence of overt heart failure, all calcium influx–blocking agents can cause further worsening of heart failure as a result of their negative inotropic effect. However, nifedipine, a potent arteriolar dilator, decreases systemic vascular resistance and left ventricular ejection impedance, which may balance the detrimental negative inotropic effect. Diltiazem has also been shown to produce beneficial effects and improvement in cardiac performance in patients with heart failure. In patients with depressed left ventricular function, therefore, nifedipine or diltiazem is preferable. In the presence of relatively low blood pressure, nifedipine can cause further deleterious lowering of blood pressure. Verapamil and diltiazem appear to produce less hypotension and may be better tolerated in these circumstances. In patients with a history of atrial tachycardia, flutter, and fibrillation, verapamil and diltiazem provide a distinct advantage because of their antiarrhythmic effects. In the digitalized patient,

verapamil should be used with caution, because it may increase digoxin blood levels through a pharmacokinetic interaction. Although increases in digoxin blood level have also been demonstrated with diltiazem and nifedipine, such interactions are less consistent than with verapamil.

Dosages and minor toxic effects of the calcium influx inhibitors are presented in Table 11–4.

BETA-ADRENOCEPTOR–BLOCKING DRUGS

Although they are not vasodilators, beta-blocking drugs (Chapter 9) are extremely useful in the management of stable and unstable angina pectoris. The beneficial effects of beta-blocking agents are related primarily to their hemodynamic effects—decreased heart rate, blood pressure, and contractility—which decrease myocardial oxygen requirements at rest and during exercise. Lower heart rate is also associated with an increase in diastolic perfusion time that may increase myocardial perfusion. It has been suggested that the beta-blocking agents can cause a favorable redistribution of coronary blood flow to the ischemic myocardium based on differential effects on the coronary vascular resistance in the relatively ischemic and nonischemic myocardial segments. However, reduction of heart rate and blood pressure—and consequently decreased myocardial oxygen consumption—appear to be the most important mechanisms for relief of angina and improved exercise tolerance.

Undesirable effects of beta-blocking agents include an increase in end-diastolic volume that accompanies slowing of the heart rate and an increase in ejection time. Increased myocardial oxygen requirements associated with increased left ventricular diastolic volume partially offset the beneficial effects of beta-blocking agents. These potentially deleterious effects of beta-blocking agents can be balanced by the concomitant use of nitrates. Indeed, combined therapy with beta blockers and nitrates is an effective way to treat angina pectoris, since these 2 agents tend to offset each other's deleterious effects on myocardial oxygen requirements. The rationale for the use of combined

Table 11–4. Dosage and toxicity of the calcium influx–blocking drugs.

Drug	Dose	Toxicity
Verapamil (Calan, Isoptin)	75–150 μg/kg intravenously; 80–160 mg every 8 hours orally.	Hypotension, myocardial depression, heart failure, dependent edema.
Nifedipine (Adalat, Procardia)	3–10 μg/kg intravenously; 10–40 mg every 8 hours orally.	Hypotension, dizziness, flushing, nausea, constipation, dependent edema.
Diltiazem (Cardizem)	75–150 μg/kg intravenously; 30–80 mg every 6 hours orally.	Hypotension, dizziness, flushing, bradycardia.

nitrates and beta blockers for treatment of angina is summarized in Table 11–5. Combined therapy reduces myocardial oxygen demand at rest and during exercise. The double rate-pressure product remains consistently lower during exercise with nitrate or beta blocker therapy, and combination therapy produces synergistic effects. However, although exercise capacity increases, there is usually no change in the myocardial ischemia threshold, ie, the rate-pressure product at which symptoms occur.

There is no evidence that any particular beta-blocking agent is better than others in the management of angina. The undesirable cardiac effects of the different types of beta-blocking agents are also quite similar. However, noncardiac side effects may differ (Chapter 9).

The effective dose of any beta blocker varies widely from patient to patient; individual titration against both rest and exercise heart rates is required along with monitoring blood pressure and cardiac function. In patients with severe effort angina, it may be necessary to decrease resting heart rate to 50–60 beats/min and maximal heart rate to 100–120 beats/min during exercise.

II. CLINICAL PHARMACOLOGY OF DRUGS USED IN THE TREATMENT OF ANGINA

Determinants of Myocardial Oxygen Demand

The major and minor determinants of myocardial oxygen requirement are set forth in Table 11–6. Unlike skeletal muscle, human cardiac muscle cannot develop an appreciable oxygen debt during stress and repay it later. As a consequence of its continuous activity, the heart's oxygen needs are relatively high, and it extracts approximately 75% of the available oxygen even under conditions of no stress. The myocardial oxygen requirement increases when there is an increase in heart rate, contractility, arterial pressure,

Table 11–5. Effects of β-adrenoceptor–blocking drugs, nitrates, and combined beta blocker–nitrate therapy in angina pectoris.

	Beta Blockers	Nitrates	Combined Nitrates and Beta Blockers
Heart rate	Decrease	Reflex increase	Decrease
Arterial pressure	Decrease	Decrease	Decrease
End-diastolic volume	Increase	Decrease	None or decrease
Contractility	Decrease	Reflex increase	None
Ejection time	Increase	Decrease	None
Diastolic perfusion time	Increase	Decrease	Increase

Table 11–6. Determinants of myocardial oxygen consumption.

Major	Minor
Wall stress	Fiber shortening
Intraventricular pressure	Activation energy
Ventricular radius (volume)	Resting metabolism
Wall thickness	
Heart rate	
Contractility	

or ventricular volume. These hemodynamic alterations frequently occur during physical exercise, which often precipitates angina in patients with obstructive coronary artery disease. The relative contributions of basal metabolism, activation of contraction, and fiber shortening to the overall myocardial oxygen consumption appear to be small, but under pathologic conditions these apparently minor determinants of myocardial oxygen consumption may become relevant.

Because in the clinical setting it is not possible to measure all of the determinants listed in Table 11–6 directly, indirect measures are often used to assess changes in myocardial oxygen demand and consumption. One commonly used index is the "triple product" (heart rate × systolic blood pressure × ejection time), a measure closely related to the tension-time index. The tension-time index is calculated by multiplying the area (in mm Hg/s) under the systolic phase of the left ventricular pressure curve by the heart rate. The "double product" or rate-pressure product (systolic blood pressure × heart rate per minute) appears to be as reliable as the triple product as an indirect measure of myocardial oxygen consumption (Fig 11–5). These indices are somewhat limited, however, because they do not include left ventricular volume or contractile state.

Determinants of Coronary Blood Flow & Myocardial Oxygen Supply

Oxygen supply is a function of myocardial delivery and extraction. Since myocardial oxygen extraction is nearly maximal at rest, there is little reserve to meet increased demands; furthermore, the oxygen content of the blood cannot be significantly increased under normal atmospheric conditions. Thus, increased myocardial demands for oxygen in the normal heart are met by augmenting coronary blood flow.

Coronary blood flow is directly related to the perfusion pressure (aortic diastolic pressure) and the duration of diastole. Because coronary flow drops to negligible values during systole, the duration of diastole becomes a limiting factor for myocardial perfusion during tachycardia. Coronary blood flow is inversely proportionate to coronary vascular bed resistance. Resistance is determined by intrinsic factors, including metabolic products and autonomic activity; by various pharmacologic agents; and by the extravascular mechanical compression of the coronary arteries. The site of autoregulation appears to be the arteriolar resistance vessels.

A. Angina of Effort (Classic Angina): When the large coronary arteries are obstructed, as in atherosclerosis, their intraluminal resistance is added to the autoregulatory resistance of the arterioles and contributes significantly to the total coronary arterial resistance to blood flow. The relation between coronary artery stenosis and distal coronary artery bed resistance is thus important in the genesis of effort angina.

In patients with angina of effort, angina threshold—ie, the magnitude of increase in myocardial oxygen demand that induces angina and the capacity to increase coronary blood flow in relation to increased metabolic demand (coronary reserve)—does not vary significantly. In fact, myocardial perfusion and coronary reserve can be enhanced only by revascularization surgery or coronary angioplasty. Pharmacologic agents produce their beneficial effects primarily by decreasing myocardial oxygen requirements. Therefore, beneficial effects of pharmacologic agents are measured as a decrease in the heart rate–blood pressure product at subanginal heart rates or as an increase in the duration of exercise tolerated before onset of angina (Fig 11–5).

B. Variant Angina: The pathogenesis of the variant form of angina pectoris is different from that of classic angina. Variant angina is characterized by cyclic recurrent chest pain at rest that is unrelated to effort but is associated with ST segment elevation on the ECG. Patients with this form of angina frequently have prolonged attacks of chest pain, which sometimes occur at the same time each day. Cardiac arrhythmias of various types occur during anginal attacks in about half of these patients. In some patients, prolonged anginal episodes may culminate in myocardial infarction and sudden death.

The primary decrease in coronary blood flow during variant angina appears to be caused by a marked increase in tone of smooth muscle in the large epicardial coronary arteries (coronary artery spasm) that is unrelated to changes in oxygen demand. Angiographic studies during spontaneous variant angina have documented coronary artery spasm and complete interruption of coronary blood flow. Localized spasm can also be provoked by intravenous injection of vasoconstrictors such as ergonovine; such spasm is usually accompanied by symptoms and electrocardiographic changes similar to those associated with the patient's spontaneous attacks. With relief of angina, restoration of flow and increase in luminal diameter of the arteries occur. The great majority of patients with variant angina also have fixed obstructive coronary artery disease; only a few have normal coronary arteries.

C. Unstable Angina: The term unstable angina applies to angina of changing intensity. The patient population with unstable angina includes individuals with prolonged angina at rest who do not have evidence of myocardial necrosis at the time of initial presentation. In most patients, the syndrome of unstable angina consists of ischemic cardiac pain at rest that is severe enough to warrant hospitalization. Both coro-

nary artery spasm and increased myocardial oxygen demand may be implicated in the pathogenesis of unstable angina.

D. Mixed Angina: In patients with mixed angina, angina occurs at variable levels of exercise. Patients may also experience rest angina with a symptom profile typical of variant angina. Symptoms may be precipitated by emotional stress and exposure to cold. Both increased coronary vascular tone and increased myocardial oxygen requirement have been suggested as underlying mechanisms for mixed angina. Therefore, concomitant reduction in coronary vascular tone (with nitrates or calcium channel blockers) and reduction in myocardial oxygen requirement (with nitrates, beta blockers, or calcium channel blockers) appear to be appropriate therapeutic strategies.

Principles of Therapy of Angina

In addition to modification of the risk factors for coronary atherosclerosis (smoking, hypertension, hyperlipidemia), the treatment of angina and other manifestations of myocardial ischemia is based on reduction of myocardial oxygen demand and increase of coronary blood flow to the potentially ischemic myocardium to restore the balance between myocardial oxygen supply and demand. In classic angina, pharmacologic agents are effective mainly in reducing myocardial oxygen demand; surgical revascularization and angioplasty are the only methods available that restore coronary blood flow and increase oxygen supply. In variant angina, some drugs are effective in preventing and reversing coronary spasm and therefore can increase oxygen supply.

MYOCARDIAL REVASCULARIZATION & TRANSLUMINAL CORONARY ANGIOPLASTY

It is now well established that myocardial revascularization by coronary artery bypass surgery is extremely effective treatment for angina. About 70% of patients become asymptomatic, and another 20% have marked symptomatic relief. In patients with significant left main coronary lesions or with triple coronary vessel disease, better survival statistics have been obtained following coronary artery bypass surgery than with medical therapy. Transluminal coronary angioplasty (percutaneous transluminal coronary angioplasty, PTCA) also provides marked improvement in angina in patients with obstructive coronary artery disease. However, angioplasty can be performed only in a few selected patients with single- or double-vessel disease with proximal lesions. Nevertheless, following successful angioplasty (as with coronary artery bypass surgery), symptomatic relief along with improvement in angina threshold or regional myocardial function occurs in most patients.

In contrast to pharmacologic interventions, coronary artery bypass surgery and coronary artery angioplasty increase the heart rate × pressure product at the appearance of angina as well as exercise tolerance in patients with effort angina. The mechanism for the increased angina threshold is related to enhanced perfusion of the relatively ischemic myocardial segments and improved regional myocardial metabolic function. Furthermore, increased regional perfusion has been documented by myocardial perfusion scintigraphy.

GENERAL MANAGEMENT OF THE PATIENT WITH ANGINA

Both pharmacologic interventions and revascularization or angioplasty are effective for management of the angina syndromes. Therapy is aimed both at providing symptomatic relief and at prolonging life. The principal prognostic determinants are the degree of left ventricular dysfunction, the extent of coronary atherosclerosis, and the severity of myocardial ischemia. In patients with chronic stable angina, the degree of left ventricular dysfunction and the severity of the obstructive coronary artery disease should be determined before a therapeutic plan is offered. Noninvasive investigations such as echocardiography and radioisotope angiography can provide significant information regarding the state of left ventricular function. Similarly, the severity and the extent of coronary atherosclerosis can be assessed in most instances by treadmill exercise tests with or without thallium 201 myocardial scintigraphy. When a high risk of myocardial infarction is suspected, coronary arteriography should be performed. If significant left main coronary artery disease or severe proximal triple-vessel disease is detected, coronary artery bypass surgery is indicated. In the absence of very high risk coronary artery lesions, the pharmacologic approach is preferable. Nitrates are the drugs of choice for the immediate relief of angina. For the long-term management of patients with chronic stable angina, a combination of nitrates and beta blockers provides substantial benefit in most patients. The addition of calcium influx–blocking drugs produces a synergistic effect and should be considered if nitrates and beta blocker therapy fail to produce a satisfactory response. If the manifestations of myocardial ischemia continue despite combined drug therapy, surgical revascularization or angioplasty should be considered.

In patients with unstable angina, immediate therapy should be directed to the relief of rest angina, which can be achieved with aggressive nitrate and beta blocker therapy in approximately 50% of patients. The addition of calcium influx–blocking agents to nitrates and beta blockers will prevent recurrence of rest angina and myocardial ischemia in an even larger proportion of patients. In patients who continue to demonstrate manifestations of myocardial ischemia despite aggressive medical therapy, coronary arteriography should be undertaken with a view to revascularization or angioplasty. In patients who obtain complete relief of angina from pharmacologic interventions, elective coronary arteriography is desirable to determine whether revascularization or angioplasty is necessary or likely to be of benefit.

Because coronary artery spasm appears to be the principal mechanism of variant angina, nitrates and calcium influx–blocking agents should be considered first. In patients with additional obstructive coronary artery disease, beta blockers may also be used concurrently. Patients who fail to respond to these pharmacologic interventions should undergo coronary arteriography to assess the presence and severity of obstructive coronary artery disease. In the absence of fixed obstructive coronary artery lesions, pharmacologic therapy should be continued. If severe fixed obstructive coronary artery lesions are present, revascularization or angioplasty should be considered.

REFERENCES

Abrams J: Nitroglycerin tolerance: Fact or fancy. *Prac Cardiol* 1978;**4**:113.

Alterhog JH, Ekelund LG, Melin AL: Effect of nifedipine on exercise tolerance in patients with angina pectoris. *Eur J Cardiol* 1975;**8**:125.

Bassenge E, Kukovetz WR: Molsidomine. Pages 177–191 in: *New Drugs Annual: Cardiovascular Drugs Vol 2*. Scriabine A (editor). Raven, 1984.

Benson H, McCallie DP Jr: Angina pectoris and the placebo effect. *N Engl J Med* 1979;**300**:1424.

Braunwald E: Mechanism of action of calcium-channel–blocking agents. *N Engl J Med* 1982;**307**:1618.

Bright GE: The effects of nitroglycerin on those engaged in its manufacture. *JAMA* 1914;**62**:201.

Carmichael P, Lieben J: Sudden death in explosives workers. *Arch Environ Health* 1963;**7**:50.

Cauvin C, Loutzenhiser R, Van Breemen C: Mechanisms of calcium antagonist–induced vasodilation. *Annu Rev Pharmacol Toxicol* 1983;**23**:373.

Chatterjee K et al: Improved angina threshold and coronary reserve following direct myocardial revascularization. *Circulation* 1975;**52(2–Suppl 1)**:82.

Cohn PF, Gorlin R: Physiologic and clinical actions of nitroglycerin. *Med Clin North Am* 1974;**58**:407.

Conti CR et al: Unstable angina pectoris: Randomized study of surgical vs. medical therapy. *Am J Cardiol* 1975;**35**:129.

Davidor ME, Mroczek WJ: The effect of sustained release nitroglycerin capsules on anginal frequency and exercise capacity. *Angiology* 1977;**28**:181.

Ganz W, Marcus HS: Failure of intracoronary nitroglycerin to alleviate pacing-induced angina. *Circulation* 1972;**46**:880.

Grunzig A: Transluminal dilation of coronary artery stenosis. *Lancet* 1978;**1**:263.

Hartman PE: Review: Putative mutagens and carcinogens in foods. 1. Nitrate/nitrite ingestion and gastric cancer mortality. *Environ Mutagen* 1983;**5**:111.

Henry PD: Comparative pharmacology of calcium antagonists; Nifedipine, verapamil, and diltiazem. *Am J Cardiol* 1980; **46**:1047.

Hiller LD, Braunwald E: Coronary artery spasm. *N Engl J Med* 1978;**299**:695.

Hoekenga D, Abrams J: Rational medical therapy for stable angina pectoris. *Am J Med* 1984;**76**:309.

Ignarro LJ et al: Mechanisms of vascular smooth muscle relaxation by organic nitrates, nitrites, nitroprusside, and nitric oxide: Evidence for the involvement of S-nitrosothiols as active intermediates. *J Pharmacol Exp Ther* 1981;**218**:739.

Kreye VAW: Direct vasodilators with unknown modes of action: The nitro-compounds and hydralazine. *J Cardiovasc Pharmacol* 1984;**6**:S646.

Kukovetz WR et al: Evidence for cyclic GMP mediated relaxant effects of nitro-compounds in coronary smooth muscle. *Naunyn Schmiedebergs Arch Pharmacol* 1979;**310**:129.

Lawrie GM, Morris GC: Survival after coronary artery bypass surgery in specific patient groups. *Circulation* 1982;**65(Suppl 2)**:43.

Levin RI et al: Nitroglycerin stimulates synthesis of prostacyclin by cultural human endothelial cells. *J Clin Invest* 1981; **67**:762.

Lindenberg BS et al: Efficacy and safety of incremental doses of diltiazem for the treatment of stable angina pectoris. *J Am Coll Cardiol* 1983;**2**:1129.

Livesley B et al: Double blind evaluation of verapamil, propran-olol, and isosorbide dinitrate against placebo in the treatment of angina pectoris. *Br Med J* 1973;**2**:375.

Muller JE, Gunther SJ: Nifedipine therapy for Prinzmetal's angina. *Circulation* 1978;**57**:137.

Reichek N et al: Sustained effects of nitroglycerin ointment in patients with angina pectoris. *Circulation* 1974;**50**:348.

Robinson BF: Relation of heart rate and systolic blood pressure to the onset of pain in angina pectoris. *Circulation* 1967; **35**:1073.

Rouleau JL et al: Mechanism of relief of pacing-induced angina with oral verapamil: Reduced oxygen demand. *Circulation* 1983;**67**:94.

Russek HI: Propranolol and isosorbide dinitrate synergism in angina pectoris. *Am J Cardiol* 1968;**21**:45.

Takaro T et al: The Veterans Administration Cooperative Study of Stable Angina: Current status. *Circulation* 1982;**65(Suppl 2)**:60.

Thadani U et al: Comparison of adrenergic beta-receptor antagonists in angina pectoris. *Br Med J* 1973;**1**:138.

Ulmsten U, Andersson K-E, Forman A: Relaxing effects of nifedipine on the nonpregnant human uterus in vitro and in vivo. *Obstet Gynecol* 1978;**52**:436.

Whitworth CG, Grant MM: Use of nitrate and vasodilators by glaucomatous patients. *Arch Ophthalmol* 1964;**71**:492.

Wyatt HL et al: Effect of graded reductions in coronary perfusion on regional and total cardiac function. *Am J Cardiol* 1975;**36**:185.

12

Cardiac Glycosides & Other Drugs Used in the Treatment of Congestive Heart Failure

Bertram G. Katzung, MD, PhD, & William W. Parmley, MD

Congestive heart failure occurs when the cardiac output is inadequate to provide the oxygen needed by the body. The cardiac glycosides comprise a group of steroid compounds that have complex primary effects on the mechanical and electrical functions of the heart. They also have effects on smooth muscle and other tissues. The principal therapeutic effect in congestive heart failure is an increase in cardiac contractility (positive inotropic action). Nevertheless, there is some doubt regarding the long-term efficacy of cardiac glycosides in patients with heart failure. On the other hand, there is general agreement that the commonly used glycosides have a narrow margin of safety and that less toxic compounds with positive inotropic actions are needed. Several agents are candidates for this role, including **amrinone** and certain **β-adrenoceptor stimulants.** Furthermore, clinical research has shown that in some types of congestive failure, reduction of vascular tone by unloading the stressed myocardium gives effective relief. Thus certain vasodilators have been used with considerable success. Such agents include **aminophylline** (which also has a positive inotropic action), **nitroprusside, nitroglycerin, captopril,** and **α-adrenoceptor antagonists.**

This chapter presents the basic pharmacology of the cardiac glycosides and amrinone, agents with primary cardiac inotropic effects. The clinical management of congestive heart failure with these agents and with vasodilators and diuretics is discussed in the second portion of the chapter.

I. BASIC PHARMACOLOGY OF DRUGS USED IN CONGESTIVE HEART FAILURE

DIGITALIS

Medicinal plants containing cardiac glycosides were known to the ancient Egyptians 3000 years ago, but these agents were used erratically and with variable success until the 18th century, when Willliam Withering, an English physician and botanist, pub-

lished a monograph describing the clinical effects of an extract of the foxglove plant (*Digitalis purpurea*, a major source of these agents). His book, *An Account of the Foxglove and Some of Its Medical Uses: With Practical Remarks on Dropsy and Other Diseases*, published in 1785, described in detail the indications for the use of cardiac glycosides and offered cautionary remarks about their toxicity. Unfortunately, many of Withering's recommendations were ignored in the subsequent enthusiastic use of these agents. It was not until about 60 years ago that the physiologic basis for the action of digitalis (the positive inotropic response) was clearly demonstrated and more rational use of the agents was reestablished.

Chemistry

All of the commonly used cardiac steroids, or cardenolides—of which **digoxin** may be considered the prototype—combine a steroid nucleus with an unsaturated lactone ring at the 17 position and a series of sugars linked to carbon 3 of the nucleus (Fig 12–1). Because they lack an easily ionizable group, their solubility is not pH-dependent.

Sources of these drugs include white and purple foxglove (*Digitalis lanata* and *D purpurea*), Mediterranean sea onion (squill), *Strophanthus gratus*, oleander, lily of the valley, milkweed, and numerous other tropical and temperate zone plants. During larval development, monarch butterflies concentrate cardenolides in their bodies from ingested milkweed—a factor that apparently protects adult butterflies from predation by birds: Since the cardenolides are potent emetics in most birds, the birds learn to avoid these butterflies. Certain toads have skin glands capable of elaborating **bufadienolides,** which differ from the cardenolides only in having a 6-membered lactone ring at the 17 position.

Structure-activity studies indicate that the lactone ring and the steroid nucleus are essential for activity. The other substituents—especially the sugar molecules in the 3 position—influence pharmacokinetic variables, including absorption, half-life, and metabolism. There is no clinical evidence that any of the natural cardenolides differs from the others in therapeutic index or maximal efficacy.

These agents are very stable if protected from

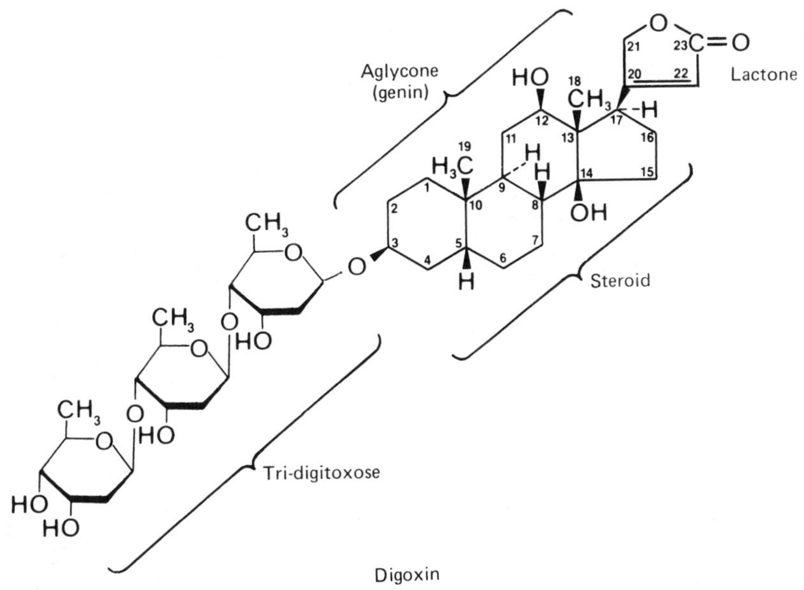

Figure 12–1. Structure of digoxin, a typical cardiac glycoside.

strong light and low pH. Their shelf-life is reported to be 1–5 years, depending on conditions of storage.

Pharmacokinetics

A. Absorption and Distribution: Cardenolides have both lipophilic (steroid nucleus) and hydrophilic (lactone ring, hydroxyl, sugar) groups. The balance of these 2 factors has an important effect on absorption, metabolism, and excretion, as shown by comparison of 3 of the most important agents: **digoxin, digitoxin, and ouabain** (Table 12–1). As noted in the table, digoxin is fairly well absorbed after oral administration. However, because of its very narrow safety margin, even minor variations in bioavailability could cause serious toxicity or loss of effect. In fact, product formulation (factors in manufacture of the tablets) can modify the bioavailability of digoxin. As a result, digoxin preparations must pass absorption tests before they can be marketed. Ouabain, because it is never used by the oral route, and digitoxin, because it is well absorbed under almost all circumstances, are not subject to this restriction. Digitalis leaf, a standardized

Table 12–1. Properties of 3 typical cardiac glycosides.

	Ouabain*	Digoxin	Digitoxin
Lipid solubility (oil/water coefficient)	Low	Medium	High
Oral availability (percentage absorbed)	0	75	>90
Half-life in body (hours)	21	40	168
Plasma protein binding (percentage bound)	0	20–40	>90
Percentage metabolized	0	<20	>80
Volume of distribution (L/kg)	18	6.3	0.6

*Ouabain is no longer in common clinical use.

preparation of the powdered plant material, contains chiefly digitoxin. Except for dosage, its properties are almost identical to those of digitoxin. Beta-methyl-digoxin, a semisynthetic derivative of digoxin, is almost completely absorbed from the gut and is metabolized to digoxin in the body.

Once absorbed into the blood, all cardiac glycosides are widely distributed to tissues, including the central nervous system. The highest concentrations—for digoxin, 10–50 times higher than plasma—are found in heart, kidney, and liver.

B. Metabolism and Excretion: Digoxin is not extensively metabolized in humans but is largely excreted unchanged by the kidneys. Its elimination half-life is significantly prolonged in patients with renal impairment, and equations are available for adjusting digoxin dosage on the basis of creatinine clearance (eg, see Jelliffe reference). In contrast, digitoxin is metabolized in the liver and excreted into the gut via the bile. Cardioactive metabolites as well as unchanged digitoxin can then be reabsorbed from the intestine, thus establishing an enterohepatic circulation that contributes to the very long half-life of this agent. Renal impairment does not significantly prolong the half-life of digitoxin, so this drug may occasionally be useful in patients with erratic or rapidly failing renal function. On the other hand, a variety of hepatic enzyme–inducing drugs (see Chapter 3) can reduce the blood level of digitoxin by accelerating its metabolism. Ouabain must be given parenterally and is therefore used only for acute therapy and rarely for more than a few doses. It is metabolized very little and excreted primarily by the kidney.

Pharmacodynamics

Digitalis has multiple direct and indirect cardiovascular effects, with both therapeutic and toxic (arrhythmogenic) consequences. In addition, it has undesirable effects on the central nervous system and gut. A small direct renal (diuretic) effect has been demonstrated but is probably of no clinical significance.

At the molecular level, all therapeutically useful cardiac glycosides *inhibit* **Na+,K+-ATPase,** the membrane-bound enzyme associated with the "sodium pump." Very low concentrations of these drugs have occasionally been observed to *stimulate* the enzyme. In contrast, inhibition over most of the dose range has been extensively documented in all tissues studied. Since the sodium pump is necessary for maintenance of normal resting potential in most excitable cells, it is generally believed that at least a portion of the toxicity of digitalis is caused by this enzyme-inhibiting action. It is also probable that this action is partly or wholly responsible for the therapeutic effect (positive inotropy) in the heart. Other molecular-level effects of digitalis have been studied in the heart and are discussed below.

A. Cardiac Effects: For clarity, the effects of digitalis on mechanical and on electrical function are discussed separately, but it must be realized that these changes occur simultaneously.

1. Mechanical effects–The therapeutic direct action of cardiac glycosides on mechanical function is to increase the intensity of the "active state" of the contractile apparatus—the interaction of the actin and myosin filaments of the cardiac sarcomere (Fig 12–2). This increased intensity is caused by increase in the free calcium concentration in the vicinity of the contractile proteins during systole, ie, by facilitation of excitation-contraction coupling. The precise mechanism by which this facilitation occurs is not fully understood. It may well be the result of inhibition of ATPase referred to above; reduced transport of sodium out of the cell (at ① in Fig 12–2) results in an increase in intracellular sodium. This increase reduces the normal transport of calcium out of the cell via the Na+/Ca2+ exchange mechanism (at ①ₐ in Fig 12–2), resulting in an increase in intracellular calcium. A second possible mechanism is facilitation of calcium entry into the cell through the voltage-gated

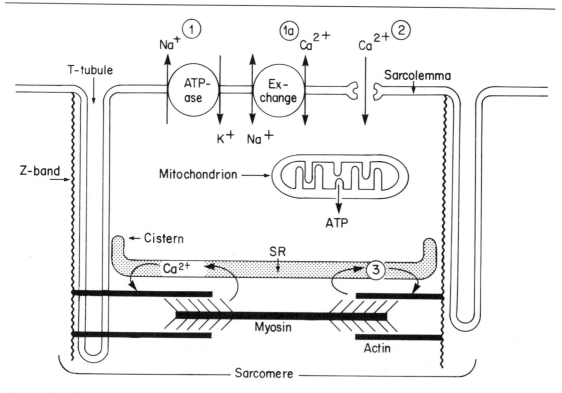

Figure 12–2. Schematic diagram of a sarcomere, the functional unit of a myocardial cell, with the possible sites of action of digitalis. Normal function involves the transduction of chemical energy (ATP, from the mitochondria) into mechanical shortening and tension development by the sliding of the thin actin filaments over the thicker myosin filaments. This reaction is brought about by an increase in free calcium ions in the vicinity of the actin strand. This calcium is released from the enlarged cisternae on the sarcoplasmic reticulum, the organelle that also sequesters calcium during relaxation. Release of the stored calcium is linked to membrane electrical activity (excitation) by "trigger calcium," which enters through membrane channels and thus couples excitation to contraction. Removal of excess calcium requires its exchange for sodium across the cell membrane and probably active pumping as well. Possible sites of digitalis action include ① Na+,K+-ATPase (the sodium pump), together with ①ₐ, the Na+/Ca2+ exchanger; ② the ionic channel permeable to calcium; and ③ the sarcoplasmic reticulum (SR).

calcium channel during the plateau of the action potential (at ② in Fig 12–2). A third hypothesis is that digitalis may increase the release of stored calcium from the sarcoplasmic reticulum (at ③ in Fig 12–2). It is possible that all 3 mechanisms participate in the action of digitalis.

The net result of the action of therapeutic concentrations of a cardiac glycoside is a distinctive increase in cardiac contractility (Fig 12–3). In isolated myocardial preparations, the rate of development of tension and of relaxation are both increased, with little or no change in time to peak tension. The duration of the contractile response is neither shortened (as in the case of β-adrenoceptor stimulation) nor prolonged (as in the case of methylxanthines such as theophylline). These effects occur in both normal and failing myocardium, but in the intact animal or patient the responses are modified by cardiovascular reflexes and the pathophysiology of congestive heart failure.

2. Electrical effects–The effects of digitalis on the electrical properties of the heart in the intact organism are a complex mixture of direct and indirect actions. Direct actions on the membranes of cardiac cells follow a well-defined progression: an early, brief prolongation of the action potential with an increase in membrane resistance, followed by a protracted period of shortening of the action potential (especially the plateau phase) associated with a decrease in membrane resistance (Fig 12–3). This decrease in membrane resistance is probably the result of increased intracellular calcium, which is known to increase membrane potassium conductance. The latter change would result in action potential shortening. (See Chapter 13 for a discussion of the effects of ionic conductances on the action potential.) All of these effects can

be observed in the absence of overt toxicity. Shortening of the action potential by direct drug action may contribute to the shortening of atrial and ventricular refractoriness (Table 12–2). With more toxic concentrations, resting membrane potential is reduced (made less negative) as a result of inhibition of the sodium pump and reduced intracellular potassium. As toxicity progresses, oscillatory depolarizing afterpotentials appear following normally evoked action potentials (Fig 12–3). The afterpotentials (also known as "delayed afterdepolarizations") are associated with overloading of the intracellular calcium stores and oscillations in the free intracellular calcium ion concentration. When below threshold, these afterpotentials may interfere with normal conduction because of the further reduction of resting potential. Eventually, an afterpotential may reach threshold, eliciting an action potential (premature ventricular depolarization or "ectopic beat") that is coupled to the preceding normal one. If afterpotentials in the Purkinje conducting system regularly reach threshold in this way, bigeminy will be recorded on the ECG. With further toxic deterioration, each afterpotential-evoked action potential will itself elicit a sizable afterpotential, and a self-sustaining arrhythmia (ventricular tachycardia) will be established. If allowed to progress, such a tachycardia may deteriorate into ventricular fibrillation.

Indirect actions of cardiac glycosides on the heart involve the autonomic nervous system and occur throughout the therapeutic and toxic dose ranges. In the lower portion of the dose range, cardioselective **parasympathomimetic** effects predominate. In fact, these atropine-blockable effects are probably responsible for a significant portion of the early electrical effects of digitalis (Table 12–2). This action involves

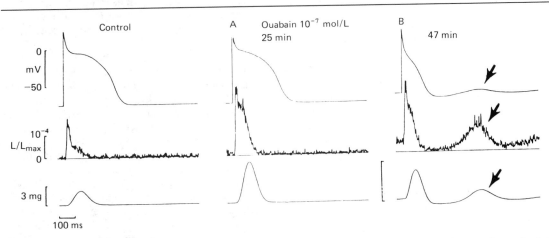

Figure 12–3. Effects of a cardiac glycoside, ouabain, on isolated cardiac tissue. The top tracing shows action potentials evoked during the control period, early in the "therapeutic" phase, and later, when toxicity is present. The middle tracing shows the light emitted by the calcium-detecting protein aequorin (relative to the maximum possible, L/L$_{max}$) and is roughly proportionate to the free intracellular calcium concentration. The bottom tracing records the tension elicited by the action potentials. The early phase of ouabain action (A) shows a slight shortening of action potential and a marked increase in free intracellular calcium concentration and contractile tension. The toxic phase (B) is associated with depolarization of the resting potential, a marked shortening of the action potential, and the appearance of an oscillatory depolarization, calcium increment, and contraction (arrows). (Unpublished data kindly provided by P Hess and H Gil Wier.)

Table 12–2. Actions of digitalis on cardiac electrical function.
(Dominant effects in boldface italic.)

Effect	Atria	Atrioventricular Node	Ventricles, Purkinje System
Direct	Shortens refractory period.	Increases refractory period.	Shortens refractory period, or no significant effect.
	No significant effect on conduction velocity.	Decreases conduction velocity.	Decreases conduction velocity.
	Decreases normal automaticity; increases abnormal automaticity.	Increases or decreases normal automaticity; increases abnormal automaticity.	Increases or decreases normal automaticity; *increases abnormal automaticity.*
Indirect (ANS) 1. Vagal	*Shortens refractory period.*	*Increases refractory period.*	
	Decreases sinoatrial rate.	*Decreases conduction velocity.*	
2. Sympathetic (toxic doses)	Increases sinoatrial rate.	Shortens refractory period.	*Increases abnormal automaticity.*
		Junctional extrasystoles.	
Effect on ECG and rhythm Early	P wave changes.	*Lengthens PR interval.*	*ST depression, T wave inversion.*
Progressive toxicity	Premature atrial beats.	Second- or third-degree block.	*Ventricular premature depolarizations.*
	Atrial fibrillation.	Junctional tachycardia.	Bigeminy.
			Ventricular tachycardia.
			Ventricular fibrillation.

sensitization of the baroreceptors, central vagal stimulation, and facilitation of muscarinic transmission at the cardiac muscle cell. Because cholinergic innervation is much richer in the atria, these actions affect atrial and atrioventricular nodal function more than Purkinje or ventricular function. Some of the cholinomimetic effects are useful in the treatment of certain arrhythmias. At toxic levels, sympathetic outflow is increased by digitalis. This effect is not essential for typical cardenolide toxicity but sensitizes the myocardium and exaggerates all of the toxic effects of the drug.

The most common cardiac manifestations of glycoside **toxicity** include atrioventricular junctional rhythm, premature ventricular depolarizations, bigeminal rhythm, and second-degree atrioventricular blockade. However, it is claimed that digitalis can cause virtually every variety of arrhythmia. The membrane cardiotoxicity of digitalis was described above as involving resting depolarization (due to sodium pump inhibition) and oscillatory afterdepolarizations (caused by overload of intracellular calcium). The first effect may be responsible for a portion of the conduction abnormalities such as atrioventricular block. The second effect is probably responsible for most glycoside arrhythmias involving abnormal automaticity, including premature ventricular depolarizations, bigeminy, and ventricular tachycardia.

B. Effects on Other Organs: Cardiac glycosides affect all excitable tissues, including smooth muscle and the central nervous system. The mechanism of these effects has not been fully explored but probably involves the inhibition of Na^+,K^+-ATPase in these tissues. The depolarization resulting from depression of the sodium pump would be expected to increase spontaneous activity both in neurons and in smooth muscle cells. In addition, an increase in intracellular calcium could predictably increase smooth muscle tone. However, it should be remembered that in most cases of congestive heart failure successfully treated with digitalis, a *decrease* in vascular tone is the net effect, resulting from a beneficial reduction of sympathetic tone (see below).

The gastrointestinal tract is the most common site of digitalis effects outside the heart. These actions include anorexia, nausea, vomiting, and diarrhea. This toxicity may be partially caused by direct effects on the gastrointestinal tract but is also the result of central nervous system actions, including chemoreceptor trigger zone stimulation.

Central nervous system effects commonly include vagal and chemoreceptor zone stimulation, as noted above. Much less often, disorientation and hallucinations—especially in the elderly—and visual disturbances are noted. The last effect may include aberrations of color perception. Agitation and even convulsions are occasionally reported in patients taking digitalis.

Gynecomastia and galactorrhea are rare effects reported in men taking digitalis; it is not certain whether these effects represent a peripheral estrogenic action of these steroid drugs or a manifestation of hypothalamic stimulation.

ATPase-dependent transport processes such as

aqueous humor and cerebrospinal fluid production, as well as sodium reabsorption in the kidney, can be shown experimentally to be inhibited by cardenolides. These effects are of no clinical significance.

C. Interactions With Potassium, Calcium, and Magnesium: The concentrations of potassium and calcium in the extracellular compartment (usually measured as serum K^+ and Ca^{2+}) have important effects on sensitivity to digitalis. Potassium and digitalis interact in 2 ways. First, they inhibit each other's binding to Na^+,K^+-ATPase; therefore, hyperkalemia reduces the enzyme-inhibiting actions of cardiac glycosides, whereas hypokalemia facilitates these actions. Second, abnormal cardiac automaticity is inhibited by hyperkalemia (see Chapter 13); thus, moderately increased extracellular K^+ reduces the effects of digitalis, especially the toxic effects. Calcium ion facilitates the toxic actions of cardiac glycosides by accelerating the overloading of intracellular calcium stores that appears to be responsible for digitalis-induced abnormal automaticity. The effects of magnesium ion, although not as well documented, appear to be directly opposite to those of calcium. These interactions mandate careful evaluation of serum electrolytes in patients with digitalis-induced arrhythmias.

OTHER POSITIVE INOTROPIC DRUGS USED IN HEART FAILURE

Bipyridines, several agents related to the methylxanthines, and a group of β-adrenoceptor stimulants are under investigation as digitalis substitutes. Aminophylline, a traditional methylxanthine compound, is sometimes used in the treatment of acute pulmonary edema; it is of no value in the treatment of chronic congestive heart failure.

BIPYRIDINES

Amrinone and **milrinone** are new bipyridine compounds that can be given orally or parenterally. They have elimination half-lives of 2–3 hours, with 10–40% being excreted in the urine.

Amrinone

Pharmacodynamics

The bipyridines increase myocardial contractility without inhibiting Na^+,K^+-ATPase or activating adrenoceptors. They appear to increase inward calcium flux during the action potential and may alter the intracellular movements of calcium as well. Biochemical

studies suggest that at least a part of their action results from inhibition of phosphodiesterase, an action similar to that of the methylxanthines. This effect would be expected to increase cAMP.

Amrinone and milrinone also have some peripheral vasodilator effects (like the methylxanthines) which may be partially responsible for increased cardiac output in patients with heart failure. When given to such patients, the bipyridines increase cardiac output and reduce pulmonary capillary wedge pressure. There is little change in the heart rate or arterial pressure. Although the acute effects are clearly beneficial, there is less certainty about sustained beneficial long-term effects.

The toxicity of the bipyridines is not fully known. Amrinone causes a relatively high incidence of nausea and vomiting; thrombocytopenia and liver enzyme changes have been reported in a smaller but significant number of patients. It is available for parenteral short-term use only. Milrinone, which has considerably higher cardiac potency, may have less toxicity than amrinone since it is used in much smaller dosage. It is still investigational. Both drugs are much less likely to cause cardiac arrhythmias than is digitalis.

METHYLXANTHINE ANALOGS

These investigational agents, typified by **sulmazole (Vardax,** AR-L-115-BS), are related to theophylline and have cardiac effects very similar to those of the bipyridines. Like the latter, they inhibit cardiac phosphodiesterase and appear to increase cAMP. They are claimed to produce less tachycardia and fewer arrhythmias than theophylline. Little is known about their long-term efficacy and toxicity in patients with congestive heart failure.

BETA-ADRENOCEPTOR STIMULANTS

The general pharmacology of these agents is discussed in Chapter 8. The search for positive inotropic drugs with less arrhythmogenic potential than digitalis and less tendency to increase heart rate than isoproterenol has led to the development of β_1-selective agents. At the same time, the successful use of vasodilators in congestive heart failure has resulted in an interest in selective β_2 agents for this condition.

Selective β_1-agonists that have been studied in patients with heart failure include **dobutamine** and **prenalterol.** These drugs produce an increase in cardiac output together with a decrease in ventricular filling pressure. Some tachycardia and increase in myocardial oxygen consumption have been reported. Thus, although these agents clearly increase cardiac contractility, it is unclear what net benefit they may have in patients with ischemic heart disease. The potential for producing angina or arrhythmias in such patients must be considered, as well as tachyphylaxis that accompanies the chronic use of any beta stimulant. Intermittent dobutamine infusion may benefit some patients with chronic heart failure (see Liang reference).

Beta$_2$-selective agonists such as **salbutamol** and **pirbuterol** have also been investigated in patients with congestive heart failure. These drugs act by relaxing smooth muscle and are effective vasodilators in some patients. They appear to be useful in increasing cardiac output and reducing pulmonary wedge pressure in such patients. How much of their effect is due to inotropic stimulation (an effect on the cardiac β_1 receptor) is unclear at present.

II. CLINICAL PHARMACOLOGY OF DRUGS USED IN CONGESTIVE HEART FAILURE

PATHOPHYSIOLOGY OF HEART FAILURE

Congestive heart failure is a syndrome with multiple causes that may involve the right ventricle, the left ventricle, or both. Its cardinal feature is that cardiac output falls short of what is required for normal tissue perfusion. Cardiac output in congestive heart failure is usually below the normal range. An intrinsic biochemical defect results in decreased cardiac contractility, which is usually responsive to positive inotropic drugs. This is typical of chronic failure resulting from coronary artery disease or hypertension or acute failure resulting from myocardial infarction. Rarely, "high-output" failure may occur. In this condition, the demands of the body are so great that even increased cardiac output is insufficient. High-output failure can result from hyperthyroidism, beriberi, anemia, and arteriovenous shunts. This form of failure responds poorly to positive inotropic agents.

The primary signs and symptoms of all types of congestive heart failure include tachycardia, decreased exercise tolerance and shortness of breath, peripheral and pulmonary edema, and cardiomegaly. Decreased exercise tolerance with rapid muscular fatigue is the major *direct* consequence of diminished cardiac output. The other manifestations result from the attempts by the body to compensate for the intrinsic cardiac defect.

Extrinsic reflex compensation involves 2 major mechanisms, as described in Chapter 5 and displayed in Fig 5–6. These are the sympathetic nervous system and the renin-angiotensin-aldosterone hormonal response. Increased sympathetic outflow causes tachycardia, increased cardiac contractility, and increased vascular tone—especially venous tone. Elevation of venous tone results in increased ventricular filling pressure, dilatation of the heart, and increased fiber stretch. Increased aldosterone secretion results in sodium and water retention with increased blood volume and, ultimately, edema.

The most important *intrinsic* compensatory mechanism is myocardial hypertrophy. This increase in muscle mass helps to maintain cardiac performance in the face of adverse effects such as pressure or volume overload, loss of tissue (myocardial infarction), or decrease in cardiac contractility.

Pathophysiology of Cardiac Performance

Cardiac performance is a function of 4 primary factors.

A. Preload: Preload refers to the diastolic loading conditions of the heart, eg, left atrial pressure (or pulmonary wedge pressure) for the left ventricle and right atrial pressure for the right. These are the "filling pressures" of their respective ventricles. The effect of altered preload on cardiovascular performance is illustrated in Fig 12–4. When some measure of left ventricular performance such as stroke volume or stroke work is plotted as a function of left ventricular filling pressure, the resulting curve is termed the **left ventricular function curve.** The ascending limb (below 15 mm Hg filling pressure) represents the classic Frank-Starling relation. Beyond approximately 15 mm Hg, there is a plateau of performance. Preloads greater than 20–25 mm Hg result in pulmonary congestion. As noted above, preload is usually increased in heart failure because of increased blood volume and venous tone. Reduction of high filling pressure is the goal of salt restriction and diuretic therapy in congestive heart failure.

B. Afterload: Afterload is the resistance against which the heart must pump blood. Systemic vascular resistance is frequently increased in patients with congestive heart failure. As cardiac output falls in chronic failure, there is a reflex increase in systemic vascular resistance, mediated in part by increased sympathetic outflow and circulating catecholamines. However, elevated vascular resistance may further reduce cardiac

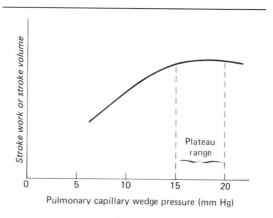

Figure 12–4. Ventricular function curve illustrating the relationship between stroke volume and left atrial (pulmonary capillary wedge) pressure. There is an increase in left ventricular performance up to a left ventricular filling pressure of about 15–20 mm Hg. At higher filling pressures, pulmonary congestion and dyspnea ensue.

ouput by increasing resistance to ejection. This sets the stage for the use of drugs that reduce arteriolar tone in congestive heart failure.

C. Contractility: Contractility is the vigor of contraction of heart muscle. In patients with chronic low-output failure, the primary defect appears to be a reduction in the intrinsic contractility of the myocardium. As contractility decreases, there is a reduction in the velocity of muscle shortening and the rate of intraventricular pressure development (dP/dt). However, the heart is still capable of an increase in contractility in response to inotropic drugs. Thus, agents such as digitalis and amrinone may be helpful in improving the depressed cardiac output.

D. Heart Rate: The heart rate is a major determinant of cardiac output. As the intrinsic function of the heart decreases in failure and stroke volume diminishes, an increase in heart rate through β-adrenoceptor activation is the first compensatory mechanism that comes into play to maintain cardiac output.

Pathophysiology of the Peripheral Vasculature in Congestive Heart Failure

The increase in systemic resistance that occurs at the arteriolar level is due to many factors. First, there is increased activity of the sympathetic nervous system, which increases resistance by α-adrenoceptor activation. Increase in plasma catecholamines is generally related to the severity of the heart failure. There is also an excessive increase in adrenergic tone during exercise, which frequently leads to a marked rise in vascular resistance.

Activation of the renin-angiotensin-aldosterone system in heart failure has also been mentioned above. Angiotensin II is a potent arteriolar vasoconstrictor that directly increases vascular resistance. Furthermore, angiotensin II facilitates sympathetic outflow. As a result of these vasoconstrictor effects and retention of sodium, congestive heart failure is associated with increased wall stiffness in peripheral arteries.

The distribution of blood to various organs changes in congestive heart failure. As cardiac output decreases, renal blood flow and urine output are also decreased. On the other hand, regional circulations with powerful autoregulatory mechanisms (like the cerebral and coronary beds) tend to maintain their blood flow in spite of moderate reductions of arterial pressure and cardiac output. As output further diminishes, vascular regions such as the skin and splanchnic bed become vasoconstricted, and blood is thus preferentially shunted to vital organs.

The venous system holds 70–75% of the blood volume and thus serves as the major capacitance or storage system for the peripheral vascular system. In congestive heart failure, there is an increase in venous tone, caused by increased sympathetic tone and circulating catecholamines, as described above. This compensatory mechanism maintains venous return to the heart but may thereby further overload the right ventricle and the pulmonary circulation. For this reason, vasodilators that selectively dilate veins (eg, nitro-

glycerin) may be useful to redistribute blood in the vascular tree and reduce right and left atrial pressures. This effect may be particularly dramatic in patients with acute left heart failure in whom venodilators can promptly relieve the signs and symptoms of pulmonary congestion.

Important changes also occur in cardiovascular reflexes. Carotid, aortic, and left atrial pressure and stretch receptors are useful homeostatic mechanisms for maintaining an appropriate arterial pressure. In heart failure, reflex effects from these receptors may be blunted. This results in less tachycardia, for example, when arterial pressure is reduced with vasodilator drugs.

DIGITALIS IN CONGESTIVE HEART FAILURE

Because it has a moderate but persistent positive inotropic effect, digitalis can, in theory, reverse all the signs and symptoms of congestive heart failure. In an appropriate case, digitalis increases stroke work and cardiac output. The increased output eliminates the stimuli evoking increased sympathetic outflow, and both heart rate and venous tone diminish. With decreased end-diastolic fiber tension (the result of increased systolic ejection and decreased filling pressure), heart size and oxygen demand decrease. Finally, increased renal blood flow improves glomerular filtration and reduces aldosterone-driven sodium reabsorption. Thus, edema fluid can be excreted, further reducing ventricular preload and the danger of pulmonary edema. It is important to note that the cardiac glycosides have the same effect on contractility in normal as in failing muscle, yet the actions of the drug in normal subjects and patients with congestive heart failure are quite different, owing to the very different reflex responses involved. In normal persons, digitalis increases cardiac contractility and ejection fraction, but homeostatic processes prevent any significant increase in cardiac output. Decreased heart rate and increased afterload are 2 contributing factors.

Administration & Dosage

Chronic treatment of a patient with digitalis requires careful attention to pharmacokinetics. Because of their long half-lives (Table 12–3), these agents accumulate in the body. According to the rules set forth in Chapter 3, it will take 3–4 half-lives to approach steady-state total body load when given at a constant dosing rate, ie, approximately 1 week for digoxin and 1 month for digitoxin. Since it is very important not to exceed the therapeutic range of plasma digitalis concentration, such a slow approach to "digitalization" is the safest dosing technique. If a more rapid effect is required, digitalization can be achieved quickly with a large loading dose (divided into 3 or 4 portions and given over 24–36 hours) followed by a maintenance dose. Typical doses used in adults are given in Table 12–3. It is essential that the patient be examined before

Table 12–3. Clinical use of cardiac glycosides. (These values are appropriate for adults with normal renal and hepatic function.)

	Digoxin	Digitoxin
Half-life	40 hours	168 hours
Therapeutic plasma concentration	0.5–2 ng/mL	10–25 ng/mL
Daily dose (slow loading or maintenance)	0.125–0.5 mg	0.05–0.2 mg
Rapid digitalizing dose	0.5–0.75 mg every 8 hours for 3 doses	0.2–0.4 mg every 12 hours for 3 doses
Time to peak effect	3–6 hours	6–12 hours

each dose when using the rapid (3-dose) method of digitalization. Sensitive plasma digoxin radioimmunoassays are available at most medical centers and should be used when patient response is not as predicted from the dosing schedule.

Interactions

Important drug interactions must be considered in patients taking cardiac glycosides. All such patients are at risk of developing serious cardiac arrhythmias if hypokalemia develops, as in diuretic therapy or diarrhea. Furthermore, patients taking digoxin are at risk if given quinidine, which displaces digoxin from tissue binding sites, markedly decreasing its volume of distribution. Quinidine may also depress renal digoxin clearance. The plasma level of the glycoside may double within a few days after beginning quinidine therapy, and toxic effects may become manifest. A similar interaction with other drugs, including nonsteroidal anti-inflammatory agents and calcium channel–blocking agents, has been reported, but clinically significant effects have not been demonstrated in humans. Quinidine does not alter volume of distribution or protein binding of digitoxin. However, it may prolong the half-life of this glycoside. Finally, agents that release catecholamines may sensitize the myocardium to digitalis-induced arrhythmias.

Reduced responsiveness to cardiac glycosides may be due to intractably severe disease or patient noncompliance. In patients concurrently taking cholestyramine (Chapter 33), digitalis absorption is reduced. The digitalis dose required for therapeutic effect must usually be increased in hyperthyroid patients because of reduction in elimination half-life.

Other Clinical Uses of Digitalis

Digitalis is useful in the management of atrial arrhythmias because of its cardioselective parasympathomimetic effects. In atrial flutter, the depressant effect of the drug on atrioventricular conduction will help control an excessively high ventricular rate. The effects of the drug on the atrial musculature may convert flutter to fibrillation, with a further decrease in ventricular rate. In atrial fibrillation, the same "vagomimetic" action helps to control ventricular rate, thereby improving ventricular filling and increasing cardiac output indirectly as well as through its ino-

tropic effect. Traditionally, digitalis was given prior to the administration of quinidine when quinidine was used to convert atrial fibrillation to normal sinus rhythm (see also Chapter 13). The atrioventricular depressant effect of the cardiac glycoside counteracts the antimuscarinic action of quinidine, which could otherwise lead to an undesirable increase in ventricular rate. Because quinidine increases the plasma concentration and toxicity of digoxin, this use of the latter drug requires caution. Digitalis is also valuable in the control of paroxysmal atrial and atrioventricular nodal tachycardia. Oral or, if necessary, cautious intravenous administration of digoxin may abruptly terminate such attacks, probably as the result of its vagomimetic action.

Although it has been recommended in the past, digitalis is not the drug of choice in the therapy of arrhythmias associated with Wolff-Parkinson-White syndrome, because it increases the probability of conduction of arrhythmic atrial impulses through the alternative rapidly conducting atrioventricular pathway. It is explicitly contraindicated in Wolff-Parkinson-White patients with atrial fibrillation (see Chapter 13).

Toxicity

In spite of its recognized hazards, digitalis is still a widely and overused drug. In a large multicenter study, 17–27% of patients admitted for all medical conditions were taking digitalis on admission, and 5–25% of the identified group showed evidence of toxicity requiring at least temporary cessation of digitalis therapy.

Therapy of digitalis toxicity manifested as visual changes or gastrointestinal disturbances generally requires no more than withholding the drug. If cardiac arrhythmia is present and can definitely be ascribed to digitalis, more vigorous therapy may be necessary. Electrolyte status should be corrected if abnormal (see p 143). For occasional premature ventricular depolarizations or brief runs of bigeminy, oral potassium supplementation and withdrawal of the glycoside may be sufficient. If the arrhythmia is more serious, parenteral potassium and antiarrhythmic drugs may be required. Of the available antiarrhythmic agents, lidocaine, phenytoin, and propranolol are favored, although quinidine and verapamil can also be shown to be effective. Serum potassium levels and the ECG should be monitored during therapy of digitalis toxicity. In very severe digitalis intoxication (which usually involves suicidal overdose), serum potassium will already be elevated at the time of diagnosis. Furthermore, antiarrhythmic agents administered in this setting may lead to cardiac arrest. Such patients are best treated with digitalis antibodies or "Fab fragments" of such antibodies. Digoxin-specific antibody is available in many centers.

Digitalis-induced arrhythmias are frequently made worse by cardioversion; this therapy should be reserved for ventricular fibrillation if the arrhythmia is glycoside-induced.

MANAGEMENT OF
CHRONIC HEART FAILURE

The major steps in the management of patients with chronic heart failure are outlined in Table 12–4. Reduction of cardiac work is a traditional form of therapy that is extemely helpful in most cases. It can be accomplished by reducing activity levels, weight reduction, and—especially important—control of hypertension. Sodium restriction is the next important step. Despite the availability of potent diuretics one should advise patients about the necessity for salt restriction and encourage them to avoid excess salt through dietary restraint.

In patients without severe edema, some authorities recommend treatment with a positive inotropic agent (digitalis) as the next step. However, considerable evidence has accumulated against the universal efficacy of digitalis in patients with heart failure who are in normal sinus rhythm. Therefore, most clinicians prefer to start drug therapy with a diuretic, even in patients with minimal visible edema.

Diuretic therapy should be started with one of the thiazides, switching to more efficacious agents as required. Furosemide and ethacrynic acid are very efficacious diuretics that should be reserved for patients with resistant edema. Sodium loss causes secondary loss of potassium, which is particularly hazardous if the patient is to be given digitalis. Therefore, serum electrolytes should be checked periodically in patients so treated. Hypokalemia can be treated with potassium supplementation or through the addition of potassium-sparing diuretics (Chapter 14).

When a positive inotropic drug is to be used in chronic heart failure, a cardiac glycoside will be chosen. It should be emphasized again that digitalis is a dangerous agent, and only about 50% of patients with normal sinus rhythm will have documentable relief of congestive failure. Better results are obtained in patients with atrial fibrillation. If the decision is made to use a cardiac glycoside, digoxin is the one chosen in the great majority of cases. (As noted in the first portion of this chapter, other glycosides are seldom needed.) When symptoms are mild, slow digitalization (Table 12–3) is safest and just as effective as the rapid method. If symptoms are moderately severe, the rapid oral method may be used, but the patient should be examined before each dose with particular attention to his cardiac rhythm. An ECG should be recorded if

Table 12–4. Steps in the treatment of chronic heart failure.

1. Reduce workload of the heart.
   a. Limit activity level.
   b. Reduce weight.
   c. Control hypertension.
2. Restrict sodium.
3. Restrict water (rarely required).
4. Diuretics.
5. Digitalis.
6. Vasodilators.
7. Newer inotropic agents.

Table 12–5. Vasodilators for use in chronic congestive heart failure.

Arteriolodilators	Combined Arteriolo- and Venodilators	Venodilators
Hydralazine	Prazosin	Nitrates
Minoxidil	Captopril	
	Trimazosin	
	Phenoxybenzamine	

there is any doubt about the nature of the pretherapy rhythm or changes during digitalization. Intravenous digitalization is rarely required in chronic heart failure; it should be used only in hospitalized patients with careful monitoring.

Determining the optimal level of digitalis effect may be difficult. In patients with atrial fibrillation, reduction of ventricular rate is the best measure of glycoside effect. In patients in normal sinus rhythm, symptomatic improvement and reductions in heart size, heart rate during exercise, venous pressure, or edema may signify optimum drug levels in the myocardium. Unfortunately, toxic effects may occur before the therapeutic end point is detected. If slow digitalization is being employed, simple omission of one dose and halving the maintenance dose will often bring the patient to the narrow range between suboptimal and toxic concentrations. Measurement of plasma digitalis levels is useful in patients who appear unusually resistant or sensitive; these assays are widely available for digoxin.

If all the above therapies are insufficient to maintain cardiovascular compensation, vasodilator drugs may be extremely helpful. A useful classification divides the drugs into selective venodilators, selective arteriolodilators, and drugs with nonselective vasodilatory effects (Table 12–5). Choice of agent should be based on the patient's signs and symptoms and hemodynamic measurements. Thus, in patients with high filling pressures in whom the principal symptom is dyspnea, the venodilators will be most helpful in reducing filling pressures and the symptoms of pulmonary congestion. In patients in whom fatigue due to low left ventricular output is a primary symptom, an arteriolodilator may be helpful in increasing forward cardiac output. In most patients with severe chronic failure that responds poorly to other therapy, the problem usually involves both elevated filling pressures and reduced cardiac output. In these circumstances, dilation of both arterioles and veins is required. To date, vasodilators have generally been used as supplements to standard therapy. Further study is required to determine whether or not vasodilator therapy may be considered as primary treatment, before digitalis or diuretics.

MANAGEMENT OF
ACUTE HEART FAILURE

Acute heart failure occurs frequently in patients with chronic failure. Such episodes are usually associated with increased exertion, emotion, salt in the diet, non-compliance with medical therapy, or increased metabolic demand occasioned by fever, anemia, etc. A particularly common and important cause of acute failure—with or without chronic failure—is acute myocardial infarction. Many of the signs and symptoms of acute and chronic failure are identical, but their therapies diverge because of the need for more rapid response and the relatively greater frequency and severity of pulmonary vascular congestion in the acute form.

Because of the need for rapid recognition and evaluation of changing hemodynamic status, it is much more important to obtain quantitative measurements in acute failure than in chronic failure. These measurements should include left ventricular filling pressure (pulmonary wedge pressure) and cardiac output in addition to heart rate, blood pressure, and heart size. The **stroke work index** (approximately stroke volume index times arterial pressure) is a useful derived variable that describes the external work performed by the heart.

Measurements of stroke work index and pulmonary capillary pressure from a large group of patients with acute myocardial infarction are illustrated in Fig 12–5. When filling pressure is greater than 15 mm Hg and stroke work index is less than 20 g-m/m² , the mortality rate is high. It is apparent, therefore, that the effects of myocardial infarction on ventricular function are not uniform and that there can be no single standard therapy for the management of congestive failure in this condition.

Subsets of Patients Following Myocardial Infarction

Patients with acute congestive failure following myocardial infarction can be usefully characterized on the basis of 3 hemodynamic measurements: arterial pressure, left ventricular filling pressure, and cardiac index. One such classification is illustrated in Table 12–6.

(1) **Hypovolemia:** Subset 1 includes patients who are relatively hypovolemic following myocardial infarction. They usually have been taking diuretics or may have had inadequate fluid intake. The primary hemodynamic abnormality is a low left ventricular filling pressure, which can be corrected by giving fluids. With an increase of filling pressure up to the optimal range of 15 mm Hg (Fig 12–4), hypotension often disappears and cardiac output increases.

(2) **Pulmonary Congestion:** The second subset—patients with severe pulmonary congestion and dyspnea—is a very large one and is also representative of other causes of acute heart failure. Several pharmacologic agents may be helpful in the management of such patients. Diuretics are helpful because they reduce intravascular volume (Chapter 14). In addition, when given intravenously, powerful diuretics such as furosemide produce an immediate increase in compliance of systemic veins. This leads to peripheral pooling of blood, which reduces central blood volume and

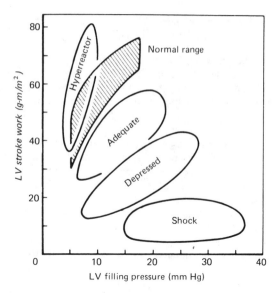

Figure 12–5. Relation of left ventricular performance to filling pressure in patients with acute myocardial infarction. The cross-hatched area is the range for normal, healthy individuals. Following infarction, there is a wide range of performance characteristics. In some patients, performance is in the normal or hypernormal range (hyperreactor). As the size of the infarct increases, however, function is shifted down and to the right. Similar depression is observed in patients with chronic congestive heart failure. (Reproduced, with permission, from Swan HJC, Parmley WW: Congestive heart failure. Page 327 in: *Pathologic Physiology.* Sodeman WA, Sodeman WA Jr [editors]. Saunders, 1979.)

decreases right and left ventricular filling pressures. Morphine sulfate also is clinically effective in the management of acute pulmonary edema. Apart from its ability to relieve the pain of infarction, the mechanisms by which it reduces pulmonary congestion are uncertain. If bronchospasm is a prominent component of the pulmonary signs, aminophylline may also be helpful, since it combines bronchodilator, vasodilator, and positive inotropic actions (Chapter 18).

(3) **Peripheral Vasodilatation:** The third subset of patients following acute myocardial infarction is relatively small. These patients are hypotensive and yet have warm extremities because of peripheral vasodilatation, usually as a consequence of drug-induced autonomic blockade. These patients may not need any therapy, since pulmonary wedge pressure is usually normal and cardiac output satisfactory. If blood pressure is extremely low, however, a vasoactive drug such as dopamine should be considered to maintain arterial perfusion pressure at the desired level.

(4) **"Power Failure":** The fourth subset represents those patients who have moderate "power failure." Hemodynamic measurements show a reduction in arterial pressure, although not to shock levels, together with an elevation of left ventricular filling pressure and a reduction of cardiac index. The goal of therapy in these patients is to increase cardiac output and reduce

Table 12–6. Therapeutic classification of subsets in acute myocardial infarction.*

Subset	Systolic Arterial Pressure (mm Hg)	Left Ventricular Filling Pressure (mm Hg)	Cardiac Index (L/min/m²)	Therapy
1. Hypovolemia	<100	<10	<2.5	Volume replacement.
2. Pulmonary congestion	100–150	>20	>2.5	Diuretics.
3. Peripheral vasodilatation	<100	10–20	>2.5	None, or vasoactive drugs.
4. Power failure	<100	>20	<2.5	Vasodilators.
5. Severe shock	< 90	>20	<2.0	Vasoactive drugs, vasodilators, circulatory assist.
6. Right ventricular infarct	<100	RVFP>10 LVFP<15	<2.5	Provide volume replacement for LVFP. Avoid diuretics.
7. Mitral regurgitation, ventricular septal defect	<100	>20	<2.5	Vasodilators, circulatory assist, surgery.

* The numerical values are intended to serve as general guidelines and not as absolute cutoff points. Arterial pressures apply to patients who were previously normotensive and should be adjusted upward for patients who were previously hypertensive. (RVFP and LVFP = right and left ventricular filling pressure.)

ventricular filling pressure without a further decrease in arterial pressure. Diuretics or nitrates are helpful in lowering filling pressures but will not increase cardiac output because the ventricle lacks sufficient power to pump against the systemic impedance. A combined venous and arteriolar dilator such as nitroprusside is extremely beneficial in such patients. Its venodilating effects reduce right and left atrial pressures by redistributing more blood into the periphery. Its arteriolar dilating properties increase forward cardiac output by reducing systemic vascular resistance. The main limiting factor in the use of nitroprusside is the reduction in arterial pressure. If the dose is titrated carefully, however, this reduction in blood pressure may be minimized. A good rule of thumb is to consider giving nitroprusside if the systolic pressure is 90 mm Hg or higher. The effects of nitroprusside depend on the level of left ventricular filling pressure. This is illustrated diagrammatically in Fig 12–6. The middle curve in the figure represents a patient with moderately severe heart failure. If the patient has a high left ventricular filling pressure (20 mm Hg), the administration of sodium nitroprusside will shift ventricular function up and to the left, as illustrated by line *A*. If, however, the patient has been given large doses of diuretics and filling pressure has thereby been reduced to 10 mm Hg, nitroprusside will produce a different result. Although the patient moves to the upper curve with nitroprusside (line *B*), there is a reduction of stroke volume because the heart is on the steep ascending limb of the curve. This will worsen hypotension and tachycardia. If the patient is volume-loaded at this point, up to the optimal filling pressure of 15 mm Hg, the beneficial effect of nitroprusside will become evident. This example illustrates the importance of filling pressure: pulmonary wedge pressure should be maintained at about 15 mm Hg by either diuresis or volume administration, as required.

(5) Severe Shock: Subset 5 represents a group of patients with cardiogenic shock following myocardial infarction. These patients have very low arterial pres-

sures, very high filling pressures, and low cardiac indices. Although diuretics may be helpful in lowering the elevated filling pressures, they will not increase cardiac output. Furthermore, the use of vasodilators in these patients is difficult, since the accompanying hypotension may be severe and may impair perfusion of vital organs. Since the mortality rate under these circumstances is high, it is often difficult to know whether any therapy is beneficial. Nevertheless, certain approaches may be helpful. If the arterial pressure

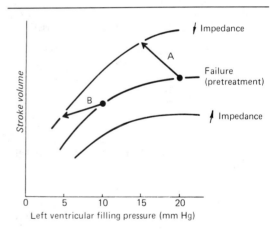

Figure 12–6. Effects of vasodilator therapy on left ventricular function. With the administration of a combined arteriolodilator and venodilator such as nitroprusside, function is shifted to a higher curve, reflecting the decreased impedance to ventricular ejection. However, the effect on stroke volume will depend on the initial filling pressure. A patient in heart failure with an initial filling pressure of 20 mm Hg will experience an increase in stroke volume along line *A*, up and to the left. If the patient was initially at a filling pressure of 10 mm Hg, nitroprusside would still shift performance to the upper curve, but this would result in a decrease of performance, along line *B*. (Reproduced, with permission, from Chatterjee K, Parmley WW: The role of vasodilator therapy in heart failure. *Prog Cardiovasc Dis* 1977;19:305.)

is extremely low, it is useful to consider use of a cate-cholamine such as dopamine. By titrating the dose of this drug, one can produce an increase in arterial pressure that is adequate for peripheral tissue perfusion. At this point, one can cautiously add nitroprusside to lower pulmonary wedge pressure. The combined effects of these 2 agents on the heart tend to be additive, since they work through different mechanisms. Dopamine directly increases cardiac contractility, while nitroprusside produces venous and arteriolar dilatation. This therapy should be combined with an attempt to optimize left ventricular filling pressure. These patients are also candidates for circulatory assist measures (intra-aortic balloon) and consideration of cardiac catheterization and possible coronary bypass surgery.

(6) Right Ventricular Infarction: Group 6 comprises a subset of patients who have an inferior myocardial infarction that predominantly involves the right ventricle. Their hypotension is due to the fact that the right ventricle is unable to deliver sufficient blood to the left side of the heart to optimize left ventricular filling pressure and cardiac output. Therefore, the primary therapeutic goal is to optimize left ventricular filling pressure. This may require volume infusion despite elevated central venous pressure. One should avoid using diuretics, since reduction of volume may lead to further reduction of filling pressure with associated hypotension and tachycardia.

(7) Mitral Regurgitation and Ventricular Septal Defect: A seventh subset is mentioned for completeness, although these patients are also found in other subsets, particularly those with shock. These are patients with mechanical abnormalities such as acute severe mitral regurgitation or a ruptured interventricular septum. Depending on the severity of the defect, cardiac surgery must be considered urgently as the most definitive form of therapy. However, vasodilator therapy such as nitroprusside may be necessary to stabilize the patient before surgery is possible.

REFERENCES

Basic Pharmacology

Antman EM, Smith TW: Digitalis toxicity. *Annu Rev Med* 1985;**36**:357.

Belz GG et al: Interaction between digoxin and calcium antagonists and antiarrhythmic drugs. *Clin Pharmacol Ther* 1983;**33**:410.

Bigger JT Jr: The quinidine-digoxin interaction. *Mod Concepts Cardiovasc Dis* 1982;**51**:73.

Bodem G, Dengler HJ (editors): *Cardiac Glycosides.* International Boehringer-Mannheim Symposia. Springer-Verlag, 1978.

Bristol JA, Evans DB: Agents for the treatment of heart failure. *Med Res Rev* 1983;**3**:259.

Jelliffe RW: An improved method of digoxin therapy. *Ann Intern Med* 1968;**69**:703.

Newer aspects of cardiac glycoside action. (Symposium.) *Fed Proc* 1977;**36**:2207.

Schwartz A, Lindenmayer GE, Allen JC: The sodium-potassium adenosine triphosphatase: Pharmacological, physiological, and biochemical aspects. *Pharmacol Rev* 1975;**27**:3.

Smith TW: Digitalis glycosides. (2 parts.) *N Engl J Med* 1973;**288**:719, 942.

Weishaar RE et al: The effect of several "new and novel" cardiotonic agents on key subcellular processes involved in the regulation of myocardial contractility: Implications for mechanism of action. *Drug Dev Res* 1983;**3**:517.

Wenger TL et al: Treatment of 63 severely digitalis-toxic patients with digoxin-specific antibody fragments. *J Am Coll Cardiol* 1985;**5**:118A.

Pathophysiology of Heart Failure

Abboud FM, Schmid PG: Circulatory adjustments to heart failure. Pages 249–260 in: *Heart Failure.* Fishman A (editor). Hemisphere Corp, 1978.

Braunwald E: Pathophysiology of heart failure. Pages 453–471 in: *Heart Disease.* Saunders, 1980.

Parmley WW: Pathophysiology of congestive heart failure. *Am J Cardiol* 1985;**56**:7A.

Swan HJC, Parmley WW: Congestive heart failure. Pages 313–334 in: *Pathologic Physiology*, 6th ed. Sodeman WA, Sodeman WA Jr (editors). Saunders, 1979.

Zelis R et al: Autonomic adjustments to congestive heart failure and their consequences. Pages 237–247 in: *Heart Failure.* Fishman AP (editor). Hemisphere Corp, 1978.

Acute Myocardial Infarction

Chatterjee K et al: Hemodynamic and metabolic responses to vasodilator therapy in acute myocardial infarction. *Circulation* 1973;**48**:1183.

Forrester JS, Chatterjee K, Swan HJC: Medical therapy of acute myocardial infarction by application of hemodynamic subsets. *N Engl J Med* 1976;**295**:1356.

Parmley W, Chatterjee K: Evaluation of cardiac function in the coronary care unit. Chap 7, pp 86–98, in: *Acute Myocardial Infarction.* Vol 4. Donoso E, Lipski J (editors). Stratton Intercontinental, 1978.

Sobel BE, Braunwald E: The management of acute myocardial infarction. Pages 1353–1386 in: *Heart Disease.* Braunwald E (editor). Saunders, 1980.

Chronic Heart Failure

Arnold SB et al: Long-term therapy improves left ventricular function in heart failure. *N Engl J Med* 1980;**303**:1443.

Chatterjee K, Parmley WW: Vasodilator therapy for acute myocardial infarction and chronic congestive heart failure. *J Am Coll Cardiol* 1983;**1**:133.

Chatterjee K, Parmley WW: Vasodilator therapy for chronic heart failure. Chap 22, pp 475–512, in: *Annual Review of Pharmacology and Toxicology.* Annual Reviews, 1980.

Lee DC-S et al: Heart failure in outpatients: A randomized trial of digoxin versus placebo. *N Engl J Med* 1982;**306**:699.

Liang C-S et al: Sustained improvement of cardiac function in patients with congestive heart failure after short term infusion of dobutamine. *Circulation* 1984;**69**:113.

Smith TW, Braunwald E: The management of heart failure. Pages 509–570 in: *Heart Disease.* Braunwald E (editor). Saunders, 1980.

White HD et al: Immediate effects of milrinone on metabolic and sympathetic responses to exercise in severe congestive heart failure. *Am J Cardiol* 1985;**56**:93.

Agents Used in Cardiac Arrhythmias

13

Luc M. Hondeghem, MD, PhD, & Jay W. Mason, MD

Cardiac arrhythmias are a frequent problem in clinical practice, occurring in up to 25% of patients treated with digitalis, 50% of anesthetized patients, and over 80% of patients with acute myocardial infarction. Arrhythmias may require treatment because too rapid, too slow, or asynchronous contractions reduce cardiac output. More importantly, some arrhythmias can precipitate more serious or even lethal rhythm disturbances—eg, early premature ventricular depolarization can precipitate ventricular fibrillation.

Arrhythmias can be treated with the drugs discussed in this chapter and with nonpharmacologic therapies such as pacemakers and cardioversion. This chapter describes the pharmacology of agents that suppress arrhythmias by a direct action on the cardiac cell membrane. Other modes of therapy are discussed briefly.

ELECTROPHYSIOLOGY OF NORMAL CARDIAC RHYTHM

The electrical impulse that triggers a normal cardiac contraction originates at regular intervals in the sinoatrial (SA) node (Fig 13–1), usually at a frequency of 60–100 beats per minute. This impulse spreads rapidly through the atria and enters the atrioventricular (AV) node, which is normally the only conduction pathway between the atria and ventricles. Conduction through the atrioventricular node is slow, requiring about 0.2 s. The impulse then propagates over the His-Purkinje system and invades all parts of the ventricles. Ventricular activation is complete in less than 0.1 s; therefore, contraction of all of the ventricular muscle is synchronous and hemodynamically effective.

Arrhythmias consist of cardiac depolarizations that deviate from the above description in one or more aspects—ie, there is an abnormality in the site of origin of the impulse, its rate or regularity, or its conduction.

Ionic Basis of Membrane Activity

The transmembrane potential of cardiac cells is determined by the concentrations of several ions—chiefly sodium (Na^+), potassium (K^+), and calcium (Ca^{2+})—on either side of the membrane and the permeability of the membrane to each ion. Ion channels—protein molecules that span the membranes—are the major routes by which ions diffuse through the membrane. These channels are relatively ion-specific, and the flux of ions through them is thought to be controlled by "gates" (probably flexible peptide chains). Each type of channel has its own type of gate (sodium and calcium channels are each thought to have 2 kinds of gates; potassium channels only one), and each kind of gate is opened and closed by specific transmembrane potential conditions.

Since movement of ions through these channels is passive and "downhill," other mechanisms must be present to maintain the average ionic concentrations inside the cell at appropriate levels. The most important of these active mechanisms is the sodium pump, Na^+,K^+-ATPase, described in Chapter 12. This pump and other active carriers of ions contribute indirectly to the transmembrane potential by maintaining the gradients necessary for diffusion through channels. In addition, they may contribute directly through electrogenic pumping.

At any given time, the potential across the cell membrane is a reflection of all the processes just described. However, under certain conditions, a useful simplification can be applied to predict the transmembrane potential. These conditions require that the cell membrane be highly permeable to one ion and relatively impermeable to all others. When this is the case, the transmembrane potential, E_m, approximates the ionic equilibrium potential, E_{ion}. The equilibrium potential is given by the **Nernst equation,** which for sodium and potassium is (at body temperature):

$$E_{ion} = 61 \log (C_e/C_i)$$

where C_e and C_i are the extracellular and intracellular concentrations, respectively, multiplied by their activity coefficients. The conditions required for application of the Nernst equation are approximated at the peak of the overshoot and during rest (phase 4, Fig 13–1) of most nonpacemaker cardiac cells.

The Resting Cell Membrane

During rest, the membrane of nonpacemaker cells is much more permeable to potassium than to other ions, so the membrane potential approaches the potassium equilibrium potential. For typical values of K_e (4 mmol/L) and K_i (150 mmol/L), the potassium equilibrium potential, E_K, is approximately −96 mV. The

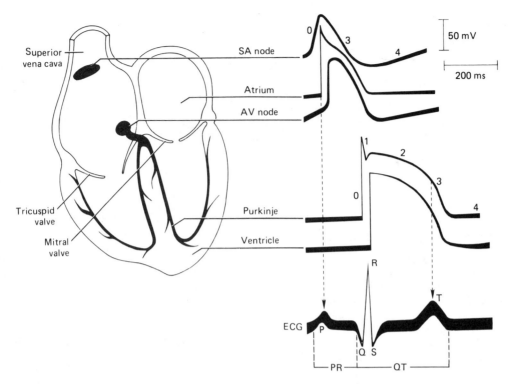

Figure 13–1. Schematic representation of the heart and normal cardiac electrical activity. Intracellular microelectrode recordings are shown for the 5 major cell types, along with an ECG recorded from the body surface. The cardiac action potential consists of 4 phases, demonstrated best in the Purkinje fiber action potential: phase 0 = upstroke, phase 1 = early fast repolarization, phase 2 = plateau, phase 3 = repolarization to the diastolic potential. Action potentials are separated by phase 4, the diastolic potential, which is stable in nonpacemaker cells such as atrial and ventricular fibers. In pacemaker cells, the membrane spontaneously depolarizes during phase 4, with the fastest depolarization occurring in the sinoatrial node, an intermediate rate in the atrioventricular node, and the slowest in Purkinje fibers. The sinoatrial and atrioventricular nodes have relatively less negative resting potentials, slower upstrokes, smaller amplitudes, and more rapid phase 4 depolarizations than other cardiac cells. Since the sinoatrial node is the fastest pacemaker, it resets latent pacemaker cells in the atrioventricular node and Purkinje system before they reach threshold. The ECG is the body surface manifestation of the depolarization and repolarization waves of the heart. The P wave reflects atrial activation; the QRS complex reflects ventricular activation; and the T wave coincides with ventricular repolarization. Thus, the PR interval is a measure of atrioventricular conduction time and the QT interval reflects the duration of the ventricular action potential.

resting potential of ventricular muscle cells is −85 to −95 mV. Small variations in K_e can markedly alter E_K and, therefore, resting E_m. For example, when extracellular K^+ concentration is 2 mmol/L, E_K is −114 mV; for K_e equal to 8 mmol/L, E_K is −77 mV. Thus, changes in extracellular potassium ion concentration have dramatic and predictable effects on resting potential in nonpacemaker cells.

The situation in pacemaker cells is more complex, because during diastole these cells have a gradually increasing ratio of sodium (or calcium) permeability to potassium permeability. As a result, the diastolic potential is closer to E_K at the beginning of diastole than at its end, and a typical diastolic pacemaker depolarization is recorded during phase 4 (see SA node tracing, Fig 13–1). Changes in extracellular potassium concentration have an effect on phase 4 depolarization in these cells in addition to that predicted by the Nernst relationship described above. Decreasing extracellular potassium decreases potassium permeability by an unknown mechanism; as a result, the membrane poten-

tial is more easily displaced from E_K toward E_{Na}, and pacemaker rate is enhanced. Conversely, increasing extracellular potassium causes an increase in potassium permeability, thus stabilizing the membrane potential close to E_K, and pacemaker rate is reduced.

Changes in resting potential occur in response to normal variations in extracellular potassium and also result from a number of pathologic conditions. The effects of these changes are described below.

The Active Cell Membrane

Normal atrial, Purkinje, and ventricular cells have sodium-dependent action potential upstrokes. The membrane events that bring about an action potential have been traditionally interpreted according to the **gating mechanism** first proposed by Hodgkin and Huxley. It is not clear that the details of the traditional interpretation apply in all cases, but the general concepts presented below provide a useful basis for understanding the action of drugs.

Depolarization to the threshold voltage results in

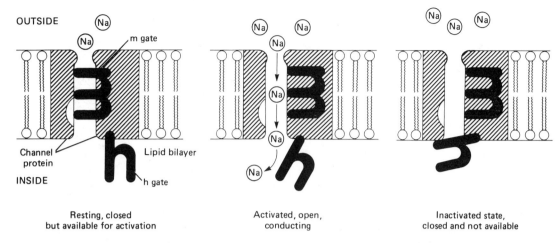

OUTSIDE

Channel protein

Lipid bilayer

INSIDE

m gate

h gate

| Resting, closed but available for activation | Activated, open, conducting | Inactivated state, closed and not available |

Figure 13–2. Schematic diagram of the cardiac sodium channel. The channel (shaded area) is a protein that spans the lipid bilayer membrane. In the resting, fully polarized membrane *(left)*, the *h* gate is open and the *m* gate is closed, preventing any movement of sodium ions through the channel. With an appropriate stimulus, the *m* gate opens, allowing a rapid influx of sodium ions *(middle)*. Approximately a millisecond later, the *h* gate closes, shutting off the sodium current *(right)*. Additional stimuli applied to the inactivated channel cannot open it (the *h* gate is already closed); therefore, it is "unavailable." The actual shapes of the channel and the gates are unknown, and those shown are purely symbolic. The light area at the lower left end of the channel is a possible location for a local anesthetic receptor.

very rapid opening of the activation *(m)* gates of sodium channels (Fig 13–2, middle panel). If the inactivation *(h)* gates of these channels have not already closed, the channels are now open or activated, and sodium permeability is markedly increased. Sodium permeability now greatly exceeds permeability to any other ion. Extracellular sodium therefore diffuses down its electrochemical gradient, and the membrane potential approaches the sodium equilibrium potential, E_{Na} (about $+50$ mV when $Na_e = 145$ mmol/L and $Na_i = 20$ mmol/L). This intense sodium current is very brief, because opening of the *m* gates upon depolarization is promptly followed by closure of the *h* gates or inactivation of the sodium channels (Fig 13–2, right panel).

The depolarization caused by the sodium current produces phase 0 of the action potential (Fig 13–1) and leads to activation of calcium channels and, more slowly, of some potassium channels. Calcium channels become activated and inactivated in what appears to be the same way as sodium channels, but in the case of calcium the transitions occur at more positive potentials and more slowly. The plateau (phases 1 and 2) reflects the turning off of sodium current, the waxing and waning of calcium current, and the slow development of a repolarizing potassium current.

Final repolarization (phase 3) of the action potential results from completion of calcium channel inactivation and the growth of potassium permeability, so that the membrane potential once again approaches the potassium equilibrium potential.

The Effect of Resting Potential on Action Potentials

A key factor in the pathophysiology of arrhythmias and the actions of antiarrhythmic drugs is the relationship between the resting potential of a cell and the action potentials that can be evoked in it (Fig 13–3). Because the inactivation gates of sodium channels in the resting membrane close over the potential range -75 to -55 mV, fewer sodium channels are "available" for diffusion of sodium ions when an action potential is evoked from a resting potential of -60 mV than when it is evoked from a resting potential of -80 mV. Important consequences of the reduction in peak sodium permeability include reduced upstroke velocity (called $\dot{V}_{max}$, for maximum rate of change of membrane voltage), reduced action potential amplitude, reduced excitability, and reduced conduction velocity.

During the plateau of the action potential (phases 1 and 2), most sodium channels are inactivated. During the latter part of phase 3 and during the subsequent phase 4 resting potential, recovery from inactivation takes place (in the terminology of Fig 13–2, the *h* gates reopen), making the channels again available for excitation. Another important effect of less negative resting potential is prolongation of this recovery time, as shown in Fig 13–3. The prolongation of recovery time is reflected in an increase in the effective refractory period, ie, the time from the start of an action potential to the time when a second action potential can be evoked and propagated.

Reduction of the resting potential,* whether brought about by hyperkalemia, sodium pump block-

---

*The steady depolarization or reduction in resting potential referred to in this section should not be confused with the abrupt depolarization involved in a normal stimulus. A brief depolarizing stimulus, whether caused by a propagating action potential or by an external electrode arrangement, causes the opening of large numbers of activation gates before a significant number of inactivation gates can close.

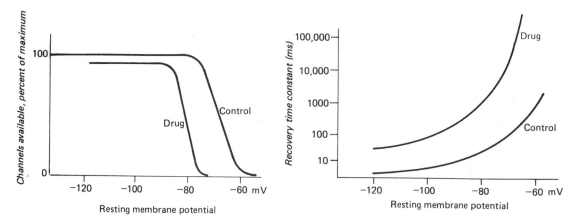

Figure 13–3. Dependence of sodium channel availability on membrane potential and time. As shown in the graph at *left*, the fraction of sodium channels "available" for opening in response to a stimulus is determined by the resting potential. The decrease in the fraction available when the resting potential is depolarized in the absence of drug (control curve) results from the closure of *h* gates in the channels. The shift in the curve illustrates the effect of a typical local anesthetic antiarrhythmic drug and may be caused by an interaction between the *h* gate and the drug molecule, or the drug may function like the *h* gate but at a more negative membrane potential. All sodium channels are inactivated during the plateau of the action potential. The time constant for recovery from inactivation after repolarization also depends on the resting potential. The graph at *right* shows that in the absence of drug, recovery occurs in less than 10 ms at normal resting potentials (−75 to −95 mV). Depolarized cells recover more slowly (note logarithmic scale). In the presence of sodium channel–blocking drugs, the time constant of recovery is increased, but the increase is far greater at depolarized potentials than at more negative ones.

ade, or ischemic cell damage, results in depressed sodium currents during the upstrokes of action potentials. Depolarization of the resting potential to levels positive to −55 mV abolishes sodium currents, since all sodium channels are inactivated. However, such severely depolarized cells have been found to support special action potentials under circumstances that increase calcium permeability or decrease potassium permeability. These "slow responses"—slow upstroke velocity and slow conduction—are important in some arrhythmias and probably constitute the normal electrical activity in the sinoatrial and atrioventricular nodes, since these tissues have a normal resting potential in the range of −50 to −70 mV.

MECHANISMS OF ARRHYTHMIAS

Many factors can precipitate or exacerbate arrhythmias: ischemia, hypoxia, acidosis or alkalosis, electrolyte abnormalities, excessive catecholamine exposure, autonomic influences, drug toxicity (eg, digitalis), overstretching of cardiac fibers, and the presence of scarred or otherwise diseased tissue. However, all arrhythmias result from (1) disturbances in impulse formation, (2) disturbances in impulse conduction, or (3) both.

Disturbances of Impulse Formation

The interval between depolarizations of a pacemaker cell is the sum of the duration of the action potential and the duration of the diastolic interval. Shortening of either duration results in an increase in pacemaker rate. The more important of the two, dias-

tolic interval, is determined by 3 factors: maximum diastolic potential, slope of phase 4 depolarization, and threshold potential (Fig 13–4). Thus, vagal discharge slows normal pacemaker rate by making the maximum diastolic potential more negative and reducing the phase 4 slope; beta receptor–blocking drugs markedly reduce phase 4 slope. Acceleration of pacemaker discharge is often brought about by increased phase 4 depolarization slope, caused by hypokalemia, beta-adrenoceptor stimulation, fiber stretch, acidosis, and partial depolarization by currents of injury.

Latent pacemakers (cells that show slow phase 4 depolarization even under normal conditions, eg, some Purkinje fibers) are particularly prone to acceleration by the above mechanisms. However, all cardiac cells, including normally quiescent atrial and ventricular cells, may show repetitive pacemaker activity when depolarized under appropriate conditions, especially hypokalemia.

A special form of pacemakerlike activity results from digitalis toxicity (Chapter 12) and other causes. Digitalis causes an increase in intracellular calcium, and this effect, if excessive, results in the triggering of oscillatory afterpotentials after each action potential (Fig 13–5). These oscillations (also called delayed afterdepolarizations) mimic phase 4 depolarization and can reach threshold, thereby evoking extrasystoles. In the severely intoxicated heart, the oscillation-extrasystole process becomes self-sustaining, and recordings show what appears to be a rapidly discharging ectopic pacemaker.

All pacemakers, normal and abnormal, are dependent upon phase 4 diastolic depolarization. Thus, hyperkalemia, because it increases potassium permeabil-

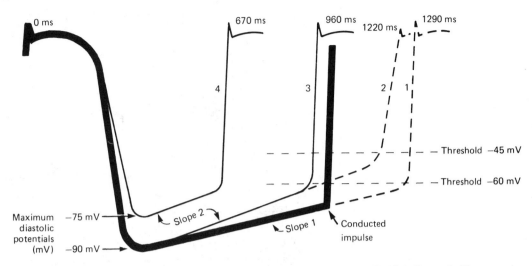

Figure 13–4. Determinants of pacemaker rate. The transmembrane potential from a Purkinje fiber cell with pacemaker capability is shown schematically. The last action potential elicited by a normally conducted sinus impulse is shown at 0 ms, and progression to the next normally conducted impulse is shown by the heavy line terminating in an upstroke at 1000 ms (large arrow). An increase in phase 4 slope (from slope 1 to slope 2) would permit the cell to reach threshold and fire spontaneously as the action potential labeled 3. If there were also a depolarization of the maximum diastolic potential from −90 mV to −75 mV, the cell would reach threshold even sooner and fire spontaneously as action potential 4. Both changes would convert the cell from a latent to the dominant pacemaker. Conversely, a change in threshold potential from −60 mV to −45 mV would delay the upstroke from 960 ms to 1220 ms and prevent this cell from becoming the dominant pacemaker.

ity, will *stabilize* the membrane close to the potassium equilibrium potential and consequently will reduce the rate of firing.* In hypokalemia, the membrane is less permeable to potassium and consequently more easily displaced from the potassium equilibrium potential, ie, spontaneous firing is facilitated.

Disturbances of Impulse Conduction

Severely depressed conduction may result in several easily recognized arrhythmias, eg, atrioventricular nodal block, bundle branch block. A more subtle and more common abnormality of conduction is **reentry,** in which one impulse reenters and excites areas of the heart more than once (Fig 13–6). In order for reentry to occur, 3 conditions must coexist: (1) There must be an obstacle (anatomic or physiologic) to homogenous conduction, thus establishing a circuit around which the reentrant wavefront can propagate; (2) there must be unidirectional block at some point in the circuit; and (3) conduction time around the circuit must be long enough so that the impulse does not enter refractory tissue as it travels around the obstacle—ie, the conduction time must exceed the effective refractory period.

Thus, reentry depends upon critically depressed conduction. If conduction is not sufficiently depressed, bidirectional conduction rather than unidirectional block will occur. In addition, even in the pres-

ence of unidirectional block, if the impulse travels around the obstacle too rapidly, it will enter tissue that is still refractory. If conduction is too depressed, bidirectional block rather than unidirectional block occurs; if the retrograde impulse is too weak, conduction may fail, or the impulse may arrive so late that it collides with the next regular impulse. Critically depressed conduction may be due to a depressed sodium current, a slow calcium current, or both. Drugs can abolish reentry either by improving critically depressed conduction (increasing the sodium or calcium current) or by further depressing it (blocking the sodium or calcium current).

Lengthening or shortening of the refractory period relative to a median value may also make reentry less likely. The longer the refractory period in tissue near the block, the greater the chance that the tissue will still be refractory when reentry is attempted. The shorter the refractory period in the depressed region, the less likely it is that unidirectional block will occur.

I. BASIC PHARMACOLOGY OF THE ANTIARRHYTHMIC DRUGS

Mechanisms of Action

Arrhythmias are caused by abnormal pacemaker activity or abnormal impulse propagation. Thus, the aim of therapy of the arrhythmias is to reduce pacemaker activity and modify critically impaired conduction. The latter objective may involve improving conduction in the depressed region or suppressing it

---

*Even though potassium depolarizes the membrane and depolarization can promote pacemaker activity, the effect of membrane *stabilization* is more important than that of the *depolarization*, so that increased potassium normally reduces pacemaker rate.

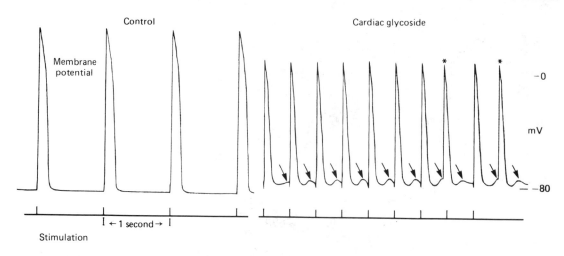

Figure 13–5. Induction of arrhythmia by a cardiac glycoside. The *left* side of the figure shows normal transmembrane action potentials in isolated cardiac muscle, produced by regular stimulation (lower tracing shows stimuli). After exposure to a toxic concentration of acetylstrophanthidin (*right* side), small oscillatory afterpotentials (arrows) occur after each action potential. Occasionally, such afterpotentials reach threshold during the regular sequence of stimuli and trigger an early action potential (first asterisk). Note that this action potential precedes the stimulus artifact (bottom tracing). After a pause in the regular driving stimulation, a second "extrasystole" (second asterisk) is evoked by an oscillatory afterpotential.

altogether. The major mechanisms for accomplishing these goals are (1) sodium channel blockade, (2) calcium channel blockade, (3) prolongation of the effective refractory period, and (4) blockade of sympathetic autonomic effects in the heart.

Antiarrhythmic drugs decrease automaticity, conduction, and excitability and increase the refractory period to a greater extent in depolarized tissue than in normally polarized tissue. This is accomplished chiefly by selectively blocking the sodium or calcium channels of depolarized cells (Fig 13–7). Therapeutically useful channel-blocking drugs have a high affinity for open channels (ie, during phase 0) or inactivated channels (ie, during phase 2) but very low affinity for rested channels. Therefore, these drugs block electrical activity when there is a fast tachycardia (many channel openings per unit time) or if there is significant loss of resting potential (many inactivated channels). Channels in normal cells that become blocked by a drug during normal activation-inactivation cycles will rapidly lose the drug from the receptors during the resting portion of the cycle. Channels in myocardium that is chronically depolarized, ie, has a resting potential more positive than −70 mV, will recover from block very slowly if at all (see Fig 13–3, right).

In cells with abnormal automaticity most of these drugs reduce the phase 4 slope (Fig 13–4) by blocking either sodium or calcium channels and thereby reducing the ratio of sodium (or calcium) permeability to potassium permeability. In addition, some agents may increase the threshold (make it more positive). Beta-adrenoceptor–blocking drugs indirectly reduce the phase 4 slope by blocking the positive chronotropic action of norepinephrine in the heart.

In critically depressed conduction with reentry,

most of the antiarrhythmic agents slow conduction further by one or both of 2 mechanisms: (1) steady-state reduction in the number of available unblocked channels, which reduces the excitatory currents to a level below that required for propagation (Fig 13–3, left); and (2) prolongation of recovery time of the channels still able to reach the rested and available state, which increases the effective refractory period (Fig 13–3, right). As a result, early extrasystoles are unable to propagate at all; later impulses propagate more slowly and are subject to bidirectional conduction block. Several agents prolong the duration of the cardiac action potential, possibly through blockade of potassium channels. Such prolongation is usually directly reflected in an increase in effective refractory period, with the same beneficial results described above.

In one special case, reentry may result from *latent* pacemaker activity, especially in Purkinje fibers. Because phase 4 depolarization in latent pacemakers results in a less negative take-off potential for any subsequent action potential, the availability of sodium channels for the upstroke of that action potential may be reduced. As illustrated by the relationship in Fig 13–3 (left), this reduction in channel availability is very steep in the potential range of −70 to −60 mV, and conduction velocity will be similarly reduced. This reduction may be sufficient to cause unidirectional block. Antiarrhythmic drugs can therefore (at least theoretically) *increase* conduction velocity in latent pacemaker cells by reduction of phase 4 depolarization in latent pacemaker cells.

By these mechanisms, antiarrhythmic drugs can suppress abnormal automaticity and conduction occurring in depolarized cells—rendering them electrically silent—while minimally affecting the electrical

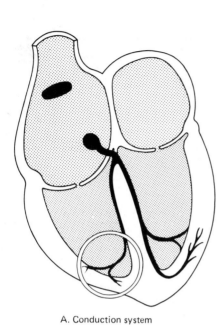

A. Conduction system

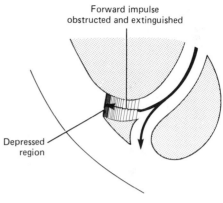

Forward impulse
obstructed and extinguished

Depressed
region

C. Decremental conduction and unidirectional
block of antegrade impulse

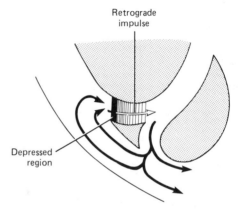

Retrograde
impulse

Depressed
region

D. Retrograde impulse conducted
across depressed region

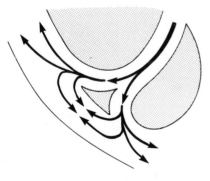

B. Normal conduction

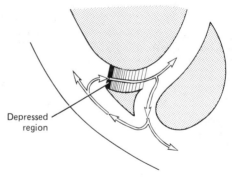

Depressed
region

E. Reentry circuit established

Figure 13-6. Unidirectional block and reentry. Panel **A** shows the heart schematically with the SA and AV nodes and the conducting system in black. A small bifurcating twig of the Purkinje system is circled where it enters the ventricular wall. Panel **B** shows the normal passage and fate of an impulse that is conducted down the twig. It splits into 2 impulses at the bifurcation, and these collide (and extinguish each other) after exciting the ventricular muscle. Panels **C–E** show the sequence of events when the normal impulse finds an area of unidirectional block (blocked depressed region) in one of the branches. As shown by the path of the impulse in the depressed region (panel **C**), this weak stimulus is unable to conduct through or to "jump over" the area of block. In contrast, the wave in the undepressed branch is able to excite the entire ventricular wall (panel **D**). Because the ventricular wall constitutes a large mass of cells, the strong ventricular depolarization is able to jump the depressed region and results in a *retrograde* impulse (shown by the open arrow, panels **D** and **E**). The retrograde impulse may be propagated if the impulse finds excitable tissue, ie, the refractory period is shorter than the conduction time. This impulse will then reexcite tissue it had previously passed through, and a reentry arrhythmia will be established in the circuit indicated by the open arrows in panel **E**.

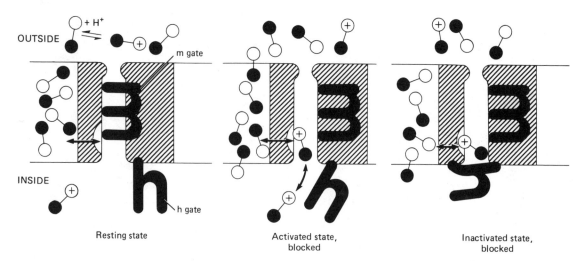

OUTSIDE

m gate

INSIDE

h gate

Resting state

Activated state,
blocked

Inactivated state,
blocked

Figure 13–7. Interaction of antiarrhythmic drugs with the cardiac sodium channel. The diagram reproduces the schematic channel model shown in Fig 13–2. Local anesthetic antiarrhythmic molecules in solution in the extracellular fluid are divided into 2 forms: uncharged (lipid-soluble) and positively charged (less lipid-soluble) according to the pH and their pK_aS. Although the lipid membrane dissolves a large amount of uncharged drug, the drug cannot easily bind to the receptor site when the channel is in the rested state. The dissociation constant is very large, ie, affinity is low. However, when the channel is open (*middle,* m gate withdrawn), drug molecules can reach the receptor site either from the lipid membrane side or from the intracellular space. The dissociation constant is now (for most antiarrhythmic drugs) relatively small. When drug is bound to the receptor, sodium ions cannot pass through the channel. When the channel is inactivated (*right,* h gate closed), drug molecules can still reach the receptor site, but only from the lipid membrane phase; access from the intracellular compartment is blocked. There may be some interaction between the h gate and the drug that is bound to the receptor. The dissociation constant for this drug-receptor combination in the inactivated channel may be extremely small for certain drugs, eg, amiodarone.

activity in normally polarized parts of the heart. However, as dosage is increased, these agents will also depress conduction in normal tissue, eventually resulting in *drug-induced* arrhythmias.

As noted above, extracellular potassium modulates the resting transmembrane potential. Therefore, hyperkalemia, by depolarizing the membrane and inactivating more channels, increases the depressant effects of antiarrhythmic drugs. When antiarrhythmic drug toxicity occurs, reduction of extracellular potassium levels (eg, by elevation of serum pH) may reverse the toxicity by hyperpolarizing the myocardium. This approach should only be considered if serum potassium is normal or high, since hypokalemia may also cause arrhythmias.

SPECIFIC ANTIARRHYTHMIC DRUGS

The antiarrhythmic agents can be divided into 4 distinct subgroups on the basis of mechanism of action: (1) Sodium channel blockers, all of which behave like local anesthetics. (In fact, the most popular parenteral antiarrhythmic drug, lidocaine, is also the most popular local anesthetic.) This is by far the most important group of antiarrhythmic drugs. (2) Calcium channel blockers, which seem to have some features in common with the local anesthetic group. (3) Drugs

that prolong effective refractory period by some mechanism other than (or in addition to) blockade of sodium channels. (4) Drugs that reduce adrenergic activity in the heart.

SODIUM CHANNEL–BLOCKING DRUGS

QUINIDINE

Although quinine was used sporadically as an antiarrhythmic drug during the 18th and 19th centuries, it was not until the early years of the 20th century that this isomer of quinine came into wide use. Quinidine is the most commonly used oral antiarrhythmic agent.

Quinidine

Cardiac Effects

Quinidine depresses the pacemaker rate (especially

of ectopic pacemakers) and depresses conduction and excitability (especially in depolarized tissue) (Table 13–1). These actions probably result to a large extent from the drug's ability to block activated sodium channels, although it may to some extent also block inactivated sodium channels. Recovery from block proceeds more slowly in depolarized channels than in fully polarized channels. Thus, quinidine lengthens the refractory period and depresses excitability and conduction in depolarized tissue more than in normal tissue.

Quinidine also lengthens the action potential duration, which is reflected in the ECG as a lengthening of the QT interval. Blockade of potassium channels with a reduction in repolarizing outward current may be responsible for this effect. It should be noted that lengthening of the action potential duration reduces the time spent at negative membrane potentials and will by itself therefore enhance the sodium-blocking efficacy of quinidine. This lengthening of the action potential duration and effective refractory period reduces the maximum reentry frequency.

Cardiac Toxicity

Quinidine has antimuscarinic actions in the heart that inhibit vagal effects. This can overcome its direct membrane effect and lead to increased sinus rate and increased atrioventricular conduction. In the presence of atrial fibrillation or flutter, the latter may result in an excessively high ventricular rate. However, this can be prevented by prior administration of digitalis (see Chapter 12).

A small percentage (1–5%) of patients given quinidine develop a syndrome called quinidine syncope, characterized by recurrent light-headedness and episodes of fainting. The symptoms are a result of a drug-induced rapid, disorganized ventricular tachycardia (torsade de pointes), resembling ventricular fibrillation, which usually terminates spontaneously but may recur incessantly or become sustained. It is associated with a striking prolongation of the QT interval.

In patients with sick sinus syndrome, quinidine may depress the pacemaker activity of the sinoatrial node. In toxic concentrations, this drug can depress cardiac electrical activity to the point of precipitating arrhythmias or asystole. These toxic effects are more likely to occur when the serum concentrations exceed 5 μg/mL and in the presence of high serum potassium levels (> 5 meq/L). Widening of the QRS duration by 30% by quinidine administration is usually considered premonitory of serious toxicity. Toxic concentrations may depress contractility and lower blood pressure.

Extracardiac Effects

Quinidine possesses alpha-adrenoceptor–blocking properties that can cause vasodilatation and a reflex increase in sinoatrial nodal rate. These effects are most prominent after intravenous administration (see below). Quinidine also has antimalarial, antipyretic, and oxytocic properties.

Extracardiac Toxicity

The most common side effects are gastrointestinal: diarrhea, nausea, and vomiting. The drug can also cause cinchonism (headache, dizziness, tinnitus).

Table 13–1. Membrane actions of antiarrhythmic drugs.

Drug	Block of Sodium Channels		Refractory Period		Calcium Channel Blockade	Effect on Pacemaker Activity	Adrenoceptor-Blocking Action
	Normal Cells	Depolarized Cells	Normal Cells	Depolarized Cells			
Amiodarone (Cordarone)	+	+++	↑↑	↑↑↑	+	↓↓	+
Bretylium (Bretylol)	0	0	↑↑↑	↑↑↑	0	↑↓*	++
Disopyramide (Norpace)	+	+++	↑	↑↑	0	↓↓	0
Encainide (investigational)	++	+++	0	↑	0	↓↓	0
Flecainide (Tambocor)	++	+++	0	↑	0	↓↓	0
Imipramine (investigational)	+	++	↑	↑↑	0	↓↓	0
Lidocaine (Xylocaine)	0	+++	↓	↑↑	0	↓↓	0
Mexiletine (Mexitil)	0	+++	0	↑↑	0	↓↓	0
Phenytoin (Dilantin)	0	+	↓	↑	+	↓	+
Procainamide (Pronestyl, others)	+	+++	↑	↑↑↑	0	↓	++
Propafenone (investigational)	+	++	↑	↑↑	+	↓↓	+
Propranolol (Inderal)	0	+	↓	↑↑	0	↓↓	+++
Quinidine (many trade names)	+	++	↑	↑↑	0	↓↓	+
Tocainide (Tonocard)	0	+++	0	↑↑	0	↓↓	0
Verapamil (Calan, Isoptin)	0	+	0	↑↑	+++	↓↓	+

*Bretylium may transiently increase pacemaker rate by causing catecholamine release.

Rarely, quinidine can cause rashes, angioneurotic edema, fever, hepatitis, and thrombocytopenia. Quinidine increases digoxin plasma levels and may precipitate digitalis toxicity in patients taking that drug (see Chapter 12).

Pharmacokinetics & Dosage

Quinidine is usually administered orally and is rapidly absorbed from the gastrointestinal tract. It is 80% bound to plasma proteins. Quinidine is hydroxylated in the liver, but 20% is excreted unchanged in the urine. Its half-life is about 6 hours (Table 13–2) and may be longer in patients with congestive heart failure or hepatic or renal disease. Urinary excretion is enhanced in acid urine. It is usually administered orally as the sulfate, gluconate, or polygalacturonate salt. The usual dose of 0.2–0.6 g of quinidine sulfate is given 4–6 times daily. The therapeutic concentration in plasma is 3–5 μg/mL.

Parenteral administration of quinidine is occasionally necessary. Quinidine is absorbed after intramuscular injection of the sulfate in oil or the aqueous gluconate preparation. Intravenous administration of quinidine can be carried out successfully if proper precautions are observed. The intravenous dose should not exceed 10 mg/kg of quinidine gluconate and should not be given at a rate exceeding 0.5 mg/kg/min. Intravenous administration of quinidine is usually associated with a decline in blood pressure as a re-

sult of its peripheral vasodilating action. Thus, when intravenous quinidine is used, blood pressure should be carefully monitored and supported when necessary with intravenous fluids.

Therapeutic Use

Quinidine is the most frequently prescribed oral antiarrhythmic agent in the USA. It is considered effective in nearly every form of arrhythmia: premature atrial contractions, paroxysmal atrial fibrillation and flutter, intra-atrial and atrioventricular nodal reentrant arrhythmias, Wolff-Parkinson-White tachycardias, premature ventricular contractions, and ventricular tachycardias.

PROCAINAMIDE

Cardiac Effects

The electrophysiologic effects of procainamide are similar to those of quinidine. It may be somewhat less effective in suppressing abnormal ectopic pacemaker activity but more effective in blocking sodium channels in depolarized cells.

Perhaps the most important difference between quinidine and procainamide is the less prominent antimuscarinic action of procainamide. Therefore, the directly depressant actions of procainamide on sinoatrial and atrioventricular nodes are not as effectively

Table 13–2. Clinical pharmacologic properties of antiarrhythmic drugs.

Drug	Effect on SA Nodal Rate	Effect on AV Nodal Refractory Period	PR Interval	QRS Duration	QT Interval	Usefulness in Arrhythmias Supra-ventricular	Ventricular	Half-Life (hours)
Amiodarone (Cordarone)	↓↓	↑↑	↑↑†	↑	↑↑↑↑	+++	+++	(weeks)
Bretylium (Bretylol)	↑↓§	↑↓§	0	0	0	0	++	4
Disopyramide (Norpace)	↑*	↑*	↑↓†	↑↑	↑↑	++	+++	6–8
Encainide (investigational)	None	↑	↑	↑↑↑	0	+**	++++	4††
Flecainide (Tambocor)	None	↑	↑	↑↑↑	0	+**	++++	20
Imipramine (investigational)	↑*	↑*	↑	↑	↑	+	+++	12
Lidocaine (Xylocaine)	None†	None	0	0	0	None‡	+++	1
Mexiletine (Mexitil)	None†	None	0	0	0	None‡	+++	12
Phenytoin (Dilantin)	None	None	0	↑	0	None‡	+	24
Procainamide (Pronestyl, others)	↑*	↑*	↑↓†	↑↑	↑↑	++	+++	4
Propafenone (investigational)	0	↑	↑	↑↑↑	0	++**	+++	7
Propranolol (Inderal)	↓↓	↑↑	↑↑	0	0	++	++	8
Quinidine (many trade names)	↑*	↑*	↑↓†	↑↑	↑↑	++	+++	6
Tocainide (Tonocard)	None†	None	0	0	0	None‡	+++	12
Verapamil (Calan, Isoptin)	↑↓	↑↑	↑↑	0	0	+++	+	7

* Anticholinergic effect partly counteracted by direct depressant action.
† May suppress diseased sinus nodes.
‡ May be effective in atrial arrhythmias caused by digitalis.
§ Initial stimulation by release of endogenous norepinephrine followed by depression.
** Especially in Wolff-Parkinson-White syndrome.
†† Half-life of active metabolites much longer.

counterbalanced by drug-induced vagolysis as in the case of quinidine. Procainamide also has ganglionic blocking properties and thus more potent negative inotropic effects than quinidine. In patients with preexisting ventricular dysfunction, procainamide may induce severe congestive heart failure.

Procainamide

Cardiac Toxicity

Procainamide's cardiotoxic effects are similar to those of quinidine. It is more likely than quinidine to produce severe or irreversible heart failure in toxic doses.

Extracardiac Effects

The ganglionic blocking effects of procainamide reduce peripheral vascular resistance and can cause hypotension. However, in therapeutic concentrations, its peripheral vascular effects are less prominent than those of quinidine. Hypotension is usually only seen during excessively rapid procainamide infusion.

Extracardiac Toxicity

The most troublesome side effect of procainamide is a syndrome resembling lupus erythematosus and usually consisting of arthralgia and arthritis. In some patients, pleuritis, pericarditis, or parenchymal pulmonary disease also occur. Renal lupus is rarely induced by procainamide. During long-term therapy, serologic abnormalities (eg, increased antinuclear antibody titer) occur in nearly all patients. Approximately one-third of patients receiving long-term procainamide therapy develop lupus-related symptoms.

Other side effects include nausea and diarrhea (about 10% of cases), rash, fever, hepatitis (less than 5%), and agranulocytosis (less than 0.1%).

Pharmacokinetics & Dosage

Procainamide can be administered safely by the intravenous and intramuscular routes and is well absorbed orally, with 75% systemic bioavailability. The major metabolite is N-acetylprocainamide. The metabolic product has antiarrhythmic activity, but some patients respond differently to the 2 substances. Either or both may be responsible for the therapeutic effect in a given patient. Some individuals rapidly acetylate procainamide and develop high levels of N-acetylprocainamide.

Procainamide's half-life is only 3–4 hours, which necessitates frequent dosing. Both procainamide and N-acetylprocainamide are eliminated chiefly by the kidneys. Thus, dosage must be reduced in patients with renal failure. The reduced volume of distribution and renal clearance associated with congestive heart failure also require reduction in dosage. The half-life of N-acetylprocainamide is considerably longer than that of procainamide, and it therefore accumulates more readily. Thus, it is important to measure plasma levels of both procainamide and N-acetylprocainamide, especially in patients with circulatory or renal impairment.

If rapid effect is needed, an intravenous loading dose of up to 12 mg/kg can be given safely at a rate of 0.3 mg/kg/min or less. This dose is followed by a maintenance dose of 2–5 mg/min, with careful monitoring of plasma levels.

Oral procainamide is frequently used improperly. If around-the-clock antiarrhythmic activity is required, the drug usually must be administered every 3 or 4 hours. In order to control ventricular arrhythmias, a total dose of 2–5 g daily is usually required. In an occasional patient who accumulates high levels of N-acetylprocainamide and in whom that compound is active, less frequent dosing may be possible. Slow-release preparations of procainamide may also allow reduction of dosing frequency.

Therapeutic Use

Like quinidine, procainamide is effective against most atrial and ventricular arrhythmias. However, many clinicians attempt to avoid long-term therapy because of the frequent dosing requirement and the common occurrence of lupus-related effects. Procainamide is the drug of second choice (after lidocaine) in most coronary care units for the treatment of ventricular arrhythmias associated with acute myocardial infarction.

DISOPYRAMIDE

Disopyramide phosphate is a relatively new drug closely related to an agent long used for its antimuscarinic properties (isopropamide).

Cardiac Effects

The electrophysiologic effects of disopyramide are nearly indistinguishable from those of quinidine. Its cardiac antimuscarinic effects are even more marked than those of quinidine. Therefore, digoxin should be administered with disopyramide in the treatment of atrial flutter or fibrillation.

Disopyramide

Cardiac Toxicity

Toxic concentrations of disopyramide can precipitate all of the electrophysiologic disturbances described under quinidine. In addition, disopyramide's negative inotropic actions are frequently troublesome in patients with preexisting left ventricular dysfunction. Moreover, in rare instances, it may produce heart failure in subjects without prior myocardial dysfunction. Because of this effect, disopyramide is not a first-line antiarrhythmic agent. It must be used with great caution in patients with congestive heart failure.

Extracardiac Effects & Toxicity

Disopyramide's atropinelike activity accounts for most of its symptomatic side effects: urinary retention in male patients with prostate hypertrophy, dry mouth, blurred vision, constipation, and worsening of preexisting glaucoma. These side effects may require discontinuation of the drug.

Pharmacokinetics & Dosage

In the USA, disopyramide is only available for oral use. Bioavailability is about 50%. The drug is extensively protein-bound, but binding sites become saturated with increasing dosage, which results in a nonlinear rise in free (active) drug levels. As a result, measurements of total plasma concentration may be misleading. The drug is excreted by the kidneys and has a half-life of approximately 6–8 hours. The usual oral dose of disopyramide is 150 mg 3 times a day, but as much as 1 g daily may be required. In patients with renal impairment, this schedule must be reduced. Because of the danger of precipitating congestive heart failure, the use of large loading doses is not recommended.

Therapeutic Use

Although disopyramide has been shown to be effective in a variety of supraventricular arrhythmias, in the USA it is only approved for the treatment of ventricular arrhythmias. It is most commonly used when quinidine and procainamide have been poorly tolerated or ineffective.

LIDOCAINE

Lidocaine is the antiarrhythmic drug most commonly used by the intravenous route. It has an unusually low incidence of toxicity and a high degree of effectiveness in arrhythmias associated with acute myocardial infarction.

Lidocaine

Cardiac Effects

Lidocaine is a potent suppressor of abnormal cardiac activity, yet it appears to act exclusively on the sodium channel. Its interaction with this channel differs substantially from that of quinidine. Whereas quinidine mostly blocks sodium channels in the open state, lidocaine blocks both activated and inactivated sodium channels. As a result, a large fraction (about 50%) of the unblocked sodium channels become blocked during each action potential in Purkinje fibers and ventricular cells, which have long plateaus. During diastole, most of the sodium channels in normally polarized cells become drug-free. Since lidocaine usually shortens the action potential duration, diastole may be prolonged, thereby extending the time available for recovery. As a result, lidocaine has few electrophysiologic effects in *normal* cardiac tissue. In contrast, depolarized (inactivated) sodium channels remain largely blocked during diastole, and more may become blocked. Thus, lidocaine suppresses the electrical activity of the depolarized, arrhythmogenic tissues while minimally interfering with the electrical activity of normal tissues. These factors appear to be responsible for the fact that lidocaine is a very effective agent for suppressing arrhythmias associated with depolarization (eg, ischemia, digitalis toxicity), but it is relatively ineffective against arrhythmias occurring in normally polarized tissues (eg, atrial flutter and fibrillation).

Cardiac Toxicity

Lidocaine is the least cardiotoxic of the currently used antiarrhythmic drugs. The drug exacerbates ventricular arrhythmias in fewer than 10% of patients (a good record). However, in diseased hearts, lidocaine does occasionally precipitate sinoatrial node standstill or worsen impaired conduction (< 1%).

In large doses, especially in patients with preexisting heart failure, lidocaine may cause hypotension—partly by depressing myocardial contractility.

Extracardiac Toxicity

Lidocaine's most common side effects—like those of other local anesthetics—are neurologic: paresthesias, tremor, nausea of central origin, light-headedness, hearing disturbances, slurred speech, and convulsions. Convulsions occur mostly in elderly or otherwise vulnerable patients and are dose-related, usually short-lived, and respond to intravenous diazepam. In general, if plasma levels above 9 $\mu g/mL$ are avoided, lidocaine is extremely well tolerated.

Pharmacokinetics & Dosage

Because of its very extensive first-pass hepatic metabolism, only 3% of orally administered lidocaine appears in the plasma. Thus, lidocaine must be given parenterally. When given by the intravenous route, lidocaine has a half-life of 0.5–4 hours. In adults, a loading dose of 150–200 mg administered over about 15 minutes should be followed by a maintenance infusion of 2–4 mg/min to achieve a therapeutic plasma level of 2–6 $\mu g/mL$. Determination of lidocaine plasma levels is of great value in adjusting the infusion rate.

In patients with congestive heart failure, lidocaine's volume of distribution and total body clearance may both be decreased. However, since these effects counterbalance each other, the half-life may not be increased as much as predicted from clearance changes alone. In patients with liver disease, plasma clearance is markedly reduced and the volume of distribution is often increased; the elimination half-life in such cases may be increased 3-fold or more. The size of the initial bolus, the maintenance infusion, and the timing of plasma level determinations must be skillfully managed in all patients.

Therapeutic Use

Lidocaine's major indication is suppression of ventricular tachycardia and prevention of fibrillation after acute myocardial infarction. Lidocaine is the agent of first choice in this setting. Impressive evidence has been obtained to justify the view that lidocaine actually reduces the incidence of ventricular fibrillation in the first few days after acute myocardial infarction. It remains controversial, however, whether lidocaine should be routinely administered to all patients after myocardial infarction.

Lidocaine is rarely effective in supraventricular arrhythmias except for those associated with Wolff-Parkinson-White syndrome or digitalis toxicity.

TOCAINIDE & MEXILETINE

Tocainide and mexiletine are congeners of lidocaine that are resistant to first-pass hepatic metabolism. Therefore they can be used by the oral route. Their electrophysiologic and antiarrhythmic actions are similar to those of lidocaine. They are useful in the treatment of ventricular arrhythmias. The therapeutic half-life of both drugs is between 8 and 20 hours, and they are administered 2 or 3 times a day. The usual daily dose of mexiletine is 600–1200 mg/d, and for tocainide 800–2400 mg/d. Both drugs cause dose-related side effects that are seen frequently at therapeutic

dosage. These are predominantly neurologic, including tremor, blurred vision, and lethargy. Nausea is also a common side effect. Rash, fever, and agranulocytosis occur in about 0.5% of patients receiving tocainide.

PHENYTOIN

Phenytoin (diphenylhydantoin) is an anticonvulsant agent with limited antiarrhythmic properties (Chapter 22). Because of its limited efficacy, it should only be considered as a second-line drug. It suppresses ectopic pacemaker activity, blocks the sodium current, and may interfere with the calcium current. It appears especially effective against digitalis-induced arrhythmias.

IMIPRAMINE

Imipramine is a tricyclic antidepressant agent that also has antiarrhythmic activity. Its electrophysiologic actions and clinical spectrum of activity are similar to those of quinidine. Like disopyramide, it also has strong atropinelike effects. Its elimination half-life is about 12 hours. The usual daily dose is 200 mg/d in 2 doses. The initial dose should be smaller, because the drug's most prominent side effect (sleepiness) is lessened by slowly increasing the dose. Imipramine is marketed as an antidepressant, and its use as an antiarrhythmic agent has not yet been approved by the FDA.

FLECAINIDE & ENCAINIDE

Flecainide and encainide are potent sodium channel blockers used primarily for therapy of ventricular arrhythmias. Flecainide has been approved and encainide is scheduled to be approved for marketing soon. Both agents have minimal effects on repolarization and neither causes antimuscarinic side effects. Both drugs are exceedingly effective in suppressing premature ventricular contractions. However, both may cause severe exacerbation of arrhythmia when higher doses are administered to patients with preexisting ventricular tachyarrhythmias. The effective dose range of encainide is 25–75 mg 3 times a day. The usual dose of flecainide is 100–200 mg twice a day.

Tocainide

Mexiletine

PROPAFENONE

Propafenone has some structural similarities to propranolol. Its spectrum of action is very similar to that of quinidine, but instead of being an antimuscarinic agent, it is a weak beta blocker. Its elimination half-life is 2–32 hours. The usual daily dosage of propafenone is 450–900 mg/d in 3 doses. The drug is

Propafenone

Amiodarone

widely used in Europe and appears to be relatively devoid of serious side effects. The most common adverse effects are a metallic taste and constipation.

AMIODARONE

Amiodarone has been widely used as an antiarrhythmic and antianginal agent in Europe, Asia, and South America, but it has only recently been approved for clinical use in the USA. It is very effective against a wide variety of arrhythmias, but its prominent side effects and unusual pharmacokinetics limit its use.

Cardiac Effects

Amiodarone has a broad spectrum of actions on the heart. It is a very effective blocker of sodium channels, but unlike quinidine it has a low affinity for activated channels, combining instead almost exclusively with channels in the inactivated state. Thus, the sodium-blocking action of amiodarone is most pronounced in tissues that have long action potentials, frequent action potentials, or less negative diastolic potentials. In therapeutic concentrations, amiodarone also markedly lengthens action potential duration by an unknown mechanism, perhaps involving blockade of potassium channels. Amiodarone is a weak calcium channel blocker as well as a noncompetitive inhibitor of beta-adrenoceptors. Perhaps as a result of this combination of potentially antiarrhythmic effects, the drug has also been shown to be a powerful inhibitor of abnormal automaticity.

Amiodarone slows the sinus rate and atrioventricular conduction, markedly prolongs the QT interval, and slightly prolongs QRS duration. It increases atrial, atrioventricular nodal, and ventricular refractory periods. Induction of new ventricular arrhythmias or worsening of preexisting ones occasionally occurs during therapy with amiodarone. In patients with Wolff-Parkinson-White syndrome, the drug delays conduction, prolongs the effective refractory period, and may even totally abolish transmission through the accessory pathways.

Amiodarone also has antianginal effects. This may result from its noncompetitive alpha- and beta-adrenoceptor–blocking properties as well as from its apparent ability to block calcium influx in coronary arterial smooth muscle.

Cardiac Toxicity

In patients with sinus or atrioventricular nodal disease, amiodarone may produce symptomatic bradycardia or heart block. It may also precipitate heart failure in susceptible patients.

Extracardiac Effects

Amiodarone causes peripheral vascular dilatation, presumably through its alpha-adrenoceptor–blocking and calcium channel–inhibiting effects. In some patients, this may be beneficial; rarely, it may require discontinuation of the drug.

Extracardiac Toxicity

Amiodarone causes a remarkable variety of extracardiac side effects. There is a log-linear relationship between toxicity and cumulative dose, which limits the utility of amiodarone for long-term therapy.

Amiodarone is deposited as microcrystals in tissue and can be found in virtually every organ. The most readily detected deposits are those in the cornea, which can be observed as yellowish-brown granules within a few weeks following initiation of therapy. These corneal deposits rarely cause visual symptoms except for an occasional halo in the peripheral visual fields, most prominent at night. Only infrequently does reduction of visual acuity occur that requires discontinuation or reduction of amiodarone dosage. Skin deposits of microcrystals can result in photodermatitis in about 25% of patients, requiring avoidance of sun exposure. In less than 5% of patients, a grayish-blue skin discoloration develops.

Thyroid dysfunction—both hypo- and hyperthyroidism—is the next most common side effect (about 5% of patients). Thyroid function should be assessed prior to and throughout the duration of therapy with amiodarone.

Neurologic side effects are common and include paresthesias, tremor, ataxia, and headaches.

Amiodarone may affect the gastrointestinal tract (eg, constipation, 20%), liver (eg, hepatocellular necrosis), or lung (eg, inflammation and fibrosis, 15%). Fatal lung fibrosis has been reported.

Drug interactions are very common, since amiodarone reduces clearance of warfarin, theophylline, quinidine, procainamide, flecainide, and other drugs. Although amiodarone is a highly effective antiarrhythmic agent, its toxicity limits its clinical usefulness.

Pharmacokinetics & Dosage

Amiodarone has an extremely long half-life (13–103 days). The effective plasma concentration is approximately 1–2 μg/mL, while the cardiac tissue concentration is about 30 times higher. It takes 15–30 days to load the body stores with sufficient amiodarone to estimate the drug's efficacy. Loading doses of 0.8–1.2 g daily for about 2 weeks are used, after which the patient is maintained on 0.2–1 g daily. Because of the drug's long half-life, once-daily dosage is adequate.

Therapeutic Use

Amiodarone is very effective against both supraventricular and ventricular arrhythmias. In general, relatively low dosages (200–400 mg/d) can be used against paroxysmal atrial fibrillation and the circus movement associated with Wolff-Parkinson-White syndrome. Amiodarone appears to be especially effective against supraventricular arrhythmias in children.

CALCIUM CHANNEL-BLOCKING DRUGS

These drugs, of which verapamil is the prototype, were first introduced as antianginal agents and are discussed in some detail in Chapter 11. However, verapamil and several newer agents in this class are very effective antiarrhythmic drugs.

Only verapamil is discussed here. Other calcium channel–blocking agents in general use are diltiazem and nifedipine. Lidoflazine and flunarizine are investigational in the USA. Nifedipine appears to have little antiarrhythmic activity, whereas diltiazem may be as effective as verapamil.

VERAPAMIL

Cardiac Effects

Verapamil blocks both activated and inactivated calcium channels. Thus, its effect is more marked in tissues that fire frequently, are less completely polarized at rest, and in which activation depends exclusively on the calcium current, such as the sinoatrial and atrioventricular nodes. Thus, it is not surprising that verapamil has marked effects on these tissues. Atrioventricular nodal conduction and effective refractory period are invariably prolonged by therapeutic concentrations. Verapamil usually slows the sinoatrial node by its direct action, but its hypotensive action may occasionally result in a small reflex increase of sinoatrial nodal rate.

Verapamil can suppress oscillatory afterpotentials resulting from digitalis toxicity and may antagonize slow responses arising in severely depolarized tissue.

Cardiac Toxicity

Verapamil's cardiotoxic effects are dose-related and usually avoidable. Its negative inotropic effects may limit its clinical usefulness in damaged hearts (see Chapter 11). Verapamil can lead to atrioventricular block when used in large doses or in patients with partial atrioventricular block. This block can be treated with atropine, beta-receptor stimulants, or calcium. In patients with sinus node disease, verapamil can precipitate sinus arrest.

Extracardiac Effects & Toxicity

Verapamil causes peripheral vasodilatation, which may be beneficial in hypertension and peripheral vasospastic disorders. Its effects upon smooth muscle provide a number of therapeutic extracardiac effects (see Chapter 11).

Minor adverse effects include constipation, lassitude, nervousness, and peripheral edema.

Pharmacokinetics & Dosage

The half-life of verapamil is approximately 7 hours. Verapamil is extensively metabolized by the liver; after oral administration, its bioavailability is only about 20%. Therefore, verapamil must be administered with great caution in patients with hepatic dysfunction. Much smaller doses are required when the drug is administered intravenously.

In adult patients without heart failure or sinoatrial or atrioventricular nodal disease, an initial bolus of 5 mg is administered over 2–5 minutes for treatment of supraventricular tachycardias, followed a few minutes later by a second 5-mg bolus if needed. Thereafter, 5- to 10-mg doses can be administered every 4–6 hours, or a constant infusion of 0.4 μg/kg/min may be used.

Effective oral dosage ranges from 120 to 600 mg daily, divided in 3 or 4 doses.

Therapeutic Use

Reentrant supraventricular tachycardia is the major indication for verapamil, and the drug is fast replacing previous treatments (propranolol, digoxin, edrophonium, vasoconstrictor agents, and cardioversion). Verapamil can also reduce the ventricular rate in atrial fibrillation and flutter. It may convert atrial flutter and fibrillation to sinus rhythm. In ventricular arrhythmias, verapamil appears to be only moderately effective.

DRUGS THAT PROLONG EFFECTIVE REFRACTORY PERIOD BY PROLONGING ACTION POTENTIAL

At present, the only agents in this category are those which have additional effects that place them in one of the other subgroups. Quinidine and especially amiodarone effectively prolong action potential duration. However, as noted above, their actions on sodium channels also contribute to the measured increase in effective refractory period. Bretylium also prolongs action potential duration and refractory period and is discussed below.

DRUGS THAT BLOCK SYMPATHETIC ACTIVITY IN THE HEART

BETA-ADRENOCEPTOR–BLOCKING DRUGS

Cardiac Effects

Propranolol and similar drugs have antiarrhythmic properties by virtue of their beta receptor–blocking action and direct membrane effects (Chapter 9). Of these drugs, some have selectivity for cardiac beta receptors (β_1 blockers); some have intrinsic sympathomimetic activity; some have marked direct membrane effects; and some prolong the cardiac action potential. The relative contributions of the beta-blocking and direct membrane effects to the antiarrhythmic effects of these drugs are not fully known. Although beta blockers are fairly well tolerated, their efficacy for suppression of ventricular ectopic depolarizations is lower than that of sodium channel blockers. However, there is growing evidence that these agents can prevent recurrent infarction and sudden death in patients recovering from acute myocardial infarction (Chapter 9). Sotalol is a non-selective beta-blocking drug that prolongs the action potential; it has been extensively investigated as an antiarrhythmic drug in Europe.

BRETYLIUM

Bretylium was first introduced as an antihypertensive agent. It interferes with the neuronal release of catecholamines but also has direct antiarrhythmic properties.

Bretylium

Cardiac Effects

Bretylium lengthens the ventricular (but not the atrial) action potential duration and effective refractory period. This effect is most pronounced in ischemic cells, which have shortened action potential durations. Thus, bretylium reverses the shortening in action potential duration precipitated by ischemia.

Experimentally, it has been shown that bretylium markedly increases the strength of electrical stimulation needed to induce ventricular fibrillation (ventricular fibrillation threshold) and delays the onset of fibrillation after acute coronary ligation. This antifibrillatory action appears to be independent of its sympatholytic properties.

Since bretylium causes an initial release of catecholamines, it has some positive inotropic actions when first administered. This action may also *precipitate* ventricular arrhythmias and must be watched for at the onset of therapy with the drug.

Extracardiac Effects

These are predictable from the drug's sympathoplegic actions. The major side effect is postural hypotension. This side effect can be almost totally prevented by concomitant administration of a tricyclic antidepressant agent such as protriptyline. Nausea and vomiting may occur after the intravenous administration of a bolus of bretylium.

Pharmacokinetics & Dosage

Bretylium is available only for intravenous use in the USA. In adults, an intravenous bolus of bretylium tosylate, 5 mg/kg, is administered over a 10-minute period. This dosage may be repeated after 30 minutes. Maintenance therapy is achieved by a similar bolus every 4–6 hours or by a constant infusion of 0.5–2 mg/min.

Therapeutic Use

Bretylium is usually used in an emergency setting, often during attempted resuscitation from ventricular fibrillation when lidocaine and cardioversion have failed. Only rarely does bretylium suppress premature ventricular contractions.

II. CLINICAL PHARMACOLOGY OF THE ANTIARRHYTHMIC AGENTS

PRINCIPLES OF ANTIARRHYTHMIC THERAPY

In addition to a thorough understanding of the pharmacokinetics and specific antiarrhythmic actions of the various antiarrhythmic agents, the clinician must employ certain basic principles and a growing number of technologic aids in treating patients with cardiac arrhythmias. The 3 main principles are (1) arrhythmia documentation, (2) drug efficacy assessment, and (3) plasma drug concentration determination. Antiarrhythmic drug therapy is rarely successful when any one of these principles is ignored.

Documentation of arrhythmias has been greatly facilitated by recent technical advances, including in-hospital, computer-assisted ECG rhythm monitoring, ambulatory ECG monitoring, patient-initiated ECG event recording, and telephonic transmission of ECG signals. With these aids, it becomes inappropriate for assumptions to be made regarding the presence, absence, or nature of an arrhythmia.

The assessment of antiarrhythmic drug efficacy in individual patients has improved markedly in the past decade. The technical developments mentioned above make it possible to confirm, with statistical validation, the efficacy or inefficacy of an antiarrhythmic drug for a specific arrhythmia in a given individual. The physician's ability to choose the appropriate antiarrhythmic drug has also been expanded. Such a choice is based first upon the known spectrum of activity of any drug under consideration. Beyond that consideration, the choice must be empiric. The conventional approach to empiric drug selection in the past required that each drug be given a full therapeutic trial, usually requiring days or weeks of therapy with dose increments. This method relies upon frequent ambulatory monitoring and entails a certain risk in patients with life-threatening cardiac arrhythmias. A protracted trial-and-error testing period before settling on the most effective drug and the optimum dose may be dangerous. A newer technique, clinical cardiac electrophysiologic testing, now permits artificial induction of clinical arrhythmias and provides a basis for immediate and rapid antiarrhythmic drug efficacy assessment in patients with sustained ventricular tachyarrhythmias. By this new technique, the patient's arrhythmia can be repeatedly induced and terminated, using temporary pacing catheters to stimulate the heart. An antiarrhythmic drug is then administered and arrhythmia induction is again attempted. Failure to induce the arrhythmia after drug administration is strongly predictive of long-term efficacy of the drug.

The third principle is antiarrhythmic drug concentration determination. Most antiarrhythmic drugs are variably absorbed and metabolized by patients, and this variability may be further exaggerated by congestive heart failure and impaired renal and hepatic function. A drug cannot be considered ineffective unless plasma concentrations have been measured and found to be in the therapeutic range. In addition, since many antiarrhythmic drugs are characterized by a narrow therapeutic concentration range, patient safety often depends upon plasma level analysis.

WHEN SHOULD ARRHYTHMIAS BE TREATED?

Deciding when antiarrhythmic therapy is indicated is a complex matter. While the need to treat immediately life-threatening rhythm disturbances is usually obvious, other situations may be less so. Rhythms that produce significant symptoms should usually be treated, regardless of their risk to the patient, unless they present a small risk *and* the likelihood of successful therapy is small (as in certain instances of atrial fibrillation).

The area of greatest controversy concerns the therapy of premature ventricular contractions. Should all premature ventricular contractions be treated? Should the goal of therapy be to *totally* eliminate them? While there is no definite answer to either question, certain reasonable guidelines can be established:

(1) The simpler therapies should not be forgotten. Many patients benefit from reduction of excessive coffee intake, cigarette use, and alcohol consumption. Exercise, emotional stress, certain foods, and other avoidable environmental factors may trigger arrhythmias in susceptible patients. Identification and elimination of such factors should always be the first step after accurate diagnosis in the management of patients with cardiac rhythm disturbances.

(2) In patients without structural heart disease, ventricular arrhythmias generally do not have to be treated unless they are causing significant symptoms or are life-threatening (eg, ventricular tachycardia).

(3) Complex ventricular arrhythmias (eg, ventricular tachycardia) should be treated with the goal of eliminating them.

In some patients, the presence of heart disease may complicate the use of antiarrhythmic drugs. Heart failure and conduction system disease are the most important problems. Most antiarrhythmic drugs depress left ventricular function to a variable, dose-related extent. Disopyramide, verapamil, and beta receptor–blocking drugs are the most frequent offenders. In patients with atrioventricular nodal disease, verapamil, digitalis, and beta blockers may cause heart block. In patients with conduction disease below the level of the atrioventricular node, therapy with disopyramide, quinidine, and procainamide and most of the experimental sodium channel–blocking drugs should only be started under careful continuous in-hospital monitoring.

Some arrhythmias do not respond to conventional or experimental drugs. In such cases, combinations of drugs may be tried. It is unwise to combine agents with similar electrophysiologic properties (eg, quinidine with procainamide, or verapamil with diltiazem). Overall, efficacy of combinations of 2 or more drugs that were ineffective when given singly in previous trials is low. If drug therapy fails, other measures may be considered (eg, pacing, cardioversion, and surgical procedures).

REFERENCES

Coraboeuf E: Ionic basis of electrical activity in cardiac tissues. *Am J Physiol* 1978;**234**:101.

Grant AO et al: The influence of pH on the electrophysiological

effects of lidocaine in guinea pig ventricular myocardium. *Circ Res* 1980;**47**:542.

Greenblatt DJ, Koch-Weser J: Clinical pharmacokinetics. (2

parts.) *N Engl J Med* 1975;**293:**702, 964.

Harrison DC, Meffin PJ, Winkle RA: Clinical pharmacology of antiarrhythmic drugs. *Prog Cardiovasc Dis* 1977;**20:**217.

Hoffman BF, Rosen MR: Cellular mechanisms of cardiac arrhythmias. *Circ Res* 1981;**49:**1.

Hoffman BF, Rosen MR, Wit AL: Electrophysiology and pharmacology of cardiac arrhythmias. 7. Cardiac effects of quinidine and procainamide. *Am Heart J* 1975;**89:**804.

Hondeghem LM, Katzung BG: Antiarrhythmic agents: Modulated receptor mechanism of action of sodium and calcium channel–blocking drugs. *Annu Rev Pharmacol Toxicol* 1984; **24:**387.

Hondeghem LM, Katzung BG: Test of a model of antiarrhythmic drug action: Effects of quinidine and lidocaine on myocardial conduction. *Circulation* 1980;**61:**1217.

Lazzara R, Hope RR, El-Sherif BJ: Effects of lidocaine on hypoxic and ischemic cardiac cells. *Am J Cardiol* 1979;**41:**872.

Mason JW, Hondeghem LM, Katzung BG: Block of inactivated sodium channels and of depolarization-induced automaticity in guinea pig papillary muscles by amiodarone. *Circ Res* 1984;**55:**278.

Mason JW, Winkle RA: Accuracy of the ventricular tachycardia-induction study for predicting long-term efficacy and inefficacy of antiarrhythmic drugs. *N Engl J Med* 1980; **303:**1073.

McDonald TF, Pelzer D, Trautwein W: On the mechanism of slow calcium channel block in heart. *Pflugers Arch* 1980; **385:**175.

Mitchell LB, Schroeder JS, Mason JW: Comparative clinical electrophysiologic effects of diltiazem, verapamil and nifedipine: A review. *Am J Cardiol* 1982;**49:**629.

Siddoway LA, Roden DM, Woosley RL: Clinical pharmacology of old and new antiarrhythmic drugs. Pages 199–248 in: *Sudden Cardiac Death.* Josephson ME (editor). Davis, 1985.

Oshita S et al: Effects of tocainide and lidocaine on the transmembrane action potentials as related to external potassium and calcium concentration in guinea pig papillary muscles. *Naunyn Schmiedebergs Arch Pharmacol* 1980;**314:**67.

Zipes DP, Troup PJ: New antiarrhythmic agents: Amiodarone, aprindine, disopyramide, ethmozin, mexiletine, tocainide and verapamil. *Am J Cardiol* 1978;**41:**1005.

Diuretics

14

David G. Warnock, MD

Drugs acting on the renal tubules are useful in a variety of clinical conditions involving abnormal electrolyte or water metabolism. Because the anatomic segments of the nephron are highly specialized in function, the actions of each agent in this group can be best understood in relation to its site of action in the nephron and the normal physiology of that segment.

RENAL TUBULE TRANSPORT MECHANISMS

PROXIMAL TUBULES

Sodium bicarbonate, glucose, amino acids, and other organic solutes are preferentially reabsorbed in the early proximal tubule. As shown in Fig 14–1, the luminal concentrations of these solutes decrease along the length of the proximal tubule. Because of the high water permeability of the proximal tubule, the luminal fluid osmolality and sodium concentration remain relatively the same along the length of the proximal tubule. The luminal chloride concentration rises along the length of the proximal tubule—in contrast to the bicarbonate concentration, which falls. Therefore, bicarbonate is preferentially reabsorbed in the early proximal tubule, at least in comparison to chloride. Bicarbonate reabsorption by the proximal tubule is known to be critically dependent upon carbonic anhydrase activity. In the later portions of the proximal tubule, the luminal fluid closely resembles a simple NaCl solution (Fig 14–2). The reabsorptive process in the late proximal tubule therefore consists of isotonic NaCl reabsorption.

Organic acid secretory systems are located in the middle third of the proximal tubule (S_2 segment). These systems secrete a variety of organic acids (uric, p-aminohippuric, diuretics, antibiotics, etc) into the luminal fluid from the bloodstream. Organic base secretory systems (creatinine, procainamide, choline, etc) are localized in the early (S_1) and middle (S_2) segments of the proximal tubules. These organic secretory systems are important determinants in delivery of diuretics to their active sites at the luminal aspects of tubule segments along the entire nephron. In addition, these sites account for several interactions between diuretics and uric acid or other exogenous organic

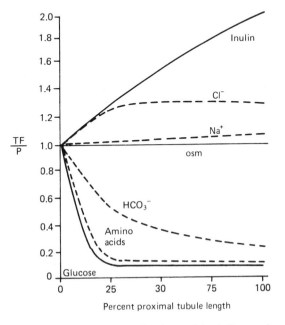

Figure 14–1. Reabsorption of various solutes in the proximal tubule in relation to tubule length. TF/P, tubular fluid to plasma concentration ratio. (Reproduced, with permission, from Ganong WF: *Review of Medical Physiology,* 12th ed. Lange, 1985.)

compounds (eg, interactions between diuretics and probenecid).

LOOP OF HENLE

Water is abstracted from the thin descending limb of the loop of Henle by osmotic forces generated in the hypertonic medullary interstitium. Solute entry (eg, NaCl, urea) may occur in some species, but water removal appears to be the dominant process in most mammalian kidneys. Any impermeant solute in the lumen will oppose water abstraction and increase the delivery of salt and water to more distal sites. Important examples of impermeant solutes include osmotic diuretics, glucose (in glycosuria), and bicarbonate (which may be present if proximal bicarbonate reabsorption has been inhibited).

The thick ascending limb of the loop of Henle is the site of an active NaCl reabsorptive system that removes salt from the lumen and adds it to the sur-

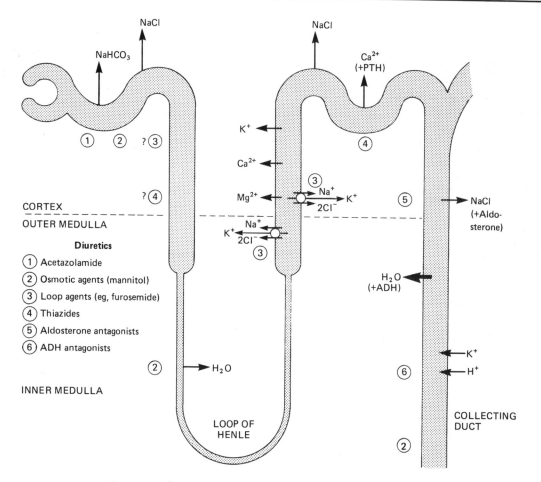

Figure 14–2. Tubule transport systems and sites of action of diuretics.

rounding interstitium. This segment is extremely impermeable to water and therefore can be regarded as a diluting segment. Medullary portions of the thick ascending limb contribute to medullary hypertonicity and thereby also play an important role in concentration of urine. In contrast, NaCl reabsorbed from the cortical portions of the thick ascending limb does not provide a driving force for water abstraction from medullary structures and therefore does not participate in concentration of the urine. The NaCl transport system in the thick ascending limb is now regarded as a sodium/potassium/2-chloride cotransport mechanism rather than an active "chloride" pump. A lumen-positive electrical potential present in this segment provides an important driving force for the reabsorption of divalent cations (Mg^{2+}, Ca^{2+}) and K^+. Inhibition of the thick ascending limb by "loop" diuretics causes an increase in urinary excretion of these cations in addition to NaCl.

DISTAL CONVOLUTED TUBULE

The distal convoluted tubule can be regarded as a cortical diluting segment that reabsorbs NaCl and ap-

pears to be impermeable to water. In contrast to more distal sites, this segment does not appear to respond to aldosterone or antidiuretic hormone (ADH). This segment does have parathyroid hormone (PTH) receptors and is a site of active Ca^{2+} reabsorption. Although the mechanism of NaCl transport in this segment has not yet been defined, it is known that the rate of NaCl reabsorption is less than in the thick ascending limb.

COLLECTING TUBULES

NaCl is reabsorbed in the collecting tubules, and this transport system is regulated by mineralocorticoid hormones. In addition, K^+ and H^+ are secreted into the lumen, especially under conditions that enhance Na^+ reabsorption. The coupling between Na^+ reabsorption and K^+ (and H^+) secretion may involve several indirect mechanisms and can be completely dissociated in certain experimental settings, ie, it is not a simple "exchange." By whatever mechanism, there does appear to be a direct relation between Na^+ delivery to these sites and the resulting secretion of H^+ and K^+. These relations are accentuated during hypermineralocorticoid conditions and when distal Na^+ delivery is accompanied by an impermeant anion such as bicarbonate, phosphate, or sulfate.

In the presence of ADH, the collecting tubule (and duct) become very permeable to water. ADH levels are elevated during antidiuresis, and a concentrated urine is excreted. On the other hand, ADH secretion is suppressed during hypotonic volume expansion and by certain drugs, and relatively large volumes of dilute urine are excreted.

I. BASIC PHARMACOLOGY OF DIURETICS

CARBONIC ANHYDRASE INHIBITORS

Carbonic anhydrase is present in many nephron sites, including the cytoplasm and the luminal and basolateral membranes, and in the red cells in the peritubular capillaries. The predominant site is in the proximal tubule, where this enzyme catalyzes the CO_2 hydration/dehydration reactions involved in bicarbonate reabsorption. Inhibitors of carbonic anhydrase cause sodium bicarbonate diuresis and a reduction in total body bicarbonate stores.

The carbonic anhydrase inhibitors were the forerunners of modern diuretics. They are unsubstituted sulfonamide derivatives and were developed when it was noted that bacteriostatic sulfonamides caused hyperchloremic metabolic acidosis with large volumes of alkaline urine. Subsequent sulfonamide diuretics (ie, thiazides) were developed to separate the natriuretic effect from the effects on bicarbonate handling.

Chemistry

The structure of acetazolamide is shown below. The $-SO_2NH_2$ (sulfamyl) group is essential for activity. Alkyl substitutions at this point completely block its effects on carbonic anhydrase activity.

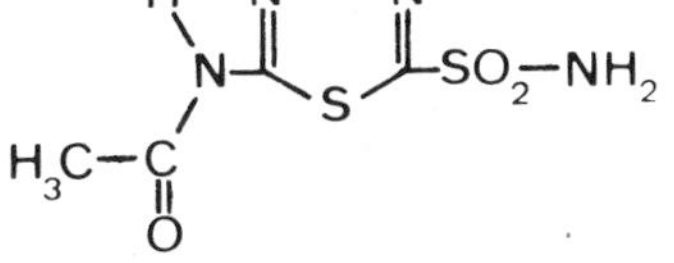

Acetazolamide

Pharmacokinetics

All of the carbonic anhydrase inhibitors are well absorbed after oral administration. Effects on urine pH are apparent within 30 minutes, are maximal at 2 hours, and persist for 12 hours after a single dose. Excretion is by tubular secretion in the S_2 segment of the proximal tubule.

Pharmacodynamics

Inhibition of carbonic anhydrase activity profoundly depresses bicarbonate reabsorption in the proximal tubule. Bicarbonate accumulates in the cells and in the luminal fluid. The discrepancy between luminal pH (which may become acid) and the elevation in the luminal bicarbonate concentration has been referred to as a "disequilibrium" pH. Nearly all of the bicarbonate-reabsorptive capacity of the superficial proximal tubule can be inhibited by acetazolamide, with an apparent IC50 (concentration for 50% inhibition) of 4 μmol/L. In contrast, substantial amounts of bicarbonate can still be absorbed at other nephron sites by one or more undefined carbonic anhydrase–independent mechanisms. The overall result of maximal acetazolamide administration is 85% inhibition of proximal bicarbonate reabsorption but only 45% inhibition of whole kidney bicarbonate reabsorption. The result is an acute bicarbonate-wasting condition. Depletion of the body stores of bicarbonate results in hyperchloremic metabolic acidosis and thereby reduces diuretic effectiveness of subsequent doses of the same drug.

An interesting effect of inhibition of proximal bicarbonate reabsorption is a parallel inhibition of chloride reabsorption in the proximal tubule. As a result, both $NaHCO_3$ and NaCl are delivered out of the proximal tubule during carbonic anhydrase inhibition. Most of the increased distal delivery of NaCl is picked up at downstream sites (ie, thick ascending limb), so the resulting natriuresis is accompanied by bicarbonate and not by chloride.

Many other secretory processes involve H^+ or HCO_3^- transport, which are mediated by carbonic anhydrase activity. Aqueous humor production is an important example, as noted below.

Clinical Indications & Dosage

A. Glaucoma: (See Table 14–1.) Aqueous humor contains a high concentration of bicarbonate ion. Inhibition of carbonic anhydrase decreases the rate of aqueous humor formation and thereby decreases intraocular pressure. This effect is of value in the chronic management of glaucoma, which is now the most common indication for use of carbonic anhydrase inhibitors.

Acetazolamide is also available in sustained-release capsules containing 500 mg and as the sodium salt in vials for parenteral administration.

B. Urinary Alkalinization: Uric acid and cystine are relatively insoluble in acid urines. Enhanced renal excretion can theoretically be achieved by increasing urinary bicarbonate excretion with carbonic anhydrase

Table 14–1. Carbonic anhydrase inhibitors used in treatment of glaucoma.

	Usual Oral Dose (1–4 Times Daily)
Acetazolamide (Diamox)	250 mg
Dichlorphenamide (Daranide, Oratrol)	50 mg

inhibitors. Similarly, renal excretion of weak acids (eg, aspirin) is increased by raising the urine pH. These effects are of relatively short duration and require bicarbonate infusion to maintain continuing bicarbonate diuresis.

C. Reduction of Total Body Bicarbonate Stores: Carbonic anhydrase inhibition will cause acute sodium bicarbonate diuresis as long as the filtered load of bicarbonate exceeds the renal capacity for bicarbonate absorption. This approach can be useful in chronic metabolic alkalosis associated with resistance to other diuretic agents. Another example is posthypercapnic metabolic alkalosis: Carbonic anhydrase inhibitors can be used to correct this condition if saline administration is ineffective or contraindicated because of elevated cardiac filling pressures.

D. Acute Mountain Sickness: Weakness, breathlessness, dizziness, and nausea can occur in mountain climbers who rapidly ascend above 3000 m and overexert themselves. The symptoms are usually mild and last for a few days. In some climbers, rapidly progressing pulmonary or cerebral edema can be life-threatening. Acetazolamide increases performance status and decreases overall symptomatology. A recent study (see Greene reference) proposed taking 500 mg (one sustained-release capsule) by mouth at night for 5 nights before a climb.

E. Other Uses: Carbonic anhydrase inhibitors have been used as adjuvants for the treatment of epilepsy, in some forms of hypokalemic periodic paralysis, and to increase urinary phosphate excretion during severe hyperphosphatemia.

Toxicity

A. Hyperchloremic Metabolic Acidosis: This is the predictable consequence of chronic reduction of body bicarbonate stores. Bicarbonate wasting will ultimately limit the diuretic efficacy of carbonic anhydrase inhibitors in direct proportion to the overall reduction in filtered load of bicarbonate.

B. Renal Stones: Phosphaturia and hypercalciuria occur during the bicarbonaturic response to carbonic anhydrase inhibition. Renal excretion of solubilizing factors (eg, citrate) may decline with chronic use. Calcium salts are relatively insoluble at alkaline pH, which means that renal stone formation can occur.

C. Renal K+ Wasting: Potassium wasting can be severe, especially during the acute bicarbonate diuresis stage. This complication may limit the usefulness of carbonic anhydrase inhibitors in chronic metabolic alkalosis associated with prior diuretic administration.

D. Other Toxicities: Drowsiness and paresthesias are common following large doses. Hypersensitivity reactions (fever, rashes, bone marrow suppression, interstitial nephritis) can also occur.

Contraindications

Carbonic anhydrase inhibitors should be avoided in hepatic cirrhosis. Alkalinization of the urine will decrease urinary trapping of NH_4^+ and may contribute to the development of hepatic encephalopathy.

LOOP AGENTS

These short-acting agents inhibit NaCl reabsorption in the thick ascending limb of the loop of Henle. Owing to the large NaCl absorptive capacity of this segment, agents that act at this site produce a diuretic effect much greater than that seen with any other diuretic group.

Chemistry

The 2 prototypical drugs of this group are furosemide and ethacrynic acid. The structures of **furosemide** and its analogs bumetanide and piretanide are shown in Fig 14–3. Like the thiazides, they are sulfonamide derivatives. These agents have a carboxyl group with a sulfamyl moiety in the meta position (carbon number 5). A halide or phenoxy substitution is present at carbon 4, and a substituted amino group is present at carbon 2 or 3.

Ethacrynic acid is not a sulfonamide and therefore is chemically distinct from the thiazides and furosemide. Ethacrynic acid is a phenoxyacetic acid derivative that also contains an adjacent ketone and methylene group. The methylene group (shaded in Fig 14–4) is fairly reactive and forms an adduct with the free sulfhydryl group of cysteine. The cysteine adduct appears to be the active form of the drug. Other members of this class (ie, phenoxyacetic acid derivatives,

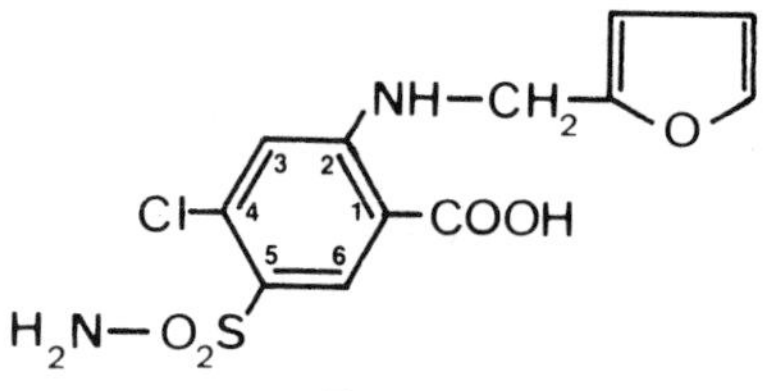

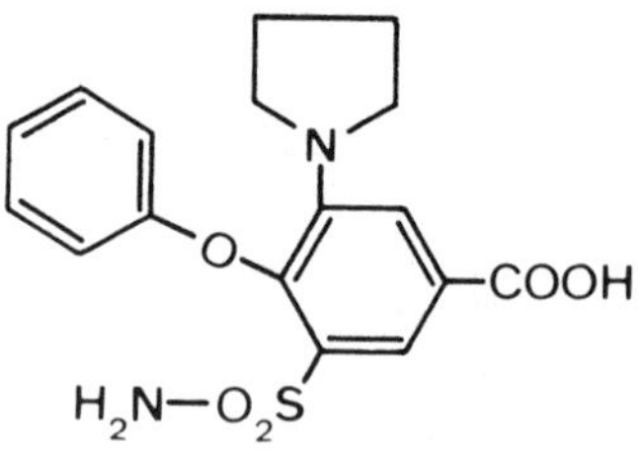

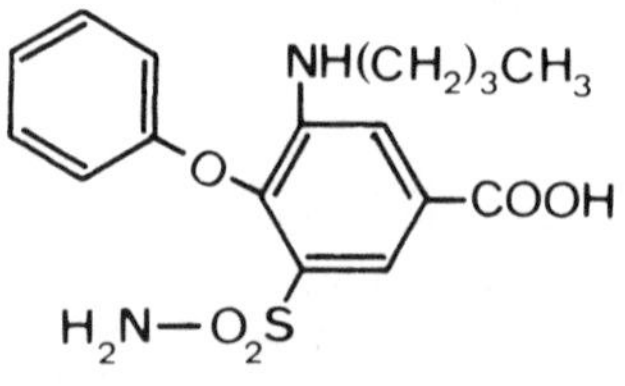

Figure 14–3. Furosemide derivatives.

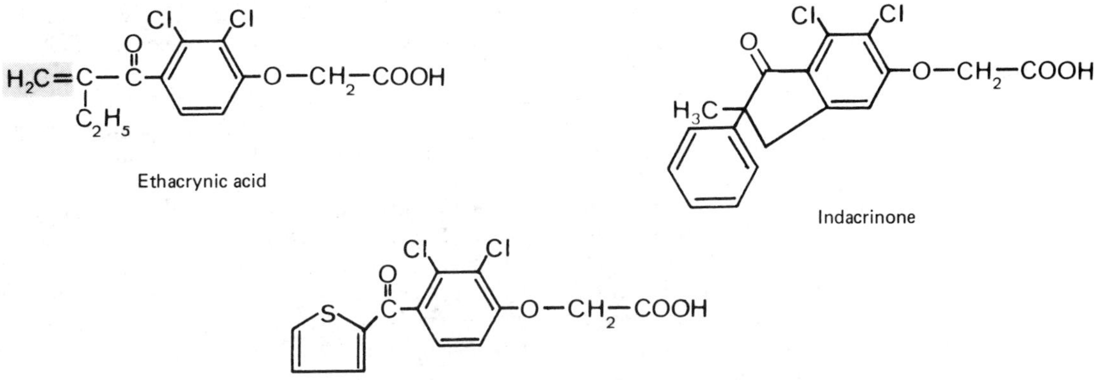

Figure 14–4. Ethacrynic acid derivatives.

Fig 14–4) are currently being developed. The analogs reveal 2 interesting features: (1) the sulfhydryl reactivity is not a requirement for diuretic activity, and (2) all members of this class have uricosuric activity. In some instances, diuretic and uricosuric effects have been associated with separate stereoisomers.

Pharmacokinetics

The loop agents are rapidly absorbed and handled by renal secretion as well as filtration. Diuretic response is usually extremely rapid following intravenous injection. The duration of effect is usually 2–3 hours. The response to furosemide correlates positively with its urinary excretion rate. Defects in the secretory component of its clearance may result from simultaneous administration of agents such as indomethacin and probenecid, which inhibit weak acid secretion in the proximal tubule. Metabolites of ethacrynic acid and furosemide have been identified, but it is not known if they have any diuretic activity.

Pharmacodynamics

These drugs inhibit NaCl transport in the thick ascending limb of the loop of Henle. The effect has been localized to a transport site at the luminal membrane. It was formerly thought that an "active" chloride pump was present in the thick ascending limb. The current view favors a coupled Na/K/2-Cl transport system that is driven by a Na^+,K^+-ATPase–dependent pump in the basolateral membrane. The loop diuretics reduce the reabsorption of both Na^+ and Cl^- and diminish the normal lumen-positive potential across the tubule. These agents at high concentrations can be shown in vivo to inhibit various ATPases and mitochondrial transport systems. These metabolic effects are probably not related to the diuretic effects of these agents.

The thick ascending limb is thought to play an important role in divalent cation handling. Inhibition of active NaCl transport causes an associated increase in Mg^{2+} and Ca^{2+} excretion, perhaps because of the diminished positive potential across the tubule. Chronic use of loop agents has been associated with Mg^{2+} wasting and severe hypomagnesemia. Calcium

excretion can be strikingly increased with loop agents and saline infusions, an effect of great usefulness in the acute management of hypercalcemia. This effect must be clearly distinguished from that of the thiazides, which *decrease* Ca^{2+} excretion.

Loop agents appear to have direct effects on blood flow through several vascular beds. Furosemide can be shown to increase renal blood flow and cause redistribution of blood flow within the renal cortex. The hemodynamic effects appear to involve the renin-angiotensin system and vasodilatory prostaglandins. However, the hemodynamic effects have not been directly linked to the diuretic response. Furosemide and ethacrynic acid have also been shown to improve pulmonary congestion and reduce left ventricular filling pressures as an acute hemodynamic effect before any measurable increase in urinary output occurs.

Clinical Indications & Dosage

A. Acute Pulmonary Edema: The therapeutic goal is rapid reduction of extracellular fluid volume and venous return so that right ventricular output and pulmonary vascular pressures are decreased. As described above, there may be an improvement in cardiac function that precedes the onset of diuresis. This response is due to an extrarenal hemodynamic response and may even be observed in anephric patients.

B. Refractory Edema: Loop diuretics are used when the patient does not respond to salt restrictions or less potent diuretics. Diuresis will ensue as long as interstitial fluid is mobilized without compromising intravascular volume. Loop agents are also useful in patients who have diminished renal function and fluid overload.

C. Hypercalcemia: Loop agents can promote a striking increase in urinary excretion of calcium with a prompt reduction in the serum calcium level. The effect is very useful in the acute treatment of hypercalcemia. Inhibition of thick ascending limb function also causes marked excretion of NaCl, water, K^+, and Mg^{2+}. Extracellular fluid volume depletion must be prevented to ensure a continued diuretic response. The usual approach is to infuse normal saline and give furosemide (80–120 mg) intravenously. Once the diuresis begins, the rate of saline infusion can be matched with the urine flow rate to avoid volume depletion. Potassium may be added to the saline infusion if clinically indicated.

D. Anion and Cation Overdose: Various electrolyte disorders may respond to increases in urine flow rate. For example, halides seem to be reabsorbed in the thick ascending limb; loop diuretics are therefore useful in treating bromide, fluoride, and iodide poisoning. Saline solution must be administered to replace urinary losses of Na^+ and to provide Cl^-, so as to avoid extracellular fluid volume depletion. Hyperkalemia is another example where renal clearance of K^+ may be increased by the use of loop agents and saline infusion. These drugs are not useful in the treatment of lithium poisoning.

E. Acute Renal Failure: Loop agents can increase the rate of urine flow in acute renal failure in both clinical and experimental circumstances. This maneuver can convert oliguric renal failure to nonoliguric failure but seems not to have any beneficial effect on overall outcome, duration of renal failure, or survival. If it is known that a large pigment load has precipitated acute renal failure or threatens to do so, loop agents may "wash out" intratubular casts and ameliorate intratubular obstruction. Loop agents may be used to increase urine flow rates if hyperkalemia complicates the course of acute renal failure.

F. Hyperuricemia: Uricosuric congeners of ethacrynic acid include **indacrinone** (MK-196) and **ticrynafen** (tienilic acid). These agents inhibit proximal reabsorption of uric acid and are therefore uricosuric. Serum uric acid levels are diminished, but acute renal insufficiency can result if the urinary load of uric acid increases too rapidly. These agents may be useful in patients with symptomatic hyperuricemia who require diuretic therapy for management of hypertension or congestive heart failure. Cholestatic jaundice occurred with the use of ticrynafen, and the drug is no longer available in the USA. Loop agents also can *cause* hyperuricemia, presumably via extracellular volume depletion and enhanced proximal reabsorption.

Toxicity

Loop agents increase delivery of salt and water to more distal segments of the nephron. The predictable consequence of this effect is enhanced renal secretion of K^+ and H^+. The clinical result is hypokalemic metabolic alkalosis. This effect reflects the potency of the diuretic agent and the extra-cellular fluid volume status. These effects will be discussed in the section on potassium-sparing diuretics.

Magnesium depletion is another predictable consequence of the effects of loop agents on the thick ascending limb. Magnesium wasting can also occur with the thiazides, but clinically important hypomagnesemia seems to occur more commonly with chronic use of loop agents. Volume status is another factor that can influence divalent cation excretion. Loop agents

are known for their calciuric effect, but clinical instances of *hypercalcemia* have been noted. This could result from volume depletion, since the proximal reabsorption of Ca^{2+} is apparently enhanced, resulting in volume contraction and hypercalcemia. Increased salt intake or use of less potent diuretics is indicated in this condition.

Ototoxicity is another well-described effect of loop agents. It is dose-related and usually (not always) reversible. This effect is seen with overzealous diuretic use in patients who have diminished renal function or are also receiving other ototoxic agents (ie, aminoglycoside antibiotics).

Contraindications

Idiosyncratic and hypersensitivity reactions occur with the use of loop agents. Acute allergic interstitial nephritis is well documented. It should be remembered that furosemide is a sulfonamide derivative and may demonstrate cross-reactivity in patients who are sensitive to other sulfonamides (ie, antimicrobial drugs used for urinary tract infections, carbonic anhydrase inhibitors, thiazides).

THIAZIDES

The thiazide diuretics emerged from efforts to synthesize more potent carbonic anhydrase inhibitors (see Fig 4–1). Chemical modification of the parent compounds changed the anion composition of the diuresis. Increased chloride, rather than bicarbonate, accompanied by sodium appeared in the urine. Subsequent work has shown that the thiazides inhibit NaCl transport independently of any effect on carbonic anhydrase activity. Some members of this group retain significant carbonic anhydrase inhibitory activity, but this effect is not related to the primary mode of action.

Chemistry

The drugs in this group are called thiazides, benzothiadiazides, or simply sulfonamide diuretics. Substitutions and the nature of the heterocyclic rings vary between the different congeners, but all of them retain, in common with the carbonic anhydrase inhibitors, an unsubstituted sulfamyl group (Fig 14–5).

The structure-activity relations of the thiazides are complex. There is a wide range of potency with regard to carbonic anhydrase inhibition. On the other hand, the diuretic potency has clearly been dissociated from the ability to inhibit carbonic anhydrase activity. Some members of the group have hyperglycemic activity, but the structural requirements for this effect differ from those of the diuresis. All of the members of this group have parallel dose-diuretic response curves and similar maximal effects on chloride excretion.

Pharmacokinetics

All of the thiazides are absorbed when given orally, but there are differences in their metabolism. Chlorothiazide, the parent of the group, is less lipid soluble

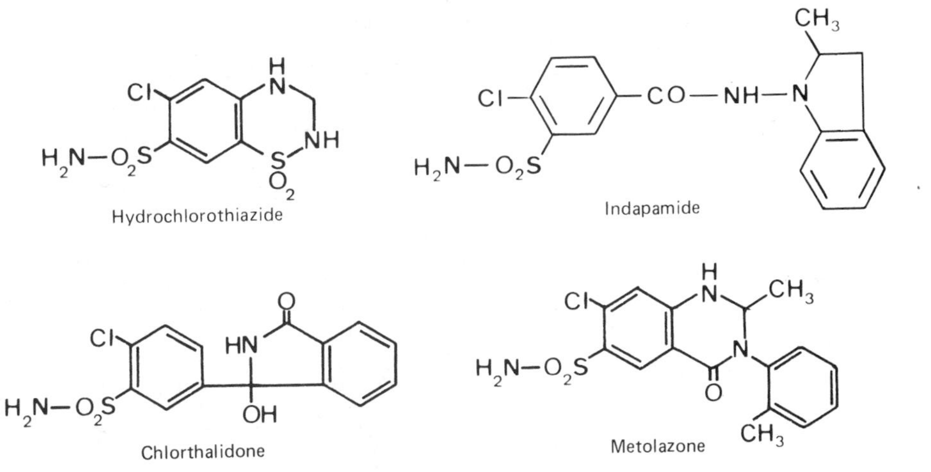

Figure 14–5. Thiazides and related agents.

and must be given in relatively large doses. Chlorthalidone is slowly absorbed and therefore appears to have a longer duration of action. Indapamide is excreted primarily by the biliary system and is useful in patients with renal insufficiency.

All of the thiazides are secreted by the organic acid secretory system and compete to some extent with the secretion of uric acid by that system. As a result, the uric acid secretory rate may be reduced, with a concomitant elevation in serum uric acid level. In the steady state, uric acid production and therefore renal excretion are not affected by the thiazides.

Pharmacodynamics

Thiazides inhibit NaCl reabsorption in the early segments of the distal tubule. Early clearance studies demonstrated an effect on NaCl reabsorption during excretion of diluted urine under water-loaded conditions. This finding suggested that the site of action was at a "cortical diluting segment," since there was no appreciable effect on urinary concentration during elaboration of hypertonic urine. More recent studies have shown that the distal convoluted tubule is the site of action of thiazides and that there is no effect on thick ascending limb function. There may also be an effect on NaCl reabsorption in the late proximal tubule, but this is not observed in the usual clinical setting. Any increase in NaCl delivery out of the proximal tubule is absorbed in the uninhibited thick ascending limb of the loop of Henle.

Very little is known about the NaCl transport system that is inhibited by thiazides. Normally, there is a lumen-negative electrical potential in the distal convoluted tubule, which is consistent with electrogenic Na^+ reabsorption. In contrast to the collecting tubule system, there does not appear to be any mineralocorticoid-dependent Na^+ transport in the distal convoluted tubule. There is an active reabsorptive process for Ca^{2+} in the distal convoluted tubule, which is modulated by parathyroid hormone (PTH). Thiazides do not inhibit Ca^{2+} reabsorption at this site. There may even

be a relative stimulation of Ca^{2+} reabsorption when thiazides inhibit NaCl reabsorption. The overall effect is NaCl diuresis with a decrease in Ca^{2+} excretion. This effect may be hidden if volume expansion (eg, increased dietary salt intake) is superimposed upon chronic thiazide therapy.

Analogs & Variants

A large number of analogs are available. Four agents merit specific mention, because they differ from other thiazides with regard to the constituents of the heterocyclic ring structure: chlorthalidone, quinethazone, metolazone, and indapamide. However, all 4 variants share with the thiazides an unsubstituted sulfonamide group.

Clinical Indications & Dosage

A. Hypertension and Congestive Heart Failure: These major indications for thiazide use are chronic conditions requiring mobilization of salt and water from interstitial compartments and reduction in "effective" circulatory volume. Dosages for some of the drugs in this group are given in Table 14–2. Lower doses of thiazides are used to treat essential hypertension than are needed to mobilize edema. This may reflect a vasodilating effect of thiazides on vascular smooth muscle. The effect is especially notable with indapamide. Thiazide diuretics are often an appropriate choice because of the mild, sustained nature of their diuretic effect. More efficacious agents—or combinations of agents—may be required if the therapeutic response to thiazides is inadequate.

B. Idiopathic Hypercalciuria: Thiazide therapy can reduce the urinary excretion of calcium and the degree to which urine is saturated with calcium salts. This effect is beneficial in calcium stone formers; a striking reduction in the incidence of new stone formation is generally seen. The reduction in urinary calcium excretion can be explained by the relative increase in calcium absorption induced by thiazides at the level of the distal convoluted tubule. This effect

Table 14–2. Thiazides and related diuretics: Dosages.

	Daily Oral Dose	Frequency of Dosage
Bendroflumethiazide (Benuron, Naturetin)	2.5–10 mg	As single dose
Benzthiazide* (Aquatag, Exna)	25–100 mg	In 2 divided doses
Chlorothiazide* (Diuril)	0.5–1 g	In 2 divided doses
Chlorthalidone† (Hygroton)	50–100 mg	As single dose
Cyclothiazide (Anhydron)	1–2 mg	As single dose
Hydrochlorothiazide* (Esidrix, Hydrodiuril, Oretic)	25–100 mg	As single dose
Hydroflumethiazide (Diucardin, Saluron)	25–100 mg	In 2 divided doses
Indapamide† (Lozol)	2.5–10 mg	As single dose
Methyclothiazide (Aquatensen, Enduron)	2.5–10 mg	As single dose
Metolazone† (Diulo, Zaroxolyn)	2.5–10 mg	As single dose
Polythiazide (Renese)	1–4 mg	As single dose
Quinethazone† (Hydromox)	50–100 mg	As single dose
Trichlormethiazide* (Metahydrin, Naqua)	2–8 mg	As single dose

*Generic preparation available. Trade name included for identification only.
†Not a thiazide but a sulfonamide qualitatively similar to the thiazides.

can be overcome by dietary salt excess, which may suppress proximal tubule reabsorption and increase urinary excretion of both Na^+ and Ca^{2+}.

C. Nephrogenic Diabetes Insipidus: Thiazide diuretics can reduce polyuria and polydipsia in patients who are not responsive to ADH. The beneficial effect is mediated through plasma volume reduction, with an attendant fall in glomerular filtration rate and enhanced proximal reabsorption of NaCl. Dietary sodium restriction can potentiate the beneficial effects of thiazides on urine volume in this setting. Lithium-induced nephrogenic diabetes insipidus may cause troublesome polyuria. Thiazides can be useful in this setting, but serum Li^+ levels must be carefully monitored, since these diuretics may *reduce* Li^+ clearance.

Toxicity

A. Weakness, Fatigability, Paresthesias: These dose-related toxic effects are similar to those of carbonic anhydrase inhibitors. Impotence has been reported as a side effect of thiazide therapy.

B. Potassium Depletion and Metabolic Alkalosis: These effects accompany the volume contraction and secondary hyperaldosteronism that occur with diuretic therapy. These issues will be discussed with the K^+-sparing diuretics.

C. Impaired Carbohydrate Tolerance: Hyperglycemia and glycosuria may occur in susceptible patients who are overtly diabetic or have abnormal glucose tolerance tests. The effect is dose-related and is the result of impaired pancreatic release of insulin or a blockade of peripheral glucose utilization.

D. Hyperuricemia and Hyperlipidemia: Serum uric acid levels usually rise when patients are given thiazide diuretics. Most patients remain asymptomatic and do not require therapy to lower their uric acid levels. Gout may be precipitated or intensified in susceptible subjects. There is no convincing evidence that hyperuricemia is a cardiovascular risk factor at present. There are associations between hypertension, hyperuricemia, and hyperlipidemia, but it is not clear if diuretics modify or effect these associations. It is

certain that effective antihypertensive therapy reduces the incidence of cardiovascular disease in hypertensive patients.

E. Hyponatremia: Life-threatening hyponatremia has occured in a very small number of patients who had recently begun diuretic therapy. This effect may be related to reduction in the diluting capacity of the kidney or sustained release of ADH. Polydipsia and K^+ depletion may play important roles in the development of hyponatremia.

F. Allergic Reactions: Skin rashes occasionally occur. Serious allergic reactions are extremely rare but do include hemolytic anemia, thrombocytopenia, acute pancreatitis, cholestatic jaundice, and acute pulmonary edema.

Contraindications

Thiazides should be used cautiously in patients with hepatic cirrhosis to avoid K^+ depletion and hepatic encephalopathy. Renal insufficiency may be intensified by overzealous diuretic use in patients with established renal failure. Digitalis toxicity may become manifest or intensified as a result of diuretic-induced K^+ depletion.

COMBINED USE OF LOOP AGENTS & THIAZIDES

Some patients are refractory to the usual doses of loop agents and are thus vulnerable to dose-related side effects (eg, ototoxicity) if abnormally large amounts of the drugs are administered. Combinations can be used as an alternative approach if it is established that renal blood flow has not been compromised by prior volume depletion.

Thiazides and loop agents can be shown to inhibit NaCl absorption in the proximal tubule. This effect appears to be independent of any carbonic anhydrase activity of these agents but requires higher luminal concentrations of the drugs than are achieved with normal clinical use.

The proximal effect of thiazides is not usually appreciated, because any increase in NaCl delivery out of the proximal tubule is simply picked up in the next downstream segment; the thick ascending limb has a large capacity to reabsorb NaCl and probably masks any proximal effect of the thiazides. As a result, the usual clinical response to the thiazides is that associated with the inhibition of NaCl reabsorption in the distal convoluted tubule, as described previously. However, when thiazides and loop agents are administered together, a true synergy occurs. Both classes may then increase NaCl delivery out of the proximal tubule. With inhibition of the thick ascending limb by the loop agents and inhibition of the distal convoluted tubule by the thiazides, the overall result is a profound diuretic effect, which is greater than that achieved with either agent alone.

Metolazone seems to be the usual choice of thiazidelike drug in patients refractory to loop agents. If a patient has not responded to a reasonable dose of furosemide (eg, 200 mg), then 5–20 mg of metolazone can be administered along with furosemide. There is no reason to prefer metolazone over any of the other members of the thiazide group. Hydrochlorothiazide, 100 mg, should be as effective as a 20-mg dose of metolazone.

Clinical Indications

Combined use of loop diuretics and thiazides is useful in managing refractory edema or other forms of fluid overload where maximal diuretic efficacy is required. The combination does lessen the dose-dependent side effects that accompany the use of loop agents alone. For this reason, the combination approach merits consideration. It can be encouraged if it decreases clinical reliance on inappropriately large doses of loop agents.

Toxicity

Very large amounts of fluid can be mobilized in patients who have been refractory to single agents. Routine outpatient use cannot be recommended because of the serious consequences of volume depletion. Potassium wasting is extremely common and requires parenteral K^+ administration with careful monitoring of the fluid and electrolyte status.

POTASSIUM-SPARING DIURETICS

The members of this group antagonize the effects of aldosterone at the cortical collecting tubule. Inhibition may occur by direct antagonism at the level of cytoplasmic mineralocorticoid receptors (spirolactones, including spironolactone and prorenone), by suppression of renin or angiotensin II generation (nonsteroidal anti-inflammatory agents, converting enzyme inhibitors), or by directly inhibiting Na^+ transport by the collecting tubule (triamterene, amiloride). These agents are used during states of mineralocorticoid excess, due either to primary hypersecretion (Conn's syndrome, ectopic ACTH production) or to secondary hyperaldosteronism. Congestive heart failure, hepatic cirrhosis, and nephrotic syndrome are conditions associated with renal salt retention and diminished "effective" extracellular volume. Use of thiazides or loop agents contributes to further volume contraction and thereby intensifies secondary hyperaldosteronism. In the setting of enhanced mineralocorticoid secretion and continuing delivery of Na^+ to distal nephron sites, renal K^+ wasting occurs owing to K^+ secretion at the level of the collecting tubule. Potassium-sparing diuretics, either direct or indirect antagonists of aldosterone, are used in this setting to blunt the K^+ secretory response and prevent depletion of the intracellular K^+ stores.

Chemistry & Pharmacokinetics

Spironolactone, prorenone, and the other spirolactones are synthetic steroids that bind to cytoplasmic mineralocorticoid receptors and prevent translocation of the receptor complex to the nucleus in the target cell. They may also inhibit the intracellular formation of active metabolites of aldosterone by inhibition of 5α-reductase activity. These agents act as competitive antagonists to aldosterone, and their structures are illustrated in Fig 14–6. Their onset and duration of action are therefore determined by the kinetics of aldosterone response in the target tissue. In addition, substantial inactivation of these agents occurs in the liver. The overall result is a rather slow onset of action, requiring several days before full therapeutic effect is achieved.

Triamterene is metabolized in the liver, but renal excretion is a major route of elimination for the active form and the metabolites. Very little is known about the diuretic effects of the metabolites. **Amiloride** is excreted unchanged in the urine. Because triamterene is extensively metabolized, it has a shorter half-life and must be given more frequently than amiloride. The structures of triamterene and amiloride are shown in Fig 14–7.

Pharmacodynamics

Overall K^+ homeostasis is controlled at the level of the aldosterone-responsive segments of the distal nephron (collecting tubules and ducts). At any given Na^+ delivery, the rate of distal K^+ secretion is strongly influenced by the prevailing levels of aldosterone. Potassium secretion is stimulated by high aldosterone levels. There appears to be a direct effect of mineralocorticoids on K^+ secretion (or inhibition of K^+ absorption), as well as a secondary effect on Na^+ transport. Sodium absorption in the collecting tubule generates an electrical potential that is lumen-negative. This electrical force facilitates K^+ secretion into the lumen and in this way increases renal K^+ excretion. Aldosterone antagonists decrease the component of K^+ secretion coupled to Na^+ reabsorption and may also inhibit any direct effects of aldosterone on K^+ handling. Similar effects seem to pertain to H^+ handling by the collecting tubule. Aldosterone stimulates H^+ secretion by a direct effect as well as by a secondary effect re-

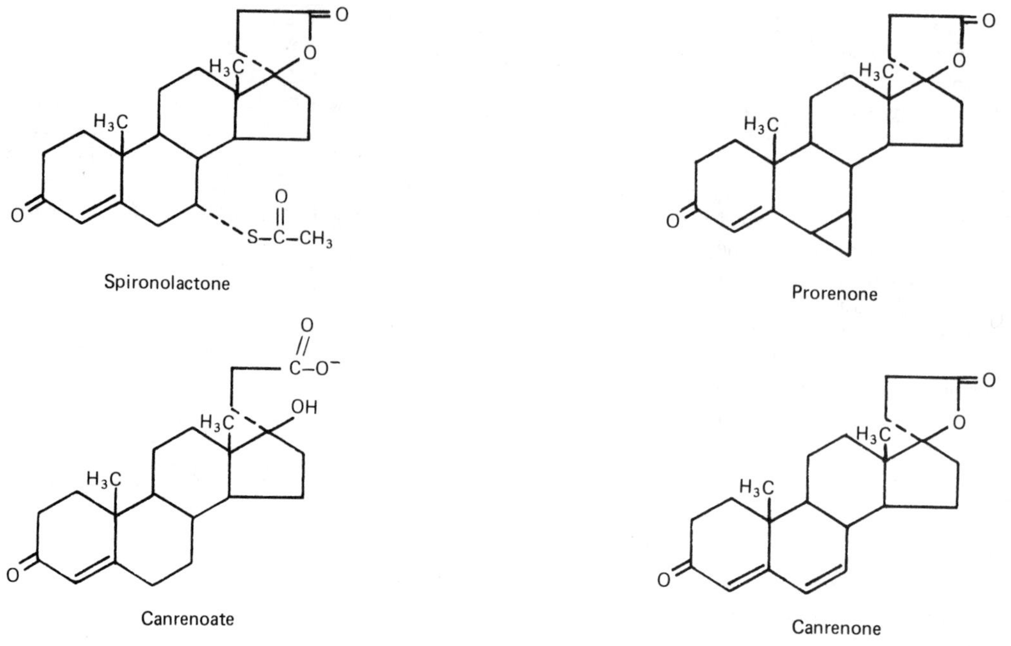

Spironolactone

Prorenone

Canrenoate

Canrenone

Figure 14–6. Spironolactones.

sulting from the effects of aldosterone on Na^+ transport in this segment.

Analogs & Variants

Converting enzyme inhibitors are discussed in Chapters 10 and 16. Although not used therapeutically as K^+-sparing diuretics, these agents do antagonize the effects of aldosterone by interfering with its secretion. The renal effects of these agents can be understood in light of the clinical toxicities of the aldosterone antagonists discussed here.

Toxicity

These agents inhibit renal K^+ and H^+ secretory systems. Hyperkalemia and hyperchloremic metabolic acidosis are dose-related effects that occur when al-

Triamterene

Amiloride

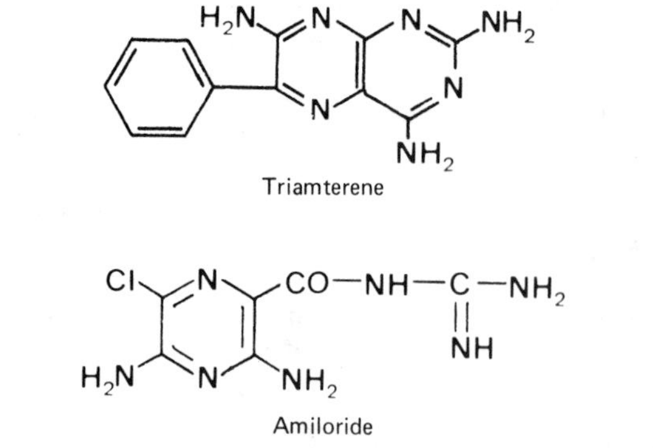

Figure 14–7. Other indirect-acting aldosterone antagonists.

dosterone antagonists are used as the sole diuretic agent. With fixed-dosage combinations of K^+-sparing and thiazide diuretics, there may be a fairly even balance, so that both the hypokalemia and the metabolic alkalosis due to the thiazide are ameliorated by the aldosterone antagonist. However, owing to variations in the bioavailability of the components of some of the fixed-dosage forms, the thiazide-associated side effects may predominate (eg, metabolic alkalosis, hyponatremia). The clinical value of these combinations has never been adequately documented.

Synthetic steroidal agents may cause endocrine abnormalities by agonist effects on other steroid receptors. Gynecomastia and androgenlike side effects have been reported with spironolactone.

A possible interaction of triamterene with indomethacin resulting in acute renal failure has been reported in a few patients. This effect has not yet been reported with other K^+-sparing agents.

Contraindications

These agents can cause severe, even fatal hyperkalemia in susceptible patients. Oral K^+ administration should be discontinued if aldosterone antagonists are administered. Patients with chronic renal insufficiency seem especially vulnerable and should not be treated with aldosterone antagonists. Patients with liver disease may have impaired metabolism of triamterene or spironolactone, and dosing must be carefully adjusted. Since triamterene and amiloride directly inhibit Na^+ transport in the collecting tubule, it follows that a diuretic response can be observed even in the absence of endogenous mineralocorticoid activity.

Table 14–3. Potassium-sparing diuretics and combination preparations.

Trade Name	Potassium-Sparing Agent	Hydrochlorothiazide	Frequency of Dosage
Aldactazide	Spironolactone 25 mg	25 mg	1–4 times daily
Aldactone	Spironolactone 25 mg	. . .	1–4 times daily
Dyazide	Triamterene 50 mg	25 mg	1–4 times daily
Dyrenium	Triamterene 100 mg	. . .	1–3 times daily
Maxzide	Triamterene 75 mg	50 mg	Once daily
Midamor	Amiloride 5 mg	. . .	Once daily
Moduretic	Amiloride 5 mg	50 mg	Once or twice daily

Dosages & Preparations

See Table 14–3.

AGENTS THAT AFFECT WATER EXCRETION

Antidiuretic hormone (ADH) acts at the collecting tubule to modulate the concentration of the final urine. ADH secretion is reduced during hypotonic volume expansion, and large volumes of dilute urine are formed. During volume contraction and in hypertonic conditions, ADH is secreted and urine is concentrated by water abstraction.

It is important to appreciate the central role of the thick ascending limb during concentration as well as dilution of the urine. Urine concentration, modulated by ADH, is driven by the hypertonicity of the medullary interstitium that is generated by the salt transport out of the thick ascending limb and the countercurrent exchange system. Dilution of the urine is accomplished by the same salt transport systems in the thick ascending limb of the loop of Henle. Therefore, *both* concentration and dilution can be reduced by loop agents, which inhibit salt transport in the thick ascending limb. Thiazides inhibit NaCl transport in segments that dilute the urine but do not contribute to the hypertonic medullary interstitium. Therefore, thiazides inhibit diluting ability but not the ability to maximally concentrate the urine. These agents are thus of some value in the treatment of **nephrogenic diabetes insipidus.** Pituitary diabetes insipidus is usually treated with ADH or its longer-acting analog **desmopressin** (DDAVP). These preparations are discussed in more detail in Chapter 36.

Two additional groups that affect the excretion of water need to be specifically considered: osmotic diuretics and ADH antagonists.

Pharmacokinetics

Mannitol is an **osmotic diuretic,** ie, it obligates the renal excretion of water by virtue of its pharmacokinetic properties. This agent is not metabolized and is handled primarily by glomerular filtration, without any important tubular reabsorption or secretion. By definition, osmotic diuretics are poorly absorbed, which means that they must be given parenterally. If given by mouth, osmotic diarrhea can result. This ef-

fect can be used to potentiate the effects of K^+-binding resins or eliminate various toxic substances from the gastrointestinal tract in conjunction with activated charcoal.

ADH antagonists include Li^+ salts and tetracycline derivatives (demeclocycline). Lithium is reabsorbed to some extent in the proximal tubule and thereafter is neither secreted nor absorbed. Demeclocycline is metabolized in the liver.

Pharmacodynamics

Osmotic diuretics primarily limit water reabsorption in those segments of the nephron that are freely permeable to water: proximal tubule, descending limb of the loop, and collecting tubule. The presence of a nonreabsorbable solute such as mannitol prevents the normal absorption of H_2O by interposing a countervailing osmotic force. As a result, urine volume increases in conjunction with mannitol excretion, but natriuresis does not necessarily occur.

ADH antagonists inhibit the effects of ADH at the collecting tubule. This effect occurs at some step following cAMP generation by ADH, since the effects of cAMP itself can be antagonized by these drugs in various model systems.

Clinical Indications & Dosage

A. To Increase Urine Volume: Osmotic diuretics are used to increase water excretion in preference to sodium excretion. This effect can be useful when renal hemodynamics are compromised or when avid Na^+ retention limits the response to conventional agents. It can be used to maintain urine volume and to prevent anuria that might otherwise result from presentation of large pigment loads to the kidney (eg, hemolysis or rhabdomyolysis). In oliguric patients, there may be no response to an osmotic diuretic. Therefore, a test dose of mannitol (12.5 g intravenously) is usually given first. Mannitol should not be continued unless there is an increase in urine flow rate to 50 mL/h during the next 3 hours. If there is a response, mannitol can then be given to maintain urine flow rates at about 100 mL/h.

B. To Reduce Intracranial and Intraocular Pressure: Osmotic diuretics reduce total body water more than total body cation content and thus reduce intracellular volume. This effect is used to reduce intracranial pressure in neurologic conditions and to reduce introcular pressure before ophthalmologic procedures. Other agents occasionally used include urea, glycerol, and sucrose.

C. Inappropriate ADH Secretion Syndrome: ADH antagonists are clinically used to manage inappropriate ADH secretion syndrome when water restriction has failed to correct the abnormality. Serum levels can be monitored directly for Li^+ therapy, with a serum concentration of 1 mmol/L as a desirable end point. Demeclocycline levels can be approximated by measurement of peak and trough levels using standard tetracycline determinations. In this way, the usual dose (900–1200 mg/d) can be adjusted to achieve a therapeutic serum level of 2 μg/mL.

Toxicity

Mannitol is rapidly distributed in the extracellular compartment and extracts water from the intracellular compartment. Hyponatremia and expansion of the extracellular fluid volume are the predictable consequences. This effect can be disastrous in patients with congestive heart failure and may produce florid pulmonary edema. Headache and nausea and vomiting are commonly observed in patients treated with osmotic diuretics.

The major complications of ADH antagonists relate to their pharmacologic effect. The syndrome of inappropriate ADH secretion is replaced by nephrogenic diabetes insipidus. Renal concentrating ability is abolished, and severe hypernatremia can result. Careful monitoring of the patient's fluid and electrolyte status is required. Side effects associated with Li^+ therapy include tremulousness, mental obtundation, leukocytosis, and renal tubular acidosis. Amiloride in large doses appears to improve the nephrogenic diabetes insipidus caused by lithium.

II. CLINICAL PHARMACOLOGY OF DIURETICS

EDEMATOUS STATES

Salt and water retention with edema formation generally occurs in response to an "ineffective" arterial blood volume. Excessive diuretic therapy in this setting may lead to further compromise of the "effective" arterial blood volume and further reduction of organ perfusion. This sequence of events will intensify the homeostatic responses that caused salt retention in the first place. Judicious use of diuretics can mobilize interstitial edema fluid and restore plasma volume. Therefore, the use of diuretics to mobilize edema requires careful monitoring of the patient's hemodynamic status and an understanding of the pathophysiology of the underlying condition.

CONGESTIVE HEART FAILURE

The primary therapeutic goal in congestive heart failure is to improve cardiac function by increasing myocardial contractility, but positive inotropic drugs have important toxicities. Reduction of pulmonary vascular congestion with diuretics may improve oxygenation and thereby improve myocardial function. On the other hand, if cardiac output is being maintained by high filling pressures, then diuretics may diminish venous return and thereby impair cardiac output. Reducing peripheral vascular resistance and improving cardiac function are more direct approaches to the underlying problem, but diuretic use in this setting should be regarded as an important part of therapy (see Chapter 12).

This issue is especially critical in right ventricular failure. Systemic rather than pulmonary vascular congestion is the hallmark of this disorder. Diuretic-induced volume contraction will predictably reduce venous return ("preload") and can severely compromise cardiac output if filling pressure is reduced below 15 mm Hg. Furthermore, diuretic-induced metabolic alkalosis may complicate an underlying compensated respiratory acidosis and produce a mixed acid-base disturbance.

HEPATIC CIRRHOSIS

Liver disease is often associated with edema and with ascites in conjunction with elevated portal hydrostatic pressures and reduced plasma oncotic pressures. Ascites fluid is much more slowly mobilized than peripheral edema. Vigorous diuretic therapy in this setting can cause marked depletion of the "effective" arterial plasma volume, hypokalemia, and metabolic alkalosis. Hepatorenal syndrome and hepatic encephalopathy are particularly unfortunate consequences of overzealous diuretic use. Diuretic therapy can be useful in initiating and maintaining diuresis but must be viewed as an adjunct to the restriction of dietary salt intake and amelioration of the underlying cause of hepatic dysfunction.

NEPHROTIC SYNDROME

Reduction of the "effective" arterial plasma volume in conjunction with reduced plasma oncotic pressures may occur in the nephrotic syndrome. Diuretic use may cause further reductions in plasma volume that can impair glomerular filtration rate and may lead to hypotension and in some cases renal vein thrombosis. Patients with nephrotic syndrome may have expanded plasma volumes and usually present with diminished glomerular filtration rate and hypertension. Diuretic therapy may be beneficial in controlling the volume-dependent component of hypertension and reducing the contribution hypertension may make to their underlying renal disease.

NONEDEMATOUS STATES

HYPERTENSION

A thiazide diuretic is usually the first drug to be used for treating mild essential hypertension. Large doses of thiazides can produce adequate control in nearly two-thirds of patients with mild essential hypertension. Careful hemodynamic measurements have demonstrated a fall in peripheral vascular resistance and a sustained fall in plasma volume in patients who respond to chronic thiazide therapy, eg, 100 mg of hydrochlorothiazide per day. Recent studies indicate that lower doses of thiazides may control hypertension in many patients without the attendant dose-related side effects (eg, K^+ wasting) seen with higher doses. Patients who do not respond to thiazides alone are often managed with one or more peripheral vasodilators. Salt and water retention is a predictable consequence of vasodilator therapy, so continued diuretic therapy is indicated.

Early studies suggested that diuretic therapy may directly reduce peripheral vascular resistance by an effect on vascular smooth muscle. These effects can be demonstrated most convincingly with parenteral administration of diuretics but are not necessarily related to the antihypertensive effect of thiazide diuretics. This issue will probably not be resolved until the cause of increased peripheral vascular resistance in essential hypertension is better understood.

It is worth reemphasizing that mild, sustained reduction of plasma volume may be a critical factor in the response to thiazide therapy. It is not practical to measure plasma volumes in all hypertensive patients. However, it may be useful to evaluate dietary salt intake and compliance in patients who do not respond to thiazides. Dietary history and urinary sodium excretion rates will identify patients who overcome the antihypertensive effects of thiazides by increasing their salt intake. Patient compliance may be enhanced by once-a-day dosing with a thiazide that has a 12- to 18-hour duration of action (eg, hydrochlorothiazide). This approach matches the diuretic effect with the normal pattern of dietary salt intake.

RENAL POTASSIUM WASTING

Increased levels of aldosterone secretion cause marked renal K^+ secretion when distal Na^+ delivery is increased by diuretics or by high dietary salt intake. Distal H^+ secretion with generation of metabolic alkalosis occurs in the same setting. Recent studies suggest that total body K^+ depletion and hypokalemia may have severe cardiovascular consequences owing to left ventricular irritability. There is considerable controversy over the long-term effects of diuretic-induced K^+ depletion in patients not taking digitalis derivatives. Potassium depletion does cause a reduction in the number of Na^+,K^+-ATPase sites in skeletal muscle and may therefore alter the disposition of cardioactive glycosides. It is well recognized that diuretic-induced K^+ depletion can increase the incidence of digitalis toxicity.

Dietary K^+ supplementation is one approach to managing diuretic-induced K^+ depletion. Unfortunately, it is relatively expensive and requires faithful patient compliance, which is particularly hard to achieve in the case of oral KCl administration.

A recent approach emphasizes the importance of dietary Na^+ intake. In the steady state, dietary Na^+ intake will be reflected in the urinary excretion of Na^+. This relationship also pertains to patients chronically taking thiazides or loop diuretics. Once the initial diuresis is completed, the patient should then maintain normal salt balance. Therefore, even in the setting of chronic diuretic therapy, daily excretion of Na^+ is an accurate index of intake. If dietary salt intake is excessive, then distal delivery of Na^+ and urinary excretion of Na^+ will be high and distal K^+ (and H^+) excretion will be stimulated. Moderate restriction of dietary Na^+ intake (60–100 meq/d) has been shown to potentiate the effects of diuretics in essential hypertension and to lessen renal K^+ wasting. Dietary Na^+ restriction is also indicated in states associated with avid renal Na^+ retention (congestive heart failure, cirrhosis, etc).

Potassium-sparing diuretics are indicated for the patient who has failed to respond to (or comply with) dietary Na^+ restriction or K^+ supplementation. Dietary counseling in the strongest terms should be tried before resorting to additional diuretic intervention. The reduced bioavailability of hydrochlorothiazide in some triamterene-hydrochlorothiazide combinations may well explain the K^+-sparing effect of the combination. Although newer formulations are now available, it may be more rational, and certainly less expensive, to simply reduce the thiazide dose in patients with hypokalemia before adding a K^+-sparing agent.

REFERENCES

General

Brenner BM, Rector FC Jr (editors): *The Kidney,* 3rd ed. Saunders, 1986.

Brooks BA, Lant AF: The use of the human erythrocyte as a model for studying the action of diuretics on sodium and chloride transport. *Clin Sci Mol Med* 1978;**54**:679.

Corvol P et al: Mechanism of the antimineralocorticoid effect of spirolactones. *Kidney Int* 1981;**20**:1.

Fries ED: Salt, volume, and hypertension. *Circulation* 1976; **53**:589.

Warnock DG, Eveloff J: NaCl entry mechanisms in the luminal membrane of the renal tubule. *Am J Physiol* 1982; **242:**561.

Specific Agents

Ames RP: Negative effects of diuretic drugs on metabolic risk factors for coronary heart disease: Possible alternative drug therapies. (Symposium.) *Am J Cardiol* 1983;**51:**632.

Araoye MA et al: Furosemide compared with hydrochlorothiazide: Long-term treatment of hypertension. *JAMA* 1978; **240:**1863.

Ashraf N, Locksley R, Arieff AI: Thiazide-induced hyponatremia associated with death or neurologic damage in outpatients. *Am J Med* 1981;**70:**1163.

Battle DC et al: Amelioration of polyuria by amiloride in patients receiving long-term lithium therapy. *N Engl J Med* 1985;**312:**408.

Bear R et al: Effect of metabolic alkalosis on respiratory function in patients with chronic obstructive lung disease. *Can Med Assoc J* 1977;**22:**900.

Block WD, Shiner PT, Roman J: Severe electrolyte disturbances associated with metolazone and furosemide. *South Med J* 1978;**71:**380.

Blume CD, Williams RL: A new antihypertensive agent: Maxzide (75 mg triamterene/50 mg hydrochlorothiazide). *Am J Med* 1984;**77(Suppl 5A):**52.

Boyer TD, Warnock DG: Use of diuretics in the treatment of cirrhotic ascites. (Editorial.) *Gastroenterology* 1983; **84:**1051.

Case DB et al: Proteinuria during long-term captopril therapy. *JAMA* 1980;**244:**346.

de Carvalho JG et al: Hemodynamic correlates of prolonged thiazide therapy: Comparison of responders and nonresponders. *Clin Pharmacol Ther* 1977;**22:**875.

DeTroyer A: Demeclocycline: Treatment for syndrome of inappropriate antidiuretic hormone secretion. *JAMA* 1977; **237:**2723.

Epstein M et al: Potentiation of furosemide by metolazone in refractory edema. *Curr Ther Res* 1977;**21:**656.

Greene MK et al: Acetazolamide in prevention of acute mountain sickness: A double-blind controlled cross-over study. *Br Med J* 1981;**283:**811.

Helgeland A et al: Serum triglycerides and serum uric acid in untreated and thiazide-treated patients with mild hypertension. *Am J Med* 1978;**64:**34.

Higashio T, Abe Y, Yamamoto K: Renal effects of bumetanide. *J Pharmacol Exp Ther* 1978;**207:**212.

Holland OB, Nixon JV, Kuhnert L: Diuretic-induced ventricular ectopic activity. *Am J Med* 1981;**70:**762.

Hollifield JW, Slaton PE: Thiazide diuretics, hypokalemia, and cardiac arrhythmias. *Acta Med Scand* 1981;**647 (Suppl):**67.

Inadapamide: A new indoline diuretic agent. (Symposium). *Am Heart J* 1983;**106:**183. [Entire issue.]

Kaplan NM et al: Two techniques to improve adherence to dietary sodium restriction in the treatment of hypertension. *Arch Intern Med* 1982;**142:**1638.

Kenyon CJ et al: Antinatriuretic and kaliuretic activities of the reduced derivatives of aldosterone. *Endocrinology* 1983; **112:**1852.

Kleinknecht D et al: Furosemide in acute oliguric renal failure: A controlled trial. *Nephron* 1976;**17:**51.

Koechel DA: Ethacrynic acid and related diuretics: Relationship of structure to beneficial and detrimental actions. *Annu Rev Pharmacol Toxicol* 1981;**21:**265.

Levy ST, Forrest JM, Heninger GR: Lithium-induced diabetes insipidus: Manic symptoms, brain and electrolyte correlates, and chlorothiazide treatment. *Am J Psychiatry* 1973;**130:**1014.

MacGregor GA et al: Double-blind randomised crossover trial of moderate sodium restriction in essential hypertension. *Lancet* 1982;**1:**351.

McLeod MD, Bell GM, Irvine WJ: Nephrogenic diabetes insipidus associated with dyazide (triamterene-hydrochlorothiazide). *Br Med J* 1981;**283:**1155.

Multicenter Diuretic Cooperative Study Group: Multiclinic comparison of amiloride, hydrochlorothiazide, and hydrochlorothiazide plus amiloride in essential hypertension. *Arch Intern Med* 1981;**141:**482.

Ram CVS, Garrett B, Kaplan NM: Moderate sodium restriction and various diuretics in the treatment of hypertension: Effects of potassium wastage and blood pressure control. *Arch Intern Med* 1981;**141:**1015.

Tan SY et al: Indomethacin-induced prostaglandin inhibition with hyperkalemia: A reversible cause of hyporeninemic hypoaldosteronism. *Ann Intern Med* 1979;**90:**783.

Tannenbaum PJ et al: The influence of dosage form on the activity of a diuretic agent. *Clin Pharmacol Exp Ther* 1968; **9:**598.

Tobert JA et al: Enhancement of uricosuric properties of indacrinone by manipulation of the enantiomer ratio. *Clin Pharmacol Ther* 1981;**29:**344.

Toth PJ, Horwitz RI: Conflicting clinical trials and the uncertainty of treating mild hypertension. *Am J Med* 1983; **75:**482.

Van Brummelen P, Woerlee M, Schalekamp MA: Long-term versus short-term effects of hydrochlorothiazide on renal haemodynamics in essential hypertension. *Clin Sci* 1979; **56:**463.

Warren SE, Blantz RC: Mannitol. *Arch Intern Med* 1981; **141:**493.

Weinberg MS et al: Anuric renal failure precipitated by indomethacin and triamterene. *Nephron* 1985;**40:**216.

Histamine, Serotonin, & the Ergot Alkaloids

15

Alan Burkhalter, PhD, & Oscar L. Frick, MD, PhD

Histamine and serotonin (5-hydroxytryptamine) are biologically active amines that are found in many tissues and have complex physiologic and pathologic effects. Together with endogenous polypeptides (Chapter 16) and prostaglandins and leukotrienes (Chapter 17), they are sometimes called **autacoids** (Greek "self-remedy") or local hormones in recognition of these properties.

The roles of histamine and serotonin in normal physiology are not completely understood, and these compounds have no clinical application in the treatment of disease. However, compounds that selectively antagonize the actions of these amines are of considerable clinical usefulness. This chapter therefore emphasizes the basic pharmacology of the agonist amines and the clinical pharmacology of the antagonists. The ergot alkaloids, compounds with partial agonist activity at serotonin (and other) receptors, are discussed at the end of the chapter.

HISTAMINE

Histamine was synthesized in 1907 and later isolated from mammalian tissues. Early hypotheses concerning the possible physiologic roles of tissue histamine were based on similarities between histamine's actions and the symptoms of anaphylactic shock and tissue injury. Marked species variation has been observed, but in humans histamine is an important mediator of immediate allergic and inflammatory reactions, has an important role in gastric acid secretion, and, according to recent evidence, functions as a neurotransmitter in certain areas of the brain.

I. BASIC PHARMACOLOGY OF HISTAMINE

Chemistry & Pharmacokinetics

Histamine is 2-(4-imidazolyl)ethylamine (Fig 15–1). It occurs in plants as well as in animal tissues and is a component of many venoms and stinging secretions.

Histamine is formed by decarboxylation of the amino acid L-histidine, a reaction catalyzed in mammalian tissues by the enzyme histidine decarboxylase (Fig 15–1). Pyridoxal phosphate is required as cofactor. Once formed, histamine is either stored or rapidly inactivated by one of 2 amine oxidase enzymes and by methylation. Very little histamine is excreted unchanged. Certain tumors (systemic mastocytosis, urticaria pigmentosa, gastric carcinoid, and occasionally myelogenous leukemia) are associated with increased numbers of mast cells or basophils and with increased excretion of histamine and its metabolites.

Although histamine is found in most tissues, it is very unevenly distributed. Most tissue histamine exists in bound form in granules in mast cells or basophils; the histamine content of many tissues is directly related to their mast cell content. The bound form of histamine is biologically inactive, but many stimuli, as noted below, can trigger the release of mast cell histamine, allowing the free amine to exert its actions on surrounding tissues.

Mast cells are especially rich at sites of potential tissue injury—nose, mouth, and feet; internal body surfaces; and blood vessels, especially at pressure points and bifurcations. Mast cells serve as "emergency repair kits." Mast cells in different tissues also differ. Some mast cells found in the gastrointestinal mucosa are similar to those found in connective tissue, but others exhibit different properties. Such mucosal or atypical mast cells have chondroitin sulfate instead of heparin sulfate in the storage granules and different sensitivities to chemicals that cause histamine release.

Non–mast cell histamine is found in several tissues including the brain. Both regional and intracellular distributions of brain histamine support the possibility of transmitter or modulator function, especially in those parts of the brain concerned with temperature regulation.

Storage and release of histamine. In human mast cells and basophils, storage granules contain histamine complexed with the sulfated polysaccharide, heparin, and an acidic protein. The bound form of histamine can be released through several mechanisms. Certain amines, including drugs such as morphine and tubocurarine, can displace histamine from the heparin-protein complex. This type of release does not require energy and is not associated with mast cell injury or degranulation. Loss of granules from the mast cell will

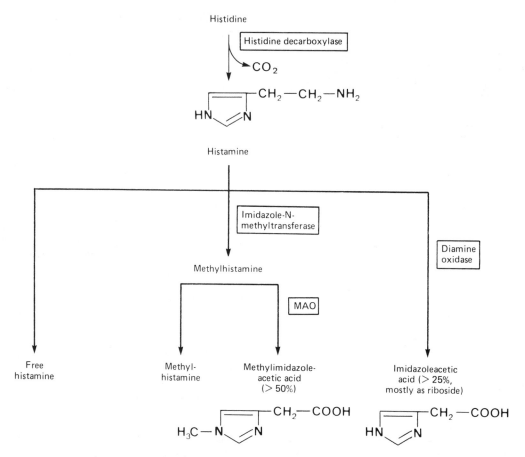

Figure 15–1. Synthesis, metabolism, and common urinary metabolites of histamine. (Modified and reproduced, with permission, from Meyers FH, Jawetz E, Goldfien A: *Review of Medical Pharmacology*, 7th ed. Lange, 1980.)

also release histamine, since sodium ions in the extracellular fluid rapidly displace the amine from the complex. Chemical and mechanical mast cell injury causes degranulation and histamine release.

More specific mechanisms also cause histamine release. Compound 48/80, a diamine polymer, specifically releases histamine from tissue mast cells by an exocytotic degranulation process requiring energy and calcium. The important pathophysiologic mechanism of histamine release is immunologic. Mast cells and basophils, if sensitized by IgE antibodies attached to their surface membranes, degranulate when exposed to the appropriate antigen. This type of release also requires energy and calcium. Degranulated mast cells will reaccumulate histamine over a period of days to weeks. Histamine released by this mechanism is a mediator in immediate (type I) allergic reactions. Substances released during IgG- or IgM-mediated immune reactions that activate the complement cascade also release histamine from mast cells and basophils.

By a negative feedback control mechanism, histamine appears to modulate the release of histamine from sensitized mast cells in some tissues. Thus, histamine may act to limit an allergic reaction by inhibiting the release of histamine and other mediators of the response (see Chapters 17 and 18). In humans, mast cells in skin and basophils show this negative feedback mechanism; lung mast cells do not.

Endogenous histamine may also have a modulating role in a variety of inflammatory and immune responses. Histamine probably plays a part in acute inflammatory responses. Upon injury to a tissue, released histamine causes local vasodilation and leakage of plasma containing mediators of acute inflammation (complement, C-reactive protein), antibodies, and inflammatory cells (neutrophils, eosinophils, basophils, monocytes, and lymphocytes). Histamine inhibits the release of lysosome contents and several T and B lymphocyte functions. Most of these actions are mediated by H_2 receptors and lead to increased intracellular cAMP. The clinical significance of these actions of histamine is not clear.

Pharmacodynamics

A. Mechanism of Action: Histamine exerts its biologic actions by combining with specific cellular receptors located in or on the surface membrane. The actions of histamine antagonists indicate that there are at least 2 distinct types of receptors: H_1 and H_2. Responses at both types of receptors may involve alterations in membrane permeability to calcium or release of calcium from internal stores. Responses mediated by H_2 receptors have been convincingly shown to involve an elevation of intracellular cAMP. Less compelling evidence suggests an association of elevated cGMP with activation of H_1 receptors. It is not known whether these cyclic nucleotide alterations represent a cause or an effect of the changes in intracellular calcium concentration.

B. Tissue and Organ System Effects of Histamine: Histamine exerts powerful effects on smooth and cardiac muscle, on certain endothelial and nerve cells, and on the secretory cells of the stomach. However, sensitivity to histamine varies greatly among species. Humans, guinea pigs, dogs, and cats are quite sensitive, while mice and rats are much less so.

1. Cardiovascular system–In humans, injection or infusion of histamine causes a decrease in systolic and diastolic blood pressure and an increase in heart rate (Fig 15–2). The acute blood pressure changes are caused by the direct vasodilator action of histamine on arterioles and precapillary sphincters; the increase in heart rate involves both stimulatory actions of histamine on the heart and a reflex tachycardia. Flushing, a sense of warmth, and headache may also occur during histamine administration, consistent with the arteriolar dilating effect. Studies with histamine receptor antagonists show that both H_1 and H_2 receptors are involved in these cardiovascular responses to high doses, since a combination of H_1 and H_2 recep-

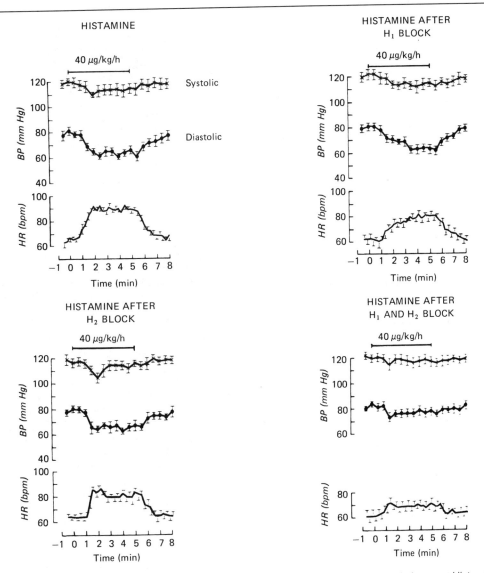

Figure 15–2. Effects of histamine and histamine antagonists on blood pressure and heart rate in humans. Histamine was infused at 40 μg/kg/h for 5 minutes as shown at the top of each panel. The H_1 antagonist was chlorpheniramine (10 mg intravenously). The H_2 antagonist was cimetidine (200 mg intravenously). (Modified and reproduced, with permission, from Torsoli A, Lucchelli PE, Brimblecombe RW [editors]: *H_2 Antagonists: H_2-Receptor Antagonists in Peptic Ulcer Disease and Progress in Histamine Research.* Excerpta Medica, 1980.)

tor–blocking agents is more effective in preventing the actions of histamine than either blocking agent alone (Fig 15–2). However, in humans, the cardiovascular effects of small doses of histamine can usually be antagonized by H_1 receptor antagonists alone.

Edema results from the action of histamine on H_1 receptors in the vessels of the microcirculation, especially the postcapillary vessels. The effect is associated with an increase in permeability of the vessel wall that has been ascribed to the separation of the endothelial cells, thus permitting the transudation of fluid and molecules as large as small proteins into the perivascular tissue. This effect is responsible for the urticaria (hives) that signals the intradermal release of histamine.

Direct cardiac effects of histamine include both increased contractility and increased pacemaker rate. These effects are mediated chiefly by H_2 receptors. In human atrial muscle, histamine can also decrease contractility; this effect is mediated by H_1 receptors. The physiologic significance of these cardiac actions is not clear.

These cardiovascular effects may also be produced by the release of endogenous histamine from mast cells. Many of the cardiovascular signs and symptoms of anaphylaxis are due to released histamine, although other mediators are also involved.

2. Gastrointestinal tract smooth muscle–Histamine causes contraction of intestinal smooth muscle, and histamine-induced contraction of guinea pig ileum is a standard bioassay for histamine. The human gut is not as sensitive as that of the guinea pig, but large doses of histamine may cause diarrhea, partly as a result of this effect. This action of histamine is mediated by H_1 receptors.

3. Bronchiolar smooth muscle–In both humans and guinea pigs, histamine causes bronchoconstriction. In the guinea pig, this effect is the cause of death from histamine toxicity, but in normal humans, bronchoconstriction following the usual doses of histamine is not marked. However, patients with bronchial asthma are very sensitive to histamine. The bronchoconstriction induced in these patients probably represents a hyperactive neural response, since they also respond excessively to many other stimuli, and the response can be blocked by autonomic blocking drugs such as ganglionic blocking agents as well as by H_1 receptor antagonists (Chapter 18). Inhalation provocation tests using increasing doses of histamine are of diagnostic value for bronchial hyperreactivity in patients with suspected asthma or cystic fibrosis. Such individuals may be 100- to 1000-fold more sensitive to histamine than normal individuals.

4. Other smooth muscle organs–In humans, histamine generally has insignificant effects on the smooth muscle of the eye and genitourinary tract. However, pregnant women who have anaphylaxis may abort as a result of histamine-induced contractions, and in some species the sensitivity of the uterus is sufficient to form the basis for a bioassay.

5. Nerve endings–Histamine is a powerful stimulant of sensory nerve endings, especially those mediating pain and itching. This H_1-mediated effect is an important component of the urticarial response and reactions to insect and nettle stings. Some evidence suggests that local high concentrations can also depolarize efferent (axonal) nerve endings (see ¶ 7, below).

6. Secretory tissue–Histamine has long been recognized as a powerful stimulant of gastric acid secretion and, to a lesser extent, of gastric pepsin and intrinsic factor production. The effect is caused by activation of H_2 receptors on the parietal cells and is associated with increased adenylate cyclase activity and cAMP concentration. Other stimulants of gastric acid secretion such as acetylcholine and gastrin do not increase cAMP even though their maximal effects on acid output can be reduced—but not abolished—by H_2 receptor antagonists.

Histamine has insignificant effects on the activity of other glandular tissue at ordinary concentrations. Very high concentrations can cause adrenal medullary discharge.

7. The "triple response"–Intradermal injection of histamine causes a characteristic wheal-and-flare response first described over 50 years ago. The effect involves 3 separate cell types: microcirculatory smooth muscle, capillary or venular endothelium, and sensory nerve endings. At the site of injection, a reddening appears owing to dilatation of small vessels, followed soon by an edematous wheal at the injection site and a red irregular flare surrounding the wheal. The flare is said to be caused by an axon reflex. As noted above, histamine stimulates nerve endings; the resulting impulses are thought to travel through other branches of the same axon, causing vasodilatation. The sensation of itch may also accompany the appearance of these effects. The wheal is due to local edema.

Similar local effects may be produced by injecting histamine liberators (compound 48/80, morphine, etc) intradermally or by applying the appropriate antigens to the skin of a sensitized person. Although most of these local effects can be blocked by prior administration of an H_1 receptor–blocking agent, H_2 receptors may also be involved.

Other Histamine Agonists

Small substitutions on the imidazole ring of histamine significantly modify the H_1 and H_2 selectivity

Betazole

Impromidine

of the compound. For example, 2-methylhistamine is relatively more specific for H_1 receptors, while 4-methylhistamine is a relatively specific H_2 agonist. The structures of 2 H_2-selective agents are shown below. **Betazole** is a drug that was used in testing gastric acid–secreting ability; **impromidine** is an experimental compound highly specific for H_2 receptors.

II. CLINICAL PHARMACOLOGY OF HISTAMINE

Clinical Uses

A. Testing Gastric Acid Secretion: Histamine and an alternative agonist, betazole (Histalog), were used as diagnostic agents in testing for gastric acid–secreting ability. However, the frequency of side effects has made their use obsolete, and pentagastrin (Peptavlon) is currently used with a much lower incidence of adverse effects.

B. Diagnosis of Pheochromocytoma: Histamine can cause release of catecholamines from adrenal medullary cells. Although this effect is not prominent in normal humans, massive release can occur in patients with pheochromocytoma. The response is caused partially by direct release of catecholamines and partly by an exaggerated overshoot in the homeostatic response to histamine-induced hypotension. This hazardous provocative test is now obsolete, since chemical assays are available for determination of the catecholamines and their metabolites in patients suspected of having this tumor.

Toxicity & Contraindications

Adverse effects following administration of histamine are dose-related. Flushing, hypotension, tachycardia, headache, wheals, bronchoconstriction, and gastrointestinal upset are noted.

Histamine should not be given to asthmatics or patients with active ulcer disease or gastrointestinal bleeding.

HISTAMINE ANTAGONISTS

The effects of histamine released in the body can be reduced in several ways. **Physiologic antagonists,** especially epinephrine, have smooth muscle actions opposite to those of histamine but act at different receptors. This is important clinically, because injection of epinephrine can be lifesaving in systemic anaphylaxis and in other conditions in which massive histamine release occurs.

Release inhibitors reduce the degranulation of mast cells that results from immunologic triggering of

antigen-IgE interaction. Cromolyn appears to have this effect (Chapter 18) and is used in the treatment of asthma. Beta$_2$-adrenoceptor stimulant agents also appear capable of reducing histamine release.

Histamine **receptor antagonists** represent a third approach to the reduction of histamine-mediated responses. For over 40 years, compounds have been available that competitively antagonize many of the actions of histamine on smooth muscle. However, not until the H_2 receptor antagonist burimamide was described in 1972 was it possible to antagonize the gastric acid–stimulating activity of histamine. The development of selective H_2 receptor antagonists has led not only to more precise definition of histamine's actions in terms of receptors involved but also to more effective therapy of peptic ulcer.

H_1 RECEPTOR ANTAGONISTS

When used without a modifying adjective, the word "antihistamine" refers to H_1 receptor antagonists. Compounds that competitively block histamine at H_1 receptor sites have been used clinically for many years, and over 30 H_1 antagonists are currently available in the USA. They are prescribed by physicians and are present in many nonprescription formulations such as "cold pills" and sleep aids (Chapter 68).

I. BASIC PHARMACOLOGY OF H_1 RECEPTOR ANTAGONISTS

Chemistry & Pharmacokinetics

The H_1 antagonists are stable lipid-soluble amines having the general structure illustrated in Fig 15–3. There are several chemical subgroups, and the structures of compounds representing different subgroups are shown in the figure. A listing of some of the available drugs is given in Table 15–1.

Most of these agents are similar with respect to absorption and distribution. They are rapidly absorbed following oral administration, with peak blood concentrations occurring in 1–2 hours. They are widely distributed throughout the body, including the central nervous system. They are extensively metabolized, primarily by microsomal systems in the liver. Most of the drugs have an effective duration of action of 4–6 hours following a single dose, but meclizine is longer-acting, with a duration of action of 12–24 hours.

Pharmacodynamics

A. Histamine Receptor Blockade: H_1 receptor antagonists block the actions of histamine by reversible, competitive antagonism at the H_1 receptor. They have negligible potency at the H_2 receptor. Therefore, the ability of these drugs to block a histamine action depends not only on the concentration of agonist and antagonist but also on the degree to which

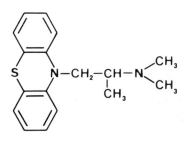

X is: C, O, or omitted

General structure

Ethers or ethanolamine derivatives

Diphenhydramine or dimenhydrinate

Ethylenediamine derivatives

Tripelennamine

Piperazine derivatives

Cyclizine

Alkylamine derivatives

Chlorpheniramine

Phenothiazine derivatives

Promethazine

Piperidine derivatives

Terfenadine

Figure 15–3. General structure of H_1 antagonist drugs and examples of the major subgroups.

the action is mediated by H_1 receptors. For example, histamine-induced contraction of bronchiolar or gastrointestinal smooth muscle can be completely blocked by these agents, while the effects of histamine on the cardiovascular system are only partly blocked because of H_2 receptor–mediated actions (Fig 15–2). H_1 receptor antagonists block most of the local tissue effects, including the increase in capillary permeability and the axon reflex–mediated flare. H_2 receptor–mediated actions such as the increase in gastric acid secretion and inhibition of histamine release from mast cells are unaffected.

B. Actions Not Caused by Histamine Receptor Blockade: The H_1 receptor antagonists have many actions not ascribable to blockade of the actions of histamine. The large number of these actions probably results from the similarity of the H_1 antagonist general structure (Fig 15–3) to the structure of drugs that have effects at muscarinic cholinoceptor, alpha-adrenoceptor, serotonin, and local anesthetic receptor sites. Some of these actions are of therapeutic value and some are undesirable.

1. Sedation–The most common side effect of H_1 antagonists is sedation, but the intensity of this action varies among chemical subgroups (Table 15–1) and among patients as well. The effect is sufficiently prominent with some agents to make them useful as

Table 15–1. Some H_1 antihistaminic drugs in clinical use.

Drug	Usual Adult Dose	Comments
Ethanolamines		
Carbinoxamine (Clistin)	4–8 mg	Slight to moderate sedation.
Dimenhydrinate (8-chlorotheophylline salt of diphenhydramine) (Dramamine, etc)	50 mg	Marked sedation; anti–motion sickness activity.
Diphenhydramine (Benadryl, etc)	25–50 mg	Marked sedation; anti–motion sickness activity.
Doxylamine (Decapryn)	1.25–25 mg	Marked sedation; now available only in OTC "sleep aids."
Ethylenediamines		
Antazoline	1–2 drops	Component of ophthalmic solutions.
Pyrilamine (Neo-Antergan)	25–50 mg	Moderate sedation; component of OTC "sleep aids."
Tripelennamine (PBZ)	25–50 mg	Moderate sedation.
Piperazine derivatives		
Cyclizine (Marezine)	25–50 mg	Slight sedation; anti–motion sickness activity.
Meclizine (Bonine, etc)	25–50 mg	Slight sedation; anti–motion sickness activity.
Alkylamines		
Brompheniramine (Dimetane, etc)	4–8 mg	Slight sedation.
Chlorpheniramine (Chlor-Trimeton, etc)	4–8 mg	Slight sedation; common component of OTC "cold" medication.
Dexchlorpheniramine (Polaramine)	2–4 mg	Slight sedation; active isomer of chlorpheniramine.
Phenothiazine derivatives		
Promethazine (Phenergan, etc)	10–25 mg	Marked sedation; antiemetic and antimuscarinic activity.
Piperidines		
Terfenadine (Seldane)	60 mg	Newer agent; little or no sedation.
Miscellaneous		
Cyproheptadine (Periactin, etc)	4 mg	Moderate sedation; also has antiserotonin activity.
Phenindamine (Thephorin)	25 mg	May cause stimulation.

"sleep aids" (Chapter 68) and unsuitable for daytime use. The effect resembles that of some antimuscarinic drugs and is considered very unlike the disinhibited sedation produced by sedative-hypnotic drugs. At ordinary dosages, children occasionally (and adults rarely) manifest excitation rather than sedation. At very high toxic dose levels, marked stimulation, agitation, and even convulsions may precede coma. Three newer H_1 antagonists are claimed to have little or no sedative action. Terfenadine is highly selective for H_1 receptors and crosses the blood-brain barrier with difficulty. The estimated half-life of terfenadine is between 16 and 23 hours. Astemizole is also highly selective for H_1 receptors and is claimed to be free of autonomic blocking effects. It is long-acting, with an estimated half-life of 104 hours. Mequitazine does not readily cross the blood-brain barrier and has less affinity for brain H_1 receptors than for peripheral H_1 receptors. The estimated half-life of this drug is about 38 hours. Astemizole and mequitazine are not yet available in the USA.

2. Nausea and vomiting–Several H_1 antagonists have significant activity in preventing motion sickness (Table 15–1). They are less effective against an episode of motion sickness already present. Certain H_1 antagonists, notably doxylamine (in Bendectin), have been used widely in the treatment of nausea and vomiting of pregnancy (see below).

3. Antiparkinsonism effects–Perhaps because of their anticholinergic effects (cf benztropine, Chapter 26), some of the H_1 antagonists have significant acute suppressant effects on the parkinsonismlike syndromes associated with certain antipsychotic drugs (Chapter 27).

4. Anticholinoceptor actions–Many of the H_1 antagonists, especially those of the ethanolamine and ethylenediamine subgroups, have significant atropine-like effects on peripheral muscarinic receptors. This action may be responsible for some of the (uncertain) benefits reported for nonallergic rhinorrhea but also may cause urinary retention and blurred vision.

5. Antiadrenoceptor actions–Weak alpha receptor–blocking effects can be demonstrated for many H_1 antagonists, especially those in the phenothiazine subgroup. This action may cause orthostatic hypotension in susceptible individuals.

6. Antiserotonin action–Strong blocking effects at serotonin receptors have been demonstrated for some H_1 antagonists, notably cyproheptadine. This drug is promoted as an antiserotonin agent and is discussed with that drug group. Nevertheless, it has a chemical structure that resembles the phenothiazine antihistamines and is a potent H_1 blocking agent.

7. Local anesthesia–Most of the H_1 antagonists are effective local anesthetics. They block sodium channels in excitable membranes in the same fashion as procaine and lidocaine. Diphenhydramine and promethazine are actually more potent as local anesthetics than is procaine. They are occasionally used to produce local anesthesia in patients allergic to the conventional local anesthetic drugs.

II. CLINICAL PHARMACOLOGY OF H₁ RECEPTOR ANTAGONISTS

Clinical Uses

A. Allergic Reactions: The H₁ antihistaminic agents are often the first drugs used to prevent allergic reactions or to treat their symptoms. In allergic rhinitis and urticaria, in which histamine is the primary mediator, the H₁ antagonists are the drugs of choice and are often quite effective. However, in bronchial asthma, which involves several mediators, the H₁ antagonists are largely ineffective (Chapter 18).

Angioedema may be precipitated by histamine-induced edema but appears to be maintained by bradykinins that are not affected by antihistaminic agents. For atopic dermatitis, antihistaminic drugs such as diphenhydramine are used mostly for their sedative side effects and for some control of the itching.

The H₁ antihistamines used for treating allergic conditions are usually prescribed with the goal of minimizing sedative side effects; in the USA, the drugs in widest use are the alkylamines. However, this effect and the therapeutic efficacy of different agents vary widely among individuals, so it is common practice to give a patient samples from each major group to determine which is the most effective with the least side effects. In addition, the clinical effectiveness of one group may diminish with continued use, and switching to another group may restore drug effectiveness for as yet unexplained reasons.

The newer H₁ blockers with lowered sedative action (terfenadine, astemizole, and mequitazine) have been widely accepted in Europe for the treatment of allergic rhinitis and chronic urticaria. Several double-blind comparisons with older agents (such as chlorpheniramine) indicated about equal therapeutic efficacy. However, sedation and interference with safe operation of machinery, which occurs in about 50% of subjects taking conventional antihistamines, occurred in only about 7% of subjects taking terfenadine or astemizole. The newer drugs are much more expensive.

B. Motion Sickness and Vestibular Disturbances: Scopolamine and certain H₁ antagonists are the most effective agents available for the prevention of motion sickness. The antihistaminic drugs with the greatest effectiveness in this application are diphenhydramine and promethazine. The piperazines also have significant activity in preventing motion sickness and are less sedative in most patients. Dosage is the same as that recommended for allergic disorders (Table 15–1). Both scopolamine and the H₁ antagonists are more effective in preventing motion sickness when combined with ephedrine or amphetamine.

It is claimed that the antihistaminic agents effective in prophylaxis of motion sickness are also useful in Meniere's syndrome.

C. Nausea and Vomiting of Pregnancy: Sev-eral H₁ antagonist drugs have been studied for possible use in treating "morning sickness." The piperazine derivatives were withdrawn from such use when it was demonstrated that they have teratogenic effects in rodents. Doxylamine, an ethanolamine H₁ antagonist, was promoted for this application as a component of Bendectin, a prescription medication that also contained pyridoxine. The question of fetal malformation resulting from this use of Bendectin is discussed below.

Toxicity

The wide spectrum of side effects of the H₁ antihistamines is described above. Several of these effects (sedation, antimuscarinic action) have been used for therapeutic purposes, especially in OTC remedies (Chapter 68). Nevertheless, these 2 effects constitute the most common undesirable actions when these drugs are used to block histamine receptors. Appropriate selection of drugs with a lower incidence of these effects (Table 15–1) and trial of several drugs by the patient are the most effective methods for minimizing both toxicities.

Less common toxic effects of systemic use include excitation and convulsions in children, postural hypotension, and allergic responses. Drug allergy is relatively common, especially after topical use of H₁ antagonists. The effects of severe systemic overdosage resemble those of atropine overdosage and are treated in the same way (Chapters 7 and 62).

Possible teratogenic effects of doxylamine were widely publicized in the lay press after 1978 as a result of case reports of fetal malformation associated with maternal ingestion of Bendectin. However, several large surveys, numbering over 60,000 pregnancies of which more than 3000 involved maternal Bendectin ingestion, disclosed no increase in the incidence of birth defects. In contrast, several case analysis studies of infants with malformations suggested a weak correlation between Bendectin use and abnormalties. One clinical epidemiologic survey, supported by an experimental study in rodents, suggested that the incidence of congenital diaphragmatic hernia might have been increased by maternal ingestion of doxylamine during the first trimester. Because of continuing controversy, adverse publicity, and lawsuits, the manufacturer of Bendectin withdrew the product from the market. Our inability to define the existence and extent of risk in this situation illustrates the difficulties involved in detecting small changes in the incidence of rare pathologic events.

H₂ RECEPTOR ANTAGONISTS

The development of H₂ receptor antagonists, beginning in 1972, led to renewed interest in possible physiologic roles for histamine and to a classification of effects and both agonists and antagonists based upon histamine receptor subtypes. The frequency of peptic ulcer disease and related gastrointestinal complaints created great interest in the therapeutic potential of H_2 receptor antagonists. The ability to reduce gastric acid secretion has made members of this class some of the most frequently prescribed drugs in the USA.

I. BASIC PHARMACOLOGY OF H_2 RECEPTOR ANTAGONISTS

Chemistry & Pharmacokinetics

The first 2 H_2 receptor antagonists, burimamide and metiamide, were imidazole compounds with long side chains containing a thiourea group. Burimamide was poorly absorbed after oral administration. Metiamide was well absorbed but, like many thiourea derivatives, caused blood dyscrasias (granulocytopenia) and was withdrawn from clinical use. Cimetidine, the third imidazole derivative of the series, lacks the thiourea moiety and appears to be relatively free of the granulocytopenic action of its predecessor. Ranitidine has neither the imidazole nor the thiourea moiety. Their long-term toxicity is not yet known (see below). Oxmetidine, famotidine, and nizatidine are newer H_2 antagonists not yet available in the USA.

Cimetidine is well absorbed following oral administration, and peak plasma levels are observed 1–2 hours following each dose. The half-life of cimetidine in humans is approximately 2 hours, and the apparent volume of distribution is 2 L/kg. The drug is widely distributed, crosses the placenta, and has been detected in breast milk. Cimetidine is excreted mostly unchanged. The pharmacokinetics of ranitidine are similar to those of cimetidine. Following oral administration, the average elimination half-life is 2.7 hours, with an average bioavailability of 52%. Most of the absorbed dose is excreted by the kidney as the parent drug. Small amounts of the N-oxide, N-desmethyl, and S-oxide metabolites are found in the urine.

Pharmacodynamics

A. Mechanism of Action: Presently available H_2 receptor antagonists reversibly compete with histamine at H_2 receptor sites. This action is quite selective in that the H_2 antagonists do not affect H_1 receptor–mediated actions. Conversely, the H_1 antagonists have no effect at H_2 receptors.

B. Organ System Effects:

1. Acid secretion and gastric motility–The most important action of H_2 receptor antagonists is to reduce the secretion of gastric acid. These drugs block the acid secretion stimulated by histamine, gastrin, cholinomimetic drugs, and vagal stimulation. The volume of gastric secretion and the concentration of pepsin are also reduced. While the ability of H_2 receptor antagonists to inhibit all phases of acid secretion has been interpreted as implicating histamine as a final common mediator of acid secretion, a more plausible hypothesis suggests that the full expression of stimuli such as gastrin and parasympathetic impulses requires the participation of histamine in some manner.

Cimetidine has little effect on gastric smooth muscle function and on lower esophageal sphincter pressure. Other gastrointestinal secretions are not significantly reduced. While there are marked potency differences among the members of this class, no agent appears to be more efficacious in reducing acid secretion.

2. Other effects related to H_2 receptor blockade–In doses that suppress gastric acid secretion, cimetidine and ranitidine have little effect on the heart or on blood pressure. This observation is consistent with the idea that histamine has little role in the normal regulation of the cardiovascular system. However, as shown in Fig 15–2, cimetidine is effective in reducing the actions of administered histamine on the heart and vessels.

It has been predicted that H_2 receptor antagonists may enhance certain immune responses by blocking histamine's ability to decrease mediator release from mast cells and basophils; *experimentally,* increases in delayed hypersensitivity reactions can be shown in some patients receiving cimetidine. However, there is no evidence that clinical hypersensitivity reactions are increased in such patients.

3. Effects not related to H_2 receptor blockade–The existing H_2 antagonists differ primarily in relative potency and pharmacokinetic characteristics

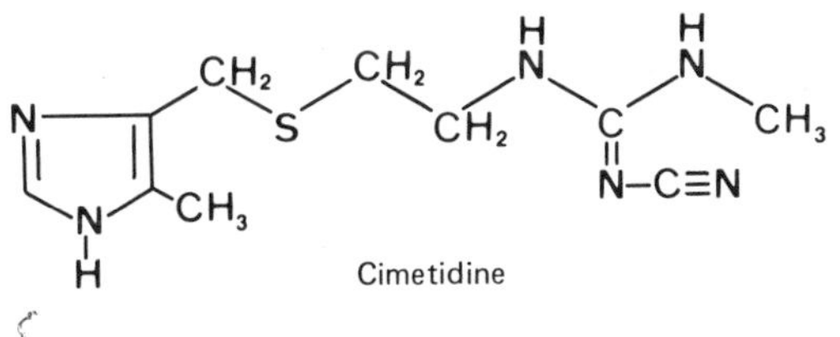

Cimetidine

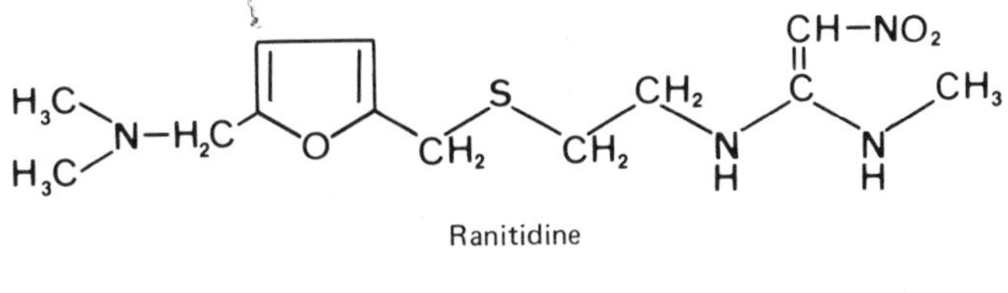

Ranitidine

when tested for their ability to block acid secretion. They also differ qualitatively with respect to actions not related to H_2 receptors. For example, cimetidine significantly inhibits the P-450 oxidative drug-metabolizing system, while ranitidine and nizatidine do not. Cimetidine—but not ranitidine, famotidine, or nizatidine—can bind to androgen receptors. These actions may have clinical significance with respect to drug interactions or adverse effects.

II. CLINICAL PHARMACOLOGY OF H_2 RECEPTOR ANTAGONISTS

Clinical Uses

A. Peptic Duodenal Ulcer: It is estimated that at least 10% of adults in the Western world will suffer an active episode of peptic ulcer disease during their lifetimes. Although the mortality rate of this condition is low, the recurrence rate is high and the socioeconomic cost is great. It has long been known that "no acid = no ulcer," and medical therapy has focused on reducing acidity by the use of antimuscarinic drugs and antacids. Antimuscarinic drugs must be used in high doses that are associated with significant adverse effects. Antacids will relieve symptoms and, in high doses, can promote healing. However, very frequent dosing is required (Chapter 66), and compliance is poor except during the acute symptomatic phase of the disease. The effectiveness of H_2 receptor antagonists in reducing gastric acidity coupled with apparent low acute toxicity represents a significant advance in the treatment of this disease. Results of many clinical trials show that these drugs are very effective in controlling symptoms during acute episodes and in promoting healing of duodenal ulcers. Prophylactic use at reduced dosage may prevent recurrence in many patients. Surgery for peptic ulcer patients is declining as a result of drug therapy.

In the short-term treatment of active duodenal ulcer, cimetidine (Tagament), 0.9–1.6 g/d, is given orally in divided doses. The dose should be less than this in elderly patients to minimize central nervous system toxicity. Following the acute phase, reduced dosage, eg, 400 mg at bedtime, may be given to prevent recurrence. The usual oral dose of ranitidine (Zantac) is 150 mg, given twice each day. This dose may be reduced in patients with significant impairment of renal function. H_2 receptor–blocking agents may be given intravenously, but hypotension and cardiac arrhythmias may occur. Patients refractory to cimetidine may respond to ranitidine.

B. Gastric Ulcer: In patients with active benign gastric ulcers, administration of H_2 receptor antagonists relieves symptoms and promotes healing. Dosage of cimetidine and ranitidine is the same as for duodenal disease.

C. Zollinger-Ellison Syndrome: In this disorder, which may be rapidly fatal, hypersecretion of acid is due to a gastrin-secreting tumor. In many patients, H_2 receptor–blocking drugs are effective in controlling symptoms related to excess acid secretion. The drugs can be used in preparation for surgery or as primary treatment when surgery is not indicated.

D. Other Hypersecretion Conditions: In patients with systemic mastocytosis or basophilic leukemia associated with high blood histamine levels, H_2 receptor–blocking drugs may be useful in controlling symptoms mediated by H_2 receptors. In other conditions in which the drugs are used, such as reflux esophagitis, hiatal hernia, stress-induced ulcers, and iatrogenic ulcers, benefit is not clearly documented in the literature. These drugs have been to an astonishing extent overprescribed.

Toxicity

These drugs are well tolerated, and adverse effects are reported in only 1–2% of patients. The most commonly reported effects are diarrhea and nausea and vomiting. Rash, headache, dizziness, and constipation have been reported in fewer than 1% of patients. Less common and more serious toxic effects are as follows:

A. Central Nervous System Dysfunction: Slurred speech, delirium, and occasionally coma appear to be most common in elderly patients.

B. Endocrine Effects: Cimetidine may cause gynecomastia in men and galactorrhea in women. The incidence approaches 1% after 6 months of therapy. In addition, a reduction in sperm count has been reported in men taking cimetidine in large doses for Zollinger-Ellison syndrome. These antiandrogenic effects are rarely troublesome if therapy with the drug is limited to 8 weeks or less. Ranitidine seems to be free of these endocrine effects.

C. Blood Dyscrasias: Cimetidine therapy has been associated with granulocytopenia and even aplastic anemia in a very few instances. The incidence is clearly far below that associated with the use of metiamide.

D. Liver Toxicity: Reversible hepatitis with or without jaundice has been reported in a few patients taking ranitidine.

Drug Interactions

Cimetidine can reduce liver blood flow and it inhibits the oxidative metabolism of other drugs, including warfarin-type anticoagulants, phenytoin, propranolol, chlordiazepoxide, diazepam, and theophylline. Patients taking warfarin-type anticoagulants should be closely monitored to avoid bleeding. The clinical significance of the interaction with other drugs has not been established. Ranitidine in ordinary therapeutic doses does not appear to inhibit the cytochrome P-450–catalyzed oxidative drug metabolism pathway, and therefore it appears less likely to cause most of the drug interactions attributed to cimetidine.

SEROTONIN
(5-HYDROXYTRYPTAMINE)

Before the identification of 5-hydroxytryptamine (5-HT), it was known that when blood is allowed to clot, a vasoconstrictor substance is released; this substance was called **serotonin**. Independent studies established the existence of a smooth muscle stimulant in intestinal mucosa; this was called **enteramine**. The synthesis of 5-hydroxytryptamine in 1951 permitted the identification of serotonin and enteramine as the same metabolite of 5-hydroxytryptophan.

I. BASIC PHARMACOLOGY OF SEROTONIN

Chemistry & Pharmacokinetics

Like histamine, serotonin is widely distributed in nature, being found in plant and animal tissues, venoms, and stings. It is an indoleethylamine formed in biologic systems from the amino acid L-tryptophan. The scheme shown in Fig 15–4 illustrates the hydroxylation of the indole ring followed by the decarboxylation of the amino acid. Hydroxylation at C5 is the rate-limiting step and can be blocked by *p*-chlorophenylalanine (PCPA, fenclonine) and by *p*-chloroamphetamine. These agents have been used experimentally to reduce serotonin synthesis in carcinoid tumor (see below).

After synthesis, the free amine is stored or is rapidly inactivated, usually by oxidation catalyzed by the enzyme monoamine oxidase. In the pineal gland, serotonin serves as a precursor of melatonin, a melanocyte-stimulating hormone. In mammals (including humans), over 90% of the serotonin in the body is found in enterochromaffin cells in the gastrointestinal tract. In the blood, serotonin is found in platelets, which lack the enzymes necessary for serotonin synthesis but are able to concentrate the amine by means of an active carrier mechanism. Serotonin is also found in the raphe nuclei cell bodies of the brain

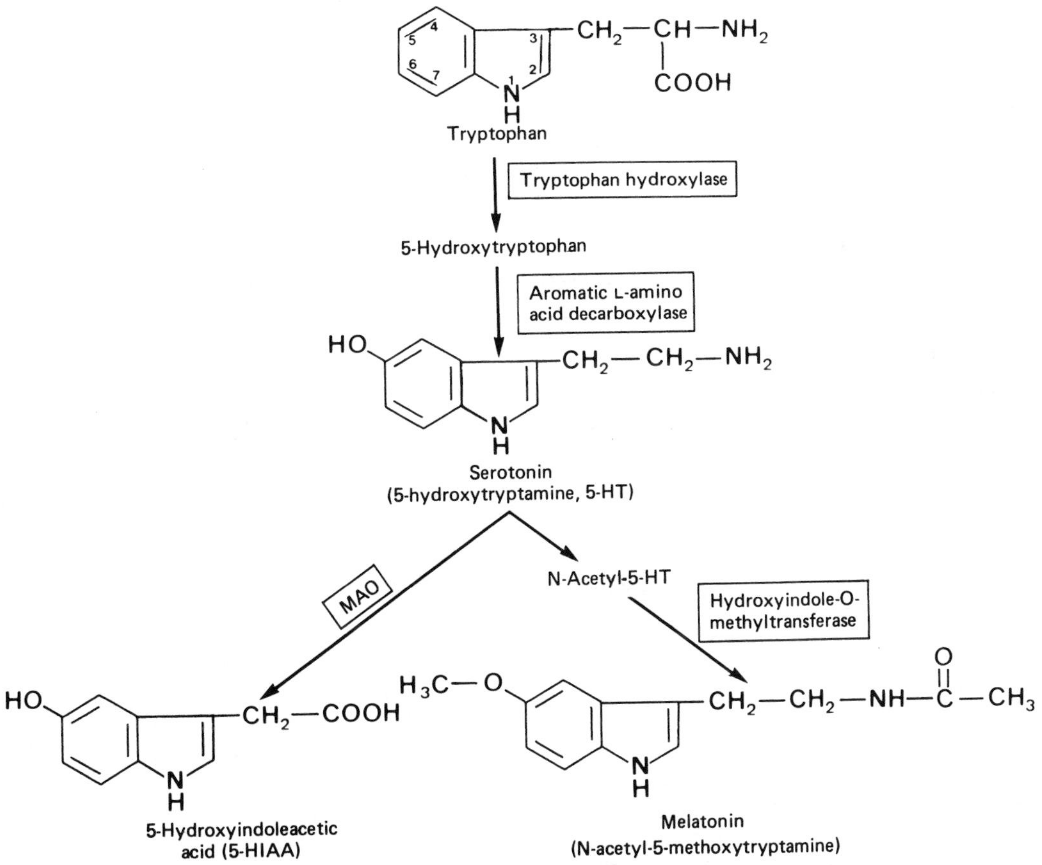

Figure 15–4. Synthesis and metabolism of serotonin. Note that the same enzyme catalyzes the decarboxylation of 5-hydroxytryptophan to serotonin and dopa to dopamine. (Modified and reproduced, with permission, from Meyers FH, Jawetz E, Goldfien A: *Review of Medical Pharmacology,* 7th ed. Lange, 1980.)

stem, which contain cell bodies of tryptaminergic (serotoninergic) neurons that synthesize, store, and release serotonin as a transmitter. Serotoninergic neurons are also found in the enteric nervous system of the gastrointestinal tract and around blood vessels. In rodents (but not in humans), serotonin is found in mast cells.

The function of serotonin in enterochromaffin cells is not clear. These cells synthesize serotonin, store the amine in a complex with ATP and with other substances in granules, and can release serotonin in response to mechanical and neuronal stimuli. Some of the released serotonin is taken up and stored in platelets.

Stored serotonin can be released by reserpine in much the same manner as this drug releases catecholamines from vesicles in adrenergic nerves (Chapter 10).

Serotonin is metabolized by monoamine oxidase, and the intermediate product, 5-hydroxyindoleacetaldehyde, is further oxidized by aldehyde dehydrogenase. When the latter enzyme is saturated, eg, by large amounts of acetaldehyde from ethanol metabolism, a significant fraction of the 5-hydroxyindoleacetaldehyde may be *reduced* in the liver to the alcohol 5-hydroxytryptophol. In humans consuming a normal diet, the excretion of 5-hydroxyindoleacetic acid is a measure of serotonin synthesis. Therefore, the 24-hour excretion of "5-HIAA" can be used as a diagnostic test for tumors that synthesize excessive quantities of serotonin, especially **carcinoid tumor.** A few foods (eg, bananas) contain large amounts of serotonin and must be prohibited during such diagnostic tests.

Pharmacodynamics

A. Mechanisms of Action: Serotonin exerts many actions, and, as in the case of histamine also, there are many species differences, making generalizations difficult. From studies with selective antagonists and results of tissue binding experiments, it appears that the actions of serotonin are mediated through receptors located in or on the surface membranes of target cells. Two subsets of serotonin receptors have been identified and designated 5-HT_1 and 5-HT_2. Most peripheral serotonin receptors (in platelets, smooth muscle) appear to be of the 5-HT_2 variety. Both 5-HT_1 and 5-HT_2 types have been identified in the brain.

The actions of serotonin on nerve and muscle cells are accompanied by changes in membrane permeability to ions such as sodium, potassium, and calcium, and stimulus-secretion coupling in enterochromaffin cells is associated with increased influx of calcium. The contraction or relaxation of smooth muscle caused by serotonin is often accompanied by elevated cGMP or cAMP, respectively, but the significance of the association between cyclic nucleotides and serotonin actions is not clear.

B. Tissue and Organ System Effects:

1. Cardiovascular system—A major direct effect of serotonin is to cause contraction of smooth muscle. In humans, serotonin is a powerful vasoconstrictor except in skeletal muscle and heart, where vessels are dilated. Serotonin can also elicit reflex bradycardia by activation of chemoreceptor nerve endings. A triphasic blood pressure response is often seen following injection of serotonin. Initially, there is a decrease in blood pressure and heart rate caused by the chemoreceptor response. Following this decrease, blood pressure increases as a result of vasoconstriction. The third phase is again a decrease in blood pressure attributed to vasodilation in vessels supplying skeletal muscle. Pulmonary and renal vessels seem especially sensitive to the vasoconstrictor action of serotonin. Serotonin also constricts veins, and venoconstriction with a resulting increased capillary filling appears responsible for the flush that is observed following serotonin administration. Serotonin has small direct positive chronotropic and inotropic effects on the heart that are probably of no clinical significance. However, continuously elevated blood levels of serotonin (which occur in carcinoid tumor) are associated with pathologic alterations in the endocardium (subendocardial fibroplasia) that may result in mechanical or electrical malfunction.

Serotonin causes aggregation of blood platelets by activating surface 5-HT_2 receptors. This response is not accompanied by release of the serotonin stored in the platelets, and its physiologic role is unclear.

2. Gastrointestinal tract—Serotonin causes contraction of gastrointestinal smooth muscle, increasing tone and facilitating peristalsis. This action is caused by the direct action of serotonin on smooth muscle plus a stimulating action on ganglion cells located in the intestinal wall. Serotonin has little direct effect on secretions, and what effects it has are generally inhibitory. It has been proposed that serotonin plays an important physiologic role as a local hormone controlling gastrointestinal motility. However, large doses of antagonists of serotonin are not associated with severe constipation. On the other hand, overproduction of serotonin—in carcinoid tumor—is associated with severe diarrhea.

3. Respiration—Serotonin has a small direct stimulant effect on bronchiolar smooth muscle in normal humans. In patients with carcinoid tumor, episodes of asthmatic bronchiolar obstruction occur in response to elevated levels of the amine. Serotonin also may cause marked hyperventilation, as a result of the chemoreceptor reflex response.

4. Nervous system—Like histamine, serotonin is a potent stimulant of pain and itch sensory nerve endings and is responsible for some of the symptoms caused by insect and plant stings. In addition, serotonin is a powerful activator of chemosensitive endings located in the coronary vascular bed. Activation of these afferent vagal nerve endings is associated with the **chemoreceptor reflex** (also known as the Bezold-Jarisch reflex). The reflex response is a triad consisting of bradycardia, hypotension, and apnea. The bradycardia is mediated by vagal outflow to the heart and can be blocked by atropine. The hypotension is a consequence of the decrease in cardiac output that results from bradycardia.

A variety of other agents are capable of activating the chemoreceptor reflex. These include nicotinic cholinoceptor stimulants and some cardiac glycosides, eg, ouabain.

Serotonin is present in a variety of sites in the brain. Its role as a neurotransmitter and its relation to the actions of drugs acting in the central nervous system are discussed in Chapters 19 and 27.

II. CLINICAL PHARMACOLOGY OF SEROTONIN

Serotonin has no clinical applications as a drug.

SEROTONIN ANTAGONISTS

The actions of serotonin, like those of histamine, can be antagonized in several different ways. Such antagonism is clearly desirable in those rare patients who have carcinoid tumor and may also be valuable in certain other conditions.

As noted above, serotonin synthesis can be inhibited by *p*-chlorophenylalanine and *p*-chloroamphetamine. However, these agents are too toxic for general use. Storage of serotonin can be inhibited by the use of reserpine, but the sympatholytic effects of this drug (Chapter 10) and the high levels of circulating serotonin that result from release prevent its use in carcinoid. Therefore, receptor blockade is the major approach to therapeutic limitation of serotonin effects.

SEROTONIN RECEPTOR ANTAGONISTS

Cyproheptadine and a number of experimental drugs have been identified as competitive serotonin receptor–blocking agents. In addition, the ergot alka-

loids discussed in the last portion of the chapter are **partial agonists** at the serotonin receptor.

Cyproheptadine (Periactin) resembles the phenothiazine antihistaminic agents in chemical structure and has potent H_1 receptor–blocking actions. The actions of cyproheptadine are predictable from its H_1 histamine and serotonin receptor affinities. It prevents the smooth muscle effects of both amines but has no effect on the gastric secretion stimulated by histamine. It has significant antimuscarinic effects and causes sedation.

The major clinical applications of cyproheptadine are in the treatment of the smooth muscle manifestations of carcinoid tumor and in the postgastrectomy dumping syndrome. The usual dosage in adults is 12–16 mg/d in 3–4 divided doses. It is also the preferred drug in cold-induced urticaria.

Ketanserin is an experimental agent that blocks 5-HT_2 receptors and has no reported H_1 receptor antagonist activity. This drug also blocks vascular α_1-adrenoceptors. The drug blocks 5-HT_2 receptors on platelets and antagonizes platelet aggregation promoted by serotonin. Interest in this compound is generated by observations that it lowers blood pressure both in hypertensive animals and in hypertensive human patients. However, the exact mechanisms involved in this hypotensive action are not clear and may involve both α_1-adrenoceptors and 5-HT_2 receptors.

THE ERGOT ALKALOIDS

Bertram G. Katzung, MD, PhD

Ergot alkaloids are produced by *Claviceps purpurea*, a fungus that infects grain—especially rye—under damp growing conditions. The ergot fungus has been called a "pharmaceutical factory," because this microorganism synthesizes histamine, acetylcholine, tyramine, and other biologically active products in addition to a score or more of ergot derivatives.

The accidental ingestion of ergot alkaloids in contaminated grain can be traced back more than 2000 years from descriptions of epidemics of the characteristic poisoning (ergotism). The most dramatic effects of poisoning are dementia with florid hallucinations; prolonged vasospasm, which may result in gangrene;

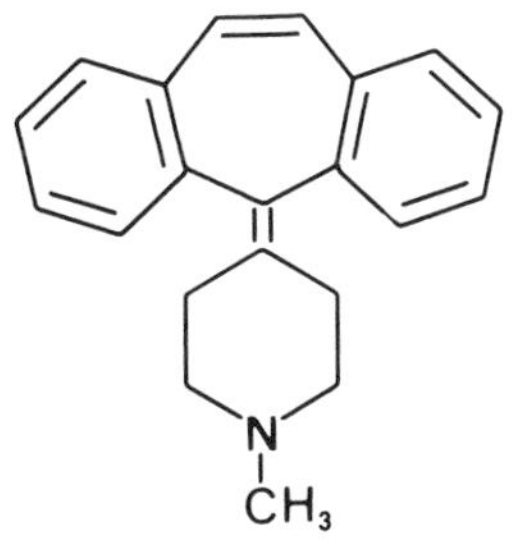

Cyproheptadine

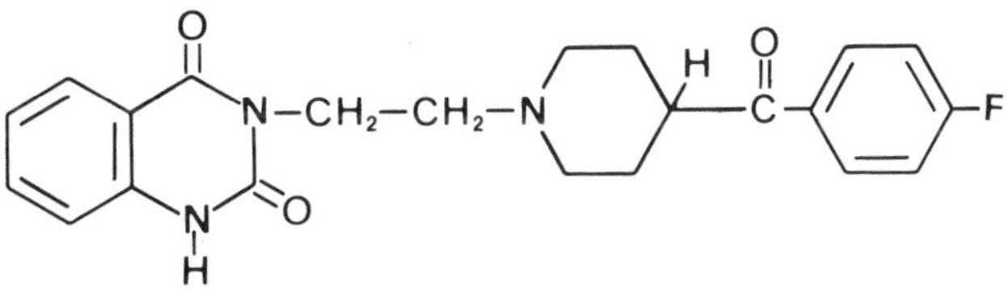

Ketanserin

and stimulation of uterine smooth muscle, which in pregnancy may result in abortion. The degree of each effect varies among reported epidemics and may represent a different mix of individual alkaloids in different crops of the fungus. In medieval times, ergot poisoning was called St. Anthony's fire after the saint whose help was sought in relieving the burning pain of vasospastic ischemia. Identifiable epidemics have occurred sporadically up to the present time (see References) and mandate continuous surveillance of all grains used for food.

In addition to the effects noted above, the ergot alkaloids produce a variety of other central nervous system and peripheral effects. Detailed structure-activity analysis and appropriate semisynthetic modifications have yielded a large number of agents with documented or potential clinical value.

I. BASIC PHARMACOLOGY OF ERGOT ALKALOIDS

Chemistry & Pharmacokinetics

Two major families of compounds that incorporate the tetracyclic **ergoline** nucleus may be identified: the amine alkaloids and the peptide alkaloids (Table 15–2). Drugs of clinical importance are found in both classes. The structures shown in Fig 15–5 compare norepinephrine, dopamine, and serotonin with the ergoline nucleus and suggest one reason for the great pharmacologic versatility of the ergot alkaloids.

The ergot alkaloids are variably absorbed from the gastrointestinal tract. The oral dose of ergotamine is about 10 times larger than the intramuscular dose, but the speed of absorption and peak blood levels after oral administration can be improved by administration with caffeine (see below). The amine alkaloids are also absorbed from the rectum, the buccal cavity, and after administration by aerosol inhaler. Absorption after intramuscular injection is slow but usually reliable. Bromocriptine is more completely absorbed from the gastrointestinal tract than is ergotamine or the amine derivatives.

The ergot alkaloids are extensively metabolized in the body. The primary metabolites are hydroxylated in the A ring, and peptide alkaloids are also modified in the peptide moiety. Most of the excretory products of methysergide are demethylated at the N1 position.

Pharmacodynamics

A. Mechanism of Action: As suggested above, the ergot alkaloids act on several types of receptors. Their effects include agonist and antagonist actions at α-adrenoceptors and serotonin receptors and agonist action at central nervous system dopamine receptors. Furthermore, some members of the ergot family have a high affinity for presynaptic receptors, while others are more selective for postjunctional receptors. There is a powerful stimulant effect on the uterus and other smooth muscle that is not clearly associated with any of the preceding receptor types. Structural variations

Table 15–2. Major ergoline derivatives (ergot alkaloids).

Amine alkaloids

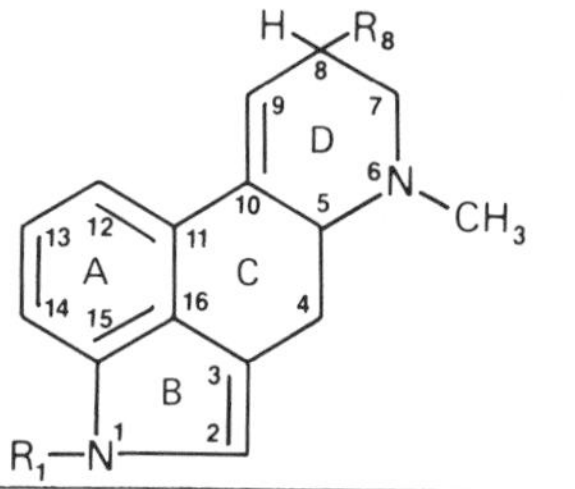

	R_1	R_8
6-Methylergoline	—H	—H
Lysergic acid	—H	—COOH
Lysergic acid diethylamide (LSD)	—H	$-\overset{\overset{\text{O}}{\|\|}}{C}-N(CH_2-CH_3)_2$
Ergonovine (ergometrine)	—H	$-\overset{\overset{\text{O}}{\|\|}}{C}-NH-CH-CH_3$ $\|$ CH_2OH
Methysergide	—CH_3	$-\overset{\overset{\text{O}}{\|\|}}{C}-NH-CH-CH_2-CH_3$ $\|$ CH_2OH

Peptide alkaloids

	R_2	R_2'	R_5'
Ergotamine	—H	—CH_3	$-CH_2-\langle\text{phenyl}\rangle$ 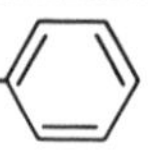
α-Ergocryptine	—H	—$CH(CH_3)_2$	$-CH_2-CH(CH_3)_2$
Bromocriptine	—Br	—$CH(CH_3)_2$	$-CH_2-CH(CH_3)_2$

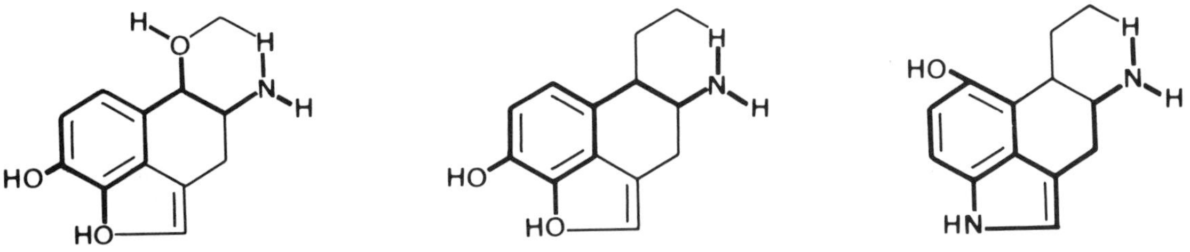

Figure 15–5. Comparison of the ergoline nucleus with several neurotransmitter amines. The ergoline nucleus is shown with light lines, the named amines with superimposed heavy lines.

increase the selectivity of certain members of the family for specific receptor types (Table 15–3); clinical use of a given agent is not inevitably associated with all of the above actions.

B. Organ System Effects:

1. Central nervous system—As indicated by traditional descriptions of ergotism, certain of the naturally occurring alkaloids are powerful hallucinogens. Lysergic acid diethylamide (LSD$_{25}$, "acid") is the semisynthetic compound that most clearly demonstrates this action. In spite of extensive research, neither the mechanism nor any clinical value has been discovered for this dramatic effect. Abuse of this drug was widespread for several decades and is discussed in Chapter 30.

Dopamine receptors in the central nervous system appear to play important roles in extrapyramidal motor control and the regulation of prolactin release. Bromocriptine has the highest selectivity for these receptors of currently available ergot derivatives. Bromocriptine directly suppresses prolactin secretion from pituitary cells by activating regulatory dopamine receptors. It competes for binding to these sites with dopamine itself and with other dopamine agonists such as apomorphine. The actions of bromocriptine on the extrapyramidal system are discussed in Chapter 26.

2. Vascular smooth muscle—The traditional view of ergot alkaloids as weak alpha-receptor antagonists and potent direct vasoconstrictor agents has given way in recent years to evidence of a much more complex pattern of vascular actions. As indicated in Table 15–3, this pattern includes agonist as well as antagonist effects at alpha receptors, since some ergot-induced vasoconstriction is blocked by conventional alpha-receptor antagonists. Both agonist and antagonist

effects also occur at serotonin receptors. Activation of vasoconstrictor tryptamine receptors has also been proposed.

Despite the presence of alpha receptor–blocking activity in the alkaloids shown in Tables 15–2 and 15–3, their dominant effect on blood vessels is vasoconstriction. This action combines the agonist effects at alpha, serotonin, and, possibly, tryptamine receptors. The remarkably specific antimigraine action of certain ergot derivatives is thought to be related to their actions on vascular or neuronal serotonin receptors. Ergotamine and methysergide are the agents most widely used for the treatment of migraine.

After overdosage with ergotamine and similar agents, vasospasm is severe and prolonged (see Toxicity, below). This vasospasm is not reversed by alpha-antagonists, serotonin antagonists, or combinations of both. Only very powerful direct-acting vasodilators such as nitroprusside have been effective in this situation.

Ergotamine is typical of the ergot alkaloids with this spectrum of action (Table 15–3). The hydrogenation of ergot alkaloids at the 9 and 10 positions (Table 15–2) yields dihydro derivatives that have much lower direct smooth muscle and serotonin effects and more selective alpha receptor–blocking action.

3. Uterine smooth muscle—Like vascular smooth muscle, the action of ergot alkaloids on the uterus appears to combine alpha-agonist, serotonin, and other effects. However, the sensitivity of the uterus to the stimulant effects of ergot varies dramatically with hormonal status. As a result, the uterus at term is more sensitive than earlier in pregnancy and far more so than the nonpregnant organ.

In small doses, ergot preparations can evoke rhyth-

Table 15–3. Effects of ergot alkaloids at several receptors.[*]

Ergot Alkaloid	Alpha-Adrenoceptor	Dopamine Receptor	Serotonin Receptor (5-HT$_2$)	Other Smooth Muscle Stimulation
Lysergic acid diethylamide (LSD)	0	+++	– – –	++
Ergonovine	+	+	– (PA)	+++
Methysergide	+/0	+/0	– – – (PA)	+
Ergotamine	– – (PA)	0	+ (PA)	+++
Bromocriptine	– –	+++	–	0

*Agonist effects are indicated by +, antagonist by –, no effect by 0. Relative affinity for the receptor is indicated by the number of + or – signs. PA means partial agonist (both agonist and antagonist effects can be detected).

mic contraction and relaxation of the uterus. At higher concentrations, these drugs induce powerful and prolonged contracture. Ergonovine is more selective than other ergot alkaloids in affecting the uterus and is the agent of choice in obstetric applications of these drugs.

4. Other smooth muscle organs–In most patients, the ergot alkaloids have no significant effect on bronchiolar smooth muscle. The gastrointestinal tract, on the other hand, varies dramatically in sensitivity among patients. Nausea, vomiting, and diarrhea may be induced by low doses in some patients but only by high doses in others. The effect is consistent with action on the central nervous system (emetic center) and on gastrointestinal serotonin receptors.

II. CLINICAL PHARMACOLOGY OF ERGOT ALKALOIDS

Clinical Uses

A. Migraine: Migraine headache in its classic form is characterized by a brief "aura" that may involve visual scotomas or even hemianopia and speech abnormalities, followed by a severe throbbing unilateral headache that lasts for a few hours to 1–2 days. The disease is familial in 60–80% of patients, more common in women, and usually has its onset in early adolescence through young adulthood, waning with advancing years. Attacks are usually precipitated by stress but often occur after rather than during the stressful episode. They vary in frequency from one attack a year to 2 or more a week.

Although the symptom pattern varies among patients, the severity of migraine headache justifies vigorous therapy in the great majority of cases.

The pathophysiology of migraine clearly includes some vasomotor mechanism, because the onset of headache is associated with a marked increase in amplitude of temporal artery pulsations, and relief of pain by administration of ergotamine is accompanied by diminution in arterial pulsation. On the other hand, these vasomotor changes may be the result of more basic processes underlying migraine, since a number of drugs with very different vascular actions are effective in migraine. Evidence strongly suggests that the onset of a migrainous aura is associated with an abnormal release of serotonin from platelets, while the arterial throbbing phase is associated with decrease of platelet and serum serotonin below normal concentrations. Other chemical triggers include falling levels of estrogen in women whose headache is linked to the menstrual cycle and elevated levels of prostaglandin E_1.

The efficacy of ergot derivatives in the therapy of migraine is so specific as to constitute a diagnostic test. Traditional therapy (ergotamine) is most effective when given during the prodrome of an attack and becomes progressively less effective if delayed. Ergotamine tartrate is available for oral, sublingual, rectal

suppository, and inhaler use. It is often combined with caffeine (100 mg caffeine for 1 mg ergotamine tartrate) to facilitate absorption of the ergot alkaloid.

The vasoconstriction induced by ergotamine is long-lasting and cumulative when the drug is taken repeatedly, as in a severe attack. Therefore, patients must be carefully informed that no more than 6 mg of the oral preparation may be taken for each attack and no more than 10 mg per week. For very severe attacks, ergotamine tartrate, 0.25–0.5 mg, may be given intravenously or intramuscularly.

Because of the cumulative toxicity of ergotamine, safer agents useful for the prophylaxis of migraine have been sought. Methysergide, a derivative of the amine subgroup (Table 15–2), has been shown to be effective in this application in about 60% of patients. Unfortunately, significant toxicity (discussed below) occurs in almost 40%. As suggested in Table 15–3, there is some evidence of a difference in the agonist:antagonist ratios of methysergide and ergotamine when assayed on serotonin receptors. Regardless of the cause, methysergide is relatively *ineffective* in treatment of impending or active episodes of migraine. The dosage of methysergide maleate (Sansert) for prophylaxis of migraine is 4–8 mg/d.

Although relatively free of the rapidly cumulative vasospastic toxicity of ergotamine, chronic use of methysergide may induce retroperitoneal fibroplasia and subendocardial fibrosis, possibly through its vascular effects. Therefore, it is important that patients taking methysergide have periodic drug holidays of 3–4 weeks every 6 months (see Toxicity).

Propranolol has also been found effective for the prophylaxis of migraine in some patients. Like methysergide, it is of no value in the treatment of acute migraine.

B. Hyperprolactinemia: Increased serum levels of the anterior pituitary hormone prolactin are associated with secreting tumors of the gland and also with the use of centrally acting dopamine antagonists, especially the antipsychotic drugs. Because of negative feedback effects, hyperprolactinemia is associated with amenorrhea and infertility in women as well as galactorrhea in both sexes.

Bromocriptine mesylate (Parlodel) is extremely effective in reducing the high levels of prolactin that result from pituitary tumors and has even been associated with regression of the tumor in some cases. The usual dosage of bromocriptine is 2.5 mg 2 or 3 times daily. Bromocriptine has also been used in the same dosage to suppress physiologic lactation.

C. Postpartum Hemorrhage: The introduction of ergot products into obstetrics in the latter part of the 18th century was accompanied by a dramatic increase in fetal and maternal mortality rates. It is now recognized that because the uterus at term is so sensitive to the stimulant action of ergot, even moderate doses produce a prolonged and powerful spasm of the muscle quite unlike natural labor. Therefore, ergot derivatives are useful only for control of late uterine bleeding and should never be given before delivery. Ergonovine maleate, 0.2 mg given usually intramuscularly, is effective within 1–5 minutes and is less toxic than other ergot derivatives for this application. It is given at the time of delivery of the placenta or immediately afterward if bleeding is significant.

D. Diagnosis of Variant Angina: Ergonovine produces prompt vasoconstriction in coronary vessels subject to spastic responses (Prinzmetal's or variant angina; see Chapter 11). Therefore, this ergot derivative may be administered by intravenous infusion during coronary angiography to diagnose variant angina.

E. Senile Cerebral Insufficiency: Dihydroergotoxine, a mixture of dihydro-α-ergocryptine and 3 similar dihydrogenated peptide ergot alkaloids,* has been promoted for many years for the relief of "senility." There is no evidence of significant benefit.

Toxicity & Contraindications

The most common toxic effects of the ergot derivatives are gastrointestinal disturbances, including diarrhea and nausea and vomiting. Activation of the medullary vomiting center and of the gastrointestinal serotonin receptors is involved. Since migraine attacks are often associated with these symptoms before therapy is begun, this side effect is rarely a contraindication to therapy of acute migraine. However, in prophylactic management with methysergide, the effect is an important factor limiting use of the drug.

A more dangerous toxic effect of overdosage with agents like ergotamine and ergonovine is prolonged vasospasm. As described above, this sign of vascular smooth muscle stimulation may result in gangrene and require amputation. Most cases involve the circulation to the arms and legs. However, bowel infarction resulting from mesenteric artery vasospasm has also been reported. Peripheral vascular vasospasm caused by ergot is refractory to most vasodilators, but infusion of large doses of nitroprusside, a powerful direct-acting vasodilator, has been successful in some cases.

Chronic therapy with methysergide is associated with development of fibroplastic changes in the retroperitoneal space, the pleural cavity, and the endocardial tissue of the heart. These changes occur insidiously over months and may present as hydronephrosis (from obstruction of the ureters) or a cardiac murmur (from distortion of the valves of the heart). Fortunately, most signs of toxicity regress when administration of the drug is halted. However, the potential for injury is such that all patients taking methysergide should have periodic drug holidays and should be carefully studied if signs or symptoms of fibroplasia occur.

Other toxic effects of the ergot alkaloids include drowsiness and, in the case of methysergide, occasional instances of central stimulation and hallucinations. In fact, methysergide has been used as a substitute for LSD by members of the "drug culture."

Contraindications to the use of ergot derivatives consist of the obstructive vascular diseases and collagen disease.

There is no evidence that ordinary use of ergotamine or methysergide for migraine is hazardous in pregnancy. However, most clinicians counsel restraint in the use of these agents in pregnant patients.

*Available as ergoloid mesylates (many trade names).

REFERENCES

Histamine

Beaven MA: *Histamine: Its Role in Physiological and Pathological Processes.* Monographs in Allergy. Vol 13. 1978.

Black JW et al: Definition and antagonism of histamine H_2-receptors. *Nature* 1972;**236**:385.

Cocco AE, Cocco DV: A survey of cimetidine prescribing. *N Engl J Med* 1981;**304**:1281.

Garg DC, Weidler DJ, Eshelman FN: Ranitidine bioavailability and kinetics in normal male subjects. *Clin Pharmacol Ther* 1983;**33**:445.

Guo Zhao-Gui et al: Inotropic effects of histamine in human myocardium: Differentiation between positive and negative components. *J Cardiovasc Pharmacol* 1985;**6**:1210.

Holmes LB: Teratogen update: Bendectin. *Teratology* 1983;**27**:277.

Howard JM et al: Famotidine, a new, potent, long-acting H_2-receptor antagonist: Comparison with cimetidine and ranitidine in the treatment of Zollinger-Ellison syndrome. *Gastroenterology* 1985;**88**:1026.

Lebert PA et al: Ranitidine kinetics and dynamics. 1. Oral dose studies. 2. Intravenous dose studies and comparison with cimetidine. (2 parts.) *Clin Pharmacol Ther* 1981;**30**:539, 545.

Lomax P, Green MD: Histamine neurons in the hypothalamic thermoregulatory pathways. *Fed Proc* 1981;**40**:2741.

MacGlashan DW et al: Comparative studies of human basophils and mast cells. *Fed Proc* 1983;**42**:2504.

Martz BL et al: Terfenadine. (Symposium.) *Arzneimittelforsch* 1982;**32**:1153.

Meredith CG, Speeg KV Jr, Schenker S: Nizatidine, a new histamine H_2-receptor antagonist, and hepatic oxidative drug metabolism in the rat: A comparison with structurally related compounds. *Toxicol Appl Pharmacol* 1985;**77**:315.

Morelock S et al: Bendectin and fetal development: A study at Boston City Hospital. *Am J Obstet Gynecol* 1982;**142**:209.

Nicholson AN: Antihistamines and sedation. *Lancet* 1983;**2**:211.

Rocklin RE, Beer DJ: Histamine and immune modulation. *Adv Intern Med* 1983;**28**:225.

Schade RR, Donaldson RMJ: How physicians use cimetidine: A survey of hospitalized patients and published cases. *N Engl J Med* 1981;**304**:1281.

Torsoli A, Lucchelli PE, Brimblecombe RW (editors): *H_2 Antagonists: H_2-Receptor Antagonists in Peptic Ulcer Disease and Progress in Histamine Research.* (Symposium.) International Congress Series 521. Excerpta Medica, 1980.

Serotonin

Cohen ML, Fuller RN, Wilkey KS: Evidence for 5-HT$_2$ receptors mediating contraction in vascular smooth muscle. *J*

Pharmacol Exp Ther 1981;**218**:421.

Cohen ML et al: Role of 5-HT$_2$ receptors in serotonin-induced contractions of nonvascular smooth muscle. *J Pharmacol Exp Ther* 1985;**232**:770.

Demoulin JC et al: 5-HT$_2$-receptor blockade in the treatment of heart failure. *Lancet* 1981;**1**:1186.

Essman WB (editor): *Serotonin in Health and Disease*. Vols 1–4. Spectrum, 1978.

Kalkman HO et al: Hypotensive activity of serotonin antagonists: Correlation with α-adrenoceptor and serotonin receptor blockade. *Life Sci* 1983;**32**:1499.

Peroutka SJ, Snyder SH: Multiple serotonin receptors and their physiological significance. *Fed Proc* 1983;**42**:213.

Pettersson A et al: Treatment of arterial hypertension with ketanserin in mono- and combination therapy. *Clin Pharmacol Ther* 1985;**38**:188.

Van Nueten JM et al: Vascular effects of ketanserin (R 41 468), a novel antagonist of 5-HT$_2$ serotonergic receptors. *J Pharmacol Exp Ther* 1981;**218**:217.

Vanhoutte PM (editor): *Serotonin and the Cardiovascular System*. Raven Press, 1985.

ERGOT ALKALOIDS

Historical

Fuller JG: *The Days of St. Anthony's Fire*. MacMillan, 1968; Signet, 1969. [A narrative account of an epidemic of ergotism in France in 1951.]

Gabbai Dr, Lisbonne Dr, Pourquier Dr: Ergot poisoning at Pont St. Esprit. *Br Med J* (Sept 15) 1951;650.

King B: Outbreak of ergotism in Wollo, Ethiopia. (Letter.) *Lancet* 1979;**1**:1411.

Basic Pharmacology

Berde B: Ergot compounds: A synopsis. *Adv Biochem Psychopharmacol* 1980;**23**:3.

Muller-Schweinitzer E. Responsiveness of isolated canine cerebral and peripheral arteries to ergotamine. *Naunyn Schmiedebergs Arch Pharmacol* 1976;**292**:113.

Saxena PR: Selective vasoconstriction in carotid vascular bed by methysergide: Possible relevance to its anti-migraine effect. *Eur J Pharmacol* 1974;**27**:99.

Clinical Pharmacology

Anderson PK et al: Sodium nitroprusside and epidural blockade in the treatment of ergotism. *N Engl J Med* 1977;**296**:1271.

Anthony M, Hinterberger H, Lance JW: Plasma serotonin in migraine and stress. *Arch Neurol* 1967;**16**:544.

Harrington E et al: Migraine: A platelet disorder. *Lancet* 1981;**2**:720.

Raskin NH: Pharmacology of migraine. *Annu Rev Pharmacol Toxicol* 1981;**21**:463.

Thorner MO et al: Hyperprolactinemia: Current concepts of management including medical therapy with bromocriptine. *Adv Biochem Psychopharmacol* 1980;**23**:165.

Polypeptides

16

Ian A. Reid, PhD

A variety of polypeptides exert important effects on vascular and other smooth muscles. These include the vasoconstrictors angiotensin II and vasopressin and several vasodilators, including bradykinin and other kinins, atrial natriuretic peptide, vasoactive intestinal peptide, substance P, and neurotensin.

ANGIOTENSIN

BIOSYNTHESIS OF ANGIOTENSIN

The pathway for the formation and metabolism of angiotensin II is summarized in Fig 16–1. The principal steps include enzymatic cleavage of angiotensin I from angiotensinogen by renin, conversion of angiotensin I to angiotensin II by converting enzyme, and degradation of angiotensin II by several peptidases.

Renin & Factors Controlling Renin Secretion

Renin specifically catalyzes hydrolytic release of the decapeptide angiotensin I from angiotensinogen. It has been classified as an acid protease and thus belongs to the same group of enzymes as pepsin and cathepsin D (which can also form angiotensin I from angiotensinogen under appropriate conditions). Renin has been purified to homogeneity and shown to be a glycoprotein with a molecular weight of 35,000–42,000. Inactive forms of renin, often referred to as "prorenins," are present in several body fluids and tissues. These can be activated by acidification, cold treatment, and various enzymes, including pepsin, cathepsin D, trypsin, and kallikrein, but the extent to which inactive renin is converted to active renin in vivo is not known.

Most (probably all) of the renin in the circulation originates in the kidneys. Enzymes with reninlike activity are present in several extrarenal tissues, including blood vessels, uterus, salivary glands, and adrenal cortex, but no physiologic role for these enzymes has been established. Within the kidney, renin is synthesized and stored in a specialized area of the nephron, the juxtaglomerular apparatus. The juxtaglomerular apparatus is composed of vascular and tubular elements. Vascular elements include the afferent and efferent arterioles and a group of mesangial cells. The afferent arteriole and, to a lesser extent, the efferent arteriole and mesangial cells contain specialized granular cells called juxtaglomerular cells that serve as the site of synthesis, storage, and release of renin. The tubular component of the juxtaglomerular apparatus is the macula densa, a specialized tubular segment closely associated with the vascular components of the juxtaglomerular apparatus. The vascular and tubular components of the juxtaglomerular apparatus, including the juxtaglomerular cells, are innervated by adrenergic neurons.

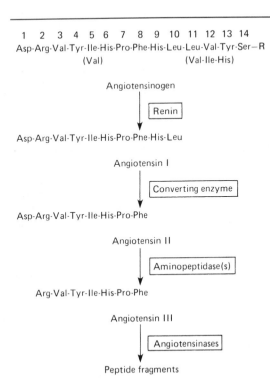

Figure 16–1. Chemistry of the renin-angiotensin system. The amino acid sequence of the amino terminal of equine and porcine angiotensinogen is shown. Bovine angiotensinogen contains Val in position 5, and human angiotensinogen contains Val-Ile-His in positions 11–13. R denotes the remainder of the protein molecule.

The rate at which renin is secreted by the kidney is the primary determinant of activity of the renin-angiotensin system. Renin secretion is controlled by a variety of factors, including a renal vascular receptor, the macula densa, the sympathetic nervous system, angiotensin II, vasopressin, and potassium.

A. Renal Vascular Receptor: The renal vascular receptor functions as a stretch receptor, decreased stretch leading to increased renin release and vice versa. The receptor is apparently located in the afferent arteriole, and it is possible that the juxtaglomerular cells themselves are sensitive to changes in stretch.

B. Macula Densa: The macula densa contains a different type of receptor, apparently sensitive to changes in the rate of delivery of sodium or chloride to the distal tubule. Decreases in distal delivery result in stimulation of renin secretion, and vice versa.

C. Sympathetic Nervous System: The sympathetic innervation of the juxtaglomerular apparatus plays an important role in the control of renin secretion. Maneuvers that increase renal neural activity cause stimulation of renin secretion, while renal denervation results in suppression of renin secretion. It appears that norepinephrine can stimulate renin secretion by a direct action on the juxtaglomerular cells. This effect is thought to be mediated by β-adrenoceptors and may involve the activation of adenylate cyclase and the formation of cAMP. At present, it is not clear if these beta receptors are of the β_1 or β_2 subtype. In some situations, norepinephrine stimulates renin secretion indirectly by way of α receptors. This stimulation apparently results from constriction of the afferent arteriole, with resultant activation of the renal vascular receptor and decreased delivery of sodium chloride to the macula densa. In other situations, α-adrenoceptor stimulation may actually inhibit renin secretion.

The rate of renin secretion is also influenced by circulating epinephrine and norepinephrine. These catecholamines may act via the same mechanisms as the norepinephrine released locally from the renal sympathetic nerves. However, there is evidence that a major component of the renin secretory response to circulating catecholamines is mediated by way of *extrarenal* beta receptors. The location of these receptors and the pathway by which they influence renin secretion remain to be determined.

D. Angiotensin, Vasopressin, and Potassium: Angiotensin II, vasopressin, and potassium all inhibit renin secretion. The inhibition of renin secretion by angiotensin II, which is thought to result from a direct action of the peptide on the juxtaglomerular cells, forms the basis of a short-loop negative feedback mechanism controlling renin secretion. Interruption of this feedback with antagonists of the renin-angiotensin system (see below) results in stimulation of renin secretion. Vasopressin inhibits renin secretion at quite low concentrations and is probably an important modulator of the rate of renin secretion. Small changes in plasma potassium concentration lead to reciprocal changes in the rate of renin secretion. Potassium appears to inhibit renin secretion indirectly by increasing the rate of delivery of sodium chloride to the macula densa.

Angiotensinogen

Angiotensinogen is the circulating protein substrate from which renin cleaves angiotensin I. Most of the angiotensinogen in the circulation originates in the liver. Angiotensinogen has been shown to be a glycoprotein with a molecular weight of 52,000–66,000. The amino acid sequence of the amino terminal of the molecule is known (Fig 16–1). In humans, the concentration of angiotensinogen in the circulation is less than the K_m (concentration for 50% of maximum reaction rate) for the renin-angiotensinogen reaction and is therefore an important determinant of the rate of formation of angiotensin. The production of angiotensinogen is increased by corticosteroids, estrogens, and angiotensin II.

The stimulation of angiotensinogen production by corticosteroids is related to their glucocorticoid activity rather than to their mineralocorticoid activity. As a consequence, plasma angiotensinogen concentration is increased in patients with Cushing's syndrome but not in those with primary aldosteronism.

Estrogens increase angiotensinogen production, and elevations in plasma angiotensinogen concentration occur during pregnancy and in women taking estrogen-containing oral contraceptives.

Angiotensin II increases angiotensinogen production, apparently by direct action on the liver. This stimulatory effect may form the basis of a positive feedback mechanism that prevents angiotensinogen levels from falling when the utilization of angiotensinogen is increased during periods of hyperreninemia.

Angiotensin I

Although angiotensin I contains the peptide sequences necessary for all of the actions of the renin-angiotensin system, it has little or no biologic activity. Instead, it must be converted to angiotensin II by converting enzyme (Fig 16–1). Angiotensin I may also be acted on by plasma or tissue aminopeptidases to form [des-Asp¹]angiotensin I; this in turn is converted to [des-Asp¹]angiotensin II (commonly known as angiotensin III) by converting enzyme.

Converting Enzyme (Peptidyl Dipeptidase, PDP, Kininase II)

Converting enzyme is a dipeptidyl carboxypeptidase that catalyzes the cleavage of dipeptides from the carboxyl terminal of certain peptides. Its most important substrates are angiotensin I, which it converts to angiotensin II; and bradykinin, which it inactivates (see below). It also cleaves enkephalins and substance P, but the physiologic significance of these effects has not been established. The action of converting enzyme is restricted by a penultimate prolyl residue, and angiotensin II is therefore not hydrolyzed by converting enzyme. Converting enzyme is distributed widely in the body, but its concentration is particularly high in the pulmonary circulation, and it is here that most conversion of angiotensin I to angiotensin II occurs. In most tissues, converting enzyme is located on the luminal surface of vascular endothelial cells and is thus in close contact with the circulation.

ACTIONS OF ANGIOTENSIN II

Angiotensin II exerts important actions at several sites in the body, including vascular smooth muscle, adrenal cortex, kidney, and brain. Through these actions, the renin-angiotensin system plays a key role in the regulation of fluid and electrolyte balance and arterial blood pressure. Overactivity of the renin-angiotensin system can result in hypertension and disorders of fluid and electrolyte homeostasis.

Effects on Blood Pressure

Angiotensin II is an extremely potent pressor agent—on a molar basis, approximately 40 times more potent than norepinephrine. The pressor response to intravenous angiotensin II is rapid in onset (10–15 seconds) and sustained during long-term infusions of the peptide. A large component of the pressor response to intravenous angiotensin II is due to direct contraction of vascular—especially arteriolar—smooth muscle. In addition, however, angiotensin II can also increase blood pressure through actions on the brain and autonomic nervous system. The central pressor effect of angiotensin II is mediated by the area postrema, a circumventricular organ located in the medulla oblongata. Like the other circumventricular organs, the area postrema lacks a blood-brain barrier and is therefore accessible to blood-borne angiotensin II. Infusion of angiotensin II into the vertebral arteries, which supply the area postrema, produces a prompt increase in blood pressure; this is abolished when a lesion is placed in the area postrema. Area postrema lesions have also been reported to decrease the pressor response to intravenous angiotensin II. The increase in blood pressure produced by intravertebral injection of angiotensin II is due to a combination of elevated total peripheral resistance resulting from increased sympathetic discharge and an increase in cardiac output secondary to withdrawal of vagal tone to the heart.

Angiotensin II also interacts with the peripheral autonomic nervous system. It facilitates sympathetic transmission by an action at adrenergic nerve terminals, increases the release of epinephrine and norepinephrine from the adrenal medulla, and stimulates autonomic ganglia. Of these actions, facilitation of adrenergic transmission is probably the most important. This effect results from both increased release and reduced reuptake of norepinephrine.

Angiotensin II also has a direct positive inotropic action on the heart. While this action may contribute to the increase in blood pressure, it is far less important than the vascular effects.

Effects on the Adrenal Cortex

Angiotensin II acts directly on the zona glomeru-losa of the adrenal cortex to stimulate aldosterone biosynthesis and secretion. In higher doses, angiotensin II also stimulates glucocorticoid secretion. The stimulation of aldosterone secretion by angiotensin II results chiefly from increased conversion of cholesterol to pregnenolone, although, during long-term exposure to the peptide, the conversion of corticosterone to aldosterone may also be facilitated. Current evidence indicates that the renin-angiotensin system is one of the major regulators of aldosterone secretion, mediating, at least in part, the increases in aldosterone secretion that occur in sodium deficiency, renal hypertension, and congestive heart failure.

Effects on the Kidney

Angiotensin II acts directly on the kidney to cause renal vasoconstriction, increase proximal tubular sodium reabsorption, and, as mentioned above, inhibit the secretion of renin. The effects of angiotensin II on renal hemodynamics and sodium reabsorption can be produced by very low doses of angiotensin II and probably represent physiologic actions of the renin-angiotensin system.

Effects on the Central Nervous System

In addition to its central effects on blood pressure, angiotensin II also acts on the central nervous system to stimulate drinking (dipsogenic effect) and increase the secretion of vasopressin and ACTH. The most impressive responses are seen when the peptide is injected into the cerebral ventricles; the responses to intravenous angiotensin II are much less impressive. Dipsogenic responses to angiotensin II are apparently mediated by 2 circumventricular organs, the subfornical organ (SFO) and the organum vasculosum of the lamina terminalis (OVLT). The relative importance of these 2 structures is not known at present. Proposed sites of action of angiotensin II on pituitary hormone secretion include the SFO for vasopressin and the median eminence and anterior pituitary for ACTH. The physiologic significance of the effects of angiotensin II on drinking and pituitary hormone secretion is not known.

ANGIOTENSIN RECEPTORS & MECHANISM OF ACTION

The presence of specific angiotensin II receptors has been demonstrated in a variety of tissues, including vascular smooth muscle, adrenal cortex, kidney, uterus, and brain. Like the receptors for other polypeptide hormones, angiotensin II receptors are located on the plasma membrane of target cells, and this permits rapid onset of the various actions of angiotensin II.

The structure-activity relationships of angiotensin II have been studied extensively. Most studies have been based on the pressor action of the peptide, but the results probably apply to all of the actions. The amino terminal (Fig 16–1) is not essential for activity, but it does influence receptor binding and duration of action. The amino acid at position 2 (arginine) also contributes to receptor affinity, but it does not influence the intrinsic activity of the peptide. The minimum structure of angiotensin II that has full intrinsic activity is the 3–8 hexapeptide. The aliphatic side chains in residues 3, 5, and 7 are necessary to stabilize the secondary structure of the molecule, while the aromatic side chains in residues 4, 6, and 8 are essential for binding to receptors. The phenyl ring in position 8 is essential for intrinsic activity.

The nature of the intracellular signal generated in response to the binding of angiotensin II to its receptors has not been definitely identified. Possible second messengers for angiotensin II include potassium, cyclic nucleotides, and calcium. Further investigation is required, but it appears likely that many of the actions of angiotensin II involve changes in intracellular calcium concentration.

METABOLISM OF ANGIOTENSIN II

Angiotensin II is removed rapidly from the circulation, with a half-life of 15–60 seconds. It is metabolized during passage through most vascular beds (a notable exception being the lung) by a variety of peptidases collectively referred to as angiotensinases. Most of the metabolites of angiotensin II are biologically inactive, but the initial product of aminopeptidase action—[des-Asp^1]angiotensin II—retains considerable biologic activity.

ANTAGONISTS OF THE RENIN-ANGIOTENSIN SYSTEM

A wide variety of agents are now available that block the formation or actions of angiotensin II. These include drugs that block renin secretion; those that block the enzymatic action of renin; those that block the conversion of angiotensin I to angiotensin II; and those that block angiotensin II receptors.

Drugs That Block Renin Secretion

A number of drugs that interfere with the sympathetic nervous system inhibit the secretion of renin. Examples are clonidine, propranolol, and methyldopa. Clonidine inhibits renin secretion by causing a centrally mediated reduction in renal neural activity, and it may also exert a direct intrarenal action. Propranolol and other β-adrenoceptor–blocking drugs act by blocking the intrarenal and extrarenal beta receptors involved in the neural control of renin secretion. The mechanism by which methyldopa inhibits renin secretion has not been established.

Renin Inhibitors

The action of renin can be blocked by pepstatin, a pentapeptide that also inhibits the action of other proteases such as pepsin and cathepsin D. The use of

pepstatin in vivo is restricted by its low solubility, but a more soluble form, N-acetylpepstatin, has been synthesized. Competitive inhibitors of renin based on the amino acid sequence around the cleavage site of angiotensinogen have been synthesized. The problem with most of these is low solubility. However, one of these peptides, Pro-His-Pro-Phe-His-Phe-Phe-Val-Tyr-Lys, is reasonably soluble and is an effective inhibitor of renin in vivo.

Converting Enzyme Inhibitors

A nonapeptide inhibitor of converting enzyme was originally isolated from the venom of the South American pit viper, *Bothrops jararaca*. The synthetic form of this peptide, (pyro)Glu-Trp-Pro-Arg-Pro-Gln-Ile-Pro-Pro, or **teprotide**, is a highly effective inhibitor of converting enzyme. However, its use is limited by the fact that it is active only when administered intravenously. A new class of converting enzyme inhibitors, directed against the active site of converting enzyme, is now available. One such inhibitor is D-3-mercapto-methylpropanoyl-L-proline, or **captopril** (Fig 16–2). Like teprotide, captopril inhibits the conversion of angiotensin I to angiotensin II in vivo; unlike teprotide, captopril is effective when administered orally. Captopril is now used clinically as an anti-hypertensive agent (see Chapter 10). A newer converting enzyme inhibitor is N-[(S)-l-(ethoxycarbonyl)-3-phenylprolyl]-L-alanyl-L-proline, or **enalapril** (see Fig 16–2). Like captopril, this inhibitor is orally active; unlike captopril, it is a non–sulfhydryl-containing agent. It should be noted that converting enzyme inhibitors not only block the conversion of angiotensin I to angiotensin II but also inhibit the degradation of bradykinin (see below). It is likely that this latter effect contributes significantly to the antihypertensive action of converting enzyme inhibitors.

Angiotensin Analogs

Substitution of aliphatic residues such as glycine, alanine, leucine, isoleucine, or threonine for the phenylalanine in position 8 of angiotensin II results in the formation of potent antagonists of the action of angiotensin II. Substitution of sarcosine (N-methylglycine) for the amino terminal aspartic acid prolongs the half-life of the peptides and thus enhances their potency. The best-known of these antagonists is [Sar^1,Val^5,-Ala^8]angiotensin-(1–8)octapeptide, or **saralasin**.

Asp-Arg-Val-Tyr-Ile-His-Pro-Phe

Angiotensin II

Sar-Arg-Val-Tyr-Val-His-Pro-Ala

Saralasin

Saralasin exhibits some agonist activity and may elicit pressor responses, particularly when circulating angiotensin II levels are low. This is true also of other angiotensin II antagonists, although some, eg, [Sar^1,-

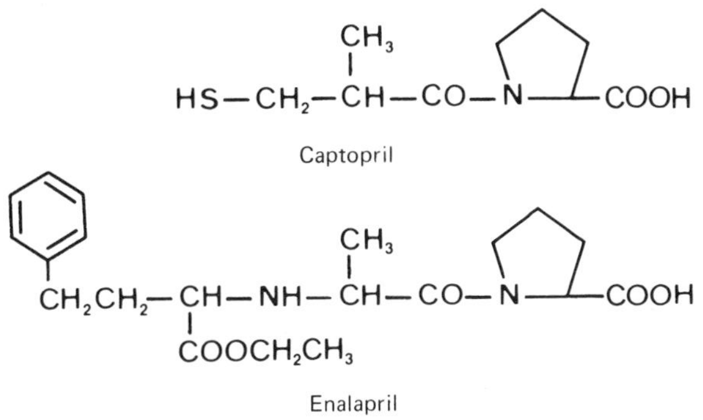

Figure 16–2. Two orally active converting enzyme inhibitors: captopril and enalapril. Enalapril is a pro-drug ethyl ester that is hydrolyzed in the body.

Thr[8]]angiotensin II, apparently have less agonist activity than saralasin. Saralasin and other angiotensin antagonists must be administered intravenously, and this severely restricts their use as antihypertensive agents. However, they have been used for the detection of renin-dependent hypertension and other hyperreninemic states. In general, angiotensin antagonists are less effective in lowering blood pressure than are converting enzyme inhibitors. This difference reflects both the agonist activity of angiotensin antagonists and the bradykinin-potentiating action of converting enzyme inhibitors.

Antibodies

Specific antibodies have been produced against renin, angiotensinogen, converting enzyme, angiotensin I, and angiotensin II. These are useful experimental tools but are not likely to have any clinical application.

KININS

BIOSYNTHESIS OF KININS

Kinins are a group of potent vasodilator peptides that are formed enzymatically by the action of enzymes known as kallikreins or kininogenases on protein substrates called kininogens. From the biochemical point of view, the kallikrein-kinin system has several features in common with the renin-angiotensin system.

Kallikreins

Kallikreins are present in plasma and in several tissues, including the kidneys, pancreas, intestine, sweat glands, and salivary glands. All kallikreins are serine proteases with active sites and catalytic properties very similar to those of enzymes such as trypsin, chymotrypsin, elastase, thrombin, plasmin, and other serine proteases. They are glycoproteins. Tissue kallikreins have molecular weights between 25,000 and

40,000; plasma kallikrein has a molecular weight of approximately 100,000.

Plasma kallikrein circulates in the blood as a precursor, prekallikrein, which is produced by the liver. Plasma kallikrein can be activated by trypsin, Hageman factor, and possibly kallikrein itself. Some glandular kallikreins exist as prekallikreins; others are present in active forms. In general, the biochemical properties of glandular kallikreins are quite different from those of plasma kallikreins. It has been shown that kallikreins can convert prorenin to active renin, but the physiologic significance of this action has not been established.

Kininogens

Kininogens—the precursors of kinins—are present in plasma, lymph, and interstitial fluid. At least 2 kininogens are present in plasma: a low-molecular-weight form (LMW kininogen) and a high-molecular-weight form (HMW kininogen). Both are acidic glycoproteins consisting of a single polypeptide chain. About 15–20% of the total plasma kininogen is in the high-molecular-weight form. It is thought that LMW kininogen crosses capillary walls and serves as the substrate for tissue kallikreins, while HMW kininogen is confined to the bloodstream and serves as the substrate for plasma kallikrein.

FORMATION OF KININS IN PLASMA & TISSUES

The pathway for the formation and metabolism of kinins is shown in Fig 16–3. Three kinins have been identified in mammals: bradykinin, lysylbradykinin (also known as kallidin), and methionyllysylbradykinin. They have the following structures:

Arg-Pro-Pro-Gly-Phe-Ser-Pro-Phe-Arg

1   2   3   4   5   6   7   8   9

Bradykinin

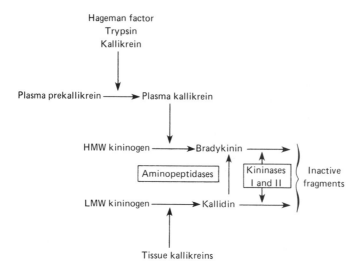

Figure 16–3. The kallikrein-kinin system. Kininase II is identical to converting enzyme peptidyl dipeptidase.

Lys-Arg-Pro-Pro-Gly-Phe-Ser-Pro-Phe-Arg

Lysylbradykinin (kallidin; Lys-bradykinin)

Met-Lys-Arg-Pro-Pro-Gly-Phe-Ser-Pro-Phe-Arg

Methionyllysylbradykinin (Met-Lys-bradykinin)

Note that each kinin contains bradykinin in its structure. Each kinin is formed from a kininogen by the action of a different enzyme. Bradykinin is released by plasma kallikrein, lysylbradykinin by glandular kallikrein, and methionyllysylbradykinin by pepsin and pepsinlike enzymes. The preferred substrate for plasma kallikrein is HMW kininogen, and the preferred substrate for tissue kallikrein is LMW kininogen. Some lysylbradykinin is converted to bradykinin by an aminopeptidase. The 3 kinins have been found in plasma, but bradykinin is the predominant type. All 3 kinins are also present in urine. Lysylbradykinin is the major urinary kinin and is probably formed by the action of renal kallikrein. Bradykinin is generated from lysylbradykinin by a renal aminopeptidase. Methionyllysylbradykinin occurs in acidified urine: acid activates uropepsinogen, which then catalyzes the release of methionyllysylbradykinin from urinary kininogens.

ACTIONS OF KININS

Effects on the Cardiovascular System

Kinins produce marked vasodilatation in several vascular beds, including the heart, kidney, intestine, skeletal muscle, and liver. In this respect, kinins are approximately 10 times more potent than histamine. The vasodilatation may result from a direct inhibitory effect of kinins on arteriolar smooth muscle or may be mediated by the release of vasodilator prostaglandins such as PGE_2 and PGI_2. In contrast, the predominant effect of kinins on veins is contraction; again, this may result from direct stimulation of venous smooth muscle or from the release of venoconstrictor prostaglandins such as $PGF_{2\alpha}$. Kinins also produce contraction of most visceral smooth muscle.

When injected intravenously, kinins produce a rapid fall in blood pressure that is due to the vasodilator action of the peptides. The hypotensive response to bradykinin is of very brief duration. Intravenous infusions of the peptide fail to produce a sustained decrease in blood pressure; prolonged hypotension can only be produced by progressively increasing the rate of infusion. The rapid reversibility of the hypotensive response to kinins is due primarily to reflex increases in heart rate, cardiac output, and myocardial contractility. In some species, bradykinin actually produces a biphasic change in blood pressure—an initial hypotensive response followed by an increase above the preinjection level. The increase in blood pressure appears to be due to a reflex activation of the sympathetic nervous system, although it is worth noting that under some conditions, bradykinin can release catecholamines from the adrenal medulla and stimulate sympathetic ganglia. Bradykinin also increases blood pressure when injected into the central nervous system, but the significance of this effect is not clear, since it is unlikely that kinins cross the blood-brain barrier. Kinins have no consistent effect on sympathetic or parasympathetic nerve endings.

The arteriolar dilatation produced by kinins causes an increase in pressure and flow in the capillary bed, thus favoring efflux of fluid from blood to tissues. This effect may be facilitated by increased capillary permeability resulting from contraction of endothelial cells and widening of intercellular junctions and by increased venous pressure secondary to constriction of veins. As a result of these changes, water and solutes pass from the blood to the extracellular fluid, lymph flow increases, and edema may result.

Effects on Endocrine & Exocrine Glands

As noted earlier, prekallikreins and kallikreins are present in several glands, including the pancreas, kidney, intestine, salivary glands, and sweat glands, and can be released into the secretory fluids of these glands. The function of the enzymes in these tissues is not known. The enzymes (or active kinins) may diffuse from the organs to the blood and act as local modulators of blood flow. Since kinins have such marked effects on smooth muscle, they may also modulate the tone of salivary and pancreatic ducts and help to regulate gastrointestinal motility. Kinins also influence the transepithelial transport of water, electrolytes, glucose, and amino acids and may regulate the transport of these substances in the gastrointestinal tract and kidney. Finally, kallikreins may play a role in the physiologic activation of various prohormones, including proinsulin and prorenin.

Role in Inflammation

There is circumstantial evidence that kinins participate in the inflammatory process. Kallikreins and kinins can produce the basic symptoms of inflammation in animals, and the production of kinins is increased in inflammatory lesions produced by a variety of methods. Nevertheless, the extent to which kinins are involved in the inflammatory process remains to be determined.

Effects on Sensory Nerves

The kinins are potent activators of sensory pain endings in the skin and the viscera.

KININ RECEPTORS & MECHANISMS OF ACTION

The biologic actions of kinins are thought to be mediated by specific receptors located on the membranes of the target tissues. There appear to be at least 2 types of receptors for bradykinin and the other kinins: B_1 receptors (eg, rabbit aorta) and B_2 receptors (eg, cat ileum and rat uterus). (Note that B stands for bradykinin, not for beta-adrenoceptor.) Bioassay studies of B_1-receptor systems indicate that Lys-bradykinin and Met-Lys-bradykinin are approximately 10 and 76 times more potent than bradykinin, respectively. The octapeptide [des-Arg^9]bradykinin is 10 times more potent while the heptapeptide [des-Phe^8-des-Arg^9]bradykinin is inactive. Structure-activity studies have resulted in the discovery of specific, competitive inhibitors of the effects of kinins on B_1 receptors. An example of such an antagonist is [Leu^8-des-Arg^9]bradykinin. Bradykinin displays the highest affinity in most B_2-receptor systems, followed by Lys-bradykinin and then by Met-Lys-bradykinin. One exception is the B_2 receptor that mediates contraction of venous smooth muscle; this appears to be most sensi-

tive to Lys-bradykinin. Pharmacologic inhibitors of the action of kinins on B_2 receptors are not yet available.

The mechanisms by which kinins produce their various effects are not well understood. As noted above, some of the actions may be mediated by generation of prostaglandins. Other responses may involve changes in the intracellular concentrations of calcium or cyclic nucleotides.

METABOLISM OF KININS

Kinins are metabolized rapidly (half-life less than 15 seconds) by nonspecific exo- or endopeptidases, commonly referred to as kininases. Two plasma kininases have been well characterized. **Kininase I**, apparently synthesized in the liver, is a carboxypeptidase that releases the carboxyl terminal arginine residue. It is a metalloprotease and is inhibited by edetate and *o*-phenanthroline. **Kininase II** is present in plasma and vascular endothelial cells throughout the body. It is identical to angiotensin-converting enzyme (peptidyl dipeptidase), discussed above. Kininase II inactivates kinins by cleaving the carboxyl terminal dipeptide phenylalanyl-arginine. Like angiotensin I, bradykinin is almost completely hydrolyzed during a single passage through the pulmonary vascular bed.

DRUGS AFFECTING THE KALLIKREIN-KININ SYSTEM

Relatively few drugs are available to modify the activity of the kallikrein-kinin system. Kinin synthesis can be inhibited with the kallikrein inhibitor **aprotinin (Trasylol)**. Competitive antagonists of the B_1-receptor subtype have been synthesized (see above), but inhibitors of B_2 receptors are not yet available. The actions of kinins mediated by prostaglandin generation can be blocked nonspecifically by inhibitors of prostaglandin synthesis. Finally, the actions of kinins can be enhanced by agents that block the degradation of these peptides. Examples of such agents are teprotide and captopril, which inhibit kininase II (angiotensin-converting enzyme). However, it is difficult to determine if the effects of these agents result from accumulation of kinins or from reduced angiotensin II formation.

VASOPRESSIN

Vasopressin (antidiuretic hormone, ADH) plays an important role in the long-term control of blood pressure through its action on the kidney to increase water reabsorption. This and other aspects of the physiology of vasopressin are discussed in Chapters 14 and 36 and will not be reviewed here.

There is now considerable evidence that vasopressin also plays an important role in the short-term regulation of arterial pressure by its vasoconstrictor action. The peptide increases total peripheral resistance when infused in doses less than those required to produce maximum urine concentration. Such doses do not normally increase arterial pressure, because the vasopressor activity of the peptide is effectively buffered by a reflex decrease in cardiac output. When the influence of this reflex is removed, pressor sensitivity to vasopressin is greatly increased. Pressor sensitivity to vasopressin is also enhanced in patients with idiopathic orthostatic hypotension. Higher doses of vasopressin increase blood pressure even when baroreceptor reflexes are intact. These doses are generally higher than those required to produce maximum urine concentration; however, pressor responses can be elicited when plasma vasopressin concentration is increased to levels reached during nonhypotensive hemorrhage.

ANALOGS OF VASOPRESSIN

Since the molecular structures of vasopressin and oxytocin were first determined, many analogs of these neurohypophyseal peptides have been synthesized. Structure-activity studies have shown that the vascular receptors for vasopressin differ markedly from the renal receptors that mediate antidiuretic responses. Using this information, it has been possible to synthesize peptides with selective pressor or antidiuretic activity. The most specific vasopressor peptide synthesized to date is [Phe^2,Ile^3,Orn^8]vasotocin. Selective antidiuretic analogs include 1-deamino[D-Arg^8]arginine vasopressin (dDAVP) and 1-deamino[Val^4,D-Arg^8]-arginine vasopressin (dVDAVP). Information on structure-activity relations has also made it possible to identify the molecular features required for binding to tissue receptors and for receptor activation. This has permitted the design of specific antagonists of the vasoconstrictor action of vasopressin. One of the most potent antagonists synthesized to date has the following structure: [1-(β-mercapto-β,β-cyclopentamethylenepropionicacid), 2-(O-methyl)tyrosine]arginine vasopressin. This compound also has antioxytocic activity but does not antagonize the antidiuretic action of vasopressin. It does not interfere with the actions of other pressor agents such as angiotensin and norepinephrine.

These vasopressor antagonists have been particularly useful for investigating the role of endogenous vasopressin in cardiovascular regulation. The antagonists have no cardiovascular effects when administered to animals in which circulating vasopressin levels are within or below the normal range. However, when they are administered to water-deprived rats or dogs in which circulating vasopressin levels are elevated, prompt decreases in arterial pressure or total peripheral resistance occur. Vasopressin blockade also decreases blood pressure in adrenal-insufficient animals and markedly impairs blood pressure regulation during hemorrhage. Taken together, these and other

observations demonstrate that, through its vasoconstrictor action, vasopressin plays an important role in cardiovascular regulation.

There is also some evidence that vasopressin plays a role in experimental hypertension in animals and may be involved in certain forms of human hypertension. Vasopressin antagonists of the type described above will be of value in the investigation of this important question.

ATRIAL NATRIURETIC PEPTIDE

The atria of mammals contain one or more peptides with potent natriuretic activity, variously referred to as atrial natriuretic peptides (ANP), cardionatrins, atriopeptins, and auriculins. They are apparently derived from the C-terminal end of a larger precursor molecule which, in the rat, is a 152-amino-acid peptide. The structure of human atrial natriuretic peptide is shown below. ANP has been measured in plasma, but little is known of the factors that regulate the biosynthesis and release of the peptides.

Ser-Leu-Arg-Arg-Ser-Ser-Cys-Phe-Gly-Gly-Arg-Met-
Asp-Arg-Ile-Gly-Ala-Gln-Ser-Gly-Leu-Gly-Cys-Asn-
Ser-Phe-Arg-Tyr

Human atrial natriuretic peptide

Administration of ANP produces prompt and marked increases in sodium and potassium excretion and urine flow. Glomerular filtration rate increases, with little or no change in renal blood flow, so that the filtration fraction increases. The ANP-induced natriuresis is largely due to the increase in glomerular filtration rate, but a direct inhibitory effect on tubular sodium reabsorption is also likely. ANP also inhibits the secretion of renin and aldosterone, and these substances may represent additional mechanisms by which the peptide increases sodium excretion. Finally, ANP decreases arterial blood pressure. The mechanism of this effect is not well understood, but antagonism of the vasoconstrictor action of angiotensin II and other vasoconstrictors may be involved.

It is clear that ANP may have important effects on the regulation of fluid and electrolyte balance and blood pressure. Nevertheless, additional investigation is required to determine the physiologic and pathologic significance of this newly discovered peptide.

VASOACTIVE INTESTINAL PEPTIDE

Vasoactive intestinal peptide (VIP) is a 28-amino-acid peptide closely related structurally to secretin and glucagon. Its structure is shown below.

His-Ser-Asp-Ala-Val-Phe-Thr-Asp-Asn-Tyr-Thr-Arg-
Leu-Arg-Lys-Gln-Met-Ala-Val-Lys-Lys-Tyr-Leu-Asn-
Ser-Ile-Leu-Asn-NH$_2$

Vasoactive intestinal peptide (VIP)

VIP was originally extracted from porcine lung and was subsequently purified from porcine duodenum. It is now known that VIP is widely distributed in the central and peripheral nervous systems of humans and several animal species. It is also present in the circulation, but most evidence suggests that VIP functions as a neurotransmitter or neuromodulator rather than as a classic hormone.

VIP produces marked vasodilatation in most vascular beds, including peripheral systemic vessels, as well as the splanchnic, pulmonary, coronary, renal, and cerebral vessels. The vasodilator action of VIP is independent of norepinephrine, acetylcholine, serotonin, and histamine receptors and apparently results from a direct action of the peptide on vascular smooth muscle. As a result of this action, arterial pressure falls and cardiac output increases. The mechanism of the vasodilator action of VIP is not fully understood. However, it has been suggested that VIP binds to specific receptors in the blood vessels and stimulates cAMP production. This effect could be produced by VIP released from the VIP-containing nerve fibers that are associated with blood vessels or by VIP in the circulation.

In addition to dilating blood vessels, VIP relaxes tracheobronchial and gastrointestinal smooth muscle, stimulates intestinal water and electrolyte secretion, promotes hepatic glycogenolysis, causes neuronal excitation, and stimulates the release of several hormones including growth hormone, prolactin, and renin. The physiologic significance of these actions remains to be defined.

SUBSTANCE P

Substance P is an undecapeptide with the following structure:

Arg-Pro-Lys-Pro-Gln-Gln-Phe-Phe-Gly-Leu-Met

Substance P

It is present in the central nervous system, where it is thought to function as a neurotransmitter; and in the gastrointestinal tract, where it may play a role as a local hormone.

Substance P is a potent vasodilator and produces a marked hypotensive action in humans and in several animal species. The vasodilatation apparently results from a direct inhibitory effect of the peptide on arteriolar smooth muscle. This action is mediated via specific receptors that differ from those mediating the actions of other vasodilators. In contrast to its effects on arteriolar smooth muscle, substance P stimulates contraction of venous, intestinal, and bronchial smooth muscle. It also causes secretion in the salivary glands, diuresis and natriuresis in the kidneys, and a variety of effects in the central and peripheral nervous systems.

The N-terminal region of substance P is not essential for activity, and several C-terminal fragments of the peptide, including the octa (4–11), hepta (5–11), and hexa (6–11) fragments, are also active. Indeed, depending on the preparation being studied, these peptides may be as potent as the intact undecapeptide or even more so. Analogs of substance P that are antagonists in vivo and in vitro have been synthesized.

NEUROTENSIN

Neurotensin is a tridecapeptide that was first isolated from the central nervous system but subsequently was found to be present in the gastrointestinal tract and in the circulation. It has the following structure:

Glu-Leu-Tyr-Glu-Asn-Lys-Pro-Arg-Arg-Pro-Tyr-Ile-
Leu

Neurotensin

When administered into the peripheral circulation, neurotensin produces a variety of effects, including vasodilatation, hypotension, increased vascular permeability, increased secretion of several anterior pituitary hormones, hyperglycemia, inhibition of gastric acid and pepsin secretion, and inhibition of gastric motility. Following administration into the cerebrospinal fluid, it produces hypothermia and analgesia. Structure-activity studies indicate that the 5–6 amino acid residues at the carboxyl terminal of the molecule are required for biologic activity. At present, the physiologic significance of the actions of neurotensin is not known.

REFERENCES

General

Iverson LL: Nonopioid neuropeptides in mammalian CNS. *Annu Rev Pharmacol Toxicol* 1983;**23**:1.

Angiotensin

Fitzsimons JT: Angiotensin stimulation of the central nervous system. *Rev Physiol Biochem Pharmacol* 1980;**87**:117.

Ganten D, Hackenthal E, Vecsei P (editors): Renin-angiotensin-aldosterone system and hypertension. (Symposium.) *Klin Wochenschr* 1978;**56(Suppl 1)**. [Entire issue.]

Genest J, Koiw E, Kuchel O (editors): *Hypertension: Physiopathology and Treatment.* McGraw-Hill, 1977.

Haber E: Specific inhibitors of renin. *Clin Sci* 1980;**59(Suppl 6):**7s.

Horovitz ZP (editor): *Angiotensin Converting Enzyme Inhibitors.* Urban & Schwarzenberg, 1981.

Johnson JA, Anderson RR: *The Renin-Angiotensin System.* Plenum Press, 1980.

Keeton TK, Campbell WB: The pharmacologic alteration of renin release. *Pharmacol Rev* 1980;**32:**81.

Laragh JH, Bühler FR, Seldin DW (editors): *Frontiers in Hypertension Research.* Springer-Verlag, 1981.

Page IH, Bumpus FM (editors): *Angiotensin.* Springer-Verlag, 1974.

Patchett AA et al: A new class of angiotensin-converting enzyme inhibitors. *Nature* 1980;**288:**280.

Peach MJ: Renin-angiotensin system: Biochemistry and mechanisms of action. *Physiol Rev* 1977;**57:**313.

Reid IA: Actions of angiotensin II on the brain: Mechanisms and physiologic role. *Am J Physiol* 1984;**246:**F533.

Reid IA, Morris BJ, Ganong WF: The renin-angiotensin system. *Annu Rev Physiol* 1978;**40:**377.

Soffer RL (editor): *Biochemical Regulation of Blood Pressure.* Wiley, 1981.

Stokes GS, Edwards KDG (editors): *Drugs Affecting the Renin-Angiotensin-Aldosterone System: Use of Angiotensin Inhibitors.* Vol 12 of: *Progress in Biochemical Pharmacology.* Karger, 1976.

Sweet CS: Pharmacological properties of the converting enzyme inhibitor enalapril maleate (MK-421). *Fed Proc* 1983;**42:**167.

Symposium: Biochemistry of the renin-angiotensin system. *Fed Proc* 1983;**42:**2722.

Zimmerman BG: Adrenergic facilitation by angiotensin: Does it serve a physiological function? *Clin Sci* 1981;**60:**343. [Editorial review.]

Kinins

Regoli D, Barabé J: Pharmacology of bradykinin and related kinins. *Pharmacol Rev* 1980;**32:**1.

Schachter M: Kallikreins (kininogenases): A group of serine proteases with bioregulatory actions. *Pharmacol Rev* 1980;**31:**1.

Vasopressin

Möhring J et al: Greatly enhanced pressor response to antidiuretic hormone in patients with impaired cardiovascular reflexes due to idiopathic orthostatic hypotension. *J Cardiovasc Pharmacol* 1980;**2:**367.

Montani J-P et al: Hemodynamic effects of exogenous and endogenous vasopressin at low plasma concentrations in conscious dogs. *Circ Res* 1980;**47:**346.

Reid IA, Schwartz J: Role of vasopressin in the control of blood pressure. Chap 5, pp 177–197, in: *Frontiers in Neuroendocrinology,* Vol 8. Martini L, Ganong WF (editors). Raven Press, 1984.

Sawyer WH, Grzonka Z, Manning M: Neurohypophysial peptides: Design of tissue-specific agonists and antagonists. *Mol Cell Endocrinol* 1981;**22:**117. [Review article.]

Vasopressin and cardiovascular regulation. (Symposium.) *Fed Proc* 1984;**43:**78.

Atrial Natriuretic Peptide

Cantin M, Genest J: The heart and the atrial natriuretic factor. *Endocr Rev* 1985;**6:**107.

Maack T et al: Atrial natriuretic factor: Structure and functional properties. *Kidney Int* 1985;**27:**607. [Editorial review.]

Needleman P et al: Atriopeptins as cardiac hormones. *Hypertension* 1985;**7:**469.

Vasoactive Intestinal Peptide

Said SI (editor): *Vasoactive Intestinal Peptide.* Raven Press, 1982.

Substance P

Caranikas S et al: Antagonists of substance P. *Eur J Pharmacol* 1982;**77:**205.

Couture R, Regoli D: Smooth muscle pharmacology of substance P. *Pharmacology* 1982;**24:**1.

Neurotensin

Nemeroff CB, Prange AJ (editors): Neurotensin: A brain and gastrointestinal peptide. *Ann NY Acad Sci* 1982;**400:**1. [Entire issue.]

Prostaglandins & Other Eicosanoids

17

Marc E. Goldyne, MD, PhD

Prostaglandins are endogenously generated fatty acid derivatives with profound physiologic effects. Their biosynthesis has been demonstrated in every major organ of the human body, albeit to varying degrees. In addition to the prostaglandins, recent research has revealed the existence of other biologically active lipids and peptidolipids, biosynthesized from the same precursors as the prostaglandins through interrelated enzymatic pathways. These other lipids include the **thromboxanes, hydroperoxyeicosatetraenoic acids (HPETEs)** and **hydroxyeicosatetraenoic acids (HETEs)**, and the **leukotrienes.** The expansion in the number of these interrelated compounds has led to the introduction of the all-inclusive term "eicosanoids," since they all derive from the same eicosaenoic (*eicosa* = 20-carbon; *enoic* = containing double bonds) acid precursors.

In the 1930s, 3 laboratories independently described a uterine smooth muscle–contracting activity deriving from semen. Von Euler named this active principle **prostaglandin** because of its assumed origin from the prostate gland. In the 1960s, Bergstrom et al showed that prostaglandin activity derived from several related compounds and named the first 2 prostaglandins E and F (PGE and PGF) because of their respective solvent partitioning into *e*ther and phosphate buffer (*f*osfat in Swedish). Today, 9 prostaglandin groups are recognized.

In 1975, Hamberg et al described substances released by aggregating platelets (thrombocytes) that derived from the same precursors as the prostaglandins but differed in that they contained an oxane ring; thus the name **thromboxane** was coined. At the same time, Hamberg et al described another series of products synthesized from the prostaglandin precursor arachidonic acid. These substances lacked a cyclic structure and contained a hydroperoxy or hydroxyl substitution on the eicosatetraenoic(arachidonic) acid backbone and were accordingly labeled **hydroperoxyeicosatetraenoic acids (HPETEs)** and **hydroxyeicosatetraenoic acids (HETEs).**

In 1978, Parker et al demonstrated that the smooth muscle–contracting principle called **slow-reacting substance of anaphylaxis (SRS-A)** was a derivative of the prostaglandin precursor arachidonic acid. Subsequently, Borgeat et al isolated arachidonic acid derivatives from rabbit leukocytes that contained a

conjugated triene bonding—hence the name **leukotrienes.** Subsequent work showed that SRS-A was in fact a combination of 2 of these leukotrienes.

Synthesis of Eicosanoids

Endogenously generated eicosanoids are synthesized by a series of membrane-bound or cytosolic enzymes (Fig 17–1). The appropriate stimulus may vary, depending on the cell type. In response to this stimulus, phospholipase A_2 or a combination of phospholipase C and diglyceride lipase catalyzes the cleavage of an esterified eicosanoid precursor, such as arachidonic acid, from the 2 position of specific glycerophospholipids that constitute part of the lipid bilayer of the cell membrane. Once free, the arachidonic acid can activate several enzyme systems that are variably distributed among different cells. One enzyme, cyclooxygenase, converts arachidonic acid to unstable endoperoxide intermediates (PGG_2 and PGH_2). These can then be further metabolized through appropriate enzymatic activity to either the prostaglandins (PGD_2 through $PGF_{2\alpha}$, and PGI_2, also called prostacyclin) or to the thromboxanes. The E prostaglandins can be further metabolized to the B prostaglandins in vivo or to the A or B prostaglandins in vitro. Another group of enzymes collectively called lipoxygenases convert arachidonic acid to a series of HPETEs, which are then further metabolized to either a series of corresponding HETEs or to the leukotrienes.

The variety of prostaglandins or related lipids synthesized is cell type–specific. For example, epidermal cells produce D, E, and F group prostaglandins and 12-HETE but not thromboxanes. Vascular endothelium synthesizes primarily prostacyclin (PGI_2), although this may vary according to the anatomic origin of the vessel. Platelets, on the other hand, synthesize primarily thromboxane A_2.

Inhibition of Eicosanoid Synthesis

Corticosteroids block all of the known pathways of eicosanoid metabolism by stimulating the synthesis of a protein called lipocortin, which in turn inhibits the activity of phospholipases, thus preventing the initial release of arachidonic acid required to activate the subsequent enzymatic pathways. The nonsteroidal anti-inflammatory drugs (eg, aspirin, indomethacin, ibuprofen) block both prostaglandin and thromboxane

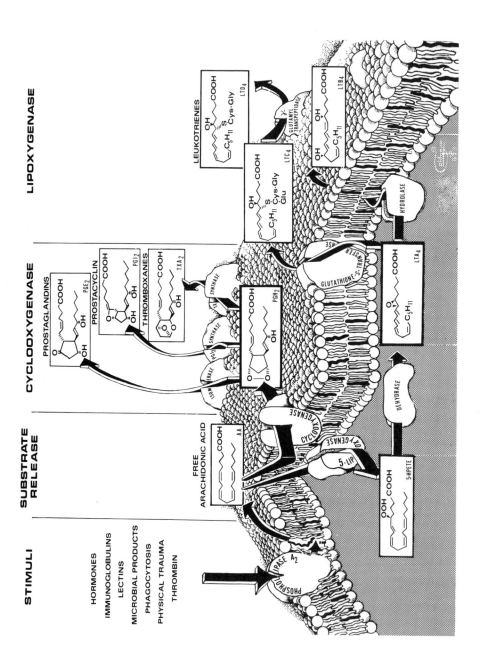

Figure 17–1. Biosynthesis of eicosanoids. The biosynthesis of prostaglandins and related lipids occurs for the most part at the cell membrane. However, the 5-lipoxygenase that catalyzes the generation of leukotrienes and 5-HETE appears to be a cytosolic enzyme. In response to an appropriate stimulus, a phospholipase is activated that cleaves arachidonic acid (a precursor of prostaglandins) from the phospholipids making up the lipid bilayer of the cell membranes. The stimuli that activate the phospholipases are often tissue- or cell-specific. The free arachidonic acid can activate several enzyme systems, depending on the enzymatic endowment of the cell(s) in question. One enzyme, cyclooxygenase, converts arachiodonic acid into an unstable endoperoxide intermediate that can be further converted, through appropriate enzymatic activity, to prostaglandins (including prostacyclin or epoprostenol) and thromboxanes. Another group of enzymes, the lipoxygenases, convert arachidonic acid to a series of hydroxy fatty acids (ie, HPETEs and HETEs) or, in conjunction with other enzymes, to the recently identified leukotrienes.

synthesis by inhibiting cyclooxygenase activity. Aspirin specifically acetylates the enzyme, whereas the exact mechanism of inhibition by the other agents is not fully understood.

Considerable effort has been made to discover selective inhibitors of thromboxane synthesis. Dazoxiben and 9,11-azoprosta-5,13-dienoic acid are investigational inhibitors of thromboxane A_2 (TXA_2) synthase. 9,11-Epoxyimino-5,13-dienoic acid is claimed to be a selective antagonist at TXA_2 receptors.

Selective inhibitors of the lipoxygenase pathway are investigational only at present. With few exceptions, the nonsteroidal anti-inflammatory drugs do not inhibit the lipoxygenase enzymes at concentrations that markedly inhibit cyclooxygenase. In fact, by blocking utilization of the eicosanoid substrates by cyclooxygenase, they may cause an increased substrate utilization through the lipoxygenase pathways leading to increased production of (for example) the smooth muscle–stimulating leukotrienes. Even among the cyclooxygenase-dependent pathways, the inhibition of synthesis of one derivative may lead to a compensatory increase in the synthesis of an enzymatically interrelated product. For example, the specific inhibition of TXB_2 synthesis by the experimental agent 9,11-azoprosta-5,13-dienoic acid leads to a compensatory increase in PGE_2 synthesis due, probably, to backing up of the shared endoperoxide intermediate $PGG(H)_2$ (Fig 17–2).

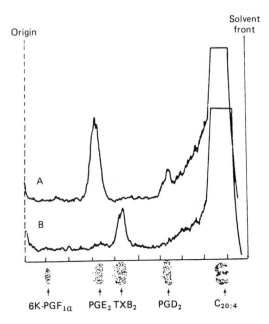

Figure 17–2. *A:* Specifically inhibiting the synthesis of TXB_2 with 9,11-azoprosta-5,13-dienoic acid (15 $\mu mol/L$) leads to increased synthesis of PGE_2. *B:* TXB_2 is the major cyclooxygenase product of these human monocytes in the absence of the inhibitor. (Reproduced, with permission, from Kennedy MS, Stobo JD, Goldyne ME: In vitro synthesis of prostaglandins and related lipids by populations of human peripheral blood mononuclear cells. *Prostaglandins* 1980;20:135.)

I. BASIC PHARMACOLOGY OF PROSTAGLANDINS & OTHER EICOSANOIDS

Chemistry of Prostaglandins

The basic structure common to all prostaglandins, referred to as "prostanoic acid," consists of a cyclopentane ring with 2 aliphatic side chains (Fig 17–3).

A. Prostaglandin Groups: There are 9 groups of prostaglandins that, with the exception of the initially discovered E and F groups, are arbitrarily assigned the letter designations A–I. They differ from each other in having substitutions at carbons 9 and 11. The 2 epimers of the F group are designated PGF_α and PGF_β. PGG and PGH are, as mentioned above, short-lived endoperoxide intermediates in the formation of all of the other prostaglandins. With the exception of PGG, which has a hydroperoxy substitution at carbon 15, all of the remaining prostaglandins possess a hydroxyl group at this position. In addition, all prostaglandins have a Δ^{13} double bond. The substitutions on the pentane ring appear responsible for the qualitative activities of the different groups, whereas the Δ^{13} bonding and carbon 15 hydroxyl group are required for full activity.

B. Prostaglandin Series: Each prostaglandin group except PGI can be classified in one of 3 series, designated by a subscript 1, 2, or 3 following the group designation. This subscript indicates the total number of double bonds in the 2 side chains of the prostaglandin molecule and reflects the fact that prostaglandins can be synthesized from 3 different eicosaenoic acids, which themselves differ in the total number of double bonds present. The 1 series derives from 8,11,14-eicosatrienoic acid (dihomo-γ-linolenic acid), the 2 series from 5,8,11,14-eicosatetraenoic acid, and the 3 series from 5,8,11,14,17-eicosapentaenoic acid. In humans, it appears that the 2 series is the most abundant. PGI exists only in the 2 and 3 series, since it requires the Δ^5 double bond for its synthesis.

Chemistry of Thromboxanes

The structure common to all thromboxanes is the presence of an oxane ring with the same 2 aliphatic side chains common to prostaglandins (Fig 17–1).

A. Thromboxane Groups: Two groups are recognized, designated TXA and TXB. TXA is a highly unstable oxane:oxetane compound with an aqueous half-life of 45 seconds. TXB is the stable spontaneous hydration derivative of TXA.

B. Thromboxane Series: Thromboxanes can also exist in any one of 3 series designated by a subscript 1, 2, or 3, depending, as with the prostaglandins, on the fatty acid precursor.

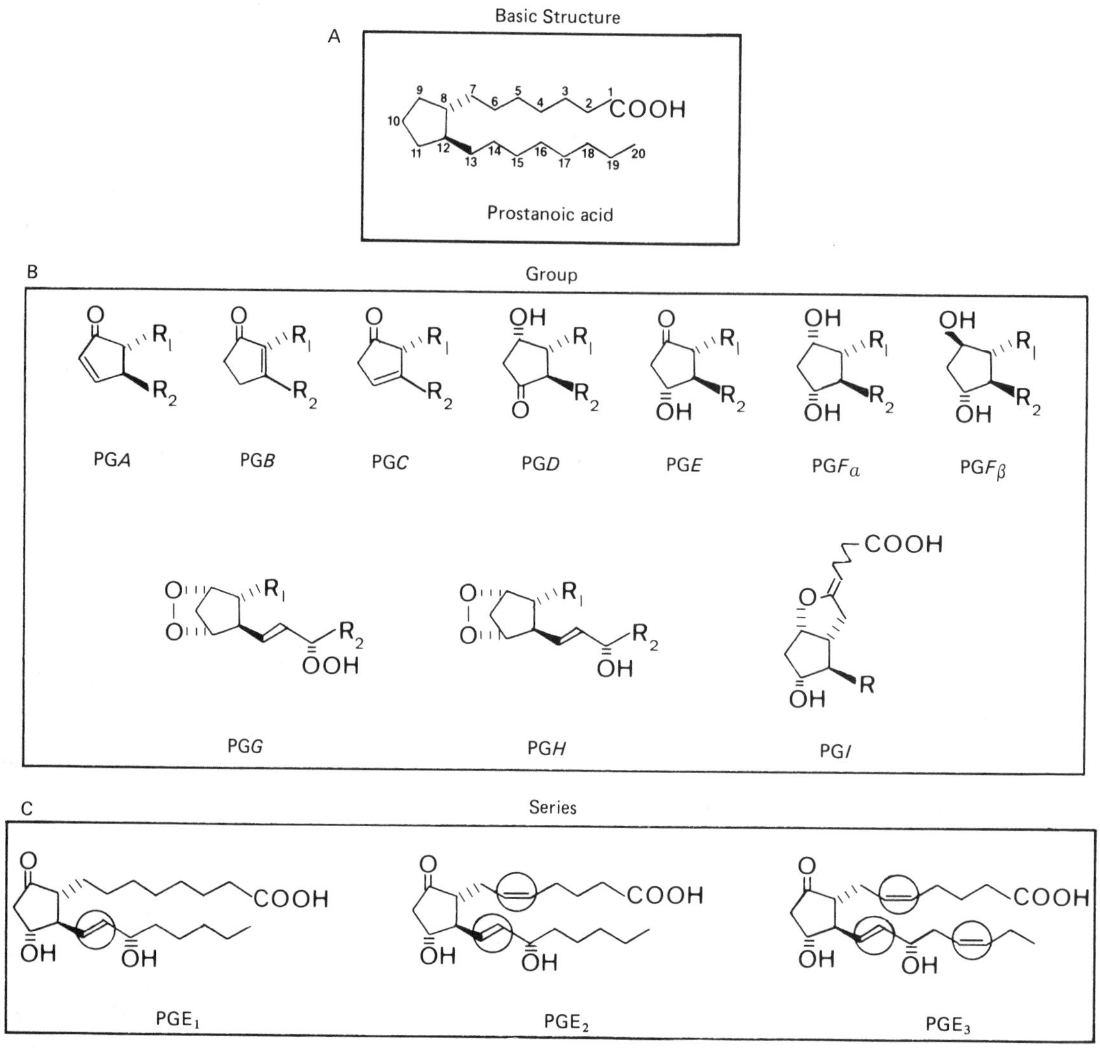

Figure 17–3. Prostaglandin groups and series. *A:* "Prostanoic acid" is the name given to the molecular skeleton common to all prostaglandins. *B:* Prostaglandin groups differ according to the substitutions on the carbon 9 and carbon 11 positions of the pentane ring and, in the case of PGG_2, on carbon 15. *C:* Prostaglandin series differ in the total number of double bonds (circled) in the side chains. Each series derives from a different unsaturated fatty acid precursor (see text). In humans, the 2 series appears to be the most abundant.

Chemistry of HPETEs & HETEs

The HPETEs derive from a different enzymatic pathway than the prostaglandins and thomboxanes and are not cyclic compounds (Fig 17–1). Their structure consists of the parent fatty acid with a hydroperoxy substituent. The position of this group is designated by a numerical prefix indicating the carbon position of the substitution (eg, 12-HPETE). The HPETEs are relatively unstable and are reduced enzymatically or nonenzymatically to the corresponding HETEs (eg, 12-HPETE → 12-HETE).

Chemistry of Leukotrienes

A. Leukotriene Groups: Five groups of leukotrienes have currently been identified, designated LTA

through LTE (Fig 17–4). LTA is an unstable epoxide intermediate that interacts with glutathione-S-transferase to produce LTC, which contains a carbon 5 hydroxyl group and a carbon 6 glutathione linked via the sulfur in the cysteinyl residue as a thioether. LTD results from the enzymatic removal of glutamic acid from glutathione. LTE is produced by the enzymatic removal of glycine from the LTD molecule. LTB is a dihydroxy derivative of 5-HPETE.

B. Leukotriene Series: As is the case with prostaglandins, there are 3 series of leukotrienes; they are designated by a subscript 3, 4, or 5 since, unlike the other eicosanoids, all of the double bonds in the parent trienoic, tetraenoic, and pentaenoic acids are retained.

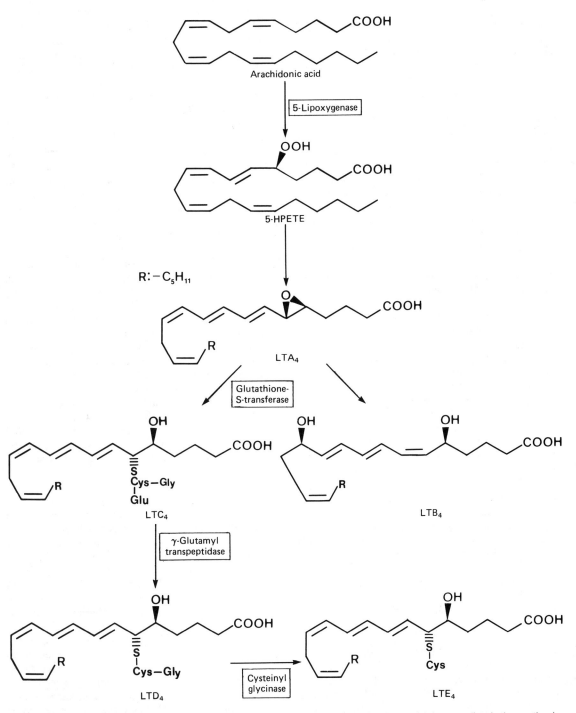

Figure 17–4. The leukotrienes synthesized from arachidonic acid. LTA_4 is an unstable epoxide intermediate in the synthesis of the remaining leukotrienes. LTC_4 and LTD_4 are the major molecules that constitute the **slow-reacting substance of anaphylaxis (SRS-A)**. LTE_4 is a less active metabolite of LTD_4. LTB_4 is a potent chemotactic substance for neutrophils and eosinophils.

Chemistry of Novel Eicosanoids

Recent research has uncovered yet another group of structurally unique metabolites of arachidonic acid generated by human leukocytes from 15-HPETE. They are trihydroxytetraenes and have been given the name lipoxins. The lipoxins retain 4 conjugated double bonds. Little is currently known about their endogenous synthesis and function.

Pharmacokinetics of Prostaglandins

The naturally occurring prostaglandins are rapidly degraded following their introduction into the systemic circulation. Whether endogenously generated or intravenously administered, PGE_2, for example, is quickly inactivated by the pulmonary, hepatic, and renal vascular beds. Such inactivation involves enzymatic oxidation of the carbon 15 hydroxyl group to a ketone (15-hydroxy prostaglandin dehydrogenase) and a reductive saturation of the Δ^{13} double bond (Δ^{13} prostaglandin reductase). In addition, there is beta and omega oxidation of the aliphatic side chains. Human studies on PGE_1 show that roughly 90% of the prostaglandin metabolites are excreted in the urine and 10% in the feces. Intravenous administration of labeled PGE_2 or $PGF_{2\alpha}$ in humans leads to rapid formation of the corresponding 15-keto-13,14-dihydro metabolites. Within 2 minutes, less than 3% of the initially administered compound remains in the blood; 40% is recovered as inactive metabolites. Within the blood, the half-life of most prostaglandins is less than 1 minute and of the metabolites about 8 minutes. Many tissues contain the enzymes necessary for prostaglandin degradation.

Pharmacokinetics of Thromboxanes

The biologically active TXA_2 is rapidly and spontaneously hydrated in the blood to TXB_2. Although the half-life of TXA_2 can be prolonged by the presence of albumin, this does not occur to a degree that would render the natural compound usable as a therapeutic agent. As with prostaglandins, thromboxane metabolites are excreted in the urine, and over 20 such metabolites have been described.

Pharmacokinetics of HPETEs & HETEs

Little is known about the metabolism of these hydroxy fatty acids, but both beta and omega oxidation probably occur.

Pharmacokinetics of Leukotrienes

The relatively recent isolation of the leukotrienes accounts for the scant information on their metabolism in humans. In porcine kidney as well as in human plasma, LTD_4, which has SRS-A activity, is converted to the less polar LTE_4, which is 8–12 times less potent as a smooth muscle stimulator. Local tissue breakdown of leukotrienes also occurs, and, as with other eicosanoids, the metabolites are probably primarily excreted in the urine.

Mechanism of Action of Eicosanoids on Smooth Muscle

Prostaglandins as well as some of the other eicosanoids appear to act on smooth muscle via specific receptors that are not blocked by conventional autonomic blocking agents (atropine, propranolol, phenoxybenzamine, hexamethonium) nor by antihistamine or antiserotonin drugs. Many of their actions appear to be associated with a change in the levels of one of the cyclic nucleotides, cAMP or cGMP, in the responding tissue. For example, venoconstriction in response to $PGF_{2\alpha}$ is associated with a rise in cGMP, whereas venodilatation induced by PGE_2 is associated with a rise in cAMP. This PGE_2-cAMP and $PGF_{2\alpha}$-cGMP association may change depending on the tissue. Nevertheless, an interaction between the prostaglandins and the cyclic nucleotides appears fairly well established for smooth muscle. This also appears to apply to the leukotrienes because both dibutyryl cAMP and aminophylline, a cAMP phosphodiesterase inhibitor, decrease the contractile response to LTC_4, LTD_4, and LTE_4. There is evidence that the peptidolipid leukotrienes may also act as calcium ionophores, directly increasing intracellular calcium concentrations; studies on isolated guinea pig tracheal smooth muscle have shown that verapamil, a calcium channel blocker, inhibited contractions normally induced by LTC_4, LTD_4, and LTE_4. Another calcium channel blocker, nifedipine, inhibits LTC_4- and LTD_4-induced contraction of human bronchial smooth muscle. The contraction of smooth muscle beds by various eicosanoids is associated with depolarization of the membrane potential, either alone or coupled with increased frequency and length of action potential bursts. Conversely, relaxation of smooth muscle by eicosanoids is associated with hyperpolarization.

Effects on Smooth Muscle
A. Vascular Smooth Muscle:

1. Prostaglandins—Prostaglandin activity is quite diverse among different vascular beds and different species. In animals, vascular smooth muscle itself synthesizes PGE_2, $PGF_{2\alpha}$, and PGI_2. In humans, PGE_2, PGI_2 (prostacyclin, epoprostenol), and PGA_2 are generally regarded as arteriolar dilators, whereas $PGF_{2\alpha}$ is a weak arteriolar dilator but an effective venoconstrictor in some vascular beds. Intravenous administration of PGE_2 in humans induces facial flushing and vasodilatation in the systemic and pulmonary vascular beds. $PGF_{2\alpha}$ administered intravenously to humans (0.1–1 $\mu g/kg/min$) does not induce facial flushing and has no effect on systemic vascular resistance but increases local peripheral vascular resistance and pulmonary vascular resistance. In contrast to its general vasodilating effects, PGE_2 constricts human umbilical cord vessels, as does $PGF_{2\alpha}$. In the dog, prostaglandins of the E and A groups dilate the coronary vessels, whereas $PGF_{2\alpha}$ has no significant effect. The local synthesis of prostaglandins in various vascular beds may contribute to maintaining normal vascular tone.

2. Thromboxanes–The instability of TXA$_2$ makes its evaluation as a vasoactive agent difficult, although it has been shown in vitro to be a potent constrictor of umbilical vessels. It may also constrict the coronary and renal vasculature when released locally from ischemic tissues. TXB$_2$ has been shown in animals to have modest constrictor activity in the pulmonary vascular bed.

3. HPETEs and HETEs–These substances do not appear to significantly affect vascular smooth muscle tone.

4. Leukotrienes–There are few data regarding the effects of leukotrienes on vascular smooth muscle in humans. In vitro, LTC$_4$ and LTD$_4$ are weak constrictors of human pulmonary artery or vein smooth muscle, whereas LTD$_4$ induces profound constriction of human coronary arteries. In other primates, intravenous injection of LTC$_4$ or LTD$_4$ (0.1 μg/kg) causes a decrease in peripheral vascular resistance; however, since LTC$_4$ and LTD$_4$ can induce PGE release from various tissues, the observed decrease may be an indirect effect. In animals, cutaneous arterioles appear to constrict initially and then relax in response to LTC$_4$ and LTD$_4$. However, regional specificity appears to exist since, in the anesthetized rat, only LTC$_4$ causes constriction of mucosal venules (LTD$_4$ is without effect).

B. Respiratory Smooth Muscle:

1. Prostaglandins–In vitro, the E prostaglandins relax tracheal or bronchial smooth muscle and antagonize the contractile response induced by agents such as bradykinin, histamine, acetylcholine, and serotonin. PGI$_2$, also formed in lung tissue, relaxes bronchiolar smooth muscle. PGF$_{2\alpha}$ and PGD$_2$ are also produced by human lung. However, they are potent constrictors of human tracheal and bronchial smooth muscle. On a molar basis, PGF$_{2\alpha}$ inhaled as an aerosol mist is several times more potent than histamine. There is some evidence that these prostaglandins may participate in regulating bronchopulmonary tone.

2. Thromboxanes–TXA$_2$ is perhaps the most potent of the eicosanoids as a bronchoconstrictor. It can be released from human lung following immunologic stimulation and may also participate with the other eicosanoids in regulating physiologic and pathophysiologic aspects of respiratory smooth muscle response.

3. HPETEs and HETEs–Various HPETEs are synthesized in the lung, and rapidly reduced to their respective HETE derivatives. 5-HETE (0.001–1 μg/mL) produces slow contractions of isolated human bronchial smooth muscle, with a potency comparable to that of histamine. In addition, if given at subthreshold doses, 5-HETE will potentiate histamine-induced contractions. 15-HETE is somewhat less potent than either 5-HETE or histamine. 12-HETE is inactive.

4. Leukotrienes–In nanogram concentrations, LTB$_4$, LTC$_4$, and LTD$_4$ cause marked constriction of human peripheral lung segments and bronchial smooth muscle in vitro (Fig 17–5). Nebulized delivery of

LTC$_4$ or LTD$_4$ induces bronchoconstriction, and comparison of FEV 1 values to expiratory flow at low lung volumes suggests that the major site of constriction is in the peripheral airways. Studies in animals show that indomethacin, a potent inhibitor of prostaglandin and thromboxane synthesis, can block the effects of the leukotrienes on airway smooth muscle, suggesting that some of the actions of leukotrienes may be mediated by the prostaglandins or thromboxanes. In fact, constriction of the guinea pig airway by LTB$_4$ appears to be mediated by the induced local release of TXA$_2$.

C. Gastrointestinal Smooth Muscle:

1. Prostaglandins–Various prostaglandins are produced throughout the gastrointestinal tract, the major ones being PGI$_2$, PGE$_2$, and PGF$_{2\alpha}$. In vitro, studies with human gastrointestinal smooth muscle show that PGE$_2$ contracts longitudinal but relaxes circular smooth muscle. PGF$_{2\alpha}$ appears to contract both longitudinal and circular smooth muscle. However, in human gallbladder, PGF$_{2\alpha}$, while contracting longitudinal smooth muscle, was without effect on circular smooth muscle. PGI$_2$, in contrast to PGE$_2$, contracts circular smooth muscle. While these observations derive from in vitro studies, oral administration of E prostaglandins to humans increases bile concentration within aspirated gastric fluid. These results are compatible with PGE-induced relaxation of the pyloric sphincter. Furthermore, intravenous administration of PGE$_2$ or PGF$_{2\alpha}$ leads to colicky cramping, suggesting that these prostaglandins increase gastrointestinal smooth muscle activity in vivo. In animals, intravenous infusion of E prostaglandins decreases lower esophageal sphincter tone, again suggesting that in vivo, the E prostaglandins relax circular smooth muscle.

2. Thromboxanes–Although TXB$_2$ has been shown to be synthesized by gastric fundal and antral mucosal cells, the effects of thromboxanes on intestinal smooth muscle are not well established.

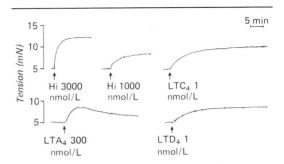

Figure 17–5. Contractions of isolated segments of human bronchi recorded after exposure to histamine (Hi) and the leukotrienes LTA$_4$, LTC$_4$, and LTD$_4$. LTC$_4$ and LTD$_4$, which together comprise SRS-A, are 300 times more potent than LTA$_4$, and 1000 times more potent than histamine. (Reproduced, with permission, from Dahlen S-E et al: Leukotrienes are potent constrictors of human bronchi. *Nature* 1980;**288**:484. Copyright © 1980 Macmillan Journals Limited.)

3. HPETEs and HETEs—The effects of these substances on gastrointestinal smooth muscle have not been well studied.

4. Leukotrienes—Before their structural elucidation, the SRS-A activity now known to be caused primarily by LTC_4 and LTD_4 was determined on smooth muscle preparations from guinea pig ileum. This smooth muscle preparation demonstrates a slow onset but prolonged contractile response. However, this effect on gastrointestinal smooth muscle in animals may be species-specific, since rat ileum fails to respond to LTC_4 or LTD_4 at concentrations causing contraction of guinea pig ileum. In contrast, the rat colon and stomach (fundus) are highly responsive to LTC_4 and LTD_4. The effects of leukotrienes on human gastrointestinal smooth muscle have not been clearly established.

D. Effects of Prostaglandins on Smooth Muscle of the Reproductive Tract: In human tissue, PGE_2 contracts the proximal quarter of the uterine tubes in vitro but relaxes the distal segments. In contrast, $PGF_{2\alpha}$ exerts a contractile effect on all segments. Intravenous injection of PGE_2 inhibits whereas $PGF_{2\alpha}$ increases tubal contractions, in keeping with the in vitro observations. Estrogens apparently enhance—whereas progesterone diminishes—the contractile response of the uterine tubes to the prostaglandins.

In the uterus, prostaglandins are synthesized primarily by the endometrium and act on myometrial smooth muscle. However, PGI_2 and TXA_2 can also be produced by the myometrium. Both PGE_2 and $PGF_{2\alpha}$ stimulate contractions of human myometrium in both pregnant and nonpregnant females. However, whereas intrauterine administration of PGE_2 in low doses (2–5 μg) produces contraction, higher doses (20–30 μg) cause relaxation. PGE_2 and PGI_2 cause re-laxation of isolated human myometrium and can antagonize $PGF_{2\alpha}$-induced contractions. However, these in vitro effects may not always reflect in vivo action.

The effects of other eicosanoids on human reproductive tract smooth muscle are not well established.

E. Summary of Effects of Eicosanoids on Human Smooth Muscle: Table 17–1 summarizes the effects of the various eicosanoids on human smooth muscle beds. It is apparent that the responses elicited vary in different types of smooth muscle. Varying the dose of eicosanoid can also change the type of response observed.

Actions of Eicosanoids on Other Tissues

The endogenously synthesized eicosanoids probably serve a far broader array of regulatory functions than simple stimulation or inhibition of smooth muscle. In fact, they probably play a role as a fine-tuning system for basic cellular functions in a variety of tissues. The rapid inactivation of most eicosanoids within the organ in which they are synthesized or within the systemic circulation permits such cell-specific effects. Thus, no definition of the roles of eicosanoids is valid unless the responding tissue or cells under study are specifically identified. For example, for the platelet, thromboxane is a signal that induces aggregation, whereas to certain smooth muscle cells it is a signal that induces contraction. In the hypothalamus, PGE_2 activates the thermoregulatory center and induces fever, whereas to some smooth muscle cells it is a signal for relaxation and to others a signal for contraction. In the kidney, PGE_2 directly stimulates renin release as well as renal sodium loss. Local prostaglandins also seem to regulate distribution of renal blood flow. To thymic-derived lymphocytes, PGE_2

Table 17–1. Effects of eicosanoids on smooth muscle in humans.
(C = contraction; R = relaxation; 0 = no effect; ? = not determined.)

	Vascular System		Respiratory System		Gastrointestinal Tract		Reproductive Tract	
	Arterial	Venous	Tracheal	Bronchial	Longitudinal	Circular	Tubal	Uterine
PGE_2	R[1]	0	R	R	C	R	C[2]	C[3]
$PGF_{2\alpha}$	R[1]	C	C	C	C	C	C	C
PGI_2 (prostacyclin, epoprostenol)	R	0	R	R	C	C	?	R
TXA_2	C	C	C	C	?	?	?	?
TXB_2	C	?	0	0	?	?	?	?
HETEs	0	0	C[4]	C[4]	?	?	?	?
LTC_4	C	C	C	C	?[5]	?[5]	?	?
LTD_4	C	C	C	C	?	?	?	?
LTE_4	0	0	C	C	?	?	?	?

[1]Both E and F prostaglandins constrict umbilical arteries.
[2]PGE_2 contracts proximal quarter but relaxes distal segment.
[3]Low-dose range (2–5 μg) contracts; high-dose range (20–30 μg) relaxes.
[4]5-HETE>15-HETE; 12-HETE is inactive.
[5]No reliable human studies.

can be a signal that either enhances or suppresses proliferation depending on the subpopulation of lymphocytes. In addition to their myotropic action, LTC_4 and LTD_4 enhance mucous secretion in isolated human airway. In the dog, the ability of LTC_4 to enhance mucous secretion in the trachea has been shown in vivo to be blocked by diphenhydramine, suggesting a possible role of histamine in this response. Such polyfunctional properties provide an explanation for the widespread and often confusing effects of eicosanoids when they are systemically administered at levels greater than can be achieved by normal endogenous metabolism. The same circumstance accounts for the difficulties inherent in using eicosanoids as therapeutic agents. Conversely, some of the side effects of drugs that block synthesis of certain eicosanoids may stem from blockade of the physiologic functions of these endogenously generated compounds. For example, the ulcer-inducing effect of corticosteroids and aspirin or indomethacin may stem from their inhibition of prostaglandin generation by the gastric mucosa, since some prostaglandins have been shown to exert a cytoprotective effect on gastrointestinal mucosa.

The leukotrienes have many actions in addition to those on smooth muscle. LTC_4 and LTD_4 cause an increase in vascular permeability at the level of the postcapillary venules and are respectively 5000- and 1000-fold more potent on a molar basis than histamine. LTB_4, on the other hand, has been shown to be one of the most potent chemoattractants for neutrophils and appears to be the source of the majority, if not all, of the neutrophil chemotactic activity present in the colonic mucosa of patients with inflammatory bowel disease. Injection of 500 ng of LTB_4 into human skin induces the local migration of neutrophils into the dermis. LTC_4 and LTD_4 do not demonstrate this chemotactic activity; however, 12-HETE, when applied to human skin, is also able to induce migration of neutrophils into the dermis. The chemoattractant property of LTB_4 is dependent on the *cis*, *trans*, *trans* configuration (see Fig 17–4) of the conjugated triene as shown by the finding that 2 isomers of LTB_4 having an all-*trans* configuration lack this chemotactic property. LTB_4 also appears capable of activating a subset of thymus-derived lymphocytes (T cells) that can suppress specific responses of other subsets of lymphocytes. It is readily apparent, therefore, that as with the other eicosanoids, it is necessary to identify the tissue or organ system under discussion in order to properly define the functions of the leukotrienes.

In addition to their individual actions, various eicosanoids may facilitate or inhibit the production or effects of other eicosanoids at the same site. For example, in some tissues LTC_4 and LTD_4 can enhance the generation of prostaglandins and thromboxanes. In human lung, $PGF_{2\alpha}$ enhances leukotriene generation. Conversely, PGE_2 appears capable of suppressing leukotriene generation. PGE_2 and PGD_2 enhance the effect of LTB_4 on neutrophil accumulation in the skin. Similarly, when PGE_2 is introduced along with LTB_4, increased vascular permeability occurs, an effect that

is not seen in response to either agent when used alone. In addition, PGE_2 appears to enhance the vascular permeability induced by LTC_4 and LTD_4. Organ specificity of some of these interactions is suggested by the observation that in the rabbit eye, in contrast to rabbit skin, PGE_2 decreases rather than increases the accumulation of neutrophils triggered by LTB_4.

II. CLINICAL PHARMACOLOGY OF PROSTAGLANDINS & OTHER EICOSANOIDS

The major clinical applications of agents in this group relate to their effects on smooth muscle. The effects of specific eicosanoids on various smooth muscle beds coupled with the knowledge of their endogenous synthesis have been used in 2 ways. The first involves direct use of prostaglandins or other eicosanoids as pharmacologic smooth muscle agonists; the second is concerned with the use of drugs that inhibit endogenous synthesis of eicosanoids and thereby modify smooth muscle activity.

EICOSANOIDS AS THERAPEUTIC AGENTS

In Gynecology
The ability of PGE_2 and $PGF_{2\alpha}$ to contract uterine smooth muscle—not only at term, as with oxytocin, but throughout pregnancy—has led to their use for inducing abortion as well as for the induction of term labor. However, since induction of term labor with these prostaglandins is accompanied by increased risks of uterine hypertonus and fetal bradycardia, their use in gynecologic practice has been primarily as abortifacients. When given intravenously, intramuscularly, or intravaginally, PGE_2 or $PGF_{2\alpha}$ is very effective in inducing second-trimester abortion. Intravaginal therapy is preferred, since this route reduces the stimulation of other smooth muscle beds that leads to side effects of nausea, vomiting, abdominal cramping, diarrhea, hypotension or hypertension, headache, and asthmalike attacks. In addition, convulsions have been observed in susceptible individuals. Three preparations have been used: (1) dinoprost tromethamine ($PGF_{2\alpha}$, Prostin F2 alpha), for intra-amniotic administration; (2) carboprost tromethamine (15-methyl $PGF_{2\alpha}$, Prostin/15M), for intramuscular injection; and (3) dinoprostone (PGE_2, Prostin E2), as vaginal suppository. These agents appear to be preferable to intra-amniotic injection of hypertonic saline because of their more rapid onset of action and the lower incidence of major complications.

In Pulmonary Disease
The bronchodilator effect of PGE_2 has led to nu-

merous studies of this prostaglandin as a possible agent to treat diseases associated with bronchoconstriction. However, inhalation of PGE compounds often causes severe irritation of the upper respiratory tract or induces paradoxic bronchoconstriction, thereby precluding its use as a therapeutically effective bronchodilator. Attempts to modify the structure of PGE_2 in order to diminish these untoward effects have so far led to a marked diminution in bronchodilator potency. This therapeutic area is still under investigation.

In Cardiovascular Disease

A significant therapeutic application of the E prostaglandins has been in the area of ductus-dependent cardiac malformations. The ability of alprostadil (PGE_1) to maintain patency of the ductus arteriosus has led to its evaluation as presurgical therapy for neonates suffering from transposition of the great arteries, pulmonary atresia, or pulmonary stenosis. Continuous infusion of $0.05-0.1$ $\mu g/kg/min$ intra-arterially or intravenously maintains ductal patency. FDA approval has been given for this use of PGE_1, and it is marketed as Prostin VR Pediatric.

PGE_1 and PGI_2 (prostacyclin, epoprostenol) have been used investigationally as vasodilators for treatment of peripheral vascular diseases. At a dose of $2-4$ $\mu g/h$, over a 10-minute period for each of 3 days, PGE_1 has in selected cases provided relief of pain and increase in skin temperature and is associated with healing of previously recalcitrant ulcers. PGI_2 infused intra-arterially or into the subclavian vein may produce a striking improvement in claudication. Muscle blood flow increased significantly in the affected extremities, and in some patients this effect lasted $4-6$ weeks after treatment. Since generation of endogenous PGI_2 by vascular endothelium is decreased in atherosclerotic areas of vessel walls, it may be that PGI_2 infusion acts by reestablishing some mechanism essential for maintenance of vascular tone as well as by clearing platelet aggregations obstructing capillary beds in the affected extremities. Synthetic prostacyclin is available as a stable freeze-dried preparation (**epoprostenol, Flolan**).

PGE_1 ($6-10$ ng/kg/min) has also been administered intravenously to patients suffering from systemic sclerosis with Raynaud's phenomenon. After administration of PGE_1 (but not of saline), increased skin temperature, improvement in cold tolerance, and reduced intensity of Raynaud attacks were reported. The improvement lasted for several weeks. Further evaluation of vasodilating prostaglandins in the treatment of occlusive vascular diseases is definitely warranted in light of these initial studies.

In Gastrointestinal Disease

A promising area of therapeutic investigation has focused on the gastrointestinal cytoprotective effect of PGE_2 and some analogs such as 16-methyl,16-hydroxy-PGE_1 (misoprostol), 15(R)-15-methyl-PGE_2 (arbostil), and dihydro-PGE_2 (enprostil). In addition to blocking gastric acid secretion, these agents, at concentrations that do not block acid secretion, appear capable of protecting the gastric mucosa from the ulcerogenic effects of aspirin, other nonsteroidal anti-inflammatory drugs, ethanol, and corticosteroids.

THERAPEUTIC INHIBITION OF ENDOGENOUS EICOSANOID SYNTHESIS

Several novel uses for the more potent nonsteroidal anti-inflammatory drugs (NSAIDs)—aspirin, indomethacin, mefenamic acid, ibuprofen, and naproxen—have been evaluated since the discovery that one of their pharmacologic effects is inhibition of prostaglandin and thromboxane synthesis.

NSAIDs & Dysmenorrhea

Current evidence strongly implicates excessive $PGF_{2\alpha}$ synthesis as an important factor in dysmenorrhea. High levels of $PGF_{2\alpha}$ are found in menstrual fluid of patients suffering from primary dysmenorrhea, and uterine cramping accompanies intravenous administration of sufficiently high doses of $PGF_{2\alpha}$. Clinical trials using indomethacin, ibuprofen, naproxen, and mefenamic acid have shown these drugs to be extremely effective in relieving the symptoms of dysmenorrhea. Aspirin is far less effective, perhaps because of the decreased sensitivity of uterine cyclooxygenase to aspirin when compared to the other NSAIDs. Typically, ibuprofen, 400 mg 4 times daily for 3 days prior to the expected menstrual period and continued for 3 days during menstruation, has produced significant relief of dysmenorrhea. Indomethacin has also been used with success when given in a dose of 50 mg at the first sign of an attack followed by no more than 2 repeat 50-mg doses over the ensuing 24 hours. Ibuprofen, naproxen, and mefenamic acid are now approved for the management of primary dysmenorrhea.

NSAIDs & Ductus Closure

Patency of the fetal ductus arteriosus is regarded as an active state caused by continual synthesis of either PGE_2 or PGI_2 by the ductal endothelium. This concept is supported by animal and human studies showing that PGE_1 and PGI_2 can maintain patency of the ductus and that agents that block prostaglandin synthesis cause closure of the ductus. Therapeutic advantage has been taken of this observation, and NSAIDs have been used to treat premature infants who develop respiratory distress due to failure of ductus closure. In such infants, administration of indomethacin ($0.3-0.6$ mg/kg/24 h) has succeeded in causing closure of the ductus, thereby precluding the need for surgical ligation (Chapter 34).

Current studies of a variety of diseases in which symptoms may derive from prostaglandin-induced smooth muscle activity offer promise of other uses for NSAIDs and other inhibitors of eicosanoid synthesis.

Sulfasalazine & Inflammatory Bowel Disease

As mentioned previously, significant quantities of the neutrophil chemoattractant LTB_4 have been recovered from the colonic mucosa of patients with inflammatory bowel disease, whereas it is virtually absent in normal colonic mucosa. Sulfasalazine, a drug with anti-inflammatory effects in patients with ulcerative colitis, has been shown to inhibit the synthesis of LTB_4. It is possible that this effect may help to explain the therapeutic benefit of sulfasalazine in this disease.

REFERENCES

Benson LN et al: Role of prostaglandin E_1 infusion in the management of transposition of the great arteries. *Am J Cardiol* 1979;**44**:691.

Borgeat P et al: Leukotrienes: Biosynthesis, metabolism, and analysis. *Adv Lipid Res* 1985; **21**:47.

Caldwell B, Behrman HR: Prostaglandins in reproductive processes. *Med Clin North Am* 1981;**65**:927.

Chan WY: Prostaglandins and nonsteroidal anti-inflammatory drugs in dysmenorrhea. *Annu Rev Pharmacol Toxicol* 1983;**23**:131.

Cohen MM et al: Protection against aspirin-induced antral and duodenal damage with enprostil. *Gastroenterology* 1985; **88**:382.

Eklund B, Carlson LA: Central and peripheral circulatory effects and metabolic effects of different prostaglandins given i.v. to man. *Prostaglandins* 1980;**20**:333.

Fischer S et al: Prostacyclin metabolism in adults and neonates. *Biochim Biophys Acta* 1983;**750**:127.

Goetzl EJ, Kaplan AP: Lipid and peptide mediators of inflammation. (Symposium.) *Fed Proc* 1983;**42**:3119.

Hirsh PD et al: Prostaglandins and ischemic heart disease. *Am J Med* 1981;**71**:1009.

Horton EW: Prostaglandins and smooth muscle. *Br Med Bull* 1979;**35**:295.

Hyman AL et al: Prostaglandins and the lung. *Med Clin North Am* 1981;**65**:789.

Johnson HG et al: Diphenhydramine blocks the leukotriene-C_4 enhanced mucus secretion in canine trachea in vivo. *Agents Actions* 1983;**13**:1.

Kohrogi H et al: Nifedipine inhibits human bronchial smooth muscle contractions induced by leukotrienes C_4 and D_4, prostaglandin $F_{2\alpha}$, and potassium. *Am Rev Respir Dis* 1985; **132**:299.

Lichtenberger LM et al: Effect of 16,16-dimethyl prostaglandin E_2 on the surface hydrophobicity of aspirin-treated canine gastric mucosa. *Gastroenterology* 1985;**88**:308.

Metz SA: Anti-inflammatory agents as inhibitors of prostaglandin synthesis in man. *Med Clin North Am* 1981;**65**:713.

Nuki G: Non-steroidal analgesic and anti-inflammatory agents. *Br Med J* 1983;**287**:39.

Rosenkranz B et al: Metabolic disposition of prostaglandin E_1 in man. *Biochim Biophys Acta* 1983;**750**:231.

Sasaki S et al: Mechanism of leukotriene-induced contraction of isolated guinea pig tracheal smooth muscle. *Lung* 1984; **162**:369.

Serhan C et al: Trihydroxytetraenes: A novel series of compounds formed from arachidonic acid in human leukocytes. *Biochem Biophys Res Commun* 1984;**118**:943.

Sirois P: Pharmacology of the leukotrienes. *Adv Lipid Res* 1985;**21**:79.

Stenson WF, Lobos E: Sulfasalazine inhibits the synthesis of chemotactic lipids by neutrophils. *J Clin Invest* 1982; **69**:494.

Vapaatalo H, Ylikorlala O (editors): Prostanoids in clinical medicine. *Ann Clin Res* 1984;**16**:225. [Editorial plus 13 review papers covering basic biology of eicosanoids as well as clinical applications in diabetes, cancer, organ transplantation, gynecology, neonatology, and cytoprotection.]

18

Bronchodilators & Other Agents Used in the Treatment of Asthma

Homer A. Boushey, MD, & Michael J. Holtzman, MD

Asthma is characterized by increased responsiveness of the trachea and bronchi to various stimuli and by widespread narrowing of the airways that changes in severity either spontaneously or as a result of therapy. The clinical hallmarks of asthma are recurrent, episodic bouts of coughing, shortness of breath, chest tightness, and wheezing. Its pathologic features are contraction of airway smooth muscle, mucosal thickening from edema and cellular infiltration, and inspissation in the airway lumen of abnormally thick, viscid plugs of mucus. Of these causes of airway obstruction, contraction of smooth muscle is most easily reversed by current therapy.

The most widely used bronchodilators are β-adrenoceptor stimulants (Chapter 8) and theophylline, a methylxanthine drug. Reversal of airway constriction can also be brought about by the use of antimuscarinic agents (Chapter 7). Two other types of drugs important in asthma are cromolyn sodium, an inhibitor of mast cell degranulation, and corticosteroids.

This chapter presents the basic pharmacology of cromolyn and methylxanthines—agents whose medical use is almost exclusively for pulmonary disease. The other classes of drugs listed above are discussed in relation to the therapy of asthma.

A rational approach to the pharmacotherapy of asthma depends on an understanding of a conceptual model for the pathogenesis of the disease. In the classic immunologic model, asthma is a disease mediated by reaginic (IgE) antibodies bound to mast cells in the airway mucosa (Fig 18–1). On reexposure to an antigen, antigen-antibody interaction takes place on the surface of the mast cells, triggering both the release of mediators stored in the cells' granules and the synthesis and release of other mediators. The agents released include histamine, slow-reacting substance of anaphylaxis (SRS-A; now known to be a group of sulfidopeptide-containing leukotrienes), eosinophil chemotactic factor (ECF), neutrophil chemotactic factor (NCF), and other compounds. These agents diffuse throughout the airway wall and cause contraction of muscle, edema, cellular infiltration, and a change in mucous secretion either by their direct actions or by altering neurohumoral regulatory mechanisms.

There are several features of asthma, however, that cannot be accounted for by this model. Most adults with asthma have no evidence of immediate hypersensitivity to antigens, and most attacks cannot be related to recent exposure to an unusual quantity of antigen. Even in patients with a history of asthma during the ragweed season and positive cutaneous and bronchial responses to ragweed antigen, the severity of symptoms correlates poorly with the quantity of antigen in the atmosphere. Furthermore, bronchospasm can be provoked by nonantigenic stimuli, such as distilled water, exercise, cold air, sulfur dioxide, and rapid respiratory maneuvers.

In healthy nonasthmatic people, inhalation of small doses of mediators of anaphylaxis (eg, histamine) does not provoke bronchoconstriction. In people with asthma, however, inhalation of even smaller doses of

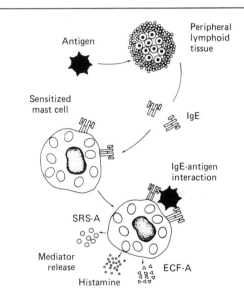

Figure 18–1. Immunologic model for pathogenesis of immediate hypersensitivity. Exposure to antigen causes synthesis of IgE, which binds to mast cells in the target organ. On reexposure to antigen, antigen-antibody interaction on mast cell surfaces triggers release of mediators of anaphylaxis. (SRS-A = slow-reacting substance of anaphylaxis; ECF-A = eosinophil chemotactic factor of anaphylaxis.) (Reproduced, with permission, from Gold WM: Cholinergic pharmacology in asthma. In: *Asthma Physiology, Immunopharmacology, and Treatment.* Austen KF, Lichtenstein LM [editors]. Academic Press, 1974.)

the same mediator provokes intense symptomatic bronchospasm. This exaggerated sensitivity of the airways is sometimes called "nonspecific bronchial hyperreactivity" to distinguish it from the bronchospasm provoked by specific antigens. Bronchial hyperactivity appears to be fundamental to asthma's pathogenesis, for it is nearly ubiquitous in patients with asthma; its degree correlates positively with the symptomatic severity of the disease; and the events that increase bronchial reactivity (viral respiratory infections, exposure to oxidizing pollutants) have often been noted to cause symptomatic worsening of disease.

The mechanism underlying bronchial hyperactivity is unknown, but it may somehow be related to inflammation of the airway mucosa. This hypothesis is supported by the observation that the agents that increase bronchial reactivity, such as ozone or allergen and infection with respiratory viruses, also cause airway inflammation. In both dogs and humans, the increase in bronchial reactivity induced by ozone is associated with an increase in the number of polymorphonuclear leukocytes found in fluid obtained by bronchial lavage or from bronchial mucosal biopsies.

How the increase in airway reactivity is linked to inflammation is uncertain. One possibility is that some of the mediators of inflammation alter smooth muscle or its innervation to enhance its responsiveness, and it has indeed been shown that eicosanoid products of arachidonic acid metabolism can alter neural and muscular function. Identification of specific mediators and their cellular sources in the asthmatic airway may ultimately lead to new specific pharmacologic therapy.

Whatever the mechanisms responsible for the overall increase in bronchomotor responsiveness of the asthmatic airway, the response itself seems to be a function of the direct effect of the mediators released and of the amplification of this effect by neural or humoral pathways activated by the mediators. Evidence for the importance of neural pathways stems largely from studies of laboratory animals. Thus, the bronchospasm provoked in dogs by histamine can be greatly reduced by pretreatment with an inhaled topical anesthetic agent, by blockade of the vagus nerves, and by pretreatment with atropine, a competitive antagonist of acetylcholine, in doses that have no effect on the responses of airway smooth muscle to histamine in vitro. Studies of humans, however, provide less unequivocal data. Pharmacologic blockage of vagal efferent pathways with aerosolized hexamethonium, a drug that inhibits transmission through parasympathetic ganglia (Chapter 7), or with atropine sulfate, a postganglionic muscarinic antagonist, causes reduction but not abolition of the bronchospastic responses to both antigenic and nonantigenic stimuli (eg, exercise, inhalation of cold air, sulfur dioxide, and distilled water). While it is possible that activity in some other neural pathway (eg, the nonadrenergic system) contributes to bronchomotor responses, the fact that responses are also partially blocked by cromolyn, a drug that appears to inhibit mast cell degranulation, suggests that both antigenic and nonantigenic stimuli

may provoke the release of mediators that contract airway smooth muscle through direct effects and through activation of parasympathetic efferent activity (Fig 18–2).

The hypothesis suggested by these studies—that asthmatic bronchospasm results from a combination of release of mediators and an exaggeration of responsiveness to their effects—suggests that asthma may be effectively treated by drugs with different modes of action. Asthmatic bronchospasm might be reversed or prevented, for example, by drugs that prevent mast cell degranulation (cromolyn, calcium channel antagonists), block the conduction along sensory or motor nerves to the airways (topical anesthetics), inhibit the effect of acetylcholine released from vagal motor nerves (muscarinic antagonists), or directly relax airway smooth muscle (sympathomimetic agents, theophylline). Some effective drugs, such as the corticosteroids, have an unknown mechanism of action and thus cannot be clearly related to this conceptual model, but they may prevent the inflammation that appears important in maintaining bronchial hyperreactivity.

I. BASIC PHARMACOLOGY OF BRONCHODILATORS & OTHER AGENTS USED IN THE TREATMENT OF ASTHMA

CROMOLYN SODIUM

Cromolyn sodium (disodium cromoglycate, Intal) differs from most antiasthmatic medications in that it is only of value when taken prophylactically. It is a stable but extremely insoluble salt (see structure below). A single dose (20–40 mg by inhalation) effectively inhibits both antigen- and exercise-induced asthma, and chronic use (20–40 mg 4 times daily) may reduce the overall level of bronchial reactivity; however, the drug has no effect on airway smooth muscle tone and is ineffective in reversing asthmatic bronchospasm. Cromolyn is poorly absorbed from the gastrointestinal tract. For use in asthma, it must be applied topically, by inhalation of a microfine powder or aerosolized solution as described below. When given by inhalation or orally, less than 10% is absorbed, and most is excreted unchanged.

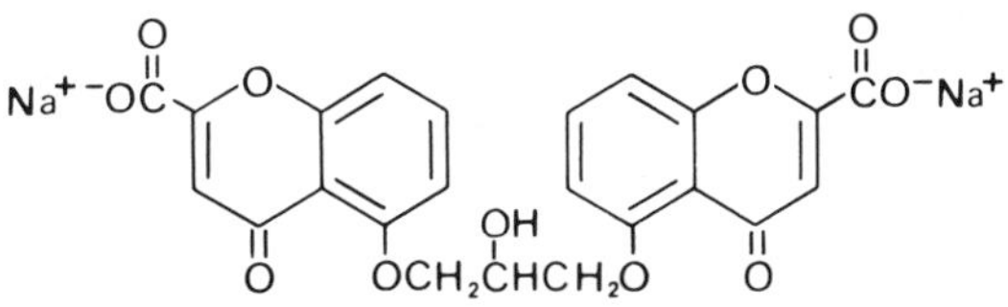

Cromolyn

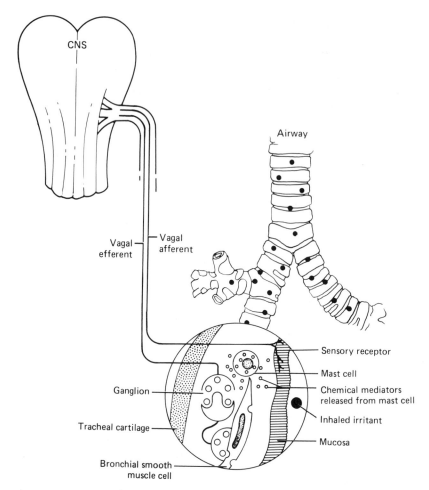

Figure 18–2. Mechanisms of response to inhaled irritants. The airway is represented microscopically by a cross section of the wall with branching vagal sensory endings lying adjacent to the lumen. Afferent pathways in the vagus nerves travel to the central nervous system; efferent pathways from the central nervous system travel to efferent ganglia. Postganglionic fibers release acetylcholine (O), which binds to muscarinic receptors on airway smooth muscle. Inhaled materials may provoke bronchoconstriction by directly stimulating smooth muscle contraction (eg, histamine, methacholine), by irritating sensory receptors and stimulating a reflex increase in parasympathetic efferent activity (eg, inert carbon particles), or by triggering release of chemical mediators from mast cells (eg, antigens) that in turn stimulate muscle contraction both directly and through activating neural reflex mechanisms.

Mechanism of Action

In vitro studies show that cromolyn prevents antigen-induced release of histamine and other mediators of anaphylaxis from sensitized mast cells and lung fragments, apparently by preventing the transmembrane influx of calcium provoked by IgE antibody-antigen interaction on the mast cell surface. This inhibitory effect appears to be specific for both cell and antibody type, for cromolyn has little inhibitory effect on mediator release from human basophils or on IgG-mediated degranulation of mast cells. It may also be specific for different organs, since cromolyn inhibits anaphylaxis in human and primate lung but not in skin. This in turn might reflect differences in mast cells found in different sites.

In vivo studies of asthmatic subjects support the concept that cromolyn inhibits mediator release. Pretreatment with cromolyn inhibits not only the bronchospasm provoked by antigen inhalation or by exercise, but it also inhibits the coincident appearance of neutrophil chemotactic factor (NCF)—a putative marker of mast cell activation—in circulating blood. This mechanism of action of cromolyn is considered by some investigators to be so well established that cromolyn has been used as a tool in studies of the mechanisms of bronchial responses. Thus, if bronchoconstriction is inhibited by cromolyn, the release of mediators from mast cells is presumed to be involved.

Other evidence, however, suggests that cromolyn's mechanism of action may not be so straightforward. The search for more effective agents has yielded many with greater potency in inhibiting mast cell degranulation in vitro, but these have been ineffective in inhibiting bronchomotor responses in vivo. Other experimental work also suggests that cromolyn may inhibit phosphodiesterase, thus increasing intracellular cAMP, and that it may alter neural pathways that influence airway smooth muscle tone.

Clinical Use of Cromolyn

In patients, the efficacy of cromolyn has been demonstrated in several circumstances. When used before exposure, the drug inhibits the immediate and delayed reactions to inhalation of antigen. Pretreatment with cromolyn also blocks exercise- and aspirin-induced bronchoconstriction and protects against the bronchospasm provoked by a variety of industrial agents, including toluene diisocyanate, wood dusts, soldering fluxes, piperazine hydrochloride, and certain enzymes. This acute protective effect of a single treatment makes cromolyn useful for administration shortly before exercise or before unavoidable exposure to an allergen.

Cromolyn is also effective in reducing the symptomatic severity and the need for bronchodilator medications in patients with perennial asthma. Not all patients benefit from chronic therapy, and although young patients with extrinsic asthma are most likely to respond favorably, some older patients with intrinsic disease are also improved. At present, the only way of determining whether a patient will respond is by a therapeutic trial of 40 mg delivered by inhalation 4 times daily for 4 weeks. In those who respond, the effectiveness of regular use of cromolyn in controlling asthmatic symptoms appears to be roughly equal to that of maintenance theophylline therapy.

It has recently been proposed that chronic treatment with cromolyn causes a decrease in bronchial hyperreactivity, possibly by protecting the airway against the inflammatory effects of the chemical mediators of anaphylaxis. At present, this concept is supported only by data from studies that are uncontrolled or involve small numbers of subjects, and the only established indication for the drug is recurrent symptomatic asthma. At present, it is not indicated for patients with only occasional asthmatic symptoms that are well controlled by "as needed" treatment with bronchodilators.

Cromolyn is absorbed poorly from the gastrointestinal tract and therefore is effective only when deposited directly into the airways. Two methods of administration are currently used. In adults, the drug is given by a Spinhaler apparatus that causes a capsule to be punctured so that its powdered contents are entrained into inspired air and deposited in the airways. The usual dose is 20 mg inhaled 4 times daily. In children, who may have difficulty coordinating the use of the Spinhaler device, cromolyn may be given by aerosol of a 1% solution.

Cromolyn solution is also useful in reducing symptoms of allergic rhinitis. Spraying a 4% solution into each nostril 6 times daily is effective in about 75% of patients with hay fever, even during the peak pollen season.

Because it is so poorly absorbed, adverse effects of cromolyn are minor and are localized in the sites of deposition. These include such symptoms as throat irritation, cough, mouth dryness, chest tightness, and wheezing. Some of these symptoms can be prevented by inhaling a β_2-agonist drug before cromolyn treatment. Serious adverse effects are rare. Reversible dermatitis, myositis, or gastroenteritis occurs in about 2% of patients, and few cases of pulmonary infiltration with eosinophilia and of anaphylaxis have been reported.

METHYLXANTHINE DRUGS

The 3 important methylxanthines are theophylline, theobromine, and caffeine. Their major source is, of course, beverages (tea, cocoa, and coffee, respectively). Theophylline is important as a therapeutic agent in the treatment of asthma.

Chemistry

As shown below, theophylline is 1,3-dimethylxanthine; theobromine is 3,7-dimethylxanthine; and caffeine is 1,3,7-trimethylxanthine. The theophylline preparation most commonly used for therapeutic purposes is the theophylline-ethylenediamine complex **aminophylline.** A synthetic analog of theophylline (dyphylline) is both less potent and shorter-acting than theophylline. The pharmacokinetics of theophylline are discussed below. The metabolic products, partially demethylated xanthines (not uric acid), are excreted in the urine.

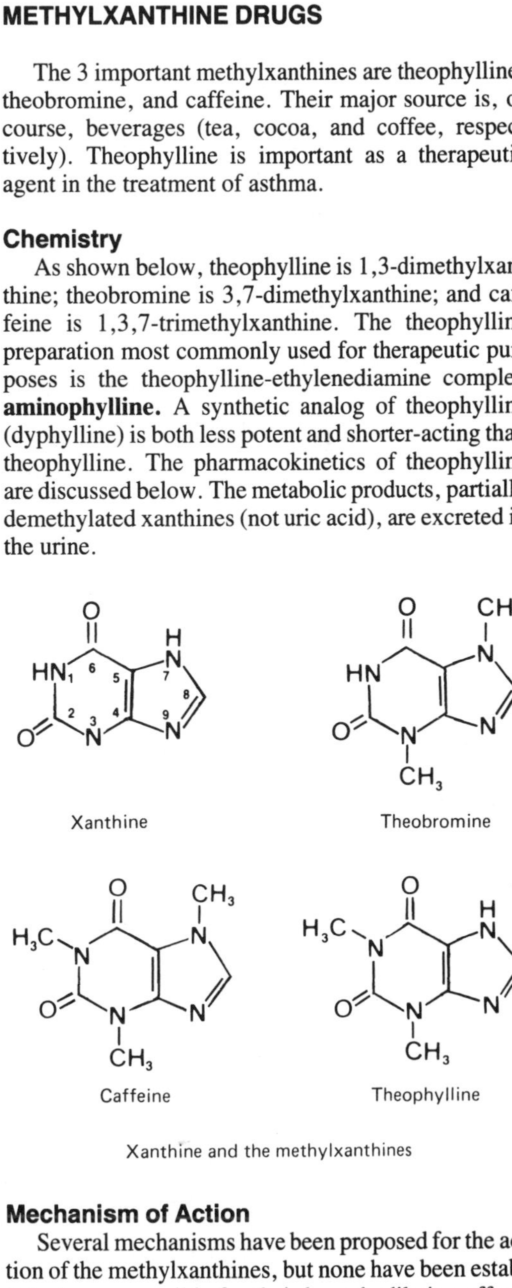

Xanthine and the methylxanthines

Mechanism of Action

Several mechanisms have been proposed for the action of the methylxanthines, but none have been established as responsible for their bronchodilating effect. They can be shown in vitro to inhibit the enzyme phosphodiesterase (Fig 18–3). Since phosphodiesterase hydrolyzes cyclic nucleotides, this inhibition results in higher concentrations of intracellular cAMP. This ef-

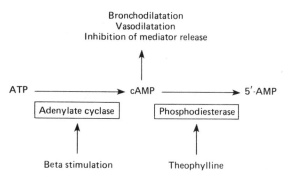

Figure 18–3. Intracellular levels of cAMP can be increased by beta-adrenoceptor agonists, which increase the rate of its synthesis by adenylate cyclase; or by phosphodiesterase inhibitors, such as theophylline, which slow the rate of its degradation.

fect could explain the cardiac stimulation and smooth muscle relaxation produced by these drugs, but it is not certain that sufficiently high concentrations are achieved in vivo to inhibit phosphodiesterase. Another proposed mechanism is the inhibition of cell surface receptors for adenosine. These receptors modulate adenylate cyclase activity, and adenosine has been shown to cause contraction of isolated airway smooth muscle and to enhance histamine release from cells present in the lung. These effects are antagonized by theophylline, an agent generally regarded as a universal antagonist of cell surface receptors for adenosine. It has also been shown, however, that xanthine derivatives devoid of adenosine-antagonistic properties (eg, enprofylline) may be many times more potent than theophylline in inhibiting bronchoconstriction in asthmatic subjects.

Pharmacodynamics of Methylxanthines

The methylxanthines have effects on the central nervous system, kidney, and cardiac and skeletal muscle as well as smooth muscle. Of the 3 agents, theophylline is most selective in its smooth muscle effects, while caffeine has the most marked central nervous system effects.

A. Central Nervous System Effects: In low and moderate doses, the methylxanthines, especially caffeine, cause mild cortical arousal with increased alertness and deferral of fatigue. In unusually sensitive individuals, the caffeine contained in beverages, eg, 100 mg in a cup of coffee, is sufficient to cause nervousness and insomnia. At very high doses, medullary stimulation and convulsions may occur. Nervousness and tremor are primary side effects in patients taking large doses of aminophylline for asthma.

B. Cardiovascular Effects: The methylxanthines have direct positive chronotropic and inotropic effects on the heart. At low concentrations, these effects appear to result from increased calcium influx, probably mediated by increased cAMP. At higher concentrations, sequestration of calcium by the sar-

coplasmic reticulum is impaired. In unusually sensitive individuals, consumption of a few cups of coffee may result in arrhythmias; but in most people, parenteral administration of higher doses of the methylxanthines produces only sinus tachycardia and increased cardiac output. Methylxanthines have occasionally been used in the treatment of pulmonary edema associated with heart failure (Chapter 12). These agents also relax vascular smooth muscle except in cerebral blood vessels, where they cause contraction.

C. Effects on Gastrointestinal Tract: The methylxanthines stimulate secretion of both gastric acid and digestive enzymes. However, even decaffeinated coffee has a potent stimulant effect on secretion, which means that the primary secretagogue in coffee is not caffeine.

D. Effects on Kidney: The methylxanthines—especially theophylline—are weak diuretics. This effect may involve both increased glomerular filtration and reduced tubular sodium reabsorption. The diuresis is not of sufficient magnitude to be therapeutically useful.

E. Effects on Smooth Muscle: The bronchodilation produced by the methylxanthines is the major therapeutic action. Tolerance does not develop, but side effects, especially in the central nervous system, may limit the dose (see below). In addition to this direct effect on the airway smooth muscle, these agents inhibit antigen-induced release of histamine from lung tissue; their effect on mucociliary transport is unknown.

F. Effects on Skeletal Muscle: The therapeutic actions of the methylxanthines may not be confined to the airways, for they also strengthen the contractions of isolated skeletal muscle in vitro and have potent effects in improving contractility and in reversing fatigue of the diaphragm in patients with chronic obstructive lung diseases. This effect on diaphragmatic performance, rather than an effect on the respiratory center, may account for theophylline's ability to improve the ventilatory response to hypoxia and to relieve dyspnea even in patients with irreversible airflow obstruction.

Clinical Use of Methylxanthines

Of the xanthines, theophylline is the most effective bronchodilator, and it has been shown repeatedly both to relieve airflow obstruction in acute asthma and to reduce the severity of symptoms and time lost from work or school in chronic asthma. Theophylline is only slightly soluble in water, so it has been administered as a number of different salts containing varying amounts of theophylline base. The 2 commonly used theophylline salts are aminophylline, which contains 86% theophylline by weight; and oxtriphylline, which contains 64% theophylline by weight. Corrections must be made to ensure equivalent doses of theophylline for different preparations. Most preparations are well absorbed from the gastrointestinal tract; their absorption is not affected significantly by food. The absorption of rectal suppositories, however, is unreliable, and these preparations should be used only in special circumstances.

Improvements in theophylline preparations have come from alterations in the physical state of the drugs rather than from new chemical formulations. For example, several companies now provide anhydrous theophylline in a microcrystalline form in which the increased surface area facilitates solubilization for complete and rapid absorption after oral administration. In addition, several sustained-release preparations (eg, Slo-Phyllin, Theo-Dur) are available and can produce therapeutic blood levels of theophylline for up to 12 hours. These preparations offer the advantages of less frequent drug administration, less fluctuation of theophylline blood levels, and, in many cases, more effective treatment of nocturnal bronchospasm.

An important advance in the use of theophylline is the availability of theophylline blood level measurements to monitor therapy. Therapeutic and toxic effects of theophylline are related to the plasma concentrations of the drug. Improvement in pulmonary function is well correlated with plasma concentration in the range of 5–20 mg/L. Anorexia, nausea, vomiting, abdominal discomfort, headache, and anxiety begin to occur at concentrations of 15 mg/L in some patients and become common at concentrations greater than 20 mg/L. Higher levels (greater than 40 mg/L) may cause seizures or arrhythmias; these may not be preceded by gastrointestinal or neurologic warning symptoms. Rational administration of theophylline, therefore, requires knowledge of its pharmacokinetics.

As described in Chapter 3, the initial or "loading" dose of a drug is determined by its volume of distribution (V_d) and the subsequent or "maintenance" dose by the rate of plasma clearance. The V_d for theophylline is proportionate to lean body weight but otherwise varies only slightly among individuals. On the average, $V_d = 0.5$ L/kg, so a plasma concentration of 10 mg/L will be achieved by a loading dose of 5 mg of theophylline per kilogram of body weight. Because aminophylline contains 86% theophylline by weight, this is approximately equivalent to 6 mg/kg of aminophylline. If administered intravenously, the loading dose should be given over 30 minutes, since rapid injection ("IV push") may result in transient toxic plasma levels with the risk of seizures or cardiac arrhythmias.

The plasma clearance of theophylline has been shown to vary widely among healthy subjects and even more so among patients. Because theophylline is metabolized by the liver, changes in hepatic function can alter the drug's half-life. For example, a decrease in hepatic function from cirrhosis or decrease in hepatic blood flow from heart failure may decrease plasma clearance and lead to toxic concentrations of the drug. Induction of hepatic enzymes by cigarette smoking or by changes in diet may increase plasma clearance and cause inadequate concentrations of drug. In normal adults, the mean plasma clearance is

0.69 mL/kg/min. Children appear to clear theophylline faster than adults (1–1.5 mL/kg/min). Neonates and young infants have the slowest clearance (Chapter 63). Even when maintenance doses are altered to correct for the above factors, plasma concentrations vary widely.

For intravenous maintenance therapy, an infusion rate of 0.7 mg/kg/h may be used in stable patients; but in acutely ill patients, it should be decreased to approximately 0.6 mg/kg/h. In the presence of liver disease or heart failure, the dose should be decreased further (approximately 0.3 mg/kg/h). Theophylline levels should be measured 24 hours after starting treatment. For oral therapy, an initial dose equivalent to 3–4 mg/kg of theophylline every 6 hours is appropriate. Changes in dosage will result in a new steady-state concentration of theophylline in 1–2 days, so the dose may be increased at intervals of 2–3 days until therapeutic plasma concentrations are achieved (10–20 mg/L) or until side effects develop.

SYMPATHOMIMETIC AGENTS

The adrenoceptor agonists, discussed in detail in Chapter 8, have several pharmacologic actions that are important in the treatment of asthma—ie, they relax airway smooth muscle and inhibit release of bronchoconstricting substances from mast cells. They may also increase mucociliary transport by increasing ciliary activity or by affecting the composition of mucous secretions. These effects may result from stimulation of adenylate cyclase, which catalyzes the formation of cAMP, although the exact role of increased intracellular concentrations of cAMP is still uncertain.

The best-characterized bronchodilator action of the adrenoceptor agonists on airways is relaxation of airway smooth muscle. Although there is no evidence for direct sympathetic innervation of human airway smooth muscle, there is evidence for the presence of adrenoceptors on airway smooth muscle. In general, stimulation of β_2 **receptors** relaxes airway smooth muscle, inhibits mediator release, and causes skeletal muscle tremor as a toxic effect.

The sympathomimetic agents most widely used in the treatment of asthma include epinephrine, ephedrine, isoproterenol, and a number of β_2-selective agents (Fig 18–4). Because epinephrine and isoproterenol cause more cardiac stimulation (mediated by β_1 receptors), they should probably be reserved for special situations (see below). Ephedrine has no advantages over more selective agents except low cost, and it should be avoided if possible.

Epinephrine is an effective, rapidly acting bronchodilator when injected subcutaneously (0.4 mL of 1:1000 solution) or inhaled as a microaerosol from a pressurized canister (320 μg per puff). Maximal bronchodilatation is achieved 15 minutes after inhalation and lasts 60–90 minutes. Because epinephrine stimulates β_1 as well as β_2 receptors, tachycardia, arrhyth-

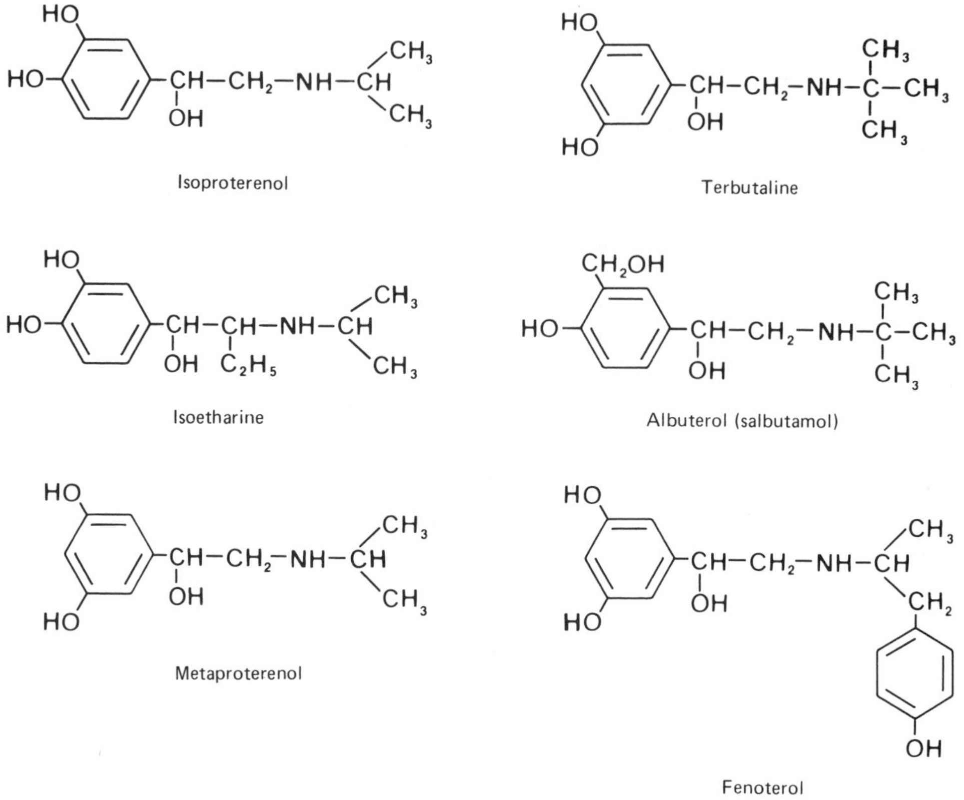

Figure 18–4. Structures of isoproterenol and several β_2-selective analogs.

mias, and worsening of angina pectoris are troublesome side effects.

Ephedrine probably has the longest history of any drug used in treating asthma, for it was used in China for more than 2000 years before it was introduced into Western medicine in 1924. Compared to epinephrine, ephedrine has a longer duration, oral activity, more pronounced central effects, and much lower potency. Because of the development of more efficacious and β_2-selective agonists, ephedrine is now used infrequently in treating asthma. It is available in 25- and 50-mg capsules and tablets but is most often prescribed in fixed-dose combination with theophylline and a sedative in commercial preparations. These fixed-dose combinations make adjustment of dosage of the individual agents impossible and should be avoided.

Isoproterenol is a potent bronchodilator; when inhaled as a microaerosol from a pressurized canister, 80–120 μg causes maximal bronchodilatation within 5 minutes. When the drug is given as an aerosolized solution from a nebulizer, the larger particle size generated results in a smaller quantity being delivered to the tracheobronchial tree, so larger doses must be given to achieve the same effect. Isoproterenol has a 60- to 90-minute duration of action. Cardiac side effects (tachycardia, arrhythmias) can occur. Cardiac arrhythmias resulting from the use of high doses of inhaled isoproterenol may have caused the increase in

mortality rate from asthma that occurred in Europe in the late 1960s. In the USA, where high-dose preparations were not available, this increase in mortality rate did not occur.

Beta$_2$-selective drugs. A new generation of adrenoceptor agonist drugs, effective after oral administration, with a long duration of action and a significant degree of β_2 selectivity, has recently become available (Fig 18–4). These agents differ structurally from epinephrine in having a larger substitution on the amino group and in the position of the hydroxyl groups on the aromatic ring. **Metaproterenol (Alupent, Metaprel), albuterol (Proventyl, Ventolin),** and **bitolterol (Tornalate)** are available as metered-dose inhalers; metaproterenol solution (5%) can be diluted in 0.3–1.5 mL of saline for delivery from a hand-held nebulizer. When given by inhalation, these agents cause bronchodilatation equivalent to that produced by isoproterenol. Bronchodilatation is maximal by 30 minutes and persists for 3–4 hours.

Metaproterenol and **terbutaline (Brethine, Bricanyl)** are prepared in tablet form (20 mg and 5 mg, respectively). One tablet 3 times daily is the usual regimen; the principal side effects of skeletal muscle tremor, nervousness, and occasional weakness may be reduced by starting the patient on half-strength tablets for the first 2 weeks of therapy.

Only terbutaline is available for subcutaneous injection (0.25 mg). The indications for this route are similar to those for subcutaneous epinephrine—severe asthma requiring treatment in hospital—but it should be remembered that terbutaline's longer duration of action means that cumulative effects may be seen after repeated injections.

Although adrenoceptor agonists may be administered by inhalation or by the oral or parenteral routes, delivery by inhalation will result in the greatest local effect on airway smooth muscle with the least systemic toxicity. Aerosol deposition depends on the particle size, the pattern of breathing (tidal volume and rate of airflow), and the geometry of the airways. Even with particles in the optimal size range of 2–5μm, 80–90% of the total dose of aerosol is deposited in the mouth or pharynx. Particles under 1–2 μm in size remain suspended and may be exhaled. Deposition can be increased by holding the breath in inspiration.

Use of sympathomimetic agents by inhalation at first raised fears about possible tachyphylaxis or tolerance to β-agonists, cardiac arrhythmias from β_1-adrenoceptor stimulation and hypoxemia, and arrhythmias from fluorinated hydrocarbons in Freon propellants. The concept that beta-agonist drugs cause worsening of clinical asthma by inducing tachyphylaxis to their own action remains unestablished. Most studies have shown only a small change in airway smooth muscle response to beta stimulation after prolonged treatment with beta-agonist drugs. Other experiments have demonstrated that arterial oxygen tension (P_{aO2}) may decrease after administration of beta-agonists if ventilation-perfusion ratios in the lung worsen. This effect may occur, however, with any class of bronchodilator drug, and the significance of such an effect will depend on the initial P_{aO2} of the patient. Supplemental oxygen may be necessary if the initial P_{aO2} is decreased markedly or if there is a large decrease in P_{aO2} during treatment with bronchodilators. Finally, there is concern over myocardial toxicity from Freon propellants contained in all of the commercially available metered-dose canisters. While fluorocarbons may sensitize the heart to toxic effects of catecholamines, such an effect occurs only at very high myocardial concentrations, which are not achieved if inhalers are used as recommended. In general, β_2-adrenoceptor agonists are safe and effective bronchodilators when given in doses that avoid systemic side effects.

MUSCARINIC ANTAGONISTS

Leaves from *Datura stramonium* have been used in treating asthma for hundreds of years. Interest in the potential value of antimuscarinic agents has recently been increased by demonstration of the importance of the vagus nerves in bronchospastic responses of laboratory animals and by the development of a potent antimuscarinic agent that is poorly absorbed after aerosol administration to the airways and that is therefore unassociated with systemic atropine effects.

Mechanism of Action in Asthma

Muscarinic antagonists competitively inhibit the effect of acetylcholine at muscarinic receptors (Chapter 7). In the airways, acetylcholine is released from efferent endings of the vagus nerves, and muscarinic antagonists can effectively block the contraction of airway smooth muscle and the increase in secretion of mucus that occurs in response to vagal activity. Very high concentrations—well above those achieved even with maximal therapy—are required to inhibit the response of airway smooth muscle to nonmuscarinic stimulation. This selectivity of muscarinic antagonists accounts for their usefulness as investigative tools in examining the role of parasympathetic pathways in bronchomotor responses but limits their usefulness in preventing bronchospasm. In the doses given, antimuscarinic agents inhibit only that portion of the response mediated by muscarinic receptors, and the involvement of parasympathetic pathways in bronchospastic responses appears to vary among individuals.

Clinical Use of Muscarinic Antagonists

Antimuscarinic agents are effective bronchodilators. When given intravenously, atropine, the prototypical muscarinic antagonist (Chapter 7), causes bronchodilatation at a lower dose than that needed to cause an increase in heart rate. The selectivity of atropine's effect can be increased further by administering the drug by inhalation. Studies of atropine sulfate aerosol have shown that it can cause an increase in baseline airway caliber—equivalent to that achieved with beta-agonist agents—and that this effect persists for 5 hours. In patients with emphysema, the bronchodilatation achieved may exceed what is obtainable with beta-agonist agents. The dose required depends on the particle size of the aerosol used. Using a nebulizer producing particles with a diameter of 1–1.5 μm, systemic effects commonly occur when 2 mg is inhaled. The initial dose, then, should be 1 mg or less. Deposition of the aerosol in the mouth frequently causes a local drying effect. Side effects due to systemic absorption include urinary retention, tachycardia, loss of visual accommodation, and agitation.

The dose of an antimuscarinic drug causing maximal change in resting airway caliber is smaller than the dose needed to maximally inhibit bronchospastic responses (Fig 18–5), probably because the quantity of acetylcholine released under resting conditions is smaller than the quantity released in response to an inhaled irritant. This is an important consideration in treating patients with asthma, for asthma is characterized by episodic bouts of bronchospasm, often occurring in response to exercise or to inhalation of antigens or irritants.

Systemic side effects limit the quantity of atropine sulfate that can be given, but the development of a more selective quaternary ammonium derivative of atropine, **ipratropium bromide (Atrovent),** permits delivery of high doses to muscarinic receptors in the airways because the compound is poorly absorbed and does not enter the central nervous system readily.

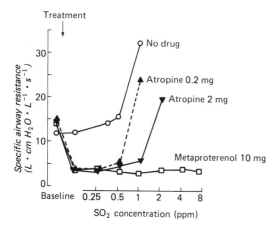

Figure 18–5. Inhibition of bronchomotor response to sulfur dioxide by 2 doses of atropine sulfate and by 10 mg of metaproterenol aerosol in one asthmatic subject. Specific airway resistance was measured after 5 minutes of eucapnic hyperpnea (40 L/min) of filtered air containing increasing amounts of SO_2. Note that all treatments caused equal changes in baseline specific resistance but different degrees of inhibition of the response to SO_2.

Studies with this agent have shown that the degree of involvement of parasympathetic pathways in bronchomotor responses varies among subjects. In some, bronchoconstriction is inhibited effectively. In others, bronchoconstriction is inhibited only modestly. That administration of higher doses of the muscarinic antagonist fails to inhibit the response further implies that mechanisms other than parasympathetic reflex pathways must be involved.

Even in the subjects least protected by this antimuscarinic agent, however, the degree of bronchodilatation and inhibition of provoked bronchoconstriction are of potential clinical value, and antimuscarinic agents may be valuable for patients intolerant of inhaled beta-agonist agents. At present, only atropine sulfate is approved for use in the USA, although ipratropium bromide is available elsewhere and is undergoing clinical trials here.

CORTICOSTEROIDS

Although corticosteroids have been used to treat asthma since 1950, their precise mechanism of action remains unknown. Like cromolyn, these drugs do not relax airway smooth muscle directly, but they may produce marked increases in airway caliber if administered for some time to asthmatic patients. Some studies suggested that corticosteroids may decrease airway obstruction by potentiating the effects of beta-receptor agonists, but most recent studies suggest that they work by inhibiting or otherwise modifying the inflammatory response in airways. For example, corticosteroids may inhibit the release of arachidonic acid from cell membranes and thereby inhibit the first step in the production of eicosanoid products from arachidonic acid. Some of these products have potent effects on airway function and may be responsible for some of the abnormalities of airway function in asthmatic patients (Chapter 17). For that reason, there has also been a renewed interest in the use of other drugs that inhibit arachidonic acid metabolism for the treatment of asthma. These other drugs, known as nonsteroidal anti-inflammatory drugs, act by inhibiting the conversion of arachidonic acid by cyclooxygenase to its oxygenation products or by inhibiting the action of the products on the target cell. However, some of these drugs (eg, aspirin) may cause at least temporary worsening of airway function in some asthmatic patients, possibly by increasing leukotriene production via the alternative lipoxygenase pathway. Therefore, the usefulness of nonsteroidal anti-inflammatory drugs in the treatment of asthma remains uncertain.

Clinical Use of Corticosteroids

In addition to uncertainty over their mechanism of action, there is controversy over the indications for corticosteroids in the treatment of asthma and their appropriate dosage schedule. Because of severe adverse effects when given chronically, corticosteroids are generally reserved for patients who do not improve adequately with bronchodilators or who experience worsening symptoms despite maintenance bronchodilator therapy. Treatment is often begun with an oral dose of 30–60 mg of prednisone per day or an intravenous dose of 1 mg/kg of methylprednisolone every 6 hours; the daily dose is decreased gradually after airway obstruction has improved. In some patients, corticosteroid therapy can be discontinued in a week or 10 days, but in other patients symptoms may worsen as the dose is decreased to lower levels. Because adrenal suppression by corticosteroids is related to dose and because secretion of corticosteroids has a diurnal variation, low doses of corticosteroids may cause less adrenal suppression if taken early in the morning. Adrenal suppression can be better avoided by alternate-day treatment. This schedule is best achieved by gradually tapering 1 day's dose while increasing the alternate day's dose by the same amount.

Another effective method of decreasing systemic side effects due to corticosteroid therapy is to administer the drug as an aerosol. The introduction of lipid-soluble corticosteroids such as beclomethasone (Beclovent, Vanceril) offers an effective method of delivering corticosteroids to the airways with minimal systemic absorption and reduced adverse effects. An average daily dose of 400 μg of the inhaled drug (2 puffs 4 times daily) is often as effective as oral corticosteroids in mild to moderate asthma and appears to be equivalent to about 10–15 mg/d of prednisone. Larger doses of inhaled steroid preparations may be more effective but may also cause a greater incidence of adrenal suppression. A special problem caused by inhaled topical corticosteroids is the occurrence of oropharyngeal candidiasis. The drug is remarkably free of other complications, but when switching from chronic oral therapy to inhaled beclomethasone, the oral therapy must be tapered slowly to avoid precipitation of adrenal insufficiency.

CALCIUM INFLUX–BLOCKING DRUGS

Each of the cell functions that may become abnormal in patients with asthma—contraction of airway smooth muscle, secretion of mucus and of various mediators, and transmission along airway nerves—depends to some degree on the movement of calcium into cells. It is not surprising, therefore, that calcium channel blockers (Chapter 11) have been tried in the treatment of asthma. So far, the results have been disappointing.

Animal studies have shown that one of the calcium channel blockers, nifedipine, given intravenously or by inhalation, has no effect on baseline airway diameter but does significantly inhibit the airway narrowing that is induced by various stimuli. Studies of asthmatic patients after administration of either nifedipine or verapamil have now led to similar findings. In these patients, neither nifedipine given sublingually nor verapamil given by inhalation had any significant effect on baseline airway diameter, but each significantly inhibited the bronchoconstriction induced by exercise, hyperventilation, or inhalation of aerosolized histamine, methacholine, or antigen. In only one study, however, was protection against bronchoconstriction completely effective. Other studies showed only partial protection and showed considerable variability in drug effect between subjects. The reasons for the small effects of calcium channel blockers are uncertain.

II. CLINICAL PHARMACOLOGY OF DRUGS USED IN ASTHMA

Patients with mild asthma and only occasional symptoms generally require no more than an inhaled β-receptor agonist (eg, metaproterenol or albuterol) on an "as needed" basis. If symptoms occur more frequently (more than 2 attacks a month) and the patient requires frequent aerosol inhalations or if nocturnal symptoms occur, maintenance treatment should include an oral theophylline compound and an inhaled β_2 agent taken at 4-hour intervals during waking hours. If symptoms remain poorly controlled or if side effects become bothersome, it is important to check the plasma level of theophylline. If the level is in the therapeutic range (10–20 mg/L) and symptoms persist, an oral β-receptor agonist (eg, terbutaline, metaproterenol) may be added, although side effects such as headache and tremor often limit the dose and usefulness of these agents. There may be a therapeutic advantage, however, in combining theophylline and adrenergic treatment in low doses in patients who develop side effects from a high dose of either drug. Thus, the addition of an oral β_2-receptor agent will

cause increased bronchodilatation in a patient with plasma levels of theophylline below 10 mg/L but will have little effect on airway caliber in a patient with plasma levels in the therapeutic range (10–20 mg/L). This observation does not imply that an aerosolized sympathomimetic agent is of no value in patients taking oral theophylline, for the inhaled drug has greater effect on large central airways, whereas the oral drug has greatest effect on smaller, more peripheral airways. The combination of oral theophylline and an inhaled β_2-receptor agonist is, in fact, standard therapy in the USA, but some investigators have suggested that the combination may have adverse myocardial effects, causing ventricular tachyarrhythmias and sudden death. There are few data in the clinical literature to substantiate this suggestion, but it is supported by studies in animals. The issue is not resolved, but these agents should be used with caution in patients with myocardial disease or ventricular ectopy.

If airway obstruction remains severe despite bronchodilator therapy, corticosteroids may be started. After initial treatment with high doses of corticosteroids (eg, 30 mg/d of prednisone for 3 weeks), these drugs should be given in the lowest dose necessary to control symptoms. If possible, patients should then be converted to alternate-day corticosteroid therapy or therapy with inhaled beclomethasone.

A therapeutic trial of cromolyn is warranted in patients who require maintenance therapy with oral theophylline and an inhaled agent and in those whose symptoms occur seasonally or after clear-cut inciting stimuli such as exercise or exposure to animal dander or irritants. In a patient whose symptoms are continuous or occur without an obvious inciting stimulus, the value of cromolyn can only be established with a therapeutic trial of 40 mg inhaled 4 times a day for 4 weeks. If the patient responds to this therapy, the dose can be reduced to 20 mg 3 times daily.

The role of inhaled muscarinic antagonists in the treatment of asthma has not been defined. When adequate doses are given, their effect on baseline airway resistance is as great as that of the sympathomimetic drugs, such as isoproterenol. The airway effects of antimuscarinic and sympathomimetic drugs given in full doses are not additive—ie, administration of a sympathomimetic drug does not cause further bronchodilatation in a person who has been treated with an antimuscarinic agent. The converse is also true: The addition of an antimuscarinic agent causes only slight additional bronchodilatation beyond that achieved with treatment with an inhaled sympathomimetic agent. Furthermore, in subgroups of patients with airflow obstruction who have been identified as more responsive to antimuscarinic than to sympathomimetic drugs, the difference is very small.

When muscarinic antagonists are used for long-term treatment, they appear to be effective bronchodilators. Although it was predicted that muscarinic antagonists might "dry up" airway secretions, direct measurements of fluid volume secretion from single airway submucosal glands in animals show that atropine decreases secretory rates only slightly; however, the drug does prevent excessive secretion caused by vagal reflex stimulation. No cases of inspissation of mucus have been reported following administration of these drugs.

MANAGEMENT OF ACUTE ASTHMA

The treatment of acute attacks of asthma in patients reporting to the hospital requires more continuous assessment and objective measurement of lung function than is necessary for chronic outpatient therapy. Repeated measurements of arterial blood gas tensions and spirometry are generally necessary. For patients with mild attacks, inhalation of a beta-receptor agonist is as effective as subcutaneous injection of epinephrine. Both of these treatments are more effective than intravenous administration of aminophylline. Severe attacks require treatment with oxygen, bronchodilators, and corticosteroids. For example, the combination of β_2-agonist drugs given subcutaneously and by aerosol, aminophylline given by continuous intravenous infusion, and intravenous corticosteroids may all be necessary in severe attacks.

REFERENCES

Atkins PC, Norman ME, Zweiman B: Antigen-induced neutrophil chemotactic activity in man: Correlation with bronchospasm and inhibition by disodium cromoglycate. *J Allergy Clin Immunol* 1978;**62**:149.

Aubier M et al: Aminophylline improves diaphragmatic contractility. *N Engl J Med* 1981;**305**:249.

Austen KF, Orange RP: State of the art: Bronchial asthma. The possible role of the chemical mediators of immediate hypersensitivity in the pathogenesis of subacute chronic disease. *Am Rev Respir Dis* 1975;**112**:423.

Bernstein IL: Cromolyn sodium in the treatment of asthma: Changing concepts. *J Allergy Clin Immunol* 1981;**68**:247.

Bernstein IL, Johnson CL, Tse CST: Therapy with cromolyn sodium. *Ann Intern Med* 1978;**89**:228.

Boushey HA et al: State of the art: Bronchial hyperreactivity. *Am Rev Respir Dis* 1980;**121**:389.

Carrina J et al: Inhibition of exercise-induced asthma by a calcium antagonist, nifedipine. *Am Rev Respir Dis* 1981;**123**:156.

Cavanaugh MJ, Cooper DM: Inhaled atropine sulfate: Dose response characteristics. *Am Rev Respir Dis* 1976;**114**:517.

Gold WM, Kessler GF, Y DYC: Role of vagus nerves in experimental asthma in allergic dogs. *J Appl Physiol* 1972;**33**:719.

Gross NJ: Sch 1000: A new anticholinergic bronchodilator. [Ipratropium.] *Am Rev Respir Dis* 1975;**112**:823.

Gross NJ, Skorodin MS: Role of the parasympathetic system in airway obstruction due to emphysema. *N Engl J Med* 1984;**311**:421.

Jackson RT et al: Mortality from asthma: A new epidemic in New Zealand. *Br Med J* 1982;**285**:771.

Kay AB, Austen KF, Lichtenstein LM (editors): *Asthma: Physiology, Immunopharmacology, and Treatment.* Academic Press, 1984.

Lee TH et al: Exercise induced release of histamine and neutrophil chemotactic factor in atopic asthmatics. *J Allergy Clin Immunol* 1982;**70**:73.

Leifer KN, Wittig HJ: The beta-2 sympathomimetic aerosols in the treatment of asthma. *Ann Allergy* 1975;**35**:69.

Mahler DA et al: Sustained-release theophylline reduces dyspnea in nonreversible obstructive airway disease. *Am Rev Respir Dis* 1985;**131**:22.

McAllen MK, Kochanowski SJ, Shaw KM: Steroid aerosols in asthma: An assessment of betamethasone valerate. *Br Med J* 1974;**1**:171.

Murciano D et al: Effects of theophylline on diaphragmatic strength and fatigue in patients with chronic obstructive pulmonary disease. *N Engl J Med* 1984;**311**:349.

Paterson JW, Woolcock AJ, Shenfield GM: State of the art: Bronchodilator drugs. *Am Rev Respir Dis* 1979;**120**:1149.

Persson CGA et al: Differentiation between bronchodilation and universal adenosine antagonism among xanthine derivatives. *Life Sci* 1982;**30**:2181.

Piafsky KM, Ogilvie RI: Dosage of theophylline in bronchial asthma. *N Engl J Med* 1975;**292**:1218.

Santa Cruz R et al: Tracheal mucous velocity in normal man and patients with obstructive lung disease: Effects of terbutaline *Am Rev Respir Dis* 1974;**109**:458.

Van Arsdel PP, Paul GH: Drug therapy in the management of asthma. *Ann Intern Med* 1977;**87**:68.

Webb-Johnson JC, Webb-Johnson DC: Bronchodilator therapy. *N Engl J Med* 1977;**297**:476.

Introduction to the Pharmacology of CNS Drugs

19

Roger A. Nicoll, MD

Drugs acting on the central nervous system (CNS) are the most widely used group of pharmacologically active agents and have extremely important medical uses. The practice of modern surgery, for example, would be impossible without general anesthetic agents. In addition to their use in therapy, drugs acting on the central nervous system are used on a daily basis without prescription to increase the sense of well-being. Caffeine, alcohol, and nicotine are socially accepted drugs in many countries, and their consumption is practiced worldwide. Because some of the drugs in this group are addictive when they are injected, ingested, or inhaled, societies have found it necessary to control their use and availability.

The mechanisms by which various drugs act on the central nervous system are not always clearly understood. Since the causes of many of the conditions for which these drugs are used (schizophrenia, anxiety, etc) are themselves poorly understood, it is not surprising that in the past much of CNS pharmacology has been purely descriptive. However, technologic advances over the past decade have led to greater understanding of how these drugs act. Studies on the mechanism of drug action have been useful not only for investigating the cellular and molecular basis of the condition for which a particular drug is given but also in providing clues about how the central nervous system normally operates. This chapter provides a broad outline of the functional organization of the central nervous system as a basis for understanding the actions of drugs on it.

ION CHANNELS

The membranes of nerve cells contain 2 types of channels defined on the basis of the mechanisms controlling their gating (opening and closing). The first mechanism is that of membrane voltage-sensitive gating; the second is that of chemically activated gating.

The voltage-sensitive sodium channel—described in Chapter 13 for the heart—is an example of the first type and is very important in the central nervous system. In nerve cells, these channels are concentrated on the initial segment and the axon and are responsible for the fast action potential, which transmits the signal from cell body to nerve terminal. There are other voltage-sensitive channels on the cell body and initial segment, which act on a much slower time scale and modulate the rate at which the neuron discharges. For example, potassium channels opened by depolarization of the cell result in slowing of further depolarization and act as a brake to limit further action potential discharge.

Chemically activated channels, sometimes called receptor-operated channels, are opened by the action of neurotransmitters and other chemical agents. The gates of these channels are insensitive to membrane potential. Neurotransmitter receptors and their ion channels are concentrated on subsynaptic membranes, eg, the nicotinic neuromuscular receptor of the skeletal muscle end-plate.

Recent evidence suggests that the traditional view of completely separate electrically gated and chemically gated channels requires modification. In particular, some neurotransmitter receptors are coupled to voltage-sensitive channels via second messenger systems.

THE SYNAPSE & SYNAPTIC POTENTIALS

It was not until the advent of glass microelectrodes that permit intracellular recording that a detailed description of synaptic transmission was possible. It is now well established that communication between neurons in the central nervous system occurs through chemical synapses in the vast majority of cases. (A few instances of electrical coupling between neurons have been documented, and such coupling may play a role in synchronizing neuronal discharge. However, it is unlikely that these electrical synapses are an important site of drug action.) The events involved in the release of transmitter from the presynaptic terminal have been studied most extensively at the vertebrate neuromuscular junction and at the giant synapse of the squid. An action potential in the presynaptic fiber propagates into the synaptic terminal and activates voltage-sensitive calcium channels in the membrane of the terminal. Calcium flows into the terminal, and the increase in intraterminal calcium concentration promotes the fusion of synaptic vesicles with the presynaptic membrane. The transmitter contained in the vesicles is released into the synaptic cleft and diffuses to the receptors on the postsynaptic membrane.

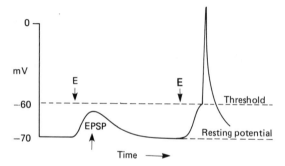

Figure 19–1. Excitatory synaptic potentials and spike generation. The figure shows a resting membrane potential of −70 mV in a postsynaptic cell. Stimulation of an excitatory pathway (E) generates transient depolarization. Increasing the stimulus strength increases the size of the depolarization, so that the threshold for spike generation is reached.

Binding of the transmitter to its receptor causes a brief change in membrane conductance (permeability to ions) of the postsynaptic cell. The time delay from the arrival of the presynaptic action potential to the onset of the postsynaptic response is approximately 0.5 ms. Most of this delay is consumed by the release process, particularly the time required for calcium channels to open.

The first systematic analysis of synaptic potentials in the central nervous system was by Eccles et al, who recorded intracellularly from spinal motoneurons in the early 1950s. When a microelectrode enters a cell, there is a sudden change in the potential recorded by the electrode, which is typically about −70 mV (Fig 19–1). This is the resting membrane potential of the neuron. Two types of pathways, excitatory and inhibitory, impinge on the motoneuron. When an excitatory pathway is stimulated, a small depolarization or excitatory postsynaptic potential (EPSP) is recorded (Fig 19–1). This potential is due to the excitatory transmitter activating a large increase in sodium and potassium permeability. The duration of these potentials is quite brief, usually less than 20 ms. Changing the stimulus intensity to the pathway and therefore the number of presynaptic fibers activated results in a graded change in the size of the depolarization. This indicates that the contribution a single fiber makes to the EPSP is quite small. When a sufficient number of excitatory fibers are activated, the EPSP depolarizes the postsynaptic cell to threshold, and an all-or-none action potential is generated.

When an inhibitory pathway is stimulated, the postsynaptic membrane is hyperpolarized, producing an inhibitory postsynaptic potential (IPSP) (Fig 19–2). A number of inhibitory synapses must be activated together to appreciably alter the membrane potential. This hyperpolarization is due to a selective increase in membrane permeability to chloride ions that flow into the cell during the IPSP. If an EPSP that under resting conditions would evoke an action potential in the post-

synaptic cell (Fig 19–2) is elicited during an IPSP, it no longer evokes an action potential, because the IPSP has moved the membrane potential farther away from the threshold for action potential generation. A second type of inhibition is termed presynaptic inhibition. In the central nervous system, this is limited to the sensory fibers entering the brain stem and spinal cord. The excitatory synaptic terminals of these sensory fibers receive synapses called axoaxonic synapses (Fig 19–4B). When activated, the axoaxonic synapses reduce the amount of transmitter released from the synapses of sensory fibers. Synaptic inhibition in an unanesthetized subject lasts tens of milliseconds.

SITES OF DRUG ACTION

Virtually all of the drugs that act on the central nervous system produce their effects by modifying some step in chemical synaptic transmission. Fig 19–3 illustrates some of the steps that can be altered. These transmitter-dependent actions can be divided into presynaptic and postsynaptic categories.

Drugs acting on the synthesis, storage, metabolism, and release of neurotransmitters fall into the presynaptic category. Synaptic transmission can be depressed by blockade of transmitter synthesis or storage. For example, *p*-chlorophenylalanine blocks the synthesis of serotonin, and reserpine depletes the synapses of monoamines by interfering with intracellular storage. Blockade of transmitter catabolism can increase transmitter concentrations and has been reported to increase the amount of transmitter released per impulse. Drugs can also alter the release of transmitter. Capsaicin induces the release of the peptide substance P from sensory neurons, and tetanus toxin blocks the release of inhibitory amino acid transmitters. After the transmitter has been released into the

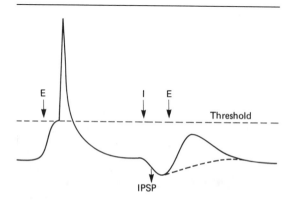

Figure 19–2. Interaction of excitatory and inhibitory synapses. On the left, a suprathreshold stimulus is given to an excitatory pathway (E). On the right, this same stimulus is given shortly after stimulating an inhibitory pathway (I), which prevents the excitatory potential from reaching threshold.

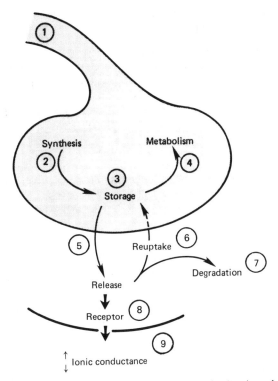

Figure 19–3. Sites of drug action. Schematic drawing of steps at which drugs can alter synaptic transmission. (1) Action potential in presynaptic fiber; (2) synthesis of transmitter; (3) storage; (4) metabolism; (5) release; (6) reuptake; (7) degradation; (8) receptor for the transmitter; (9) receptor-induced increase or decrease in ionic conductance.

ion channels, and receptor activation typically results in a brief (a few milliseconds to tens of milliseconds) opening of the channel. Drugs can act directly on the ion channel. For example, barbiturates enter and block the channel coupled to many excitatory neurotransmitter receptors. In other cases, receptors are coupled to enzymes, and receptor activation can lead to metabolic changes in the postsynaptic cell, most often as a consequence of elevations of cyclic nucleotide levels. Such metabolic changes can alter neuronal function by blocking voltage-sensitive ion channels. These effects can persist long after the transmitter has left the receptor, ie, tens of seconds to minutes. The methylxanthines are the best-known examples of drugs that can modify neurotransmitter responses mediated through cAMP. At high concentrations, the methylxanthines elevate the level of cAMP by blocking its metabolism and thereby prolong its action in the postsynaptic cell.

General anesthetics and ethanol are not thought to produce their effects by binding to specific receptors. Their actions are closely correlated with their hydrophobicity. These drugs are believed to decrease transmitter release and postsynaptic responsiveness by interacting with membrane lipids as well as membrane proteins.

As should be clear from the above discussion, the selectivity of drug action is based almost entirely on the fact that different transmitters are used by different groups of neurons. Furthermore, these various transmitters are often segregated into neuronal systems that subserve broadly different CNS functions. Without such segregation, it would be impossible to selectively modify CNS function even if one had a drug that operated on a single neurotransmitter system. It is not entirely clear why the central nervous system has relied on so many neurotransmitters and segregated them into different neuronal systems, since the primary function of a transmitter is either excitation or inhibition; this could be accomplished with 2 transmitter substances or perhaps even one. That such segregation does occur has provided neuroscientists with a powerful pharmacologic approach for analyzing CNS function and treating pathologic conditions.

IDENTIFICATION OF CENTRAL NEUROTRANSMITTERS

Since drug selectivity is based on the fact that different pathways utilize different transmitters, it is a primary goal of neuropharmacologists to identify the transmitters in CNS pathways. Establishing that a chemical substance is a transmitter has been far more difficult for central synapses than for peripheral synapses. In theory, to identify a transmitter it is sufficient to show that stimulation of a pathway releases enough of the substance to produce the postsynaptic response. In practice, this experiment cannot be done satisfactorily for at least 2 reasons. First, the anatomic complexity of the central nervous system prevents the selective activation of a single set of synaptic terminals. Second, available techniques for measuring the

synaptic cleft, its action is terminated either by uptake or degradation. For most neurotransmitters, there are uptake mechanisms into the synaptic terminal and also into surrounding neuroglia. Cocaine, for example, blocks the uptake of catecholamines at adrenergic synapses and thus potentiates the action of these amines. However, acetylcholine is inactivated by enzymatic degradation. Anticholinesterases block the degradation of acetylcholine and thereby prolong its action. No uptake mechanism has been found for any of the numerous recently discovered CNS peptides, and it has yet to be demonstrated whether specific enzymatic degradation terminates the action of peptide transmitters.

In the postsynaptic region, the transmitter receptor provides the primary site of drug action. Drugs can act either as neurotransmitter agonists, such as the opiates, which mimic the action of enkephalin, or they can block receptor function. Receptor antagonism is a common mechanism of action for CNS drugs. An example is strychnine's blockade of the receptor for the inhibitory transmitter glycine. This block is thought to be the mechanism underlying strychnine's convulsant action. Receptors are generally coupled to one of 2 transduction mechanisms. The receptors at most synapses in the central nervous system are coupled to released transmitter and applying the transmitter are not sufficiently precise to satisfy the quantitative requirements. Therefore, the following criteria have been established for transmitter identification.

Localization

A number of approaches have been used to prove that a suspected transmitter resides in the presynaptic terminal of the pathway under study. These include biochemical analysis of regional concentrations of suspected transmitters, often combined with interruption of specific pathways, and microcytochemical techniques. Immunocytochemical techniques have proved very useful in localizing peptides and enzymes that synthesize or degrade nonpeptide transmitters.

Release

To determine whether the substance can be released from a particular region, local collection (in vivo) of the extracellular fluid can sometimes be accomplished. In addition, in vitro slices of brain tissue can be stimulated electrically or chemically and the released substances measured. To determine if the release is relevant to synaptic transmission, it is important to establish that the release is calcium-dependent. As mentioned above, anatomic complexity often prevents identification of the synaptic terminals responsible for the release, and the amount collected in the perfusate is a small fraction of the amount actually released.

Synaptic Mimicry

Finally, application of the suspected substance should produce a response that mimics the action of the transmitter released by nerve stimulation. Microiontophoresis, which permits highly localized drug administration, has been a valuable technique in assessing the action of suspected transmitters. In practice, this criterion has 2 parts: physiologic and pharmacologic identity. To establish physiologic identity of action, the substance must be shown to initiate the same change in ionic conductance in the postsynaptic cell as synaptically released transmitter. This requires intracellular recording and determination of the reversal potential and ionic dependencies of the responses. However, since different transmitters can elicit identical ionic conductance changes, this finding is not sufficient. Thus, selective pharmacologic antagonism is used to further establish that the suspected transmitter is acting in a manner identical to synaptically released transmitter. Pharmacologic antagonism can be studied with extracellular recording and can therefore be used in those instances when it is technically impossible to obtain intracellular recordings.

CELLULAR ORGANIZATION OF THE BRAIN

Neuronal systems in the central nervous system can be divided in many instances into 2 broad categories: hierarchical systems and nonspecific or diffuse neuronal systems.

Hierarchical Systems

These systems include all of the pathways directly involved in sensory perception and motor control. The pathways are generally clearly delineated, being composed of large myelinated fibers that can often conduct action potentials in excess of 50 m/s. The information is typically phasic, and in sensory systems the information is processed sequentially by successive integrations at each relay nucleus on its way to the cortex. A lesion at any link will incapacitate the system. Within each nucleus and in the cortex, there are 2 types of cells: relay or projection neurons and local circuit neurons (Fig 19–4A). The projection neurons that form the interconnecting pathways transmit signals over long distances. The cell bodies are relatively large, and their axons emit collaterals that arborize extensively in the vicinity of the neuron. These neurons are excitatory, and their synaptic influences are very short-lived. The excitatory transmitter released from these cells is not known, but aspartate and glutamate are leading candidates at many sites. Local circuit neurons are typically smaller than projection neurons, and their axons arborize in the immediate vicinity of the cell body. The vast majority of these neurons are inhibitory, and they release either gamma-aminobutyric acid (GABA) or glycine. They synapse primarily on the cell body of the projection neurons but can also synapse on the dendrites of projection neurons as well as with each other. A special class of local circuit neurons in the spinal cord forms axoaxonic synapses on the terminals of sensory axons (Fig 19–4B). Two common types of pathways for these neurons (Fig 19–4A) include recurrent feedback pathways and feed-forward pathways. In many sensory pathways, local circuit neurons may actually lack an axon and release neurotransmitter from dendritic synapses in a graded fashion in the absence of action potentials. Some pathways involving presynaptic dendrites of local circuit neurons are shown in Fig 19–4C.

Although there is a great variety of synaptic connections in these hierarchical systems, the fact that a limited number of transmitters are utilized by these neurons indicates that any major pharmacologic manipulation of this system will have a profound effect on the overall excitability of the central nervous system. For instance, selectively blocking GABA receptors with a drug such as picrotoxin results in generalized convulsions. Thus, while the mechanism of action of picrotoxin is quite specific in blocking the effects of GABA, the overall functional effect appears to be quite nonspecific, since GABA-mediated synaptic inhibition is so ubiquitous.

Nonspecific or Diffuse Neuronal Systems

Those neuronal systems that contain one of the monoamines—norepinephrine, dopamine, or 5-hydroxytryptamine (serotonin)—provide typical exam-

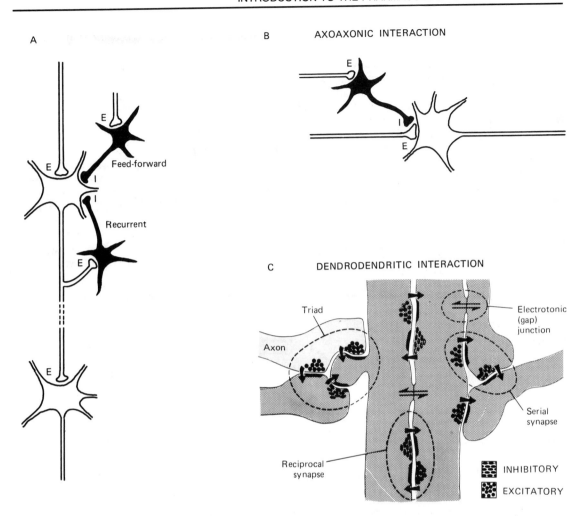

Figure 19–4. Pathways in the central nervous system. *A* shows 2 relay neurons and 2 types of inhibitory pathways, recurrent and feed-forward. The inhibitory neurons are shown in black. *B* shows the pathway responsible for presynaptic inhibition in which the axon of an inhibitory neuron synapses on the axon terminal of an excitatory fiber. *C:* Diagram illustrating that dendrites may be both pre- and postsynaptic to each other, forming reciprocal synapses, 2 of which are shown between the same dendrite pair. In triads, an axon synapses on 2 dendrites, and one of these dendrites synapses on the second. In serial synapses, a dendrite may be postsynaptic to one dendrite and presynaptic to another, thus connecting a series of dendrites. Dendrites also interact through low-resistance electrotonic ("gap") junctions (2 of which are shown). Except for one axon, all structures shown in *C* are dendrites. (Reproduced, with permission, from Schmitt FO, Dev P, Smith BH: Electrotonic processing of information by brain cells. *Science* 1976;**193:**114 Copyright © 1976 by the American Association for the Advancement of Science.)

ples in this category. Certain other pathways emanating from the reticular formation and possibly some peptide-containing pathways also fall into this category. These systems differ in fundamental ways from the hierarchical systems, and the noradrenergic systems will serve to illustrate the differences.

Noradrenergic cell bodies are found primarily in a compact cell group called the locus ceruleus located in the caudal pontine central gray matter. The number of neurons in this cell group is quite small, approximately 1500 on each side of the brain in the rat. The axons of these neurons are very fine and unmyelinated. Indeed, they were entirely missed with classic anatomic techniques. It was not until the mid 1960s,

when the formaldehyde fluorescence histochemical technique was applied to the study of CNS tissues, that the anatomy of the monoamine-containing systems was described. Because these axons are fine and unmyelinated, they conduct very slowly, in the range of 0.5 m/s. The axons branch repeatedly and are extraordinarily divergent. Branches from the same neuron can innervate several functionally different parts of the central nervous system. In the neocortex, these fibers have a tangential organization and therefore can monosynaptically influence large areas of cortex. The pattern of innervation in the cortex and nuclei of the hierarchical systems is diffuse, and the fibers form a very small percentage of the total number in the area.

In addition, the axons are studded with periodic enlargements called varicosities that contain large numbers of vesicles. In many instances, these varicosities do not form synaptic contacts, suggesting that norepinephrine may be released in a rather diffuse manner, as occurs with the noradrenergic innervation of smooth muscle. This indicates that the cellular targets of these systems will be determined largely by the location of the receptors rather than the location of the release sites. Based on all of these observations, it is clear that the monoamine systems cannot be conveying specific topographic types of information—rather, vast areas of the central nervous system must be affected simultaneously and in a rather uniform way. It is not surprising, then, that these systems have been implicated in such global functions as sleeping and waking, attention, appetite, and emotional states.

CENTRAL NEUROTRANSMITTERS

A number of small molecules have been isolated from brain (Table 19–1), and studies using a variety of approaches suggest that these agents may be neurotransmitters. A brief summary of the evidence for some of these compounds follows.

Amino Acids

The amino acids of primary interest to the pharmacologist fall into 2 categories: the neutral amino acids glycine and gamma-aminobutyric acid (GABA), and the acidic amino acids glutamate and aspartate. All of these compounds are present in high concentrations in the central nervous system and are extremely potent in modifying neuronal excitability. The neutral amino acids are inhibitory and increase membrane perme-

Table 19–1. Summary of nonpeptide neurotransmitter pharmacology in the central nervous system.

Transmitter	Anatomy	Receptor Subtypes and Preferred Agonists	Antagonists	Receptor Mechanisms*
Acetylcholine	Cell bodies at all levels; long and short connections.	Muscarinic (M_1): muscarine, McN-A-343	Pirenzepine, atropine	Excitatory: decrease in K^+ conductance.
		Muscarinic (M_2): muscarine	Atropine	Inhibitory: increase in K^+ conductance.
	Motoneuron–Renshaw cell synapse.	Nicotinic: nicotine	Dihydro-β-erythroidine	Excitatory: increase in cation conductance.
Dopamine	Cell bodies at all levels; short, medium, and long connections.	D_1	Phenothiazines	Inhibitory: (?), increases cAMP.
		D_2: apomorphine	Phenothiazines, butyrophenones	Inhibitory: (?), does not increase cAMP.
GABA	Supraspinal interneurons; spinal interneurons involved in presynaptic inhibition.	$GABA_A$: muscimol	Bicuculline, picrotoxin	Inhibitory: increase in Cl^- conductance.
		$GABA_B$: baclofen		Inhibitory (presynaptic): possibly due to decrease in Ca^{2+} conductance. Inhibitory (postsynaptic): increase in K^+ conductance.
Glutamate; aspartate	Relay neurons at all levels.	N-Methyl-D-aspartate	2-Amino-5-phosphonovalerate	Excitatory: increase in cation conductance.
		Quisqualate	Glutamate diethylester	
		Kainate		
Glycine	Spinal interneurons and some brain stem interneurons.	Taurine, β-alanine	Strychnine	Inhibitory: increase in Cl^- conductance.
5-Hydroxytryptamine (serotonin)	Cell bodies in midbrain and pons project to all levels.	$5\text{-}HT_1$: LSD	Metergoline	Inhibitory: increase in K^+ conductance.
		$5\text{-}HT_2$: LSD	Ketanserin	Excitatory: (?)
Norepinephrine	Cell bodies in pons and brain stem project to all levels.	Alpha$_1$: phenylephrine	Prazosin	Excitatory: decrease in K^+ conductance.
		Alpha$_2$: clonidine	Yohimbine	Inhibitory: increase in K^+ conductance.
		Beta: isoproterenol	Propranolol, practolol	Excitatory: decrease in K^+ conductance mediated by cAMP. Inhibitory: may involve increase in electrogenic sodium pump.

*Predicted in some cases on the basis of peripheral actions.

ability to chloride ions, thus mimicking the IPSP. Glycine concentrations are particularly high in the gray matter of the spinal cord, and destruction of the neurons in this area results in a marked fall in the concentration of glycine. In addition, strychnine, which is a potent spinal cord convulsant and has been used in some rat poisons, selectively antagonizes both the action of glycine and the IPSPs recorded in spinal cord neurons. Thus, it is generally agreed that glycine is released from spinal cord inhibitory local circuit neurons involved in postsynaptic inhibition. There is also good evidence that GABA is a widespread postsynaptic inhibitory transmitter in the brain. The IPSPs in most regions of the brain are blocked by the GABA antagonists picrotoxin and bicuculline, which both cause generalized convulsions. Immunohistochemical studies indicate that a large majority of the local circuit neurons synthesize GABA. A special class of local circuit neuron localized in the dorsal horn of the spinal cord also synthesizes GABA. These neurons form axoaxonic synapses with primary sensory nerve terminals and are responsible for presynaptic inhibition (Fig 19–4B).

Both glutamate and aspartate are also present in very high concentrations in the central nervous system. Virtually all neurons that have been tested are strongly excited by these 2 amino acids. This excitation is due primarily to an increase in sodium permeability. However, the lack of selective antagonists has greatly limited research in this area. Thus, the evidence has come primarily from biochemical studies which have shown either (1) that glutamate or aspartate concentrations in a particular region fall when specific excitatory pathways to the region are cut, or (2) that the calcium-dependent release of either amino acid is reduced after such lesions.

Acetylcholine

Acetylcholine was the first compound to be identified pharmacologically as a transmitter in the central nervous system. Eccles showed in the early 1950s that excitation of Renshaw cells by motor axon collaterals was blocked by nicotinic antagonists. Furthermore, Renshaw cells were extremely sensitive to nicotinic agonists. These experiments were remarkable for 2 reasons. First, this early success at identifying a transmitter for a central synapse was followed by disappointment, because it remained the sole pathway for which the transmitter was known until the late 1960s, when comparable data became available for the neutral amino acids. Second, the motor axon collateral synapse remains the only clearly documented example of a cholinergic nicotinic synapse in the mammalian central nervous system. Most acetylcholine-sensitive neurons in the central nervous system appear to be excited primarily through a muscarinic receptor. The muscarinic effects have a much slower time course than either nicotinic effects on Renshaw cells or the effect of amino acids. Furthermore, this muscarinic excitation is unusual in that acetylcholine produces it by *decreasing* the membrane

ion permeability to potassium, ie, the opposite of conventional transmitter action. A number of pathways contain acetylcholine, including neurons in the neostriatum, the medial septal nucleus, and the reticular formation. Until recently, progress in their investigation has been hampered by the lack of precise histochemical techniques. The introduction of monoclonal antibodies that bind to the synthetic enzyme choline acetyltransferase has greatly improved the histochemical localization of this transmitter. Cholinergic pathways appear to play an important role in cognitive functions, especially memory. It has been found that presenile dementia of the Alzheimer type is associated with a profound and relatively selective loss of cholinergic neurons.

Monoamines

These include the catecholamines (dopamine and norepinephrine) and 5-hydroxytryptamine (serotonin). Although these compounds are present in very small amounts in the central nervous system, extremely sensitive histochemical methods are available for localizing them. The methods include formaldehyde-induced fluorescence of the monoamines and immunohistochemical methods for localizing the individual synthetic enzymes.

A. Dopamine: The major pathways containing dopamine are the projection linking the substantia nigra to the neostriatum and the projection linking the ventral tegmental region to limbic structures, particularly the limbic cortex. The therapeutic action of the antiparkinsonism drug levodopa is associated with the former area, whereas the therapeutic action of the antipsychotic drugs is thought to be associated with the latter area. Dopamine-containing neurons are also present in the tuberobasal ventral hypothalamus and play an important role in regulating hypothalamo-hypophyseal function. Dopamine generally exerts a slow inhibitory action on CNS neurons, and this effect may be mediated through cAMP.

B. Norepinephrine: This system has already been discussed. Most noradrenergic neurons are located in the locus ceruleus or the lateral tegmental area of the reticular formation. Although the density of fibers innervating various sites differs considerably, most regions of the central nervous system receive diffuse noradrenergic input. When applied to neurons, norepinephrine produces a slow inhibition of spontaneous activity accompanied by hyperpolarization. In spite of this inhibitory effect, norepinephrine actually enhances excitatory inputs; this effect often predominates, so that the overall effect is to facilitate transmission. This enhancement of excitatory input occurs by both indirect and direct mechanisms. The indirect mechanism involves disinhibition, ie, inhibition of inhibitory local circuit neurons. The direct mechanism involves blockade of a potassium conductance that acts as a brake on neuronal discharge. This direct action is mediated by cAMP. Facilitation of excitatory synaptic transmission is in accordance with many of the behavioral processes thought to involve noradrenergic pathways—attention, arousal, etc.

C. 5-Hydroxytryptamine (Serotonin): Most 5-HT pathways originate from neurons in the raphe or midline regions of the pons and upper brain stem. 5-Hydroxytryptamine is contained in unmyelinated fibers that diffusely innervate most regions of the central nervous system, but the density of the innervation varies. In most areas of the central nervous system, 5-hydroxytryptamine has a strong inhibitory action. This is associated with membrane hyperpolarization that is due to an increase in potassium conductance. On some cell types, 5-hydroxytryptamine causes a slow excitation, which may be due to a blockade of potassium channels. Considerable speculation exists regarding the possible involvement of 5-hydroxytryptamine pathways in the hallucinations induced by LSD, since this compound can antagonize the peripheral actions of 5-hydroxytryptamine. However, LSD does not appear to be a 5-hydroxytryptamine antagonist in the central nervous system, and typical LSD-induced behavior is still seen in animals after destruction of raphe nuclei. Other proposed regulatory functions of 5-hydroxytryptamine–containing neurons include sleep, temperature, appetite, and neuroendocrine control.

D. Peptides: A great many CNS peptides have been discovered that produce dramatic effects both on animal behavior and on the activity of individual neurons. Some of the better known peptides have been mapped with immunohistochemical techniques and include opioid peptides (enkephalin, endorphins, etc), neurotensin, substance P, somatostatin, vasoactive intestinal polypeptide, and thyrotropin-releasing hormone. A particularly intriguing finding is that a peptide can coexist with a conventional nonpeptide transmitter in the same neuron. A good example of the approaches used to define the role of these peptides in the central nervous system comes from studies on substance P and its association with sensory fibers. Immunohistochemical studies have found substance P to be present in some of the small unmyelinated primary sensory neurons of the spinal cord and brain stem. In addition, stimulation of the sensory neurons releases substance P from the spinal cord. Application of substance P to neurons in the spinal cord excites neurons that are excited by painful stimuli. Painful stimuli are known to selectively activate unmyelinated sensory fibers. Thus, it is believed that substance P may be an excitatory transmitter released from unmyelinated fibers that respond to painful stimulation. Substance P is certainly involved in many other functions, since it is found in many areas of the central nervous system that are unrelated to pain pathways.

REFERENCES

Aghajanian GK, Rogawski MA: The physiological role of α-adrenoceptors in the CNS: New concepts from single-cell studies. *Trends Pharmacol Sci* 1983;**4:**315.

Bloom FE: The endorphins: A growing family of pharmacologically pertinent peptides. *Annu Rev Pharmacol Toxicol* 1983;**23:**344.

Bloom FE: The functional significance of neurotransmitter diversity. *Am J Physiol* 1984;**246(3–Part 1):**C184.

Bowery NG et al: Heterogeneity of mammalian GABA receptors. Pages 81–108 in: *Actions and Interactions of GABA and Benzodiazepines.* Bowery NG (editor). Raven Press, 1984.

Cooper JR, Bloom FE, Roth RH: *The Biochemical Basis of Neuropharmacology,* 2nd ed. Oxford Univ Press, 1978.

Costa E et al: Coexistence of neuromodulators: Biochemical and pharmacological consequences. (Symposium.) *Fed Proc* 1983;**42:**2910.

Coyle JT, Price DL, DeLong MR: Alzheimer's disease: A disorder of cortical cholinergic innervation. *Science* 1983;**219:**1184.

Creese I: Dopamine receptors explained. *Trends Neurosci* 1982;**5:**40.

Eccles JC: *The Physiology of Synapses.* Academic Press, 1964.

Hokfelt T et al: Peptidergic neurons. *Nature* 1980;**284:**515.

Iversen LL: Nonopioid neuropeptides in mammalian CNS. *Annu Rev Pharmacol Toxicol* 1983;**23:**1.

Iversen SD, Iversen, LL: *Behavioral Pharmacology,* 2nd ed. Oxford Univ Press, 1979.

Krieger DT: Brain peptides: What, where, and why? *Science* 1983;**222:**975.

Krnjević K: Acetylcholine receptors in vertebrate CNS. Pages 97–125 in: *Handbook of Psychopharmacology.* Vol 6. Iversen LL, Iversen SD, Snyder SH (editors). Plenum Press, 1975.

Krogsgaard-Larsen P, Honore T: Glutamate receptors and new glutamate agonists. *Trends Pharmacol Sci* 1983;**4:**31.

Lipton ME, Killam KC, DiMascio A (editors): *Psychopharmacology: A Generation of Progress.* Raven Press, 1978.

McGreer PL, Eccles JC, McGreer EG: *Molecular Neurobiology of the Mammalian Brain.* Plenum Press, 1978.

Moore RY, Bloom FE: Central catecholamine neuron systems: Anatomy and physiology. *Annu Rev Neurosci* 1978;**2:**113.

Nestler EJ, Greengard P: Protein phosphorylation in the brain. *Nature* 1983;**305:**583.

Nicoll RA: Neurotransmitters can say more than just "yes" or "no." *Trends Neurosci* 1982;**5:**369.

Nicoll RA, Schenker C, Leeman SE: Substance P as a transmitter candidate. *Annu Rev Neurosci* 1980;**3:**227.

Rakic P: Local circuit neurons. *Neurosci Res Program Bull* 1975;**13:**293.

Shepherd GM: *Neurobiology.* Oxford Univ Press, 1983.

Snyder SH: Drug and neurotransmitter receptors in the brain. *Science* 1984;**224:**22.

Watkins JC, Evans RH: Excitatory amino acid transmitters. *Annu Rev Pharmacol Toxicol* 1981;**21:**165.

Sedative-Hypnotics

20

Anthony J. Trevor, PhD, & Walter L. Way, MD

I. BASIC PHARMACOLOGY OF SEDATIVE-HYPNOTICS

Drug classifications are often based on clinical uses rather than on similarities in chemical structures or mechanisms of action. Assignment of a particular compound to the sedative-hypnotic class of drugs indicates that its major therapeutic use is to cause sedation (with concomitant relief of anxiety) or to encourage sleep. These clinical uses are of such magnitude that sedative-hypnotics are among the most frequently prescribed drugs worldwide.

An effective **sedative** (or anxiolytic agent) should reduce anxiety and exert a calming effect with little or no effect on motor or mental functions. The degree of central nervous system depression caused by a sedative should be the minimum consistent with therapeutic efficacy. A **hypnotic** drug should produce drowsiness and encourage the onset and maintenance of a state of sleep that as far as possible resembles the natural sleep state. Hypnotic effects involve more pronounced depression of the central nervous system than sedation, and this can be achieved with most sedative drugs simply by increasing the dose.

Graded dose-dependent depression of central nervous system function is a characteristic of sedative-hypnotics. However, individual sedative-hypnotic drugs may differ in the relationship between the dose and the degree of central nervous system depression. Two examples of such dose-response relationships are shown in Fig 20–1. The linear slope for drug A is typical of many of the older sedative-hypnotics, particularly drugs in the barbiturate class. An increase in dose above that needed for hypnosis may lead to a state of general anesthesia. At still higher doses, such sedative-hypnotics may depress respiratory and vasomotor centers in the medulla, leading to coma and death. Deviations from a linear dose-response relationship, as shown for drug B, will require proportionately greater dosage increments in order to achieve central nervous system depressant effects more profound than those required for hypnosis. This appears to be the case for most drugs of the benzodiazepine class, and the greater margin of safety this offers is an important reason for their extensive clinical use to treat anxiety states and disorders of sleep.

Chemical Classification

The benzodiazepines (Fig 20–2) are the most important sedative-hypnotics. All of the structures shown are 1,4-benzodiazepines, and most contain a carboxamide group in the 7-membered heterocyclic ring structure. A substituent in the 7 position, such as a halogen or a nitro group, is required for sedative-hypnotic activity. The structures of triazolam and alprazolam include 1,2-annelation of a triazole ring, and such drugs are sometimes referred to as triazolobenzodiazepines.

The chemical structures of some less commonly used sedative-hypnotics are shown in Fig 20–3. The barbiturates have been regarded as prototypes of the class because of their extensive use since their introduction approximately 80 years ago. The motivation to develop other sedative-hypnotics can be attributed to efforts to avoid certain undesirable features of the barbiturates, including their potential for addiction and physical dependence. Unfortunately, such efforts have not always been successful. For example, the piperidinediones such as glutethimide, introduced as "nonbarbiturates," are in fact chemically related and virtually indistinguishable from barbiturates in their pharmacologic properties. Because of the huge market

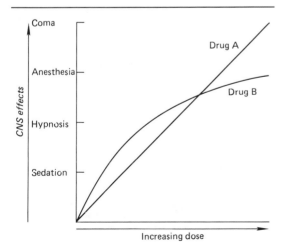

Figure 20–1. Theoretical dose-response curves for sedative-hypnotics.

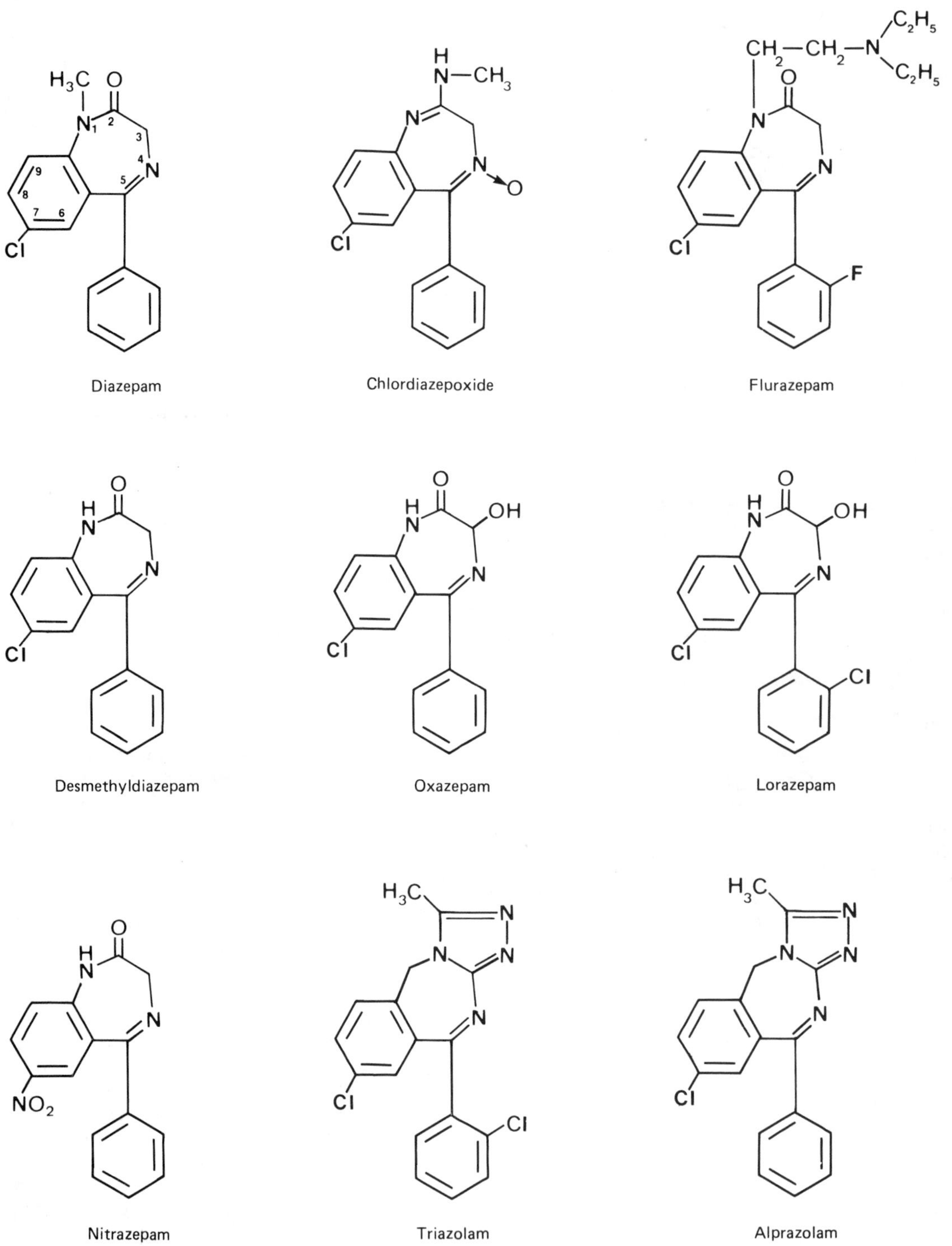

Figure 20–2. Chemical structures of benzodiazepines.

for sedative-hypnotics, such "failed attempts" have often been commercially successful. The propanediol carbamates such as meprobamate are of distinctive chemical structure but are practically equivalent to barbiturates in their pharmacologic effects, and their clinical use is rapidly declining. The sedative-hypnotic class also includes compounds of simple chemical structure, including alcohols (ethanol, chloral hydrate) and the cyclic ethers. Chloral hydrate and its congeners, such as trichloroethanol, together with paraldehyde (not shown), continue to be used, particularly in institutionalized patients.

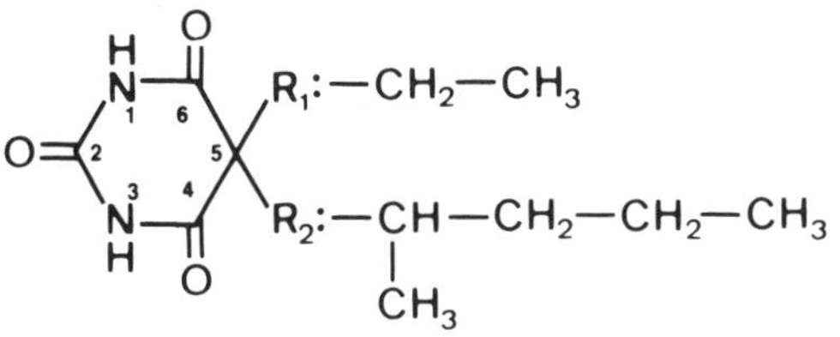

Pentobarbital

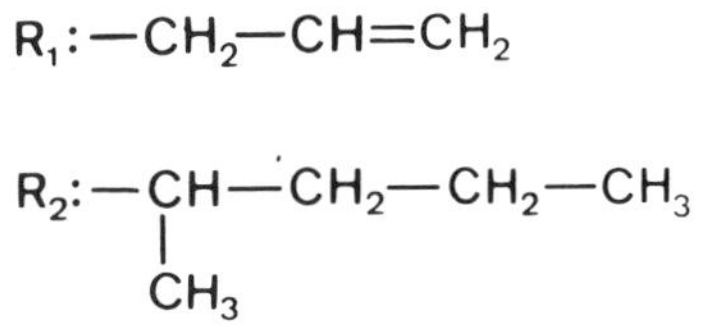

Secobarbital

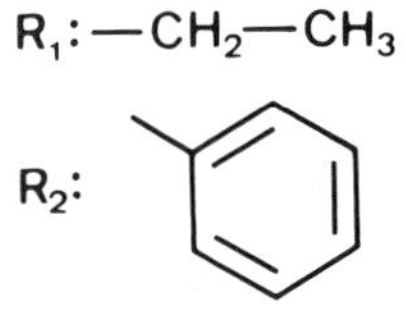

Phenobarbital

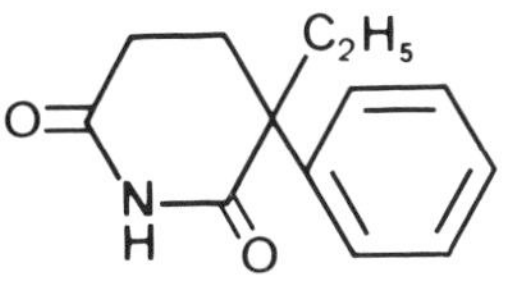

Glutethimide

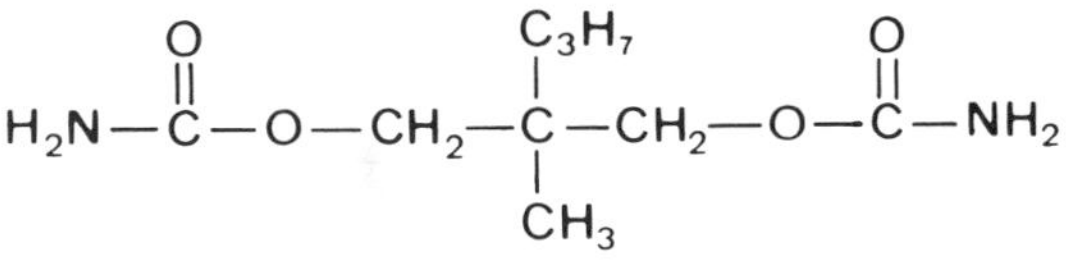

Meprobamate

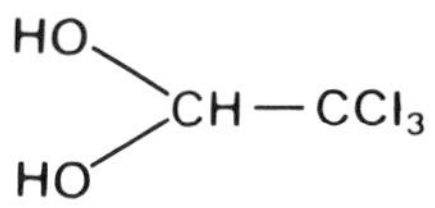

Chloral hydrate

$HO-CH_2-CCl_3$

Trichloroethanol

Figure 20–3. Chemical structures of barbiturates and other sedative-hypnotics.

Other classes of drugs not included in Fig 20–3 may exert sedative effects. For example, beta-blocking drugs are effective in certain anxiety states and functional disorders, particularly those in which somatic and autonomic symptoms are prominent. Sedative effects can also be obtained with the antipsychotic tranquilizers, the tricyclic antidepressant drugs, and antihistaminic agents. As discussed in other chapters, these agents are different from conventional sedative-hypnotics in both their effects and their major therapeutic uses. Most importantly, they do not produce general anesthesia and have low addiction liability. Since they commonly exert marked effects on the peripheral autonomic nervous system, they are sometimes referred to as "sedative-autonomic" drugs. Compounds of the antihistaminic type are present in a number of over-the-counter sleep preparations, and their autonomic properties as well as their long duration of action can result in unwanted side effects.

Pharmacokinetics

A. Absorption: When used to treat anxiety or sleep disorders, drugs of this class are usually given orally. The rates of oral absorption of sedative-hypnotics differ depending on a number of factors. Weakly basic drugs such as the benzodiazepines are absorbed most effectively at the high pH found in the duodenum, which may explain their somewhat slower onset of effect in comparison with that of the barbiturates (see below). Oral absorption of diazepam and the active metabolite of clorazepate is more rapid than that of the other commonly used benzodiazepines, whereas oxazepam is absorbed at the slowest rate. The benzodiazepine clorazepate is converted to its active form, desmethyldiazepam, by acid hydrolysis in the stomach. In the stomach (pH 1–2), weakly acidic drugs such as the barbiturates and the piperidinediones are nonionized and, since they are lipid-soluble, are usually absorbed very rapidly into the blood. One exception is glutethimide, which, because of its limited solubility in the aqueous gastric contents, may be absorbed slowly and erratically. The bioavailability of several benzodiazepines, including chlordiazepoxide and diazepam, may be unreliable after intramuscular injection.

B. Distribution: Transport of a sedative-hypnotic in the blood is a dynamic process in which drug molecules enter and leave tissues at rates dependent upon blood flow, concentration gradients, and permeabilities. Lipid solubility plays a major role in determining the rate at which a particular sedative-hypnotic enters the central nervous system. Diazepam is more lipid-soluble than chlordiazepoxide and lorazepam; thus, the central nervous system effects of the latter drugs may be slower in onset. The thiobarbiturates (eg, thiopental), in which the oxygen on C2 is replaced by sulfur, are very lipid-soluble, and a high rate of entry into the central nervous system contributes to the rapid onset of their central effects (see Chapter 23), whereas meprobamate has quite low solubility in lipids and penetrates the brain slowly even when given intravenously.

Redistribution of drug from the central nervous system to other tissues is an important feature of the biodisposition of sedative-hypnotics. Classic studies on the thiobarbiturates have shown that they are rapidly redistributed from the brain, first to highly perfused tissues such as skeletal muscle and subsequently to poorly perfused adipose tissue. These processes contribute to the termination of their major central nervous system effects. This may also be the case for other sedative-hypnotics, including the benzodiazepines, where the rate of metabolic transformation and elimination is much too slow in humans to account for the relatively short time required for dissipation of major pharmacologic effects.

Administration of sedative-hypnotics during pregnancy should be done with the recognition that the placental barrier to lipid-soluble drugs is incomplete and that all of these agents are capable of reaching the fetus. The rate of achievement of equilibrium between maternal and fetal blood is slower than that for the maternal blood and central nervous system, partly because of lower blood flow to the placenta. Nonetheless, if sedative-hypnotics are given in the predelivery period, they may contribute to the depression of neonatal vital functions.

Many sedative-hypnotics bind extensively to drug-binding sites on plasma proteins. For example, the binding of benzodiazepines to plasma albumin ranges between 80 and 97%. Since only free (nonbound) drug molecules have access to the central nervous system, the displacement of a sedative-hypnotic from plasma binding sites by another drug could modify its effects and possibly lead to drug interactions between this class and other pharmacologic agents. However, very few clinically significant interactions involving sedative-hypnotic drugs appear to be based on competition for common binding sites on the plasma proteins. One exception is chloral hydrate, which increases the anticoagulant effects of warfarin by its displacement from such binding sites.

C. Biotransformation: As noted above, redistribution to tissues other than the brain may be as important as biotransformation in terminating the central nervous system effects of many sedative-hypnotics. However, metabolic transformation to more water-soluble metabolites is necessary for final clearance from the body of almost all drugs in this class. The microsomal drug-metabolizing enzyme systems of the liver are most important in this regard. Since few sedative-hypnotics are excreted from the body unchanged, the elimination half-life ($t_{1/2\beta}$) of most drugs in this class depends mainly on the rate of their metabolic transformation.

1. Benzodiazepines–Hepatic metabolism accounts for the clearance or elimination of all benzodiazepines. The 2 major pathways involved are microsomal oxidation, including N-dealkylation or aliphatic hydroxylation, and subsequent conjugation by glucuronyl transferases to form glucuronides that are excreted in the urine. The patterns and rates of metabolism depend on the individual drugs. One important feature of benzodiazepine metabolism is formation of active metabolites with central nervous system effects, some of which may be long-lived. As shown schematically in Fig 20–4, desmethyldiazepam, which has an elimination half-life of 40–140 hours, is an active metabolite of chlordiazepoxide, diazepam, prazepam, and clorazepate. Desmethyldiazepam in turn is biotransformed to the active compound oxazepam. Other active metabolites of chlordiazepoxide include desmethylchlordiazepoxide and

demoxepam. While diazepam is metabolized mainly to desmethyldiazepam, it is also converted to temazepam (not shown in Fig 20–4) which is further metabolized in part to oxazepam. Flurazepam, which is used mainly for hypnosis, is oxidized by hepatic enzymes to 3 active metabolites, desalkylflurazepam, hydroxyethylflurazepam, and flurazepam aldehyde (not shown), which have elimination half-lives ranging from 30 to 100 hours. This may result in unwanted central nervous system depression, including daytime sedation. The triazolobenzodiazepines alprazolam and triazolam undergo α-hydroxylation, and the resulting metabolites appear to exert pharmacologic effects.

The formation of active metabolites has complicated studies on the pharmacokinetics of the benzodiazepines in humans because the elimination half-life of the parent drug may have little relationship to the time course of pharmacologic effects. Those benzodiazepines for which either the parent drug or active metabolites have long half-lives are more likely to cause cumulative effects with multiple doses. Cumulative and residual effects such as excessive drowsiness should be less of a problem with such drugs as oxazepam and lorazepam, which have shorter half-lives and are metabolized directly to inactive glucuronides. Some biodispositional properties of selected benzodiazepines are given in Table 20–1.

2. Barbiturates–With the exception of phenobarbital, only insignificant quantities of the barbiturates are excreted intact. The major metabolic pathways involve oxidation by hepatic enzymes of chemical groups attached to C5, which are different for the individual barbiturates. The alcohols, acids, and ketones formed appear in the urine as glucuronide conjugates. Another type of metabolic reaction, glycosylation, involves direct attachment of glucose to N1 or N3 to form more water-soluble derivatives that can then be eliminated via the kidney. With very few exceptions, the metabolites of the barbiturates lack pharmacologic activity. The overall rate of hepatic metabolism in humans depends on the individual drug but (with the exception of the thiobarbiturates) is usually slow. The range of elimination half-life of secobarbital and pentobarbital is from 18 to 48 hours. The elimination half-life of phenobarbital in humans may be as long as 4–5 days. Multiple dosing with barbiturates with longer half-lives can lead to cumulative effects.

3. Other sedative-hypnotics–Most other sedative-hypnotics, including the piperidinediones and meprobamate, are biotransformed to more water-soluble compounds by hepatic enzymes. Trichloroethanol is the pharmacologically active metabolite of chloral hydrate and has a half-life of 6–10 hours. However, its toxic metabolite, trichloroacetic acid, is cleared very slowly and can accumulate with the nightly administration of chloral hydrate.

D. Excretion: The water-soluble metabolites of benzodiazepines and other sedative-hypnotics are excreted mainly via the kidney. In most cases, changes in renal function do not have a marked effect on the elimination of parent drugs. Phenobarbital is excreted

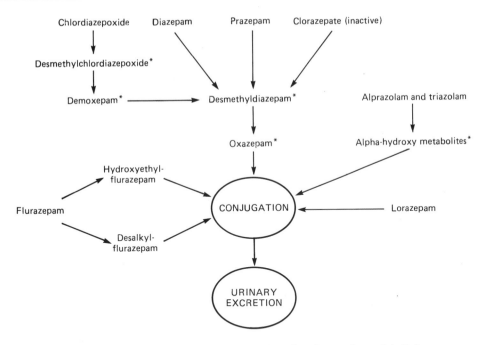

Figure 20–4. Biotransformation of benzodiazepines (* = active metabolite).

unchanged in the urine to a certain extent (20–30% in humans), and its elimination rate can be increased significantly by alkalinization of the urine. This is partly due to increased ionization at alkaline pH, since phenobarbital is a weak acid with pK_a of 7.2. Only trace amounts of the benzodiazepines and less than 10% of a hypnotic dose of meprobamate appear in the urine unchanged.

E. Factors Affecting Biodisposition: The biodisposition of sedative-hypnotics can be influenced by several factors, particularly those that change rates of metabolic clearance. These include alterations in hepatic function resulting from disease, old age, or drug-induced increases or decreases in microsomal enzyme activities.

Generally, decreased hepatic function results in reduction of the clearance rates of drugs metabolized via oxidative pathways. This group includes many of the benzodiazepines, almost all of the barbiturates, the piperidinediones, and meprobamate. In very old patients or those with severe liver disease, the elimination half-lives of these drugs are usually increased significantly. If given in such cases, multiple normal doses of these sedative-hypnotics can often result in cumulative or enhanced central nervous system effects. Surprisingly, there are only a few clinical studies that document this. However, it seems prudent to lower the dose of such sedative-hypnotics in patients who are elderly or who may have limited hepatic function. Metabolism involving glucuronide conjugation appears to be less affected than oxidative metabolism by old age or liver disease.

The activity of hepatic microsomal drug-metabolizing enzymes may be increased in patients exposed to certain sedative-hypnotics on a chronic basis (en-

zyme induction; see Chapter 3), especially the barbiturates and carbamates. Drugs with long elimination half-lives such as phenobarbital and meprobamate are most likely to cause this effect and result in an increase in the rate of their own hepatic metabolism as well as that of certain other drugs. Self-induction of metabolism is a possible but not well-documented mechanism that contributes to the development of tolerance to sedative-hypnotics. Increased biotransformation of other pharmacologic agents by sedative-hypnotics is a potential mechanism underlying drug interactions. (See Appendix I.) The benzodiazepine group of sedative-hypnotics is less likely than the barbiturates to change hepatic drug-metabolizing enzyme activity with continuous use.

Mechanisms of Action

A unitary hypothesis regarding the mechanisms of action of sedative-hypnotics has been slow to develop. As the role of gamma-aminobutyric acid (GABA) as an important inhibitory neurotransmitter in the central nervous system has been elucidated, it has become more probable that modification of its functions underlie the pharmacologic effects of several classes of drugs, including the benzodiazepines and barbiturates. Electrophysiologic studies have shown that benzodiazepines potentiate GABA-ergic neurotransmission at all levels of the neuroaxis, including the spinal cord, hypothalamus, hippocampus, substantia nigra, cerebellar cortex, and cerebral cortex. Benzodiazepines appear to increase the efficiency of GABA-ergic synaptic inhibition, which leads to a decrease in the firing rate of critical neurons in many regions of the brain. The benzodiazepines do not appear to substitute for GABA but require the presence of the neurotrans-

Table 20–1. Biodispositional properties of benzodiazepines in humans.

Drug	Elimination Half-Life Range (hours)	Metabolites	Comments
Alprazolam	12–15	Active: α-hydroxyalprazolam	Rapid oral absorption.
Chlordiazepoxide	5–30	Active: desmethyl derivative, demoxepam, oxazepam	Poor intramuscular bioavailability.
Clorazepate	50–100 (metabolites)	Active: desmethyldiazepam, oxazepam	Hydrolyzed to active form in stomach.
Diazepam	50–150	Active: desmethyldiazepam, temazepam, oxazepam	Poor intramuscular bioavailability.
Flunitrazepam	12–24	Active: desmethylflunitrazepam	Large volume of distribution.
Flurazepam	24–100 (metabolites)	Active: desalkyl derivative and others	Long elimination half-lives of active metabolites.
Lorazepam	10–18	Inactive: glucuronides	Elimination not much affected by age or liver disease.
Nitrazepam	24–36	Probably inactive	Large volume of distribution.
Oxazepam	4–10	Inactive: glucuronides	Slow oral absorption may delay onset of effects.
Prazepam	30–120	Active: desmethyldiazepam	Slow oral absorption.
Temazepam	5–8	Possibly active	Slow oral absorption.
Triazolam	3–5	Active: α-hydroxytriazolam	Rapid oral absorption.

mitter to elicit a response. This has led to the concept that benzodiazepines indirectly enhance GABA-ergic neurotransmission at the level of postsynaptic receptors without direct activation of GABA receptors or the associated chloride channels. The change in chloride ion conductance induced by the interaction of GABA with its receptors is enhanced by benzodiazepines, resulting in an increase in the frequency of channel-opening events. Barbiturates also facilitate the inhibitory actions of GABA at multiple sites in the central nervous system, but electrophysiologic studies show that—in contrast to benzodiazepines—they prolong rather than intensify GABA responses. At high concentrations, the barbiturates may also be GABA-mimetic, directly activating chloride ion channels. Barbiturates appear to be less selective in their actions than benzodiazepines, since they also depress the actions of excitatory neurotransmitters and exert nonsynaptic membrane effects in parallel with their effects on GABA neurotransmission. This multiplicity of sites of action of barbiturates may be the basis for their ability to induce full surgical anesthesia and for their more pronounced central depressant effects (which results in their low margin of safety) compared to benzodiazepines. The actions of other sedative-hypnotics such as meprobamate have been less well studied electrophysiologically but do not appear to be related to GABA neurotransmission.

Neurochemical studies during recent years have complemented and extended the electrophysiologic evidence for the modulation of GABA neurotransmission by benzodiazepines. High-affinity receptor sites for benzodiazepines have been demonstrated in many regions of the central nervous system, including the spinal cord, brain stem, hypothalamus, limbic structures, cerebellar cortex, and cerebral cortex. Such benzodiazepine receptors are located at GABA-ergic synapses and are functionally coupled to GABA-responsive chloride channels but are separate macromolecules from either the GABA receptor or the chloride ionophore. Possible physical and functional relationships between these components are schematically illustrated in Fig 20–5. The macromolecular complex also includes a polypeptide GABA-modulin that may modulate coupling between the GABA receptor and the benzodiazepine receptor protein. In addition, a barbiturate receptor protein (which may be identical to the chloride channel protein) is a component of the macromolecular complex. This component also contains binding sites for certain convulsant drugs such as picrotoxin.

The identification of benzodiazepine receptors in the brain has led to the characterization of 3 main types of benzodiazepine receptor ligands: (1) The clinically useful benzodiazepines which exert anxiolytic, hypnotic, and anticonvulsant effects and which appear to act as classic receptor agonists. (2) Benzodiazepine receptor *antagonists* (including the imidazodiazepine Ro 15-1788) that selectively block the actions of benzodiazepines without pharmacologic effects of their own. These molecules do not block the actions of other sedative-hypnotics such as barbiturates, meprobamate, or ethanol. Members of this second class of ligands appear to be classic antagonists, and they have potential clinical application in the treatment of benzodiazepine intoxication and overdosage. (3) A third group of *anxiogenic* benzodiazepine receptor ligands is represented by various β-carbolines, some of

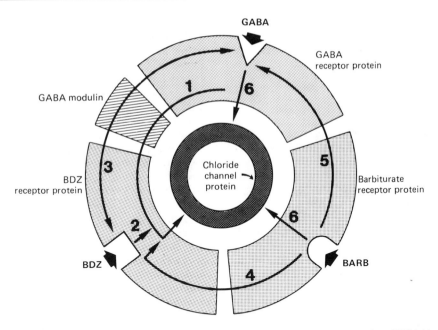

Figure 20–5. Proposed model of the GABA-benzodiazepine-chloride channel receptor complex. GABA binding to its receptor activates the chloride channel through a coupling mechanism involving GABA-modulin and the benzodiazepine (BDZ) receptor protein (1). Binding of benzodiazepines (BDZ) enhances this coupling function (2) and increases GABA binding in a reciprocal relationship (3). Binding of barbiturates (BARB) also enhances the coupling function (4), increases the affinity of GABA for its receptor (5), and may directly activate the chloride channel at high concentrations (6). GABA= gamma-aminobutyric acid.

which are naturally occurring. These molecules can block the effects of benzodiazepine agonists, and when administered alone produce such effects as anxiety reaction, proconvulsant activity, and seizures. Such ligands have been termed "inverse agonists" and are of interest in terms of their possible role as natural endogenous mediators of anxiolytic responses.

Newer Anxiolytic Drugs

Although the benzodiazepines continue to be the agents of choice in the treatment of anxiety, their pharmacologic effects include sedation and drowsiness and synergistic central nervous system depression with other drugs, especially alcohol. Anxiolytic drugs with reduced propensity for such actions would be desirable. Several nonbenzodiazepines are presently under active investigation, including the pyrazolopyridine tracazolate, the piperazinyl pyrimidine derivative buspirone, and certain triazolopyridazines. These drugs have minimal potentiating effects on the actions of ethanol. Buspirone appears to be "anxioselective" in that it relieves anxiety with minimum sedative and muscle relaxing effects. Buspirone does not appear to

exert its effects through the GABA receptor–benzodiazepine receptor–chloride ionophore complex but may interact with brain dopamine receptors. The drug is metabolized by hepatic enzymes to 1-(2-pyrimidinyl)piperazine, which also has anxiolytic effects but is without dopaminergic actions. These drugs are currently undergoing clinical evaluation.

Pharmacodynamics

A. Sedation: Sedation can be defined as a decrease in responsiveness to a constant level of stimulation, with decrease in spontaneous activity and ideation. These behavioral changes occur at the lowest effective doses of the sedative-hypnotics. It is not yet clear whether antianxiety actions seen clinically are equivalent to or different from sedative effects. In experimental animal models, the sedative-hypnotic drugs are able to release punishment-suppressed behavior, and this disinhibition has been equated with antianxiety effects. However, the release of previously suppressed behavior may be more relevant to behavioral disinhibitory effects of these drugs, including euphoria, impaired judgment, and loss of self-control,

Buspirone

which occur at doses slightly higher than those used to cause sedation. All sedative-hypnotic drugs are capable of releasing punishment-suppressed behavior in animals, but the benzodiazepines exert such effects at doses that do not cause general central nervous system depression. Phenothiazine antipsychotic drugs and tricyclic antidepressants are not effective in this experimental model.

B. Hypnosis: By definition, all of the sedative-hypnotics will induce sleep if high enough doses are given. Normal sleep is considered to consist of distinct stages, based on 3 physiologic measures: the electroencephalogram, the electromyogram, and the electrooculogram (a measure of lateral movements of the eye). Based on the latter, 2 major categories can be distinguished: non–rapid eye movement (NREM) sleep, which represents approximately 70–75% of total sleep; and rapid eye movement (REM) sleep. REM and NREM sleep occur cyclically over an interval of about 90 minutes. The REM sleep stage is that in which most recallable dreams occur. NREM sleep progresses through 4 stages (1–4), with the greatest proportion (50%) of sleep being spent in stage 2. This is followed by delta or slow-wave sleep (stages 3 and 4), in which somnambulism and night terrors have been noted to occur.

The effects of drugs on the sleep stages have been studied extensively, although often with normal volunteer subjects rather than patients with sleep disorders. In the case of sedative-hypnotics, effects depend on several factors, including the specific drug, the dose, and the frequency of its administration. While some exceptions exist, the effects of sedative-hypnotics on patterns of normal sleep are as follows: (1) the latency of sleep onset is decreased (time to fall asleep); (2) the duration of stage 2 NREM sleep is increased; (3) the duration of REM sleep is decreased; and (4) the duration of slow-wave sleep is decreased.

More rapid onset of sleep and prolongation of stage 2 are presumably clinically useful effects. However, the significance of effects on REM and slow-wave sleep is not clear. Use of sedative-hypnotics for more than a week or so leads to some tolerance to their effects on sleep patterns. Withdrawal after continued use can result in a "rebound" increase in the frequency of occurrence and duration of REM sleep. It is important to recognize that claims have often been made for superiority of one sedative-hypnotic over another based on differential actions on one stage of sleep or another. Since little is known about the function of any sleep stage, statements about the desirability of a particular drug based on its effects on sleep patterns can have no validity. Clearly, clinical criteria of efficacy in alleviating a particular sleeping problem are more useful. The ideal hypnotic—one that would promote sleep without any change in its natural pattern—has yet to be introduced.

C. Anesthesia: As shown in Fig 20–1, sedative-hypnotics in high doses will depress the central nervous system to a point known as stage III or general anesthesia (see Chapter 23). However, the suitability of a particular agent as an adjunct in anesthesia depends mainly on the physicochemical properties that determine its rapidity of onset and duration of effect. Among the barbiturates, thiopental and methohexital are very lipid-soluble, penetrating brain tissue rapidly following intravenous administration. Rapid tissue redistribution accounts for the short duration of action of these drugs, which are therefore useful in anesthesia practice (see Fig 23–5).

Although certain of the benzodiazepines have been used intravenously in anesthesia, none of them have proved successful as induction agents capable of producing surgical anesthesia by themselves. This statement is supported by the fact that the MAC (minimum alveolar concentration) of another anesthetic cannot be reduced to zero by the substitution of a benzodiazepine. Diazepam and midazolam have been studied in this regard and are incapable of producing adequate surgical anesthesia. Not surprisingly, most of the benzodiazepines given in large doses may cause a persistent postanesthetic depression. This is probably related to their relatively long half-lives and the formation of active metabolites. It is possible that newer benzodiazepines with much shorter half-lives will be more useful in clinical practice.

D. Anticonvulsant Effects: Most of the sedative-hypnotics are capable of inhibiting the development and spread of epileptiform activity in the central nervous system, but some selectivity exists in that certain drugs do so without marked central nervous system depression, so that normal mentation and activity are relatively unaffected. Of the barbiturates, phenobarbital and metharbital (converted to phenobarbital in the body) are effective in the treatment of grand mal and jacksonian epilepsy. Certain benzodiazepines also have selective actions: diazepam is used in status epilepticus and in the treatment of seizures induced by local anesthetics, and nitrazepam is used in certain infantile spasms and myoclonic seizures (see Chapter 22).

E. Muscle Relaxation: Some sedative-hypnotics, particularly members of the carbamate and benzodiazepine groups, exert inhibitory effects on polysynaptic reflexes and internuncial transmission, and at high doses may depress transmission at the skeletal myoneural junction. Selective actions of this type leading to muscle relaxation can be readily demonstrated in animals, and this has led to claims of usefulness for relaxing contracted voluntary muscle in joint disease or muscle spasm. Unfortunately, there is little clinical evidence to support such claims at dose levels that do not also cause significant depression of the central nervous system, leading to changes in mental or motor functions. What positive evidence does exist concerns specialized clinical situations such as the treatment with diazepam of spasticity in patients with cerebral palsy.

F. Effects on Respiration and Cardiovascular Function: At hypnotic doses in healthy patients, the effects of sedative-hypnotics on respiration are comparable to changes during natural sleep. However, sedative-hypnotics even at therapeutic doses can produce significant respiratory depression in patients with obstructive pulmonary disease. Effects on respiration are dose-related, and depression of the medullary respiratory center is the usual cause of death due to overdose of sedative-hypnotics.

At doses up to those causing hypnosis, no significant effects on the cardiovascular system are observed in healthy patients. However, in hypovolemic states, congestive heart failure, or other diseases impairing cardiovascular function, normal doses of sedative-hypnotics may cause cardiovascular depression, probably as a result of actions on the medullary vasomotor centers. At toxic levels, myocardial contractility and vascular tone may both be depressed by central and peripheral effects, leading to circulatory collapse. Respiratory and cardiovascular effects become more apparent when sedative-hypnotics are given intravenously.

Tolerance; Psychologic & Physical Dependence

Tolerance, a decrease in responsiveness to a drug following continuous exposure, is a common feature of the sedative-hypnotics. In some instances, it may result in a need to increase the dose to maintain symptomatic improvement or to promote sleep. It is important to recognize that **cross-tolerance** occurs between the sedative-hypnotics described here and also with ethanol (Chapter 21)—a feature of some clinical importance, as explained below. The mechanisms of development of tolerance to sedative-hypnotics are not well understood. An alteration in rates of metabolic inactivation with chronic administration may be partly responsible (metabolic tolerance), but changes in responsiveness of the central nervous system (pharmacodynamic tolerance) are more important.

The perceived desirable properties of relief of anxiety, euphoria, disinhibition, and promotion of sleep have led to the compulsive misuse of virtually all of the drugs classed as sedative-hypnotics. (See Chapter 30 for a detailed discussion of drug abuse.) The consequences of abuse of these agents can be defined in both psychologic and physiologic terms. The psychologic component may initially parallel simple neurotic behavior patterns hard to differentiate from those of the inveterate coffee drinker or cigarette smoker. When the pattern of sedative-hypnotic use becomes compulsive, more serious complications develop, including physical dependence and tolerance.

Physical dependence can be described as an altered physiologic state that requires continuous drug administration to prevent the appearance of an abstinence or withdrawal syndrome. As described more fully later, in the case of sedative-hypnotics this syndrome is characterized by states of increased excitability that may even progress to convulsions. All sedative-hypnotics are capable of causing physical dependence when used on a chronic basis. However, the severity of withdrawal symptoms differs between individual drugs and depends also on the magnitude of the dose used immediately prior to cessation of use. When higher doses of sedative-hypnotics are used, abrupt withdrawal will lead to more serious withdrawal signs. Differences in the severity of withdrawal symptoms between individual sedative-hypnotics relate in part to biodisposition properties, since drugs with long half-lives are eliminated slowly enough to accomplish gradual withdrawal with few physical symptoms. The use of drugs with very short half-lives for hypnotic effects may lead to signs of withdrawal even between doses. For example, triazolam, a benzodiazepine with a half-life of about 4 hours, has been reported to cause daytime anxiety when used to treat sleep problems.

II. CLINICAL PHARMACOLOGY OF SEDATIVE-HYPNOTICS

TREATMENT OF ANXIETY STATES

Throughout history, the psychologic and behavioral responses to stress have been a significant part of human experience, and many ingenious approaches have been devised for relieving the various symptoms of anxiety. Before considering the clinical use of sedative-hypnotics, it is important to analyze the patient's symptoms carefully. If the patient presents with anxiety as a primary complaint, other psychiatric problems must be suspected. These may best be managed by psychotherapy or, when the situation warrants, by the use of pharmacologic agents such as the tricyclic antidepressants or antipsychotic drugs. Frequently, however, anxiety is secondary to organic disease states— acute myocardial infarction, angina pectoris, gastrointestinal ulcers, etc—which themselves require specific therapy. Another class of secondary anxiety states (situational anxiety) results from circumstances that may only have to be dealt with once or a few times, including anticipation of frightening medical or dental procedures and family illness or other tragedy. Even though situational anxiety tends to be self-limiting, the *short-term* use of sedative-hypnotics may be appropriate for the treatment of this and certain disease-associated anxiety states. Similarly, the acute use of a sedative-hypnotic as a premedicant prior to surgery or some unpleasant medical procedure is rational and proper (Table 20–2).

Historically, the rationale for the treatment of anxiety with sedative-hypnotics was quite empiric, since evidence for efficacy from well-controlled, blind clinical studies did not become available until the last decade. Difficulties in establishing efficacy can be related to many nonpharmacologic factors that influence the success of therapy, including personal expectations, personality of the therapist, environmental factors, and the placebo response. Although anxiety symptoms can now be ameliorated by drug therapy, it is difficult to demonstrate the superiority of one drug

Table 20-2. Clinical uses of sedative-hypnotics.

For relief of anxiety.
Hypnosis.
For sedation and amnesia before medical and surgical procedures.
Treatment of epilepsy and seizure states.
Intravenous administration, as a component of balanced anesthesia.
For control of ethanol or other sedative-hypnotic withdrawal states.
For muscle relaxation in specific neuromuscular disorders.
As diagnostic aids or for treatment in psychiatry.

over another. Thus, a preference for a particular drug for a specific situation is based on factors other than pharmacologic effect.

Although phenobarbital, meprobamate, and certain sedative-autonomic drugs (hydroxyzine, diphenhydramine) continue to be used, the most commonly used drugs for treatment of anxiety are the benzodiazepines. The selection of benzodiazepines is based on several sound pharmacologic principles: (1) a relatively high therapeutic index (see drug B in Fig 20–1), since hypnotic and anesthetic doses are considerably higher than those causing sedation; (2) a low risk of drug interactions based on enzyme induction; (3) slow elimination rates, which may favor persistence of useful central nervous system effects; and (4) a low risk of physical dependence, with minor withdrawal symptoms.

Disadvantages of the benzodiazepines include the tendency to develop psychologic dependence, the formation of active metabolites, and their higher cost. *As is true of all drugs of the sedative-hypnotic class, the benzodiazepines exert additive central nervous system depression when administered with other drugs, including ethanol.* The patient should be warned of this possibility to avoid impairment of performance of any task requiring mental alertness and motor coordination.

Perhaps the most important guide to therapy is to use the drug selected with appropriate restraint to minimize adverse effects. A dose should be prescribed that does not impair mentation or motor functions during working hours. Some patients may tolerate the drug better if most of the daily dose is given at bedtime, with smaller doses during the day. Prescriptions should be written for short periods, since there is little justification for long-term therapy. The physician should make an effort to assess the efficacy of therapy from the patient's subjective responses. Plasma drug concentrations are too variable to be useful as a guide to dosage. Combinations of antianxiety agents should be avoided, and people taking sedatives should be cautioned about drinking alcohol and concurrent use of over-the-counter medications (see Chapter 69).

TREATMENT OF SLEEP PROBLEMS

The complaint of insomnia embraces a wide variety of sleep problems that include difficulty in falling asleep, frequent awakenings, short duration of sleep,

and "unrefreshing" sleep. Insomnia is a serious complaint calling for careful evaluation to uncover possible causes (organic, psychologic, situational, etc) that can perhaps be managed without hypnotic drugs. Nonpharmacologic therapies sometimes useful include proper diet and exercise, avoiding stimulants before retiring, assuring a comfortable sleeping place, and retiring at a regular time each night. In some cases, however, the patient will need and should be given a sedative-hypnotic for a limited period. It should be noted that the discontinuance of any drug in this class can lead to rebound insomnia. *Note: Long-term use of hypnotics is irrational and dangerous medical practice.*

The hypnotic drug selected should be one that provides sleep of fairly rapid onset (decreased sleep latency) and sufficient duration, with minimal "hangover" effects such as drowsiness, dysphoria, and mental or motor depression. Drugs with a favorable therapeutic index such as benzodiazepines are generally preferred. However, many benzodiazepines have slow elimination rates and are biotransformed to active metabolites—properties that are undesirable because they lead to cumulative and hangover effects. If hypnotics are used every night, tolerance can occur, leading to dose increases by the patient to produce the desired effect. It should be recalled that if physical dependence develops, the shorter-acting drugs are associated with more intense withdrawal signs when discontinued. The drugs commonly used for sedation and hypnosis are listed in Table 20–3 together with recommended doses.

OTHER THERAPEUTIC USES

Table 20–2 summarizes several other important clinical uses of drugs in the sedative-hypnotic class. Drugs used in the management of seizure disorders and for intravenous anesthesia are discussed in Chapters 22 and 23. For sedative and possible amnestic effects during medical or surgical procedures such as endoscopy and bronchoscopy, as well as premedication prior to anesthesia, oral formulations of shorter-acting drugs are preferred. When drug administration is under close supervision, the danger of accidental or intentional overdosage is less than in the outpatient situation, and a barbiturate may be as appropriate as any sedative-hypnotic. Meprobamate and, more recently, the benzodiazepines have frequently been used as central muscle relaxants, though evidence for general efficacy without accompanying sedation is lacking. Sedative-hypnotics are occasionally used as diagnostic aids in neurology and psychiatry.

CLINICAL TOXICOLOGY OF SEDATIVE-HYPNOTICS

Direct Toxic Actions

Many of the common adverse effects of drugs in

Table 20–3. Dosages of drugs used commonly for sedation and hypnosis.

Sedation		Hypnosis	
Drug	Dosage	Drug	Dosage (at Bedtime)
Alprazolam (Xanax)	0.25–0.5 mg 2–3 times daily	Chloral hydrate	500–1000 mg
Chlordiazepoxide (Librium)	10–20 mg 2–3 times daily	Flurazepam (Dalmane)	15–30 mg
Clorazepate (Tranxene)	5–7.5 mg twice daily	Lorazepam (Ativan)	2–4 mg
Diazepam (Valium)	5 mg twice daily	Methaqualone* (Quaalude)	150–250 mg
Lorazepam (Ativan)	1–2 mg once or twice daily	Pentobarbital	100–200 mg
Oxazepam (Serax)	15–30 mg 3–4 times daily	Secobarbital	100–200 mg
Phenobarbital	15–30 mg 2–3 times daily	Temazepam (Restoril)	10–30 mg
Prazepam (Centrax)	10–20 mg 2–3 times daily	Triazolam (Halcion)	0.5–1 mg

*Methaqualone has been discontinued, but illicit use of the drug will probably continue.

this class are those resulting from dose-related depression of central nervous system functions. In ambulatory patients, relatively low doses may lead to drowsiness, impaired judgment, and diminished motor skills, sometimes with a significant impact on driving skills, job performance, and personal relationships. Hangover effects are not uncommon following use of drugs with long half-lives for sleep problems in such patients. The most common reversible cause of confusional states in the elderly is overuse of sedative-hypnotics. At higher doses, toxicity may present as lethargy or a state of exhaustion or, alternatively, gross symptoms equivalent to those of ethanol intoxication. The titration of useful therapeutic effects against such side effects is usually more difficult with sedative-hypnotics that exhibit steep dose-response relationships of the type shown in Fig 20–1 (drug A), including the barbiturates and piperidinediones. Unwanted depression of central nervous system functions also occurs more frequently when therapy is continued for longer periods and when drugs with long half-lives and active metabolites are used. The physician should be aware of variability among patients in terms of doses causing adverse effects. A relatively small dose in one individual may result in unwanted central nervous system depression that would require 2 or 3 times that dose in another patient. Variability is even more common in patients with cardiovascular or respiratory disease and hepatic impairment or in old age.

Sedative-hypnotics are the drugs most frequently involved in deliberate overdosage situations, in part because of their general availability as the most commonly prescribed pharmacologic agents. The benzodiazepines are generally considered to be "safer" drugs in this respect, since they have flatter dose-response curves. Epidemiologic studies on the incidence of drug-related deaths support this general assumption— eg, 0.3 deaths per million tablets of diazepam prescribed versus 11.6 deaths per million capsules of secobarbital in a recent study. Of course, many factors other than the specific sedative-hypnotic could influence such data—particularly the presence of other central nervous system depressants, including ethanol. In fact, most serious cases of drug overdosage,

intentional or accidental, do involve polypharmacy; and when combinations of agents are taken, the practical "safety" of benzodiazepines may be less than the foregoing would imply.

The lethal dose of any sedative-hypnotic is variable (Chapter 62). If discovery of the ingestion is made early and a conservative treatment regimen is started, the outcome is rarely fatal, even following very high doses. On the other hand, for most sedative-hypnotics, with the exception of benzodiazepines, a dose as low as 10 times what is required for hypnosis may be fatal if the patient is not discovered or does not seek help in time. With severe toxicity, the respiratory depression from central actions of the drug may be complicated by aspiration of gastric contents in the unattended patient—an even more likely occurrence if ethanol is present. Loss of brain stem vasomotor control, together with direct myocardial depression, further complicates successful resuscitation. In such patients, treatment consists of mechanical respiration; maintenance of plasma volume, renal output, and cardiac function; and perhaps use of a positive inotropic drug such as dopamine, which preserves renal blood flow. Hemodialysis or hemoperfusion may be used to hasten elimination of some of these drugs (see Table 62–7).

Adverse effects of the sedative-hypnotics that are not referable to their central nervous system actions occur infrequently. Hypersensitivity reactions, including skin rashes, occur only occasionally with most drugs of this class. Reports of teratogenicity leading to fetal deformation following use of piperidinediones and certain benzodiazepines justify caution in the use of these drugs during pregnancy. Because barbiturates enhance porphyrin synthesis, they are absolutely contraindicated in patients with a history of acute intermittent porphyria.

Alterations in Drug Response

Depending on dosage and duration of use, tolerance may occur to many of the pharmacologic effects of sedative-hypnotics. This can be demonstrated experimentally in humans by changes in the effects of chronic use of these drugs on the electroencephalogram and other characteristics of the stages of sleep. Clearly, it must occur with respect to other effects, since it is known that chronic abusers sometimes ingest quantities of sedative-hypnotics many times the conventional dosage without experiencing severe toxicity. However, it should not be assumed that the degree of tolerance achieved is identical for all pharmacologic effects, and there is evidence that lethal dose ranges are not altered significantly with chronic use of sedative-hypnotics. Cross-tolerance between the different sedative-hypnotics, including ethanol, could lead to an unsatisfactory therapeutic response when standard doses of a drug are used in a patient with a recent history of abuse of these agents.

With chronic use of sedative-hypnotics, especially as doses are increased, a state of physical dependence can occur. This may develop to a degree unparalleled by chronic use of any other drug group, *including the opiates,* since withdrawal from a sedative-hypnotic can have severe and life-threatening manifestations. Withdrawal symptoms range from restlessness, anxiety, weakness, and orthostatic hypotension to hyperactive reflexes and generalized seizures. The severity of withdrawal symptoms depends to a large extent on the dosage range used immediately prior to discontinuance but also on the particular drug. For example, barbiturates such as secobarbital or pentobarbital (in doses less than 400 mg/d) or diazepam (less than 40 mg/d) may produce only mild symptoms of withdrawal when discontinued. On the other hand, the use of more than 800 mg/d of barbiturates or 50–60 mg/d of diazepam for 60–90 days is likely to result in seizures if abrupt withdrawal is attempted. Symptoms of withdrawal are usually more severe following discontinuance of sedative-hypnotics with shorter half-lives. Symptoms are less pronounced with longer-acting drugs, which may partly accomplish their own withdrawal by virtue of their slow elimination. Cross-dependence, defined as the ability of one drug to suppress abstinence symptoms from discontinuance of another drug, is quite marked among sedative-hypnotics. This provides the rationale for therapeutic regimens in the management of withdrawal states. Thus, longer-acting drugs such as phenobarbital and diazepam can be used to alleviate withdrawal symptoms of shorter-acting drugs, including ethanol.

Drug Interactions

The most frequent drug interactions involving sedative-hypnotics are interactions with other central nervous system depressant drugs, leading to additive effects. These interactions have some therapeutic utility with respect to the use of these drugs as premedicants or anesthetic adjuvants. However, they can lead to serious adverse effects, including enhanced depression with concomitant use of many other drugs. Obvious additive effects can be predicted with use of alcoholic beverages, narcotic analgesics, anticonvulsants, phenothiazines, and other sedative-hypnotic drugs. Less obvious but just as important is enhanced central nervous system depression with a variety of antihistamines, antihypertensive agents, and antidepressant drugs of the tricyclic class.

Interactions involving changes in the activity of hepatic drug-metabolizing enzyme systems can occur, especially following continuous use of barbiturates and meprobamate. For example, in humans, barbiturates have been shown to increase metabolic degradation rates of dicumarol, phenytoin, digitalis compounds, and griseofulvin, effects that could lead to decrease in response to these agents. Cimetidine has recently been reported to double the elimination half-life of diazepam, presumably via inhibition of hepatic metabolism. As mentioned above, chloral hydrate may displace warfarin from plasma proteins to cause enhanced anticoagulant effects.

REFERENCES

Allquander C: Dependence on sedative and hypnotic drugs. *Acta Psychiatr Scand [Suppl]* 1978;**270**:1.

Breimer DD: Clinical pharmacokinetics of hypnotics. *Clin Pharmacokinet* 1977;**2**:93.

Burrows GD, Norman TR, Davies B: *Antianxiety Agents.* Vol 2 of: *Drugs in Psychiatry.* Elsevier, 1984.

Choi DW, Farb DH, Fischbach GD: Chlordiazepoxide selectively potentiates GABA conductance of spinal cord and sensory neurons in culture. *J Neurophysiol* 1981;**45**:621.

Consensus Conference: Drugs and insomnia: The use of medications to promote sleep. *JAMA* 1984;**251**:2410.

Council on Scientific Affairs: Hypnotic drugs and treatment of insomnia report. *JAMA* 1981;**245**:749.

Danneberg P, Weber KH: Chemical structure and biological activity of the diazepines. *Br J Clin Pharmacol* 1983;**16**:2315.

Goldberg ME et al: Novel non-benzodiazepine anxiolytics. *Neuropharmacology* 1983;**22**:1499.

Greenblatt DJ et al: Benzodiazepines: A summary of pharmacokinetic properties. *Br J Clin Pharmacol* 1981;**11(Suppl 1)**:11S.

Greenblatt DJ et al: Clinical pharmacokinetics of the newer benzodiazepines. *Clin Pharmacokinet* 1983;**8**:233.

Greenblatt DJ et al: Current status of benzodiazepines. *N Engl J Med* 1983;**309**:354.

Haefely W, Polc P: Electrophysiological studies on the interaction of anxiolytic drugs with GABAergic mechanisms. Pages 113–145 in: *Anxiolytics: Neurochemical, Behavioral and Clinical Perspectives.* Malick JB, Enna SJ, Yamamura HI (editors). Raven Press, 1983.

Mendelson WB: *The Use and Misuse of Sleeping Pills: A Clinical Guide.* Plenum Press, 1980.

Middlemiss DN et al: Beta-adrenoreceptor antagonists in psychiatry and neurology. *Pharmacol Ther* 1981;**12**:419.

Mohler H, Richards JG: Receptors for anxiolytic drugs. Pages

15–40 in: *Anxiolytics: Neurochemical, Behavioral and Clinical Perspectives*. Malick JB, Enna SJ, Yamamura HI (editors). Raven Press, 1983.

Olsen RW: GABA-benzodiazepine-barbiturate receptor interactions. *J Neurochem* 1981;**37**:1.

Rosenbaum JF: The drug treatment of anxiety. *N Engl J Med* 1982;**306**:401.

Sepinwall J, Cook L: Behavioral pharmacology of antianxiety drugs. Chap 6, pp 345–393, in: *Biology of Mood and Antianxiety Drugs*. Vol 13 of: *Handbook of Psychopharmacology*. Iversen LL, Iversen SD, Snyder SH (editors). Plenum Press, 1978.

Skolnick P, Paul SM: The mechanism(s) of action of the benzodiazepines. *Med Res Rev* 1981;**1**:3.

Snyder SH: Drugs and neurotransmitter receptors in the brain. Science 1984;**224**:22.

Solomon F et al: Sleeping pills, insomnia, and medical practice. *N Engl J Med* 1979;**300**:803.

Study RE, Barker JL: Diazepam and (–)pentobarbital: Fluctuation analysis reveals different mechanisms for potentiation of GABA responses in cultured central neurons. *Proc Natl Acad Sci USA* 1981;**78**:7180.

Tallman JF et al: Receptors for the age of anxiety: Pharmacology of the benzodiazepines. *Science* 1980;**207**:274.

21

The Alcohols

Nancy M. Lee, PhD, & Charles E. Becker, MD

Ethyl alcohol (ethanol) is a sedative-hypnotic consumed as a social drug. Alcohol abuse (alcoholism) is a complex disorder whose natural history and basic causes are not well-defined. It is a major medical and public health problem in many societies.

Many other alcohols with potentially toxic effects are used in chemical industries, some in enormous quantities. Methanol and ethylene glycol toxicity occur with sufficient frequency to warrant some discussion in this chapter.

I. BASIC PHARMACOLOGY OF ALCOHOLS

ETHANOL

Pharmacokinetics

Ethanol (CH_3CH_2OH) is a small water-soluble molecule that is absorbed rapidly and completely from the gastrointestinal tract. Ethanol vapor can also be readily absorbed in the lungs. After ingestion of alcohol in the fasting state, peak blood levels are reached within 40 minutes. The presence of food in the gut delays absorption. Distribution is rapid, with tissue levels rapidly approximating the blood concentration. The volume of distribution is 0.7 L/kg.

Over 90% of alcohol consumed is oxidized in the liver; the rest is excreted through the lungs and in urine. The rate of oxidation follows zero-order kinetics, ie, it is independent of time and concentration of the drug. The amount of alcohol oxidized per unit time is approximately proportionate to body weight or liver weight, and the rate of disappearance of alcohol from the body is markedly reduced or halted entirely by hepatectomy or liver damage. However, the typical adult can metabolize 7–10 g of alcohol per hour. Two pathways of alcohol metabolism to acetaldehyde have been proposed. Acetaldehyde is then oxidized by a third metabolic process.

A. Alcohol Dehydrogenase Pathway: The main pathway for alcohol metabolism involves alcohol dehydrogenase, a cytosolic enzyme that contains zinc and catalyzes the conversion of alcohol to acetaldehyde, according to the following reaction:

$$\boxed{\text{Alcohol dehydrogenase}}$$

$$CH_3CH_2OH + NAD^+ \longrightarrow CH_3CHO + NADH + H^+$$

This enzyme is located mainly in the liver; however, trace amounts can be found in other organs such as brain and testes.

In the reaction shown above, hydrogen ion is transferred from alcohol to the cofactor nicotinamide adenine dinucleotide (NAD) to form NADH. As a net result, alcohol oxidation generates an excess of reducing equivalents in the liver, chiefly as NADH. There is some controversy over whether chronic alcohol consumption affects the activities of hepatic alcohol dehydrogenase. Actually, alcohol dehydrogenase itself is not rate-limiting, but the velocity of oxidation may depend on the availability of the cofactor NAD; therefore, the increased rate of blood alcohol clearance in alcoholics is probably not due to increased alcohol dehydrogenase activity.

B. Microsomal Ethanol Oxidizing System (MEOS): This enzyme system, also known as the mixed function oxidase system (Chapter 3), uses NADPH instead of NAD as cofactor in the following reaction:

$$\boxed{\text{MEOS}}$$

$$CH_3CH_2OH + NADPH + H^+ + O_2 \longrightarrow CH_3CHO + NADP^+ + H_2O$$

Since the K_m varies from 0.26 to 2 mmol/L for alcohol dehydrogenase and from 8 to 10 mmol/L for microsomal ethanol oxidizing system, it is thought that at low concentrations of alcohol, alcohol dehydrogenase is the main oxidizing system while at higher alcohol concentrations MEOS plays the more significant role. This may have important implications for the known interactions of alcohol (especially at high concentrations) with a host of other drugs also metabolized by this system. During chronic alcohol consumption, MEOS activity increases significantly. As described in Chapter 3, this induction of enzyme activity is associated with an increase in various constituents of the smooth fraction of the membranes involved in drug metabolism. Other "inducing" drugs such as barbiturates may also enhance the rate of blood alcohol clearance.

C. Acetaldehyde Metabolism: It is now generally accepted that over 90% of the acetaldehyde formed from alcohol is also oxidized in the liver. While several enzyme systems may be responsible for this reaction, observations that acetaldehyde levels in the liver after ethanol administration are only 100–350 μmol have led to the conclusion that mitochondrial NAD–dependent **aldehyde dehydrogenase** (the apparent K_m for acetaldehyde is $\sim$10 μmol/L) is the main pathway for acetaldehyde oxidation. The product of this reaction is acetate, which can be further metabolized to CO_2 and water. Chronic alcohol consumption results in a decreased rate of acetaldehyde oxidation in intact mitochondria, although the enzyme activity is unaffected.

Tolerance & Physical Dependence

The consumption of alcohol over a long period may result in tolerance and physical dependence. Tolerance to the intoxicating effects of alcohol is a complex process involving changes in metabolism and poorly understood changes in the nervous system. Acute tolerance may occur after a few hours of drinking; this may occur in both alcoholics and social drinkers. Although minor degrees of metabolic tolerance after chronic alcohol use have been demonstrated in which the subject's capacity to metabolize the drug increases, the maximal increase in alcohol metabolism does not account for the magnitude of the observed clinical effect. Finally, as with other sedative-hypnotic drugs, there is a limit to tissue tolerance, so that only a relatively small increase in the lethal dose occurs with increasing doses.

Chronic alcohol drinkers, when forced to reduce or discontinue alcohol, experience a withdrawal syndrome, which indicates the existence of physical dependence. Although the mechanism of physical dependence on sedative-hypnotic drugs and alcohol is not known, it is recognized that both the rate of alcohol consumption and the duration determine the intensity of the withdrawal syndrome. When consumption has been very high, merely reducing the rate of consumption may lead to signs of withdrawal.

Although tolerance and physical dependence are important components of alcohol abuse, the spectrum of illness associated with abuse of alcohol is so broad that it is difficult to contrive a simple definition of the phenomenon.

Pharmacodynamics of Acute Ethanol Abuse

A. Central Nervous System: The central nervous system is more markedly affected by acute alcohol consumption than any other organ system. Alcohol can lead to sedation and relief of anxiety, slurred speech, ataxia, impaired judgment, uninhibited behavior, or what is loosely called drunkenness.

Ethanol may affect a large number of molecular processes, but it is now generally accepted that one of its most significant sites of action is the cell membrane. More than a decade ago, it was pointed out that small organic molecules such as ethanol can readily dissolve in the lipid bilayer of cell membranes. Since then, studies have confirmed that ethanol reduces the viscosity of ("fluidizes") the membrane of many types of cells and even of artificial systems such as liposomes. Fluidization is thus a general response to ethanol of virtually all biologic membranes and one that is likely to contribute to the great diversity of the drug's effects. The fluidizing effect of ethanol has been related to changes in specific membrane functions, including neurotransmitter receptors for dopamine, norepinephrine, glutamate, and opioids; enzymes such as Na^+, K^+-ATPase, Ca^{2+}-ATPase, $5'$-nucleotidase, acetylcholinesterase, and adenylate cyclase; the mitochondrial electron transport chain; and ion channels such as those for Ca^{2+} (see Lee and Smith reference).

Ethanol may also have direct effects on receptor and transport molecules associated with the cell membrane. For example, acute ethanol exposure has been reported to increase the number of GABA receptors, which is consistent with the ability of GABA-mimetics to intensify many of the acute effects of alcohol. There is also evidence that ethanol has effects on sodium-dependent calcium uptake not accounted for by changes in bulk membrane fluidity.

Alcohol also has diverse effects at the cellular and tissue levels, particularly in the nervous system. In trigeminal motoneurons, both intracellular and extracellular application of ethanol depressed action potentials and excitatory and inhibitory postsynaptic potentials (EPSPs and IPSPs); intracellular application also depolarized the membrane, while extracellular application resulted in biphasic potential shifts. Similarly, ethanol has been reported to both reduce and enhance function at the neuromuscular junction.

In cerebellar Purkinje cells and in the dopamine-containing neurons in the substantia nigra, pars compacta, and striate nucleus, low concentrations of ethanol enhance the firing rate while higher doses inhibit it. In other systems, including the lateral geniculate nucleus, the locus ceruleus, the midbrain raphe nucleus, and hippocampal neurons in culture, only inhibitory effects were observed. More complex neuronal responses are similarly affected. For example, both the after-discharge following high-frequency stimulation of hippocampal neurons and the frog spinal reflex are enhanced by low doses of ethanol and inhibited by higher doses (see Lee and Smith reference).

B. Heart: Significant depression of myocardial contractility has been observed in individuals who consume only moderate amounts of alcohol, ie, at a blood concentration of 100 mg/dL. Myocardial biopsies in humans before and after infusion of small amounts of alcohol have shown ultrastructural changes that may be associated with impaired myocardial function. Acetaldehyde is implicated as a cause of heart abnormalities by altering myocardial stores of catecholamines.

C. Smooth Muscle: Ethanol is a vasodilator, probably as a result of both central nervous system effects (depression of the vasomotor center) and direct smooth muscle relaxation caused by its metabolite, acetaldehyde. In cases of severe overdose, hypothermia consequent to vasodilatation may be marked. Ethanol also relaxes the uterus and has been used intravenously for the suppression of premature labor. However, the acute maternal toxicity of ethanol and the hazard to the fetus should relegate this therapeutic application to history, since other drugs (β_2-adrenoceptor stimulants and calcium influx inhibitors) appear to be more effective.

Consequences of Chronic Alcohol Consumption

The literature on alcoholism contains only limited data relating to precise dose-response relationships between chronic alcohol ingestion and injury of vital organ systems. However, several major studies with appropriate controls have demonstrated that the threshold for increased mortality rate is in the range of admitted regular alcohol intake of 3–5 drinks a day. The risk rises sharply at 6 or more drinks a day. Deaths linked to alcohol consumption are caused by liver disease, cancer, accidents, and suicide.

A. Liver and Gastrointestinal Tract: Alcohol in large doses creates a metabolic cascade effect, resulting in liver and gastrointestinal tract injury. The increased NADH/NAD ratio described above produces a change in the ratio of those metabolites that is dependent on the availability of NAD. It has been proposed that this altered ratio of NADH to NAD leads to a number of metabolic abnormalities in the liver, including reduced gluconeogenesis, hypoglycemia and ketoacidosis, and accumulation of fat in the liver parenchyma. Other factors such as heredity, associated disease, and the amount and duration of alcohol intake probably determine the severity of liver injury. Acetaldehyde also adversely affects liver function. Since metabolism of acetaldehyde via aldehyde dehydrogenase results in the generation of NADH, some of the acetaldehyde effects may be attributable to NADH excess. Acetaldehyde, however, is a very reactive compound that may have toxic effects of its own.

In some cases, nutritional factors are critical in alcohol-induced liver disease. It has been suggested that essential factors such as glutathione may be decreased in a malnourished alcoholic, thus removing a valuable scavenger of toxic free radicals that otherwise will injure the liver. Clinically significant alcoholic liver disease may be insidious in onset and progress without evidence of overt nutritional abnormalities. Alcoholic fatty liver may progress to alcoholic hepatitis and finally to **cirrhosis.** Hepatic failure may be the cause of death.

Other portions of the gastrointestinal tract may also be injured. Ingestion of alcohol increases gastric and pancreatic secretion and alters mucosal barriers that may enhance the risk of gastritis and pancreatitis. Acute gastrointestinal bleeding is often caused by alcoholic gastritis. The acute effects of alcohol on the stomach are related primarily to the toxic effect of ethanol on the mucosal membranes and have relatively little to do with increased production of gastric acid. Chronic alcoholics are prone to develop gastritis and increased susceptibility to blood and plasma protein loss during drinking, which may contribute to anemia and protein malnutrition. Alcohol also injures the small intestine, leading to diarrhea, weight loss, and multiple vitamin deficiencies.

The statement sometimes made that malnutrition of alcoholic patients is due simply to dietary deficiency is probably not justified. **Malabsorption of vitamins,** especially water-soluble ones, contributes to the clinical abnormalities. Although deficiencies in water-soluble vitamins were proposed in the past to account for most of the pathologic effects of alcohol, replacement doses of the vitamins do not protect against the injurious effects of alcohol. Thiamine deficiency, associated with Wernicke-Korsakoff syndrome, peripheral neuropathy, and beriberi heart disease, occurs in alcoholic patients, yet these nutritional deficiency syndromes are relatively rare in the alcoholic population.

B. Nervous System: As noted above, chronic ethanol consumption produces tolerance and physical dependence; when forced to reduce or discontinue the drug, the subject experiences withdrawal symptoms, which may consist of discomfort and hyperexcitability in mild cases and convulsions, toxic psychosis, and delirium tremens in severe ones. Consumption of large amounts of alcohol over extended periods (usually years) can also result in a number of neurologic deficits. The patient may have impairment of intellectual and motor functions, emotional lability, reduced perceptual acuity, and amnesia.

The most frequent neurologic abnormality in chronic alcoholism is a generalized symmetric peripheral nerve injury that begins with distal paresthesias of the hands and feet. While this is a diagnosis of exclusion requiring absence of other factors known to cause peripheral neuropathy, such neuropathies are commonly related to chronic alcohol use.

Wernicke-Korsakoff syndrome is a relatively uncommon but important entity characterized by paralysis of the external eye muscles, ataxia, and altered mentation, with amnesia and impairment of memory function. It is apparently associated with thiamine deficiency but is rarely seen in the absence of alcoholism. Wernicke-Korsakoff disease may be difficult to distinguish from the acute confusional state created by acute alcohol intoxication, which later blends in with the perceptual and behavioral problems associated with alcohol withdrawal. A distinguishing feature is the longer duration of the confusional state in Korsakoff's disease and the relative absence of the agitation that would be expected during withdrawal. Because of the importance of this pathologic condition, all patients suspected of Korsakoff's disease should receive thiamine therapy (50 mg intravenously once and 50 mg intramuscularly repeated daily until a normal diet is resumed).

Alcohol may also impair visual acuity, with painless bilateral blurring that occurs over several weeks of heavy alcohol consumption. Examination may reveal scotomas and reduced visual acuity for near and distant objects. Changes are usually bilateral and symmetric and may be followed by optic nerve degeneration. Ingestion of ethanol substitutes such as methanol (see below) causes severe visual disturbances.

C. Blood: Mild **anemia** resulting from alcohol-related folic acid deficiency is the most common hematologic disorder resulting from chronic alcohol abuse. Iron deficiency anemia may result from gastrointestinal bleeding, but sideroblastic anemia has also been described in alcoholic patients. Alcohol has also been implicated as a cause of several hemolytic syndromes, some of which are associated with hyperlipidemia and severe liver disease. Alcohol directly inhibits the proliferation of all cellular elements in bone marrow.

Abnormalities in platelets and leukocytes have been described in alcoholics. These effects may account for some of the hemostatic impairment and increased frequency of infection in these individuals.

D. Cardiovascular System: Alcohol alters the cardiovascular system in many ways. Direct injury to the myocardium resulting from alcohol abuse was thought to be caused by thiamine deficiency or by contaminants in alcoholic beverages. Alcohol cardiomyopathy is now thought to occur in many men with a history of heavy drinking episodes over prolonged periods regardless of vitamin or other dietary deficiencies. Arrhythmias have been reported in association with "social" drinking and during the alcohol abstinence syndrome.

The amount of alcohol intake is apparently directly related to elevated systolic and diastolic blood pressure, independent of obesity, salt intake, coffee drinking, or cigarette smoking. Although magnesium deficiency has also been associated with changes in blood pressure and alcohol intake, convincing data are not yet available to link these 2 observations. Current data do not establish the threshold of alcohol administration that causes alterations of electrolyte balance.

Curiously, the incidence of coronary heart disease has been reported to be lower in moderate consumers of alcohol (1–3 drinks a day) than in those who totally abstain. Evidence also suggests that alcohol elevates plasma levels of the HDL_3 fraction of high-density lipoproteins. However, HDL_2, which is less dense, is epidemiologically associated with reduction of heart disease risk, while the denser HDL_3 is not clearly related to heart disease. When alcohol use is associated with liver disease, HDL fractions decrease. The clinical significance of this information is not understood.

Patients undergoing alcohol withdrawal can develop severe arrhythmias that may reflect metabolic abnormalities of hypokalemia or alterations in magnesium metabolism. Seizures and syncope as well as sudden death during alcohol withdrawal may be due to these arrhythmias.

E. Endocrine System: Chronic alcohol use has important effects on the endocrine system and mineral and fluid electrolyte balance. Clinical reports of gynecomastia and testicular atrophy in alcoholics with cirrhosis suggest a derangement in steroid hormone balance. Gynecomastia and testicular atrophy have also been noted in alcoholics who have limited evidence of liver disease.

Alcoholics with chronic liver disease may have disorders of fluid and electrolyte balance, including ascites, edema, and effusions. These factors may be related to decreased protein synthesis and portal hypertension. Alterations of whole body potassium induced by vomiting and diarrhea, as well as severe secondary hyperaldosteronism, may contribute to muscle weakness and can be worsened by diuretic therapy. Abnormalities of trace metals such as zinc may also contribute to metabolic difficulties and infertility. Some alcoholic patients develop hypoglycemia, probably as a result of impaired hepatic gluconeogenesis. Some alcoholics also develop ketosis, caused by excessive lipolytic factors, especially increased cortisol and growth hormone.

F. Fetal Alcohol Syndrome: Chronic maternal alcohol abuse during pregnancy is associated with important teratogenic effects on the offspring. The abnormalities that have been characterized as fetal alcohol syndrome include (1) retarded body growth; (2) microencephaly (small head size relative to body size); (3) poor coordination; (4) underdevelopment of midfacial region (appearing as a flattened face); and (5) minor joint anomalies. More severe cases may include congenital heart defects and mental retardation. It is likely that heavy drinking in the first trimester of pregnancy has the greatest effect on fetal maldevelopment; heavy alcohol consumption near term may have a greater effect on fetal nutrition and birth weight. Although the extent to which alcohol alone causes these abnormalities is not clear, alcohol use during pregnancy appears to be a preventable cause of some fetal abnormalities.

G. Increased Risk of Cancer: Chronic alcohol use increases the risk for cancer of the mouth, pharynx, larynx, esophagus, and liver. Although the methodologic problems of studies relating cancer to alcohol use have been formidable, the consistency of results is impressive. Much more information is required before a threshold level for alcohol consumption as it relates to cancer can be established. In fact, alcohol itself does not appear to be a carcinogen in most test systems. However, alcoholic beverages may carry potential carcinogens produced in fermentation or processing.

Alcohol-Drug Interactions

Interactions between ethanol and other drugs can have important clinical effects that result from alterations in the pharmacokinetics or pharmacodynamics of the second drug. The interaction with disulfiram is discussed on p 259.

The most frequent pharmacokinetic alcohol-drug interactions occur as a result of alcohol-induced proliferation of the smooth endoplasmic reticulum of liver cells as described in Chapter 3. Thus, prolonged intake of alcohol without damage to the liver may enhance the metabolic biotransformation of other drugs. In contrast, *acute* alcohol use may *inhibit* metabolism of other drugs. This inhibition may be due to alteration of metabolism or alteration of liver blood flow. This acute alcohol effect may contribute to the commonly recognized danger of mixing alcohol with other drugs when performing activities requiring some skill, especially driving. Phenothiazines, tricyclic antidepressants, and sedative-hypnotic drugs are the most important drugs that may interact with alcohol by this mechanism.

Pharmacodynamic alcohol interactions are also of great clinical significance. Additive interaction with other sedative-hypnotics is most important. Alcohol also potentiates the pharmacologic effects of many nonsedative drugs including vasodilators and oral hypoglycemic agents. Alcohol also enhances the antiplatelet action of aspirin.

II. CLINICAL PHARMACOLOGY OF ETHANOL

Ethanol is probably the least potent drug consumed by humans, yet it is the cause of more preventable morbidity and mortality than all other drugs combined with the exception of tobacco.

Although the disorder known as alcoholism is difficult to define, epidemiologic studies of alcohol consumption provide important information for predicting health-related factors that predispose to physical and psychologic problems. Approximately 80% of adults in the USA consume alcoholic beverages. It is estimated that 5–10% of the adult male population have alcohol-related problems at some time in their lives. Recent studies in almost 90,000 men and women who participated in multiphasic health examinations and were observed over a 10-year period disclosed a twice-normal mortality rate in persons who admitted to having 6 or more drinks a day; those taking 3–5 drinks a day had a rate 40–50% higher than normal. Cancer, hepatic cirrhosis, and accidents contributed significantly to the excessive mortality rate of heavy drinkers. Smoking, which is common in alcoholics, is also a possible mortality risk factor in heavy drinkers. The results of the study suggest that there is a threshold for increased mortality risk in the range of 2–3 drinks a day and that this risk rises sharply at a level of 6 or more drinks a day. There is also evidence that small amounts of alcohol (one beer a day) place patients at less risk of myocardial infarction than individuals who never consume alcohol.

The search for specific etiologic factors or the identification of significant predisposing variables for alcohol abuse has generally given disappointing results. Personality type, severe life stresses, psychiatric disorders, and parental role models are not reliable predictors of alcohol abuse. Comparisons of differences in alcohol metabolism are unreliable, and markers of disordered alcohol metabolism are not sufficiently predictive. It is clear that alcohol abuse is not equally distributed in all social groups, and its abuse appears to occur at a higher rate among relatives of alcoholics than in the general population. The rate of alcoholism in persons with an alcoholic biologic parent is almost 4 times that of a selected control group—a finding that has now been confirmed by several studies. It is difficult to distinguish between contributing factors of familial learning experiences and genetic variables, but current evidence suggests that genetic factors play a role in defining human alcohol use and medical complications. Genetic control of alcohol preference in animals has been clearly established. However, the nature of the genetic factors involved is still unknown.

MANAGEMENT OF ACUTE ALCOHOLIC INTOXICATION

Nontolerant individuals who consume alcohol in large quantities develop typical effects of acute sedative-hypnotic drug overdose, along with the cardiovascular effects described above (vasodilatation, tachycardia) and gastrointestinal irritation. Since tolerance is not absolute, even chronic alcoholics may become severely intoxicated. The degree of intoxication depends upon 3 factors: the blood ethanol concentration, the rapidity of the rise of the alcohol level, and the time during which the blood level is maintained. The pattern of drinking, the state of the absorptive surface of the gastrointestinal tract, and the presence in the body of other medications also affect the apparent degree of intoxication.

The most important goal in the treatment of acute alcohol intoxication is to prevent severe respiratory depression and aspiration of vomitus. Even with very high blood ethanol levels, survival is possible as long as the respiratory and cardiovascular systems can be supported. The lethal dose of alcohol varies widely because of varying degrees of tolerance. A normal nontolerant adult individual can metabolize 7–10 g of alcohol per hour (the ethanol content of 30 mL of 80-proof whiskey). The legal definition of intoxication in the USA varies in different states, but a blood level of 100 mg/dL or higher is often regarded as evidence of impaired judgment and performance sufficient for conviction of driving while intoxicated. The average blood alcohol concentration in fatal cases is about 400 mg/dL.

Metabolic alterations may require treatment of hypoglycemia and ketosis by administration of glucose. Alcoholic patients who are dehydrated and vomiting should also receive electrolyte solutions. If vomiting is severe, large amounts of potassium may also be required as long as renal function is normal. Especially important is recognition of decreased phosphate stores, which may be aggravated by glucose administration. Low phosphate stores may contribute to poor wound healing, neurologic deficits, and increased risk of infection.

MANAGEMENT OF ALCOHOL WITHDRAWAL SYNDROME

When alcohol ingestion is abruptly discontinued, the characteristic syndrome of motor agitation, anxiety, insomnia, and reduction of seizure threshold occurs. The severity of the alcohol withdrawal syndrome is usually proportionate to the dose and the duration of alcohol abuse. However, this can be greatly modified by the use of other sedatives as well as by associated medical (eg, diabetes) or surgical factors (injury). In its mildest form, the alcohol withdrawal syndrome of tremor, anxiety, and insomnia occurs 6–8 hours after alcohol is stopped. These effects usually abate in 1–2 days. In some patients, more severe withdrawal reactions occur in which visual hallucinations, total disorientation, and marked abnormalities of vital signs occur. The more severe the withdrawal syndrome, the greater the need for meticulous investigation of possible underlying medical or surgical complications. The mortality risks of severe alcohol withdrawal have been overstated in the past. The prognosis is probably related chiefly to the underlying medical and surgical complications.

The major objective of drug therapy in the alcohol withdrawal period is prevention of seizures, delirium, and arrhythmias. Restoration of potassium, magnesium, and phosphate balance should be achieved rapidly if renal function is normal. Thiamine therapy is initiated in more severe cases. Persons in mild alcohol withdrawal do not need any other pharmacologic assistance.

Specific drug treatment for detoxification in severe cases involves 2 basic principles: substituting a long-acting sedative-hypnotic drug for alcohol and then gradually reducing ("tapering") the dose of the long-acting drug. Unfortunately, the most widely used "treatment" for alcohol withdrawal is renewed alcohol intake. Although alcohol can be slowly tapered, it is psychologically undesirable to maintain the patient on alcohol. Currently, benzodiazepines are preferred for this purpose. The benzodiazepines chlordiazepoxide and diazepam have pharmacologically active metabolites that may accumulate. Oxazepam is rapidly converted to inactive water-soluble metabolites that will not accumulate and is especially useful in alcoholic patients with liver disease. Most benzodiazepines are poorly absorbed from intramuscular sites; when rapid clinical effects are required, the intravenous route is preferred.

Phenothiazine medications for alcohol withdrawal have potentially serious side effects (eg, increasing seizures) that probably outweigh their benefits. Antihistaminic medications have been used but with little justification.

Phenytoin (diphenylhydantoin) may be effective in preventing seizures in alcoholic patients with a history of seizures. Since phenytoin is poorly absorbed from intramuscular sites, the drug should be given by mouth or intravenously. A loading dose of 12–15 mg/kg is given, and the patient is maintained on 300 mg/d with monitoring of blood levels.

After the alcohol withdrawal syndrome has been treated acutely, sedative-hypnotic medications must be tapered slowly over several weeks. Complete detoxification is probably not achieved within a few days of sobering up. Several months may be required for restoration of normal nervous system function.

Disulfiram

Disulfiram (tetraethylthiuram), a widely used antioxidant in the rubber industry, has been shown to cause extreme discomfort to patients who drink alcoholic beverages. Disulfiram given by itself to nondrinkers has little effect; however, flushing, throbbing headache, nausea, vomiting, sweating, hypotension, and confusion occur within a few minutes after taking a drink. The effect may last 30 minutes in mild cases or several hours in severe ones. After the symptoms wear off, the patient is usually exhausted and may sleep for several hours.

Disulfiram acts by inhibiting **aldehyde dehydrogenase.** Thus, alcohol is metabolized as usual, but acetaldehyde is accumulated. The symptoms resulting from disulfiram plus alcohol are typical for acetaldehyde toxicity; the reaction is reproduced by acetaldehyde infusion in humans.

Disulfiram is rapidly and completely absorbed from the gastrointestinal tract; however, a period of 12 hours is required for its full action. Its elimination rate is very slow, so that the action may persist for several days after the last dose. The drug interacts with many other therapeutic agents.

Disulfiram should be considered as a pharmacologic adjunct in the treatment of alcoholism and should only be used in conjunction with behavioral therapies. When the drug is prescribed, the alcohol content of common nonprescription medications should be considered and communicated to the patient; some of these are listed in Table 68–3. Management with disulfiram should be initiated only when the patient has been free of alcohol for at least 24 hours. The safety of disulfiram in pregnancy has not been demonstrated. The duration of disulfiram treatment should be individualized and determined by the patient's responsiveness and clinical improvement. The usual oral dose is 250 mg daily taken at bedtime. Mandated use of disulfiram by court order is probably not efficacious.

Many other drugs, eg, metronidazole, have disulfiramlike effects on ethanol metabolism (see Stockley reference).

III. OTHER ALCOHOLS

Other alcohols related to ethanol have wide applications as industrial solvents and occasionally cause severe poisoning.

Methanol (CH_3OH; methyl alcohol, wood alcohol) is derived from the destructive distillation of wood. Methanol is used as a gasoline additive, as a home heating material, as an industrial solvent, as a solvent in xerographic copier solutions, and as a feedstock for bacterial synthesis of protein. Methanol is most frequently found in the home in the form of "canned heat" or in windshield washing materials. It can be absorbed through the skin or from the respiratory or gastrointestinal tracts. It is rapidly absorbed from the gastrointestinal tract and distributed in body water. The primary mechanism of elimination of methanol in humans is by oxidation to formaldehyde, formic acid, and CO_2:

$$CH_3OH \longrightarrow HCH \longrightarrow HCOH \longrightarrow CO_2 + H_2O$$

Methanol may also be removed by induced vomiting, and small amounts are excreted in the breath, sweat, and urine. Methanol does not bind to charcoal.

Various animal species show great variability in mean lethal doses of methanol. The special susceptibility of humans to methanol toxicity is probably due to the formate metabolite of methanol and not to methanol itself or to formaldehyde, the intermediate metabolite.

The enzyme chiefly responsible for methanol oxidation in the liver is alcohol dehydrogenase. Ethanol has a higher affinity than methanol for alcohol dehydrogenase; thus, saturation of alcohol dehydrogenase with ethanol can reduce formate production and is often used as treatment for acute methanol toxicity. Another agent known to inhibit alcohol dehydrogenase, 4-methylpyrazole, alone or in combination with ethanol, is probably of therapeutic value in methanol as well as ethylene glycol poisoning (see below).

Polyhydric alcohols such as **ethylene glycol** (CH_2OHCH_2OH) are used as heat exchangers, in antifreeze formulations, and as industrial solvents. Owing to the low volatility of the glycols, they produce little vapor hazard at ordinary temperatures. However, since they are used as antifreeze mixtures and as heat exchangers, they may be encountered in vapor or mist form, particularly if the temperature is high. Ethylene glycol appears to be considerably more toxic to humans than to many other animal species. As with other alcohols, ethylene glycol is metabolized by alcohol dehydrogenase to aldehydes, acids, and oxalate. The oxalate may be deposited in the renal tubules, causing acute renal failure. Prompt administration of ethanol or treatment with 4-methylpyrazole may prevent the development of metabolic acidosis.

MANAGEMENT OF INTOXICATION WITH OTHER ALCOHOLS

Methanol Intoxication

Severe methanol poisoning is usually encountered in chronic alcoholics and may not be recognized unless characteristic symptoms are noted in a group of patients. Because methanol and its metabolite formate are much more potent toxins than ethanol, it is essential that patients with methanol poisoning be recognized and treated as soon as possible.

The most important initial symptom in methanol poisoning is a visual disturbance frequently described as "like being in a snowstorm." Visual disturbances are a universal complaint in epidemics of methanol poisoning. A complaint of blurred vision with a relatively clear sensorium should strongly suggest the diagnosis of methanol poisoning. In severe cases, the odor of formaldehyde may be present on the breath or in the urine. The development of bradycardia, prolonged coma, seizures, and resistant acidosis all indicate a poor prognosis.

Physical findings in methanol poisoning are generally nonspecific. Fixed dilated pupils have been described in severe cases. Optic atrophy is a late finding. The cause of death in fatal cases is sudden cessation of respiration.

It is critical that the blood methanol level be determined as soon as possible if the diagnosis is suspected. If the clinical suspicion of methanol poisoning is high, treatment should not be delayed. Methanol levels in excess of 50 mg/dL are probably an absolute indication for hemodialysis and ethanol treatment, although formic acid blood levels may be a better indication of clinical pathology. Additional laboratory evidence includes metabolic acidosis with an elevated anion gap and osmolar gap (see Chapter 62). Ethylene glycol, paraldehyde, and salicylates may also cause an anion gap. A decrease in serum bicarbonate is a uniform feature of severe methanol poisoning. Ethylene glycol toxicity (see below) usually results in central nervous system excitation, increase in muscle enzymes, and hypocalcemia but not visual symptoms. Salicylate intoxication can be readily determined from salicylate levels in the blood.

The first treatment for methanol poisoning, as in all critical poisoning situations, is to establish respiration, with an artificial airway if necessary. Emesis can be induced if the patient is not comatose, is not having seizures, and has not lost the gag reflex. If any of these contraindications exists, the patient should be endotracheally intubated and gastric lavage carried out with a large-bore tube.

There are 3 "specific" modalities of treatment for severe methanol poisoning: suppression of metabolism by alcohol dehydrogenase to toxic products, dialysis to enhance removal of methanol and its toxic products, and alkalinization to counteract metabolic acidosis.

Because ethanol competes for alcohol dehydrogenase, which is responsible for metabolizing methanol to formic acid, it is essential to saturate this enzyme with the less toxic ethanol. The dose-dependent characteristics of ethanol metabolism and the variability induced by chronic ethanol intake require frequent monitoring of blood ethanol levels to ensure appropriate alcohol concentration. Ethanol may be given intravenously as a 10% solution.

With initiation of dialysis procedures, ethanol will also be eliminated in the dialysate, requiring alterations in the dose of ethanol. Hemodialysis is discussed in Chapter 62.

Because of profound metabolic acidosis in methanol poisoning, treatment with bicarbonate may be necessary. Quantities of bicarbonate to be administered should be based on estimated sodium intake, potassium balance, and cardiovascular status.

Since folate-dependent systems are probably responsible for the oxidation of formic acid to CO_2 in humans, it would probably be useful to administer folic acid to patients poisoned with methanol, although this has never been tested in clinical studies. 4-Methylpyrazole, by inhibiting alcohol dehydrogenase, may also be a useful adjunct in methanol poisoning when it becomes available for human use.

A special diagnosic problem occurs if a patient has a relatively low methanol level but visual symptoms are present. In this situation, laboratory tests for methanol itself should be repeated and confirmed with osmolality estimates. If visual impairment is present, hemodialysis should be started in spite of low methanol levels.

Ethylene Glycol Intoxication

Few clinical cases of ethylene glycol poisoning have been reported. As with methanol poisoning, there may be a delay in the onset of acidosis and renal insufficiency. Three stages of ethylene glycol overdose have been recognized. Initially, there is transient excitation followed by central nervous system depression. Severe acidosis then develops, and finally delayed renal insufficiency occurs. Ophthalmoscopic examination is usually normal, although occasional cases of papilledema have been described. Oxalate crystals are usually present in urine. Ethylene glycol–intoxicated patients have no detectable odor of alcohol on their breath. In severe cases, increased muscle enzyme and decreased calcium have been found in the plasma. The key to the diagnosis of ethylene glycol poisoning is the recognition of anion gap acidosis, osmolar gap, and oxalate crystals in the urine in a patient without visual symptoms. As with methanol poisoning, early alcohol infusion and dialysis are required. 4-Methylpyrazole therapy will also be of use in this situation when it becomes commercially available.

REFERENCES

Becker CE: Alcohol and drug use: Is there a "safe" amount? *West J Med* 1984;**141**:884.

Becker CE: The alcoholic patient is a toxic emergency. *Emerg Med Clin North Am* 1983;**1**:51.

Becker CE: Methanol poisoning. *J Emerg Med* 1983;**2**:47.

Becker CE, Roe RL, Scott RA: *Alcohol as a Drug: A Curriculum on Pharmacology, Neurology and Toxicology.* RE Kreiger, 1979.

Brien JF, Loomis CW: Pharmacology of acetaldehyde. *Can J Physiol Pharmacol* 1983;**61**:1.

Goekas MC et al: Ethanol: The liver and the gastrointestinal tract. *Ann Intern Med* 1981;**95**:198.

Interactions of drugs with alcohol. *Med Lett Drugs Ther* (April 3) 1981;**23**:33.

Klatsky AR, Friedman JD, Siegelaub AB: Alcohol and mortality: A ten year Kaiser Permanente experience. *Ann Intern Med* 1981;**95**:139.

Lee NM, Smith AS: Ethanol. In: *Toxicology of CNS Depressants.* Ho IK (editor). CRC Press, 1986.

Meagher RC, Sieber F, Spivak JL: Suppression of hematopoietic-progenitor-cell proliferation by ethanol and acetaldehyde. *N Engl J Med* 1982;**307**:845.

Neurobiological correlates of intoxication and physical dependence upon ethanol. (Symposium.) *Fed Proc* 1981;**40**:2048.

Stockley IH: Drugs, foods, and environmental chemical agents which can initiate Antabuse-like reactions with alcohol. *Pharmacy Int* 1983;**4**:12.

22

Antiepileptic Drugs

Roger J. Porter, MD, & William H. Pitlick, PhD

Approximately 1% of the population of the USA has epilepsy, the second most common neurologic disorder after stroke. Although standard therapy permits control of seizures in 80% of these patients, 500,000 people in the USA have uncontrolled epilepsy. Epilepsy is a heterogeneous symptom complex—a chronic disorder characterized by recurrent seizures. Seizures are finite episodes of brain dysfunction resulting from abnormal discharge of cerebral neurons. The causes of seizures are many and include the gamut of neurologic diseases from infection to neoplasm to head injury. In only a few subgroups has heredity been proved to be a major contributing factor. The antiepileptic drugs described in this chapter are also used in patients with febrile seizures or with seizures occurring as part of an acute illness such as meningitis, even though the term epilepsy is not usually applied to such patients unless they later develop chronic seizures. Occasionally, seizures are caused by an acute underlying toxic or metabolic disorder, in which case appropriate therapy should be directed toward the specific abnormality, eg, hypocalcemia. In most cases of epilepsy, however, the choice of medication depends on the empirical seizure classification.

Before discovery of the antiepileptic drugs, treatment of epilepsy consisted of trephining, cupping, and the use of herbal medicines and animal extracts. In 1857, Sir Charles Locock reported the successful use of potassium bromide in the treatment of what is now known as catamenial epilepsy. In 1912, phenobarbital was first used for epilepsy, and in the next 25 years, 35 analogs of phenobarbital were studied as anticonvulsants. In 1938, phenytoin was found to be effective against experimental seizures in cats.

Between 1935 and 1960, tremendous strides were made both in the development of experimental models and in methods for screening and testing new antiepileptic drugs. During that period, 13 new antiepileptic drugs were developed and marketed. Following the enactment of requirements for proof of drug efficacy in 1962, antiepileptic drug development slowed dramatically. In the last 25 years, only 5 new antiepileptic drugs have reached the marketplace.

For a long time it was assumed that a single drug could be developed for treatment of all forms of epilepsy. It now appears unlikely that the wide variety of epileptic seizures can be managed successfully with just one drug. More than one mechanism may be re-

sponsible for the various seizures, and drugs useful for one seizure type may occasionally aggravate other types.

Drugs used in the treatment of the 2 major types of seizures (partial and generalized; Table 22–1) are quite distinct in their clinical effects and also fall into 2 pharmacologic classes, even though seizures may be induced experimentally by a wide variety of methods. The clinical aspects of generalized seizures, especially absence seizures, are highly correlated with experimental seizures produced in animals by subcutaneous administration of pentylenetetrazol (sometimes also called the Metrazol test). Likewise, partial seizures in humans correlate positively with experimental seizures elicited by the maximal electroshock (MES) test. In general, antiepileptic drugs effective against maximal electroshock seizures alter ionic transport across excitable membranes. Phenytoin, for example, is effective against partial seizures and maximal electroshock but with the exception of generalized tonic-clonic seizures is not effective against generalized seizures or those induced by subcutaneous pentylenetetrazol (scMet); it affects membrane potentials through its action on Ca^{2+} and Na^+ fluxes. On the other hand, ethosuximide, which is active against certain generalized seizures and pentylenetetrazol, has little or no direct effect on ion fluxes across excitable membranes. The effectiveness of ethosuximide can be diminished by lipophilic substitution, in which more anti–maximal electroshock and less antipentylenetetrazol activity is observed. It is notable that the 2 dis-

Table 22–1. Classification of seizure types.

Partial seizures
Simple partial seizures.
Complex partial seizures.
Partial seizures secondarily generalized.

Generalized seizures
Generalized tonic-clonic (grand mal) seizures.
Absence (petit mal) seizures.
Tonic seizures.
Atonic seizures.
Clonic and myoclonic seizures.
Infantile spasms.*

*Infantile spasms is an epileptic syndrome rather than a specific seizure type; drugs useful in infantile spasms will be reviewed separately.

tinct classes of antiepileptic drugs have apparently different mechanisms of action in spite of marked structural similarities between many of the drugs in the 2 groups. These differences in potency are indicated below in terms of ED50s for the 2 standard tests.

I. BASIC PHARMACOLOGY OF ANTIEPILEPTIC DRUGS

Chemistry

Approximately 16 major antiepileptic drugs are presently available. Thirteen of them can be classified into 5 very similar chemical groups: barbiturates, hydantoins, oxazolidinediones, succinimides, and acetylureas. These groups have in common a similar heterocyclic ring structure with a variety of substituents (Fig 22–1). The remaining 3 drugs are carbamazepine, valproic acid, and the benzodiazepines—all structurally dissimilar from one another.

For drugs with the basic structure shown in Fig 22–1, the substituents on the heterocyclic ring determine the pharmacologic class, either anti–maximal electroshock or antipentylenetetrazol. Very small changes in structure can alter the mechanism of action and clinical properties of a drug significantly. For example, the presence of a phenyl group at the R_1 position, as in phenytoin, produces activity against partial seizures; whereas an alkyl group, as in ethosuximide, produces activity against certain generalized seizures.

The development of new drugs involves structural modification based on knowledge of structure-activity relationships in the hope that a specific receptor exists for a drug with a particular spatial conformation. Even though a great many modifications and corresponding pharmacologic data exist, especially with such drugs as phenytoin and phenobarbital, only unproved hypotheses can be offered in an attempt to explain the nature of the drug receptors. Phenytoin, for example, has at least 3 major pharmacologic actions—it affects membrane conductances, alters reuptake of neuro-

transmitters, and changes hormonal balance—and it is not known which of these (if any) is responsible for the drug's anticonvulsant activity. In spite of these limitations, however, some generalizations regarding the structural requirements for anticonvulsant activity are possible. Common stereochemical features have been identified; most antiepileptic drugs possess 2 hydrophobic regions. When 2 antiepileptic drugs are compared and these regions are superimposed, 2 electron donor groups are found with similar orientation and position. The distances between these electron donor groups are critical for anticonvulsant activity. The 2,4-benzodiazepines, for example, which match the stereochemistry of known anticonvulsants, are more active than the 1,3-benzodiazepines. In general, to be active against partial seizures, the drug must have at least one phenyl ring as a hydrophobic region. Unfortunately, addition of hydrophobic groups reduces solubility, and diphenylbarbituric acid, which is effective against experimental seizures, is not useful clinically because of its very low solubility.

Pharmacokinetics

As a class, antiepileptic drugs exhibit many similar pharmacokinetic properties, even though their structural and chemical properties are often quite diverse. Although many of these compounds are only sparingly soluble, absorption is usually good, with 80–100% of the dose reaching the circulation. Bioavailability is a problem with phenytoin, in which both the rate and extent of absorption are highly dependent on the formulation.

Except for phenytoin, the benzodiazepines, and valproic acid, anticonvulsants are not highly bound to plasma proteins. Only the 3 named drugs are able to displace other highly bound drugs, and such drugs may also displace other anticonvulsants.

Antiepileptic drugs have low extraction ratios (see Chapter 3). An increase in the percentage of free drug will not change free concentrations but will reduce total drug concentrations and may lead the clinician to increase the dose; this increase in dose will result in higher free drug levels and possible drug toxicity. Sodium valproate is unique in that the fraction of drug bound is a function of the concentration of both the drug and the free fatty acids in plasma.

Antiepileptic drugs are cleared chiefly by hepatic mechanisms. Many, such as primidone and the benzodiazepines, are converted to active metabolites that are also cleared by the liver. The intrinsic ability of the liver to metabolize anticonvulsant drugs is generally low and, with the exception of phenytoin, independent of concentration. These drugs are predominantly distributed into total body water. Plasma clearance is relatively slow; many anticonvulsants are therefore considered to be medium- to long-acting. For most, half-lives are usually greater than 12 hours. The intrinsic clearance of antiepileptic drugs is sensitive both to those drugs and to other drugs. Phenobarbital and carbamazepine are potent inducers of hepatic microsomal enzyme activity.

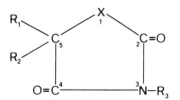

Figure 22–1. Antiepileptic heterocyclic ring structure. The "X" varies as follows: hydantoin derivatives, –N–; barbiturates, –C–N–; oxazolidinediones, –O–; succinimides, –C–; acetylureas, –NH$_2$ (N connected to C2). R_1, R_2, and R_3 vary within each subgroup.

DRUGS USED IN PARTIAL SEIZURES & GENERALIZED TONIC-CLONIC SEIZURES

The major drugs for partial and generalized tonic-clonic seizures are phenytoin (and congeners), carbamazepine, and the barbiturates.

PHENYTOIN

Phenytoin (Dilantin) is the oldest nonsedative antiepileptic drug, introduced in 1938 following a systematic evaluation of compounds such as phenobarbital that altered electrically induced seizures in laboratory animals. It was known for decades as diphenylhydantoin (DPH).

Chemistry
Phenytoin is a diphenyl-substituted hydantoin with the structure shown below. Alkyl substituents at the 5 position result in sedative properties.

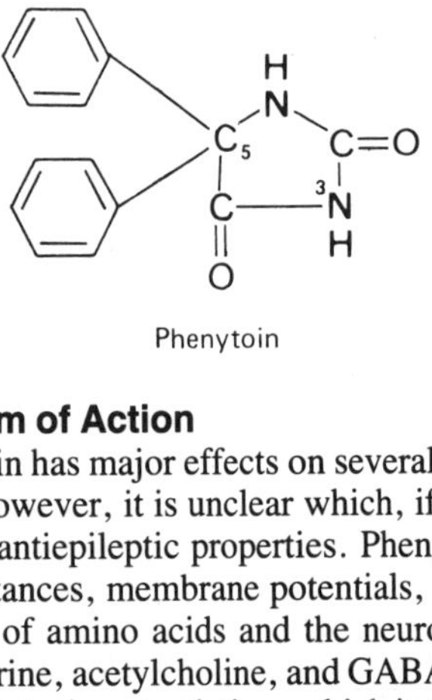

Phenytoin

Mechanism of Action
Phenytoin has major effects on several physiologic systems. However, it is unclear which, if any, are related to its antiepileptic properties. Phenytoin affects ion conductances, membrane potentials, and the concentrations of amino acids and the neurotransmitters norepinephrine, acetylcholine, and GABA. Phenytoin blocks posttetanic potentiation, which is thought to be the basis for its inhibition of the development and spread of epileptiform discharges, probably by raising membrane potentials and suppressing burst activity and repetitive firing.

Early studies indicated that phenytoin suppresses repetitive action potentials, in part by blocking sodium channels and decreasing the inward flux of sodium—similar to that observed with local anesthetics and tetrodotoxin. However, these effects are seen only at high concentrations and may not be related to the therapeutic effects of phenytoin. In addition, phenytoin paradoxically causes excitation in some cerebral neurons. The reduction of calcium permeability, with inhibition of calcium influx across the cell membrane, may explain the ability of phenytoin to inhibit a variety of calcium-induced secretory processes, including release of hormones and neurotransmitters.

At high concentrations, phenytoin also inhibits the release of serotonin and norepinephrine, promotes the uptake of dopamine, and inhibits monoamine oxidase activity. The drug interacts with membrane lipids; this binding might promote the stabilization of the membrane. The significance of these biochemical actions and their relationship to phenytoin activity are unclear.

Recent studies provide evidence that phenytoin may affect GABA-mediated inhibition through indirect effects. The drug seems to decrease GABA uptake, induce proliferation of GABA receptors, suppress excitatory amino acid neurotransmitter release, increase the breakdown of acetylcholine, and increase the function of glial Na^+, K^+-ATPase; it may antagonize glutamic acid.

The mechanism of phenytoin's action probably involves a combination of actions at several levels. Evidence seems to indicate that at therapeutic concentrations, the major actions of phenytoin are to decrease excitatory neurotransmission and potentiate GABA-mediated inhibition. The ED50 of phenytoin against maximal electroshock in mice is 9.5 mg/kg; phenytoin has no activity against pentylenetetrazol seizures.

Clinical Use
Phenytoin is one of the most effective drugs against partial seizures and generalized tonic-clonic seizures. In the latter, it appears to be effective against attacks that are either primary or secondary to another seizure type.

Pharmacokinetics
Absorption of phenytoin is highly dependent on the formulation of the dosage form. Particle size and pharmaceutical additives affect both the rate and extent of absorption. Oral absorption of phenytoin sodium is nearly complete in most patients, although the time to peak may range from 3 hours to 12 hours. Absorption after intramuscular injection is unpredictable, and some drug precipitation in the muscle occurs; this route of administration is not recommended.

Phenytoin is highly bound to plasma proteins. It appears certain that the total plasma level decreases when the percentage that is bound decreases, as in uremia or hypoalbuminemia, but correlation of free levels with clinical states remains uncertain. Drug concentration in cerebrospinal fluid is proportionate to the free plasma level. Phenytoin is highly bound to brain proteins and is also reversibly stored in fat.

Phenytoin is metabolized primarily by parahydroxylation to 5-(p-hydroxyphenyl)-5-phenyl hydantoin (HPPH), which is subsequently conjugated with glucuronic acid. The metabolites are clinically inactive and are excreted in the urine. Only a very small portion of phenytoin is excreted unchanged.

The pharmacokinetics of phenytoin are dose-dependent. At very low blood levels, phenytoin metabolism is proportionate to the rate at which the drug is presented to the liver, ie, first-order metabolism. However, as blood levels rise within the therapeutic range, the maximum capacity of the liver to metabolize phenytoin is approached (Fig 22–2). Further increases in dose, even though relatively small, may produce very large changes in phenytoin concentrations. In such cases, the half-life of the drug increases markedly, steady state is not achieved (since the plasma level continues to rise), and patients quickly develop symptoms of toxicity.

The half-life of phenytoin varies from 12 to 36 hours, with an average of 24 hours for most patients in the low to mid therapeutic range. Much longer half-lives are observed at higher concentrations. At low blood levels, it takes 5–7 days to reach steady-state blood levels after every dosage change; at higher levels it may be 4–6 weeks before blood levels are stable.

Therapeutic Levels & Dose

The therapeutic plasma level of phenytoin for most patients is between 10 and 20 μg/mL. A loading dose can be given either orally or intravenously; the latter is the method of choice for convulsive status epilepticus (discussed later). When oral therapy is started, it is common to begin adults at a dosage of 300 mg/d regardless of body weight. While this may be acceptable in some patients, it frequently yields steady-state blood levels below 10 μg/mL, the minimum therapeutic level for most patients. If seizures continue, higher doses are usually necessary to achieve plasma levels in the upper therapeutic range. Because of its dose-dependent kinetics, some toxicity may occur with only small increments in dose; the phenytoin dosage should be increased each time by only 25–30 mg in adults, and ample time should be allowed for the new steady

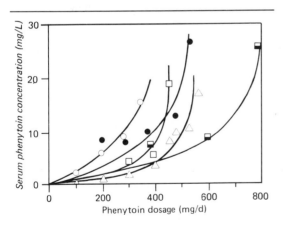

Figure 22–2. Nonlinear effect of phenytoin dosage on plasma concentration. Five different patients (identified by different symbols) received increasing dosages of phenytoin by mouth, and the steady-state serum concentration was measured at each dosage. The curves are not linear, since, as the dosage increases, the first-pass effect is proportionately less marked. Note also the marked variation among patients in the serum levels achieved at any dosage. (Modified, with permission, from Jusko WJ: Bioavailability and disposition kinetics of phenytoin in man. Pages 115–136 in: *Quantitative Analytic Studies in Epilepsy.* Kellaway P, Peterson I [editors]. Raven Press, 1977.)

state to be achieved before further increasing the dose. A common clinical error is to increase the dose directly from 300 mg/d to 400 mg/d; toxicity frequently occurs at a variable time thereafter. In children, a dose of 5 mg/kg/d should be followed by readjustment after steady-state plasma levels are obtained.

Two types of oral phenytoin sodium are currently available in the USA, differing in their respective rates of dissolution; one is absorbed rapidly and one more slowly. Only the latter can be given in a single daily dose, and care must be used when changing brands. Although a few patients being given phenytoin on a chronic basis have been proved to have low blood levels either from poor absorption or rapid metabolism, the most common cause of low levels is poor compliance.

Drug Interactions & Interference With Laboratory Tests

Drug interactions involving phenytoin are primarily related either to protein binding or to metabolism. Since phenytoin is highly bound, other highly bound drugs, such as phenylbutazone, sulfonamides, benzodiazepines, or anticoagulants, can displace phenytoin from its binding site, causing an increase in free drug levels and intoxication when efforts are made to maintain total drug levels in the therapeutic range. The protein binding of phenytoin is markedly decreased in the presence of renal disease. A binding inhibitor, irreversible in the presence of uremia, may cause this displacement of phenytoin. The drug has an affinity for thyroid-binding globulin (TBG), which confuses some tests of thyroid function; the most reliable screening test of thyroid function in patients on phenytoin appears to be measurement of TSH.

Phenytoin has been shown to induce microsomal enzymes responsible for the metabolism of a number of drugs. Autostimulation of its own metabolism, however, appears to be insignificant. Other drugs, notably phenobarbital and carbamazepine, cause decreases in phenytoin steady-state concentrations through induction of hepatic microsomal enzymes. On the other hand, isoniazid inhibits the metabolism of phenytoin, resulting in increased steady-state concentrations when the 2 drugs are given together.

Toxicity

Dose-related side effects caused by phenytoin are unfortunately similar to other antiepileptic drugs in this group, making differentiation difficult in patients receiving multiple drugs. Nystagmus occurs early, as does loss of smooth extraocular pursuit movements, but neither is an indication for decreasing the dose. Diplopia and ataxia are the most common dose-related side effects requiring dose adjustment; sedation usually occurs only at considerably higher levels. Gingival hyperplasia and hirsutism occur to some degree in most patients; the latter can be especially unpleasant in females. Long-term chronic use is associated in some patients with coarsening of facial features and with mild peripheral neuropathy, usually manifested by diminished deep tendon reflexes in the lower extremities. Chronic use may also result in abnormalities of vitamin D metabolism leading to osteomalacia. Low folate levels and megaloblastic anemia have been reported, but the clinical importance of this observation is unknown.

Idiosyncratic reactions to phenytoin are relatively rare. Most commonly, a typical skin rash heralds the hypersensitivity of the patient to the drug, which is then appropriately discontinued. Fever may also occur, and in rare cases the skin lesions may be severe and exfoliative. Lymphadenopathy may be difficult to distinguish from malignant lymphoma, and although some studies suggest a causal relationship between phenytoin and Hodgkin's disease, the data are far from conclusive. Hematologic complications are exceedingly rare, although agranulocytosis has been reported in combination with fever and rash.

MEPHENYTOIN, ETHOTOIN, & PHENACEMIDE

Many congeners of phenytoin have been synthesized, but only 3 are marketed in the USA, and these are used to a limited extent. Mephenytoin (Mesantoin) has a methyl group at the 3 position of the heterocyclic ring, and one of the phenyl groups at the 5 position is replaced by an ethyl group (Fig 22–1). Ethotoin (Peganone) has an ethyl group at the 3 position of the heterocyclic ring and only one phenyl group at the 5 position. The third analog, phenacemide (Phenurone), is similar to phenytoin except that only one phenyl ring is present at carbon 5 and the heterocyclic ring has been opened to form a straight-chain phenylacetylurea compound. The ED50 of mephenytoin against maximal electroshock in mice is 61 mg/kg; its antipentylenetetrazol ED50 is 30 mg/kg. The anti–maximal electroshock ED50 of ethotoin is 86; its antipentylenetetrazol ED50 is 48.

In spite of their anti–maximal electroshock:antipentylenetetrazol ratios, mephenytoin and ethotoin, like phenytoin, appear to be most effective against generalized tonic-clonic seizures and partial seizures. No well-controlled clinical trials have documented their effectiveness. The incidence of severe reactions such as dermatitis, agranulocytosis, or hepatitis is higher for mephenytoin than for phenytoin.

Ethotoin may be recommended for patients hypersensitive to phenytoin, but larger doses are required. The side effects and toxicity are generally less severe than those associated with phenytoin, but the drug appears to be less effective.

The pharmacokinetics of ethotoin and mephenytoin are not well established, but both drugs share with phenytoin the property of saturable metabolism within the therapeutic dosage range. Careful monitoring of the patient during dosage alterations with either drug is essential. Mephenytoin is metabolized to 5,5-ethylphenylhydantoin via demethylation. This metabolite, nirvanol, contributes most of the antiepileptic

activity of mephenytoin. Both mephenytoin and nirvanol are hydroxylated and undergo subsequent conjugation and excretion.

Therapeutic levels for mephenytoin range from 5 to 16 μg/mL, and levels above 20 μg/mL are considered toxic. Therapeutic blood levels of nirvanol are between 25 and 40 μg/mL. A therapeutic range for ethotoin has not been established.

Phenacemide, the straight-chain analog of phenytoin, is a toxic drug of last resort for refractory partial seizures. It is active against both maximal electroshock and pentylenetetrazol seizures. Its mechanism of action is unknown. It is well absorbed and completely metabolized. The relationship between blood levels and effect has not been established. Serious and sometimes fatal side effects have been reported in association with the use of phenacemide. Dose-related effects include behavioral changes, including psychosis and depressive reactions. Reactions of an idiosyncratic nature, including hepatitis, nephritis, and aplastic anemia, appear to be more frequent than with other antiepileptic drugs.

CARBAMAZEPINE

Closely related to imipramine and other antidepressants, carbamazepine (Tegretol) is a tricyclic compound effective in treatment of bipolar depression. It was initially marketed for the treatment of trigeminal neuralgia but has proved useful for epilepsy as well.

Chemistry

Although they are not obvious from a 2-dimensional representation of its structure (Fig 22–3), carbamazepine has many similarities to phenytoin. The ureide moiety (–N–CO–NH$_2$) present in the hetero-

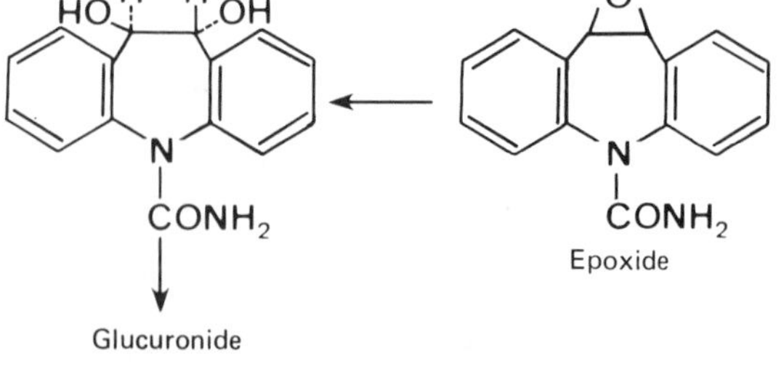

Figure 22–3. Carbamazepine and its metabolites. Carbamazepine is oxidized to the epoxy intermediate, which opens to form the dihydroxy derivative.

cyclic ring of most antiepileptic drugs is also present in carbamazepine. Three-dimensional structural studies indicate that its spatial conformation is similar to that of phenytoin.

Mechanism of Action

The mechanism of action of carbamazepine is unknown. Like phenytoin, carbamazepine shows activity against maximal electroshock seizures. Studies on membrane permeability indicate that carbamazepine, like phenytoin, diminishes sodium and, to a lesser degree, potassium conductance. Unlike phenytoin, however, carbamazepine has no significant effect on posttetanic potentiation. Carbamazepine also inhibits uptake and release of norepinephrine from brain synaptosomes but does not influence gamma-aminobutyric acid (GABA) uptake in brain slices, suggesting that its action is probably independent of the GABA-ergic system. Carbamazepine antagonizes ouabain-mediated stimulation by adenosine of adenylate cyclase. The ED50 of carbamazepine against maximal electroshock in mice is 9 mg/kg; it has no antipentylenetetrazol activity.

Clinical Use

Carbamazepine is considered the drug of choice for partial seizures, and many physicians also use it first for generalized tonic-clonic seizures. It is used with phenytoin in many patients who are difficult to control. Carbamazepine is nonsedative in its usual therapeutic range. The drug is also very effective in some patients with **trigeminal neuralgia,** although older patients may tolerate higher doses poorly, with ataxia and unsteadiness. Some of these patients require specific surgical intervention.

Pharmacokinetics

The rate of absorption of carbamazepine varies widely among different patients, though almost complete absorption apparently occurs in all. Peak levels are usually achieved 6–8 hours after administration. Slowing absorption by giving the drug after meals helps the patient tolerate larger total daily doses.

Distribution is slow and generally limited to highly perfused tissues, and volume of distribution is roughly 1 L/kg of body weight. The drug is only 70% bound to plasma proteins; no displacement of other drugs from protein binding has been observed.

Carbamazepine has a very low systemic clearance of approximately 1 L/kg/d. The drug has a notable ability to induce microsomal enzymes. In several studies of epileptic patients or volunteers on dosage regimens exceeding 1 month, the clearance of carbamazepine increased 2-fold over initial treatment. Typically, the half-life of 36 hours observed in subjects following an initial single dose decreases to much less than 20 hours in subjects receiving continuous therapy. Considerable dosage adjustments are thus to be expected during the first weeks of therapy. These changes in dose may further alter the microsomal enzyme capacity. Carbamazepine also alters the clearance of other drugs. For example, carbamazepine has been shown to increase the clearance and decrease the half-life and steady-state blood levels of several other antiepileptic drugs such as phenytoin, primidone, valproic acid, or clonazepam.

Carbamazepine is completely metabolized in humans, in part to the 10,11-dihydro derivative, which is subsequently conjugated. The dihydro derivative is formed by way of a stable epoxide, carbamazepine-10,11-epoxide, which has been shown to have anticonvulsant activity (Fig 22–3). The contribution of this and other metabolites in the clinical activity of carbamazepine is unknown.

Therapeutic Levels & Dose

Carbamazepine is considered the drug of choice in partial seizures. It is available only in oral form. The drug is effective in children, in whom a dose of 15–25 mg/kg is appropriate. In adults, doses of 1 g or even 2 g are tolerated. Higher doses are achieved by giving multiple doses daily. In patients receiving 3 or 4 daily doses, in whom the blood is drawn just before the morning dose (trough level), the therapeutic level is usually 4–8 μg/mL; although many patients complain of diplopia above 7 μg/mL, others can tolerate levels above 10 μg/mL. When blood samples are drawn randomly, levels are frequently above 8 μg/mL, but fluctuations related to absorption make long-term comparisons difficult.

Drug Interactions

Drug interactions involving carbamazepine are almost exclusively related to the enzyme-inducing properties of this drug. As noted previously, the increased metabolic capacity of the hepatic enzymes may cause a reduction in steady-state carbamazepine concentrations and an increased rate of metabolism of primidone, phenytoin, ethosuximide, valproic acid, and clonazepam. Other drugs such as propoxyphene, troleandomycin, and valproic acid may inhibit carbamazepine clearance and increase steady-state carbamazepine blood levels. Other anticonvulsants, however, such as phenytoin and phenobarbital, may decrease steady-state concentrations of carbamazepine through enzyme induction. No clinically signifi-cant protein binding interactions have been reported.

Toxicity

The most common dose-related side effects of carbamazepine are diplopia and ataxia. The diplopia often occurs first and may last less than an hour during a particular time of day. Rearrangement of the divided daily dose can often remedy this complaint. Other dose-related complaints include mild gastrointestinal upsets, unsteadiness, and, at much higher doses, drowsiness. Hyponatremia and water intoxication have occasionally occurred and may be dose-related.

Considerable concern exists regarding the occurrence of idiosyncratic blood dyscrasias with carbamazepine, including fatal cases of aplastic anemia and agranulocytosis. Most of these have been in elderly patients with trigeminal neuralgia, and most have occurred within the first 4 months of treatment. A mild persistent leukopenia is also seen in some patients; this is not necessarily an indication to stop treatment but obviously requires careful monitoring. The most common idiosyncratic reaction is an erythematous skin rash; other idiosyncratic responses such as hepatic dysfunction are unusual.

PHENOBARBITAL

Aside from the bromides, phenobarbital is the oldest of the currently available antiepileptic drugs. Although it has long been considered one of the safest of the antiepileptic agents, the use of other medications with lesser sedative effects has been urged. Many consider the barbiturates (phenobarbital and primidone) the drugs of choice only for seizures in infants.

Chemistry
The 4 derivatives of barbituric acid clinically useful as antiepileptic drugs are phenobarbital, mephobarbital, metharbital, and primidone. The first 3 are so similar that they will be considered together. Metharbital is methylated barbital, and mephobarbital is methylated phenobarbital; both are demethylated in vivo. The pK$_a$s of these 3 compounds range from 7.3 to 7.9. Slight changes in the normal acid-base balance, therefore, can cause significant fluctuation in the ratio of the ionized/un-ionized species. This is particularly important for phenobarbital, the most commonly used barbiturate, whose pK$_a$ of 7.3 is quite close to the plasma pH of 7.4.

X-ray crystallographic analysis of the structure of phenobarbital and its congeners indicates that the distance between the phenyl ring and the heterocyclic ring and the distance between ketonic oxygen atoms in the heterocyclic ring is critical for anticonvulsant activity. The 3-dimensional conformations of phenobarbital and N-methylphenobarbital are virtually identical to that of phenytoin. Both compounds possess a phenyl ring and are active against partial seizures.

Mechanism of Action
The exact mechanism of action of phenobarbital is unknown. It markedly prolongs posttetanic potentiation and enhances presynaptic inhibition. Recent data indicate that phenobarbital may act only on abnormal neurons, inhibiting the spread and suppressing firing from the foci. Like phenytoin, phenobarbital decreases sodium and potassium conductance, but only at high concentrations. Phenobarbital may exert its effect by binding to the dihydropicrotoxinin sites on the GABA receptor, thereby enhancing chloride conductance. However, direct activation of GABA receptors appears to correlate better with the hypnotic effect than with the anticonvulsant action of phenobarbital. At therapeutic concentrations, phenobarbital antagonizes glutamate excitation while at the same time greatly enhancing GABA inhibition. The ED50 of

phenobarbital against maximal electroshock in mice is 21 mg/kg; its antipentylenetetrazol ED50 is 15 mg/kg.

Clinical Use
Phenobarbital is useful in the treatment of partial seizures and generalized tonic-clonic seizures, although the drug is often tried for virtually every seizure type, especially when attacks are difficult to control. There is little evidence for its effectiveness in generalized seizures such as absence, atonic attacks, or infantile spasms; it may worsen certain patients with these seizure types.

Some physicians prefer either metharbital (Gemonil) or mephobarbital (Mebaral)—especially the latter—to phenobarbital because of supposed decreased side effects. Only anecdotal data are available for such comparisons.

Pharmacokinetics
See Chapter 20.

Therapeutic Levels & Dose
The therapeutic levels of phenobarbital in most patients range from 10 to 40 μg/mL. Documentation of effectiveness is best in febrile seizures, and levels below 15 μg/mL appear ineffective for prevention of febrile seizure recurrence. The upper end of the therapeutic range is more difficult to define, as many patients appear to tolerate chronic levels above 40 μg/mL.

Drug Interactions
See Chapter 20.

Toxicity
See Chapter 20.

PRIMIDONE

Primidone (Mysoline), or 2-desoxyphenobarbital (Fig 22–4), was marketed in the early 1950s. It was later reported that primidone was metabolized to phenobarbital and phenylethylmalonamide (PEMA). All 3 compounds are active anticonvulsants.

Mechanism of Action
Although primidone is converted to phenobarbital, the mechanism of action of primidone itself may be more like that of phenytoin, according to some recent studies. This may partially account for the increased use of primidone rather than phenobarbital in the treatment of complex partial seizures. The ED50 of primidone against maximal electroshock in mice is 11 mg/kg; the ED50 against pentylenetetrazol is 59 mg/kg.

Clinical Use
Primidone, like its metabolites, is effective against partial seizures and generalized tonic-clonic seizures and may be more effective than phenobarbital. It was previously considered to be the drug of choice for

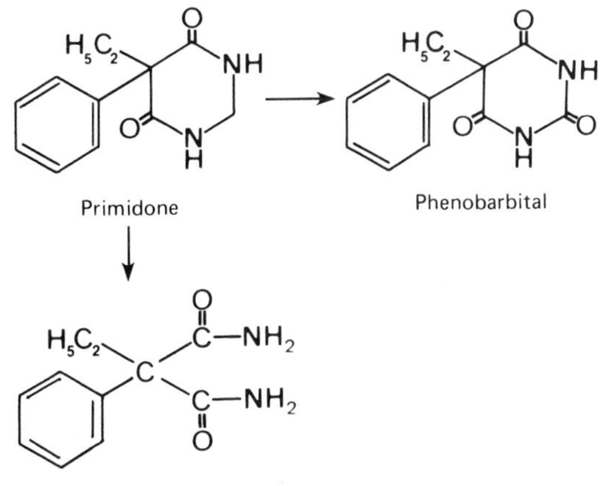

Figure 22–4. Primidone and its active metabolites.

complex partial seizures, but the latest studies of partial seizures in adults strongly suggest that carbamazepine and phenytoin are superior to primidone. Recent attempts to determine the relative potencies of the parent drug and its 2 metabolites have concentrated on newborn infants, in whom drug-metabolizing enzyme systems are very immature and in whom primidone is only slowly metabolized. Primidone has been shown to be effective in controlling seizures in this group, as well as in patients just beginning treatment with primidone; the latter show seizure control before phenobarbital concentrations reach the therapeutic range. Finally, animal studies suggest that greater protection against maximal electroshock seizures occurs with primidone than with phenobarbital alone, supporting the notion that primidone possesses independent activity. Nevertheless, the clinical use is similar to that of phenobarbital.

Pharmacokinetics

Primidone is absorbed slowly but completely. The time required to reach peak concentrations after oral administration is about 3 hours, but considerable variation has been reported.

Primidone is generally confined to total body water, with a volume of distribution of 0.6 L/kg of body weight. It is not highly bound to plasma proteins; approximately 70% circulates as unbound drug.

Primidone is metabolized by oxidation to phenobarbital, which accumulates very slowly, and by scission of the heterocyclic ring to form PEMA (Fig 22–4). Both primidone and phenobarbital are also hydroxylated at the para position of the phenyl ring and undergo subsequent conjugation and excretion.

Primidone has a larger clearance than other antiepileptic drugs (2 L/kg/d), corresponding to a half-life of 6–8 hours. PEMA clearance is approximately half that of primidone, but phenobarbital has a very low clearance. The appearance of phenobarbital corresponds to the disappearance of primidone. Phenobarbital therefore accumulates very slowly but eventually reaches therapeutic concentrations in most patients when therapeutic doses of primidone are administered. Phenobarbital levels derived from primidone are usually 2–3 times higher than primidone levels. PEMA, which probably makes a minimal contribution to the efficacy of primidone, has a half-life of 8–12 hours and therefore reaches steady state more rapidly than phenobarbital.

Therapeutic Levels & Dose

Primidone is most efficacious when plasma levels are in the range of 8–12 μg/mL. Concomitant levels of its metabolite, phenobarbital, at steady state will usually vary from 15 to 30 μg/mL. Doses of 10–20 mg/kg/d are necessary to obtain these levels. It is very important, however, to start primidone at low doses and gradually increase over days to a few weeks to avoid prominent sedation and gastrointestinal complaints. When adjusting doses of the drug, it is important to remember that the parent drug will rapidly reach steady state (30–40 hours), but the active metabolites phenobarbital (20 days) and phenylethylmalonamide (3–4 days) will reach steady state much more slowly.

Toxicity

The toxic side effects of primidone are similar to those of its metabolite, phenobarbital, except that drowsiness occurs early in treatment and may be prominent if the initial dose is too large; gradual increments are indicated when starting the drug in either children or adults.

DRUGS USED IN GENERALIZED SEIZURES

ETHOSUXIMIDE

Ethosuximide (Zarontin) was introduced in 1960 as the third of 3 marketed succinimides in the USA. Ethosuximide has very little activity against maximal electroshock but remarkable efficacy against pentylenetetrazol seizures and was introduced as a "pure petit mal" drug. Its popularity continues, based on its safety and efficacy; its role as the "first choice" antiabsence drug remains undiminished, in part because of the idiosyncratic hepatotoxicity of the alternative drug, valproic acid.

Chemistry

Ethosuximide is the last antiepileptic drug to be marketed whose origin is in the antiepileptic heterocyclic ring structure. The 3 antiepileptic succinimides marketed in the USA are ethosuximide, phensuximide (Milontin), and methsuximide (Celontin). All 3 are substituted at the 2 position. (See structure below, and note difference in numbering relative to Fig 22–1.) Methsuximide and phensuximide have phenyl substituents, while ethosuximide is 2-ethyl-2-methylsuccinimide. Many other substituted succinimides have antiepileptic activity, and several studies have demonstrated the optimal structural properties. Two substituents are optimal at the 2 position. If these substituents are small dialkyl groups, the compound will have antipentylenetetrazol activity. A phenyl group at the 2 position results in activity against maximal electroshock seizures but reduces activity against pentylenetetrazol seizures. Diphenyl compounds have no antipentylenetetrazol effects. Ethosuximide has an ED50 against maximal electroshock in mice of greater than 1000 mg/kg; its antipentylenetetrazol activity is 130 mg/kg.

Ethosuximide

Mechanism of Action

The mechanism of action of the succinimides is undetermined. Ethosuximide inhibits Na^+,K^+-ATPase, depresses the cerebral metabolic rate, and inhibits GABA transaminase. However, none of these actions are seen at therapeutic concentrations. Ethosuximide does not inhibit the calcium influx into nervous tissue stimulated by maximal electroshock. Its lack of effect on membranes may be due to its hydrophilic nature. Addition of a phenyl group, which increases lipophilicity, results in increased anti–maximal electroshock activity. Other studies have shown that while ethosuximide can stimulate GABA release from presynaptic terminals, it does not elevate brain GABA levels, and most data suggest that the mechanism of action is not related to GABA-mediated inhibition.

Clinical Use

Ethosuximide is particularly effective against absence seizures, as might be expected from its activity in laboratory models. Documentation of its effectiveness required specific advances in quantitation of absence seizures; this was accomplished in the 1970s when the characteristic generalized 3/s spike-wave electroencephalographic abnormality was correlated with a decrement in consciousness, even when the abnormality occurs for only a few seconds. Long-term electroencephalographic recordings, therefore, provided the necessary quantitative method for determining the frequency of absence attacks and allowed rapid and effective evaluation of the efficacy of anti-absence drugs. Although ethosuximide was marketed in advance of the federal requirements for efficacy, these techniques were applied to later drugs such as clonazepam and valproic acid in documentation of their efficacy. This was accomplished by comparison with ethosuximide.

Pharmacokinetics

Absorption is complete following administration of the oral dosage forms. Peak levels are observed 3–7 hours after oral administration of the capsules. Animal studies indicate that chronic administration of the solution may prove irritating to the gastric mucosa.

Ethosuximide is uniformly distributed throughout perfused tissues and does not penetrate fat. Consequently, the volume of distribution approximates that of total body water, ie, 0.7 L/kg. It is not protein-bound, and spinal fluid concentrations are therefore equal to plasma concentrations.

Ethosuximide is completely metabolized, principally by hydroxylation. Four hydroxylated metabolites have been identified. These metabolites undergo subsequent conjugation and excretion. There is no evidence that these metabolites are pharmacologically active.

Ethosuximide has a very low total body clearance (0.5 L/kg/d). This corresponds to a half-life of approximately 40 hours, although values from 18 to 72 hours have been reported.

Therapeutic Levels & Dose

Therapeutic levels of 60–100 μg/mL can be achieved in adults with doses of 750–1500 mg/d, though lower or higher doses may be necessary. Some authors report that higher levels (up to 125 μg/mL) are needed in certain patients to achieve efficacy; such patients may tolerate the drug without apparent toxicity at these levels. Ethosuximide has a linear relationship between dose and steady-state plasma levels, and no change in pharmacokinetic parameters with age has been reported. The drug might be administered as a single daily dose were it not for its gastrointestinal side effects; twice-a-day dosage is common. The time of day at which the level is measured is not particularly critical for ethosuximide, as its half-life is relatively long. No parenteral dosage form for ethosuximide is available.

Drug Interactions

Administration of ethosuximide with valproic acid results in a decrease in ethosuximide clearance and higher steady-state concentrations due to inhibition of metabolism. No other important drug interactions have been reported for the succinimides.

Toxicity

The most common dose-related side effect of ethosuximide is gastric distress, including pain, nausea, and vomiting. This can often be avoided by starting therapy at a low dose, with gradual increases into the therapeutic range. When the side effect does occur, temporary dosage reductions may allow adaptation. Ethosuximide is a highly efficacious and safe drug for absence seizures; the appearance of relatively mild, dose-related side effects should not immediately deter the physician from its use. Other dose-related side effects include transient lethargy or fatigue and, much less commonly, headache, dizziness, hiccup, and euphoria. Behavioral changes are usually in the direction of improvement.

Non–dose-related or idiosyncratic side effects of ethosuximide are extremely uncommon. Skin rashes have been reported, including at least one case of Stevens-Johnson syndrome. A few patients have had eosinophilia, thrombocytopenia, leukopenia, or pancytopenia; in none was it entirely certain that ethosuximide was the causal agent. The development of systemic lupus erythematosus has also been reported, but other drugs may have been involved.

PHENSUXIMIDE & METHSUXIMIDE

Phensuximide (Milontin) and methsuximide (Celontin) are phenylsuccinimides that were developed and marketed before ethosuximide. They are used primarily as anti-absence drugs. Methsuximide is generally considered more toxic—and phensuximide less effective—than ethosuximide. Unlike ethosuximide, these 2 compounds have activity against maximal electroshock seizures, and methsuximide has been used for partial seizures by some investigators. The toxicity and lack of effectiveness of phensuximide when compared to methsuximide has been investigated, and the failure of the desmethyl metabolite to accumulate in the former probably explains its relatively weak effect. The desmethyl metabolite of methsuximide, however, has a half-life of 25 hours or more and exerts the major antiepileptic effect.

VALPROIC ACID & SODIUM VALPROATE

Valproic acid (Depakene), also available as the sodium salt, sodium valproate, was found to have antiepileptic properties when it was used as a solvent in the search for other drugs effective against seizures. It was marketed in France in 1969 but was not licensed in the USA until 1978.

Chemistry

Valproic acid is one of a series of fatty or carboxylic acids that have antiepileptic activity; this activity appears to be greatest for carbon chain lengths of 5–8 atoms. Branching and unsaturation do not significantly alter the drug's activity but may increase its lipophilicity, thereby increasing its duration of action. The amides and esters of valproic acid are also active antiepileptic agents.

$$CH_3 - CH_2 - CH_2$$
$$CH_3 - CH_2 - CH_2 \!\!\!\searrow\!\! CH - COOH$$

Valproic acid

Mechanism of Action

The time course of anticonvulsant activity appears to be poorly correlated with blood or tissue levels of the parent drug, an observation giving rise to considerable speculation regarding both the active species and the mechanism of action of valproic acid. Valproic acid is active against both pentylenetetrazol and maximal electroshock seizures. Its ED50 in mice against pentylenetetrazol is 149 mg/kg; the ED50 against maximal electroshock is 272 mg/kg. As expected, it has little or no effect on sodium conductance, but at very high concentrations it increases potassium conductance. The greatest area of interest, however, has been the effects of valproic acid on GABA. Several studies have shown increased levels of GABA in the brain after administration of valproic acid, though the mechanism for this increase remains unclear. Doubt about the relevance of this increase in GABA to the therapeutic effect is raised by the fact that anticonvulsant effects are observed before GABA brain levels are elevated. If the effect of valproic acid is related to the enzymes necessary for either the production or breakdown of GABA, the drug may have a greater effect on inhibiting GABA transaminase (GABA-T) than on facilitating glutamic acid decarboxylase (GAD). At very high concentrations, valproic acid inhibits GABA-T in the brain, thus increasing levels of GABA by blocking conversion of GABA to succinic semialdehyde. However, at the relatively low doses of valproic acid needed to abolish pentylenetetrazol seizures, brain GABA levels may remain unchanged. Many investigators think the changes in brain GABA do not represent a direct action of valproic acid but are instead due to an active metabolite. Some have proposed that valproic acid potentiates postsynaptic GABA responsiveness. However, these findings have not been validated at therapeutic concentrations and at physiologic pH.

At high concentrations, valproic acid has been shown to increase membrane potassium conductance. Furthermore, low concentrations of valproic acid tend to hyperpolarize membrane potentials. These findings have led to speculation that valproic acid may exert its action through a direct effect on the potassium channels of the membrane.

Another postulated mechanism of action relates to the acidic properties of the drug. Valproic acid might cause a whole-body shift toward metabolic acidosis by stimulation of beta oxidation of fatty acids, resulting in an increase in circulating ketone bodies. These ketones could then be utilized to increase brain glycogen, which might protect against seizures induced by transient stimulation.

Clinical Use

Valproic acid is very effective against absence seizures and might be considered the drug of choice in this seizure type were it not for its hepatotoxicity. Because of this toxicity, ethosuximide is preferred. Valproic acid is unique in its ability to control certain types of myoclonic seizures; in some cases, the effect can be very dramatic. The drug has some effectiveness against generalized tonic-clonic seizures, and a few patients with atonic attacks may also respond. There is no convincing evidence that the drug is effective in partial seizures or infantile spasms.

Pharmacokinetics

Valproic acid is well absorbed following an oral dose, with bioavailability greater than 80%. Peak blood levels are observed within 2 hours. Food may delay absorption, and decreased toxicity may result if the drug is given after meals.

Valproic acid has a pK_a of 4.7 and is therefore completely ionized at physiologic plasma pH. The drug is also 90% bound to plasma proteins, though the fraction bound is somewhat reduced at blood levels greater than 150 $\mu g/mL$. Since it is both highly ionized and highly protein-bound, its distribution is essentially confined to extracellular water, with a volume of distribution of approximately 0.15 L/kg.

Approximately 20% of the drug is excreted as a direct conjugate of valproic acid. The remainder is metabolized by beta and omega oxidation to a number of compounds; these are also subsequently conjugated and excreted.

Clearance for valproic acid is very low, corresponding to the small volume of distribution and accounting for a half-life of 9–18 hours. At very high blood levels, the clearance of valproic acid is dose-dependent. There appear to be offsetting changes in the intrinsic clearance and protein binding at higher doses.

The sodium salt of valproate is marketed in Europe as a tablet protected by aluminum foil, as it is quite hygroscopic. In Central and South America, the magnesium salt is available, which is considerably less hygroscopic. The free acid of valproate was first marketed in the USA in a capsule containing corn oil; the sodium salt is also used, in syrup, primarily for pediatric use. A calcium salt may also become available. There is little evidence that any of these various forms have any advantage over the other, with the possible exception of increased gastrointestinal side effects of the capsules of valproic acid. An enteric-coated tablet (Depakote) is also marketed. This product, a 1:1 mixture of valproic acid and sodium valproate, is as bioavailable as the capsule but is absorbed much more slowly and is preferred by many patients. Peak concentrations following administration of the enteric-coated tablets are seen in 3–4 hours.

Therapeutic Levels & Dose

Doses of 25–30 mg/kg/d may be adequate in some patients, but others may require 60 mg/kg or even more. Therapeutic levels of valproic acid range from 50 to 100 $\mu g/mL$. The drug should not be abandoned until morning "trough" levels of at least 80 $\mu g/mL$ have been attained; some patients may require and may tolerate levels in excess of 100 $\mu g/mL$.

Drug Interactions

As noted above, the clearance of valproic acid is dose-dependent, caused by changes in both the intrinsic clearance and protein binding. Valproic acid in-hibits its own metabolism at low doses, thus decreasing intrinsic clearance. At higher doses, there is an increased free fraction of valproic acid, resulting in lower total drug levels than expected. It may be clinically useful, therefore, to measure both total and free drug levels. Valproic acid also displaces phenytoin from plasma proteins. In addition to binding interactions, valproic acid inhibits the metabolism of several drugs, including phenobarbital, phenytoin, and carbamazepine, leading to higher steady-state concentrations. The inhibition of phenobarbital metabolism may cause levels of the barbiturate to rise precipitously, causing stupor or coma. The inhibition of phenytoin metabolism may partially offset the reduction in total drug levels caused by displacement from plasma proteins.

Toxicity

The most common dose-related side effects of valproic acid are nausea, vomiting, and other gastrointestinal complaints such as abdominal pain and "heartburn." The drug should be started gradually to avoid these symptoms; a temporary reduction in dose can usually alleviate the problems, and the patient will eventually tolerate higher doses. Sedation is uncommon with valproic acid alone but may be striking when valproate is added to phenobarbital. A fine tremor is frequently seen at higher levels. Other reversible side effects, seen in a small number of patients, include weight gain, increased appetite, and hair loss.

The idiosyncratic toxicity of valproic acid is largely limited to hepatotoxicity, but this may be severe. Although most cases have been patients who are also taking other antiepileptic drugs, there seems little doubt that the hepatotoxicity of valproic acid has been responsible for more than 50 fatalities. The effect does not appear to be dose-related, nor is the age of the patient important, though most fatalities are pediatric because of the high utilization of the drug in this age group. Initial SGOT values may not be elevated in susceptible patients, though these levels do eventually become abnormal. Most fatalities have occurred within 4 months after initiation of therapy. Careful monitoring of liver function is obviously mandatory when starting the drug; the hepatotoxicity is reversible in some cases if the drug is withdrawn. The other observed idiosyncratic response with valproic acid is thrombocytopenia, though documented cases of abnormal bleeding are lacking. It should be noted that valproic acid is an effective and popular antiepileptic drug and that only a very small number of patients have had severe toxic effects from its use.

Recent studies of valproate suggest an increased incidence of spina bifida in the offspring of women who took the drug during pregnancy. In addition, an increased incidence of cardiovascular, orofacial, and digital abnormalities has been reported. These observations, although based on a small number of cases, must be strongly considered in the choice of drugs during pregnancy.

OXAZOLIDINEDIONES

Trimethadione (Tridione), the first oxazolidine-dione, was introduced as an antiepileptic drug in 1945 and remained the drug of choice for absence seizures until the introduction of succinimides in the 1950s. The use of the oxazolidinediones (trimethadione, paramethadione, and dimethadione) is now very limited.

Chemistry

The oxazolidinediones contain as a heterocyclic ring the oxazolidine ring (Fig 22–1) and are similar in structure to other antiepileptic drugs introduced before 1960. The structure includes only short-chain alkyl substituents on the heterocyclic ring, with no attached phenyl group.

Trimethadione

Mechanism of Action

As expected, these compounds are active against pentylenetetrazol-induce seizures. Trimethadione has an ED50 against maximal electroshock in mice of 627 mg/kg; its antipentylenetetrazol ED50 is 301 mg/kg. A number of other physiologic effects of these drugs have been observed, the most notable of which is a reduction in synaptic transmission in the spinal cord during repetitive stimulation without affecting single-impulse transmission through monosynaptic pathways. In the brain, trimethadione increases the after-discharge threshold in the cortex. Some of these effects may be related to action of trimethadione on pre- and postsynaptic inhibition in synapses that utilize GABA as the neurotransmitter. Trimethadione may also contribute to an increase in GABA levels.

Pharmacokinetics

Trimethadione is rapidly absorbed, with peak levels reached within an hour after drug administration. It is distributed to all perfused tissues, with a volume of distribution that approximates that of total body water. It is not bound to plasma proteins. Trimethadione is completely metabolized in the liver by demethylation to 5,5-dimethyl-2,4-oxazolidine-dione (dimethadione), which may exert the major antiepileptic activity. The drug has a relatively low clearance (1.6 L/kg/d), corresponding to a half-life of approximately 16 hours. The demethylated metabolite, however, is very slowly cleared and accumulates to a much greater extent than the parent drug. The clearance of dimethadione is 0.08 L/kg/d, reflected in a smaller volume of distribution and an extremely long half-life (240 hours).

Therapeutic Levels & Dose

The therapeutic plasma level range for trimetha-dione has never been established, though trimetha-dione blood levels above 20 μg/mL and dimethadione levels above 700 μg/mL have been suggested. A dose of 30 mg/kg/d of trimethadione is necessary to achieve these levels in adults.

Drug Interactions

Relatively few drug interactions involving the oxazolidinediones have been reported, although trimetha-dione may competitively inhibit the demethylation of other drugs such as metharbital.

Toxicity

The most notable dose-related side effect of the oxazolidinediones is sedation. An unusual side effect is hemeralopia, a glare effect in which visual adaptation is impaired; it is reversible upon cessation of the drug. Accumulation of dimethadione has been reported to cause a very mild metabolic acidosis. Trimethadione has been associated with idiosyncratic dermatologic reactions, including rashes and exfoliative dermatitis, as well as toxic reactions involving the blood-forming organs; these have ranged from mild alterations in cell counts to fulminating pancytopenia. Other idiosyncratic reactions include reversible nephrotic syndrome, which may involve an immune reaction to the drug, as well as a myasthenic syndrome.

OTHER DRUGS USED IN MANAGEMENT OF EPILEPSY

Some drugs are not classifiable by application to seizure type and will be discussed separately in this section.

BENZODIAZEPINES
(See also Chapter 20.)

Five benzodiazepines play prominent roles in the therapy of epilepsy, but their roles cannot be classified under a single seizure group. Although many benzodiazepines are quite similar chemically, subtle structural alterations result in differences in activity. Electronegative substituents in the 7 position are necessary for anticonvulsant activity; both Cl and NO_2 are effective. A phenyl group at the 5 position gives maximum anticonvulsant potency. Although they are quite different structurally from other antiepileptic drugs, the spatial conformation of the benzodiazepines is very similar to that of phenytoin. Possible mechanisms of action are discussed in Chapter 20.

Diazepam (Valium) intravenously is the drug of choice for stopping continuous seizure activity, especially generalized tonic-clonic status epilepticus (see below). The drug is marketed as an adjunct to therapy and is occasionally given orally on a chronic basis, though it is not considered very effective in this application, probably because of the rapid development of tolerance. In mice, the anti–maximal electroshock ED50 for diazepam is 19 mg/kg, whereas the antipentylenetetrazol ED50 is 0.2 mg/kg.

Lorazepam (Ativan) is a newer benzodiazepine that, when given intravenously, appears in some studies to be more effective and longer-acting than diazepam in the treatment of status epilepticus.

Clonazepam (Clonopin) is a long-acting drug with documented efficacy against absence seizures and one of the most potent antiepileptic agents known. It is also effective in some cases of myoclonic seizures and has been tried in infantile spasms. Sedation is prominent, especially on initiation of therapy; starting doses should be small. Maximal tolerated doses are usually in the range of 0.1–0.2 mg/kg, but many weeks of gradually increasing daily dosage may be needed to achieve these doses in some patients. Therapeutic blood levels are usually less than 0.1 μg/mL and are not routinely measured in most laboratories. In mice, the ED50 against maximal electroshock is 87 mg/kg; the ED50 against pentylenetetrazol is 0.01 mg/kg.

Nitrazepam (Mogadon) is not marketed in the USA but is used in many other countries, especially for infantile spasms and myoclonic seizures. It is less potent than clonazepam, and whether it has any clinical advantages over clonazepam remains unclear.

Clorazepate dipotassium (Tranxene) is a benzodiazepine approved in the USA as an adjunct to treatment of complex partial seizures in adults. Drowsiness and lethargy are common side effects, but as long as the drug is increased gradually, doses as high as 45 mg/d can be given.

The pharmacokinetic properties of the benzodiazepines in part determine their clinical use. In general, the drugs are well absorbed, widely distributed, and extensively metabolized, with many active metabolites. The rate of distribution of benzodiazepines within the body is different from that of other antiepileptic drugs. Diazepam and lorazepam in particular are rapidly and extensively distributed to the tissues, with volumes of distribution between 1 and 3 L/kg. The onset of action, therefore, is also very rapid. Total body clearance of parent drug and metabolites, however, is very low, corresponding to half-lives of 40–50 hours.

Two prominent aspects of benzodiazepines limit their usefulness. The first is their pronounced sedative effect, which is unfortunate both in the treatment of status epilepticus and in chronic therapy. Children may manifest a paradoxic hyperactivity, as with barbiturates. The second problem is tolerance, in which seizures may initially respond, but within a few months the initial improvement may diminish. The remarkable antiepileptic potency of these compounds often cannot be realized because of these limiting factors.

ACETAZOLAMIDE

Acetazolamide (Diamox) is a diuretic whose main action is the inhibition of carbonic anhydrase (see Chapter 14). It has been proposed that the accumulation of carbon dioxide in the brain is the mechanism by which the drug exerts its antiepileptic activity. Acetazolamide has been used for all types of seizures but is severely limited by the rapid development of tolerance, with return of seizures usually within a few weeks. The drug may have a special role in epileptic women who experience seizure exacerbations at the time of menses; seizure control may be improved and tolerance may not develop, because the drug is not administered continuously. The usual dose is approximately 10 mg/kg up to a maximum of 1000 mg/d.

Another carbonic anhydrase inhibitor, **sulthiame,** was not found to be effective in clinical trials in the USA. It is marketed in some other countries.

BROMIDE

Bromide was introduced by Locock in 1857 and was the first antiepileptic drug with any measurable efficacy. Though largely discarded in favor of phenobarbital after the turn of the century, bromide is still occasionally useful, such as in management of epilepsy in patients with porphyria, in whom other drugs may be contraindicated. Its half-life is approximately 12 days, and it is given in doses of 3–6 g/d in adults to obtain plasma levels of 10–20 meq/L. The mechanism of action of bromide as an antiepileptic agent is unknown. Major toxic problems are unfortunately frequent, including skin rashes, sedation, and behavioral changes.

II. CLINICAL PHARMACOLOGY OF ANTIEPILEPTIC DRUGS

SEIZURE CLASSIFICATION

The type of medication utilized for epilepsy is dependent upon the empirical nature of the seizure. For this reason, considerable effort has been made to classify seizures so that clinicians will be able to make a "seizure diagnosis" and thereby prescribe appropriate therapy. Errors in seizure diagnosis cause use of the wrong drugs, and an unpleasant cycle ensues in which poor seizure control is followed by increasing drug doses and medication toxicity. As noted above, seizures are divided into two groups: partial and generalized. Drugs used for partial seizures are more or less the same for the entire group, but drugs used for generalized seizures are determined by the individual seizure type. A shortened version of the international classification of epileptic seizures is presented in Table 22–1.

Partial Seizures

Partial seizures are those in which a localized onset of the attack can be ascertained, either by clinical observation or by electroencephalographic recording; the attack begins in a specific locus in the brain. There are 3 types of partial seizures, determined to some extent by the degree of brain involvement by the abnormal discharge.

The least complicated partial seizure is the elementary or **simple partial seizure,** characterized by minimal spread of the abnormal discharge such that normal consciousness and awareness are preserved. For example, the patient may have a sudden onset of clonic jerking of an extremity lasting 60–90 seconds; residual weakness may last for 15–30 minutes after the attack. The patient is completely aware of the attack and can describe it in detail. The EEG may show an abnormal discharge highly localized to the involved portion of the brain.

The **complex partial seizure** also has a localized onset, but the discharge becomes more widespread (usually bilateral) and almost always involves the limbic system. Most (not all) complex partial seizures arise from one of the temporal lobes, possibly because of the susceptibility of this area of the brain to insults such as hypoxia or infection. Clinically, the patient may have a brief warning followed by an alteration of consciousness during which some patients may stare and others may stagger or even fall. Most, however, demonstrate fragments of integrated motor behavior called automatisms for which the patient has no memory. Typical automatisms are lip smacking, swallowing, fumbling, scratching, or even walking about. After 30–120 seconds, the patient makes a gradual recovery to normal consciousness but may feel tired or ill for several hours after the attack.

The last type of partial seizure is the **secondarily generalized attack,** in which a partial seizure immediately precedes a generalized tonic-clonic (grand mal) seizure. This seizure type is described below.

Generalized Seizures

Generalized seizures are those in which there is no evidence of localized onset. The group is quite heterogeneous.

Generalized tonic-clonic (grand mal) seizures are the most dramatic of all epileptic seizures and are characterized by tonic rigidity of all extremities, followed in 15–30 seconds by a tremor that is actually an interruption of the tonus by relaxation. As the relaxation phases become longer, the attack enters the clonic phase, with massive jerking of the body. The clonic jerking slows over 60–120 seconds, and the patient is usually left in a stuporous state. The tongue or cheek may be bitten, and urinary incontinence is common. Primary generalized tonic-clonic seizures begin without evidence of localized onset, whereas secondary generalized tonic-clonic seizures are preceded by another seizure type, usually a partial seizure. The medical treatment of both primary and secondary generalized tonic-clonic seizures is the same and utilizes drugs appropriate for partial seizures.

The **absence (petit mal) seizure** is characterized by both sudden onset and abrupt cessation. Its duration is usually less than 10 seconds and rarely more than 45 seconds. Consciousness is altered; the attack may also be associated with mild clonic jerking of the eyelids or extremities, with postural tone changes, autonomic phenomena, and automatisms. The occurrence of automatisms can complicate the clinical differentiation from complex partial seizures in some patients. Absence attacks begin in childhood or adolescence and may occur up to hundreds of times a day. The EEG during the seizure shows a highly characteristic 2.5–3.5 Hz spike-and-wave pattern. Atypical absence patients have seizures with postural changes that are more abrupt, and the patients are often mentally retarded; the EEG may show a slower spike-and-wave discharge, and the seizures may be more refractory to therapy.

Myoclonic jerking is seen, to a greater or lesser extent, in a wide variety of seizures, including generalized tonic-clonic seizures, partial seizures, absence seizures, and infantile spasms. Treatment of seizures that include myoclonic jerking should be directed at the primary seizure type rather than at the myoclonus. Some patients, however, have myoclonic jerking as the major seizure type, and some have frequent myoclonic jerking and occasional generalized tonic-clonic seizures without overt signs of neurologic deficit. In patients with the severe genetic syndrome of Unverricht-Lundborg, the myoclonus is progressive, severe, and associated with generalized tonic-clonic seizures and dementia. Many other kinds of myoclonus exist, and much effort has gone into the attempt to classify this entity. Further discussion is beyond the scope of this text.

Atonic seizures are those in which the patient has sudden loss of postural tone. If standing, the patient falls suddenly to the floor and may be injured. If seated, the head and torso may suddenly drop forward; the patient's face typically falls directly into a plate of food set on the table. Although most often seen in children, this seizure type is not unusual in adults. Many patients with atonic seizures wear helmets to prevent severe injury.

Infantile spasms are an epileptic syndrome and not a seizure type. The attacks, though sometimes fragmentary, are most often bilateral and are included for pragmatic purposes with the generalized seizures. These attacks are most often characterized clinically by brief, recurrent myoclonic jerks of the body with sudden flexion or extension of the body and limbs; the forms of infantile spasms are, however, quite heterogeneous. Ninety percent of affected patients have their first attack before the age of 1 year. Most patients are mentally retarded, presumably from the same origin as the spasms. The cause is unknown in many patients, but such widely disparate disorders as infection, kernicterus, tuberous sclerosis, and hypoglycemia have been implicated. In some cases, the EEG is characteristic. Drugs used to treat infantile spasms are effective only in some patients; there is no evidence that the mental retardation is alleviated by therapy, even when the attacks disappear.

THERAPEUTIC STRATEGY

For antiepileptic drugs, relationships between blood levels and therapeutic effects have been characterized to a particularly high degree. The same is true for the pharmacokinetics of these drugs. These relationships provide significant advantages in the development of therapeutic strategies for the treatment of epilepsy. Decisions on therapy are aided by blood level determinations, and decisions on dosage adjustments are based on pharmacokinetic data. The therapeutic index for most antiepileptic drugs is low, and toxicity is not uncommon. Thus, effective treatment of seizures requires an awareness of the therapeutic levels and pharmacokinetic properties as well as the characteristic toxicities of each agent. Measurements of antiepileptic drug plasma levels are extremely useful when combined with clinical observations and pharmacokinetic data (Table 22–2).

MANAGEMENT OF EPILEPSY

PARTIAL SEIZURES & GENERALIZED TONIC-CLONIC SEIZURES

The choice of drugs is usually limited to phenytoin, carbamazepine, or barbiturates. There has been a strong tendency in the past few years to limit the use of sedative antiepileptic drugs such as barbiturates and benzodiazepines to patients who cannot tolerate other

medications. The trend has been to increase the use of carbamazepine. In patients with resistant partial seizures, the combination of phenytoin and carbamazepine is preferred.

GENERALIZED SEIZURES

The drugs used for generalized tonic-clonic seizures are the same as for partial seizures; in addition, valproate may be useful.

Three drugs are effective against absence seizures. Two are nonsedative and therefore preferred: ethosuximide and valproic acid. Clonazepam is also highly effective but has disadvantages of dose-related side effects and development of tolerance. The drug of choice is ethosuximide, even though valproic acid is effective in some ethosuximide-resistant patients. The major drawback in the use of valproic acid is its hepatotoxicity.

Specific myoclonic syndromes are usually treated with valproic acid. It is nonsedative and can be dramatic in its effect. Other patients respond to clonazepam or other benzodiazepines, though high doses may be necessary, with accompanying sedation and drowsiness. A highly specific myoclonic syndrome, "intention myoclonus," which occurs after severe hypoxia, is characterized by myoclonus associated with volitional activity. Although further studies are needed, improvement in some patients with this unusual disorder has been reported using 5-hydroxytryptophan.

Atonic seizures are often refractory to all available medications, although some reports suggest that valproic acid may be beneficial. Benzodiazepines have been reported to improve seizure control in some patients but may worsen the attacks in others. If the loss of tone appears to be part of another seizure type (such as absence or complex partial seizures), every effort should be made to treat the other seizure type vigorously, hoping for simultaneous alleviation of the atonic component of the seizure.

DRUGS USED IN INFANTILE SPASMS

The treatment of infantile spasms is unfortunately limited to improvement of control of the seizures rather than other features of the disorder, such as retardation. Most patients receive a course of intramuscular corticotropin, though some clinicians note that prednisone may be equally effective and can be given orally. Clinical trials have thus far been unable to settle the matter. In either case, therapy must often be discontinued because of side effects. If seizures recur, repeat courses of corticotropin or corticosteroids can be given, or other drugs may be tried. Other drugs widely used are the benzodiazepines such as clonazepam or nitrazepam, though their efficacy in this heterogeneous syndrome is unknown.

The basic mechanism of action of corticosteroids or

Table 22–2. Effective plasma levels of 6 antiepileptic drugs.*

Drug	Effective Level (µg/mL)	High Effective Level† (µg/mL)	Toxic Level (µg/mL)
Carbamazepine	4–10	7	> 8
Primidone	5–15	10	> 12
Phenytoin	10–20	18	> 20
Phenobarbital	10–40	35	> 40
Ethosuximide	50–100	80	> 100
Valproate	50–100	80	> 100

*Reprinted, with permission, from Porter RJ: *Epilepsy: 100 Elementary Principles.* Saunders, 1984.

†Level that should be achieved, if possible, in patients with refractory seizures, assuming that the blood samples are drawn before administration of the morning medication.

corticotropin in the treatment of infantile spasms is unknown. It is known that glucocorticoids decrease septal-hippocampal excitability and thereby elevate convulsive thresholds of these limbic structures. It is not clear whether these agents interact directly with intracellular receptors involved in infantile spasms.

In spite of more than 20 years experience with corticosteroids and corticotropin for infantile spasms, the optimal dosage and duration of therapy have not been established. Initial studies suggested periods up to 12 weeks; most patients who responded showed improvement within 2–3 weeks and were continued on therapy for the full 12 weeks. With corticotropin, dosages were increased by 2–5 units daily until a level of 40–50 units daily was reached. Currently, a broad range of dosages are utilized, although most patients are treated with 25–40 units of corticotropin daily. A very few investigators recommend up to 240 units daily. In the 60% of patients who respond, seizure reduction is usually reported within 1–5 weeks. Corticotropin therapy may be continued for 3 months or more unless toxicity requires cessation. For corticosteroids, doses of 2 mg/kg of prednisolone or 0.3 mg/kg of dexamethasone have been utilized.

The toxic effects of corticotropin include hypertension, cushingoid obesity, gastrointestinal disturbances, skin changes, osteoporosis, and electrolyte imbalance.

STATUS EPILEPTICUS

There are many forms of status epilepticus. The most common, generalized tonic-clonic status epilepticus, is a life-threatening emergency, requiring immediate cardiovascular, respiratory, and metabolic management as well as pharmacologic therapy. The latter virtually always requires intravenous administration of antiepileptic medications. Diazepam is the most effective drug in most patients for stopping the attacks and is given directly by intravenous push to a maximum total dose of 20–30 mg in adults. Intravenous diazepam may depress respiration (less frequently cardiovascular function), and facilities for resuscitation must be immediately at hand during its administration. The effect of diazepam is not lasting, but the 30- to 40-minute seizure-free interval allows more definitive therapy to be initiated. For patients who are not actually in the throes of a seizure, diazepam therapy can be omitted and the patient treated at once with a long-acting drug such as phenytoin.

The mainstay of continuing therapy for status epilepticus is intravenous phenytoin, which is effective and nonsedative. It should be given as a loading dose of 13–18 mg/kg in adults; the usual error is to give too little of the drug. Administration should be at a maximum rate of 50 mg/min. It is safest to give the drug directly by intravenous push, but it can also be diluted in saline; it precipitates rapidly in the presence of glucose. Especially in elderly people, careful monitoring of cardiac rhythm and blood pressure is necessary. At least part of the cardiotoxicity is from the diluent, propylene glycol, in which the phenytoin is dissolved.

In previously treated epileptic patients, the administration of a large loading dose of phenytoin may cause some dose-related toxicity such as ataxia. This is usually a relatively minor problem during the acute status episode and is easily alleviated by later adjustment of plasma levels.

For patients who do not respond to phenytoin, phenobarbital can be given in large doses: 100–200 mg intravenously to a total of 400–800 mg. Respiratory depression is a common complication, especially if diazepam has already been given, and there should be no hesitation in instituting intubation and ventilation.

Other drugs have been recommended for the treatment of generalized tonic-clonic status epilepticus, including intravenous lorazepam or lidocaine. General anesthesia may be necessary in highly resistant cases.

SPECIAL ASPECTS OF THE TOXICOLOGY OF ANTIEPILEPTIC DRUGS

TERATOGENICITY

The potential teratogenicity of antiepileptic drugs is a controversial and important area. It is important because teratogenicity resulting from chronic drug treatment of millions of people throughout the world may have a profound effect even if the effect occurs in only a small percentage of cases. It is controversial because both epilepsy and antiepileptic drugs are heterogeneous and often inseparable in their effects. Furthermore, patients with severe epilepsy, in whom genetic factors rather than drug factors may be of greater importance in the occurrence of fetal malformations, are often receiving multiple antiepileptic drugs in high doses.

In spite of these limitations, it appears—from whatever cause—that children born to mothers taking antiepileptic drugs have an increased risk, perhaps 2-fold, of congenital malformations. One drug, phenytoin, has been implicated in a specific syndrome called **fetal hydantoin syndrome,** though not all investigators are convinced of its existence and a similar syndrome has been attributed to phenobarbital. Valproate, as noted above, has also been implicated in a specific malformation, spina bifida. It is estimated that a pregnant woman taking valproic acid or sodium valproate has a 1–2% risk of having a child with spina bifida (see *MMWR* reference).

In dealing with the clinical problem of a pregnant woman with epilepsy, most students of epilepsy agree that while it is important to minimize antiepileptic drugs, both in numbers and doses, it is also important not to allow maternal seizures to go unchecked.

WITHDRAWAL

Withdrawal of antiepileptic drugs, whether by accident or by design, can cause increased seizure frequency and severity. There are 2 factors to consider: the effects of the withdrawal itself and the need for continued drug suppression of seizures in the individual patient. In many patients, both factors must be considered and dealt with. It is important to note, however, that the abrupt discontinuation of antiepileptic drugs ordinarily does not cause seizures in nonepileptic patients, provided that the drug levels are not above the usual therapeutic range when the drug is stopped.

Some drugs are more easily withdrawn than others. In general, withdrawal of anti-absence drugs is easier than withdrawal of drugs needed for partial or generalized tonic-clonic seizures. Barbiturates and benzodiazepines are the most difficult to discontinue; weeks or months may be required, with very gradual dosage decrements, to accomplish their complete removal, especially if the patient is not hospitalized.

Because of the heterogeneity of epilepsy, consideration of the complete removal of antiepileptic drugs is an especially difficult problem. If a patient is seizure-free for 3 or 4 years, gradual discontinuation is usually warranted. Children whose seizures have always been infrequent and whose EEGs are normal are candidates for gradual removal of drugs after 4 seizure-free years.

OVERDOSE

Antiepileptic drugs are real or potential central nervous system depressants but are rarely lethal. Very high blood levels are usually necessary before overdoses can be considered life-threatening. The most dangerous effect of antiepileptic drugs after large overdoses is respiratory depression, which may be potentiated by other agents, such as alcohol. Treatment of antiepileptic drug overdose is supportive; stimulants should not be used. Efforts to hasten removal of antiepileptic drugs, such as urine alkalinization, are usually ineffective. Lipid dialysis has also been attempted; the data are too scanty to interpret its efficacy.

REFERENCES

Bjerkedal T et al: Valproic acid and spina bifida. *Lancet* 1982;**2**:1096.

Dalessio DJ: Current concepts: Seizure disorders and pregnancy. *N Engl J Med* 1985;**312**:559.

Delgado-Escueta AV et al: Current concepts in neurology: Management of status epilepticus. *N Engl J Med* 1982;**306**:1337.

Emerson R et al: Stopping medication in children with epilepsy: Predictors of outcome. *N Engl J Med* 1981;**304**:1125.

Glaser GH, Penry JK, Woodbury DM (editors): *Antiepileptic Drugs: Mechanisms of Action.* Raven Press, 1980.

Glazko AJ: Antiepileptic drugs: Biotransformation, metabolism, and serum half-life. *Epilepsia* 1975;**16**:367.

Hvidberg EF, Dam M: Clinical pharmacokinetics of anticonvulsants. *Clin Pharmacokinet* 1976;**1**:161.

Mattson RH et al: Comparison of carbamazepine, phenobarbital, phenytoin, and primidone in partial and secondarily generalized tonic-clonic seizures. *N Engl J Med* 1985;**313**:145.

Meldrum BS, Porter RJ (editors): *New Anticonvulsant Drugs.* John Libbey, 1986.

Morselli PL, Lloyd KG: Mechanism of action of antiepileptic drugs. Chap 3, pp 40–81, in: *The Epilepsies.* Porter RJ, Morselli PL (editors). Butterworth, 1985.

Porter RJ: *Epilepsy: 100 Elementary Principles.* Saunders, 1984.

Porter RJ, Penry JK, Lacy JR: Diagnostic and therapeutic reevaluation of patients with intractable epilepsy. *Neurology* 1977;**27**:1006.

Porter RJ et al: Antiepileptic Drug Development Program. *Cleve Clin Q* 1984;**51**:293.

Richens A: Interactions with antiepileptic drugs. *Drugs* 1977;**13**:266.

Theodore WH, Porter RJ: Removal of sedative-hypnotic antiepileptic drugs from the regimens of patients with intractable epilepsy. *Ann Neurol* 1983;**13**:320.

Theodore WH et al: Barbiturates reduce human cerebral glucose metabolism. *Neurology* 1986;**36**:60.

Valproate: A new cause of birth defects: Report from Italy and follow-up from France. *MMWR* 1983;**32**:438.

Woodbury DM, Penry JK, Pippenger CE (editors): *Antiepileptic Drugs.* Raven Press, 1983.

General Anesthetics 23

Anthony J. Trevor, PhD, & Ronald D. Miller, MD

I. BASIC PHARMACOLOGY OF GENERAL ANESTHETICS

The attempted suppression of the pain of surgical procedures by the use of drugs dates from ancient times and includes the oral administration of ethanol and opiates. The first scientific demonstration of drug-induced anesthesia during surgery was in 1846, when William Morton used diethyl ether in Boston. Within a year, chloroform was introduced by James Simpson in Scotland, and this was followed 20 years later by the successful demonstration of the anesthetic properties of nitrous oxide, which had been first suggested by Davy in the 1790s. Modern anesthesia dates from the 1930s, during which period the intravenous barbiturate thiopental was introduced. A decade later, curare was used in anesthesia to ensure adequate skeletal muscle relaxation. The first modern halogenated hydrocarbon, halothane, was introduced as an inhaled anesthetic in 1956 and has become the standard for comparison for several other more recently developed inhaled anesthetic drugs.

The state of "general anesthesia" usually includes analgesia, amnesia, loss of consciousness, inhibition of sensory and autonomic reflexes, and skeletal muscle relaxation. It can be produced by some but not all sedative-hypnotics (Chapter 20). The extent to which any individual anesthetic drug can exert these effects is variable. It is desirable to be able to induce anesthesia smoothly and rapidly as well as to ensure rapid recovery from the effects of the anesthetic. An ideal anesthetic drug would also possess a wide margin of safety and be devoid of adverse effects. No *single* anesthetic agent is capable of achieving all of these desirable effects without some disadvantages when used alone. Thus, the modern practice of anesthesia involves the use of combinations of drugs, taking advantage of their individual desirable properties while attempting to minimize their potential for harmful actions. **Balanced anesthesia** includes the administration of medications preoperatively for sedation and analgesia, the use of neuromuscular blocking drugs intraoperatively, and the use of both intravenous and inhaled anesthetic drugs.

TYPES OF GENERAL ANESTHETICS

General anesthetics are usually given by inhalation or by intravenous injection.

Inhalational Agents

The chemical structures of the 5 most commonly used inhalational agents are shown in Fig 23–1. Nitrous oxide, a gas at ambient temperature and pressure, continues to be an important component of many anesthesia regimens. Halothane, enflurane, isoflurane, and methoxyflurane are volatile liquids. Other inhalational agents (not shown) include ether, cyclopropane, and chloroform, which have limited current use for reasons that include potential flammability (ether, cyclopropane) and organ toxicity (chloroform).

Intravenous Agents

Several drugs are used intravenously to achieve anesthesia:

(1) Thiobarbiturates (thiopental, methohexital).

(2) Opioid analgesics and neuroleptics.

(3) Arylcyclohexylamines (ketamine), which produce a state called dissociative anesthesia.

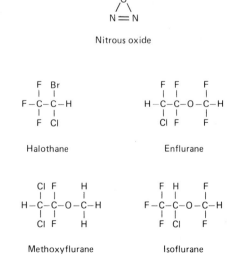

Figure 23–1. Inhalational anesthetics.

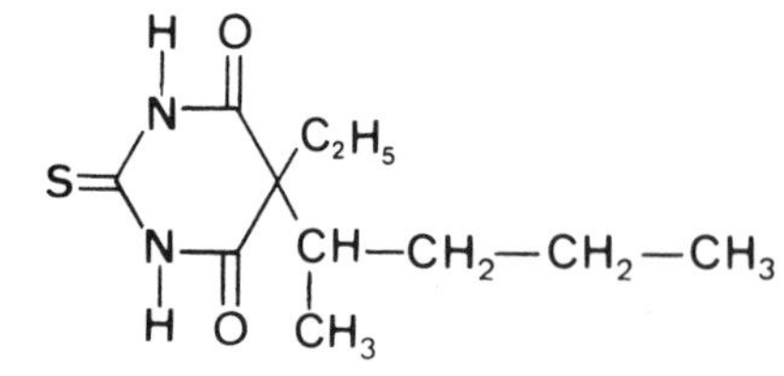

Thiopental

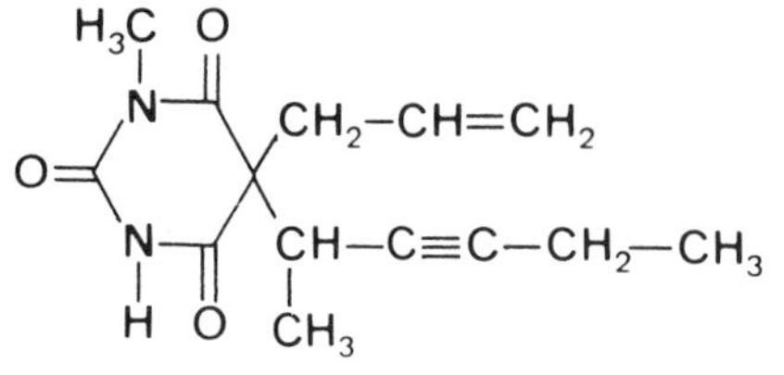

Methohexital

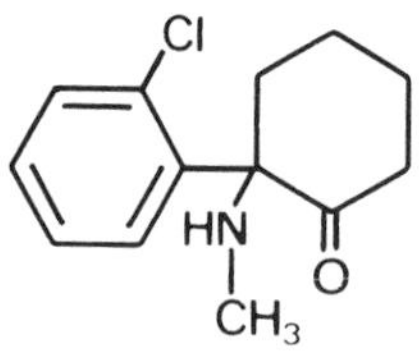

Ketamine

Figure 23–2. Intravenous anesthetics.

(4) Miscellaneous drugs (etomidate, steroid anesthetics, propanidid), most of which are not currently available in the USA.

Fig 23–2 shows the structures of 2 commonly used barbiturates and ketamine.

SIGNS & STAGES OF ANESTHESIA

Since the introduction of general anesthetics, attempts have been made to correlate their observable effects or signs with the *depth* of anesthesia. Descriptions of the signs and stages of anesthesia (Guedel's signs) originate mainly from observations of the effects of diethyl ether, which has a slow onset of central action due to its high solubility in blood. These stages and signs may not occur so readily with the more rapidly acting modern inhaled anesthetics and are unusual with intravenous agents. Many of the signs refer to the effects of anesthetic agents on respiration, reflex activity, and muscle tone. Traditionally, anesthetic effects are divided into 4 stages of increasing depth of CNS depression.

I. Stage of analgesia: The patient initially experiences analgesia without amnesia. However, later in stage I, both analgesia and amnesia ensue.

II. Stage of excitement: During this stage, the patient often appears to be delirious and excited but definitely is amnesic. Respiration is irregular both in volume and rate, and retching and vomiting may oc-

cur. Incontinence and struggling sometimes occur. For these reasons, efforts are made to limit the duration and severity of this stage, which ends with the reestablishment of regular breathing.

III. Stage of surgical anesthesia: With the beginning of regular respiration, this stage extends to complete cessation of spontaneous respiration. Four planes of stage III have been described in terms of changes in ocular movements, eye reflexes, and pupil size, which under specified conditions may represent signs of increasing depth of anesthesia.

IV. Stage of medullary depression: When spontaneous respiration ceases, stage IV is present. This stage of anesthesia obviously includes severe depression of the respiratory center in the medulla and the vasomotor center as well. Without full circulatory and respiratory support, coma and death rapidly ensue.

In modern anesthesia practice, the distinctive signs of each of the 4 stages described above are often obscured. Reasons for this include the relatively rapid onset of action of many inhaled anesthetics compared to that of diethyl ether and the fact that pulmonary ventilation is often controlled with the aid of a mechanical ventilator. In addition, the presence of other pharmacologic agents given pre- or intraoperatively can also influence the signs of anesthesia. Atropine, used to decrease secretions, also dilates pupils; drugs such as tubocurarine and succinylcholine affect muscle tone; and the opioid analgesics exert depressant effects on respiration. The most reliable indications that stage III (surgical anesthesia) has been achieved are loss of the eyelash reflex and establishment of a respiratory pattern that is regular in rate and depth. The adequacy of ensuing depth of anesthesia for the particular surgical situation is assessed mainly by changes in respiratory and cardiovascular responses to stimulation.

MECHANISMS OF ACTION

A common neurophysiologic action of general anesthetics is to *increase the threshold* of cells to firing, resulting in decreased activity. Almost all anesthetics also *reduce the rate of rise of the action potential* by interfering with sodium influx. One interpretation of this effect is that the physical presence of anesthetic molecules blocks or distorts neuronal membrane channels involved in sodium conductance. Current theories of the possible mechanisms by which anesthetics interfere with the sodium channel include consideration of their molecular interactions with the lipid matrix of the membrane and with hydrophobic regions of specific membrane proteins. This interpretation is encouraged by several facts: (1) There are few, if any, characteristics of chemical structure common to all general anesthetic molecules (compare structures shown in Figs 23–1 and 23–2). This suggests that "receptor sites" for these drugs, if they exist, are quite nonselective. (2) The potency of general anesthetics is well correlated with their lipid solubility

(Meyer-Overton principle). (3) The interaction of anesthetics with artificial lipid membranes causes changes in the physicochemical characteristics of these membranes suggestive of a reduction of structural order in the lipid matrix. These changes in the lipid matrix could alter the function of proteins in the membrane—eg, reducing sodium conductance. Conversely, in experimental animals, general anesthesia can be reversed quite rapidly by high pressure (eg, 50–100 atm), which increases the ordering of lipids in the membrane bilayer. This has led to suggestions that as the anesthetic molecule dissolves in the neuronal membrane, it causes a small expansion that distorts the sodium channel. High pressure restores the membrane to its former state to permit the normal influx of sodium that occurs during generation of the action potential.

The neuropharmacologic basis for the effects that characterize the stages of anesthesia appears to be a **differential sensitivity** to the anesthetics of specific neurons or neuronal pathways. Cells of the substantia gelatinosa in the dorsal horn of the spinal cord are very sensitive to relatively low anesthetic concentration in the central nervous system. A decrease in the activity of the dorsal horn interrupts sensory transmission in the spinothalamic tract, including that concerning nociceptive stimuli. These effects contribute to stage I, or analgesia. The disinhibitory effects of general anesthetics (stage II), which occur at higher brain concentrations, result from complex neuronal actions including blockade of many small inhibitory neurons such as Golgi type II cells, together with a paradoxic facilitation of excitatory neurotransmitters. A progressive depression of ascending pathways in the reticular activating system occurs during stage III, or surgical anesthesia, together with suppression of spinal reflex activity that contributes to muscle relaxation. Neurons in the respiratory and vasomotor centers of the medulla are relatively insensitive to the effects of the general anesthetics, but at high concentrations their activity is depressed, leading to cardiorespiratory collapse (stage IV).

PHARMACOKINETICS OF INHALED ANESTHETICS

Depth of anesthesia is determined by the concentrations of anesthetics in the central nervous system. The rate at which an effective brain concentration is reached (the rate of induction of anesthesia) depends on multiple pharmacokinetic factors that influence the uptake and distribution of the anesthetic. These factors determine the different rates of transfer of the inhaled anesthetic from the lung to the blood and from the blood to the brain and other tissues. These factors also influence the rate of recovery from anesthesia when inhalation of the anesthetic is terminated.

Uptake & Distribution

The **concentration** of an individual gas in a mixture of gases is proportionate to its **partial pressure** or **tension.** These terms are often used interchangeably in discussing the various transfer processes of anesthetic gases in the body. Achievement of a brain concentration of an anesthetic adequate to cause anesthesia requires transfer of that anesthetic from the alveolar air to blood and then to brain. The rate at which a given concentration of anesthetic in the brain is reached depends on the solubility properties of the anesthetic, its concentration in the inspired air, pulmonary ventilation rate, pulmonary blood flow, and the concentration gradient of the anesthetic between arterial and mixed venous blood.

A. Solubility: One of the most important factors influencing the transfer of an anesthetic from the lungs to the arterial blood is its solubility. The blood:gas partition coefficient is a useful index of solubility and defines the relative affinity of an anesthetic for the blood compared to air. This partition coefficient may be as low as 0.5 for anesthetics such as nitrous oxide or cyclopropane, which are quite insoluble in blood. Alternatively, the value may be higher than 10 for agents such as diethyl ether or methoxyflurane, which are very soluble in blood (Table 23–1). When an anesthetic with low blood solubility diffuses from the lung into the arterial blood, relatively few molecules are required to raise its partial pressure, and the arterial tension rises quickly. Conversely, for anesthetics with moderate to high solubility, more molecules dissolve before partial pressure is changed, and arterial tension of the gas will increase slowly. This inverse relationship between the blood solubility of an anesthetic and rate of rise of its tension in arterial blood is illustrated in Fig 23–3. The blood:gas partition coefficients for nitrous oxide, halothane, and methoxyflurane are 0.47, 2.3, and 12, respectively. Nitrous oxide, with low solubility in blood, reaches high arterial tensions rapidly, which in turn results in more rapid equilibrium with the brain and faster induction of anesthesia. In contrast, even after 40 minutes, methoxyflurane has reached only 20% of the equilibrium concentration.

B. Anesthetic Concentration in the Inspired Air: The concentration of an inhaled anesthetic in the

Table 23–1. Properties of inhalational anesthetics.

Anesthetic	Blood:Gas Partition Coefficient	Brain:Blood Partition Coefficient	Minimum Alveolar Concentration (percent)
Nitrous oxide	0.47	1.1	> 100
Isoflurane	1.40	2.6	1.40
Enflurane	1.80	1.4	1.68
Halothane	2.30	2.9	0.75
Methoxyflurane	12.00	2.0	0.16

Partition coefficients (at 37 °C) are from multiple literature sources. Minimum alveolar concentration (MAC) is the anesthetic concentration that produces immobility in 50% of patients exposed to a noxious stimulus.

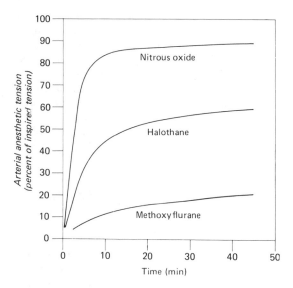

Figure 23–3. Tensions of anesthetic gases in arterial blood.

inspired gas mixture has direct effects on both the maximum tension that can be achieved in the alveoli and the rate of increase in its tension in arterial blood. Increases in the inspired anesthetic concentration will increase the rate of induction of anesthesia by increasing the rate of transfer into the blood. Advantage is taken of this effect in anesthetic practice with inhaled anesthetics of moderate blood solubility such as enflurane or halothane, which have a relatively slow onset. For example, a 3–4% concentration of halothane may be inspired initially to increase the rate of induction, and this is reduced to 1–2% for maintenance when adequate anesthesia is achieved.

C. Pulmonary Ventilation: The rate of rise of anesthetic gas tension in arterial blood is directly dependent on both the rate and depth of ventilation, ie, minute ventilation. The magnitude of the effect varies according to the blood:gas partition coefficient. An increase in pulmonary ventilation is accompanied by only a slight increase in arterial tension of an anesthetic with low blood solubility or low coefficient but can significantly increase tension of agents with moderate or high blood solubility (Fig 23–4). For example, a 4-fold increase in ventilation rate may double the arterial tension of halothane during the first 10 minutes of anesthesia, with little effect on the arterial tension of nitrous oxide. Hyperventilation by mechanical control of respiration or by CO_2 stimulation increases the speed of induction of anesthesia with inhaled anesthetics that would normally have a slow onset. Depression of respiration by other pharmacologic agents, including opioid analgesics, may slow the onset of anesthesia of some inhaled anesthetics if ventilation is not controlled.

D. Pulmonary Blood Flow: Changes in the rates of blood flow to and from the lungs influence transfer processes of the anesthetic gases. An increase in pulmonary blood flow (increased cardiac output) *slows*

the rate of rise in arterial tension, particularly for those anesthetics with moderate to high blood solubility. This is because increased pulmonary blood flow exposes a larger volume of blood to the anesthetic; thus, blood "capacity" increases and tension rises slowly. A decrease in pulmonary blood flow has the opposite effect and increases the rate of rise of arterial tension of inhaled anesthetics. In a patient with circulatory shock, the combined effects of decreased cardiac output (decreased pulmonary flow) and increased ventilation may accelerate the induction of anesthesia with some anesthetics. This is least likely to occur with nitrous oxide because of its low solubility.

E. Arterial-Venous Concentration Gradient: The anesthetic concentration gradient between arterial and mixed venous blood is dependent mainly on uptake of the anesthetic by the tissues; depending on the rate and extent of tissue uptake, venous blood returning to the lungs may contain significantly less anesthetic than that present in arterial blood. The greater this difference in tensions, the more time it takes to achieve equilibrium. Anesthetic entry into tissues is influenced by factors similar to those that determine transfer from lung to blood, including tissue:blood partition coefficient, rates of blood flow to the tissues, and concentration gradients.

During the induction phase of anesthesia, the tissues that exert greatest influence on the arterial-venous anesthetic concentration gradient are those which are highly perfused. These include the brain, heart, liver, kidneys, and splanchnic bed, which together receive over 75% of the resting cardiac output. In the case of anesthetics with relatively high solubility in these tissues, venous blood concentration will initially be very low, and equilibrium with arterial blood is achieved slowly.

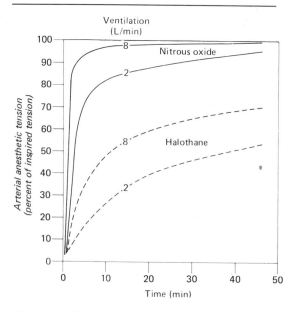

Figure 23–4. Ventilation rate and arterial anesthetic tensions.

During maintenance of anesthesia with inhaled anesthetics, there may continue to be transfer of these drugs between various tissues at rates dependent on solubility and blood flow. Muscle and skin, which together constitute 50% of body mass, accumulate anesthetics more slowly than the richly vascularized tissues, since they receive only one-fifth of the blood flow of the latter group. Although most anesthetic gases have high solubility in adipose tissues, low blood perfusion rates to these tissues delay accumulation, and equilibrium is unlikely to occur with anesthetics such as halothane and enflurane during the time anesthetics are usually required for surgery.

Elimination

The time to recovery from inhalational anesthesia depends on the rate of elimination of anesthetics from the brain after the inspired concentration of anesthetic has been decreased. Many of the processes of anesthetic transfer during recovery are similar to those that occur during induction of anesthesia. Factors controlling rate of recovery include the pulmonary blood flow and the magnitude of ventilation as well as solubility of the anesthetic in the tissues and the blood and in the gas phase in the lung. Two features of recovery, however, are quite different from what happens during induction of anesthesia. First, while transfer of an anesthetic from the lungs to blood can be enhanced by increasing its concentration in inspired air, the reverse transfer process cannot be enhanced, since the concentration in the lungs cannot be reduced below zero. Second, at the beginning of recovery, the anesthetic gas tension in different tissues may be quite variable, depending on the specific agent and the duration of anesthesia. With induction of anesthesia, the initial anesthetic tension in all tissues is zero.

Inhaled anesthetics that are relatively insoluble in blood and brain are eliminated at faster rates than more soluble anesthetics. For example, the "washout" of nitrous oxide occurs at a fast rate, which leads to a rapid recovery from its anesthetic effects. Halothane is approximately twice as soluble in brain tissue and 5 times more soluble in blood than nitrous oxide; its elimination therefore takes place more slowly, and recovery from halothane anesthesia is less rapid. The duration of exposure to the anesthetic can have a marked effect on the time of recovery, especially in the case of more soluble anesthetics such as methoxyflurane. Accumulation of agents in tissues, including muscle, skin, and fat, increases with continuous inhalation; and blood tension may decline slowly during recovery as the anesthetic gradually leaves such tissues. Thus, if exposure to the anesthetic is short, recovery may be rapid. After prolonged anesthesia, recovery may be delayed even with anesthetics of modest solubility such as halothane.

Clearance of inhaled anesthetics by the lung into the expired air is the major route of their elimination from the body. However, metabolism by enzymes of the liver and other tissues may also contribute to the elimination of anesthetics. For example, the washout

of halothane during recovery is more rapid than that of enflurane, which would not be predicted from their respective solubilities. However, 15–20% of inspired halothane is metabolized during an average anesthetic procedure, while only 2–3% of enflurane is metabolized over the same period. Oxidative metabolism of halothane results in the formation of trifluoroacetic acid and release of bromide and chloride ions. Under conditions of low oxygen tension, halothane is metabolized to the chlorotrifluoroethyl free radical, which is capable of reacting with hepatic membrane components. The slow rate of metabolism of enflurane results in the formation of difluoromethoxydifluoroacetic acid and fluoride ion, which do not reach toxic levels. Methoxyflurane is metabolized by the liver at a faster rate than any other inhaled anesthetic and releases fluoride ions at levels that can be nephrotoxic. Nitrous oxide is metabolized to a very small extent.

MINIMUM ALVEOLAR ANESTHETIC CONCENTRATIONS

Inhaled anesthetics are delivered to the lungs in gas mixtures in which concentrations and flow rate are easy to measure and control. However, achievement of an anesthetic state depends on the concentration of the anesthetic in the brain, and that concentration is impossible to measure under clinical conditions. During general anesthesia, the partial pressure of the anesthetic in the brain equals that in the lung when steady state is reached. At this point, the measurement of the alveolar concentrations of different anesthetics provides a comparison of their relative potencies. The **minimum alveolar anesthetic concentration (MAC)** of an anesthetic is defined as that concentration which results in immobility in 50% of patients when exposed to a noxious stimulus such as surgical incision. Table 23–1 shows such concentrations for the common inhaled anesthetics, permitting comparison of their relative anesthetic potencies. The MAC value greater than 100% for nitrous oxide shows that it is the least potent, since not even 1 MAC can be reached at normal barometric pressures. Furthermore, the dose administered can be stated in multiples of MAC. While a dose of 1 MAC of any agent prevents movement in response to surgical incision in 50% of patients, individual patients may required from 0.5 to 1.5 MAC. In general, however, the dose-response relationship for inhaled anesthetics is steep; thus, over 95% of patients may fail to respond to a noxious stimulus at 1.1 MAC. The measurement of MAC values under controlled conditions has permitted quantitation of the effects of a number of variables on anesthetic requirements. For example, MAC values decrease in elderly patients but are not affected greatly by sex, height, and weight. Of particular importance is the presence of adjuvant drugs, which can change anesthetic requirement greatly. For example, when drugs such as the opioid analgesics or sedative-hypnotics are present, MAC is decreased, which means that the inspired concentration of anesthetic should be decreased accordingly.

II. CLINICAL PHARMACOLOGY OF GENERAL ANESTHETICS

INHALED ANESTHETICS

General Overview of Clinical Use

Of the inhaled anesthetics available, nitrous oxide, halothane, enflurane, and isoflurane are most commonly used in the USA. As indicated previously, nitrous oxide lacks sufficient potency to produce surgical anesthesia by itself and therefore is usually used in combination with another inhaled or intravenous anesthetic to produce the total anesthetic state. Methoxyflurane is occasionally used, especially in obstetrical anesthesia, but not for prolonged procedures because of its nephrotoxicity, which is described below. Chloroform is not used because of its hepatotoxicity. Although cyclopropane and diethyl ether were the most commonly used anesthetics before 1960, they are rarely used now because of their flammable and explosive characteristics.

General Pharmacologic Effects

A. Effects on Cardiovascular System: Halothane, enflurane, and isoflurane all decrease mean arterial pressure in direct proportion to their alveolar concentration. With halothane and enflurane, the reduced arterial pressure appears to be caused by a reduction in cardiac output, since there is little change in systemic vascular resistance. In contrast, isoflurane has a depressant effect on arterial pressure as a result of a marked decrease in systemic vascular resistance; it has little effect on cardiac output.

Older anesthetics such as cyclopropane, diethyl ether, and fluroxene generally do not reduce arterial blood pressure or significantly change cardiac output. In fact, diethyl ether and cyclopropane often increase arterial blood pressure as a result of their ability to liberate catecholamines.

Inhaled anesthetics change heart rate either by altering the rate of sinus node depolarization directly or by shifting the balance of autonomic nervous system activity. Bradycardia is often seen with halothane and may be a result of direct depression of atrial rate. In contrast, methoxyflurane, enflurane, and isoflurane increase heart rate. All of these changes in heart rate have been determined in normal subjects undergoing surgery. The patient's excited state preoperatively or the stimulation of surgery intraoperatively will often alter the heart rate response to inhaled anesthetics.

All inhaled anesthetics tend to increase right atrial pressure in a dose-related fashion that reflects depression of myocardial function. In general, enflurane and halothane are very depressant to the myocardium, but cyclopropane, diethyl ether, and fluroxene are not. Inhaled anesthetics reduce myocardial oxygen consumption, primarily by decreasing those variables that control oxygen demand, such as arterial blood pressure and contractile force. Although certainly less depressant than the other inhaled anesthetics, nitrous oxide has also been found to depress the myocardium in a dose-dependent manner. However, nitrous oxide alone or in combination with potent inhaled anesthetics produces sympathetic stimulation that may obscure any cardiac depressant effects of the inhaled anesthetic. The combination of nitrous oxide plus halothane or enflurane, for example, appears to produce less depression at a given level of anesthesia than either more potent anesthetic given alone.

B. Effects on Respiratory System: With the exception of nitrous oxide and diethyl ether, all inhaled anesthetics cause a decrease in tidal volume and an increase in respiratory rate. However, the increase in rate is insufficient to compensate for the decrease in volume, resulting in a decrease in minute ventilation. All inhaled anesthetics are respiratory depressants, as gauged by the reduced response to various levels of carbon dioxide. The degree of ventilatory depression varies with anesthetic agents, with isoflurane and enflurane being the most depressant and diethyl ether the least depressant. All inhaled anesthetics except diethyl ether increase the resting level of $P_{a_{CO_2}}$ (the partial pressure of carbon dioxide in arterial blood). Because diethyl ether is a respiratory irritant, ventilation may remain sufficiently high to maintain normal $P_{a_{CO_2}}$. However, if the patient is challenged with increasing inspired concentrations of carbon dioxide, the respiratory depressant effect of diethyl ether will become apparent. The ventilatory depressant effects of anesthetics are overcome by assisting or controlling ventilation via a mechanical ventilator during surgery. Inhaled anesthetics also depress mucociliary function in the airway. Thus, prolonged anesthesia may lead to pooling of mucus and then result in atelectasis and respiratory infections. On the other hand, inhaled anesthetics tend to be bronchodilators, with halothane probably one of the most potent. This effect has been utilized in the treatment of asthma.

C. Effects on Brain: Inhaled anesthetics decrease the metabolic rate of the brain. Nevertheless, most of them *increase* cerebral blood flow because they decrease cerebral vascular resistance. The increase in cerebral blood flow is often clinically undesirable. For example, in patients who have an elevated intracranial pressure because of brain tumor or head injury, the administration of an inhaled anesthetic may increase cerebral blood flow, which in turn will increase cerebral blood volume and further increase intracranial pressure.

Of the inhaled anesthetics, nitrous oxide increases cerebral blood flow the least, although when 60% nitrous oxide is added to halothane anesthesia, cerebral blood flow usually increases more than with halothane alone. Halothane, enflurane, and isoflurane in low doses have similar effects on cerebral blood flow. At higher doses, enflurane and isoflurane increase cerebral blood flow less than does halothane. If the patient is hyperventilated before the anesthetic is given, increase in intracranial pressure from inhaled anesthetics can be minimized.

Halothane, isoflurane, and enflurane have similar effects (eg, burst suppression) on the EEG up to doses of 1–1.5 MAC. At higher doses, the cerebral irritant effects of enflurane may lead to the development of a spike-and-wave pattern during which auditory stimuli can precipitate mild generalized muscle twitching that is augmented by hyperventilation. This seizure activity has never been shown to have any adverse clinical consequences. The effect is not seen clinically with the other inhaled anesthetics.

D. Effects on Kidney: To varying degrees, all inhaled anesthetics decrease glomerular filtration rate and effective renal plasma flow and increase filtration fraction. All the anesthetics tend to increase renal vascular resistance. Since renal blood flow decreases during general anesthesia in spite of well-maintained or even increased perfusion pressures, autoregulation of renal flow is probably impaired.

E. Effects on Liver: All inhaled anesthetics cause a decrease in hepatic blood flow, ranging from 15 to 45% of the preanesthetic flow. Despite transient changes in liver function tests intraoperatively, rarely does permanent change of liver function occur from the use of these agents. The possible hepatotoxicity of halothane is discussed below.

F. Effects on Uterine Smooth Muscle: Nitrous oxide appears to have little effect on uterine musculature. However, isoflurane, halothane, and enflurane are potent uterine muscle relaxants. This pharmacologic effect can be used to advantage when profound uterine relaxation is required for intrauterine fetal manipulation during delivery. In contrast, during dilatation and curettage for therapeutic abortion, these anesthetics may cause increased bleeding.

Toxicity

A. Hepatotoxicity (Halothane): Postoperative hepatitis is usually associated with factors such as blood transfusions, hypovolemic shock, and other surgical stresses rather than anesthetic toxicity. However, halocarbons can cause liver damage, and chloroform was identified as a hepatotoxin in the first decade of this century. Halothane was introduced into clinical practice in 1956; by 1963, several cases of postoperative jaundice and liver necrosis associated with halothane had been reported. However, several retrospective studies in which halothane was compared with other anesthetics showed no increased incidence in postoperative hepatic damage with halothane. In 1966, the United States National Halothane Study undertook a retrospective review of the incidence of fatal massive hepatic necrosis in a population of about 850,000 surgical patients. Results of the study were inconclusive and did not identify halothane clearly as a hepatotoxin. The incidence of massive necrosis associated with halothane was 7 out of 250,000 halothane administrations, or about one in 35,000 (not one in 10,000, as sometimes reported). Because halothane is such a valuable anesthetic, it is important to establish whether it is indeed a significant hepatotoxin before limiting its use. Unlike chloroform and fluroxene, which can produce fatty infiltration, centrilobular necrosis, and elevated transaminase concentrations, prolonged exposure of animals to halothane produces little evidence of liver damage. Several animal models have been developed to help define possible halothane-mediated hepatotoxicity. When rats are pretreated with phenobarbital and then exposed to hypoxic conditions with an inspired oxygen concentration of 7–14%, hepatotoxicity from halothane (as well as other inhalational agents) will occur. The mechanism underlying hepatotoxicity in the animals remains unclear, although these models suggest that it may depend on the production of a reactive metabolite (eg, a free radical) that either causes direct hepatocellular damage or initiates an immune-mediated response. Although this model is reproducible and well-defined, its clinical applicability is uncertain because hypoxia is a necessary precondition for production of liver damage.

B. Nephrotoxicity (Methoxyflurane): In 1966, vasopressin-resistant polyuric renal insufficiency was first reported in 13 of 41 patients receiving methoxyflurane anesthesia for abdominal surgery. Subsequently, the causative agent was shown to be inorganic fluoride, an end product of the biotransformation of methoxyflurane.

C. Chronic Toxicity:

1. Mutagenicity–Under normal conditions, most modern and many previously used inhaled anesthetics are not mutagens and probably not carcinogens. On the other hand, anesthetics that contain the vinyl moiety (fluroxene and divinyl ether) may be mutagens.

2. Carcinogenicity–Several epidemiologic studies have suggested an increase in the cancer rate in operating room personnel who may be exposed to trace concentrations of anesthetic agents. However, no study has demonstrated the existence of a cause-and-effect relationship between anesthetics and cancer. Many other factors might account for the questionably positive results seen after a careful review of epidemiologic data. Most operating room theaters remove trace concentrations of anesthetics released from anesthetic machines via vents to the atmosphere.

3. Effects on reproduction–The most consistent finding reported from surveys conducted to determine the reproductive performance of female operating room personnel has been a higher than expected incidence of miscarriages. There are several problems in interpreting these studies, but in general it can be stated that the evidence is not strong.

On the other hand, the association of obstetric problems with surgery and anesthesia in pregnant patients is not open to question. In the USA, at least 50,000 pregnant women each year undergo anesthesia and surgery during pregnancy for indications unrelated to the pregnancy. The risk of abortion is clearly higher following this experience. It is not obvious whether the underlying disease, surgery, anesthesia, or a combination of these factors is the cause of the increased risk.

Another concern not yet substantiated is that anesthetics during pregnancy may lead to an increased incidence of congenital anomalies. If anesthetics are teratogenic, the risk must be very small.

INTRAVENOUS ANESTHETICS

ULTRA–SHORT-ACTING BARBITURATES

Although there are several ultra–short-acting barbiturates, thiopental is the one most commonly used for induction of anesthesia, often in combination with inhaled anesthetics. The general pharmacology of the barbiturates is discussed in Chapter 20.

Following intravenous administration, thiopental crosses the blood-brain barrier and, if given in sufficient dosage, produces hypnosis in one circulation time. Similar effects occur with other ultra–short-acting barbiturates, eg, thiamylal and methohexital. With all of these barbiturates, plasma:brain equilibrium occurs rapidly (in approximately 1 minute) because of high lipid solubility. Thiopental rapidly diffuses out of the brain and other vascular tissues and is redistributed to muscle, fat, and eventually all body tissues (Fig 23–5). It is because of this rapid removal from brain tissue that a single dose of thiopental is so short-acting.

Metabolism following thiopental administration is much slower than redistribution and takes place primarily in the liver. Less than 1% of an administered dose of thiopental is excreted unchanged by the kidney. Thiopental is metabolized at the rate of 12–16% per hour in humans following a single dose.

With large doses, thiopental causes dose-dependent decreases in arterial blood pressure, stroke volume, and cardiac output. This is due primarily to its myocardial depressant effect; there is little change in total peripheral resistance. However, thiopental also markedly increases venous vessel compliance, resulting in pooling of blood and impaired venous return to the heart.

Thiopental, like other barbiturates, is a potent respiratory depressant, lowering the sensitivity of the medullary respiratory center to carbon dioxide.

Cerebral metabolism and oxygen utilization are decreased after thiopental administration in proportion to the degree of cerebral depression. Cerebral blood flow is also decreased but much less so than oxygen consumption. This makes thiopental a much more desirable drug for use in patients with cerebral swelling than the inhaled anesthetics, since intracranial pressure and blood volume are not increased.

Thiopental may reduce hepatic blood flow and glomerular filtration rate, but it produces no lasting effects on hepatic and renal function.

OPIOID ANALGESIC ANESTHESIA & NEUROLEPTANESTHESIA

During the past 10 to 15 years there has been an increasing use of large doses of opioid (narcotic) analgesics to achieve general anesthesia, particularly in patients undergoing cardiac surgery or other major surgery when circulatory reserve is minimal. Intravenous morphine, 1 mg/kg, and subsequently the high-potency drug fentanyl, 50 μg/kg, have been used in such situations with minimal evidence of circulatory deterioration. Despite such high doses (see Table 29–2 for conventional analgesic doses), awareness during anesthesia or postoperative recall has occurred. In addition, postoperative respiratory depression requiring assisted ventilation may be a problem. One approach to reducing postoperative respiratory effects is the lowering of opioid analgesic dose with simultaneous administration of short-acting barbiturates or benzodiazepines, usually with nitrous oxide to achieve "balanced anesthesia." Several short-acting congeners of fentanyl including sufentanil and alfentanil are presently being evaluated for their usefulness as intravenous agents in shorter surgical procedures.

Neuroleptanesthesia is a term used to characterize a state in which the patient becomes completely disinterested and detached from the environment without loss of consciousness or the ability to obey commands or communicate with others. The desire to move or change body position is also lost. The most common drug combination used to produce this state is Innovar, which is a combination of droperidol, a butyrophenone, and fentanyl, an opioid analgesic. This drug combination is usually used with nitrous oxide to produce complete general anesthesia.

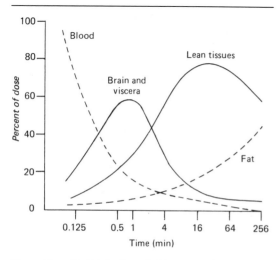

Figure 23–5. Redistribution of thiopental after an intravenous bolus administration.

KETAMINE

Ketamine (Fig 23–2) produces "dissociative anesthesia," characterized by catatonia, amnesia, and analgesia. Although it is a desirable anesthetic in many respects, ketamine has been associated with disorientation, sensory and perceptual illusions, and vivid dreams following anesthesia, effects that are termed "emergence phenomena." Diazepam, 0.2–0.3 mg/kg intravenously 5 minutes before administration of ketamine, reduces the incidence of these phenomena.

Ketamine, a lipophilic drug, is rapidly distributed into highly vascular organs, including the brain, and subsequently redistributed to less perfused tissues with concurrent hepatic metabolism and both urinary and biliary excretion.

Besides being a powerful analgesic, ketamine is the only intravenous anesthetic that routinely produces cardiovascular stimulation. Heart rate, arterial blood pressure, and cardiac output are usually significantly increased. The peak increases in these variables occur 2–4 minutes after intravenous injection and then slowly decline to normal over the next 10–20 minutes. Ketamine produces its cardiovascular stimulation by excitation of the central sympathetic nervous system. Increases in plasma epinephrine and norepinephrine levels occur as early as 2 minutes after intravenous ketamine and return to control levels 15 minutes later.

Ketamine markedly increases blood flow, cerebral oxygen consumption, and intracranial pressure. Like most inhaled anesthetics, it is therefore a potentially dangerous drug when intracranial pressure is elevated.

In most patients, ketamine decreases the respiratory rate slightly for 2–3 minutes. Upper airway muscle tone is well maintained, and upper airway reflexes are usually (not always) active. Ketamine produces little other change in organ systems.

Because of the high incidence of postoperative psychic phenomena associated with its use, ketamine is not commonly used in general surgery in the USA, except for poor-risk geriatric patients and patients in shock, because of its cardiostimulatory properties. Because ketamine tends not to depress respiration and is short-acting, it is used quite often in outpatient anesthesia and in children undergoing dressing changes on burned tissue.

ETOMIDATE

Etomidate is a carboxylated imidazole first synthesized in 1965. It causes rapid induction of anesthesia with minimal cardiovascular and respiratory changes. The compound has been studied extensively in Europe and was recently approved for use in the USA. Distribution of etomidate is rapid, with a biphasic concentration curve showing distribution half-lives of 2.6 and 28.7 minutes. The drug is lipid-soluble and has a large volume of distribution (about 4.5 L/kg of body weight). Preliminary studies in humans indicate that almost 90% of the drug—of which only 2% is unchanged—eventually appears in the urine. This suggests that the total clearance of etomidate represents mostly metabolic clearance; the liver is the primary site of metabolism. Etomidate produces hypnosis within seconds, with no effect on heart rate, slight hypotension, and a low frequence of apnea. Unfortunately, it causes a high incidence of myoclonia and half of patients report pain during injection. The myoclonic movements are not associated with epileptiform discharges on the EEG. Etomidate may also cause adrenocortical suppression, via inhibitory effects on steroidogenesis.

BENZODIAZEPINES

Certain members of this class of sedative-hypnotic drugs have found clinical use in anesthesia, including diazepam, lorazepam, and midazolam. (For the basic pharmacology of benzodiazepines, see Chapter 20.) Diazepam and lorazepam are not water-soluble, and their intravenous use necessitates nonaqueous vehicles, which may be irritating. Compared to the intravenous barbiturates, the onset of central nervous system effects of the benzodiazepines is slower, and the extent of central depression appears to reach a plateau short of a true anesthetic state. Used intravenously, the benzodiazepines appear to prolong the postanesthetic recovery period and cause a high incidence of amnesia. The benzodiazepines are most useful in anesthesia as premedication, but they can also be used for intraoperative sedation and with other drugs as part of balanced anesthesia.

PROPANIDID

Propanidid produces anesthesia with about the same rapidity as thiopental. Recovery is more complete and accumulation less likely with propanidid than with thiopental, since it is rapidly degraded by cholinesterase into inactive metabolites.

Propanidid causes hypotension, chiefly due to peripheral vasodilatation and a negative inotropic effect on the heart. Because of rapid recovery, an apparent lack of cumulative effect, and minimal cardiorespiratory effects, propanidid was at one time considered a promising anesthetic. However, numerous adverse reactions have been reported: Major epileptiform convulsions occur occasionally in patients with or without epilepsy, and severe hypotension with rash has occurred after injection.

DIISOPROPYLPHENOL

2,6-Diisopropylphenol—propofol or disoprofol (Diprivan)—produces anesthesia at a rate similar to that of the intravenous barbiturates, and recovery is equally rapid. After intravenous administration, distribution of this investigational drug occurs with a half-life ($t_{1/2\alpha}$) of 2–3 minutes and the elimination half-life ($t_{1/2\beta}$) of disoprofol is approximately 1 hour. Total body clearance of the anesthetic occurs at a rate greater than that of hepatic blood flow, suggesting that its elimination includes other mechanisms in addition to metabolism by liver enzymes.

Effects on the cardiovascular system are minimal at usual anesthetic doses. Disoprofol appears to cause a relatively high incidence of nausea, vomiting, and dreaming. Muscle movements, hypotonus, and, rarely, tremors have also been reported following its use. Hyposensitivity reactions involving hypotension, flushing, and bronchospasm have occurred with preparations of disoprofol dissolved in a vehicle.

REFERENCES

Baden JM, Rice SA: Metabolism and toxicity of inhaled anesthetics. Page 701 in: *Anesthesia,* 2nd ed. Miller RD (editor). Churchill Livingstone, 1986.

Cohen EN: Toxicity of inhalational anesthetic agents. *Br J Anaesth* 1978;**50**:665.

Eger EI II: *Anesthetic Uptake and Action.* Williams & Wilkins, 1974.

Eger EI II, Saidman LJ, Brandstater B: Minimum alveolar anesthetic concentration: A standard of anesthetic potency. *Anesthesiology* 1965;**26**:756.

Evans JM, Keogh JAM: Adverse reactions to intravenous induction agents. *Br J Med* 1977;**2**:235.

Grogono AW, Seltzer JL: A guide to drug interactions in anesthetic practice. *Drugs* 1980;**19**:279.

Judge SE: Effects of general anesthetics on synaptic ion channels. *Br J Anaesth* 1983;**55**:191.

Kay B, Stephenson DK: ICI 35868 (Diprivan): A new intravenous anesthetic. *Anaesthesia* 1980;**37**:536.

Koblin DD, Eger EI II: Theories of narcosis. *N Engl J Med* 1979;**301**:1222.

Mazze R: Nephrotoxicity of fluorinated anesthetic agents. Page 469 in: *Clinics in Anaesthesiology.* Mazze R (editor). Saunders, 1983.

Ngai SH: Effects of anesthestics on various organs. *N Engl J Med* 1980;**302**:564.

Prys-Roberts C, Hug CC Jr: *Pharmacokinetics of Anesthesia.* Blackwell, 1984.

Reves JG et al: Midazolam: Pharmacology and uses. *Anesthesiology* 1985;**62**:310.

Richards CD: Actions of general anesthetics on synaptic transmission in the CNS. *Br J Anaesth* 1983;**55**:201.

Sakai T, Takaori M: Biodegradation of halothane, enflurane and methoxyflurane. *Br J Anaesth* 1978;**50**:785.

Stanski DR, Watkins WD: *Drug Disposition in Anesthesia.* Grune & Stratton, 1982.

Trudell JR: Biophysical concepts in molecular mechanisms of anesthesia. Page 261 in: *Molecular Mechanisms of Anesthesia.* Fink BR (editor). Raven Press, 1980.

Van Dyke RA: Halogenated anesthetic hepatoxicity. Page 485 in: *Clinics in Anaesthesiology.* Mazze R (editor). Saunders, 1983.

Vessey MP: Epidemiological studies of the occupational hazards of anaesthesia. *Anaesthesia* 1978;**33**:430.

White PF, Way WL, Trevor AJ: Ketamine: Its pharmacology and therapeutic uses. *Anaesthesiology* 1982;**56**:119.

Local Anesthetics

24

Luc M. Hondeghem, MD, PhD, & Ronald D. Miller, MD

Local anesthetics reversibly block impulse conduction along the axon. This action can be used to block pain sensation from—or sympathetic vasoconstrictor impulses to—specific areas of the body. Cocaine, the first such agent, was isolated by Niemann in 1860. It was introduced into clinical use by Koller in 1884 as an ophthalmic anesthetic. It was soon found to have strongly addicting central nervous system actions but was widely used, nevertheless, for 30 years, since it was the only local anesthetic drug available. In an attempt to improve the properties of cocaine, Einhorn in 1905 synthesized procaine, which became the dominant local anesthetic for the next 50 years. Since 1905, many local anesthetic agents have been synthesized. The goals of these efforts were reduction of local irritation and tissue damage, minimization of systemic toxicity, shorter onset of action, and longer duration of action. Lidocaine, currently the most popular agent, was synthesized in 1943 by Löfgren and may be considered the prototype local anesthetic agent.

I. BASIC PHARMACOLOGY OF LOCAL ANESTHETICS

Chemistry

Most local anesthetic agents consist of a lipophilic group (frequently an aromatic ring) connected by an intermediate chain (commonly including an ester or amide) to an ionizable group (usually a tertiary amine; Table 24–1). Optimal activity requires a delicate balance between the lipophilic and hydrophilic strengths of these groups. In addition to the general physical properties of the molecules, specific stereochemical configurations can also be important; ie, differences in the potency of stereoisomers have been documented for a few compounds. Since ester links (as in procaine) are more prone to hydrolysis than amide links, esters usually have a shorter duration of action.

Local anesthetics are weak bases. For therapeutic application, they are usually made available as salts for reasons of solubility and stability. In the body, they exist either as the uncharged base or as a cation. The relative proportions of these 2 forms is governed by their pK_a and the pH of the body fluids according to the Henderson-Hasselbalch equation:

$$\log \frac{\text{Cationic form}}{\text{Uncharged form}} = pK_a - pH$$

Since the pK_a of most local anesthetics is in the range of 8–9, the larger fraction in the body fluids at physiologic pH will be the charged, cationic form. The cationic form is thought to be the most active form at the receptor site (cationic drug cannot readily leave closed channels), but the uncharged fraction is very important for rapid penetration of biologic membranes: the local anesthetic receptor is not accessible from the external side of the cell membrane (Fig 13–7). This partly explains why dentists and surgeons observe that local anesthetics are much less effective in infected tissues; these tissues have a low extracellular pH, so that a very low fraction of nonionized local anesthetic is available for diffusion into the cell.

Pharmacokinetics

Local anesthetics are usually administered by injection into the area of the nerve fibers to be blocked. Thus, absorption and distribution are not as important in controlling the onset of effect as in determining the rate of offset of anesthesia and the likelihood of central nervous system and cardiac toxicity. Topical application of local anesthetics, on the other hand, requires drug diffusion to its intracellular site of action for both onset and offset of anesthetic effect.

A. Absorption: Systemic absorption of injected local anesthetic from the site of administration is modified by several factors, including dosage, site of injection, drug-tissue binding, the presence of vasoconstricting substances, and the physiochemical and pharmacologic properties of the drug. Application of a local anesthetic to a highly vascular area such as the tracheal mucosa results in more rapid absorption and thus higher blood levels than if the local anesthetic had been injected into a poorly perfused area, such as tendon. For regional anesthesia involving block of large nerves, maximum blood levels of local anesthetic decrease according to site of administration in the following order: intercostal (highest) > caudal > epidural > brachial plexus > sciatic nerve (lowest).

Vasoconstrictor substances such as epinephrine reduce systemic absorption of local anesthetics from the depot site by decreasing regional blood flow in these areas. This is especially true for drugs with intermedi-

Table 24–1. Structure and properties of some ester and amide local anesthetics.*

	Lipophilic Group	Intermediate Chain	Amine Substituents	Potency (Procaine = 1)	Duration of Action
Esters					
Cocaine				2	Medium
Procaine (Novocain)				1	Short
Tetracaine (Pontocaine)				16	Long
Benzocaine				Surface use only	
Amides					
Lidocaine (Xylocaine, etc)				4	Medium
Mepivacaine (Carbocaine, Isocaine)				2	Medium
Bupivacaine (Marcaine)				16	Long
Etidocaine (Duranest)				16	Long
Prilocaine (Citanest)				3	Medium

*Other chemical types are available including ethers (pramoxine), ketones (dyclonine), and phenetidin derivatives (phenacaine).

ate and short durations of action such as procaine, lidocaine, and mepivacaine (but not prilocaine). Neuronal uptake of the drug is presumably enhanced by the higher local drug concentration, and the systemic toxic effects of the drug are reduced, since blood levels are lowered by as much as one-third. The combination of reduced systemic absorption and enhanced uptake by the nerve is responsible for prolonging the local anesthetic effect by about 50%. Vasoconstrictors are less effective in prolonging anesthetic properties of the more lipid-soluble, long-acting drugs (bupiva-

caine, etidocaine), possibly because these molecules are highly tissue-bound. In addition, catecholamines may also alter neuronal function in such a way as to promote analgesia. As noted below, cocaine is a special case owing to its sympathomimetic properties (Table 5–3).

B. Distribution: The amide local anesthetics are widely distributed after intravenous bolus administration. There is evidence that sequestration occurs in storage sites, possibly fat tissue. After an initial rapid distribution phase, which probably indicates uptake into highly perfused organs such as the brain, liver, kidney, and heart, a slower distribution phase occurs with uptake into moderately well perfused tissues, such as muscle and gut.

C. Metabolism and Excretion: Because of the extremely short plasma half-lives of the ester type agents (see below), their tissue distribution has not been studied. The local anesthetics are converted in the liver or in plasma to more water-soluble metabolites and then excreted in the urine. Since local anesthetics in the unchanged form diffuse readily through lipid, little or no urinary excretion of neutral form occurs. Acidification of urine will promote ionization of the tertiary base to the more water-soluble charged form, which is more readily excreted since it is not so easily reabsorbed by renal tubules.

Ester type local anesthetics are hydrolyzed very rapidly in the plasma by plasma cholinesterase. Therefore, they typically have very short half-lives, eg, less than 1 minute for procaine and chloroprocaine.

The amide linkage of amide local anesthetics is hydrolyzed by liver microsomal enzymes. There is considerable variation in the rate of liver metabolism of individual amide compounds, the approximate order being prilocaine (fastest) > etidocaine > lidocaine > mepivacaine > bupivacaine (slowest). As a result, toxicity from the amide type of local anesthetic is more likely to occur in patients with liver disease. For example, the average half-life of lidocaine may be increased from 1.8 hours in normal patients to over 6 hours in patients with liver disease.

Decreased hepatic removal of local anesthetics should also be anticipated in patients with reduced hepatic blood flow. For example, the hepatic elimination of lidocaine in animals anesthetized with halothane is slower than that measured in animals receiving nitrous oxide and curare. The reduced elimination may be related to decreased hepatic blood flow and to halothane-induced depression of hepatic microsomes. Propranolol may also prolong the half-life of amide local anesthetics such as lidocaine.

Pharmacodynamics

A. Mechanism of Action: The excitable membrane of nerve axons, like the membrane of cardiac muscle (Chapter 13) and neuronal cell bodies (Chapter 19), maintains a transmembrane potential of -90 to -60 mV. During excitation, the sodium channels open and a fast inward sodium current quickly depolarizes the membrane toward the sodium equilibrium potential ($+40$ mV). As a result of depolarization, the sodium channels close (inactivate) and potassium channels open. The outward flow of potassium repolarizes the membrane toward the potassium equilibrium potential (about -95 mV); repolarization returns the sodium channels to the rested state. The transmembrane ionic gradients are maintained by the sodium pump. These characteristics are similar to those of heart muscle, and local anesthetics have similar effects in both tissues (Chapter 13).

When progressively increasing concentrations of a local anesthetic are applied to a nerve fiber, the threshold for excitation increases, impulse conduction slows, the rate of rise of the action potential declines, the action potential amplitude decreases, and, finally, the ability to generate an action potential is abolished. All of these effects result from the binding of the local anesthetic to sodium channels; binding results in blockade of the sodium current. If the sodium current is blocked over a critical length of the nerve, propagation across the blocked area is no longer possible. At the minimum dose required to block propagation, the resting potential is not significantly affected.

The blockade of sodium channels by most local anesthetics is strongly *voltage-* and *time-dependent:* Channels in the rested state (which predominate at more negative membrane potentials) have a much lower affinity for local anesthetics than activated (open state) and inactivated channels (which predominate at more positive membrane potentials). Thus, the effect of a given drug concentration is more marked in rapidly firing axons than in resting fibers (Fig 24–1).

Between depolarizations of the axon, the sodium channels recover from local anesthetic block. The recovery from drug-induced block is 10–1000 times slower than the recovery of channels from normal inactivation, as shown for the cardiac membrane in Fig 13–3. As a result, the refractory period is lengthened and the nerve can conduct fewer impulses.

Elevated extracellular calcium partially antagonizes the action of local anesthetics. This reversal is caused by the calcium-induced increase of the surface potential on the membrane, which favors the low-affinity rested state. Conversely, elevation of extracellular potassium depolarizes the membrane potential and favors the inactivated state. This enhances the effect of local anesthetics.

Structure-activity characteristics of local anesthetics. The smaller and more lipophilic the molecule, the faster the rate of interaction with the sodium channel receptor. Potency is also positively correlated with lipid solubility, as long as the agent remains to some extent water-soluble, since water solubility is required for diffusion to the site of action. Lidocaine, procaine, and mepivacaine are more water-soluble than tetracaine, etidocaine, and bupivacaine. The latter agents are more potent and have longer durations of action. They also bind more extensively to proteins and will displace or be displaced from these binding sites by other drugs.

B. Actions:

1. Differential nerve block–Since local anesthetics are capable of blocking all nerves, their actions are not usually limited to the desired loss of sensation. Although motor paralysis may at times be desirable, it may also limit the ability of the patient to cooperate, eg, during obstetric delivery. During spinal anesthesia, motor paralysis may impair respiratory activity and autonomic nerve blockade may lead to hypotension. However, different types of nerve fibers differ significantly in their susceptibility to local anesthetic blockade on the basis of size and myelination (Table

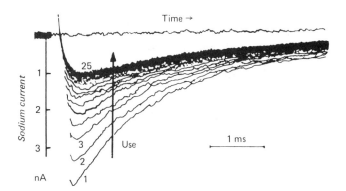

Figure 24–1. Effect of repetitive activity on the block of sodium current produced by a local anesthetic in a myelinated axon. A series of 25 pulses was applied, and the resulting sodium currents are superimposed. Note that the current produced by the pulses rapidly decreased from the first to the 25th pulse. A long rest period following the train resulted in recovery from block, but the block could be reinstated by a subsequent train. nA = nanoamperes. (Modified slightly and reproduced, with permission, from Courtney KR: Mechanism of frequency-dependent inhibition of sodium currents in frog myelinated nerve by the lidocaine derivative GEA. *J Pharmacol Exp Ther* 1975;**195:**225.)

24–2). Upon application of a local anesthetic to a nerve root, the smaller B and C fibers are blocked first. The small type A delta fibers are blocked next. Thus, pain fibers are blocked first; other sensations disappear next; and motor function is blocked last.

Local anesthetics preferentially block small fibers because the distance over which such fibers can passively propagate an electrical impulse (related to the space constant) is shorter. During the onset of local anesthesia, when short sections of nerve are blocked, the small-diameter fibers are the first to fail to conduct. For the same reason, they will recover last upon washout of the drug. Myelinated nerves tend to become blocked before unmyelinated nerves of the same diameter. For this reason, the preganglionic beta fibers may be blocked before the smaller unmyelinated C fibers.

Another important reason for preferential blockade of sensory fibers follows directly from the state-dependent mechanism of action of local anesthetics. Block by these drugs is more marked at higher frequencies of depolarization and with longer depolarizations. Sensory fibers, especially pain fibers, have a high firing rate and a relatively long action potential duration (up

to 3 ms). Motor fibers fire at a slower rate and have a shorter action potential duration (less than 0.5 ms).

An anatomic circumstance that sometimes creates exceptions to the above rules for differential nerve block is the location of the fiber in the peripheral bundle. In large nerve trunks, motor nerves are usually located circumferentially—hence, they are exposed first to the drug. Therefore, it is not uncommon that motor nerve block occurs before sensory block in large mixed nerves. In the extremities, proximal sensory fibers are located in the mantle of the nerve trunk, whereas the distal sensory innervation is in the core of the nerve. Thus, during infiltration block of a large nerve, anesthesia first develops proximally and then spreads distally as the drug penetrates the core of the nerve.

2. Effects on other excitable membranes–Local anesthetics have weak neuromuscular blocking effects that are of little clinical importance. However, their effects on cardiac cell membranes are of major clinical significance. Some are useful antiarrhythmic agents (see Chapter 13) at concentrations lower than those required to produce nerve block.

Table 24–2. Relative size and susceptibility to block of types of nerve fibers.

Fiber Type	Function	Diameter (μm)	Myelination	Conduction Velocity (m/s)	Sensitivity to Block
Type A					
Alpha	Proprioception, motor	12–20	Heavy	70–120	+
Beta	Touch, pressure	5–12	Heavy	30–70	++
Gamma	Muscle spindles	3–6	Heavy	15–30	++
Delta	Pain, temperature	2–5	Heavy	12–30	+++
Type B	Preganglionic autonomic	< 3	Light	3–15	++++
Type C					
Dorsal root	Pain	0.4–1.2	None	0.5–2.3	++++
Sympathetic	Postganglionic	0.3–1.3	None	0.7–2.3	++++

II. CLINICAL PHARMACOLOGY OF LOCAL ANESTHETICS

Local anesthetics can provide temporary but complete analgesia of well-defined parts of the body after topical application, after injection in the vicinity of peripheral nerve endings and major nerve trunks, or after instillation within the epidural or subarachnoid spaces surrounding the spinal cord. In addition, block of autonomic sympathetic fibers can be used to evaluate the role of sympathetic tone in patients with peripheral vasospasm.

The choice of local anesthetic for a specific procedure is usually based on the duration of action required. Procaine (Novocain) and chloroprocaine (Nesacaine) are short-acting; lidocaine (Xylocaine, etc), mepivacaine (Carbocaine, Isocaine), and prilocaine (Citanest) have an intermediate duration of action; tetracaine (Pontocaine), bupivacaine (Marcaine), and etidocaine (Duranest) are long-acting drugs (Table 24–1).

As noted above, the anesthetic effect of the agents with short and intermediate durations of action can be prolonged by increasing the dose or by adding a vasoconstrictor agent, such as epinephrine or phenylephrine. The vasoconstrictor retards the removal of drug from the injection site. In addition, it decreases the blood level and hence the chance of toxicity.

The onset of local anesthesia is sometimes accelerated by the use of solutions saturated with carbon dioxide ("carbonated"). The high tissue level of CO_2 results in intracellular acidosis (CO_2 crosses membranes readily), which in turn results in intracellular accumulation of the cationic form of the local anesthetic.

Repeated injection of local anesthetics during epidural anesthesia results in loss of effectiveness (tachyphylaxis). This is probably a consequence of local extracellular acidosis. Local anesthetics are commonly marketed as hydrochloride salts (pH 4–6). After injection, the salts are buffered in the tissue to physiologic pH, thereby providing sufficient free base for diffusion through axonal membranes. However, repeated injections deplete the local available buffer. The ensuing acidosis increases the extracellular cationic form, which diffuses poorly into axons. The clinical result is apparent tachyphylaxis, especially in areas of limited buffer reserve, such as the cerebrospinal fluid.

Toxicity

Ultimately, local anesthetic agents are absorbed from the site of administration. If blood levels rise too high, effects on several organ systems may be observed.

A. Central Nervous System: Since prehistoric times, the natives of Peru have chewed the leaves of the indigenous plant *Erythroxylon coca,* the source of cocaine, to obtain a feeling of well-being and reduce fatigue. Intense central nervous system effects can be achieved by sniffing cocaine powder and smoking cocaine base. This abuse of the drug has recently gained in popularity (see Chapter 30). Other local anesthetics have been thought to lack the euphoriant effects of cocaine. However, recent studies indicate that some habitual cocaine users cannot differentiate between intranasal cocaine and lidocaine given by the same route.

Other central nervous system effects include sleepiness, light-headedness, visual and auditory disturbances, and restlessness. At higher concentrations, nystagmus and shivering may occur. Finally, overt tonic-clonic convulsions followed by central nervous system depression and death may occur with all local anesthetics, including cocaine. Local anesthetics apparently lead to depression of cortical inhibitory pathways, thereby allowing unopposed activity of excitatory components. This transitional stage of unbalanced excitation may be followed by generalized central nervous system depression if higher blood levels of local anesthetic are reached.

Most serious toxic reactions to local anesthetics are due to convulsions from excessive blood levels. These are best prevented by administering the smallest dose of local anesthetic required for adequate anesthesia. When large doses must be administered, premedication with a benzodiazepine, eg, diazepam, 0.1–0.2 mg/kg parenterally, probably provides significant prophylaxis against seizures. If seizures do occur, it is essential to prevent hypoxemia. Although administration of oxygen is recommended in the treatment of convulsions from local anesthesia, oxygen inhalation does not prevent seizure activity. However, hyperoxemia after onset of seizures appears to be beneficial. Conversely, hypercapnia and acidosis appear to promote the occurrence of seizures. Thus, hyperventilation is recommended during treatment of seizures. Hyperventilation elevates blood pH, which in turn lowers extracellular potassium. This hyperpolarizes the transmembrane potential of axons, which favors the rested or low-affinity state of the sodium channels, resulting in decreased local anesthetic toxicity.

Seizures induced by local anesthetics can also be treated with small doses of short-acting barbiturates, eg, thiopental, 1–2 mg/kg intravenously, or diazepam, 0.1 mg/kg intravenously. The muscular manifestations can be suppressed by a short-acting neuromuscular blocking agent, eg, succinylcholine, 0.5–1 mg/kg intravenously. It should be emphasized that succinylcholine does not obliterate cortical manifestations on the EEG. In especially severe cases of convulsions, intubation of the trachea combined with succinylcholine administration and mechanical ventilation can prevent pulmonary aspiration of gastric contents and facilitate hyperventilation therapy.

B. Peripheral Nervous System (Neurotoxicity): When applied at excessively high concentrations, all local anesthetics can be toxic to nerve tissue. Several case reports document prolonged sensory and motor deficits following accidental spinal anesthesia with large volumes of chloroprocaine. Whether chloroprocaine is more neurotoxic than other local anesthetics has not been determined.

C. Cardiovascular System: The cardiovascular effects of local anesthetics result partly from direct effects upon the cardiac and smooth muscle membranes and from indirect effects upon the autonomic nerves. As described in Chapter 13, local anesthetics block cardiac sodium channels and thus depress abnormal cardiac pacemaker activity, excitability, and conduction. They also depress the strength of cardiac contraction and cause arteriolar dilatation—except for cocaine, which causes vasoconstriction—both leading to hypotension. Although cardiovascular collapse and death usually occur only after large doses, they may result occasionally from the small amounts used for infiltration anesthesia.

As noted above, cocaine differs from the other local anesthetics in its cardiovascular effects. The blockade of norepinephrine reuptake results in vasoconstriction and hypertension. It may also precipitate cardiac arrhythmias. The vasoconstriction produced by cocaine can lead to ischemia of the nasal mucosa and, in chronic users, to ulceration of the mucous membrane and even damage to the septum. This vasoconstrictor property of cocaine can be used clinically to decrease bleeding from mucosal damage such as occurs with epistaxis.

Bupivacaine is more cardiotoxic than other local anesthetics. Several case reports have appeared indicating that accidental intravenous injection of bupivacaine may lead not only to seizure but also to cardiovascular collapse, from which resuscitation may be extremely difficult or unsuccessful. Several experimental animal studies have confirmed the idea that bupivacaine is indeed more toxic when given intravenously than most other agents. This reflects the fact that bupivacaine block of sodium channels is greatly potentiated by the very long action potential duration of cardiac cells (as compared to nerve fibers) and, unlike lidocaine blockade, cumulates markedly at normal heart rates. Subsequent studies have shown that the most common electrocardiographic finding in patients with bupivacaine intoxication is slow idioventricular rhythm with broad QRS complexes and electromechanical dissociation. Resuscitation has been successful with standard cardiopulmonary support and aggressive administration of epinephrine, atropine, and bretylium.

D. Blood: The administration of large doses (>10 mg/kg) of prilocaine during regional anesthesia may lead to accumulation of the metabolite *o*-toluidine, an oxidizing agent capable of converting hemoglobin to methemoglobin. When sufficient methemoglobin is present (3–5 mg/dL), the patient may appear cyanotic and the blood chocolate-colored. Such levels of methemoglobinemia are tolerated by healthy individuals but may cause decompensation in patients with cardiac or pulmonary disease and require immediate treatment. Reducing agents such as methylene blue or, less satisfactorily, ascorbic acid may be given intravenously to rapidly convert methemoglobin to hemoglobin.

E. Allergic Reactions: The ester type local anesthetics are metabolized to *p*-aminobenzoic acid derivatives. These metabolites are responsible for allergic reactions in a small percentage of the population. Amides are not metabolized to *p*-aminobenzoic acid, and allergic reactions to agents of the amide group are extremely rare.

REFERENCES

Albright GA: Cardiac arrest following regional anesthesia with etidocaine or bupivacaine. *Anesthesiology* 1979;**51**:285.

Clarkson CW, Hondeghem LM: Evidence for a specific receptor site for lidocaine, quinidine, and bupivacaine associated with cardiac sodium channels in guinea pig ventricular myocardium. *Circ Res* 1985;**56**:496.

Courtney KR: Structure-activity relations for frequency-dependent sodium channel block in nerve by local anesthetics. *J Pharmacol Exp Ther* 1980;**213**:114.

Covino BG, Vassallo HG: *Local Anesthetics: Mechanisms of Action in Clinical Use.* Grune & Stratton, 1976.

Covino BG et al: Prolonged sensory/motor deficits following inadvertent spinal anesthesia. (Editorial.) *Anesth Analg (Cleve)* 1980;**59**:399.

Fink BR (editor): *Progress in Anesthesiology: Molecular Mechanisms of Anesthesia.* Vol 2. Raven Press, 1980.

Hille B: Local anesthetics: Hydrophilic and hydrophobic pathways for the drug-receptor reactions. *J Gen Physiol* 1977;**69**:497.

Kasten GW, Martin ST: Successful cardiovascular resuscitation after massive intravenous bupivacaine overdosage in anesthetized dogs. *Anesth Analg* 1985;**64**:491.

Mather LE, Cousins MJ: Local anesthetics and their current clinical use. *Drugs* 1979;**18**:185.

Ravindran RS et al: Prolonged neural blockade following regional anesthesia with 2-chloroprocaine. *Anesth Analg (Cleve)* 1980;**59**:447.

Savarese JJ, Covino BG: Pharmacology of local anesthetics. Page 563 in: *Anesthesia.* Miller RD (editor). Churchill Livingstone, 1981.

Tucker GT, Mather LE: The clinical pharmacokinetics of local anesthetics. *Clin Pharmacokinet* 1979;**4**:241.

Skeletal Muscle Relaxants

25

Ronald D. Miller, MD

Drugs that affect skeletal muscle function fall into 2 major therapeutic groups: those used during surgical procedures to cause paralysis (neuromuscular blockers) and those used to reduce spasticity in a variety of neurologic conditions (spasmolytics). Members of the first group, as their name implies, interfere with transmission at the neuromuscular end-plate and are not CNS-active drugs. However, because they are used almost exclusively as an adjunct to general anesthesia, they are often discussed in connection with central nervous system agents. Drugs in the second group have traditionally been called "centrally acting" muscle relaxants. However, at least one of its important members (dantrolene) has no central effects, so the traditional name is somewhat inappropriate.

NEUROMUSCULAR BLOCKING DRUGS

History

During the 16th century, European explorers found that natives of the Amazon Basin of South America were using an arrow poison that produced death by skeletal muscle paralysis. This poison later became the subject of intense investigation. **Curare,** the active crude material, formed the basis for some of the earliest scientific studies in pharmacology. The active principle from curare, **tubocurarine (d-tubocurarine),** and its synthetic derivatives have had a tremendous influence on the practice of anesthesia and have been useful also in defining normal neuromuscular physiologic mechanisms.

Normal Neuromuscular Function

Theoretically, muscular relaxation and paralysis can occur from interruption of function at several sites, including the central nervous system, myelinated somatic nerves, unmyelinated motor nerve terminals, the acetylcholine receptor, the motor end-plate, and the muscle membrane or contractile apparatus (Fig 25–1). The mechanism of neuromuscular transmission at the end-plate is similar to that described in Chapter 5, with arrival of an impulse at the motor nerve terminal, influx of calcium, and release of acetylcholine (Fig 25–1). Acetylcholine then diffuses across the synaptic cleft to the nicotinic receptor located on the motor end-plate. When the receptor and acetylcholine interact, permeability of the membrane

in the end-plate region increases to sodium primarily but also to potassium. Sodium moves from outside to inside the cell, and the membrane depolarizes. This change in voltage is termed the end-plate potential. The magnitude of the end-plate potential is directly related to the amount of acetylcholine released. If the potential is small, the permeability and the end-plate potential return to normal without an impulse being propagated from the end-plate region to the rest of the muscle membrane. However, if the end-plate potential is large, the muscle membrane is depolarized, and the impulse will be propagated along the entire muscle fiber. Muscle contraction is then initiated by the process known as excitation-contraction coupling. The released acetylcholine is removed from the end-plate region by diffusion and rapid enzymatic destruction by acetylcholinesterase.

Blockade of normal end-plate function can occur by 2 mechanisms. Pharmacologic blockade of the agonist, acetylcholine, is characteristic of *antagonist* drugs like curare. Block of transmission can also be produced by an excess of depolarizing *agonist*. (This paradoxic effect also occurs at the ganglionic nicotinic acetylcholine receptor.) The prototype depolarizing blocking drug is succinylcholine, although a similar

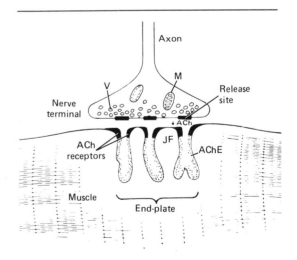

Figure 25–1. Schematic representation of the neuromuscular junction. V = transmitter vesicle; M = mitochondrion; ACh = acetylcholine; AChE = acetylcholinesterase; JF = junctional folds. (Reproduced, with permission, from Drachman DB: Myasthenia gravis. *N Engl J Med* 1978;**298**:135.)

depolarizing block can be produced by acetylcholine itself.

I. BASIC PHARMACOLOGY OF NEUROMUSCULAR BLOCKING DRUGS

Chemistry

All of the neuromuscular blocking drugs are structurally similar to acetylcholine. Often this resemblance is to 2 acetylcholine molecules linked end-to-end. In fact, succinylcholine is such a compound (Fig 25–2). In contrast to the single linear structure of depolarizing drugs such as succinylcholine, the nondepolarizing agents conceal the "double-acetylcholine" structure in a variety of bulky, relatively rigid ring systems (Figs 25–2 and 25–3). Another feature common to all useful drugs in this class except vecuronium is

Acetylcholine

Succinylcholine
(Anectine)

Pancuronium
(Pavulon)

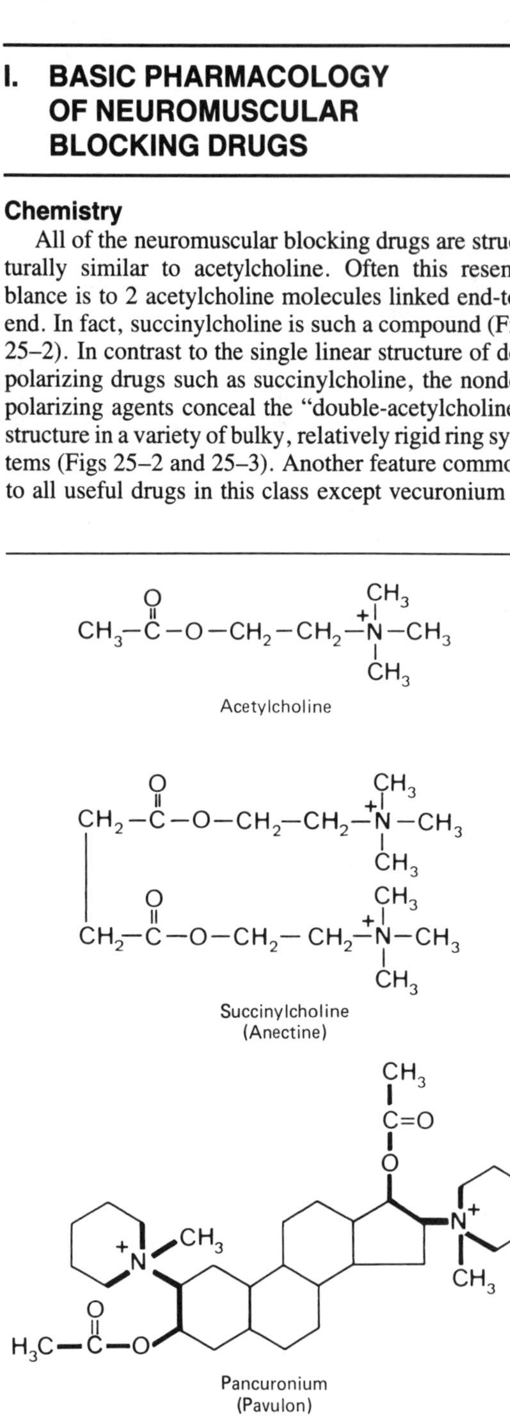

Figure 25–2. Structural relationship of succinylcholine, a depolarizing agent, and pancuronium, a nondepolarizing agent, to acetylcholine, the neuromuscular transmitter. Succinylcholine, originally called diacetylcholine, is simply 2 molecules of acetylcholine linked through the acetate methyl groups. Pancuronium may be viewed as 2 acetylcholinelike fragments *(outlined in dark print)* oriented on a steroid nucleus.

the quaternary nitrogen, which makes them poorly soluble in lipid. Agents currently available for use in the USA are shown in Figs 25–2 and 25–3.

Pharmacokinetics of Neuromuscular Blocking Drugs

A. Nondepolarizing Drugs: The rate of disappearance of a nondepolarizing neuromuscular blocking drug from blood is characterized by a rapid initial disappearance followed by a slower decay (Fig 25–4). Distribution to tissues is the major cause of the initial decrease, whereas the slower decay is due to excretion. Because neuromuscular blocking drugs are highly ionized, they do not cross membranes well and have a limited volume of distribution—80–140 mL/kg, not much larger than blood volume.

Tubocurarine, metocurine (dimethyltubocurarine), and gallamine (Fig 25–3) are not metabolized. Gallamine is entirely dependent on the kidney for its elimination. In contrast, only about 50–60% of an injected dose of tubocurarine or metocurine is excreted in the urine over a 24-hour period in humans. The exact route of excretion of the remainder of these agents in humans is unclear, though it is presumed that biliary excretion accounts for most of it. Although the kidney is the major route of excretion for pancuronium, this drug is also metabolized (15–25%) to 3-hydroxy-, 17-hydroxy-, and 3,17-dihydroxypancuronium. Most of the remaining drug is excreted unchanged in the urine. 3-Hydroxypancuronium has about half the potency of its parent drug, pancuronium. Although the remaining metabolites also have neuromuscular blocking properties, they are very weak.

Vecuronium (Fig 25–3) is a short-acting neuromuscular blocking drug. It has a steroid nucleus like pancuronium, differing only in that the nitrogen at position 2 is tertiary rather than quaternary and in the presence of methyl groups at positions 10 and 13 of the nucleus. Despite the small structural differences, vecuronium has distinctly different pharmacologic properties. Vecuronium has a shorter duration of action (eg, 30 minutes versus 60 minutes), minimal cardiovascular effects, and is not heavily dependent upon the kidney for its elimination. Only about 15% of an injected dose of this agent is eliminated by the kidney; presumably, the remainder is eliminated in the bile. It is not known to what extent it is metabolized. Atracurium (Fig 25–3) is another short-acting nondepolarizing muscle relaxant with many of the same characteristics as vecuronium. Atracurium probably undergoes a form of spontaneous breakdown (Hofmann elimination) of the quaternary group by which it is inactivated, rather than being dependent on renal or hepatic mechanisms for the termination of its action. The main breakdown products are laudanosine and a related quaternary acid, neither of which has neuromuscular blocking properties. However, laudanosine is very slowly metabolized by the liver and has a long elimination half-life (ie, 150 minutes) in comparison with its parent compound, atracurium. It readily crosses the blood-brain barrier and at high blood con-

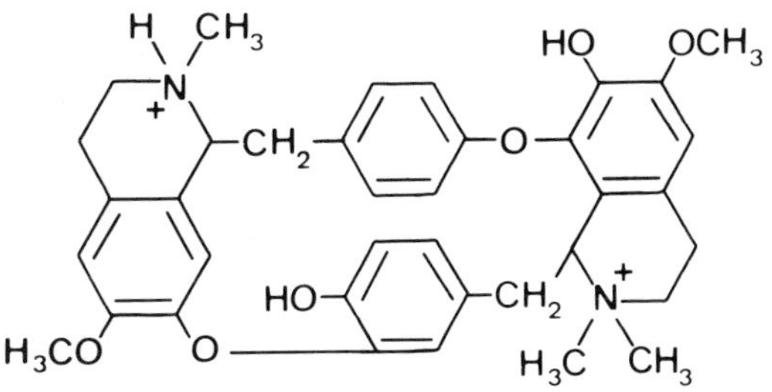

Tubocurarine

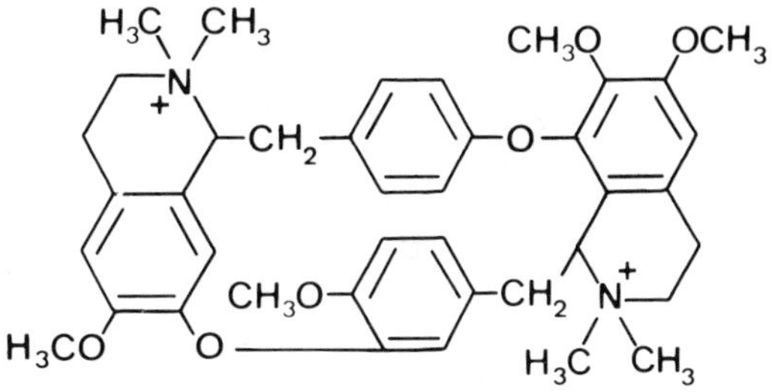

Dimethyltubocurarine
(Metubine)

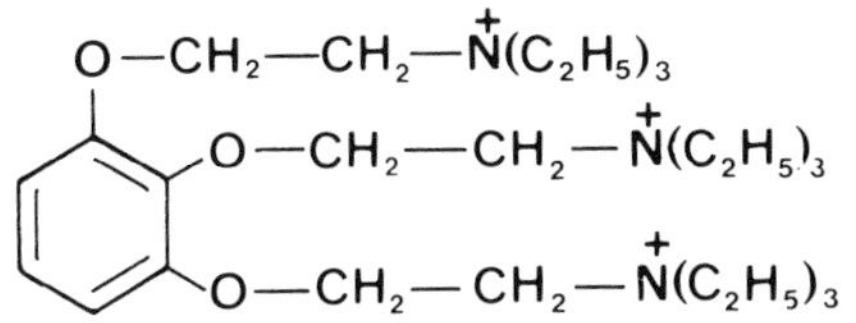

Gallamine
(Flaxedil)

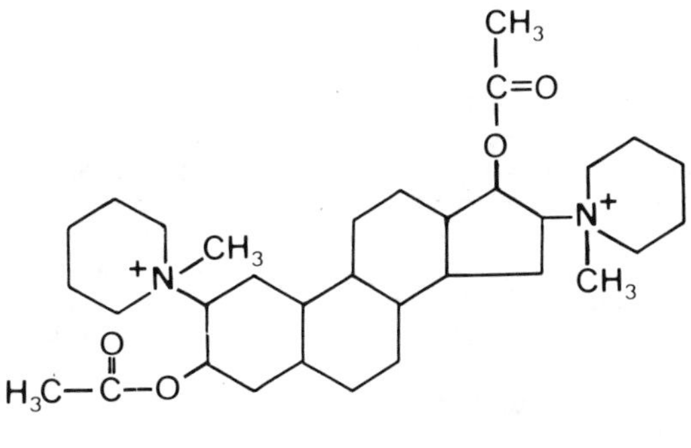

Pancuronium
(Pavulon)

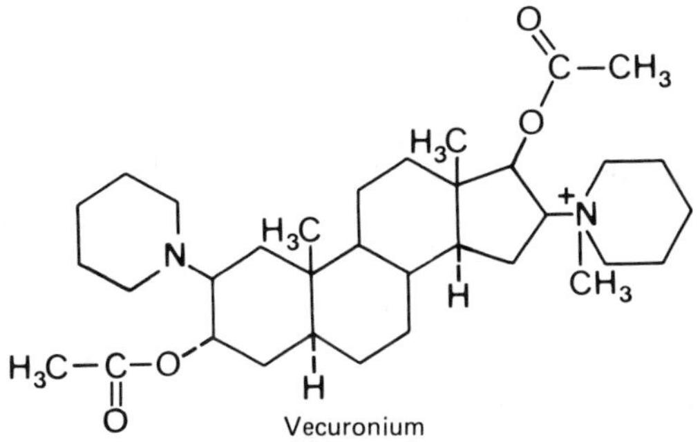

Vecuronium
(Norcuron)

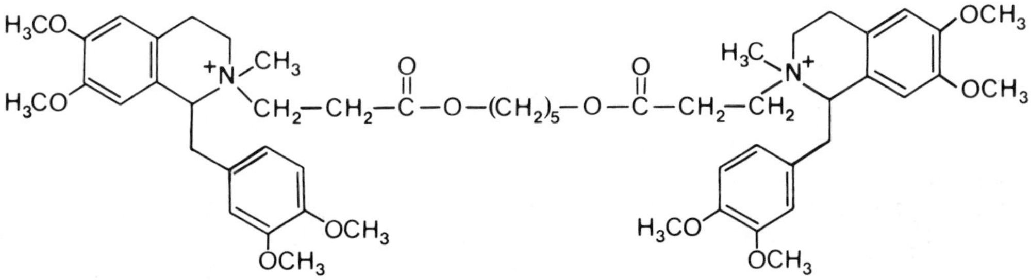

Atracurium
(Tracrium)

Figure 25–3. Chemical formulas of nondepolarizing blocking drugs currently available in the USA.

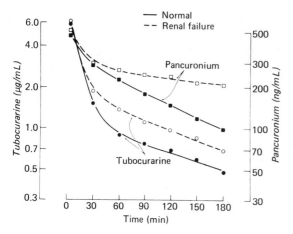

Figure 25-4. Rates at which the plasma concentrations of tubocurarine and pancuronium decrease in patients with and without renal failure. Note that the decay rates are about the same in patients with normal renal function. However, the decay rate is much slower in patients with renal failure receiving pancuronium than in those receiving tubocurarine. (Reprinted, with permission, from Miller RD, Savarese JJ: Pharmacology of muscle relaxants, their antagonists, and monitoring of neuromuscular function. In: *Anesthesia.* Miller RD [editor]. Churchill Livingstone, 1981.)

centrations (ie, 17 μg/mL) may cause seizures. At much lower blood concentrations (0.2–0.8 μg/mL), laudanosine causes about a 30% increase in anesthetic requirement. Blood concentrations that have been documented in patients who have received atracurium range from 0.1 to 5 μg/mL. Thus, it is unlikely that laudanosine could reach levels sufficient to cause seizures, but the metabolite certainly can cause an increase in anesthetic requirement.

B. Depolarizing Drugs: The extremely brief duration of action of succinylcholine (5–10 minutes) is due chiefly to its rapid hydrolysis by pseudocholinesterase, an enzyme of the liver and plasma. The initial metabolite, succinylmonocholine, is a much weaker neuromuscular blocker. It in turn is metabolized to succinic acid and choline. Pseudocholinesterase has an enormous capacity to hydrolyze succinylcholine at a very rapid rate; as a result, only a small fraction of the original intravenous dose reaches the neuromuscular junction. Since there is little or no pseudocholinesterase at the motor end-plate, the neuromuscular blockade of succinylcholine is terminated by its diffusion away from the end-plate into extracellular fluid. Pseudocholinesterase, therefore, influences the duration of action of succinylcholine by controlling the rate at which the latter is hydrolyzed before it reaches the end-plate.

Neuromuscular blockade by succinylcholine may be prolonged in patients with an abnormal variant of pseudocholinesterase of genetic origin. The "dibucaine number"—a test for ability to metabolize succinylcholine—can be used to identify such patients. Under standardized test conditions, dibucaine inhibits the normal enzyme about 80% and an abnormal enzyme only 20%. Many genetic variants of pseudocholinesterase have been identified, although the dibucaine-related variants are the most important.

Mechanism of Action

Recently the interactions of drugs with the acetylcholine receptor and the end-plate channel have been described on a molecular level. Several modes of action of drugs on the receptor appear to be possible and are illustrated in Fig 25–5.

A. Nondepolarizing Blocking Drugs: Neuromuscular blocking drugs classified as nondepolarizing

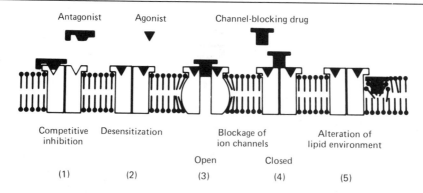

Figure 25-5. Schematic diagram of the interactions of drugs with the acetylcholine receptor and the end-plate channel. From left to right: *(1)* Binding of a competitive inhibitor to the receptor, preventing acetylcholine-induced activation (eg, nondepolarizing muscle relaxants). *(2)* Desensitization produced by long exposure to an agonist of the receptor (eg, depolarizing muscle relaxants). Some channels enter a prolonged closed state that cannot be opened by acetylcholine. *(3)* Drug-induced blockade of open ion channels, preventing not only the closing of the channels but also the flow of ions. Several drugs block open ion channels, including local anesthetics, some antibiotics, and succinylcholine. The latter drug can open the channel and then block it once it has opened. *(4)* Binding of drugs to the ion channel in its closed conformation, preventing opening of the channels. *(5)* Alteration of the lipid environment of the receptor, thereby changing the channel properties (eg, alcohols and volatile anesthetics).

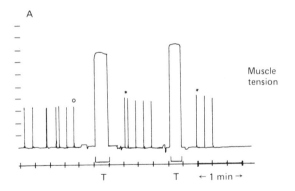

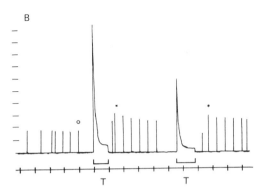

Figure 25–6. Effects of tubocurarine on neuromuscular transmission in humans. Panel *A* shows the twitch response induced by stimulation of the ulnar nerve in an anesthetized patient before curare was administered. The tetanic contractions (T) were evoked by stimulation at 50 pulses per second and were well maintained. A small increase (compare twitches marked by [*] with pretetanus twitch [○]) in twitch amplitude followed each tetanus. Panel *B* shows the effects of a small dose of tubocurarine in the same patient. The single stimulus twitch responses were reduced about 50%. The responses to tetanic stimulation showed a strong initial contraction followed by a rapid decline of tension ("fade"). The twitch responses following tetanic stimulation were increased by almost 80% (posttetanic potentiation).

antagonists—tubocurarine and metocurine (from curare), pancuronium, gallamine, vecuronium, and atracurium—produce a surmountable blockade. In very low doses and at low frequencies of stimulation, nondepolarizing muscle relaxants act predominantly at the *nicotinic receptor site* to compete with acetylcholine. There is now considerable evidence that at higher doses, the drugs also enter the *ion channel* of the end-plate to cause channel blockade. This further weakens neuromuscular transmission and diminishes the ability of acetylcholinesterase inhibitors (eg, neostigmine) to antagonize nondepolarizing muscle relaxants. Nondepolarizing relaxants may also block prejunctional sodium—but not calcium—channels. As a result, these muscle relaxants interfere with the mobilization of acetylcholine from synthesis sites to release sites. They do not interfere with acetylcholine release, which is calcium-dependent.

One consequence of the surmountable nature of the postsynaptic blockade produced by these agents is the fact that tetanic stimulation, by releasing a large quantity of acetylcholine, is followed by a transient posttetanic breakthrough or relief of the block (Fig 25–6). An important clinical consequence of the same principle is the ability to cholinesterase inhibitors to reverse the blockade.

The characteristics of a nondepolarizing muscular blockade are summarized in Table 25–1.

B. Depolarizing Drugs:

1. Phase I block (depolarizing)–Succinylcholine is the only depolarizing neuromuscular blocking drug commonly used clinically. Its neuromuscular effects can be conveniently thought of as almost identical to those of acetylcholine, except that the former produces a longer effect. Succinylcholine reacts with a receptor to open the channel and cause depolarization of the end-plate, and this in turn spreads to and depolarizes adjacent membranes, causing generalized disorganized contraction of muscle motor units. Because succinylcholine is not metabolized as rapidly as acetylcholine, the depolarized membranes remain depolarized and unresponsive to additional impulses. Because excitation-contraction coupling requires repolarization ("repriming") and repetitive firing to maintain muscle tension, a flaccid paralysis results. Phase I block is potentiated, not reversed, by cholinesterase inhibitors.

Characteristics of a depolarizing blockade are summarized in Table 25–1.

2. Phase II block (desensitization)–With continued exposure to succinylcholine, the initial depolarization decreases; in other words, the membrane becomes repolarized. Despite this repolarization, the membrane cannot be depolarized again by acetyl-

Table 25–1. Comparison of a typical nondepolarizing muscle relaxant (tubocurarine) and a depolarizing muscle relaxant (succinylcholine).

	Tubocurarine	Succinylcholine	
		Phase I	Phase II
Administration of tubocurarine	Additive	Antagonistic	Augmented*
Administration of succinylcholine	Antagonistic	Additive	Augmented*
Effect of neostigmine	Antagonistic	Augmented*	Antagonistic
Initial excitatory effect on skeletal muscle	None	Fasciculations	None
Response to a tetanic stimulus	Unsustained	Sustained†	Unsustained
Posttetanic facilitation	Yes	No	Yes
Rate of recovery	30–60 min‡	4–8 min	> 20 min‡

*It is not known whether this interaction is additive or synergistic (superadditive).

†The amplitude is decreased, but the response is sustained.

‡The rate depends on the dose and on the completeness of neuromuscular blockade.

choline as long as succinylcholine is present. The mechanism for the development of a phase II block is unknown. One hypothesis is that a nonexcitable area develops in the investing muscle membrane (immediately surrounding the end-plate) which becomes repolarized shortly after the arrival of succinylcholine. This area presumably impedes centrifugal spread of impulses initiated by the action of acetylcholine on the receptor. Because the end-plate is partially repolarized and still does not respond to acetylcholine, the membrane is said to be desensitized to the effects of acetylcholine. Therefore, this block has also been called a "desensitization block." Whatever the mechanism, the channels behave as if they are in a prolonged closed state (Fig 25–5).

The characteristics of a phase II block are nearly identical to those of a nondepolarizing block, ie, a nonsustained response to a tetanic stimulus and reversal by acetylcholinesterase inhibitors.

II. CLINICAL PHARMACOLOGY OF NEUROMUSCULAR BLOCKING DRUGS

Skeletal Muscle Paralysis

Before the introduction of neuromuscular blocking drugs, adequate skeletal muscle relaxation could only be achieved by deep anesthesia that was often associated with hazardous depressant effects on various organ systems, especially the cardiorespiratory system. The drugs have made it possible to achieve adequate muscle relaxation for all surgical requirements without the depressant effects of deep anesthesia.

A. Nondepolarizing Drugs: During anesthesia, the intravenous administration of tubocurarine, 0.12–0.4 mg/kg, will first cause motor weakness; ultimately, skeletal muscles become totally flaccid and nonexcitable to stimulation (Fig 25–7). Muscles capable of rapid movement, such as those of the jaw and eye, are paralyzed before the larger muscles of the limbs and trunk. Lastly, the diaphragm is paralyzed and respiration ceases. If ventilation is controlled, no adverse effects occur. Recovery of muscles usually occurs in reverse order, with the diaphragm regaining function first. The above dose of tubocurarine usually lasts 30–60 minutes by gross evaluation; more subtle evidence of paralysis may last for another hour. Pancuronium and vecuronium are about 6 times more potent than tubocurarine, metocurine about 4 times more potent, and gallamine about one-fifth as potent. Atracurium is slightly more potent than tubocurarine.

B. Depolarizing Drugs: Following the intravenous administration of succinylcholine, 0.5–1 mg/kg, transient muscle fasciculations occur, especially over the cheeks and abdomen, although general anesthesia tends to attenuate them (Fig 25–8). As paralysis develops, the arm, neck, and leg muscles are involved at a time when there is only slight weakness of the facial and pharyngeal muscles. Respiratory muscle weakness follows. The onset of neuromuscular blockade from succinylcholine is very rapid, usually within 1 minute. Because of its rapid hydrolysis by pseudocholinesterase in the plasma and liver, the duration of neuromuscular block from this dose usually is 5–10 minutes.

Cardiovascular Effects

All of the currently used nondepolarizing muscle relaxants produce cardiovascular effects. Many of these effects are mediated by autonomic and histamine

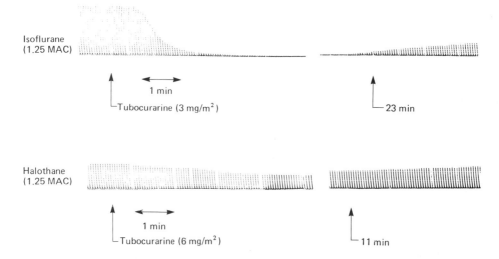

Figure 25–7. Neuromuscular blockade from tubocurarine during isoflurane and halothane anesthesia. Note that at equivalent levels of anesthesia, isoflurane augments the block far more than does halothane.

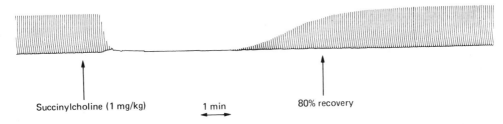

Figure 25–8. Neuromuscular blockade from succinylcholine during anesthesia. Fasciculations are not seen, because the anesthetic obliterated them.

receptors (Table 25–2). Tubocurarine and, to a much lesser extent, metocurine produce hypotension. This hypotension probably results from the liberation of histamine and, in larger doses, from ganglionic blockade. Premedication with promethazine, an antihistamine drug, will attenuate tubocurarine-induced hypotension. Pancuronium causes a moderate increase in heart rate and to a lesser extent cardiac output, with little or no change in systemic vascular resistance. Although the tachycardia is primarily due to a vagolytic action, release of norepinephrine from adrenergic nerve endings and blockade of neuronal uptake of norepinephrine have been suggested as secondary mechanisms. Gallamine increases heart rate by both vagolytic action and sympathetic stimulation. The latter involves the release of norepinephrine from adrenergic nerve endings in the heart by an unknown mechanism.

Succinylcholine-induced cardiac arrhythmias are many and varied. The drug stimulates all autonomic cholinoceptors: nicotinic receptors in both sympathetic and parasympathetic ganglia and muscarinic receptors in the sinus node of the heart. In low doses, both negative inotropic and chronotropic responses occur that can be attenuated by administration of atropine. With large doses, positive inotropic and chronotropic effects may result. Bradycardia has been repeatedly observed when a second dose of the drug is given approximately 5 minutes after the first dose. This bradycardia can be prevented by thiopental, atropine, ganglionic blocking drugs, and nondepolarizing muscle relaxants. Direct myocardial effects, increased muscarinic stimulation, and ganglionic stimulation may all be involved in the bradycardia response.

Other Effects

A. Hyperkalemia: Some patients respond to succinylcholine by an exaggerated release of potassium into the blood, occasionally of such magnitude that cardiac arrest occurs. Patients with burns, nerve damage or neuromuscular disease, closed head injury and other trauma, peritoneal infections, and renal failure are especially susceptible. The mechanism of the hyperkalemic response has not been established, but it may be related to depolarization in association with the increased number of receptors that occur extrajunctionally in a denervated muscle or one that is not used.

B. Intraocular Pressure: Administration of succinylcholine is followed by an increase in intraocular pressure that is manifested 1 minute after injection, maximal at 2–4 minutes, and subsides after 5 minutes. The mechanism for this effect has not been clearly defined, but it may involve contraction of tonic myofibrils or transient dilatation of choroidal blood vessels. Despite the increase in pressure, the use of succinylcholine for eye operations is not contraindicated unless the anterior chamber is to be opened.

C. Intragastric Pressure: In some patients, especially muscular ones, the fasciculations associated with succinylcholine will cause an increase in intragastric pressure ranging from 5 to 40 cm of water. This may make emesis more likely, with the potential hazard of aspiration of gastric contents.

D. Muscle Pain: The incidence of muscle pain following succinylcholine administration varies from 0.2 to 8.9%. It occurs more frequently in ambulatory than in bedridden patients. The pain is thought to be secondary to damage produced in muscle by the unsynchronized contractions of adjacent muscle fibers just before the onset of paralysis. Muscle damage has been verified by the occurrence of myoglobinuria following the use of succinylcholine.

Interactions With Other Drugs

A. Anesthetics: Inhaled anesthetics augment the neuromuscular block from nondepolarizing muscle relaxants in dose-dependent fashion. Of the drugs that have been studied, inhaled anesthetics augment the effects of muscle relaxants in the following order:

Table 25–2. Autonomic effects of neuromuscular blocking drugs.

Drug	Effect on Autonomic Ganglia	Effect on Cardiac Muscarinic Receptors	Effect on Histamine Release
Succinylcholine	Stimulates	Stimulates	Slight
Tubocurarine	Blocks	None	Moderate
Metocurine	Blocks weakly	None	Slight
Gallamine	None	Blocks strongly	None
Pancuronium	None	Blocks moderately	None
Vecuronium	None	None	None
Atracurium	None	None	Slight

Isoflurane and enflurane augment more than halothane, which in turn augments more than nitrous oxide–barbiturate–opioid anesthesia (Fig 25–7). The most important factors involved in this interaction are the following: (1) Depression at sites proximal to the neuromuscular junction, ie, the central nervous system. (2) Increased muscle blood flow, which allows a larger fraction of the injected muscle relaxant to reach the neuromuscular junction. This is probably a factor only with isoflurane. (3) Decreased sensitivity of the postjunctional membrane to depolarization.

B. Antibiotics: Over 140 reports of enhancement of neuromuscular blockade by antibiotics, especially aminoglycosides, have appeared in the literature. Many of the antibiotics have been shown to cause a depression of evoked release of acetylcholine similar to that caused by magnesium. The same antibiotics also have postjunctional activity.

C. Local Anesthetics and Antiarrhythmic Drugs: In large doses, most local anesthetics block neuromuscular transmission; in smaller doses, they enhance the neuromuscular block from both nondepolarizing and depolarizing muscle relaxants.

In low doses, local anesthetics depress posttetanic potentiation, and this is thought to be a neural prejunctional effect. With higher doses, local anesthetics block acetylcholine-induced muscle contractions. This stabilizing effect is the result of blockade of the ionic channels linked to the nicotinic receptors.

Most antiarrhythmic drugs, including quinidine, enhance the block produced by nondepolarizing muscle relaxants. Quinidine appears to act at the prejunctional membrane, as judged by its lack of effect on acetylcholine-evoked twitch. However, large nonclinical doses of quinidine given intra-arterially produce a neuromuscular blockade of the depolarizing type that is augmented by edrophonium.

Effects of Disease & Aging on Drug Response

Several diseases can diminish or augment the neuromuscular blockade produced by nondepolarizing muscle relaxants. Myasthenia gravis augments the neuromuscular blockade from these drugs. Advanced age is often associated with a prolonged duration of action from nondepolarizing relaxants, probably owing to decreased clearance of drugs by the liver and kidneys. As a result, the dose of neuromuscular blocking drugs should probably be reduced in elderly patients.

Conversely, patients with severe burns and those with upper motor neuron disease are resistant to nondepolarizing muscle relaxants. This is probably because of the proliferation of extrajunctional receptors, which requires additional nondepolarizing muscle relaxant to block sufficient receptors to produce neuromuscular blockade.

Reversal of Nondepolarizing Neuromuscular Blockade

The cholinesterase inhibitors effectively antagonize neuromuscular blockade by nondepolarizing drugs. Their general pharmacology is discussed in Chapter 6. Neostigmine and pyridostigmine antagonize nondepolarizing neuromuscular blockade by increasing the availability of acetylcholine at the muscle end-plate, mainly by inhibition of acetylcholinesterase. To a lesser extent, these agents also increase release of transmitter from the motor nerve terminal. In contrast, edrophonium antagonizes neuromuscular blockade purely by inhibiting acetylcholinesterase.

Other Uses of Neuromuscular Blocking Drugs

A. Control of Ventilation: In patients who have ventilatory failure from various causes, such as obstructive airway disease, it is often desirable to control ventilation to provide adequate volumes and expansion of lungs. To eliminate chest wall resistance and ineffective spontaneous ventilation, paralysis is sometimes induced by administration of neuromuscular blocking drugs.

B. Treatment of Convulsions: Neuromuscular blocking drugs are sometimes used to attenuate or eliminate the peripheral manifestations of convulsions from such causes as epilepsy or local anesthetic toxicity. Although this approach is effective in eliminating the muscular manifestations of the conditions, it has no effect on the central processes involved, since neuromuscular blocking drugs do not cross the blood-brain barrier.

SPASMOLYTIC DRUGS

Bertram G. Katzung, MD, PhD

Spasticity is characterized by an increase in tonic stretch reflexes and flexor muscle spasms together with muscle weakness. It is often associated with cerebral palsy, multiple sclerosis, and stroke. These conditions often involve abnormal function of the bowel and bladder, as well as skeletal muscle. In this section, only skeletal muscle spasticity is considered. The mechanisms underlying clinical spasticity appear to involve not the stretch reflex arc itself but higher centers ("upper motor neuron lesion"), with damage to descending pathways that results in hyperexcitability of alpha motoneurons in the cord. Nevertheless, drug therapy may ameliorate some of the symptoms of spasticity by modifying the stretch reflex arc or by interfering directly with skeletal muscle excitation-contraction coupling. The components involved in these processes are shown in Fig 25–9.

Drugs modifying this reflex arc may modulate excitatory or inhibitory synapses (Chapter 19). Thus, to reduce the hyperactive stretch reflex, it is desirable to reduce the activity of the Ia fibers that excite the primary motoneuron or enhance the activity of the inhibitory internuncial neurons. These structures are shown in greater detail in Fig 25–10.

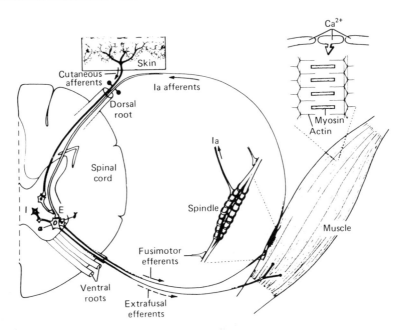

Figure 25–9. Diagram of the structures involved in the stretch reflex arc. I is an inhibitory interneuron; E indicates an excitatory presynaptic terminal; Ia is a primary intrafusal afferent fiber; Ca^{2+} denotes activator calcium stored in the sarcoplasmic reticulum of skeletal muscle. (Reproduced, with permission, from Young RR, Delwaide PJ: Drug therapy: Spasticity. *N Engl J Med* 1981;**304**:28.)

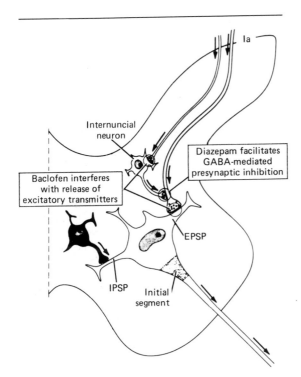

Figure 25–10. Postulated sites of spasmolytic action of diazepam and baclofen in the spinal cord. (Reproduced, with permission, from Young RR, Delwaide RJ: Drug therapy: Spasticity. *N Engl J Med* 1981;**304**:28.)

A variety of compounds used in the past can be loosely described as depressants of spinal "polysynaptic" reflex arcs (barbiturates: phenobarbital; glycerol ethers: mephenesin). However, it is clear from Fig 25–10 that nonspecific depression of synapses involved in the stretch reflex could reduce desirable inhibitory activity as well as excitatory transmission. In fact, in clinical use, phenobarbital and mephenesin have little specific spasmolytic effect, and such relief as may be produced appears to be the result of marked sedation. During the past decade, more specific therapy has become available. Unfortunately, the lack of a precisely quantifiable measure of clinical response—or, alternatively, an accurate experimental model—has prevented definitive comparison of the agents promoted for use in this heterogeneous group of conditions.

DIAZEPAM

As described in Chapter 20, benzodiazepines facilitate the action of gamma-aminobutyric acid (GABA) in the central nervous system. Diazepam has useful antispastic activity. Diazepam apparently acts at all GABA synapses, but its site of action in reducing spasticity is at least partly in the spinal cord, because it is effective in patients with cord transection. It can be used in patients with muscle spasm of almost any origin, including local muscle trauma. However, it produces sedation in most patients at the doses required to significantly reduce muscle tone. Dosage is usually begun at 4 mg/d and gradually increased to a maximum of 60 mg/d.

BACLOFEN
(Lioresal)

Baclofen (*p*-chlorophenyl GABA) was designed to be an orally active GABA-mimetic agent. The structure is shown below.

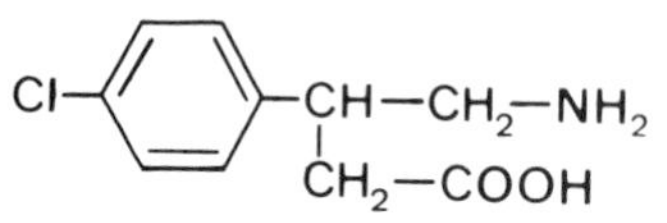

Baclofen

Baclofen is an active spasmolytic, and it displaces GABA from certain bicuculline-insensitive sites (GABA_B receptors). It seems probable that the drug acts as a GABA agonist at these receptors. It has been suggested that these receptors may serve a presynaptic inhibitory function, probably by reducing calcium influx, to reduce the release of excitatory transmitters in both the brain and the spinal cord. Baclofen may also reduce pain in patients with spasticity, possibly by inhibiting the release of substance P in the spinal cord.

Baclofen is at least as effective as diazepam in reducing spasticity but causes much less sedation. In addition, it does not reduce general muscle strength, as does dantrolene. It is rapidly and completely absorbed after oral administration and has a plasma half-life of 3–4 hours. Dosage is started at 15 mg twice daily, increasing, if tolerated, to as much as 100 mg daily. Toxicity of this drug includes drowsiness, to which the patient may become tolerant. Increased seizure activity has been reported in epileptic patients.

OTHER DRUGS THAT ACT IN THE SPINAL CORD

Progabide and **glycine** have been found in preliminary studies to reduce spasticity in some patients. Progabide is a GABA_A and GABA_B agonist and has active metabolites, including GABA itself. Glycine is another inhibitory neurotransmitter amino acid (Chapter 19). It appears to be active when given orally and readily passes the blood-brain barrier. These drugs are investigational.

DANTROLENE
(Dantrium)

Dantrolene is a hydantoin derivative (like phenytoin) but with a unique mechanism of spasmolytic ac-

tion outside the central nervous system. Its structure is shown below.

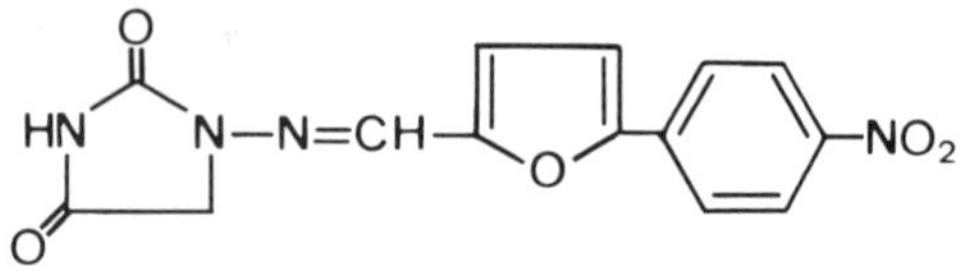

Dantrolene

Dantrolene reduces skeletal muscle strength by interfering with excitation-contraction coupling in the muscle fiber. The normal contractile response involves release of activator calcium from its stores in the sarcoplasmic reticulum of the sarcomere. This calcium brings about the tension-generating interaction of actin with myosin. Dantrolene interferes with the release of activator calcium from the sarcoplasmic reticulum. Thus, the action of this drug involves neither central synapses nor the neuromuscular junction; it is intracellular at the effector organ. Motor units that contract rapidly are more sensitive to the drug than are slow units. Cardiac muscle and smooth muscle are depressed only slightly, perhaps because the release of calcium from their sarcoplasmic reticulum (smooth muscle has very little) involves a somewhat different process.

Only about one-third of an oral dose of dantrolene is absorbed; the half-life of the drug is about 8 hours. Treatment is usually begun with 25 mg daily as a single dose, increasing to a maximum of 100 mg 4 times daily if necessary and tolerated. Major adverse effects are generalized muscle weakness, sedation, and occasionally hepatitis.

A special application of dantrolene is in the treatment of **malignant hyperthermia,** a rare disorder that can be triggered by a variety of stimuli, including general anesthesia and neuromuscular blocking drugs. Patients with this condition have a hereditary impairment of the ability of the sarcoplasmic reticulum to sequester calcium. A trigger event results in sudden and prolonged release of calcium, with massive muscle contraction, lactic acid production, and increased body temperature. Prompt treatment is essential to control acidosis and body temperature and to reduce calcium release. The latter is accomplished with intravenous dantrolene, starting with 1 mg/kg and repeating as necessary to a maximum of 10 mg/kg.

REFERENCES

Neuromuscular Blockers

Dreyer F: Acetylcholine receptor. *Br J Anaesth* 1982;**54:**115.

Katz B, Miledi R: A re-examination of curare action at the motor endplate. *Proc R Soc Lond* 1978;**211:**119.

Kitz RJ: Molecular pharmacology of acetylcholinesterase. Page 333 in: *A Guide to Molecular Pharmacology and Tox-*

icology. Featherstone RM (editor). Marcel Dekker, 1977.

Lambert JJ, Durant NN, Henderson EG: Drug-induced modification of ionic conductance at the neuromuscular junction. *Annu Rev Pharmacol Toxicol* 1983;**23:**505.

Miller RD, Agoston S, Booij LDHJ: The comparative potency and pharmacokinetics of pancuronium and its metabolites in anesthetized man. *J Pharmacol Exp Ther* 1978; **207**:539.

Miller RD, Savarese JJ: Pharmacology of muscle relaxants and their antagonists. In: *Anesthesia*. Miller RD (editor). Churchill Livingstone, 1985.

Miller RD et al: Clinical pharmacology of vecuronium and atracurium. *Anesthesiology* 1984;**61**:444.

Owen RT: Resistance to competitive neuromuscular blocking agents in burn patients: A review. *Methods Find Exp Clin Pharmacol* 1985;**7**:203.

Schoner PJ, Brown RL, Kirksey TD: Succinylcholine-induced hyperkalemia in burned patients. *Anesth Analg (Cleve)* 1969;**48**:764.

Waud BE, Waud DR: Physiology and pharmacology of neu-romuscular blocking agents. Page 1 in: *Muscle Relaxants*. Katz RL (editor). Excerpta Medica, 1975.

Spasmolytics

Davidoff RA: Antispasticity drugs: Mechanisms of action. *Ann Neurol* 1985;**17**:107.

Giesser B: Multiple sclerosis: Current concepts in management. *Drugs* 1985;**29**:88.

Pinder RM et al: Dantrolene sodium: A review of its pharmacological properties and therapeutic efficacy in spasticity. *Drugs* 1977;**3**:3.

Young RR, Delwaide PJ: Drug therapy: Spasticity. (2 parts.) *N Engl J Med* 1981;**304**:28, 96.

26

Pharmacologic Management of Parkinsonism & Other Movement Disorders

Michael J. Aminoff, MD, FRCP

Many of the movement disorders have been attributed to disturbances of the basal ganglia, but the precise function of these anatomic structures is not yet clearly understood, and it is not possible to relate individual symptoms to involvement at specific sites.

Several different types of abnormal movement are recognized. **Tremor** consists of a rhythmic oscillatory movement around a joint and is best characterized by its relation to activity. Tremor present at rest is characteristic of parkinsonism, when it is often associated with rigidity and an impairment of voluntary activity. Tremor may occur during maintenance of sustained posture (postural tremor) or during movement (intention tremor). A conspicuous postural tremor is the cardinal feature of benign essential or familial tremor. Intention tremor occurs in patients with a lesion of the brain stem or cerebellum, especially when the superior cerebellar peduncle is involved, and may also occur as a manifestation of toxicity from alcohol or certain other drugs.

Chorea consists of irregular, unpredictable, involuntary muscle jerks that may occur in different parts of the body and impair voluntary activity. In some instances, the proximal muscles of the limbs are most severely affected, and because the abnormal movements are then particularly violent, the term **ballismus** has been used to describe them. Chorea may be hereditary or may occur as a complication of a number of general medical disorders and of therapy with certain drugs.

Abnormal movements may be slow and writhing in character (**athetosis**) and in some instances are so sustained that they are more properly regarded as abnormal postures (**dystonia**). Athetosis or dystonia may occur with perinatal brain damage, with focal or generalized cerebral lesions, as an acute complication of certain drugs, as an accompaniment of diverse neurologic disorders, or as an isolated phenomenon of uncertain cause known as idiopathic torsion dystonia or dystonia musculorum deformans. Its pharmacologic basis is uncertain, and treatment is unsatisfactory.

Tics are sudden coordinated abnormal movements that tend to occur repetitively, particularly about the face and head, especially in children, and can be suppressed voluntarily for short periods of time. Common tics include, for example, repetitive sniffing or shoulder shrugging. Tics may be single or multiple and transient or chronic. Gilles de la Tourette's syndrome is characterized by chronic multiple tics; its pharmacologic management is discussed at the end of this chapter.

PARKINSONISM
(Paralysis Agitans)

Parkinsonism is characterized by a combination of rigidity, bradykinesia, tremor, and postural instability that can occur for a wide variety of reasons but is usually idiopathic. The course is generally progressive, leading to increasing disability unless effective treatment is provided. The normally high concentration of dopamine in the basal ganglia of the brain is reduced in parkinsonism, and pharmacologic attempts to restore dopaminergic activity with levodopa and dopamine agonists have been successful in alleviating many of the clinical features of the disorder. An alternative but complementary approach has been to restore the normal balance of cholinergic and dopaminergic influences on the basal ganglia with antimuscarinic drugs.

LEVODOPA
(Larodopa)

Dopamine does not cross the blood-brain barrier and therefore has no therapeutic effect in parkinsonism. However, (−)-3-(3,4-dihydroxyphenyl)-L-alanine (levodopa), the immediate metabolic precursor of dopamine, does penetrate the brain, where it is decarboxylated to dopamine. Several dopamine agonists have also been developed and may lead to clinical benefit, as discussed below.

Dopamine receptors can be classified according to various biochemical and pharmacologic features. They have, for example, been subdivided according to whether they are linked to an adenylate cyclase. Cyclic adenosine monophosphate (cAMP) is formed with activation of this cyclase and may well be responsible for mediating certain tissue-specific responses to dopamine. Other responses to dopamine apparently do not involve the stimulation of an adenylate cyclase or accumulation of cAMP. The designation D_1 has been proposed for those receptors linked to adenylate cyclase and D_2 for those that are not.

Dopamine receptors of the D_1 type are located in the zona compacta of the substantia nigra and presynaptically on striatal axons coming from cortical neurons and from dopaminergic cells in the substantia nigra. The D_2 receptors are located postsynaptically on striatal neurons and presynaptically on axons in the substantia nigra belonging to neurons in the basal ganglia. The benefits of dopaminergic antiparkinsonism drugs appear to depend on stimulation of the D_2 receptors. Dopamine agonist or partial agonist ergot derivatives such as lergotrile or bromocriptine that are powerful stimulators of the D_2 receptors have antiparkinsonism properties, whereas certain dopamine blockers that are selective D_2 antagonists can induce parkinsonism.

Chemistry

As discussed in Chapter 5, dopa is the precursor of dopamine and norepinephrine. Its structure is shown in Fig 26–1. Levodopa is the levorotatory stereoisomer of dopa.

Pharmacokinetics

Levodopa is rapidly absorbed from the small intestine, but its absorption depends on the rate of gastric emptying and the pH of the gastric contents. Food will delay the appearance of levodopa in the plasma. Moreover, certain amino acids from ingested food can compete with the drug for absorption from the gut and for transport from the blood to the brain. Plasma concentrations usually peak between 1 and 2 hours after an oral dose, and the plasma half-life is usually between 1 and 3 hours, though it varies considerably between individuals. About two-thirds of the dose appears in the urine as metabolites within 8 hours of an oral dose, the main metabolic products being 3-methoxy-4-hydroxyphenylacetic acid (homovanillic acid, HVA) and dihydroxyphenylacetic acid (DOPAC). Unfortunately, only about 1–3% of administered levodopa actually enters the brain unaltered, the remainder being metabolized extracerebrally, predominantly by decarboxylation to dopamine, which does not penetrate the blood-brain barrier. This means that levodopa must be given in large amounts when it is used alone. However, when it is given in combination with a dopa decarboxylase inhibitor that does not penetrate the blood-brain barrier, the peripheral metabolism of levodopa is reduced, plasma levels of levodopa are higher, plasma half-life is longer, and more dopa is available for entry into the brain. Indeed, concomitant administration of a peripheral dopa decarboxylase inhibitor may reduce the daily requirements of levodopa by approximately 75%

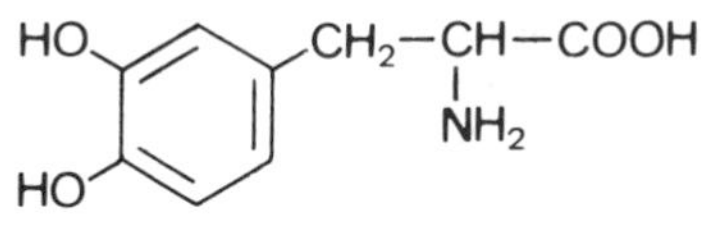

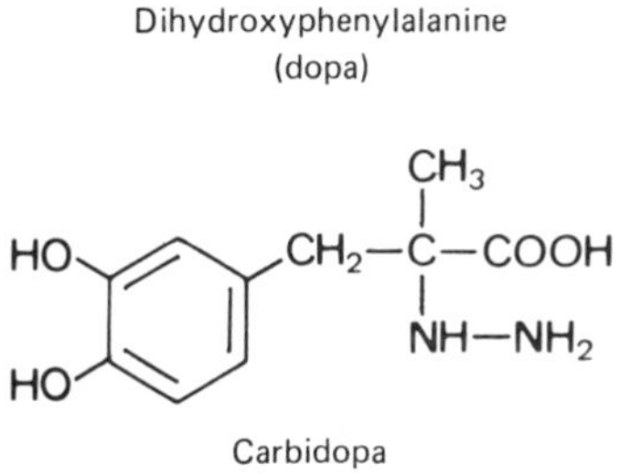

Clinical Use

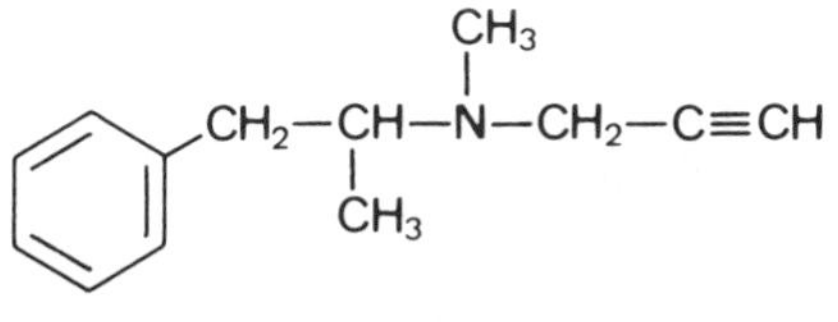

In considering the use of levodopa in patients with parkinsonism, it is important to appreciate that the best results are obtained in the first few years of treatment. This is sometimes because the daily dose of levodopa must be reduced with time in order to avoid side effects at doses that were well tolerated at the outset. The reason that side effects develop in this way is unclear, but selective denervation or drug-induced supersensitivity may be responsible. Some patients also become less responsive to levodopa, so that previously effective doses eventually fail to produce any therapeutic benefit. It is not clear whether this relates to disease progression or to duration of treatment. Responsiveness to levodopa may ultimately be lost completely, perhaps because of the disappearance of dopaminergic nigrostriatal nerve terminals or some pathologic process directly involving the striatal dopamine receptors. For such reasons, the benefits of levodopa treatment often begin to diminish after about 3 or 4 years of therapy irrespective of the initial therapeutic response. Moreover, levodopa therapy does not stop the progression of parkinsonism, and long-term therapy may lead to a number of problems in management such as development of the on-off phenomenon discussed below. It may therefore be better practice to reserve levodopa therapy until there is significant functional disability and to use other drugs for early management, but this is controversial.

When levodopa is used, it is generally given in combination with carbidopa (Fig 26–1), a peripheral decarboxylase inhibitor, for the reasons set forth

Figure 26–1. Some drugs used in the treatment of parkinsonism.

above. **Sinemet** is a preparation containing carbidopa and levodopa in fixed proportion (1:10 or 1:4). Treatment is started with a small dose, eg, Sinemet-25/100 (carbidopa 25 mg, levodopa 100 mg) 3 times daily, and gradually increased depending upon the therapeutic response and development of side effects. Most patients ultimately require Sinemet-25/250 (carbidopa 25 mg, levodopa 250 mg) 3 or 4 times daily.

Levodopa can ameliorate all of the clinical features of parkinsonism, but it is particularly effective in relieving bradykinesia and any disabilities resulting from it. When it is first introduced, about one-third of patients respond very well and one-third less well. Most of the remainder either are unable to tolerate the medication or simply fail to respond at all.

Side Effects

A. Gastrointestinal Effects: When levodopa is given without a peripheral decarboxylase inhibitor, anorexia and nausea and vomiting occur in about 80% of patients. These side effects can be minimized by taking the drug in divided doses, with or immediately after meals, and by increasing the total daily dose very slowly; antacids taken 30–60 minutes before levodopa may also be beneficial. The vomiting has been attributed to stimulation of an emetic center located in the brain stem but outside the blood-brain barrier to dopamine and to peripheral decarboxylase inhibitors. Fortunately, tolerance to this emetic effect develops in many patients after several months. Antiemetics such as phenothiazines are sometimes given but may reduce the antiparkinsonism effects of levodopa.

When levodopa is given in combination with carbidopa to reduce its extracerebral metabolism, gastrointestinal side effects are much less frequent and troublesome, occurring in fewer than 20% of cases, so that patients can tolerate proportionately higher doses.

B. Cardiovascular Effects: A variety of cardiac arrhythmias have been described in patients receiving levodopa, including tachycardia, ventricular extrasystoles, and, rarely, atrial fibrillation. This effect has been attributed to increased catecholamine formation peripherally. The incidence of such arrhythmias is low, even in the presence of established cardiac disease, and may be reduced still further if the levodopa is taken in combination with a peripheral decarboxylase inhibitor. In parkinsonism patients who also have heart disease, the anticipated benefits of levodopa, especially when combined with carbidopa, generally outweigh the slight risk of inducing a cardiac arrhythmia.

Postural hypotension is common, often asymptomatic, and tends to diminish with continuing treatment. Hypertension may also occur, especially in the presence of monoamine oxidase inhibitors or other sympathomimetics or when massive doses of levodopa are being taken.

C. Dyskinesias: Dyskinesias occur in about 80% of patients receiving levodopa therapy for long periods. The development of dyskinesias is dose-related, but there is considerable individual variation in the dose required to produce them. Dyskinesias seem to occur more commonly in patients receiving levodopa combined with a peripheral decarboxylase inhibitor than in those receiving levodopa alone. Moreover, with continuing treatment, dyskinesias may develop at a dose of levodopa that previously was well tolerated. They can be alleviated or reversed by lowering the daily dose of levodopa, but usually at the expense of reduced antiparkinsonism benefit; many patients are therefore willing to tolerate even a marked dyskinesia, because their mobility is so greatly improved by the medication. In some instances, dyskinesias are less marked if levodopa is prescribed alone rather than in combination with carbidopa; in other instances, a drug holiday (see below) may help control the problem. Pharmacologic attempts to counteract the dyskinesia with drugs used to treat chorea have generally not been successful or require the use of drugs that tend to worsen the parkinsonism.

The form and nature of dopa dyskinesias vary widely in different patients but tend to remain constant in character in individual patients. Chorea, ballismus, athetosis, dystonia, myoclonus, tics, and tremor may occur individually or in any combination in the face, trunk, or limbs. Choreoathetosis of the face and distal extremities is the most common presentation.

D. Behavioral Effects: A wide variety of mental side effects have been reported including depression, anxiety, agitation, insomnia, somnolence, confusion, delusions, hallucinations, nightmares, euphoria, and other changes in mood or personality. Such side effects are more common in patients taking levodopa in combination with a decarboxylase inhibitor rather than levodopa alone, presumably because higher levels are reached in the brain. They may be precipitated by intercurrent illness or operation. The only treatment is to reduce or withdraw the medication if necessary. A drug holiday (see below) may also lead to improvement of mental side effects.

E. Fluctuations in Response: Unpredictable fluctuations in clinical response to levodopa occur with increasing frequency as treatment continues. They occur in more than 50% of patients after 5 years of treatment. In some patients, these fluctuations relate to the timing of levodopa intake, and they are then referred to as wearing-off reactions or end-of-dose akinesia. In other instances, fluctuations in clinical state are unrelated to the timing of doses (on-off phenomenon). In the on-off phenomenon, off-periods of marked akinesia alternate over the course of a few hours with on-periods of improved mobility but often marked dyskinesia. The phenomenon is most likely to occur in patients who responded well to treatment initially. The exact mechanism is unknown, but the off-period can sometimes be shown to relate to falling plasma levels of levodopa. Patients may benefit from taking their medication at more frequent intervals in smaller doses during the day or from the addition of dopamine agonists such as bromocriptine (see below) to the drug regimen. Alternatively, a brief holiday from levodopa under careful medical supervision may help in restoring its effectiveness, although any benefit is usually temporary.

F. Miscellaneous Side Effects: Mydriasis may occur and may precipitate an attack of acute glaucoma in some patients. Other reported but rare side effects include various blood dyscrasias; a positive Coombs test with evidence of hemolysis; hot flushes; aggravation or precipitation of gout; abnormalities of smell or taste; brownish discoloration of saliva, urine, or vaginal secretions; priapism; and mild—usually transient—elevations of blood urea nitrogen and of serum transaminases, alkaline phosphatase, and bilirubin.

Drug Holidays

A drug holiday may help in alleviating some of the neurologic and behavioral side effects of levodopa but is usually of little help in the management of the on-off phenomenon. Patients must be under close medical supervision. Levodopa medication is withdrawn gradually, since abrupt cessation of treatment may lead to a severely akinetic state. The optimal duration of a break in treatment with levodopa is unclear, but it has varied from 3 to 21 days in different studies. Up to about two-thirds of patients show improved responsiveness to levodopa when the drug is reinstituted, and, because they can be managed on lower doses than before, mental side effects and dyskinesias are less troublesome. Fluctuations in response (on-off phenomenon) are reduced in many instances, but any benefit in this regard is usually short-lived. Unfortunately, there is no way of predicting which patients will respond satisfactorily to the holiday.

Drug Interactions

Pharmacologic doses of pyridoxine (vitamin B$_6$) enhance the extracerebral metabolism of levodopa and may therefore prevent its therapeutic effect unless a peripheral decarboxylase inhibitor is also taken. Levodopa should not be given to patients taking monoamine oxidase A inhibitors or within 2 weeks of their discontinuation, because such a combination can lead to hypertensive crises.

Contraindications

Levodopa should not be given to psychotic patients, as it may exacerbate the mental disturbance. It is also contraindicated in patients with angle-closure glaucoma, but those with chronic open-angle glaucoma may be given levodopa if intraocular pressure is well controlled and can be monitored. It is best given combined with carbidopa to patients with cardiac disease, but even so there is a slight risk of cardiac dysrhythmia. Patients with active peptic ulcer must also be managed carefully, since gastrointestinal bleeding has occasionally occurred with levodopa. Because levodopa is a precursor of skin melanin and conceivably may activate malignant melanoma, its use should be avoided in patients with a history of melanoma or with suspicious undiagnosed skin lesions.

BROMOCRIPTINE
(Parlodel)

The enzymes responsible for synthesizing dopamine are depleted in the brains of parkinsonism patients, and drugs acting directly on dopamine receptors may therefore have a beneficial effect additional to that of levodopa. Moreover, drugs specifically affecting certain (but not all) dopamine receptors may have more limited side effects than levodopa. There are a number of dopamine agonists with antiparkinsonism activity. Some, such as apomorphine, piribedil, and lergotrile, have such serious side effects that they cannot be used clinically, but others may have a role in treatment of parkinsonism.

The most promising group of dopamine agonists currently being evaluated are ergot derivatives. Several ergot derivatives have been used experimentally in the treatment of parkinsonism; unlike other dopaminelike drugs, these drugs appear to be partial agonists at presynaptic dopamine D$_2$ receptors. Lisuride and pergolide both appear to be helpful but are not yet available for general use in the USA, and so **bromocriptine** (structure shown in Chapter 15) is the only one in widespead use. It has also been used to treat certain endocrinologic disorders, especially hyperprolactinemia (see Chapters 15 and 36), but in lower doses than those required to counteract parkinsonism. The drug is absorbed to a variable extent from the gastrointestinal tract, peak plasma levels being reached within 1–2 hours after an oral dose. It is excreted in the bile and feces.

It is not clear whether bromocriptine itself has a role as a first-line drug in the treatment of parkinsonism nor whether its use in this disease is associated with a lower incidence of the side effects commonly seen with long-term levodopa therapy. In any case, bromocriptine is an expensive drug best reserved for parkinsonism patients taking levodopa who have end-of-dose akinesia or on-off phenomena or who are becoming refractory to treatment with levodopa. Partial replacement of levodopa with bromocriptine may then be valuable. Optimal results are obtained by a combination of levodopa and bromocriptine in doses less than the maximum tolerated doses of each. The results of bromocriptine treatment are generally disappointing in patients totally unresponsive to levodopa, and addition of bromocriptine to patients receiving optimal levodopa therapy may cause intolerable side effects. Bromocriptine does not complicate treatment with antimuscarinic drugs or amantadine, and these drugs can be continued without change in dosage in patients who are to be given bromocriptine as well.

Clinical Use

The usual daily dose of bromocriptine in parkinsonism is between 10 and 40 mg, but in about one-fourth to one-half of cases therapeutic doses either fail to provide sustained benefit or cannot be tolerated. In order to minimize adverse effects, the dose of bromocriptine should be built up slowly over about 2 or 3 months from a starting level of 1.25 mg twice daily after meals; the dose of levodopa taken concurrently may have to be gradually lowered to about half of that previously required. However, because occasional patients are very sensitive to the hypotensive effect of bromocriptine and may even collapse within an hour of the first dose, a test dose of 1 mg should be given initially, with food and with the patient in bed. If vascular collapse occurs, recovery is usually rapid and spontaneous, and patients often tolerate subsequent doses well. Treatment with bromocriptine should be stopped if it leads to psychiatric disturbances, cardiac dysrhythmia, erythromelalgia, ergotism, or other intolerable side effects.

Toxicity

A. Gastrointestinal Effects: Anorexia and nausea and vomiting are especially common when bromocriptine therapy is introduced and can be minimized by taking the medication with meals. Other gastrointestinal side effects include constipation, dyspepsia, and symptoms suggestive of reflux esophagitis. Bleeding from peptic ulceration has also been reported.

B. Cardiovascular Effects: Postural hypotension is fairly common, especially at the initiation of therapy. Painless digital vasospasm is a complication of long-term treatment that can be reversed by lowering the dose. Cardiac arrhythmias may also occur with bromocriptine and are an indication for discontinuing treatment.

C. Dyskinesias: Abnormal movements similar to those induced by levodopa can also be produced by bromocriptine. Treatment consists of reducing the total dose of dopaminergic drugs being taken.

D. Mental Disturbances: Confusion, hallucinations, delusions, and other psychiatric reactions are established complications of dopaminergic treatment of parkinsonism. They are more common and severe with bromocriptine than with levodopa itself. Such effects clear on withdrawal of the offending medication.

E. Miscellaneous Side Effects: Headache, nasal congestion, increased arousal, pulmonary infiltrates, and erythromelalgia are other reported side effects of bromocriptine. Erythromelalgia consists of red, tender, painful, swollen feet and, occasionally, hands, at times associated with arthralgia; symptoms and signs clear within a few days of withdrawal of bromocriptine.

Contraindications

Bromocriptine treatment is contraindicated in patients with a history of psychiatric illness or recent myocardial infarction. It is best avoided in patients with peripheral vascular disease or peptic ulceration.

MONOAMINE OXIDASE INHIBITORS

Two types of monoamine oxidase have been distinguished. Monoamine oxidase A metabolizes norepinephrine and serotonin; monoamine oxidase B metabolizes dopamine. **Deprenyl** (Fig 26–1), a selective inhibitor of monoamine oxidase B, retards the breakdown of dopamine; in consequence, it enhances and prolongs the antiparkinsonism effect of levodopa and may reduce mild on-off or wearing-off phenomena. Its use for this purpose is experimental at present. Deprenyl has no useful therapeutic effect on parkinsonism when given alone, but recent studies in animals suggest that it may reduce disease progression.

The combined administration of levodopa and an inhibitor of both forms of monoamine oxidase must be avoided, since it may lead to hypertensive crises, probably because of the peripheral accumulation of norepinephrine.

AMANTADINE
(Symmetrel)

Amantadine, an antiviral agent, was by chance found to have antiparkinsonism properties. Its mode of action in parkinsonism is unclear, but it may potentiate dopaminergic function by influencing the synthesis, release, or reuptake of dopamine. Release of catecholamines from peripheral stores has been documented.

Pharmacokinetics

Peak plasma concentrations of amantadine are reached 1–4 hours after an oral dose. The plasma half-life is between 2 and 4 hours, most of the drug being excreted unchanged in the urine.

Clinical Use

Amantadine is less potent than levodopa, and its benefits may be short-lived, often disappearing after only a few weeks of treatment. Nevertheless, during that time it may favorably influence the bradykinesia, rigidity, and tremor of parkinsonism. The standard dose is 100 mg orally twice daily.

Side Effects

Amantadine has a number of central nervous system side effects that can be reversed by stopping the drug. These include restlessness, depression, irritability, insomnia, agitation, excitement, hallucinations, and confusion. Overdosage may produce an acute toxic psychosis. With doses several times higher than recommended, convulsions have occurred.

Livedo reticularis sometimes occurs in patients taking amantadine and usually clears within a month after the drug is withdrawn. Other dermatologic reactions have also been described. Peripheral edema, another well-recognized complication, is not accompanied by signs of cardiac, hepatic, or renal disease and responds to diuretics. Other adverse reactions include headache, congestive heart disease, postural hypotension, urinary retention, and gastrointestinal disturbances (eg, anorexia, nausea, constipation, and dry mouth).

Table 26–1. Some drugs with antimuscarinic properties used in parkinsonism.

Drug	Usual Daily Dose (mg)
Benztropine mesylate (Cogentin)	1–6
Biperiden (Akineton)	2–12
Chlorphenoxamine (Phenoxene)	150–400
Ethopropazine (Parsidol)	150–300
Orphenadrine (Disipal, Norflex)	150–400
Procyclidine (Kemadrin)	7.5–30
Trihexyphenidyl (Artane)	6–20

Contraindications

The drug should be used with caution in patients with a history of seizures or congestive heart failure.

ACETYLCHOLINE-BLOCKING DRUGS

A number of centrally acting antimuscarinic preparations are available that differ in their potency and in their efficacy in different patients.

Clinical Use

Treatment is started with a low dose of one of the drugs in this category, the level of medication gradually being increased until benefit occurs or side effects limit further increments. Antimuscarinic drugs may improve the tremor and rigidity of parkinsonism but have little effect on bradykinesia. If patients fail to respond to one drug, a trial with another is certainly warranted and may be successful. Some of the more commonly used drugs are listed in Table 26–1.

Side Effects

Antimuscarinic drugs have a number of central nervous system side effects, including drowsiness, mental slowness, inattention, restlessness, confusion, agitation, delusions, hallucinations, and mood changes. Such side effects are sometimes precipitated by intercurrent infections and usually subside within a few days after withdrawal of the offending substance. Other common side effects include dryness of the mouth, blurring of vision, mydriasis, urinary retention, nausea and vomiting, constipation, tachycardia, tachypnea, increased intraocular pressure, palpitations, and cardiac arrhythmias. Dyskinesias occur in rare cases. Acute suppurative parotitis sometimes occurs as a complication of dryness of the mouth.

If medication is to be withdrawn, this should be accomplished gradually rather than abruptly in order to prevent acute exacerbation of parkinsonism.

Contraindications

Acetylcholine-blocking drugs should be avoided in patients with prostatic hypertrophy, obstructive gastrointestinal disease (eg, pyloric stenosis or paralytic ileus), or angle-closure glaucoma. In parkinsonism patients receiving antimuscarinic medication, concomitant administration of other drugs with antimuscarinic properties—eg, tricyclic antidepressants or antihistamines—may precipitate some of the complications mentioned above.

DL-THREO-3,4-DIHYDROXY-PHENYLSERINE (DOPS)

Regional cerebral deficits of norepinephrine (as well as of dopamine) have been found in patients with parkinsonism, and it has recently been proposed that norepinephrine lack is responsible for the clinical phenomenon of sudden transient freezing-up or arrest of movement observed in some patients with advanced disease who respond unpredictably to levodopa. Administration of DL-threo- 3,4-dihydroxyphenylserine (DOPS), a precursor of norepinephrine, has been reported to improve such phenomena in some studies but not in others.

GENERAL COMMENTS ON DRUG MANAGEMENT OF PATIENTS WITH PARKINSONISM

There is no means of influencing the course of idiopathic parkinsonism. Moreover, the benefits of levodopa therapy often seem to diminish with time; certain side effects may complicate long-term levodopa treatment; and there are a number of controversies concerning treatment with this drug. In particular, it has been suggested that levodopa therapy may accelerate disease progression and that high-dose levodopa therapy is associated with more long-term side effects than low-dose therapy. Such impressions have still to be established with certainty. Nevertheless, pharmacologic treatment of mild parkinsonism is probably best avoided until there is some degree of disability or until symptoms begin to have a significant impact on the patient's life-style. When treatment becomes necessary, it is best to start with amantadine or an antimuscarinic drug, reserving levodopa until there is definite incapacity. In patients with more severe parkinsonism, levodopa is usually prescribed in combination with carbidopa as Sinemet, and amantadine or an antimuscarinic drug (or both) may be necessary as well for optimal benefit. Physical therapy is also helpful in improving mobility. In patients with severe parkinsonism and long-term complications of levodopa therapy, such as the on-off phenomenon, a trial of treatment with bromocriptine may be worthwhile. All patients require continual support and encouragement to maintain an independent existence.

DRUG-INDUCED PARKINSONISM

Reserpine and the related drug tetrabenazine deplete biogenic monoamines from their storage sites, while haloperidol and the phenothiazines block dopaminergic receptors. These drugs may therefore produce a parkinsonian syndrome, usually within 3 months after introduction, which is related to high dosage and clears over a few weeks or months after withdrawal. If treatment is necessary, antimuscarinic are preferred. Levodopa is of no help if neuroleptic drugs are continued and may in fact aggravate the mental disorder for which antipsychotic drugs were prescribed originally.

Recently, a drug-induced form of parkinsonism has been discovered in individuals who attempted to synthesize and use a narcotic drug related to meperidine but actually synthesized and self-administered: 1-methyl-4-phenyl-1,2,5,6-tetrahydropyridine. This compound (MPTP) selectively destroys dopaminergic neurons in the substantia nigra and induces a severe form of parkinsonism in animals as well as in humans. The experimental use of this drug has provided a model that could assist in the development of new drugs for this disease.

OTHER MOVEMENT DISORDERS

Tremor

Tremor consists of rhythmic oscillatory movements. Physiologic postural tremor is enhanced in amplitude by anxiety, fatigue, thyrotoxicosis, and intravenous epinephrine or isoproterenol. Propranolol reduces its amplitude, and, if administered intra-arterially, prevents the response to isoproterenol in the perfused limb, presumably through some peripheral action. Certain drugs—especially the bronchodilators, tricyclic antidepressants, and lithium—may produce a dose-dependent exaggeration of the normal physiologic tremor that is readily reversed by discontinuing the drug. Although the tremor produced by sympathomimetics such as terbutaline (a bronchodilator) is blocked by propranolol, which antagonizes both β_1 and β_2 receptors, it is not blocked by metoprolol, a β_1-selective antagonist, suggesting that such tremor is mediated mainly by the β_2 receptors.

Essential tremor is a postural tremor, sometimes familial, that is clinically similar to physiologic tremor. Dysfunction of β_1 receptors has been implicated in some instances, since the tremor may respond dramatically to standard doses of metoprolol as well as to propranolol. The most useful approach is with propranolol, but whether the response depends on a central or peripheral action is unclear. The pharmacokinetics, pharmacologic effects, and adverse reactions of propranolol are discussed in Chapter 9. Daily doses of propranolol on the order of 120 mg (60–240 mg) are usually required, and reported side effects have been few. Propranolol should be used with caution in patients with congestive cardiac failure, heart block, asthma, or hypoglycemia. Patients can be instructed to take their own pulse and call the physician if significant bradycardia develops. Metoprolol, a relatively selective β_1 blocker, is sometimes useful in treating tremor when patients have concomitant pulmonary disease that contraindicates use of propranolol. Primidone (an antiepileptic drug; see Chapter 22), in gradually increasing doses up to 250 mg 3 times daily, is also effective in providing symptomatic control in some cases. Patients with tremor are very sensitive to primidone and often cannot tolerate the doses used to treat siezures; they should be started on 50 mg once daily and the daily dose increased by 50 mg every 2 weeks depending on response. Small quantities of alcohol may suppress essential tremor, but only for a short time and by an unknown mechanism. Diazepam, chlordiazepoxide, mephenesin, and antiparkinsonism agents have been advocated in the past but are generally worthless.

Intention tremor—tremor present during movement but not at rest—sometimes occurs as a toxic manifestation of alcohol or drugs such as phenytoin. Withdrawal or reduction in dosage provides dramatic relief. There is no satisfactory pharmacologic treatment for intention tremor due to other neurologic disorders.

Rest tremor is usually due to parkinsonism.

Huntington's Disease

This dominantly inherited disorder is characterized by progressive dementia and chorea that usually begin in adulthood. The development of chorea seems to be related to an imbalance of dopamine, acetylcholine, gamma-aminobutyric acid (GABA), and perhaps other neurotransmitters in the basal ganglia. Pharmacologic studies indicate that chorea results from functional overactivity in dopaminergic nigrostriatal pathways, perhaps because of increased responsiveness of postsynaptic dopamine receptors or deficiency of a neurotransmitter that normally antagonizes dopamine. Drugs that impair dopaminergic neurotransmission, either by depleting central monoamines (eg, reserpine, tetrabenazine) or by blocking dopamine receptors (eg, phenothiazines, butyrophenones), often alleviate chorea, whereas dopaminelike drugs such as levodopa tend to exacerbate it.

Both GABA and the enzyme (glutamic acid decarboxylase) concerned with its synthesis are markedly reduced in the basal ganglia of patients with Huntington's disease, and GABA receptors are usually implicated in inhibitory pathways. There is also a significant decline in concentration of choline acetyltransferase, the enzyme responsible for synthesizing acetylcholine, in the basal ganglia of these patients. These findings may be of pathophysiologic significance and have led to attempts to alleviate chorea by enhancing central GABA or acetylcholine activity. Unfortunately, such pharmacologic manipulations have been disappointing, yielding no consistently beneficial response, and as a consequence the most commonly used drugs for controlling dyskinesia in patients with Huntington's disease are still those that interfere with dopamine activity. With all of the latter drugs, however, reduction of abnormal movements may be associated with iatrogenic parkinsonism.

Reserpine depletes cerebral dopamine by preventing intraneuronal storage; it is introduced in low doses (eg, 0.25 mg daily), and the daily dose is then built up gradually (eg, by 0.25 mg every week) until benefit occurs or side effects become troublesome. A daily dose of 2–5 mg is often effective in suppressing abnormal movements, but side effects may include hypotension, depression, sedation, diarrhea, and nasal congestion. Tetrabenazine resembles reserpine in depleting cerebral dopamine and has less troublesome side effects, but it is available in the USA only on an experimental basis. Treatment with postsynaptic dopamine receptor blockers such as phenothiazines and butyrophenones may also be helpful. Haloperidol is started in a small dose, eg, 1 mg twice daily, and increased every 4 days depending upon the response. If haloperidol is not helpful, treatment with increasing doses of perphenazine up to a total of about 20 mg daily sometimes helps. The pharmacokinetics and clinical properties of these drugs are considered in greater detail elsewhere in this book.

It has recently been reported that low doses of a dopamine agonist may reduce the choreiform movements of patients with Huntington's disease, perhaps because of activation of presynaptic or self-inhibitory dopamine receptors whose stimulation results in inhibition of the activity of dopaminergic neurons. Such an approach remains experimental at this time but may prove to have some useful therapeutic application in the future.

Other Forms of Chorea

Treatment is directed at the underlying cause when chorea occurs as a complication of general medical disorders such as thyrotoxicosis, polycythemia vera rubra, systemic lupus erythematosus, hypocalcemia, and hepatic cirrhosis. Drug-induced chorea is managed by withdrawal of the offending substance, which may be levodopa, an antimuscarinic drug, amphetamine, lithium, phenytoin, or an oral contraceptive. Neuroleptic drugs may also produce an acute or tardive dyskinesia (discussed below). Sydenham's chorea is temporary and usually so mild that pharmacologic management of the dyskinesia is unnecessary, but dopamine-blocking drugs are effective in suppressing it.

Ballismus

The biochemical basis of ballismus is unknown, but the pharmacologic approach to management is the same as for chorea. Treatment with haloperidol, perphenazine, or other dopamine-blocking drugs may be helpful.

Athetosis & Dystonia

The pharmacologic basis of these disorders is unknown, and there is no satisfactory medical treatment for them. Occasional patients with dystonia may respond to diazepam, amantadine, antimuscarinic drugs (in high dosage), levodopa, carbamazepine, baclofen, haloperidol, or phenothiazines. A trial of these pharmacologic approaches is worthwhile even though often not successful.

Tics

The pathophysiologic basis of tics is unknown. Chronic multiple tics (Gilles de la Tourette's syndrome) may require treatment if the disorder is severe or is having a significant impact on the patient's life. The most effective pharmacologic approach is with haloperidol, and patients are better able to tolerate this drug if treatment is started with a small dose (eg, 0.25 or 0.5 mg daily) and then increased very gradually over the following weeks. Most patients ultimately require a total daily dose of 3–8 mg. If haloperidol is not helpful, fluphenazine, clonazepam, clonidine, or carbamazepine should be tried. The pharmacologic properties of these drugs are discussed elsewhere in this book. Recently, pimozide, an oral dopamine blocker, has been approved for use in the USA and may help patients intolerant or unresponsive to haloperidol, but the long-term safety of the drug is unclear.

Drug-Induced Dyskinesias

The pharmacologic basis of the acute dyskinesia or dystonia sometimes precipitated by the first few doses of a phenothiazine is not clear. In most instances, parenteral administration of an antimuscarinic drug such as benztropine (2 mg intravenously) or biperiden (2–5 mg intravenously or intramuscularly) is helpful, while in other instances diazepam (10 mg intravenously) alleviates the abnormal movements.

Tardive dyskinesia is a disorder characterized by a variety of abnormal movements that develop after long-term neuroleptic drug treatment. A reduction in dose of the offending medication, a dopamine receptor blocker, commonly worsens the dyskinesia, while an increase in dose may suppress it. These clinical observations, and the exacerbation in the movement disorder that is produced by levodopa, suggest that tardive dyskinesia relates to increased dopaminergic function, but its precise pharmacologic basis is unclear. It would seem, therefore, that phenothiazines cause a short-term reversible blockade of dopamine receptors but that over the long term they increase dopaminergic function. Whether this latter effect depends upon the development of denervation supersensitivity, increased dopamine synthesis, or diminished reuptake of dopamine at central synapses is not known.

There is some evidence that GABA is involved in a striatonigral feedback loop modulating the activity of dopaminergic cells in the substantia nigra, and GABA efferents also pass from the striatum to the globus pallidus and thalamus. GABA-mediated activity may diminish the activity of nigrostriatal dopaminergic cells and thereby decrease involuntary movements. **Muscimol,** a semirigid structural analog of GABA, has been given to a small number of patients with tardive dyskinesia, and at oral doses of 5–9 mg daily consistently attenuated their involuntary movements in one study. However, muscimol has behavioral side effects that limit any role for it in the treatment of tardive dyskinesia. Other attempts to increase central GABA activity (eg, with benzodiazepines or sodium valproate) have not yielded consistent benefit. Attempts to restore the balance between dopaminergic and cholinergic activity by increasing the latter with oral choline or lecithin have been helpful in some instances but not in others, and the same was true of treatment with deanol acetamidobenzoate, a drug related to acetylcholine and now discontinued. The drugs most likely to provide immediate symptomatic benefit are those interfering with dopaminergic function, either by depletion (eg, reserpine, tetrabenazine) or receptor blockade (eg, phenothiazines, butyrophenones). Paradoxically, the receptor-blocking drugs are the very ones that also cause the dyskinesia, and they are probably best avoided to prevent the development of a spiral phenomenon in which continuing aggravation of the dyskinesia by the drugs used to control it necessitates increasingly higher doses for its temporary suppression.

Because tardive dyskinesia developing in adults is usually irreversible and has no satisfactory treatment, care must be taken to reduce the likelihood of its occurrence. Antipsychotic medication should be prescribed only when necessary and should be withheld periodically to assess the need for continued treatment and to unmask incipient dyskinesia. Thioridazine, a phenothiazine with a piperidine side chain, is an effective antipsychotic that seems less likely than most to cause extrapyramidal reactions, perhaps because it has little effect on dopamine receptors in the striatal system. Finally, antimuscarinic drugs should not be prescribed routinely in patients receiving neuroleptics, since the combination may increase the likelihood of dyskinesia.

Wilson's Disease

Wilson's disease, a recessively inherited disorder of copper metabolism, is characterized biochemically by reduced serum copper and ceruloplasmin concentrations, pathologically by markedly increased concentration of copper in the brain and viscera, and clinically by signs of hepatic and neurologic dysfunction. Treatment involves the removal of excess copper, followed by maintenance of copper balance. The most satisfactory agent currently available for this purpose is **penicillamine** (dimethylcysteine), a chelating agent that forms a ring complex with copper. It is readily absorbed from the gastrointestinal tract and rapidly excreted in the urine. A common starting dose in adults is 500 mg 3 or 4 times daily. After remission occurs, it may be possible to lower the maintenance dose, generally to not less than 1 g daily, which must thereafter be continued indefinitely. Side effects include nausea and vomiting, nephrotic syndrome, a lupuslike syndrome, pemphigus, myasthenia, arthropathy, optic neuropathy, and various blood dyscrasias. Treatment should be monitored by frequent urinalysis and complete blood counts. Dietary copper should also be kept below 2 mg daily by the exclusion of chocolate, nuts, shellfish, liver, mushrooms, broccoli, and cereals; and distilled or demineralized water may have to be provided if tap water contains more than 0.1 mg of copper per liter. Potassium disulfide, 20 mg 3 times daily with meals, reduces the intestinal absorption of copper and should also be prescribed.

REFERENCES

Calne DB: Progress in Parkinson's disease. *N Engl J Med* 1984; **310:**523.

Fahn S: High dosage anticholinergic therapy in dystonia. *Neurology* 1983;**33:**1255.

Findley LJ, Calzetti S: Double-blind controlled study of primidone in essential tremor: Preliminary results. *Br Med J* 1982; **285:**608.

Gopinathan G et al: Lisuride in parkinsonism. *Neurology* 1981; **31:**371.

Langston JW et al: Chronic parkinsonism in humans due to a product of meperidine-analog synthesis. *Science* 1983; **219:**979.

Langston JW et al: Selective nigral toxicity after systemic administration of 1-methyl-4-phenyl-1,2,5,6-tetrahydropyridine (MPTP). *Brain Res* 1984;**292:**390.

Lesser RP et al: Analysis of the clinical problems in parkinsonism and the complications of long-term levodopa therapy. *Neurology* 1979;**29:**1253.

Lieberman AN, Goldstein M: Bromocriptine in Parkinson disease. *Pharmacol Rev* 1985;**37:**217.

Lieberman AN et al: Further studies with pergolide in Parkinson disease. *Neurology* 1982;**30:**1181.

Lieberman AN et al: Long-term efficacy of bromocriptine in Parkinson disease. *Neurology* 1980;**32:**518.

Markham CH, Diamond SG: Evidence to support early levodopa therapy in Parkinson disease. *Neurology* 1981; **31:**125.

Nutt JG, Fellman JH: Pharmacokinetics of levodopa. *Clin Neuropharmacol* 1984;**7:**35.

Nutt JG et al: The "on-off" phenomenon in Parkinson's disease. *N Engl J Med* 1984;**310:**483.

Parkes JD: Adverse effects of antiparkinsonian drugs. *Drugs* 1981;**21:**341.

Quinn NP: Anti-parkinsonian drugs today. *Drugs* 1984;**28:**236.

Seeman P: Brain dopamine receptors. *Pharmacol Rev* 1981; **32:**229.

Antipsychotics & Lithium

27

Leo Hollister, MD

ANTIPSYCHOTICS

The term **antipsychotics** is one of several applied to a group of drugs that have been used mainly for treating schizophrenia but are effective in some other psychoses and agitated states. The preferred term in Europe is **neuroleptics,** connoting the capacity of these drugs to affect several integrating systems of the brain, including the ability to cause movement disorders. The term **major tranquilizers** has fortunately fallen into disuse, since it confounds these drugs with **minor tranquilizers** (actually sedative-hypnotics), which they resemble only superficially.

History

No acceptable forms of drug treatment were available for treating schizophrenia until the early 1950s, when both reserpine and chlorpromazine appeared almost simultaneously. Chlorpromazine had been developed as an antihistamine and reserpine as an antihypertensive agent. Fortuitous observations of their calming properties led to trials in psychiatric patients. Initial clinical trials were enthusiastically reported. Over the years, reserpine became obsolete as an antipsychotic drug, since it was not believed to be as effective as chlorpromazine and was more likely to produce mental depression. The success of chlorpromazine led to the introduction of numerous phenothiazine derivatives. During the past 30 years, many different chemical structures have been shown to share the spectrum of pharmacologic activities associated with antipsychotic activity.

Nature of Psychosis & Schizophrenia

The term "psychosis" denotes a variety of mental disorders. Schizophrenia is a particular kind of psychosis characterized mainly by a clear sensorium but a marked thinking disturbance. The pathogenesis is unknown.

Largely as a result of research stimulated by the discovery of antipsychotic drugs, it has been proposed that genetic predisposition is a necessary but not always sufficient condition underlying the psychotic disorders. The ensuing abnormality is thought to reside primarily, but not exclusively, in overactivity of do-

paminergic pathways of the brain, particularly in the mesolimbic-frontal dopaminergic system (Fig 27–1). Whether the overactivity is due to excessive synthesis and release of dopamine presynaptically or impaired metabolism or enhanced postsynaptic receptor sensitivity is uncertain. The "dopamine hypothesis" of schizophrenia is based on 3 circumstantial lines of evidence: (1) virtually all antipsychotic drugs block postsynaptic dopamine receptors; (2) increasing dopaminergic activity by administering levodopa sometimes produces a schizophreniform psychosis; and (3) abuse of sympathomimetic stimulants, which increase release of dopamine, produces a paranoid state resembling paranoid schizophrenia.

More recently, evidence has been adduced that some schizophrenic patients show brain atrophy as measured by CT scan and that these patients are gener-

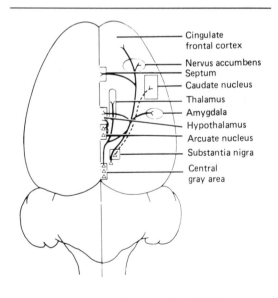

Dopamine (mesolimbic) ——
Dopamine (nigrostriatal) - - -

Figure 27–1. Diagrammatic section of brain showing the 2 principal dopaminergic tracts of the mesolimbic-frontal system and the nigrostriatal system. (Reproduced, with permission, from Hollister LE: *Clinical Pharmacology of Psychotherapeutic Drugs,* 2nd ed. Monographs in Clinical Pharmacology. Vol 1. Churchill Livingstone, 1983.)

ally refractory to treatment with drugs, following a deteriorating course. On the other hand, patients without this structural abnormality may have a functional abnormality of the dopamine system that is corrected by antipsychotic drugs. Even in the latter instance, the amelioration of schizophrenia is at best partial, manifested by clearer thinking, more acceptable behavior, and some degree of social and vocational rehabilitation.

I. BASIC PHARMACOLOGY OF ANTIPSYCHOTIC DRUGS

Chemical Types

A number of chemical structures have been associ-

ated with antipsychotic properties. The drugs can be classified into 4 major groups as shown in Fig 27–2.

A. Phenothiazine Derivatives: Three subfamilies of phenothiazines, based primarily on the side chain of the molecule, are in use. Aliphatic derivatives (eg, chlorpromazine) and piperidine derivatives (eg, thioridazine) are the least potent. Piperazine derivatives are more potent in the sense that they are effective in lower milligram doses. However, the piperazine derivatives are also more specific in their pharmacologic effects.

B. Thioxanthene Derivatives: This group of drugs is exemplified primarily by thiothixene. In general, this group of compounds is slightly less potent than its phenothiazine homologs.

C. Butyrophenone Derivatives: This rapidly growing group, of which haloperidol is the most

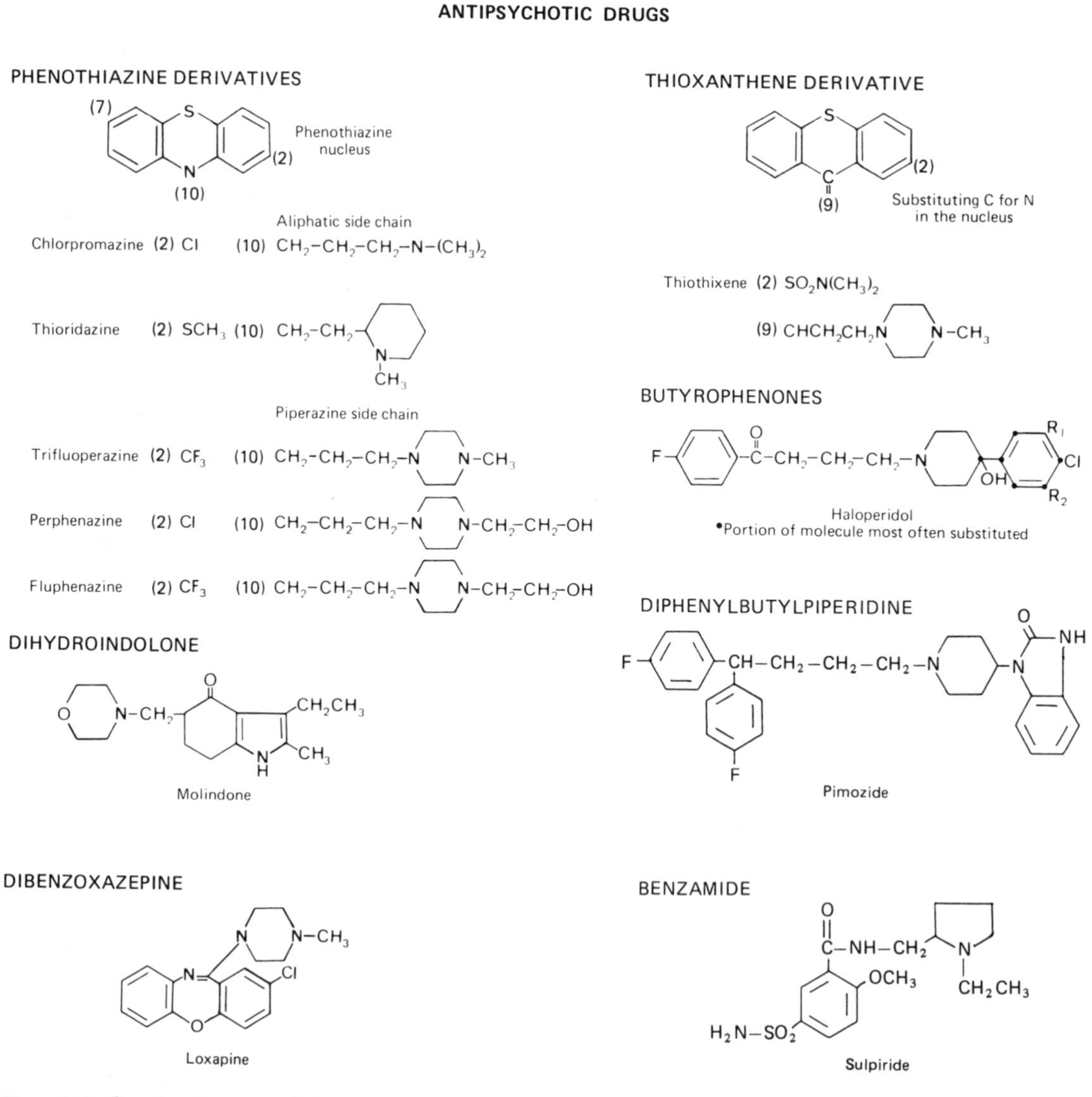

ANTIPSYCHOTIC DRUGS

Figure 27–2. Structural formulas of phenothiazines, thioxanthenes, butyrophenones, and a miscellaneous group of antipsychotics. Only representative members of each type are shown.

widely used, has a very different structure from those of the 2 preceding groups. Diphenylbutylpiperidines are closely related compounds.

D. Miscellaneous Structures: These include dihydroindolone derivatives (molindone), some tricyclic structures with a 6–7–6 ring structure (loxapine), and a benzamide (sulpiride) that is related to metoclopramide.

Pharmacokinetics

A. Metabolism: Chlorpromazine may have one of the most complicated routes of metabolism of any drug, with 60 or so identified metabolites. Various routes include nuclear transformations of the tricyclic portion (hydroxylations with subsequent conjugation as well as sulfoxidation of the sulfur atom) and transformations of the aliphatic side chain (demethylations, N-oxidation, and deamination). Some of the metabolites may be active, especially the 7-hydroxy metabolite.

Thioridazine produces 2 active metabolites, mesoridazine and sulforidazine, both from sulfoxidations on the thiomethyl ring substituent. Ring sulfoxidation results in an inactive metabolite. Trifluoperazine has metabolic pathways similar to those of chlorpromazine, with the addition of opening of the piperazine moiety and formation of a free amine. The thioxanthenes are metabolized like the phenothiazines. Metabolism of haloperidol involves N-dealkylation, oxidation, and conjugation. Although an active hydroxy metabolite is formed, its concentrations are inconsequential.

B. Distribution and Excretion: Most antipsychotics are highly lipid-soluble and protein-bound (92–99%). Thus, they tend to have large volumes of distribution (usually more than 7 L/kg). Bioavailability following oral administration is quite variable, tending to be low (25–35%) with drugs such as chlorpromazine that are extensively metabolized and higher with drugs such as haloperidol (50–85%) that have simpler metabolic pathways. The plasma half-lives tend to be short, ranging from 10 to 20 hours, but the clinical duration of the antipsychotic action is much longer than the short plasma half-life would indicate. Urinary metabolites of chlorpromazine may be found weeks after the last dose of chronically administered drug, suggesting that a large amount of the drug is sequestered in tissues. The importance of active metabolites in determining the clinical effects of these drugs is not known.

Pharmacologic Effects

A. Effects on Dopaminergic Synapses: Experiments showing block of dopamine's effects on electrical activity in central synapses, production of cAMP by adenylate cyclase, and specific receptor binding all suggest that these drugs should be considered **dopamine antagonists.** Blockade of postsynaptic dopamine receptors in the mesolimbic system of the brain probably accounts for their ability to ameliorate schizophrenia, while the same action in the nigrostriatal pathway may account for the unwanted parkinsonism symptoms that result from prolonged administration (Fig 27–3A). Blockade of dopamine receptors in the tuberoinfundibular dopamine pathway releases prolactin from the tonic inhibitory control of dopamine, resulting in hyperprolactinemia. Thus, the same pharmacodynamic action may have distinct psychiatric, neurologic, and endocrine consequences.

Despite their ability to block postsynaptic dopamine receptors, these drugs are only partially effective in schizophrenia. Furthermore, their effects can be easily antagonized by administering dopamine precursors, such as levodopa, or dopamine receptor agonists, such as apomorphine. These findings suggest either that dopamine receptor blockade is incomplete or that part of the antipsychotic action is due to some other mechanism, possibly in conjunction with the effect at dopamine synapses.

With continued use of antipsychotics, some pa-

A. Postsynaptic dopamine receptor block by antipsychotic drugs

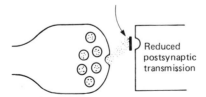

Antipsychotic effects (mesolimbic)

Extrapyramidal reactions (nigrostriatal)

B. Denervation supersensitivity

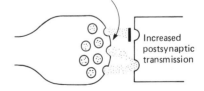

Initial disappearance of Parkinson's syndrome

Onset of tardive dyskinesia

Figure 27–3. *A:* Postsynaptic dopamine receptor blockade by antipsychotic drugs produces 2 actions: antipsychotic effects and extrapyramidal reactions. *B:* Continued treatment is thought to lead to increased dopamine stores and turnover presynaptically, and new and supersensitive receptors postsynaptically. Compensatory mechanisms may eliminate initial extrapyramidal reactions (parkinsonism), but if overcompensation occurs, the symptoms may be replaced by those of tardive dyskinesia. (Reproduced, with permission, from Hollister LE: *Clinical Pharmacology of Psychotherapeutic Drugs,* 2nd ed. Monographs in Clinical Pharmacology. Vol 1. Churchill Livingstone, 1983.)

tients develop supersensitivity of dopamine receptors, especially in the nigrostriatal system, that leads to the clinical manifestation called **tardive dyskinesia,** characterized by choreoathetoid movements resembling those associated with Huntington's disease. This change apparently occurs as a compensatory mechanism against the blockade of dopamine receptors (Fig 27–3B). Whether such supersensitivity of receptors in the mesolimbic system leads to tolerance to the antipsychotic effects of these drugs is still under investigation.

B. Effects on Other Neurotransmitters: Although some antipsychotics have antiserotonin or antiadrenoceptor actions, it is uncertain how these contribute to the therapeutic effects. Some investigators have suggested that the antiadrenoceptor action may be related to their ability to control excitement as well as their peripheral effects such as orthostatic hypotension. Many antipsychotics also show evidence of central blockade of histamine H_1 receptors, an action that may relate to their sedative effects. All have varying degrees of antimuscarinic action, thioridazine being most potent. This action may reduce the intensity of parkinsonism, but it is also manifested peripherally by many common side effects, such as dry mouth, blurred vision, constipation, and difficulty in urination. Some of these effects are summarized in Table 27–1.

C. Psychologic Effects: Most antipsychotic drugs cause unpleasant reactions in nonpsychotic individuals; the combination of sleepiness, restlessness, and autonomic effects creates experiences unlike those associated with more familiar sedatives or hypnotics. Performance is impaired as judged by a number of psychomotor and psychometric tests. Such responses occur in nonpsychotic persons. Psychotic individuals, on the other hand, may actually show improvement in their performance as the psychosis is alleviated.

D. Neurophysiologic Effects: Antipsychotic drugs produce shifts in the pattern of electroencephalographic frequencies, chiefly in the direction of

Table 27–1. Unwanted pharmacologic effects of antipsychotic drugs.

Type	Manifestations	Mechanism
Autonomic nervous system	Loss of accommodation, dry mouth, difficulty urinating, constipation.	Muscarinic cholinoceptor blockade.
	Orthostatic hypotension, impotence, failure to ejaculate.	Alpha-adrenoceptor blockade.
Central nervous system	Parkinson's syndrome, akathisia, dystonias.	Dopamine receptor blockade.
	Tardive dyskinesia.	Supersensitivity of dopamine receptors.
	Toxic-confusional state.	Muscarinic blockade.
Endocrine system	Amenorrhea-galactorrhea, infertility, impotence.	Dopamine receptor blockade resulting in hyperprolactinemia.

slowing and increased synchronization. The slowing (hypersynchrony) is sometimes focal or unilateral, which may lead to erroneous diagnostic interpretations. Both the frequency and the amplitude changes induced by psychotropic drugs are readily apparent and can be quantitated by sophisticated electronic techniques.

Electroencephalographic changes associated with antipsychotic drugs appear first in subcortical electrodes, supporting the view that their chief action is exerted at subcortical sites. The hypersynchrony produced by these drugs may account for their activating effect on the EEG in epileptic patients, as well as their occasional elicitation of seizures in patients with no history of seizure disorders.

E. Endocrine Effects: Antipsychotic drugs produce striking side effects on the reproductive system. Amenorrhea-galactorrhea, false-positive pregnancy tests, and increased libido have been reported in women, whereas men have been troubled by decreased libido and gynecomastia. Some of these effects are secondary to loss of the tonic inhibition of prolactin secretion by dopamine; others may be due to increased peripheral conversion of androgens to estrogens.

F. Cardiovascular Effects: Orthostatic hypotension and high resting pulse rates frequently result from use of the "high-dose" phenothiazines. Mean arterial pressure, peripheral resistance, and stroke volume are decreased, and pulse rate is increased. These are predictable from the autonomic actions of these agents (Table 27–1).

Abnormal ECGs have been observed, especially with thioridazine. Changes include prolongation of the QT interval and abnormal configurations of the ST segment and T waves, the latter being rounded, flattened, or notched. These changes are readily reversible upon withdrawal of the drug.

G. Animal Screening Tests: Inhibition of conditioned (but not unconditioned) avoidance behavior is one of the tests most predictive of antipsychotic action. Another is the inhibition of amphetamine- or apomorphine-induced stereotyped behavior. This inhibition no doubt is related to the dopamine receptor-blocking action of the drugs, countering these 2 dopamine agonists. Other tests that may predict antipsychotic action are reduction of exploratory behavior without undue sedation, induction of a cataleptic state, inhibition of intracranial stimulation of reward areas, and prevention of apomorphine-induced vomiting. It is difficult to relate most of these tests to any model of clinical psychosis.

II. CLINICAL PHARMACOLOGY OF ANTIPSYCHOTIC DRUGS

Indications

A. Psychiatric Indications: Schizophrenia is the primary indication for these drugs, which presently constitute the only clearly efficacious treatment. Unfortunately, some patients do not respond at all, and virtually none show a complete response. Because some schizophrenics have a favorable course with prolonged remission after an initial episode, most physicians recommend discontinuing drug therapy after remission has been achieved following the first episode.

Schizoaffective disorders may be more similar to affective disorders than to schizophrenia. Nonetheless, the psychotic aspects of the illness require treatment with antipsychotics, which may be used in combination with other drugs, such as antidepressants or lithium.

The manic episode in bipolar affective disorder is most effectively treated with antipsychotics, although lithium alone may suffice in milder cases. As mania subsides, the antipsychotic drug may be withdrawn. Nonmanic excited states may also be managed by antipsychotics, but attempts to define the diagnosis should not be abandoned.

Psychoses associated with old age, notably Alzheimer's disease, may show some symptomatic improvement with antipsychotics. Disturbed behavior, emotional lability, and abnormal sleep-wake cycles may be improved, but the basic disorder is untouched.

Gilles de la Tourette's syndrome, characterized by unpredictable barking tics and outbursts of foul language, has been successfully managed with haloperidol and pimozide.

The use of antipsychotics as primary treatment for depression is controversial. Because of the danger of tardive dyskinesia, most clinicians would use them only adjunctively in patients with agitated or psychotic depressions.

Acute brain syndromes during withdrawal from alcohol or other drugs should not be treated with antipsychotics. Substitution of a pharmacologically equivalent drug, stabilization on that drug, and subsequent gradual withdrawal are the time-honored principles of management. Acute adverse reactions associated with the use of other social drugs may be aggravated by antipsychotics but can be managed with simple sedatives. Overdoses of amphetamine and related stimulants are best managed with haloperidol, which is also likely to help the delirium of medically or surgically ill patients.

Antipsychotics in small doses have been (wrongly) promoted for relief of anxiety associated with minor emotional disorders. The antianxiety sedatives (Chapter 20) are far better in every respect, including safety and acceptability to patients.

B. Nonpsychiatric Indications: Most antipsychotic drugs, with the exception of thioridazine, have a strong antiemetic effect. This action is due to dopamine receptor blockade, both centrally (in the chemoreceptor trigger zone of the medulla) and peripherally (on receptors in the stomach). Some drugs, such as prochlorperazine and benzquinamide, are promoted solely as antiemetics. Phenothiazines with shorter side chains have considerable H_1 receptor-

blocking action and have been used for relief of pruritus or, in the case of promethazine, as preoperative sedatives. The butyrophenone droperidol is used in combination with a meperidinelike drug, fentanyl, in "neuroleptanesthesia." The use of these drugs for nonpsychiatric indications is described in Chapter 23.

Choice of Drug

A rational choice of antipsychotic drugs may be based on differences between chemical structures and the attendant pharmacologic differences, since the differences between groups are greater than the differences within groups. Thus, one might choose to be familiar with one member of each of the 3 subfamilies of phenothiazines, a member of the thioxanthene and butyrophenone group, and perhaps 2 members of the miscellaneous group. A possible selection is shown in Table 27–2.

No basis exists for choosing drugs for use against "target symptoms," as there is no evidence of specificity in their effects. The physician whose practice often or sometimes requires prescribing drugs for long-term managment of psychotic disorders does not need to know all of the drugs but should become familiar with the effects—including the side effects—of one or 2 drugs in each class. The best guide for selecting a drug for individual patients is their past responses to drugs. The trend in recent years has been away from the "low-potency" agents such as chlorpromazine and thioridazine to the "high-potency" drugs such as thiothixene, haloperidol, and fluphenazine. Chlorpromazine, in fact, should probably now be considered obsolete in view of its high incidence of side effects (see below).

Doses

The range of effective doses among various antipsychotics is quite broad. Even with individual drugs in each class, a wide range of doses may be used, since therapeutic margins are substantial. Assuming that doses are equivalent, there is no evidence that any antipsychotic drug is superior in overall efficacy to any other. However some patients who fail to respond to one drug may respond to another, and for this reason, several drugs may have to be tried to find the one most effective for an individual patient. Some seemingly refractory patients have responded to larger-than-usual doses of the more potent antipsychotics, such as 100 mg/d of haloperidol or 200–300 mg/d of thiothixene. Before it is concluded that a patient will not respond to drug therapy, such doses should be tried on an experimental basis.

Some dose relationships between various antipsychotic drugs, as well as possible therapeutic ranges, are shown in Table 27–3.

Plasma Concentrations & Clinical Effects

Attempts to define a therapeutic range of plasma concentrations of antipsychotic agents are beset by many difficulties. A range of 150–300 ng/mL has

Table 27–2. Some representative antipsychotic drugs.

Drug Class	Drug	Advantages	Disadvantages
Phenothiazines Aliphatic	Chlorpromazine[1]	Generic.	Many side effects; probably should not be used (obsolete).
Piperidine	Thioridazine[2] (Mellaril)	Slight extrapyramidal syndrome.	800 mg/d limit; no parenteral form; (?) cardiotoxicity.
Piperazine	Fluphenazine[3] (Permitil, Prolixin)	Depot form also available (enanthate, decanoate).	(?) Increased tardive dyskinesia.
Thioxanthene	Thiothixene[4] (Navane)	Parenteral form also available; (?) decreased tardive dyskinesia.	Uncertain.
Butyrophenone	Haloperidol (Haldol)	Parenteral form also available.	Severe extrapyramidal syndrome.
Dibenzoxazepine	Loxapine (Loxitane)	(?) No weight gain.	Uncertain.
Dihydroindolone	Molindone (Moban)	(?) No weight gain.	Uncertain.

[1]Other aliphatic phenothiazines: promazine (Sparine, generic); triflupromazine (Vesprin).
[2]Other piperidine phenothiazines: piperacetazine (Quide), mesoridazine (Lidanar, Serentil).
[3]Other piperazine phenothiazines: acetophenazine (Tindal), perphenazine (Trilafon), carphenazine (Proketazine), prochlorperazine (Compazine, generic), trifluoperazine (Stelazine).
[4]Other thioxanthenes: chlorprothixene (Taractan).

been suggested for chlorpromazine, but the evidence is tenuous. Ranges of 7–20 ng/mL have been suggested for haloperidol, although some very refractory patients may benefit from levels up to 50 ng/mL. Clinical monitoring of plasma concentrations of these drugs, although technically feasible, is not warranted at this time.

Pharmaceutical Preparations

Well-tolerated parenteral forms of the high-potency drugs are available for rapid initiation of treatment as well as for maintenance treatment in noncompliant patients. Since the parenterally administered drugs may have much greater bioavailability than the oral forms, doses should be only a fraction of what might be given orally. Fluphenazine decanoate is the drug most widely used for parenteral maintenance

therapy. A single intramuscular dose of this drug may be adequate for long periods (1–4 weeks). However, the release characteristics of such preparations are somewhat uncertain. While their value in maintenance treatment is established for noncompliant patients, these preparations offer no advantage over oral doses in compliant patients. Thus, they should not be used routinely.

Dosage Schedules

Antipsychotics may be given in divided daily doses initially while an effective dose level is being sought. They need not always be equally divided doses, even when given orally. After an effective daily dose has been defined for an individual patient, doses can be given less frequently. Once-daily doses, usually given at night, are feasible for many patients during chronic maintenance treatment. Simplification of dosage schedules leads to better compliance. Maximum dose units of many drugs are being increased by manufacturers to meet the needs of once-daily dosing.

Table 27–3. Dose relationships of antipsychotics.

	Minimum Effective Therapeutic Dose (mg)	Usual Range of Daily Doses (mg)
Chlorpromazine (Thorazine)	100	100–1000
Thioridazine (Mellaril)	100	100–800
Mesoridazine (Lidanar, Serentil)	50	50–400
Piperacetazine (Quide)	10	20–160
Trifluoperazine (Stelazine)	5	5–60
Perphenazine (Trilafon)	10	8–64
Fluphenazine (Permitil, Prolixin)	2	2–20
Thiothixene (Navane)	2	2–120
Haloperidol (Haldol)	2	2–20
Loxapine (Loxitane)	10	20–160
Molindone (Lidone, Moban)	10	20–200

Benefits & Limitations of Drug Treatment

The impact of these drugs on psychiatry and on psychiatric patients has been great. First, they have shifted the care of patients from mental institutions to the community. For many patients, this shift has provided a more meaningful life under more humane circumstances. For others, the tragedy of a fruitless life is now being played out in the streets of our inner cities rather than in mental institutions.

Second, they have markedly shifted psychiatric thinking to a more biologic orientation. Despite a great amount of research done by highly competent persons from many disciplines, schizophrenia remains as much a scientific mystery and a personal disaster as ever. While most schizophrenic patients obtain some degree of benefit from these drugs, none are well.

Maintenance Treatment

A small minority of schizophrenic patients may remit from an acute episode and require no further drug therapy for prolonged periods. In most cases, however, schizophrenia is a chronic disorder that only partially remits, so that drug therapy must be continued indefinitely.

One issue is whether treatment should be continuous or intermittent. Advocates of "drug holidays" maintain that once remission has been achieved with drugs, many patients do not relapse for substantial periods after treatment is stopped, and that such interruptions in treatment diminish the total amount of exposure to drugs and lessen the likelihood of tardive dyskinesia. The contrary view is that there is no way of predicting who will relapse early; that it is better to maintain doses at minimal levels to reduce total exposure to drugs; and that rapid and unexpected relapse may undo much of the hard-won rehabilitative gains afforded by a good treatment program.

Drug Combinations

Combining antipsychotic drugs confounds evaluation of the efficacy of the drugs being used. Tricyclic antidepressants may be used with antipsychotics, but only for clear symptoms of depression complicating schizophrenia. They are of no proved efficacy for alleviating the social withdrawal and blunted affect of the psychotic. Lithium is sometimes added with benefit to antipsychotic agents when patients fail to respond to the latter drugs alone. It is uncertain whether such instances represent misdiagnosed cases of mania. Sedative drugs may be added for relief of anxiety or insomnia not controlled by antipsychotics.

The drugs most frequently combined with antipsychotics are antiparkinsonism agents (see below).

Adverse Reactions

Most of the unwanted effects of antipsychotics are extensions of their known pharmacologic actions, but a few are allergic and some are idiosyncratic.

A. Behavioral Effects: Antipsychotic drugs are unpleasant to take—the more so the less psychotic the patient. Many patients stop taking their drug because of the unpleasant side effects, which may be mitigated by giving small doses during the day and the major portion at bedtime. A "pseudodepression" that may be due to akinesia from these drugs usually responds to treatment with antiparkinsonism drugs. Other "pseudodepressions" may be due to using higher doses than needed in a partially remitted patient, in which case decreasing the dose may relieve the symptoms. Toxic-confusional states may occur with very high doses of drugs that have prominent antimuscarinic actions. The development of supersensitivity of receptors that are blocked by the antipsychotic agents could result in tolerance to the drugs or even a drug-resistant form of psychosis. This is a matter of current concern.

B. Neurologic Effects: Extrapyramidal reactions occurring early during treatment include typical Parkinson's syndrome, akathisia (uncontrollable restlessness), and acute dystonic reactions (spastic retrocollis or torticollis). Parkinson's syndrome can be treated, when necessary, with conventional antiparkinsonism drugs of the antimuscarinic type or, in rare cases, by amantadine. Parkinson's syndrome may be self-limiting, so that an attempt to withdraw antiparkinsonism drugs should be made every 3–4 months. Akathisia and dystonic reactions will also respond to such treatment, but many prefer to use a sedative antihistamine with anticholinergic properties, eg, diphenhydramine, which can be given either parenterally or orally as capsules or elixir. Prophylactic use of oral diphenhydramine may be useful in patients at high risk of developing acute dystonic reactions, such as children or young adults being treated with substantial doses of high-potency drugs. Parenteral administration may be effective in reversing acute dystonia after it has occurred.

Tardive dyskinesia, as the name implies, is a late-occurring syndrome of abnormal choreoathetoid movements. It is the most important unwanted effect of antipsychotics. It has been proposed that it is caused by a relative cholinergic deficiency secondary to supersensitivity of dopamine receptors in the caudate-putamen. Older women treated for long periods are most susceptible to the disorder, although it can occur at any age and in either sex. The prevalence varies enormously, but tardive dyskinesia is estimated to occur in 20–40% of chronically treated patients. Early recognition is important, since advanced cases may be difficult to reverse. Many treatments have been proposed, but their evaluation is confounded by the fact that the course of the disorder is variable and sometimes self-limited. Most authorities agree that the first step would be to try to decrease dopamine receptor sensitivity by discontinuing the antipsychotic drug or by reducing the dose. A logical second step would be to eliminate all drugs with central anticholinergic action, particularly antiparkinsonism drugs and tricyclic antidepressants. These 2 steps are often enough to bring about improvement. If they fail, the addition of diazepam in doses as high as 30–40 mg/d may add to the response. The use of reserpine may also be considered, although one runs the risk of increasing receptor sensitivity. Other treatments that have been proposed include precursors of acetylcholine, such as lecithin or choline, propranolol, lithium, and many others.

C. Autonomic Nervous System Effects: Most patients become tolerant to the antimuscarinic side effects of antipsychotic drugs. Those who are made too uncomfortable or who are impaired, as with urinary retention, should be given bethanechol, a peripherally acting cholinomimetic. Orthostatic hypotension or impaired ejaculation, common complications of therapy with chlorpromazine or mesoridazine, should be managed by switching to drugs with less marked adrenoceptor-blocking actions.

D. Metabolic and Endocrine Effects: Weight gain is common and requires monitoring of food intake. Hyperprolactinemia in women results in the amenorrhea-galactorrhea syndrome and infertility;

in men, loss of libido, impotence, and infertility may result.

E. Toxic or Allergic Reactions: Agranulocytosis is no longer a major risk except with low-potency drugs, eg, chlorpromazine. Clozapine, a promising drug several years ago, produced the greatest epidemic of drug-induced agranulocytosis in medical history and is now seldom used. Cholestatic jaundice is now rare, even with chlorpromazine.

F. Ocular Complications: Deposits in the anterior portion of the eye (cornea and lens) are a common complication of chlorpromazine therapy. They may accentuate the normal processes of aging of the lens. Thioridazine is the only antipsychotic drug that causes retinal deposits, which in advanced cases may resemble retinitis pigmentosa. The deposits are usually associated with "browning" of vision. The maximum daily dose of thioridazine has been limited to 800 mg/d to reduce the possibility of this complication.

G. Cardiac Toxicity: Thioridazine in doses exceeding 300 mg daily is almost always associated with minor abnormalities of T waves that are easily reversible. Overdoses of thioridazine are associated with major ventricular arrhythmias, cardiac conduction block, and sudden death; it is not certain whether thioridazine can cause these same disorders when used in therapeutic doses. In view of possible additive antimuscarinic and quinidinelike actions with various tricyclic antidepressants, thioridazine should not be combined with the latter drugs.

H. Use in Pregnancy; Dysmorphogenesis: Although the antipsychotic drugs appear to be relatively safe in pregnancy, a small increase in risk could be missed. Questions about whether to use these drugs during pregnancy and whether to abort a pregnancy in which the fetus has already been exposed must be decided individually.

I. Malignant Neuroleptic Syndrome: This complication of treatment appears to be an idiosyncratic response. It often follows an initial large dose of antipsychotic drug. High fever, mutism, extrapyramidal disturbances, and autonomic signs are characteristic. Death occurs unless cooling and rehydration are prompt and vigorous. Dantrolene, a skeletal muscle relaxant, has been reported to be effective in this type of hyperthermia (see p 304). Bromocriptine, a dopamine agonist, has also been used successfully, suggesting that the mechanism of the syndrome is underactivity of dopaminergic systems. This syndrome is somewhat different from the "heat stroke" that may occur during chronic treatment with these drugs during periods of high ambient temperature.

Unconventional Drugs

The efficacy of propranolol as treatment for schizophrenia remains uncertain after 15 years of study. Patients with marked agitation, hostility, and belligerence may be controlled by the addition of propranolol to conventional antipsychotic drugs. High-dose treatment with diazepam may control disturbed behavior, just as amobarbital sodium did 35 years ago.

Levodopa, thyrotropin-releasing hormone, endorphins, and apomorphine have been ineffective. Megavitamin therapy has been discredited scientifically, but adherents still persist.

Drug Interactions

Pharmacodynamic interactions are more frequent than pharmacokinetic ones and are of greater importance clinically. The most important pharmacodynamic interaction of the antipsychotics is an additive depressant effect when they are used along with various other central nervous system depressants. Such drugs include conventional sedative-hypnotics, antihistamines, opiates, and alcohol. Neuroleptics have relatively little respiratory depressant action when taken by themselves, but they may have a modest additive effect when taken with other drugs that also depress respiration.

Autonomic interactions can be largely predicted from their antimuscarinic and alpha-blocking actions. In addition, chlorpromazine may reverse the antihypertensive effects of drugs that work on sympathetic neurons, such as guanethidine, clonidine, bethanidine, debrisoquin, and possibly methyldopa.

Thioridazine has quinidinelike effects perhaps related to its cardiotoxicity. Other drugs with such actions include quinidine and procainamide, tricyclic antidepressants, and hydroxyzine. The use of thioridazine with any of these classes of drugs should be avoided.

Pharmacokinetic interactions are of less importance. Colloidal antacids, kaolin, and activated charcoal adsorb chlorpromazine and probably also other phenothiazines and tricyclic antidepressants. It would seem desirable to separate by at least 1–2 hours the ingestion of such antacids and the subsequent administration of any drug.

The hydroxylation of imipramine and nortriptyline is inhibited by chlorpromazine, perphenazine, haloperidol, chlorprothixene, and thioridazine, and the reverse is true to some extent. Thus, concurrent administration of both types of drugs may lead to elevated plasma concentrations of both. This interaction—at least between nortriptyline and perphenazine—seems to occur only with large doses of either drug.

A possible interaction between phenothiazines (specifically thioridazine) and phenytoin might be of greater consequence. Inhibition of metabolism of phenytoin, which has a narrow therapeutic range, has led to serious clinical toxicity.

Overdoses

Poisonings with antipsychotics are rarely fatal, with the exception of those due to mesoridazine and thioridazine. In general, drowsiness proceeds to coma, with an intervening period of agitation. Neuromuscular excitability may be increased and proceed to convulsions. Pupils are miotic, and deep tendon reflexes are decreased. Hypotension and hypothermia are the rule, although fever may be present later in the course. The lethal effects of mesoridazine and thioridazine are related to their actions on the heart.

Patients should be monitored in an intensive care setting for the usual vital signs, venous pressure, arterial blood gases, and electrolytes. Attempts at gastric lavage should be made even if several hours have elapsed since the drug was taken, since gastrointestinal motility is decreased. Activated charcoal effectively binds most of these drugs, following which a saline cathartic may be given. Hypotension often responds to fluid replacement. If a pressor agent is to be used, norepinephrine or dopamine is preferred to epinephrine, whose unopposed β-adrenoceptor–stimulant action in the presence of alpha blockade may cause vasodilatation. Seizures may be treated with either diazepam or phenytoin, the latter being given with an initial loading dose. Management of overdoses of thioridazine and mesoridazine, which are complicated by cardiac arrhythmias, is similar to that for tricyclic antidepressants (Chapter 28).

LITHIUM

Lithium is often referred to as an "antimanic" drug, but some cases of depression also seem to respond. In many parts of the world, lithium is referred to as a "mood-stabilizing" agent because of its primary action of preventing mood swings in patients with bipolar affective (manic-depressive) disorder. Other drugs possibly effective in preventing mood swings include carbamazepine, clonidine, and spironolactone.

Nature of Bipolar Affective Disorder

Bipolar affective (manic-depressive) disorder is a frequently diagnosed and very serious emotional disorder. Patients with cyclic attacks of mania have many symptoms of paranoid schizophrenia (grandiosity, bellicosity, paranoid thoughts, and overactivity). The gratifying response to lithium therapy of patients with bipolar disorder has made such diagnostic distinctions important.

Bipolar disorder has a strong genetic component and seems to be biologically determined. The episodes of mood swings are generally unrelated to life events. The exact biologic disturbance has not been identified, but a preponderance of catecholamine-related activity is thought to be present. Drugs that increase this activity tend to exacerbate mania, whereas those that reduce activity of dopamine or norepinephrine relieve mania. Acetylcholine may also be involved. The nature of the abrupt switch from mania to depression experienced by some patients is uncertain.

Drugs for Bipolar Affective Disorder

When mania is mild, lithium alone may be effective treatment. In more severe cases, it is almost always necessary to give one of the antipsychotic drugs also. After mania is controlled, the antipsychotic drug

may be stopped and lithium continued as maintenance therapy.

Unlike antipsychotic or antidepressant drugs, which exert several actions on the central or autonomic nervous system, lithium ion produces only mild sedation and is devoid of autonomic blocking effects. Since it is a small inorganic ion, lithium is easily measured in body fluids such as plasma, urine, or saliva, is distributed in body water, and is not metabolized. Thus, its kinetics can be studied much more easily, and plasma or tissue concentrations can be correlated with clinical effects. A third attribute of considerable interest has been the prophylactic use of lithium in preventing both mania and depression. It is indeed remarkable that a so-called functional psychosis can be controlled so easily by such a simple chemical as lithium carbonate.

Lithium may be combined with antipsychotics when mania breaks through a prophylactic treatment program, or with antidepressants when depression becomes apparent. Although haloperidol was alleged to be a poor drug to combine with lithium, it seems in retrospect to be no different from other neuroleptics. All neuroleptics may produce more severe extrapyramidal syndromes when combined with lithium.

Carbamazepine has emerged as a reasonable alternative to lithium when the latter is less than optimal. It may be used not only to treat acute mania but also for prophylactic therapy. Side effects are no greater and sometimes are less than those associated with lithium. The mode of action of carbamazepine is unclear, but it may reduce the sensitization of the brain to repeated episodes of mood swing. Such a mechanism might be similar to its anticonvulsant effect. Doses are similar to those used for treating epilepsy—roughly 800–1000 mg/d.

I. BASIC PHARMACOLOGY OF LITHIUM

No single mechanism accounts for the therapeutic effect of lithium. Its effects on neurotransmitters, cell membranes, cations, and water have been the major avenues of inquiry.

Lithium is thought to accelerate the presynaptic destruction of catecholamines, to inhibit release of transmitters at the synapse, and to decrease the sensitivity of the postsynaptic receptor. All of these actions would tend to correct the overactivity of catecholaminergic systems presumed to occur in mania. However, many of these actions of lithium are acute and have not been demonstrated to be sustained during chronic treatment.

Presynaptic and postsynaptic regulation of neurotransmission is intimately involved with various cations of physiologic importance, eg, sodium, potassium, magnesium, and calcium. Neurotransmitter release is probably calcium-dependent, while the con-

Table 27–4. Pharmacokinetics of lithium.

Absorption	Rapid. Virtually complete within 6–8 hours; peak plasma levels in 30 minutes to 2 hours.
Distribution	In total body water; slow entry into intracellular compartment. Apparent volumes of distribution of 0.5–0.9 L/kg body weight; some sequestration in bone. No protein binding.
Metabolism	None.
Excretion	Virtually entirely in urine. Lithium clearance about 20% of creatinine. Plasma half-life about 20 hours.

figuration of postsynaptic receptors may be altered by sodium. The passage of lithium into cells, where it exerts its major action, is intimately concerned with these ions as well.

Both calcium and magnesium are required for stabilization of cell membranes, tending to make them less fluid. Displacement by lithium of either calcium or magnesium might increase membrane permeability.

In extracellular fluid, lithium acts similarly to potassium and stimulates sodium efflux from cells, both by cation exchange and by stimulation of the Na^+-K^+ pump mechanism. Lithium also enhances the entry of choline into cells, but the significance of this action is uncertain.

The rather simple pharmacokinetic properties of lithium are summarized in Table 27–4.

II. CLINICAL PHARMACOLOGY OF LITHIUM

Bipolar Affective Disorder

Agreement is almost universal that lithium carbonate is the preferred treatment for bipolar disorder, especially in the manic phase. Because its onset of action is slow, concurrent use of antipsychotic drugs may be required for severely manic patients. The success rate for attaining remission from the manic phase of bipolar disorder is about 60–80%. Maintenance (prophylactic) therapy in patients with classic bipolar disorder is now well accepted. In general, control with maintenance lithium is about 60% effective.

Some clinicians find that depressive episodes during typical bipolar illness may respond better when a tricyclic antidepressant is added to lithium maintenance during this period. Rapidly cycling manic-depressive episodes have been linked to treatment with tricyclic antidepressants. Carbamazepine may be useful in such situations, or in those patients whose manic episodes are not controlled by lithium alone.

Other Applications

Acute endogenous depression is not generally considered to be an indication for treatment with lithium. On the other hand, recurrent endogenous depressions with a cyclic pattern are controlled by lithium and imipramine, both of which are superior to a placebo.

Schizoaffective disorders are characterized by a mixture of schizophrenic symptoms and altered affect in the form of depression or excitement. Antipsychotic drugs alone or combined with lithium are used in the excited phase; tricyclic antidepressants are used if depression is present.

Alcoholism is commonly believed to have a high association with depression and mania. When the 2 conditions exist, lithium may be useful in reducing drinking. Lithium has no established efficacy in the absence of affective symptoms.

Lithium is not regarded as useful for schizophrenia. Whether lithium added to antipsychotic drugs can enhance their efficacy in ordinary schizophrenia is an unsettled question.

An interesting application of lithium currently being investigated is the management of aggressive, violent behavior in prisoners. These men, both in and out of prison, have explosive responses to minimal provocation, possible brain damage with nonspecific abnormal EEGs, and long histories of violent criminal behavior. Sufficient studies are available to suggest that this may be an important indication for the use of lithium.

Doses & Dosage Schedules

Before treatment is started, one should obtain laboratory data such as a complete blood count, urinalysis, common biochemical tests, tests of thyroid function, and an ECG. Patients over 50 years of age should also have a creatinine clearance test. These tests serve as baseline measurements in assessing possible complications of treatment.

The patient's age and body weight and renal function should be considered in determining initial appropriate doses of lithium carbonate. The initial volume of distribution of lithium will be the same as body water, or about 0.5 L/kg body weight for women and 0.55 L/kg for men. The proportion of body water may decrease slightly in older individuals. What is more important in older patients is a subtle decrease in renal function. Any patient over 50 years of age is likely to have a decreased creatinine clearance, which may reach 50% or less of the usual normal values without abnormal elevation of serum creatinine.

A daily lithium dose of 0.5 meq/kg will produce the desired serum lithium concentration in the range of 0.9–1.4 meq/L after a week of treatment if renal function is normal. Each 300-mg dose unit of lithium carbonate contains approximately 8 meq of lithium. Daily doses of lithium may range between 600 and 3600 mg among different individuals. The majority require between 1500 and 1800 mg/d.

It is almost always necessary to give lithium in divided doses to avoid gastric distress. Medication is best taken with or shortly after meals.

Monitoring Treatment

Clinicians have relied heavily on measurements of

plasma concentrations for assessing both the dose required for satisfactory treatment of acute mania and the adequacy of maintenance treatment. These measurements are customarily taken 10–12 hours after the last dose, so all data in the literature pertaining to these concentrations reflect this interval.

An initial determination of serum lithium concentration should be obtained about 5 days after start of treatment, at which time steady-state conditions should obtain for the dose chosen. If the clinical response suggests a change in dosage, a simple arithmetic adjustment (present dose times desired blood level divided by present blood level) should produce the desired level. The serum concentration attained with the adjusted dose can be checked in another 5 days. Once the desired concentration has been achieved, levels can be measured at increasing intervals unless intercurrent illness or the introduction of a new drug into the treatment program intervenes.

Maintenance Treatment

The decision to use lithium as *prophylactic* treatment depends on many factors: the frequency and severity of previous episodes, a crescendo pattern of appearance, and the degree to which the patient is willing to follow a program of indefinite maintenance therapy. If the present attack was the patient's first or if the patient is unreliable, one might prefer to terminate treatment after it has subsided. Patients who have one or more episodes of illness per year are candidates for maintenance treatment. Maintenance treatment can often be achieved with lower levels than those required initially, probably as low as 0.5–0.6 meq/L.

Drug Interactions

Renal clearance of lithium is reduced about 25% in the presence of oral diuretics, and doses may have to be reduced by a similar amount. A similar reduction in lithium clearance has been noted with several of the newer nonsteroidal anti-inflammatory drugs that block synthesis of prostaglandins. It is not known whether this interaction extends to aspirin.

Side Effects & Complications

Many side effects associated with lithium treatment occur at varying times after treatment is started. Some are harmless, but it is important to be alert to side effects that may signify impending serious toxic reactions.

A. Neurologic and Psychiatric Side Effects: Tremor is one of the most frequent side effects of lithium treatment, occurring at therapeutic dose levels. Propranolol, which has been reported to be effective in essential tremor, also alleviates lithium-induced tremor. Other neurologic abnormalities that have been reported include choreoathetosis, motor hyperactivity, ataxia, dysarthria, and aphasia. Psychiatric disturbances are generally marked by mental confusion and withdrawal or bizarre motor movements. Appearance of any new neurologic or psychiatric symptoms or signs is a clear indication for temporarily

stopping treatment with lithium and close monitoring of serum levels.

B. Effects on Thyroid Function: Lithium probably decreases thyroid function in most patients exposed to the drug, but the effect is reversible or nonprogressive. Some patients develop frank thyroid enlargement, but only about 15% show symptoms of hypothyroidism.

C. Renal Side Effects: Polydipsia and polyuria are frequent but reversible concomitants of lithium treatment, occurring at therapeutic serum concentrations. The principal physiologic lesion involved is loss of the ability of the distal tubule to conserve water under the influence of antidiuretic hormone, resulting in excessive free water clearance. Resistance of lithium-induced **nephrogenic diabetes insipidus** to vasopressin has led to other attempts at therapy. Thiazide diuretics may be used, but the dose of lithium should be reduced by about 25% if such treatment is started.

An extensive literature has been concerned with **chronic interstitial nephritis** during long-term lithium therapy. The damage to the renal interstitium seems to be dependent both on the serum lithium concentration and the duration of treatment. However, similar changes have been found in manic-depressive patients who have not received lithium.

Although the kidney tubule is most vulnerable to lithium, the glomerulus has been involved in a few cases of **minimal change glomerulopathy** with nephrotic syndrome. Some instances of decreased glomerular filtration rate have been encountered but no instances of marked azotemia or renal failure.

Patients receiving lithium should avoid dehydration with the consequent increased concentration of lithium in urine. Periodic tests of renal concentrating ability should be carried out to detect changes.

D. Edema: Edema is a frequent side effect of lithium treatment and may be related to some effect of lithium on sodium retention. Although weight gain may be expected in patients who become edematous, water retention alone probably does not account for all of it.

E. Cardiac Side Effects: Reduced amplitude of T waves is a frequent finding during lithium treatment if the electrocardiographic tracing is examined carefully. No evidence of myocardial damage can be found when enzyme tests are done during periods of T wave abnormality, and the effect seems to be readily reversible. The sinus node may also be susceptible to toxic effects of lithium, with depression of its normal pacemaker function. The drug is definitely contraindicated in the "sick sinus" syndrome.

F. Use During Pregnancy: Renal clearance of lithium increases during pregnancy and reverts to lower levels immediately after delivery. A patient whose serum lithium concentration is in a good therapeutic range during pregnancy may develop toxic levels following delivery. Special care in monitoring lithium levels is needed at these times. Lithium is transferred to nursing children through breast milk, in which it has a concentration about one-third to one-half that of serum. Lithium toxicity in newborns is manifested by lethargy, cyanosis, poor suck and Moro reflexes, and possibly hepatomegaly.

The issue of dysmorphogenesis is not settled. One report suggests an alarming increase in the frequency of cardiac anomalies, especially Ebstein's anomaly, in lithium babies.

G. Miscellaneous Side Effects: Transient acneiform eruptions have been noted early in lithium treatment. Some of them subside with temporary discontinuation of treatment and do not recur with its resumption. Folliculitis is less dramatic and probably occurs more frequently. Leukocytosis is always present during lithium treatment, probably reflecting a direct effect on leukopoiesis rather than mobilization from the marginal pool. This "side effect" has now become a therapeutic effect in patients with low leukocyte counts. Disturbed sexual function has been reported in men treated with lithium.

Overdoses

Therapeutic overdoses are more common than those due to deliberate or accidental ingestion of the drug. Therapeutic overdoses are usually due to accumulation of lithium resulting from some change in the patient's status, such as diminished serum sodium, use of diuretics, fluctuating renal function, or pregnancy. Since the tissues will have already equilibrated with the blood, the plasma concentrations of drugs may not be excessively high in proportion to the degree of toxicity; any value over 2 meq/L must be considered as indicating potential toxicity.

A primary consideration is to rid the patient of the drug. Because of the physically large amounts of drug involved in cases of acute deliberate overdosage (one may be dealing with 30–60 g), absorption is slow. Lavage should be done with a wide-bore tube, as the material tends to clump and may be difficult to remove through smaller tubes. Saline cathartics should follow lavage. Charcoal is not an effective adsorbent in this instance. As lithium is a small ion, it is dialyzed readily. Both peritoneal dialysis and hemodialysis are effective, though the latter is preferred. Dialysis should be continued until the plasma concentrations fall below the usual therapeutic range.

REFERENCES

Antipsychotics

Branchey MH et al: High- and low-potency neuroleptics in elderly psychiatric patients. *JAMA* 1978;**239**:1860.

Carlsson A: Antipsychotic drugs, neurotransmitters and schizophrenia. *Am J Psychiatry* 1978;**135**:164.

Carlton PL, Manowitz P: Dopamine and schizophrenia: An analysis of the theory. *Neurosci Biobehav Rev* 1984;**8**:137.

Chouinard G, Jones BD: Neuroleptic-induced supersensitivity psychosis: Clinical and pharmacologic characteristics. *Am J Psychiatry* 1980;**137**:16.

Crow TJ: Molecular pathology of schizophrenia: More than one disease process? *Br Med J* 1980;**280**:66.

Donlon PT, Tupin JP; Successful suicides with thioridazine and mesoridazine. *Arch Gen Psychiatry* 1977;**34**:955.

Hamblin M, Creese I: Receptor binding and the discovery of psychotherapeutic drugs. *Drug Dev Res* 1981;**1**:343.

Hashimoto F, Sherma CB, Jeffery WH: Neuroleptic malignant syndrome and dopaminergic blockade. *Arch Intern Med* 1984;**144**:629.

Hollister LE: Drug treatment of schizophrenia. *Psychiatr Clin North Am* 1984;**7**:435.

Lehmann HE, Wilson WH, Deutsch M: Minimal maintenance medication: Effects of three dose schedules on relapse rates and symptoms in chronic schizophrenic outpatients. *Compr Psychiatry* 1983;**24**:293.

O'Connor SE, Brown RA: The pharmacology of sulpiride: A dopamine receptor antagonist. *Gen Pharmacol* 1982;**13**:185.

Rome HP: The classification of schizophrenia: A historical review. *Psychiatr Ann* 1979;**9**:12.

Schooler NR et al: Prevention of relapse in schizophrenia. *Arch Gen Psychiatry* 1980;**37**:16.

Simpson GM, Pi EH, Stramek JJ Jr: Management of tardive dyskinesia: Current update. *Drugs* 1982;**23**:381.

Stevens JR: Schizophrenia and dopamine regulation in the mesolimbic system. *Trends Neurosci* 1979;**1**:102.

Tarsy D, Baldessarini RJ: The pathophysiologic basis of tardive dyskinesia. *Biol Psychiatry* 1977;**12**:431.

Thompson LT, Moran MG, Nies AS: Psychotropic drug use in the elderly. (2 parts.) *N Engl J Med* 1983;**308**:134, 194.

Lithium

Amdisen A: Serum lithium monitoring and clinical pharmacokinetics of lithium. *Clin Pharmacokinet* 1977;**2**:73.

Bunney WE Jr et al: Mode of action of lithium. Some biological considerations. *Arch Gen Psychiatry* 1979;**36**:898.

Goodwin FW (editor): Lithium ion. *Arch Gen Psychiatry* 1979;**36**:833.

Hansen HE: Renal toxicity of lithium. *Drugs* 1981;**22**:461.

Hansen HE, Amdisen A: Lithium intoxication: Report of 23 cases and review of 100 cases from the literature. *Q J Med* 1978;**186**:123.

Jefferson JW, Greist JH: *Primer of Lithium Therapy.* Williams & Wilkins, 1977.

Kishimoto A et al: Longterm prophylactic effects of carbamazepine in affective disorder. *Br J Psychiatry* 1983; **143**:327.

Prien RF et al: Drug therapy for the prevention of recurrences in unipolar and bipolar affective disorders: Report of the NIMH Collaborative Study Group comparing lithium carbonate, imipramine and a lithium carbonate-imipramine combination. *Arch Gen Psychiatry* 1984;**41**:1096.

Report of the APA Task Force: The current status of lithium therapy. *Am J Psychiatry* 1975;**132**:997.

Vestergaard P, Amdisen A, Schou M: Clinically significant side effects of lithium treatment: A survey of 237 patients in long-term treatment. *Acta Psychiatr Scand* 1980;**62**:193.

Antidepressants

28

Leo Hollister, MD

Nature of Depression

Depression is readily diagnosed when it is the chief complaint, but unfortunately it rarely is; a host of complaints may mask the true underlying disorder. Patients with vague complaints that resist explanation as manifestations of somatic disorders and those who may be called "neurotics" or "crocks" should be suspected of being depressed.

Depression and anxiety are symptoms that usually occur together. The initial complaints of depressed patients are often physical; and some manifestations, such as fatigue, headache, insomnia, and gastrointestinal disturbances, resemble those of simple anxiety. Other complaints may be more distinctive: anorexia and weight loss, bad taste in the mouth, chronic pain, loss of interest, inactivity, loss of sexual desire, and a general feeling of despondency. The constellation of fatigue, musculoskeletal complaints, sleep disorder, and loss of joy in living is characteristic of depression. Guilt as a symptom is almost unique to depression; if anger is directed outward rather than inward, hostility rather than depression may dominate the clinical picture.

Depression is a heterogeneous disorder that has been characterized and classified in a variety of ways. According to the current classification of the *Diagnostic and Statistical Manual of Mental Disorders (DSM-III)* of the American Psychiatric Association, several diagnoses of affective disorders are possible, based on the presence or absence of mania, as well as the severity of the depression. A simplified classification based on presumed origin is as follows: (1) "reactive" or "secondary" depression (most common; over 60%), occurring in response to real stimuli such as grief, illness, etc; (2) "endogenous" depression, a genetically determined biochemical disorder manifested by inability to cope with ordinary stress (about 25%); and (3) depression associated with bipolar affective (manic-depressive) disorder (about 10–15%). Drugs discussed in this chapter are used chiefly in management of the second type. Table 28–1 indicates how the 3 types may be differentiated.

I. BASIC PHARMACOLOGY OF ANTIDEPRESSANTS

Chemistry

A variety of different chemical structures have been found to have antidepressant activity. The number is constantly growing, but as yet no group has been found to have a clear therapeutic advantage over the others. Table 28–4 lists some clinically used antidepressants and their trade names.

A. Tricyclics: (Fig 28–1.) Tricyclic antidepressants—so called because of the characteristic 3-ring nucleus—have been used clinically for over 2 decades. They closely resemble the phenothiazines chemically and, to a lesser extent, pharmacologically. Like the latter drugs, they were first thought to be use-

Table 28–1. Differentiation of types of depression.

Type	Diagnostic Features	Comments
Reactive	Loss (adverse life events). Physical illness (myocardial infarct, cancer). Drugs (antihypertensives, alcohol, hormones). Other psychiatric disorders (senility).	More than 60% of all depressions. Core depressive syndrome: depression, anxiety, bodily complaints, tension, guilt. May respond spontaneously or to a variety of ministrations.
Major depressive (endogenous)	Precipitating life event not adequate for degree of depression. Autonomous (unresponsive to changes in life). May occur at any age (childhood to old age). Biologically determined (family history).	About 25% of all depressions. Core depressive syndrome plus "vital" signs: abnormal rhythms of sleep, motor activity, libido, appetite. Usually responds specifically to antidepressants or electroconvulsive therapy. Tends to recur throughout life.
Bipolar affective (manic-depressive)	Characterized by episodes of mania. Cyclic; mania alone, rare; depression alone, occasional; mania-depression, usual.	About 10–15% of all depressions. May be misdiagnosed as endogenous if hypomanic episodes are missed. Lithium carbonate stabilizes mood. Mania may require antipsychotic drugs as well; depression managed with antidepressants.

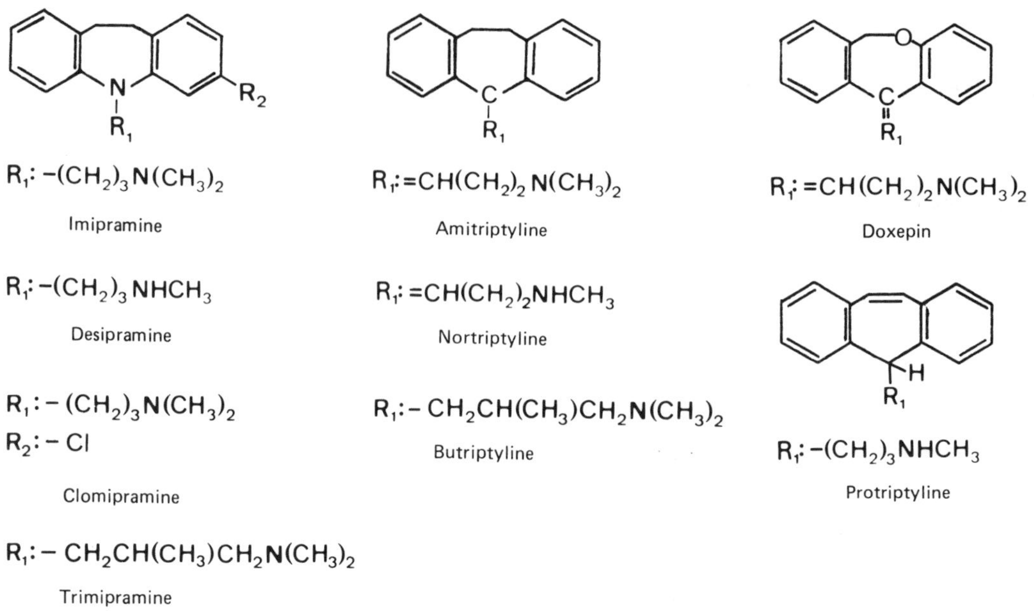

R_1: $-(CH_2)_3 N(CH_3)_2$

Imipramine

R_1: $-(CH_2)_3 NHCH_3$

Desipramine

R_1: $-(CH_2)_3 N(CH_3)_2$
R_2: $-Cl$

Clomipramine

R_1: $-CH_2CH(CH_3)CH_2N(CH_3)_2$

Trimipramine

R_1: $=CH(CH_2)_2 N(CH_3)_2$

Amitriptyline

R_1: $=CH(CH_2)_2NHCH_3$

Nortriptyline

R_1: $-CH_2CH(CH_3)CH_2N(CH_3)_2$

Butriptyline

R_1: $=CH(CH_2)_2N(CH_3)_2$

Doxepin

R_1: $-(CH_2)_3NHCH_3$

Protriptyline

Figure 28–1. Structural relationships between various tricyclic antidepressants.

ful as antihistamines and later as antipsychotics. The discovery of their antidepressant properties was a fortuitous clinical observation. Imipramine and amitriptyline are the prototypical drugs of the class and the most commonly used.

B. Monoamine Oxidase (MAO) Inhibitors: (Fig 28–2.) MAO inhibitors may be classified as hydrazides, exemplified by the C–N–N moiety, as in phenelzine and isocarboxazid; or nonhydrazides,

Phenelzine: $-CH_2-CH_2-NH-NH_2$

Tranylcypromine

Dextroamphetamine: $-CH_2-CH-NH_2$ / CH_3

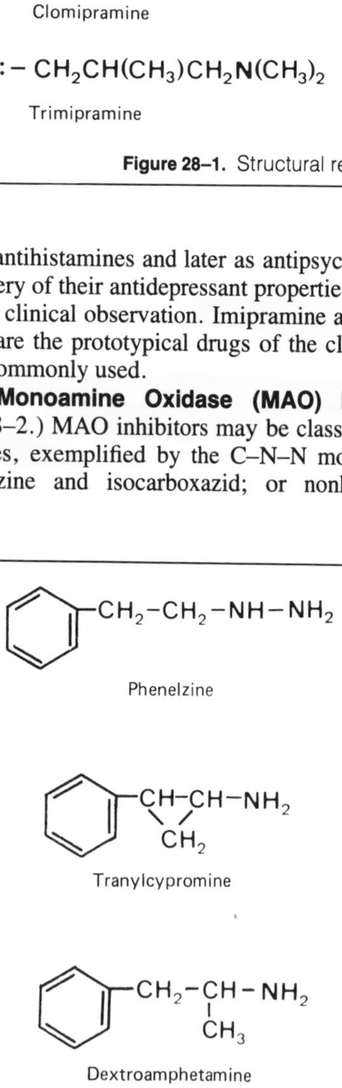

Figure 28–2. Some monoamine oxidase inhibitors. Phenelzine has a hydrazide configuration, while tranylcypromine has a cyclopropyl amine side chain compared with the isopropyl amine side chain of dextroamphetamine.

which lack such a moiety, as in tranylcypromine. Tranylcypromine bears a close resemblance to dextroamphetamine, which is itself a weak inhibitor of MAO. It retains some of the sympathomimetic characteristics of the amphetamines. The hydrazides appear to combine irreversibly with the enzyme, while tranylcypromine has a prolonged duration of effect even though it is not bound irreversibly. Both types inhibit MAO-A and MAO-B nonselectively.

C. Sympathomimetic Stimulants: Dextroamphetamine, other amphetamines, and amphetamine surrogates such as pipradrol and methylphenidate are occasionally used as antidepressants. Although the action of amphetamines in blocking MAO has generally been regarded as too weak to confer significant antidepressant action, it may contribute to an antidepressant action in some people.

D. "Second-Generation" Drugs: Three new antidepressant drugs (amoxapine, maprotiline, and trazodone) are currently available in the United States, and several more may soon be approved for marketing (Fig 28–3). **Nomifensine**, which was used for several years in other countries, has no sedative effects but rather seems to be a mild stimulant. Neither does it have any effect on cardiovascular functions, which would make it acceptable for patients with these disorders. However, nomifensine was withdrawn in 1986 because hemolytic anemia was reported in a significant number of cases. Nausea, vomiting, restlessness, and aggravation of psychosis have occurred. Overdoses have been marked by drowsiness, tremor, and tachycardia, but no arrhythmias or convulsions.

Bupropion is of interest in that it seems to work primarily through dopamine-related mechanisms. The drug also lacks most of the sedative, antimuscarinic,

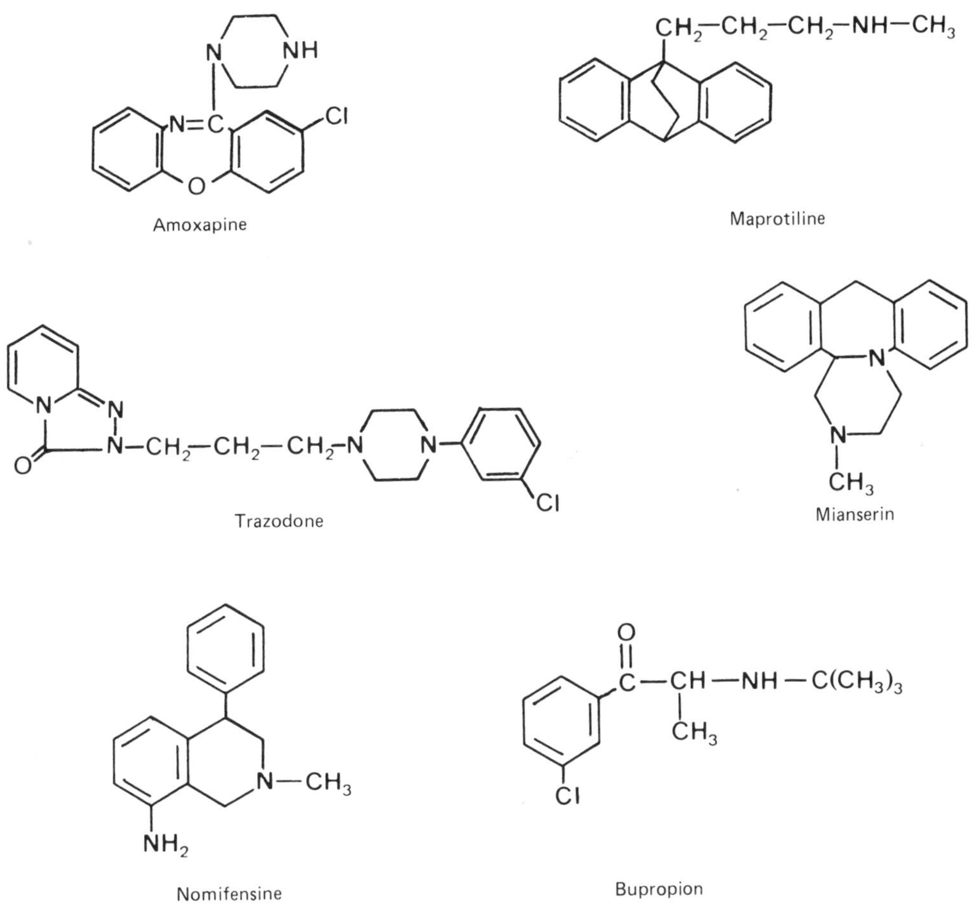

Figure 28–3. Some "second-generation" antidepressants.

and cardiovascular side effects of the tricyclics, although it is equally effective. Overdoses have caused convulsions and have halted marketing of this compound.

Other drugs that may appear as "second-generation" antidepressants are **alprazolam, mianserin**, and **viloxazine**. **Zimeldine** (now withdrawn because of side effects), **fluoxetine**, and several other compounds constitute another group of antidepressants that selectively block serotonin uptake by nerve endings. These drugs are said to be devoid of effects on muscarinic, alpha, and 5HT$_2$ receptors.

Some of the drugs in this category have unconventional structures, and some differ greatly in their pharmacologic effects from tricyclics, especially in their actions on aminergic neurotransmitters. No claim for increased efficacy over tricyclics has been substantiated, but claims are made that to varying degrees, these newer agents may work more quickly or have fewer adverse effects.

1. Amoxapine–Amoxapine is a metabolite of the antipsychotic drug loxapine and retains some of its antipsychotic action. A combination of antidepressant and antipsychotic actions might make it a suitable drug for psychotically depressed patients. On the other

hand, the antipsychotic action may cause akathisia, parkinsonism, amenorrhea-galactorrhea syndrome, and perhaps tardive dyskinesia. In addition to these new side effects, it retains much of the sedative and antimuscarinic effects of tricyclics. The drug lacks cardiotoxicity when taken in overdose but has dangerous neurotoxicity.

2. Maprotiline–Maprotiline (a "tetracyclic" drug) is most like desipramine, even to the point of some structural resemblance. Like the latter drug, it may have less sedative and antimuscarinic actions than the older tricyclics. Its major disadvantage is that it tends to evoke seizures at the top range of therapeutic doses.

3. Trazodone–Trazodone is the most novel drug of the lot. Clinical experience has indicated unpredictable efficacy: some patients do remarkably well, while others obtain scarcely any benefit. Sedation can be troublesome for some patients, but atropinelike side effects are minimal. Overdoses have been easily managed without cardiac or neurologic toxicity.

Pharmacodynamics

Drugs used to treat mental depression are not central nervous system stimulants and are actually contraindicated in organic or drug-induced central nervous system depression. Studies of the mode of action of antidepressants have largely focused on the effects on various amine neurotransmitters in the brain.

A. Amine Hypothesis: Soon after the introduction of reserpine in the early 1950s, it became apparent that the drug could induce depression in patients being treated for hypertension and schizophrenia as well as in normal subjects. Within the next few years, pharmacologic studies revealed that the principal mechanism of action of reserpine was to inhibit the storage of amine neurotransmitters such as serotonin and norepinephrine in the vesicles of presynaptic nerve endings. Reserpine induced depression and depleted stores of amine neurotransmitters; therefore, it was reasoned, depression must be associated with decreased functional amine-dependent transmission. This simple syllogism provided the basis for what became known as the amine hypothesis of depression.

B. Action of Antidepressants on Biogenic Amine Neurotransmitters: The amine hypothesis was buttressed by studies on the mechanism of action of various types of antidepressant drugs. Tricyclics block the amine reuptake pump, the "off switch" of amine neurotransmission (see Table 28–2 and Chapter 5). Such an action presumably permits a longer sojourn of neurotransmitter at the receptor site. MAO inhibitors block a major degradative pathway for the amine neurotransmitters, which presumably permits more amines to accumulate presynaptically and more to be released. Amphetaminelike sympathomimetics also block the amine pump but are thought to act chiefly by increasing the release of catecholamine neurotransmitters. Thus, these 3 classes of antidepressant drugs might remedy a deficiency in amine neurotransmission, although by somewhat different mechanisms. Some of the "second-generation" antidepressants have similar effects on amine neurotransmitters,

while others have mild or minimal effects. The apparent ability of zimeldine and fluoxetine to block serotonin uptake by nerve endings without inhibiting norepinephrine uptake contrasts with the ability of most of the tricyclic agents to block norepinephrine uptake at doses that have negligible effects on serotonin uptake. Since both groups of drugs are antidepressant, a *dual* mechanism, involving both transmitter systems, is suggested.

C. Consequences of Increased Amine-Dependent Neurotransmission: Increased amine neurotransmitters in the synapse were long thought to *increase* postsynaptic responses in a deficient system. Such conclusions were based on observations of the results of acute dosage. Clinically, however, drugs are given chronically for their antidepressant action. When they are administered chronically to animals and the postsynaptic consequences are measured by the generation of cAMP, *subsensitivity* of the postsynaptic receptor is observed. Thus, the evidence now strongly suggests that downstream neurotransmission is *decreased* rather than increased.

D. Peripheral Effects: See Adverse Effects, below.

Pharmacokinetics

A. Tricyclics: Absorption of most tricyclics is incomplete, and there is significant first-pass metabolism. As a result of high protein binding and relatively high lipid solubility, volumes of distribution tend to be very large. Tricyclics are metabolized by 2 major routes: transformation of the tricyclic nucleus and alteration of the aliphatic side chain. The former route involves ring hydroxylation and conjugation to form glucuronides; the latter, primarily demethylation of the nitrogen. Monodemethylation of tertiary amines leads to active metabolites, such as desipramine and nortriptyline (Fig 28–1). The proportion of monodemethylated metabolites formed varies from one patient to another. In general, the proportion of amitriptyline to its metabolite nortriptyline favors the parent drug. The converse is the case with imipramine and its metabolite desipramine. The pharmacokinetic parameters of various antidepressants are summarized in Table 28–3.

B. Monoamine Oxidase Inhibitors: These drugs produce an inhibition of MAO that persists even after the drug is no longer detectable in plasma. In following the effectiveness of a dosage regimen, it has been more useful to measure the inhibition of MAO activity in platelets than to measure the plasma levels of the drug directly. Present feeling is that optimal antidepressant effect from these drugs requires about 60–80% inhibition of the enzyme—a degree achieved with doses of approximately 1 mg/kg/d of phenelzine.

C. Second-Generation Drugs: The pharmacokinetics of these drugs and of the tricyclics are similar. Although the claim for many second-generation drugs is faster onset of clinical action, neither a pharmacokinetic nor a pharmacodynamic explanation for this clinical effect is apparent. Some of these drugs are

Table 28–2. Pharmacologic differences among several tricyclic antidepressants.*

| Drug | Sedative | Antimuscarinic | Block of Amine Pump For: | | |
			Serotonin	Norepinephrine	Dopamine
Amitriptyline	+++	+++	+++	+	0
Amoxapine	++	+	+	++	+
Bupropion	0	0	0	++	++
Desipramine	+	+	0	+++	0
Doxepin	+++	+++	++	+	0
Imipramine	++	++	++	++	0
Maprotiline	++	++	0	+++	0
Nomifensine	0	0	0	++	++
Nortriptyline	++	++	+	++	0
Protriptyline	0	++	?	+++	?
Trazodone	+++	0	+	0	0

*0 = none; + = slight; ++ = moderate; +++ = high; ? = uncertain.

Table 28–3. Pharmacokinetic parameters of various antidepressants.

Drug	Bioavailability (percent)	Protein Binding (percent)	Plasma $t_{1/2}$ (hours)	Active Metabolites	Volume of Distribution (L/kg)	Therapeutic Plasma Concentrations (ng/mL)
Amitriptyline	31–61	82–96	31–46	Nortriptyline	5–10	80–200 total
Amoxapine	*	*	8	7-,8-Hydroxy	*	*
Bupropion	*	85	11–14	Several (?)	*	25–100
Clomipramine	*	*	22–84	Desmethyl	7–20	240–700
Desipramine	60–70	73–90	14–62	*	22–59	145†
Doxepin	13–45	*	8–24	Desmethyl	9–33	30–150
Imipramine	29–77	76–95	9–24	Desipramine	15–30	> 180 total
Maprotiline	66–75	88	21–52	Desmethyl	15–28	200–300
Nomifensine	*	*	2–4; active metabolites longer	Several (?)	*	*
Nortriptyline	32–79	93–95	18–93	10-Hydroxy	21–57	50–150
Protriptyline	77–93	90–95	54–198	*	19–57	70–170
Trazodone	*	*	4–9	m-Chlorophenyl-piperazine	*	*

*No data available.
†Lower concentrations may be effective, but no data are available.

said to have less cardiotoxicity than tricyclics when taken in overdose quantities.

Clinical Indications

The major indication for these drugs is to treat depression, but a number of other uses have been established by clinical experience.

A. Depression: This indication has been kept broad deliberately, even though evidence from clinical studies strongly suggests that the drugs are specifically useful only in major depressive episodes. Major depressive episodes are diagnosed not so much by their severity as by their quality. Formerly, they were referred to as "endogenous," "vital," or "vegetative"—reflecting the characteristic disturbances of major body rhythms of sleep, hunger and appetite, sexual drive, and motor activity. The diagnosis of major depression may be uncertain in individual patients, so that on balance it is probably better to treat too many patients with tricyclics than to miss treating those who might benefit.

B. Enuresis: Enuresis is an established indication for tricyclics. Proof of efficacy for this indication is substantial, but drug therapy is not the preferred approach. The beneficial effect of drug treatment lasts only as long as drug treatment is continued.

C. Chronic Pain: Clinicians in pain clinics have found tricyclics to be especially useful for treating a variety of chronically painful states that often cannot be definitely diagnosed. Whether such painful states represent depressive equivalents or whether such patients become secondarily depressed after some initial pain-producing insult is not clear. It is even possible that the tricyclics (sometimes phenothiazines are also used in combination) work directly on pain pathways.

D. Other Indications: Less frequent and less well documented indications include obsessive compulsive phobic states, cataplexy associated with narcolepsy, acute panic attacks, school phobia, and attention deficit disorder in children.

II. CLINICAL PHARMACOLOGY OF ANTIDEPRESSANTS

Choice of Drug

Controlled comparisons of the available antidepressants have usually led to the conclusion that they are roughly equivalent drugs. Although this may be true for groups of patients, individual patients may for uncertain reasons fare better on one drug than on another. Thus, finding the right drug for the individual patient must be accomplished empirically at present. The past history of the patient's drug experience, if available, is the most valuable guide. At times such a history may lead to the exclusion of tricyclics, as in the case of patients who have responded well in the past to MAO inhibitors.

Tricyclic antidepressant drugs are apt to be most successful in patients with clearly "vegetative" characteristics, including psychomotor retardation, sleep disturbance, poor appetite and weight loss, and loss of libido. MAO inhibitors in adequate doses may also be useful for such patients.

Tricyclics differ mainly in the degree of sedation (amitriptyline, doxepin, and trazodone cause the most, protriptyline the least) and the amount of antimuscarinic effects (amitriptyline and doxepin have the greatest, trazodone the least) (Table 28–2). Although it is often argued that more sedative drugs are preferable for markedly anxious or agitated depressives while the least sedative drugs are preferable for patients with psychomotor withdrawal, this hypothesis has not been tested.

MAO inhibitors are helpful in patients described as having "atypical" depressions—a nonspecific designation scarcely helpful in their identification. Depressed patients with considerable attendant anxiety, phobic features, and hypochondriasis are the ones who respond best to these drugs. Either phenelzine or tranylcypromine may be used.

None of the second-generation antidepressants have been shown to be more effective overall than the tricyclics with which they have been compared. The major claims are: (1) a faster onset of action, (2) less sedative and autonomic side effects, and (3) less toxicity when overdoses are taken. Solid evidence to support a claim of more rapid onset of action has been difficult to obtain. Amoxapine and maprotiline seem to have as many sedative and autonomic actions as most tricyclics; some of the other drugs, such as trazodone, may have fewer. Amoxapine and maprotiline are at least as dangerous as the tricyclics when taken in overdoses. Thus, the advantages of the newer drugs appear to be restricted and must be weighed against the proved efficacy of tricyclics and MAO inhibitors.

Few clinicians use lithium, an antimanic agent, as primary treatment for depression. However, some have found that lithium along with one of the other antidepressants may achieve a favorable response not obtained by the antidepressant alone. Another potential use of lithium is to prevent relapses of depression.

Doses

The usual dose ranges of antidepressants are shown in Table 28–4. Doses are almost always determined empirically; the patient's acceptance of side effects is the usual limiting factor. Tolerance to some of the objectionable side effects may develop, so that the usual pattern of treatment has been to start with small doses, increasing either to a predetermined daily dose, or to one that produces relief of depression, or to the maximum tolerated dose. The effective dose of an antidepressant varies widely depending upon many factors. Undertreatment has been thought to be a frequent cause of apparent failure of drug therapy to relieve depression.

Dosage Schedules for Treating the Acute Episode

The initial doses of a tricyclic may vary from 10 to 75 mg on the first day of treatment, depending on the patient's size and tolerance for the acute effects. If a first goal is to attain a daily dose of 150 mg, increments of 25 mg may be added every second or third day until this level is reached.

The sedative and antimuscarinic actions of these drugs are less bothersome when the drug is taken in the evening. However, the patient should be warned of

Table 28–4. Usual daily doses of antidepressant drugs.

Drug	Dose (mg)
Tricyclics	
Amitriptyline (Elavil, etc)	75–200
Clomipramine (Anafranil)	75–300
Desipramine (Norpramin, Pertofrane)	75–200
Doxepin (Adapin, Sinequan)	75–300
Imipramine (Tofranil, etc)	75–200
Nortriptyline (Aventyl, Pamelor)	75–150
Protriptyline (Triptil, Vivactil)	20–40
Trimipramine (Surmontil)	75–200
Monoamine oxidase inhibitors	
Isocarboxazid (Marplan)	20–50
Phenelzine (Nardil)	45–75
Tranylcypromine (Parnate)	10–30
Second-generation drugs	
Amoxapine (Asendin)	150–300
Maprotiline (Ludiomil)	75–300
Trazodone (Desyrel)	50–600

these side effects and should construe them as evidence of the action of the drug.

Maintenance Treatment

Whether or not to undertake long-term maintenance treatment of a depressed patient depends entirely on the natural history of the disorder. If the depressive episode was the patient's first and if it responded quickly and satisfactorily to drug therapy, it is rational to gradually withdraw treatment over a period of a few months. If relapse does not occur, drug treatment can be stopped until the next attack occurs, which is unpredictable but nearly certain. On the other hand, a patient who has had several previous attacks of depression, especially if each succeeding attack was more severe and more difficult to treat, is a prime candidate for maintenance therapy.

Considerable controversy exists concerning the proper duration of treatment of a major depressive episode. Most clinicians treat with full dosage for 2–6 months, after which some discontinue therapy; others reduce the dose to one-half or one-third of the initial level. Some patients have been on maintenance treatment for years with apparent good control of their illness and no long-term adverse effects. Members of the household should be instructed in how to detect early signs of relapse; the patients themselves may be poor judges of that.

Monitoring Plasma Concentrations

Routine monitoring of plasma concentrations of antidepressants, while technically feasible for most drugs, is still of uncertain value. Experience with monitoring of plasma concentrations of tricyclics suggests that about 20% of patients become noncompliant at some time or other. Thus, a "poor response" in a patient for whom an adequate dosage of drug has been prescribed may be shown by measurement of the plasma drug concentration to be due merely to failure to take the drug. Blood for plasma drug level determination should be obtained in the postabsorptive state, about 10–12 hours after the last dose. Even when sampling time is constant, the same patient may show variation in both the total plasma concentration and the proportion of parent drug versus metabolites while on a constant dose at steady-state conditions. Under no circumstances should the laboratory test results be permitted to overrule the physician's clinical judgment.

Unresponsive Patients

Almost one-third of patients receiving tricyclic antidepressants fail to respond. In evaluating a patient's resistance to treatment, one should consider the five *d's:* diagnosis, drug, dose, duration of treatment, and different treatment. Failure to respond to 2 or 3 weeks of treatment with most tricyclics at a daily dose of 150 mg, with plasma concentrations within the presumed therapeutic range, suggests the need for reassessment of the diagnosis. If the patient is actually bipolar, lithium may be added. On the other hand, a patient with an adjustment disorder with depressed mood (reactive depression) may be overly sensitive to the side effects of the drugs and be better managed without them. It is often said that failure to respond to one tricyclic calls for a trial of therapy with another tricyclic, but there is no evidence to support that view unless the problem is related to poor tolerance of side effects. Some patients unresponsive to tricyclics are responsive to MAO inhibitors, which should be considered in all such cases. A few patients, especially elderly ones, seem to respond specifically to direct sympathomimetic stimulants such as dextroamphetamine. Second-generation drugs might be tried after failure with both tricyclics and MAO inhibitors. Finally, some patients may need a completely different type of treatment. Patients with adjustment disorders with depressed mood (reactive depression) need to deal with the precipitating event.

Noncompliance is an important cause of lack of response. Patients should be warned also that noticeable improvement may be slow, perhaps taking 3 weeks or more. Inability to tolerate side effects and discouragement with treatment are 2 major causes for noncompliance and for failure of tricyclics to relieve depression.

Electroconvulsive therapy (ECT) is often viewed as a treatment of last resort for endogenous depressions, but it should not be withheld from patients with this disorder who cannot be helped by drug therapy.

Combination therapy using tricyclics and MAO inhibitors has been recommended, although recent controlled trials do not suggest any special virtues for such combinations. Tricyclics should be combined with lithium or antipsychotics for treating psychotic depressions or the depressed phase of bipolar affective (manic-depressive) disorder.

Adverse Effects

Adverse effects of various antidepressants are summarized in Table 28–5. Most common unwanted effects are minor, but they may seriously affect the acceptance of drug treatment by the patient; the more

Table 28–5. Side effects of antidepressants.

Type	Minor, Early	Major
Sedation	Lassitude, fatigue.	Sleepiness; impaired consciousness with alcohol and other drugs.
Sympathomimetic	Tachycardia, tremor, sweating.	Agitation, insomnia, aggravation of psychosis.
Antimuscarinic	Blurred vision, constipation, urinary hesitancy, fuzzy thinking.	Aggravation of glaucoma, paralytic ileus, urinary retention, delirium.
Cardiovascular	Orthostatic hypotension, electrocardiographic abnormalities.	Delayed cardiac conduction, arrhythmias, cardiomyopathy, sudden death.
Psychiatric	Confusion.	Central antimuscarinic syndrome, withdrawal.
Neurologic	Tremor, paresthesias, electroencephalographic alterations.	Seizures, neuropathy.
Allergic/toxic		Cholestatic jaundice, agranulocytosis.
Metabolic/endocrine	Weight gain, sexual disturbances.	Gynecomastia, amenorrhea.
Birth defects		Uncertain.
Hematologic		Hemolytic anemia (nomifensine).

seriously depressed the patient is, the more likely it is that unwanted effects will be tolerated. Most normal persons find that even moderate doses of these drugs cause disagreeable symptoms.

A. Sedation: Although we think of antidepressants as "activators," tricyclics—with the possible exception of protriptyline—are strongly sedative. Complaints of lassitude, fatigue, and loss of energy are common, especially early in treatment. If doses are too high, the patient may sleep at inappropriate times. Sedative effects are less bothersome when a single daily dose is taken at night. MAO inhibitors, especially those with sympathomimetic actions such as tranylcypromine, may produce mild degrees of stimulation.

B. Sympathomimetic Actions: These effects of various antidepressants are usually obscured by other more prominent actions on the autonomic nervous system. However, tremor is extremely common (see Neurologic Effects, below).

C. Atropinelike Effects: Dry mouth, constipation, urinary hesitancy, and loss of visual accommodation are the most frequent antimuscarinic side effects. More extensive antimuscarinic action may result in paralytic ileus or urinary retention, especially in elderly patients. Treatment with bethanechol, a peripherally acting cholinomimetic, may counter the peripheral antimuscarinic action of the tricyclics.

D. Cardiovascular Effects: Palpitation, tachycardia, and orthostatic hypotension were recognized early as unwanted effects of these drugs. Later, arrhythmias and electrocardiographic abnormalities were described. Congestive heart failure and sudden death are rare complications.

E. Psychiatric Effects: Some patients may become agitated and manic with tricyclics, but one should always consider the possibility that they are really bipolar. Confusional reactions are most often seen in patients over 40 years of age. The situation may be made worse if the patient is also receiving other drugs with antimuscarinic action, such as antipsychotics or antiparkinsonism drugs.

A central antimuscarinic syndrome consisting of delirium, anxiety, hyperactivity, hallucinations, disorientation, and seizures has been described for many drugs with antimuscarinic action, especially when they are taken in combination. A good general rule is that any patient showing new or bizarre mental symptoms while receiving antidepressant medication should have the drug discontinued until the situation can be appraised. Most cases respond quickly to simple discontinuation of the drug.

F. Neurologic Effects: Tremor is more similar to essential tremor than to the tremor of Parkinson's disease. Treatment with a beta-blocking drug such as propranolol or nadolol may be helpful. Paresthesias are less common and may herald the rare development of peripheral neuropathy. Other neurologic abnormalities are usually signs of therapeutic overdoses. Although Parkinson's syndrome has been reported, it is extremely rare. Tardive dyskinesia has not occurred.

G. Allergic or Toxic Reactions: Skin rashes are uncommon. Cholestatic jaundice and agranulocytosis have been reported but are now so rare as to hardly merit consideration. Nomifensine was withdrawn because of its association with a high incidence of hemolytic anemia.

H. Metabolic and Endocrine Effects: Weight gain is frequent with these drugs, just as it is with the phenothiazines. It may be due in part to increased appetite with remission of depression, but a central action is probably responsible also. Some patients report a craving for sweets, and beverages containing sugar are often used to relieve dry mouth.

The syndrome of inappropriate secretion of antidiuretic hormone has been reported with various tricyclics.

I. Birth Defects: As is the case with so many drugs, it is not clear whether or not the antidepressant drugs have been responsible for birth defects in infants born to mothers taking the drugs early in pregnancy. The evidence is not very persuasive, and the results of national surveys are equivocal.

Drug Interactions

A. Pharmacodynamic Interactions: Many of the pharmacodynamic interactions of antidepressants with other drugs have already been discussed. Sedative effects may be additive with other sedatives, especially alcohol. Patients taking tricyclics should be warned that use of alcohol may lead to greater than usual impairment of driving ability. MAO inhibitors, by increasing stores of catecholamines, sensitize the patient to indirectly acting sympathomimetics such as tyramine, which is found in many fermented foods and beverages, and to sympathomimetic drugs that may be administered therapeutically, such as diethylpropion or phenylpropanolamine.

B. Pharmacokinetic Interactions: Reversal of the antihypertensive action of guanethidine is a dramatic interaction (see Chapter 10). The blood pressure not only returns quickly to high levels but may overshoot to dangerously high levels. Guanethidine is concentrated in sympathetic nerve endings by the same amine pump that is blocked by tricyclics. Thus, it is prevented from reaching its site of action. A similar reversal of action of other antihypertensives, such as methyldopa and clonidine, has been described. Although doxepin is less likely than other tricyclics to produce this interaction, because it is less potent in blocking the amine pump, interaction can occur with high doses of the drug. MAO inhibitors predictably prolong the half-lives of the many drugs that are oxidatively deaminated.

Overdoses

A. Tricyclic Drugs: Tricyclics are extremely dangerous when taken in overdose quantities, and depressed patients are more likely than others to be suicidal. Prescriptions should therefore be limited to amounts less than 1.25 g, or 50 dose units of 25 mg, on a "no refill" basis. If suicide is a serious possibility, the tablets should be entrusted to a family member. The drugs must be kept away from children.

Both accidental and deliberate overdoses are frequent and are a serious medical emergency. Major symptoms include (1) coma with shock and sometimes metabolic acidosis; (2) respiratory depression with a tendency to sudden apnea; (3) agitation or delirium both before and after consciousness is obtunded; (4) neuromuscular irritability and seizures; (5) hyperpyrexia; (6) bowel and bladder paralysis; and (7) a great variety of cardiac manifestations, including conduction defects and arrhythmias.

Management of cardiac problems is difficult. Antiarrhythmic drugs having the least depressant effect on cardiac conduction should be used. Lidocaine, propranolol, and phenytoin have been used successfully, but quinidine and procainamide are contraindicated. Physostigmine given in small (0.5-mg) intravenous boluses to a total dose of 3–4 mg may awaken the patient and reverse a rapid supraventricular arrhythmia. It is *unlikely* to be effective for ventricular arrhythmias. Continual cardiac monitoring is essential, and facilities must be at hand for resuscitation if needed. Arterial blood gases and pH should be measured frequently, since both hypoxia and metabolic acidosis predispose to arrhythmias. Sodium bicarbonate and intravenous potassium chloride may be required to restore acid-base balance and to correct hypokalemia. Electrical pacing must be used in refractory cases.

Other treatment is entirely supportive. After placement of a cuffed endotracheal tube, attempts should be made to remove residual drug from the gastrointestinal tract. Absorption may be slow because of the strong antimuscarinic effects. Activated charcoal may be used to bind the drug, which may subsequently be removed by catharsis. Ventilatory assistance is of prime importance. Shock is best treated with fluids or plasma expanders, since adrenoceptors may be blocked. Hyperpyrexia is treated by cooling. Seizures may be treated with intravenous phenytoin (which may also double as an antiarrhythmic agent) or diazepam. Patients should not be discharged until they have been conscious for a day or 2 and most abnormal signs have disappeared. Measurement of plasma concentrations of the drug may be helpful in deciding about the safety of discharge. Virtually all patients who survive recover completely with no permanent sequelae.

Intoxication with MAO inhibitors is unusual. Agitation, delirium, and neuromuscular excitability are followed by obtunded consciousness, seizures, shock, and hyperthermia. Supportive treatment is usually all that is required, although sedative phenothiazines with alpha-adrenoceptor–blocking action, such as chlorpromazine, may be useful.

B. Second-Generation Drugs: Overdoses of amoxapine are characterized by severe neurotoxicity with seizures that are difficult to control. Overdoses of maprotiline also have a tendency to cause seizures as well as cardiotoxicity. Overdoses of the other second-generation drugs appear to create only minor problems and can usually be managed with purely supportive measures.

REFERENCES

American Psychiatric Association: *Diagnostic and Statistical Manual of Mental Disorders (DSM-III)*, 3rd ed. American Psychiatric Association, 1980.

Blackwell B: Antidepressant drugs. Pages 24–61 in: *Meyler's Side Effects of Drugs.* Dukes MNG (editor). Elsevier, 1984.

Coccaro EF, Siever LJ: Second generation antidepressants: A comparative review. *J Clin Psychopharmacol* 1985;**25**:241.

Costa E et al: Molecular mechanisms in the action of imipramine. *Experientia* 1983;**39**:855.

Davis JM: Overview: Maintenance therapy in psychiatry. 2. Affective disorders. *Am J Psychiatry* 1976;**133**:1.

Garver DL, Davis JM: Biogenic amine hypothesis of affective disorders. *Life Sci* 1979;**24**:383.

Hollister LE: Monitoring tricyclic antidepressant plasma concentrations. *JAMA* 1979;**241**:2530.

Hollister LE: Treatment of depression with drugs. *Ann Intern Med* 1978;**89**:78.

Jarvik LF, Kakkar PR: Aging and response to antidepressants. Chap 4, pp 49–77, in: *Clinical Pharmacology and the Aged Patient.* Jarvik LF et al (editors). Raven Press, 1982.

Lemberger L, Fuller RW, Zerbe RL: Use of specific serotonin uptake inhibitors as antidepressants. *Clin Neuropharmacol* 1985;**8**:299.

Maxwell RA: Second-generation antidepressants: The pharmacological and clinical significance of selected examples. *Drug Dev Res* 1983;**3**:203.

Morris JB, Beck AT: The efficacy of antidepressant drugs. *Arch Gen Psychiatry* 1974;**30**:667.

Potter WZ: Psychotherapeutic drugs and biogenic amines: Current concepts and therapeutic implications. *Drugs* 1984;**28**:127.

Shaw DM: The practical management of affective disorders. *Br J Psychiatry* 1977;**130**:432.

Sugrue MF: Do antidepressants possess a common mechanism of action? *Biochem Pharmacol* 1983;**32**:1811.

Sulser F: Antidepressant treatments and regulation of norepinephrine receptor–coupled adenylate cyclase systems in the brain. *Adv Biochem Psychopharmacol* 1984;**39**:249.

Tang SW, Seeman P: Effect of antidepressant drugs on serotonergic and adrenergic receptors. *Naunyn Schmiedebergs Arch Pharmacol* 1980;**311**:255.

Veith RC et al: Cardiovascular effects of tricyclic antidepressants in depressed patients with chronic heart disease. *N Engl J Med* 1982;**306**:954.

29

Opioid Analgesics & Antagonists

Walter L. Way, MD, & E. Leong Way, PhD

Even today, the black bag carried by physicians would almost certainly contain an opioid analgesic, probably morphine sulfate. One hundred years ago, morphine would without question have been the most important drug in the bag; since there were no antibiotics, hormonal agents, or antipsychotic drugs, the practitioner depended heavily on drugs that would at least provide symptomatic relief. Not only could opium and its derivatives be counted upon to allay severe pain of different origins, it would also control diarrhea, cough, anxiety, and insomnia. For these reasons, Sir William Osler called morphine "God's own medicine."

Compounds similar to morphine that produce pain relief and sedation have traditionally been called narcotic analgesics to distinguish them from the antipyretic analgesics such as aspirin and acetaminophen (Chapter 34). However, the term "narcotic" is an imprecise one, since narcosis signifies a stuporous state whereas the opiates produce analgesia without loss of consciousness. The terms "opiate" and "opioid analgesic" are more appropriate, but established usage of a word is always difficult to extinguish. Consequently, "narcotic analgesics" are usually understood to include natural and semisynthetic alkaloid derivatives from opium as well as their synthetic surrogates with actions that mimic those of morphine. In 1954, it was found that nalorphine, an antagonist of morphine, itself had analgesic effects. In recent years, more potent analgesics that also possess morphine *antagonist* properties have found extensive applications in clinical situations where morphine might be used. Moreover, the recent discovery of endogenous peptides with analgesic properties suggests that synthetic peptides with opiate characteristics may in the future also be included in this group. In this chapter, "opioid analgesic" will be used as the general term for this group of analgesic drugs. Among the opioids we include the **opiates** (derived from the opium alkaloids), **synthetic** compounds (such as meperidine and methadone) that have rather different structures but similar effects, and the **opiopeptins** (such as β-endorphin and the enkephalins). Morphine is considered the prototypical agonist.

History

The source of opium, the crude substance, and morphine, one of its purified constituents, is the opium poppy, *Papaver somniferum*. The plant may have been used as much as 6000 years ago, and there are ac-

counts of it in ancient Egyptian, Greek, Roman, and Chinese documents. It was not until the 18th century that the addiction liability of opium began to cause concern. Until quite recently, opiates were used indiscriminately for analgesia and sedation and to control diarrhea and cough.

The modern basis of pharmacology was established by Sertürner, a German pharmacist, who described the isolation of a pure active alkaline substance from opium in 1803. This first isolation in chemically pure form of an active principle from a plant was a landmark event in that it made it possible to derive a standardized potency for a natural product. Sertürner ingested the substance himself and gave it to his friends to produce a deep narcotic state. He proposed the name "morphine" for the compound—after Morpheus, the Greek god of dreams.

I. BASIC PHARMACOLOGY OF THE OPIOID ANALGESICS

Source

Opium is obtained from the opium poppy by incision of the seed pod after the petals of the flower have dropped. The white latex that oozes out turns brown and hardens on standing. This sticky brown gum is opium. It is scraped off and kneaded into a homogeneous mass that contains about 20 alkaloids, including morphine, codeine, thebaine, and papaverine. Thebaine and papaverine are not analgesic agents, but thebaine is the precursor of several semisynthetic opiate agonists (eg, etorphine, an experimental agent 500–1000 times as potent as morphine) and antagonists (naloxone). Papaverine is a vasodilator with no established clinical applications that nevertheless inspired the development of verapamil, an important calcium channel-blocking drug (Chapter 13). The principal alkaloid in opium is morphine, present in a concentration of about 10%. Codeine is present in less than 0.5% concentration; it is synthesized commercially from morphine. Cultivation of the opium poppy is now restricted by international agreement, but illicit production of opium is difficult to control.

Chemistry

Since the early discoveries in alkaloid chemistry, many compounds with opiate agonist activity have

336

been synthesized. Several different families may be identified, all bearing a common "backbone" as shown in Fig 29–1. Several important members of these families are shown in Table 29–1, and some of their properties are summarized in Table 29–2. Relatively small molecular alterations may drastically change the action of these compounds, converting an agonist to an antagonist or to a compound with both agonist and antagonist effects—a "mixed agonist-antagonist."

Antagonist properties are associated with replacement of the methyl substituent on the nitrogen atom with larger groups—allyl in the case of nalorphine and naloxone; methylcyclopropane or methylcyclobutane for several other agents.

Substitutions at the C3 and C6 hydroxyl groups of morphine significantly alter pharmacokinetic properties. Methyl substitution at the phenolic hydroxyl at C3 reduces susceptibility to first-pass hepatic inactivation of the molecule by glucuronide conjugation. Therefore, drugs such as codeine and oxycodone have a higher ratio of oral:parenteral potency. Acetylation of both hydroxyl groups of morphine yields heroin, which penetrates the blood-brain barrier much more rapidly than morphine. It is rapidly hydrolyzed in the brain to monoacetylmorphine and morphine. In Table 29–1, compounds are listed according to their agonist,

mixed agonist-antagonist, or antagonist properties. The pharmacologic basis for their different properties is discussed below.

Pharmacokinetics

A. Absorption: Most opioid analgesics are well absorbed from subcutaneous and intramuscular sites as well as from the mucosal surfaces of the nose and gastrointestinal tract. However, although absorption from the gastrointestinal tract may be rapid, the pharmacologic potency of some compounds taken by this route may be considerably less than after parenteral administration, because of significant first-pass metabolism in the liver after absorption. Therefore, the oral dose required to elicit a therapeutic effect for such compounds may be considerably higher than that required when parenteral administration is used (Chapter 3). Opioid analgesics with a free hydroxyl group (eg, morphine) are usually metabolized by conjugation with glucuronic acid. Since the amount of the enzyme responsible for this reaction varies considerably in different individuals, the effect of a specified oral dose of a compound that will be metabolized by conjugation is difficult to predict.

Examples of compounds that have high oral:parenteral potency ratios are codeine and oxycodone.

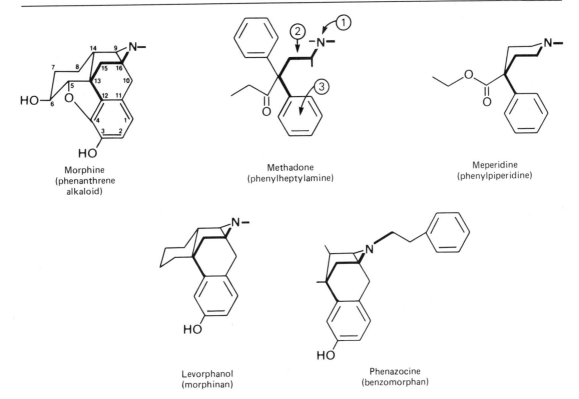

Figure 29–1. The chemical structures of an opium alkaloid and 4 examples of synthetic opioid analgesics written to emphasize the structure common to all: (1) a tertiary nitrogen; (2) a short hydrocarbon chain held in a plane perpendicular to the page; (3) a flat aryl group held in the plane of the page. (Modified and reproduced, with permission, from Meyers FH, Jawetz E, Goldfien A: *Review of Medical Pharmacology*, 7th ed. Lange, 1980.)

Table 29–1. Chemical structures of opioid analgesics and antagonists.

Basic Structure	Strong Agonists	Mild to Moderate Agonists	Mixed Agonist-Antagonists	Antagonists
Phenanthrenes	Morphine	Codeine	Nalbuphine (Nubain)	Nalorphine (Nalline)*
	Hydromorphone (Dilaudid)	Oxycodone (Percodan)	Buprenorphine (Temgesic)	Naloxone (Narcan)
	Oxymorphone (Numorphan)	Hydrocodone (Hycodan)		Naltrexone (Trexan)
Phenylheptylamines	Methadone	Propoxyphene (Darvon)		

Phenylpiperidines			
Meperidine (Demerol)	Diphenoxylate		Levallorphan (Lorfan)*
Fentanyl (Sublimaze)		Butorphanol (Stadol)	
		Pentazocine (Talwin)	

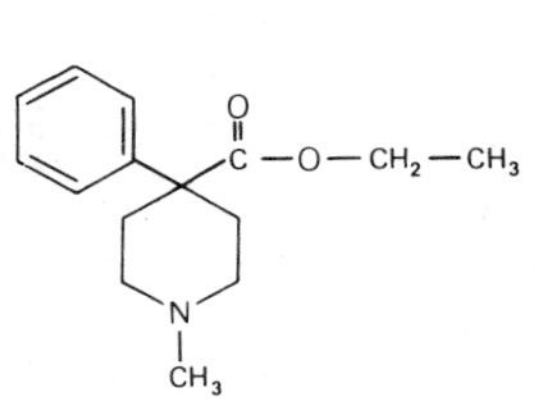

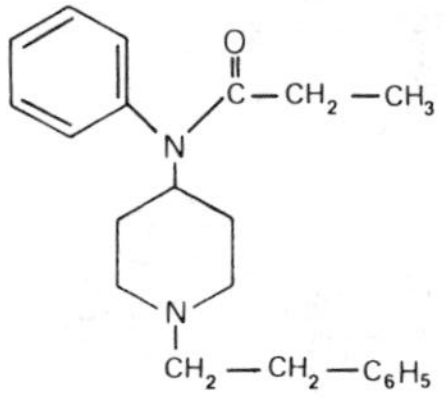

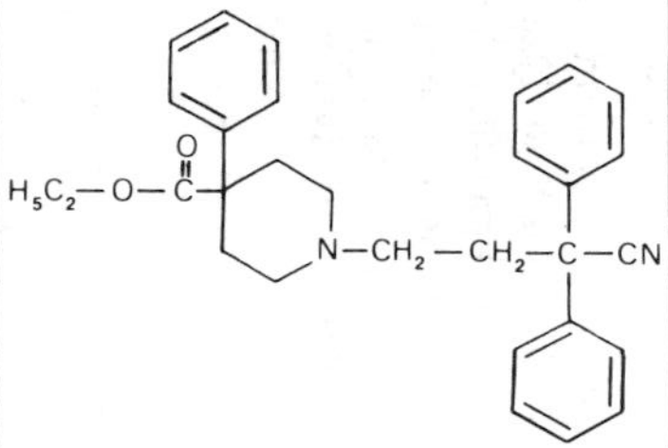

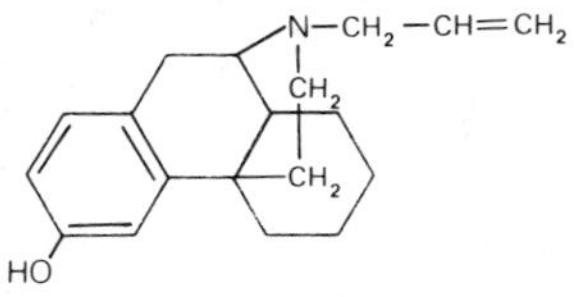

Morphinans

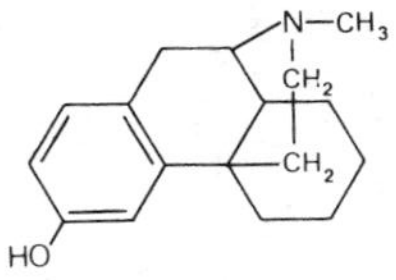

Levorphanol (Levo-Dromoran)

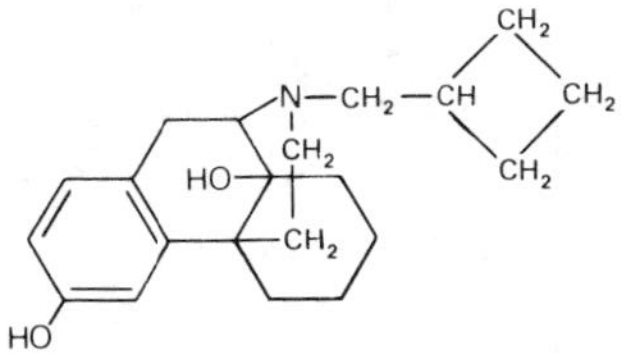

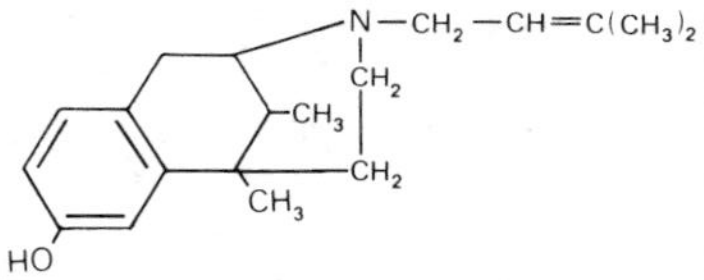

Benzomorphans

*Not a pure antagonist. See text for explanation.

Table 29-2. Useful opioid analgesics.

Generic Name	Proprietary Name	Approximate Dose (mg)	Oral:Parenteral Potency Ratio	Duration of Analgesia (hours)	Maximum Efficacy	Addiction/Abuse Liability
Morphine		10	Low	4–5	High	High
Hydromorphone	Dilaudid	1.5	Low	4–5	High	High
Oxymorphone	Numorphan	1.5	Low	3–4	High	High
Methadone	Dolophine	10	High	4–6	High	High
Meperidine	Demerol	60–100	Medium	2–4	High	High
Alphaprodine	Nisentil	30–50	Parenteral use only	1–2	High	High
Fentanyl	Sublimaze	0.2	Parenteral use only	1–1½	High	High
Levorphanol	Levo-Dromoran	2–3	High	4–5	High	High
Codeine		30–60[†]	High	3–4	Low	Medium
Oxycodone*	Percodan	4.5[†]	Medium	3–4	Moderate	Medium
Dihydrocodeine*	Drocode	16[†]	Medium	3–4	Moderate	Medium
Propoxyphene	Darvon	60–120[†]	Oral use only	4–5	Very low	Low
Pentazocine	Talwin	30–50[†]	Medium	3–4	Moderate	Low
Nalbuphine	Nubain	0.5–1	Parenteral use only	3–6	High	Low
Buprenorphine	Temgesic	0.3	Parenteral use only	4–8	High	Low
Butorphanol	Stadol	2	Parenteral use only	3–4	High	Low

*Available only in tablets containing aspirin, etc.
[†]Analgesic efficacy at this dose not equivalent to 10 mg of morphine. See text for explanation.

Their greater effectiveness by the oral route is thought to result from a decrease in first-pass metabolism, because their conjugation is prevented by a methyl group on the aromatic hydroxyl group.

B. Distribution: The uptake of opiates by various organs and tissues is a function of both physiologic and chemical factors. Although all opiate analgesics bind to plasma proteins with varying degrees of affinity after absorption, the compounds rapidly leave the blood and localize in highest concentrations in parenchymatous tissues such as lungs, liver, kidneys, and spleen. Although drug concentrations in skeletal muscle may be much lower, this tissue serves as the main reservoir for the drug because of its greater bulk. However, accumulation in fatty tissue can also become important, particularly after frequent high-dose administration of highly lipophilic opiates that are slowly metabolized, eg, fentanyl. Brain concentrations of opiate analgesics are usually relatively low in comparison to most other organs, although the blood-brain barrier is traversed readily by compounds in which the aromatic hydroxyl at C3 is substituted, as in heroin and codeine. Difficulty in gaining access to the brain appears to be greater with amphoteric agents such as morphine. However, this barrier is lacking in the infant. Since the opioid analgesics also traverse the placenta, their use for obstetric analgesia can result in the delivery of an infant with depressed respiration.

C. Metabolism: The opiates are converted in large part to polar metabolites, which are then readily excreted by the kidneys. Compounds that have free hydroxyl groups are readily conjugated with glucuronic acid; examples are morphine and levorphanol.

Esters (eg, meperidine, heroin) are rapidly hydrolyzed by common tissue esterases. Heroin is hydrolyzed to monoacetylmorphine and finally to morphine, which is then conjugated with glucuronic acid. The opiate analgesics are also N-demethylated by the liver, but this is a minor pathway. In the presence of liver or kidney disease, therapeutic blood levels can probably be achieved with lower than usual doses of these compounds.

D. Excretion: The polar metabolites of the opiates are excreted mainly in the urine. Small amounts of the unchanged drug may also be excreted in the urine. Glucuronide conjugates are also excreted in the bile, but enterohepatic circulation represents only a small portion of the excretory process.

Pharmacodynamics

A. Mechanism of Action: Morphine and its surrogates combine selectively at many recognition sites throughout the body to produce pharmacologic effects. Brain loci involved in the transmission of pain and in the alteration of reactivity to nociceptive (painful) stimuli appear to be primary but not the only sites at which opioids act. In general, sites that display a high affinity for exogenous opioid ligands such as morphine also contain high concentrations of endogenous peptides having opiatelike properties. Although there are many shared features in the chemistry and pharmacology of these peptides, there are distinct differences with respect to their biochemical and neuronal pathways. The generic name used for these substances has been **endorphins,** a blend of the words "endogenous" and "morphine." However, this term has caused considerable confusion because of its association with one principal opioid peptide prototype, β-endorphin. Of all the native peptides, the pharmacologic profile of this latter compound appears to be most similar to that of morphine. As a consequence, the term **"opiopeptins"** has been suggested as the generic name for the native opioid peptides, and the term endorphin is being reserved for the peptide type closely related to β-endorphin.

The smallest peptides possessing direct opioid activity are 2 pentapeptides: **methionine-enkephalin** (met-enkephalin) and **leucine-enkephalin** (leu-enkephalin). With the exception of the methionine or leucine terminal group, the amino acid sequence of both enkephalins is identical (tyrosine, glycine, glycine, phenylalanine). One or both of these 2 peptides are contained in 3 principal precursor proteins having similar numbers of amino acids (between 257 and 265) with different repetitive peptide sequences.

Pro-enkephalin A contains 6 copies of met-enkephalin and one copy of leu-enkephalin that are part of several larger peptides with potent opioid activity. Pro-dynorphin (or pro-enkephalin B), on processing, yields several active peptides that contain leu-enkephalin as a fragment. The most potent appears to be a 17-amino-acid peptide, **dynorphin;** others include the neo-endorphins, dynorphin B (rimorphin), and certain smaller fragments of dynorphin. The third precursor protein, pro-opiomelanocortin (POMC), contains met-enkephalin, but the latter compound is not one of the processing end products. The most important fragment having general opiatelike properties is **β-endorphin,** a 31-amino-acid peptide with met-enkephalin at its carboxy terminus. Any reduction in the chain length of β-endorphin results in a great reduction in opioid activity. Other important peptides are contained in POMC but are devoid of opiatelike properties; these include melanocyte-stimulating hormone (MSH) and ACTH. Thus, a natural system is present in the body that can selectively release various opiopeptins in response to pain and other stimuli. Morphine and the other opioid analgesics apparently mimic the action of these endogenous ligands by binding with their receptors; this interaction gives rise to pharmacologic effects.

1. Receptor types—Several types of opioid receptors have been identified at various sites in the central and peripheral nervous systems. Exogenous and endogenous ligands bind at these loci to varying degrees, and the predominance and nature of the combination between a particular substance and a specific receptor give rise to a characteristic pharmacologic profile.

Analgesia at the supraspinal level as well as the euphoriant, respiratory depressant, and physical dependence properties of morphine (typical agonistlike effects) result principally from combination with μ (mu) receptors. The κ (kappa) receptors are responsible primarily for the expression of analgesia at the spinal level, miosis, and sedation. The σ (sigma) receptor seems related to the dysphoric, hallucinogenic, and cardiac stimulant effects. The δ (delta) and other receptors have been postulated based mainly on in vitro experiments, but their significance in vivo is unclear.

2. Receptor distribution—Opioid binding or recognition sites have been identified by radioligand binding, autoradiographic, and immunohistochemical techniques. A high density of binding sites is present in the dorsal horn of the spinal cord and certain subcortical regions of the brain. Some of the brain opioid binding sites that are concerned with pain transmission include the nucleus raphe magnus and locus ceruleus of the brain stem, the midbrain periaqueductal gray area, and several hypothalamic and thalamic nuclei. Binding of an opioid at these supraspinal sites greatly augments the effect at the spinal level to reduce nociceptive input and thereby raise the pain threshold. Certain spinal cord cells containing opioid analgesic binding sites have been identified as short interneurons terminating on pain-transmitting primary central sensory afferents containing the peptide transmitter substance P (Chapter 19). Substance P neurons have been hypothesized to transmit pain, and opioids and opiopeptins have been shown to inhibit the release of substance P.

The brain sites involved in altering reactivity to pain are less well identified. It has been suggested that pathways between the diencephalon and the frontal cortex are involved, since the effects of opioid analgesics bear some resemblance to those occurring after prefrontal lobotomy. The individual is aware of pain but states that it is no longer bothersome. Some support for such a postulate is provided by the fact that several nuclei of the thalamus and hypothalamus have been found to have a high density of opioid binding sites.

3. Neurochemical effects—Electrical activity in specific areas of the nervous system is inhibited by opioid analgesics, and the reduction in neuronal firing is accompanied by a general decrease in the release of certain neurotransmitters. Since the release of transmitter substances is known to be coupled with the entry of calcium into the neuron, it has been suggested that the action of opioids depends upon their ability to selectively interfere with calcium influx and lower brain calcium. This reduction in intracellular calcium in specific neurons where opioids act causes a deficiency in neurotransmitter release with decreased activation of their postsynaptic sites.

In contrast to the depression of calcium entry into neurons caused by a single exposure to opioids, chronic exposure, which is associated with tolerance and physical dependence, causes an elevation of intracellular calcium content in neurons.

Another recent hypothesis attempts to relate opioid analgesic effects to an inhibitory action on adenylate cyclase. The postulate is based principally on the effects of opioids on hybrid neuroblastoma cells in culture. Opioid effects on calcium and adenylate cyclase may be closely related, but definitive experiments to establish this relationship have not been carried out.

The release of several neurotransmitters is inhibited by opioid analgesics; these transmitters include acetylcholine, norepinephrine, dopamine, 5-hydroxy-tryptamine, and substance P. Earlier attempts to explain opioid action by linking certain effects with a single neurotransmitter have not been successful, mainly because no one neurotransmitter can account for all of the varied effects of the opioid analgesics.

4. Tolerance and physical dependence–With frequently repeated administration of therapeutic doses of morphine or its surrogates, there is a gradual loss in effectiveness, called **tolerance.** To reproduce the original response, a larger dose must be administered. With the development of tolerance, **physical dependence** occurs, so that continued administration of the drug becomes necessary to prevent a characteristic withdrawal or abstinence syndrome (Chapter 30).

The mechanism of development of tolerance and physical dependence is not related to pharmacokinetic factors but is a true cellular adaptive response. It has been suggested that the accumulation of neuronal calcium following frequent opioid administration may be partially responsible, since the ability to sequester calcium increases with chronic opioid administration and calcium readily antagonizes opioid effects. Discontinuing the opioid would then result in loss of the ability to sequester calcium and in enhanced release of a number of neurotransmitters. The increased transmitter release may be the immediate cause of the abstinence syndrome.

The clinical aspects of tolerance and physical dependence are discussed below.

B. Organ System Effects of Morphine and Its Surrogates: The actions given below for morphine, the prototype agonist opioid, are also observed with all of the other agonists (Table 29–1). The agonist-antagonist agents, when given to a patient who has not recently received an agonist agent, also produce analgesia, but with minor variations in effects as noted below. Characteristics of specific members of these 2 groups are discussed below.

The pure antagonists and the agonist-antagonists, when given to a subject who has received an agonist, will have very different effects, as noted at the end of this chapter.

1. Central nervous system effects–The principal effects of the opioid analgesics with affinity for μ receptors are on the central nervous system; the more important ones include analgesia, euphoria, sedation, and respiratory depression. With repeated use, a high degree of tolerance occurs to all of these effects (Table 29–3).

a. Analgesia–A painful sensation, no matter what its origin, consists of the noxious input plus the reaction of the organism to the stimulus. The analgesic properties of the opioids are related to their ability to change both pain *perception* and the *reaction* of the patient to pain. Experimental and clinical studies indicate that opioid analgesics can effectively raise the threshold for pain, but their effects on the reactive component can only be inferred from subjective effects on the patient. In the presence of effective anal-

Table 29–3. Extent of tolerance developed to some of the effects of the opiates.

High Degree of Tolerance	Moderate Degree of Tolerance	Minimal or No Tolerance
Analgesia	Bradycardia	Miosis
Euphoria, dysphoria		Constipation
Mental clouding		Convulsions
Sedation		
Respiratory depression		Antagonist actions
Antidiuresis		
Nausea and vomiting		
Cough suppression		

gesia, pain may still be noted or perceived by the patient, but even very severe pain is no longer an all-consuming and destructive sensory input.

b. Euphoria–After a dose of morphine, a patient in pain or an addict experiences a pleasant floating sensation and freedom from anxiety and distress. However, other patients and some normal subjects (not in pain) experience dysphoric rather than pleasant effects after a dose of opioid analgesic. Dysphoria is a disquieted state accompanied by both restlessness and a feeling of malaise. In general, if a real indication exists for administration of an opioid analgesic, the most common affective response is euphoria.

c. Sedation–Drowsiness and clouding of mentation are frequent concomitants of opioid action, and there may be some impairment of reasoning ability. There is little or no amnesia. Sleep is induced by opiates more frequently in the elderly than in young, healthy individuals. Ordinarily, the patient can be easily aroused from sleep. However, the combination of morphine with other central depressant drugs, such as the sedative-hypnotics, may result in profound depression. Marked sedation occurs more frequently with compounds closely related to the phenanthrene derivatives and less frequently with the synthetic agents such as meperidine and fentanyl. In contrast to humans, a number of species (cats, horses, cows, pigs) manifest excitation rather than sedation when given opioids. The reason for this difference is unknown.

d. Respiratory depression–All of the opioid analgesics can produce significant respiratory depression by inhibiting brain stem respiratory mechanisms. Alveolar P_{CO_2} may increase, but the most significant aspect of this depression is decreased responsiveness to carbon dioxide. Many well-designed studies have demonstrated this effect, chiefly as a depressed response to a carbon dioxide challenge. The respiratory depression is dose-related and is influenced significantly by the degree of other sensory input occurring at the same time. For example, it is possible to partially overcome the opioid-induced respiratory depression by stimulation of various sorts. When strongly painful stimuli that have prevented the depressant action of a large dose of an opioid are relieved, respiratory depression may suddenly become marked. A small to moderate decrease in respiratory function, as measured by P_{CO_2} elevation, may be well tolerated in the patient without prior respiratory impairment. However, in individuals with increased intracranial pressure, asthma, chronic obstructive pulmonary disease, or cor pulmonale, this decrease may not be tolerated.

e. Cough suppression–Suppression of the cough reflex is a well-recognized action of opioid analgesics. Codeine in particular has been used to good advantage in persons suffering from pathologic cough and in patients in whom it is necessary to maintain ventilation via an endotracheal tube. However, cough suppression by opiates may allow accumulation of secretions and thus lead to airway obstruction and atelectasis. Tolerance develops to the cough suppressant action of opioid analgesics (Table 29–3).

f. Miosis–Constriction of the pupils is seen with virtually all of the opioid agonists. Miosis is also a pharmacologic action to which little or no tolerance develops; thus, it is valuable in the diagnosis of opiate overdose, since even highly tolerant addicts will have miosis. The action can be blocked by atropine and by opioid antagonists.

g. Truncal rigidity–An intensification of tone in the large trunk muscles has been noted with a number of opioids. It is believed that this is the result of an action of the opioids at the spinal cord level. Truncal rigidity reduces thoracic compliance and thus interferes with ventilation. This action may be overcome by administration of a opioid antagonist.

h. Emesis–The opioid analgesics can activate the brain stem chemoreceptor trigger zone to produce nausea and vomiting. There may be another component to these effects in that ambulation seems to increase the incidence of nausea and vomiting, perhaps by an action on the vestibular apparatus.

2. Peripheral effects–

a. Cardiovascular system–Most opioid analgesics have no significant direct effects on the heart and no major effects on cardiac rate or rhythm or on blood pressure. Exceptions to this generalization will be noted below as the specific drugs are discussed. Blood pressure is usually well maintained in subjects receiving opiates unless the cardiovascular system is stressed, in which case hypotension may occur. This hypotensive effect is probably due to peripheral arterial and venous dilatation, which has been attributed to a number of mechanisms including release of histamine and central depression of vasomotor-stabilizing mechanisms. No consistent effect on cardiac output is seen, and the ECG is not significantly altered. However, caution should be exercised in patients with decreased blood volume, since the above mechanisms make these patients quite susceptible to blood pressure decreases. Opioid analgesics affect cerebral circulation minimally except when P_{CO_2} rises as a consequence of respiratory depression. Increased P_{CO_2} leads to cerebral vascular dilatation and a concomitant decrease in cerebral vascular resistance, increase in cerebral blood flow, and increase in cerebrospinal fluid pressure (intracranial pressure).

b. Gastrointestinal tract–Constipation has long been recognized as an effect of opioid analgesics,

although the effects of the opioids on smooth muscle of the gut are generally stimulatory. There is considerable variation in the response at different levels of the gut. The effects are mediated through an action on the central nervous system as well as a local one. In the stomach, motility may be decreased but tone may increase—particularly in the central portion; gastric secretion of hydrochloric acid is decreased. Small intestine resting tone is increased, with periodic spasms, but the amplitude of nonpropulsive contractions is markedly decreased. In the large intestine, propulsive peristaltic waves are diminished and tone is increased; this delays passage of the fecal mass and allows increased absorption of water, which leads to constipation. The large bowel actions are the basis for the use of opioids in management of diarrhea. There is a clinical impression that the benzomorphans (eg, pentazocine) cause less constipation than other opioids.

c. Biliary tract–The opioids constrict biliary smooth muscle, which may result in biliary colic. The sphincter of Oddi may constrict, resulting in reflux of biliary and pancreatic secretions and elevated plasma amylase and lipase levels.

d. Genitourinary tract–Renal function is depressed by opioids. It is believed that in humans this is chiefly due to decreased renal plasma flow. This contrasts with animal studies, in which reduced urine output seems to result from increased secretion of antidiuretic hormone as well as reduced renal perfusion. Ureteral and bladder tone is increased by therapeutic doses of the opioid analgesics. Increased urethral sphincter tone may precipitate urinary retention, especially in postoperative patients. Occasionally, ureteral colic caused by a renal calculus is made worse by the increase in ureteral tone.

e. Uterus–The opioid analgesics may prolong labor. The mechanism for this action is unclear, but both peripheral and central effects of the opioids may reduce uterine tone.

f. Neuroendocrine–Opioid analgesics stimulate the release of antidiuretic hormone, prolactin, and somatotropin but inhibit the release of luteinizing hormone. These effects are of importance in that they may reflect regulatory roles in these systems by endogenous opioid peptides and are probably mediated by effects in the hypothalamus.

g. Miscellaneous–Therapeutic doses of the opioid analgesics will produce flushing and warming of the skin accompanied sometimes by sweating and itching; central effects and histamine release may be responsible for these reactions.

C. Effects of Agonist-Antagonists: Pentazocine and other agonist-antagonist drugs usually produce sedation in addition to analgesia when given in therapeutic doses. At higher doses, sweating, dizziness, and nausea are common, but severe respiratory depression may be less common than with pure agonists. When it does occur, respiratory depression may be reversed by naloxone but not reliably by other agonist-antagonists such as nalorphine. Psychotomimetic effects, with hallucinations, nightmares, and anxiety, have been reported following the use of agonist-antagonist agents.

II. CLINICAL PHARMACOLOGY OF THE OPIOID ANALGESICS

Management of pain is essential to good medical practice and requires careful consideration of proper dose, type of drug, and the disease being treated. There are many situations in which analgesia must be provided before a definitive diagnosis can be reached. Indeed, in some acute situations relief of pain may actually facilitate history taking and physical examination and thus speed the diagnostic process.

Use of these drugs in acute situations may be contrasted to their use in chronic pain management, where other factors must be considered—particularly tolerance and physical dependence. In all instances, the factors that should enter into the decision about choice of drug include the following: (1) Is analgesia needed? (2) Will the opioid analgesic obscure or alter the signs and symptoms of the underlying disorder? (3) Are the pharmacologic effects of the opioid liable to worsen the condition for which they are being used, eg, by increasing cerebrospinal fluid pressure or producing respiratory depression? (4) Do the opioid agent's adverse effects impose a significant hazard? (See Table 29–4.) (5) Is there a possibility of significant drug interaction between the opioid agent and other drugs the patient is receiving? (See Table 29–5.) (6) Are tolerance and drug dependence likely to develop?

Table 29–2 shows the variability in agonist efficacy of different opioid drugs. It is therefore necessary to select a drug appropriate to the type and severity of pain being treated to make certain that adequate analgesia is provided. The level of pain associated with various disease states also varies; thus, the postoperative pain of a forearm fracture may be adequately treated with codeine; the severe pain of a kidney stone may not. Each drug has a therapeutic ceiling, and to attempt to raise the ceiling with higher doses creates a risk of significant drug side effects and therapeutic failure.

Clinical Use of Opioid Analgesics

A. Analgesia: Severe, *constant* pain is usually

Table 29–4. Toxic effects of the opioid analgesics.

Behavioral restlessness, tremulousness, hyperactivity (in dysphoric reaction).
Respiratory depression.
Nausea and vomiting.
Increased intracranial pressure.
Postural hypotension accentuated by hypovolemia.
Constipation.
Urinary retention.
Itching around nose, urticaria (more frequent with parenteral administration).

Table 29–5. Opioid drug interactions.

Sedative-hypnotics: Increased central nervous system depression, particularly respiratory depression.

Antipsychotic tranquilizers: Increased sedation. Variable effects on respiratory depression. Accentuation of cardiovascular effects (antimuscarinic and alpha-blocking actions).

MAO inhibitors: Absolute contraindication to all opioid analgesics because of the high incidence of hyperpyrexic coma; hypertension has also been reported.

relieved with the more efficacious opioids, but sharp, intermittent pain does not appear to be as amenable to relief. An attempt should be made to quantify the pain; this information should be used to select the proper agent and to monitor its effects. In this evaluation and selection process, such considerations as route of administration (oral versus parenteral administration), duration of action, ceiling effect (maximal efficacy), duration of therapy, and past experience with opioids are of obvious importance.

The pain associated with cancer and other terminal illnesses must be treated adequately, and concerns about tolerance and dependence should be set aside in favor of making the patient as comfortable as possible. Research by workers in the hospice movement has demonstrated that fixed-interval administration of opioid medication (a regular dose at a regular time) is more effective in achieving pain relief than dosing on demand. In addition, drugs such as the amphetamines have been shown to enhance the actions of the opioids and thus may be very useful adjuncts in the patient with chronic pain.

Opioid analgesics are often employed during obstetric labor. Because all of the opioids cross the placental barrier and reach the fetus, care must be taken to minimize neonatal opioid depression. If this occurs, immediate injection of naloxone will reverse the depression. The phenylpiperidine drugs (eg, meperidine) appear to produce less depression in newborn infants than does morphine; this may justify their use in obstetric practice.

The acute, severe pain of renal and biliary colic often requires a strong agonist opioid for adequate relief. However, the increase in smooth muscle tone may cause a paradoxic *increase* in pain secondary to increased spasm around the stone. An increase in the dose of opioid is usually successful in providing analgesia.

B. Acute Pulmonary Edema: The relief produced by intravenous morphine in dyspnea from pulmonary edema associated with left ventricular failure is truly remarkable. The mechanism is not clear but probably involves a reduction in *perception* of shortness of breath and the anxiety associated with it as well as a reduction in cardiac preload (reduced venous tone) and afterload (decreased peripheral resistance). (See also Chapter 12.)

C. Cough: Suppression of cough can be obtained

at doses lower than those needed for analgesia. However, in recent years the use of opioid analgesics to allay cough has diminished largely because a number of effective synthetic compounds have been developed that are neither analgesic nor addictive. These agents are discussed in the section on antitussives.

D. Diarrhea: Diarrhea from almost any cause can be controlled with the opioid analgesics, but if diarrhea is associated with infection such use must not substitute for appropriate chemotherapy. Opium preparations (eg, paregoric) have long been used to control diarrhea, but in recent years opiates with more selective gastrointestinal effects have been developed, eg, diphenoxylate. Formulations are cited below that have been prepared specifically for this purpose.

E. Applications in Anesthesia: The opioids are frequently used as premedicant drugs before anesthesia and surgery because of their sedative, anxiolytic, and analgesic properties. The opioids are also used intraoperatively both as adjuncts to other anesthetic agents and, in high doses (eg, 1–3 mg/kg of morphine, or 0.02–0.075 mg/kg of fentanyl), as the primary anesthetic agent (see Chapter 23), most commonly in cardiovascular surgery and other types of high-risk surgery where a primary goal is to minimize cardiovascular depression. In such situations, mechanical respiratory assistance must be provided.

Recently, there has been great interest in the use of opioids as regional analgesics by administration into the epidural or subarachnoid spaces of the spinal column. This interest is based on the laboratory finding that there is a spinal component of opiate action and that there are a great many opioid receptors in the dorsolateral horn of the spinal cord. Theoretically, therefore, the epidural application of opioids might selectively produce analgesia without impairment of motor, autonomic, or sensory functions other than pain. A number of studies have, in the main, confirmed these expectations. Long-lasting analgesia (6–30 hours) with minimal side effects can be achieved by epidural administration of 3–5 mg of morphine. However, respiratory depression may occur hours after the drug is injected. This adverse effect may require reversal with naloxone. Other side effects such as pruritus and nausea and vomiting are common after epidural and subarachnoid administration of opioids and may also be reversed with naloxone if necessary.

Toxicity & Undesired Effects

Direct toxic effects of the opioid analgesics that are extensions of their acute pharmacologic actions include the adverse effects of nausea, vomiting, constipation, and respiratory depression (Table 29–4). In addition, the following must be considered.

A. Tolerance and Dependence: Drug dependence of the opioid type is marked by tolerance, a relatively specific withdrawal or abstinence syndrome, and pronounced craving or psychologic dependence. Just as there are pharmacologic differences between the various opioids, there are also differences in

abuse potential and the severity of withdrawal effects. For instance, administration of an opioid antagonist to a methadone-dependent person is followed by severe withdrawal symptoms. Propoxyphene, a related compound, causes less marked dependence, and the withdrawal syndrome appears to be milder although qualitatively similar to that of other opioids. The addiction liabilities of the mixed agonist-antagonist opioids appear to be considerably less than those of the agonist drugs. Heroin addicts usually resort to pentazocine only when agonists are not available.

1. Tolerance–As mentioned above, repeated administration of therapeutic doses of any opioid results in a gradual loss of effectiveness. Although development of tolerance begins with the first dose of an opioid, tolerance generally does not become clinically manifest until 2–3 weeks of frequent experience with ordinary therapeutic doses. Tolerance develops most readily when large doses are given at short intervals and is minimized by giving small amounts of drug with larger intervals between doses. Thus, compulsive abusers of opioids may develop tolerance very rapidly.

Depending on the compound and the effect measured, the degree of tolerance may be as great as 35-fold. Marked tolerance usually develops to the analgesic, euphoriant, and respiratory depressant effects. It is possible to produce respiratory arrest in a nontolerant person with a dose of 60 mg of morphine, whereas in addicts maximally tolerant to opioids as much as 2000 mg of morphine taken over a 2- or 3-hour period may not produce significant respiratory depression. Tolerance also develops to the antidiuretic, emetic, and hypotensive effect but not to the miotic, convulsant, and constipating actions (Table 29–3).

Tolerance to the euphoriant and respiratory effects of the opioids dissipates within a few days after the drugs are discontinued. Tolerance to the emetic effects may persist for several months after withdrawal of the drug. The rates at which tolerance appears and disappears, as well as the degree of tolerance, may also differ considerably among the different opioid analgesics. For instance, tolerance to methadone develops more slowly and to a lesser degree than to morphine.

Cross-tolerance is an extremely important characteristic of the opioids, ie, patients tolerant to morphine are also tolerant to all other agonist opioids. Morphine, meperidine, methadone, and their congeners exhibit cross-tolerance not only with respect to their analgesic actions but also to their euphoriant, sedative, and respiratory effects.

Tolerance develops also to the agonist-antagonist analgesics but to a much lesser extent than to the agonists. Such effects as hallucinations, sedation, hypothermia, and respiratory depression are reduced after repeated administration of the agonist-antagonist drugs. However, tolerance to agonist-antagonist agents does not generally include cross-tolerance to the agonist opioids. It is also important to note that tolerance does not develop to the antagonist actions of the mixed agonist-antagonists nor to those of the pure antagonists.

2. Physical dependence–The development of physical dependence on an opioid of the μ type after its repeated administration is an invariable accompaniment of tolerance. Failure to continue administering the drug results in a characteristic withdrawal or abstinence syndrome that reflects an exaggerated rebound from the acute pharmacologic effects of the opioid. The signs and symptoms of withdrawal include rhinorrhea, lacrimation, yawning, chills, goose pimples, hyperventilation, hyperthermia, mydriasis, muscular aches, vomiting, diarrhea, anxiety, and hostility (see also Chapter 30). The number and intensity of the signs and symptoms are largely dependent on the degree of physical dependence that has developed. Administration of an opioid suppresses abstinence signs and symptoms almost immediately. The time of onset, the intensity, and the duration of the abstinence effects depend on the drug used and may be related to its biologic half-life. With morphine or heroin, withdrawal signs usually start within 6–10 hours after the last dose. Peak effects are seen at 36–48 hours, after which most of the signs and symptoms gradually subside. By 5 days, most of the effects have disappeared, but some may persist for months. In the case of meperidine, the withdrawal syndrome largely subsides within 24 hours, whereas with methadone several days are required to reach the peak of abstinence syndrome, and it may last as long as 2 weeks. The slower subsidence of methadone effects is associated with a less intense immediate syndrome, and this is the basis for its use in the detoxification of heroin addicts.

A transient, explosive abstinence syndrome—antagonist-precipitated withdrawal—can be induced in a subject physically dependent on opioids by administering naloxone or other antagonist. Within 5 minutes after injection of the antagonist, signs and symptoms similar to those seen after abrupt discontinuance appear, peaking in 10–20 minutes and largely subsiding after 1 hour. In contrast to the relatively mild abstinence syndrome that results from methadone withdrawal (cessation of drug administration), antagonist-precipitated methadone abstinence syndrome may be very severe.

In the case of the agonist-antagonist agents, withdrawal signs and symptoms can be induced after repeated administration followed by abrupt discontinuance of pentazocine, cyclazocine, or nalorphine, but the syndrome appears to be quite different from that produced by morphine and other agonists. Anxiety, loss of appetite and body weight, tachycardia, chills, increase in body temperature, and abdominal cramps have been noted.

3. Psychologic dependence–The euphoria, indifference to stimuli, and sedation usually caused by the opioid analgesics, especially when injected intravenously, tend to promote their compulsive use. In addition, the addict experiences abdominal effects that have been likened to an intense sexual orgasm. These factors constitute the primary reasons for opioid abuse

liability and are strongly reinforced by the development of physical dependence, since the drug user rationalizes continued use of the drug as the means of preventing abstinence symptoms, ie, to remain "normal."

Under no circumstances should adequate pain relief be denied simply because an opioid exhibits potential for abuse or because laws complicate the process of prescribing narcotics. However, there are certain principles that can be followed by the clinician to avoid the problems presented by tolerance and dependence when using opioid analgesics: (1) Establish therapeutic goals before starting opioid therapy. This tends to limit the potential for physical dependence. (2) When drugs equivalent to morphine must be used, attempt to limit both the dosage and duration of administration. (3) Instead of opioid analgesics, especially in chronic management, consider using other types of analgesics or compounds exhibiting less pronounced withdrawal symptoms on discontinuance.

B. Diagnosis and Treatment of Opioid Overdosage: The diagnosis of opioid overdosage may be very simple (known addict, needle marks, brought to hospital by friends who appear to be using drugs), or it may be very difficult—as in any comatose patient for whom no past history is available. Intravenous injection of naloxone, 0.2–0.4 mg, can provide quick information about whether coma is due to opiate overdose. Treatment is with the same drug, 0.4–0.8 mg given intravenously, and repeated every 2–3 minutes for 2–3 doses. In using naloxone in the severely depressed newborn, it is important to start with doses of 5–10 μg/kg and to consider a second dose of up to a total of 25 μg/kg if no response is noted. Use of the antagonist should not, of course, delay the institution of other therapeutic measures, especially respiratory support.

C. Contraindications and Cautions in Therapy:

1. Use of pure agonists with mixed agonist-antagonists–When a mixed agonist-antagonist agent such as pentazocine is given to a patient also receiving an agonist (eg, morphine), the possibility of diminishing analgesia or perhaps inducing a state of withdrawal is present; combining agonist with agonist-antagonist opiates should be done cautiously, if at all.

2. Use in patients with head injuries–Carbon dioxide retention caused by respiratory depression results in cerebral vasodilatation; in patients with elevated intracranial pressure, this may lead to lethal alterations in brain functions.

3. Use during pregnancy–In pregnant women who are chronically using opioids, the fetus may become addicted in utero and may manifest withdrawal symptoms in the early postpartum period. A daily dose as small as 6 mg of heroin (or equivalent) will result in a mild withdrawal syndrome in the infant, and twice that much may result in severe signs and symptoms, including irritability, shrill crying, diarrhea, or even seizures. Recognition of the problem is aided by a careful history and physical examination.

OPIOID ANALGESICS & ANTAGONISTS / **347**

Initial treatment of the neonate may consist of giving paregoric, 0.12–0.24 mL/kg orally (1 mL of paregoric is equivalent to 0.4 mg of morphine) or methadone, 0.1–0.5 mg/kg orally. Large intravenous doses of the piperidine derivatives (meperidine, fentanyl, etc) should be avoided, since they cause central nervous system stimulation, particularly in infants and children. More recently, diazepam, 0.1 mg/kg intravenously, has been used in the treatment of neonatal withdrawal syndrome. The pharmacologic basis for this is unclear, since diazepam is a sedative and does not bind to opiate receptors.

4. Use in patients with impaired pulmonary function–In patients with borderline respiratory reserve, the depressant properties of the opioid analgesics may lead to acute respiratory failure.

5. Use in patients with impaired hepatic function–Morphine and its congeners are metabolized primarily by conjugation to glucuronides in the liver; their use in patients in prehepatic coma may thus be questioned.

6. Use in patients with endocrine disease–Patients with adrenal insufficiency (Addison's disease) and those with hypothyroidism (myxedema) may have prolonged and exaggerated responses to opioids.

Drug Interactions

Because seriously ill or hospitalized patients may require a large number of drugs, there is always a possibility of drug interactions when the opioid analgesics are administered. Table 29–5 lists some of these drug interactions and the reasons for not combining the named drugs with opioids.

SPECIFIC AGENTS

The following section describes the most important widely used opioid analgesics, along with features peculiar to specific agents. Data about doses approximately equivalent to 10 mg of intramuscular morphine, oral:parenteral efficacy, duration of analgesia, maximum efficacy, and addiction and abuse liability are presented in Table 29–2.

STRONG AGONISTS

PHENANTHRENES

Morphine, hydromorphone, and **oxymorphone** are strong agonists useful in treating severe pain. These prototypic agents have been described in detail above. **Heroin** is a potent and fast-acting narcotic, but its use is prohibited by legislation in the USA. In recent years there has been considerable agitation to revive its use. However, double-blind studies have not supported the claim that heroin is more effective than morphine in relieving severe chronic pain.

PHENYLHEPTYLAMINES

Methadone has a pharmacodynamic profile very similar to that of morphine but is somewhat longer-acting. Acutely, its analgesic potency and efficacy are at least equal to those of morphine. Methadone gives reliable effects when administered orally. Tolerance and physical dependence develop more slowly with methadone than with morphine. As noted above, the withdrawal signs and symptoms occurring after abrupt discontinuance of methadone are milder, although more prolonged, than those of morphine. These properties make methadone a useful drug for detoxification and for maintenance of the chronic relapsing heroin addict. For detoxification of a heroin-dependent addict, low doses of methadone (5–10 mg orally) are given twice or 3 times daily for 2 or 3 days. Upon discontinuing methadone, the addict experiences a mild but endurable withdrawal syndrome. For maintenance therapy of the opioid recidivist, tolerance to 50–100 mg/d of oral methadone is deliberately produced; in this state, the addict exhibits cross-tolerance to heroin that prevents most of the addiction-reinforcing effects of heroin. The rationale of maintenance programs is that blocking the reinforcement obtained from abuse of illicit opioids removes the motive for criminal activity and makes the addict more amenable to psychiatric and rehabilitative therapy. The pharmacologic basis for the use of methadone in maintenance programs is sound and the sociologic basis is rational, but some methadone programs fail because nonpharmacologic management is inadequate.

PHENYLPIPERIDINES

Meperidine, fentanyl, and **alphaprodine** are the most widely used agents in this family. Fentanyl is used chiefly as part of the anesthesia regimen during surgery. Meperidine has significant antimuscarinic effects, which may be a contraindication if tachycardia would be a problem. It is also reported to have a negative inotropic action on the heart. Alphaprodine is largely used in obstetrics and dentistry, because of its rapid absorption from subcutaneous injection sites.

MORPHINANS

Levorphanol is a synthetically prepared opioid analgesic closely resembling morphine in its action but offering no advantages.

MILD TO MODERATE AGONISTS

PHENANTHRENES

Codeine, oxycodone, dihydrocodeine, and **hydrocodone** are all somewhat less potent than morphine or have side effects that limit the maximum tolerated dose when one attempts to achieve analgesia comparable to that of morphine. These compounds are rarely used alone but are combined in formulations containing aspirin or acetaminophen and other drugs.

PHENYLHEPTYLAMINES

Propoxyphene is chemically related to methadone but has low analgesic activity. Various studies have reported its potency at levels ranging from no better than placebo to half as potent as codeine, ie, 120 mg propoxyphene = 60 mg codeine. Its true potency probably lies somewhere between these extremes, and its analgesic effect is additive to that of an optimal dose of aspirin. However, its low efficacy makes it unsuitable, even in combination with aspirin, for severe pain. Although propoxyphene has a low abuse liability, the increasing incidence of deaths associated with its misuse in recent years has caused it to be scheduled as a controlled substance with low potential for abuse.

PHENYLPIPERIDINES

Diphenoxylate is not used for analgesia but for the treatment of diarrhea. It is not scheduled for control because the likelihood of its abuse is remote. The poor solubility of the compound limits its use for parenteral injection. As an antidiarrheal drug, it is usually used in combination with atropine (Lomotil, other names).

Loperamide (Imodium) is another phenylpiperidine derivative used to control diarrhea. Its potential for abuse is low because of its limited ability to gain access to the brain. The usual dose is 4 mg to start and then 2 mg after each diarrheal stool.

MIXED AGONIST-ANTAGONISTS

PHENANTHRENES

Nalbuphine is a κ agonist and μ antagonist; it is given parenterally. At doses higher than usual, there seems to be a definite ceiling—not noted with morphine—to the respiratory depressant effect. Unfortunately, when respiratory depression does occur, it may be relatively resistant to naloxone reversal.

Buprenorphine is a potent and long-acting phenanthrene derivative that behaves like a mixed agonist-antagonist at the μ receptor. Its clinical applications are much like those of nalbuphine.

MORPHINANS

Butorphanol produces analgesia equivalent to nalbuphine and buprenorphine but appears to produce more sedation at equianalgesic dose. Butorphanol is considered to be a κ agonist.

BENZOMORPHANS

Pentazocine is also a κ agonist and is the oldest mixed agonist-antagonist available. It may be used orally or parenterally. However, because of its irritant properties, the injection of pentazocine subcutaneously is not recommended. As with all of the agonist-antagonists, care should be taken not to administer them to patients receiving pure agonist drugs because of the unpredictability of both drugs' effects.

ANTITUSSIVES

As noted above, the opioid analgesics are among the most effective drugs available for the suppression of cough. This effect is often achieved at doses below those necessary to produce analgesia. Furthermore, the antitussive effect is also produced by the stereoisomers of opioid molecules, which are devoid of analgesic effects and addiction liability. The receptors involved in the antitussive effect appear to differ from those associated with the other actions of opioids.

The physiologic mechanism of cough is a complex one, and little is known about the specific mechanism of action of the opioid antitussive drugs. It is likely that both central and peripheral effects come into play.

The opioid derivatives most commonly used as antitussives are dextromethorphan, codeine, levopropoxyphene, and noscapine. While these agents (other than codeine) are largely free of the side effects associated with the opiates, none of them should be used in patients taking MAO inhibitors (see Table 29–5).

Dextromethorphan is the dextrorotatory stereoisomer of a methylated derivative of levorphanol. It is essentially free of analgesic and addictive properties and produces less constipation than codeine. The usual antitussive dose is 15–30 mg 3–4 times daily. It is available in many over-the-counter products.

Codeine, as noted above, has a useful antitussive action at doses lower than those required for analgesia. Thus, 15 mg is usually sufficient to relieve cough.

Levopropoxyphene is the stereoisomer of the weak opioid agonist dextropropoxyphene. It is devoid of opioid effects, although sedation has been described as a side effect. The usual antitussive dose is 50–100 mg every 4 hours.

Noscapine is, like papaverine, a nonanalgesic benzylisoquinoline opium alkaloid. It is used only as an antitussive and is claimed to be as effective in this application as codeine. The usual dose is 15–30 mg every 6 hours.

THE OPIOID ANTAGONISTS

The pure opioid antagonist drugs **naloxone** and **naltrexone** are morphine derivatives with larger substituents at the N position. These agents have a relatively high affinity for opioid binding sites of the μ receptor type. Their affinity for κ receptors is about one-twentieth of that for μ receptors and probably even less for δ receptors.

Pharmacokinetics

Naloxone has poor efficacy when given by the oral route and a short duration of action (1–4 hours) when given by injection. Metabolic disposition is chiefly by glucuronide conjugation, like that of the agonist opioids. Naltrexone is well absorbed after oral administration but may undergo rapid first-pass metabolism. It has a half-life of 10 hours, and a single oral dose of 100 mg will block the effects of injected heroin for up to 48 hours.

Pharmacodynamics

When given in the absence of an agonist drug, these antagonists are almost inert at doses that produce marked antagonism of agonist effects.

When given to a morphine-treated subject, the antagonist will completely reverse the opioid effects within 1–2 minutes. This constitutes one of the most dramatic examples of pharmacologic antagonism in medicine. In individuals who are acutely depressed by an overdose of an opioid, the antagonist will effectively normalize respiration, level of consciousness, pupil size, bowel activity, etc. In dependent subjects who appear normal while taking opioids, naloxone or naltrexone will almost instantaneously precipitate an abstinence syndrome, as described previously.

There is no tolerance to the antagonistic action of these agents, nor does withdrawal after chronic administration precipitate an abstinence syndrome.

Clinical Use

Naloxone is a pure antagonist and is preferred over earlier weak agonist-antagonist agents that had been used primarily as antagonists, eg, nalorphine and levallorphan.

The major application of naloxone is in the treatment of acute opioid overdose, as described above; it is the specific antidote for this condition (see also Chapter 62). It is very important that the relatively short duration of action of naloxone be borne in mind when using it for this purpose, since a severely depressed patient may recover after a single dose of naloxone and appear normal, only to relapse into coma after 1–2 hours. The usual dose of naloxone is 0.1–0.4 mg intravenously, which can be repeated as necessary.

Because of its long duration of action, naltrexone has been proposed as a "maintenance" drug for addicts in treatment programs. A single dose given on alternate days blocks virtually all of the effects of a dose of heroin. It might be predicted that this approach to rehabilitation would not be popular with a large percentage of drug users unless they are motivated to become drug-free.

Recent experimental studies suggest that naloxone may be of value in the treatment of shock. Experimental animals with hemorrhagic, endotoxin-induced, and spinal transection shock respond to naloxone with an increase in blood pressure and improved survival rates. The mechanism for this effect is not known, but elevated concentrations of opiopeptins can be detected in the blood of animals in shock. Similarly, it has been used in cerebrovascular disease, eg, stroke, where the regional ischemic effects appear to be lessened.

REFERENCES

Akil H et al: Endogenous opioids: Biology and function. *Annu Rev Neurosci* 1984;**7**:233.

Beaver WT: A clinical comparison of the analgesic effects of intramuscular nalbuphine and morphine in patients with postoperative pain. *J Pharmacol Exp Ther* 1978;**204**:487.

Belleville JW et al: Influence of age on pain relief from analgesics. *JAMA* 1971;**217**:1835.

Bloom FE: The endorphins: A growing family of pharmacologically pertinent peptides. *Annu Rev Pharmacol Toxicol* 1983; **23**:151.

Braude MC et al (editors): *Narcotic Antagonists*. Raven Press, 1974.

Frederickson RCA, Geary LE: Endogenous opioid peptides: Review of physiological, pharmacological, and clinical aspects. *Prog Neurobiol* 1982;**19**:19.

Holaday J: Cardiovascular effects of endogenous opiate systems. *Annu Rev Pharmacol Toxicol* 1983;**23**:541.

Höllt V: Multiple endogenous opioid peptides. *Trends Neurol Sci* 1983;**6**:24.

Houde RW: Analgesic effectiveness of the narcotic agonist-antagonists. *Br J Clin Pharmacol* 1979;**7(Suppl 3)**:297S.

Houde RW, Wallenstein SL, Beaver WT: Clinical measurement of pain. Pages 75–122 in: *Analgetics*. De Stevens G (editor). Academic Press, 1965.

Iwamoto ET, Martin W: Multiple opiate receptors. *Med Res Rev* 1981;**1**:411.

Kuhar MJ, Pasternak GW (editors): *Analgesics: Neurochemical, Behavioral, and Clinical Perspectives*. Raven Press, 1984.

Smith AP, Loh HH: The opiate receptor. In: *Hormonal Proteins and Peptides: β-Endorphin*. Vol 10. Li CH (editor). Academic Press, 1981.

Way EL: Review and overview of four decades of opiate research. Chapter 1 in: *Neurochemical Mechanisms of Opiates and Endorphins*. Loh HH, Ross DH (editors). Vol 20 of: *Advances in Biochemical Psychopharmacology*. Raven Press, 1979.

Way EL, Adler TK: The pharmacologic implications of the fate of morphine and its surrogates. *Pharmacol Rev* 1968;**12**:383.

30

Drugs of Abuse

Leo Hollister, MD

The term "drug abuse" is unfortunate because it connotes social disapproval and may have different meanings to different people. One must also distinguish drug abuse from drug "misuse." Abuse of a drug might be construed as any use of a drug for nonmedical purposes, almost always for altering consciousness. To misuse a drug might be to take it for the wrong indication, in the wrong dosage, or for too long a period, to mention only a few obvious examples. In the context of drug abuse, the drug itself is of less importance than the pattern of use. For example, taking 50 mg of diazepam to heighten the effect of a daily dose of methadone is an abuse of diazepam. On the other hand, taking the same excessive daily dose of the drug but only for its sedative effect is misusing diazepam.

Dependence is a biologic phenomenon. **Psychic dependence** is manifested by compulsive drug-seeking behavior in which the individual uses the drug repetitively for personal satisfaction. Heavy cigarette smoking is an example. **Physical dependence** is present when withdrawal of the drug produces symptoms and signs that are frequently the opposite of those sought by the user. It has been suggested that the body adjusts to a new level of homeostasis during the period of drug use and reacts in opposite fashion when the new equilibrium is disturbed. Alcohol withdrawal syndrome is perhaps the best-known example, but milder degrees of withdrawal may be observed in people who drink a lot of coffee every day. Psychic dependence almost always precedes physical dependence but does not inevitably lead to it. **Addiction** is usually taken to mean a state of physical and psychic dependence, but the word is too imprecise to be useful.

Tolerance signifies a decreased response to the effects of the drug, necessitating ever larger doses to achieve the same effect. Tolerance is closely associated with the phenomenon of physical dependence. It is largely due to compensatory responses that mitigate the drug's pharmacodynamic action. **Metabolic tolerance** due to increased disposition of the drug after chronic use is occasionally reported. **Behavioral tolerance**, an ability to compensate for the drug's effects, is another possible mechanism of tolerance. Most other tolerance is due to a decreased pharmacodynamic action of the drug.

A number of experimental techniques have been devised to predict the ability of a drug to produce dependence and to assess its likelihood for abuse. Most of these techniques employ self-administration of the drug by animals. The rates of reinforcement can be altered so as to make the animal work harder for each dose of drug, providing a semiquantitative measure as well. Comparisons are made against a standard drug in the class, eg, morphine among the opioids. Withdrawal of dependent animals from drugs can be used to assess the nature of the withdrawal syndrome as well as to test drugs that might cross-substitute for the standard drug. Most agents with significant potential for psychic or physical dependence can be readily detected by these techniques. The actual abuse liability, however, is difficult to predict, since variables enter into the decision to abuse drugs.

Cultural Considerations

Each society accepts certain drugs as licit and condemns others as illicit. In the USA and most of Western Europe, the "national drugs" are caffeine, nicotine, and alcohol. In the Middle East, cannabis may be added to the list of licit drugs, while alcohol is forbidden. Among certain American Indian tribes, peyote, a hallucinogen, may be used licitly for religious purposes. In the Andes of South America, cocaine is used to allay hunger and enhance the ability to perform arduous work at high altitude. Thus, which drugs are licit or illicit or—to use other terminology—"used" or "abused" depends on a social judgment. A major social cost of relegating any substance to the illicit category is the criminal activity that often results, since purveyors of the substance are lured into illegal traffic by the opportunity to make enormous profits while dependent users may resort to robbery, prostitution, and other types of antisocial behavior to support their habits.

Current USA attitudes to drugs of this type are reflected in the Schedule of Controlled Substances (Table 30–1). This schedule is quite similar to those published by international control bodies. They affect principally ethical and law-abiding manufacturers of the drugs and have had little deterrent effect on underground manufacturers or suppliers.

Any use of mind-altering drugs is based on a complicated interplay between 3 factors: the user, the setting in which the drug is taken, and the drug. Thus, the personality of the user and the setting may have a strong influence on what the user experiences. Nonetheless, it is usually possible to identify a pharmacologic "core" of drug effects that will be experienced by almost anyone under almost any circumstances if dosage is adequate.

Table 30–1. Illustrations from Schedule of Controlled Substances, United States Drug Enforcement Agency. Note that the criteria given by the agency do not always reflect the actual pharmacologic properties of the drugs (see text).

Schedule	Criteria	Examples*
I	No medical use; high addiction potential.	Hallucinogens Marihuana Heroin
II	Medical use; high addiction potential.	Morphine, most other opioid analgesics Cocaine Amphetamines Sedatives such as pentobarbital sodium
III	Medical use; moderate potential for dependence.	Codeine in combination Paregoric Glutethimide, sodium butabarbital
IV	Medical use; low abuse potential.	Phenobarbital Chloral hydrate Benzodiazepines Other sedatives

*List not complete.

SPECIFIC TYPES OF DRUGS OF ABUSE

OPIATES & OPIOIDS

History

The nepenthe (Greek, "free from sorrow") mentioned in the *Odyssey* probably contained opium. Opium smoking was widely practiced in China and the Near East until recently. Isolation of active opium alkaloids as well as the introduction of the hypodermic needle, allowing parenteral use of morphine, increased opiate use in the West. The first of several "epidemics" of opiate use in the USA followed the Civil War. Relief of pain with liberal doses of opiates was one of the few forms of treatment army physicians could offer the gravely wounded, and those lucky enough to survive often found themselves physically dependent. About 4% of adults in the USA used opiates regularly during the postbellum period. By the 1900s, the number had dropped to about one in 400 people in the USA, but the problem was still considered serious enough to justify passage of the Harrison Narcotic Act just before World War I. A new epidemic of opiate use started around 1964 and has remained unabated ever since. Present estimates are that the number of opiate-dependent people in the USA has recently stabilized at between 400,000 and 600,000.

Chemistry & Pharmacology

The most commonly abused drugs in this group are heroin, morphine, oxycodone, and (among health professionals) meperidine. The chemistry and general pharmacology of these agents are presented in Chapter 29.

Tolerance to the mental effects of opiates develops with chronic use. The need for ever-increasing amounts of drug to sustain the desired euphoriant effects—as well as avoid the discomfort of withdrawal—has the expected consequence of strongly reinforcing dependence once it has started. The role of endogenous opioids (endorphins) in opiate dependence is uncertain.

Clinical Aspects

Curiosity and social pressure are the strongest factors in initiating opiate use. Intravenous administration is routine not only because it is the most efficient route but also because it produces a bolus of high concentration of drug that reaches the brain to produce a "rush," followed by euphoria, a feeling of tranquility, and sleepiness ("the nod"). Most doses of heroin available on the street are less than 25 mg and produce effects that last 3–5 hours. Thus, several doses a day are required to forestall manifestations of withdrawal in dependent persons. The trouble and expense of meeting these dose requirements put the dependent person always "on the hustle," either to get money to buy the drug or to find a "connection" with something to sell. Since supplies of heroin are of widely varying potency, the risk of overdosage is always present. And sooner or later in the lives of most heroin abusers, the money runs out or the supplies run out, and the withdrawal syndrome then begins.

Symptoms of opiate withdrawal begin 8–10 hours after the last dose. Many of these symptoms resemble those of increased activity of the sympathetic nervous system. Lacrimation, rhinorrhea, yawning, and sweating appear first. Restless sleep followed by weakness, chills, gooseflesh ("cold turkey"), nausea and vomiting, muscle aches, and involuntary movements ("kicking the habit"), hyperpnea, hyperthermia, and hypertension occur in later stages of the withdrawal syndrome. The acute course of withdrawal may last 7–10 days. A secondary phase of protracted abstinence lasts for 26–30 weeks and is characterized by hypotension, bradycardia, hypothermia, mydriasis, and decreased responsiveness of the respiratory center to carbon dioxide.

Besides the ever-present risk of fatal overdose, a number of other serious complications are associated with opiate dependence. Hepatitis B and other viral infections, such as that with human T cell leukemia virus (HTLV-III/LAV/ARV), which causes acquired immunodeficiency syndrome (AIDS), are complications of sharing contaminated hypodermic syringes. Bacterial infections lead to septic complications such as meningitis, osteomyelitis, and abscesses in various organs. Homicide, suicide, and accidents are more prevalent among heroin abusers than in the general population.

Treatment

Treatment of acute overdoses of opiates and opioids may be lifesaving and is described in Chapters 29 and 62.

Pharmacologic or psychosocial approaches may be used, either separately or together in long-term treatment of opiate-dependent persons. Widely different opinions have been vigorously expounded about which is the preferred type of treatment. Because each treatment method has a self-selected patient population, it is difficult to compare results. Chronic users tend to prefer pharmacologic approaches; those with shorter histories of drug abuse are more amenable to psychosocial interventions.

Pharmacologic treatment is most often used for detoxification. The principles of detoxification are the same for all drugs: to substitute a longer-acting, orally active, pharmacologically equivalent drug for the abused drug, stabilize the patient on that drug, and then gradually withdraw the substituted drug. **Methadone** is admirably suited for such use in opiate-dependent persons. More recently, clonidine, a centrally acting sympathoplegic agent, has been used for detoxification. By reducing the outflow of norepinephrine, clonidine might be expected to mitigate many of the signs of sympathetic overactivity. A presumed advantage of clonidine is that it has no narcotic action and is not addicting.

While it is easy to detoxify patients, the recidivism rate (return to abuse of the agent) is extraordinarily high. Methadone maintenance therapy, which substitutes a long-acting orally active opioid for heroin, has been effective in some settings. A single dose can be given each day, with the possibility of even less frequent than once-a-day doses for long-term patients. Methadone saturates the opiate receptors and prevents the desired sudden onset of central nervous system effects normally produced by intravenous administration. An even longer-acting methadone homolog, methadyl acetate, may offer additional technical advantages if it proves to be safe.

Use of a narcotic antagonist is rational therapy because blocking the action of self-administered opiates should eventually extinguish the habit. **Naltrexone**, a long-acting orally active pure narcotic antagonist, has been extensively studied. It can be given 3 times a week once dosage reaches levels of 100–150 mg/d. The greatest drawback is that few addicts will accept naltrexone as permanent treatment.

Psychosocial approaches include a variety of techniques. Drug-free communities are based on the assumption that drug use is a symptom of some emotional disturbance or inability to cope with life's stresses. The most common technique employs peer group pressures, emphasizing confrontation. Other techniques include variations on group or individual psychotherapy, didactic approaches, alternative lifestyles through work or communal living, and a variety of types of meditation. Treatment may have to be continued for months or years, with costs depending on the degree to which professional staff is used. Many addicts eventually tire of their habit or "burn out," even without therapy.

BARBITURATES & OTHER SEDATIVES

History

Alcohol, the oldest and most widely abused drug of any kind, is discussed in Chapter 21.

Bromides were first used as sedatives and anticonvulsants in 1857. They are now obsolete because they cause excessive drowsiness, must be given in doses close to toxic levels, have a slow onset of action, and have the unwanted effect of replacing chloride ion with bromide ion, leading to toxic delirium. Misuse of bromides was common when the drugs were available, but abuse was not.

Chloral hydrate was introduced in 1869 as a hypnotic. Its action is mediated by an active metabolite, trichloroethanol. Although it has the disadvantages of causing gastric irritation and an unpleasant breath odor, it is still used. Possibly because of these drawbacks, chloral hydrate was not widely abused.

Barbiturates were introduced in 1903. Short-acting members of this group have been—and still are—widely abused. Meprobamate was introduced in 1954 as a nonbarbiturate sedative presumably lacking the disadvantages of the older drugs. It turned out to have more similarities to barbiturates than differences. In fact, some of the nonbarbiturate sedative-hypnotics—examples are glutethimide and methaqualone—were worse than barbiturates in many respects, including abuse potential. The current era of **benzodiazepines** began in 1960. In the opinion of many authorities, these drugs are now the sedative-hypnotics of therapeutic choice. Abuse and physical dependence have been reported but are probably less frequent than with barbiturates.

Chemistry & Pharmacology

The chemical relationships among this class of drugs are reviewed in Chapter 20.

Depending on the dose, these drugs produce sedation, hypnosis, anesthesia, coma, and death. The exact mechanism by which they produce psychic and physical dependence is unclear.

Both barbiturates and benzodiazepines can be classified pharmacokinetically into short- and long-acting compounds. Experience with barbiturates was that most nonmedical use involved short-acting drugs, eg, secobarbital or pentobarbital sodium, and not long-acting ones, eg, phenobarbital. Whether this pattern will be repeated with the benzodiazepines remains to be seen. What has become evident is that the abruptness of onset of withdrawal syndromes as well as their severity is a function of the half-life of the drug. Drugs with half-lives in the range of 8–24 hours produce a rapidly evolving, severe withdrawal syndrome, while those with longer half-lives, such as 48–96 hours, produce a withdrawal syndrome that is slower in onset and less severe but longer in duration. Drugs with half-lives longer than 96 hours usually have a built-in tapering-off action that reduces the possibility of withdrawal reactions. Drugs with very short half-lives (less than 4 hours) generally cannot be taken frequently enough to sustain high concentrations of the drug and are rarely associated with withdrawal reactions.

Clinical Aspects

No one knows how many persons are dependent on sedatives. Much of the presumed dependence is psychologic, possibly based on the need for these drugs as a form of "replacement therapy." Physical dependence of the classic type (see below) has been relatively rare with benzodiazepines considering the extensive use these agents have had. It usually occurs following long-term treatment with doses of 40 mg/d or more of diazepam or the equivalent dose of another drug. During the past several years, much interest has developed in the phenomenon of "therapeutic dose dependence." Many patients with this syndrome have never taken more than normal medical doses (15–30 mg/d) of diazepam or other benzodiazepine. Abrupt withdrawal may be followed by some of the same symptoms observed in classic withdrawal but is characterized by weight loss, changes in perception, paresthesias, and headache. Such a syndrome almost always follows months or years of continual use. This phenomenon may be related to some adaptive change in benzodiazepine receptors following long-term exposure to the drug. All patients who have been taking these drugs for substantial periods of time should have them withdrawn slowly.

Several patterns of sedative abuse have emerged. People with severe emotional disorders may use these drugs to seek escape into oblivion. Most abusers of sedatives use them to produce an altered mental state with disinhibition in the same way other people—or they themselves—use alcohol. One sometimes sees a pattern of alternating use of sedatives and stimulants, one type of drug being used to counter the effects of the other. A growing trend has been to use sedatives in a pattern of polydrug abuse, which includes most drugs of abuse.

The effects sought by the user are similar to those produced by alcohol—an initial disinhibition followed by drowsiness. Speech may be slurred and incoordination evident. As the goal seems to be to repeat such intoxications frequently, drugs that are eliminated rapidly are preferred.

As these drugs are usually taken orally and the pills or capsules are consistent in drug content, inadvertent fatal overdoses of single agents are rare. Tolerance may develop to the sedative effect but not to the respiratory depressant effect. Thus, if these drugs are used with large amounts of alcohol, another respiratory depressant, fatalities can occur.

The withdrawal syndrome from sedatives is so much like that from alcohol that the 2 types of dependence are classified together (alcohol-barbiturate type). Symptoms and signs of chronic intoxication

from short-acting drugs may improve during the first 8 hours after withdrawal but are followed by increasing anxiety, tremors, twitches, and nausea and vomiting for the next 16 hours. Propanolol may be of value in reducing some of these effects. Convulsions may occur 16–48 hours after withdrawal. Severe cases are associated with delirium, hallucinations, and other psychosislike manifestations.

In the case of long-acting drugs, the withdrawal syndrome is attenuated. No symptoms may appear for 2–3 days, and initial symptoms may suggest a recrudescence of those originally treated. Only by the fourth or fifth day can one be sure that a withdrawal reaction is under way. Convulsions are a late manifestation when they do occur—often not until the eighth or ninth day. Following this, the syndrome subsides. This slow evolution may allow some patients to recognize what is happening and to abort the syndrome by resuming their drug. As withdrawal is generally mild, other patients may go through the syndrome, knowing that something is wrong but not being entirely sure what is happening.

Treatment

The time-honored principles of treating abstinence syndromes hold for sedative withdrawal as well. If short-acting drugs have been abused, phenobarbital is substituted as the pharmacologically equivalent agent. If long-acting drugs have been used, the same drug may be restarted. The patient is stabilized on whatever dose is required to cause signs and symptoms to abate, and the drug is then gradually withdrawn. The rate of decrement may be 15–25% of the daily dose early in treatment, with later decrements of 5–10%. Complete detoxification can usually be achieved in less than 2 weeks.

No specific treatment programs have been developed for sedative abusers. The problem is so often complicated by abuse of other drugs that it may be more expeditious to put the patient in a program designed for alcoholics or opiate-dependent persons. Patients with psychiatric disorders that can be defined, especially those with depression, may be treated with specific drug treatment for the underlying disorder.

STIMULANTS

History

Caffeine is probably the most widely used social drug worldwide. Most people do not consider it to be a drug, although many, especially as they age, experience disturbing effects on sleep and heart rhythm from too much coffee. A withdrawal syndrome characterized by lethargy, irritability, and headache has been recognized in users of more than 600 mg/d (roughly 6 cups of coffee).

Cocaine has been used for at least 1200 years in the custom of chewing coca leaves by natives of the South American Andes. Coca was first imported to Europe from the western hemisphere in 1580. Cocaine was isolated as the active material in 1860. Its anesthetic properties, especially its topical anesthetic action, were discovered in the 1870s and 1880s. Sigmund Freud was intrigued by the drug and thought it might even be a panacea, but his enthusiasm was dampened by its disastrous effects on a friend who became addicted. A colleague of Freud's, Karl Koller, is credited with first using the drug as a topical anesthetic for eye surgery, a use that still prevails.

Amphetamine was synthesized in the late 1920s and was introduced into medical practice in 1936. Dextroamphetamine is the major member of the class, although many other amphetamines and amphetamine surrogates, such as methamphetamine (Methedrine, "speed"), phenmetrazine (Preludin), and methylphenidate (Ritalin), were subsequently introduced.

The closely related natural alkaloid *cathinone* is found in the leaves of *Catha edulis*, or khat, a plant found and cultivated in the Middle East and Africa. Chewing of freshly harvested khat leaves results in effects indistinguishable from those of the amphetamines.

Chemistry & Pharmacology

The chemical relationships of the various stimulants are shown in Fig 30–1. Despite their remarkably similar actions, caffeine, cocaine, and amphetamine have very different structures.

Caffeine is thought to increase cAMP concentration by blocking the catabolic enzyme phosphodiesterase, thus increasing the effects of catecholamine neurotransmitters. Another possible mode of action is interaction with receptors for adenosine, a purine neurotransmitter structurally similar to caffeine. Cocaine appears to facilitate catecholaminergic neurotransmission by increasing its release and reducing reuptake, and a similar mode of action has been proposed for amphetamines. In addition, amphetamines are weak inhibitors of monoamine oxidase, an action that would increase catecholaminergic activity.

Although psychic dependence is strong (cocaine is one of the most strongly reinforcing drugs in self-administration paradigms in animals), it was thought for some time that physical dependence occurred only rarely. However, recent patterns of abuse of these drugs, especially of amphetaminelike agents, have revealed a typical pattern of withdrawal manifested by signs and symptoms opposite to those produced by the drug. Users become sleepy, have a ravenous appetite, are exhausted, and may suffer mental depression. This syndrome may last for several days after the drug is withdrawn. Tolerance develops quickly, so that abusers may take monumental doses compared with those used medically, eg, as anorexiants.

Clinical Aspects

Amphetamine abuse began in the 1940s. The substance was present in substantial amounts in inhalers promoted as nasal decongestants. During World War II, amphetamines were frequently used by military personnel. A huge supply of amphetamines became available to young people in Japan in the postwar period, resulting in an epidemic of abuse that was ultimately curbed by draconian punishments. Meanwhile, in the USA the drug continued to be used in relatively small oral doses, often alternating with barbiturates. In the 1960s, the pattern changed. Methamphetamine became the preferred drug (largely because it was more easily synthesized illicitly), and the preferred route of administration became intravenous injection.

One pattern of amphetamine abuse is called a "run." Repeated intravenous injections are self-administered (as with opiates) to obtain a "rush"—an orgasmlike reaction—followed by a feeling of mental alertness and marked euphoria. Total daily doses as high as 4000 mg have been reported. After several days of such spree use, subjects may enter a paranoid schizophrenialike state. Typically, they develop delusions that bugs are crawling under their skin, which leads to characteristic discrete excoriations. Finally,

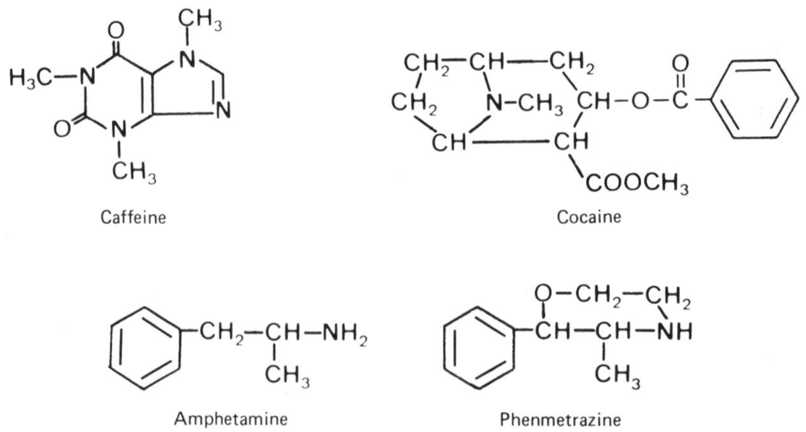

Figure 30–1. Chemical structures of some popular stimulants.

the spree is terminated by exhaustion from lack of sleep and lack of food, followed by the withdrawal syndrome mentioned above.

As is so often the case with social drugs, a pattern of stimulant use has developed in which the drug is thought to enhance sexual pleasure. Although reports are anecdotal and largely unsubstantiated, a better case is made for stimulants in this application than for other agents. Sexual intercourse may be markedly prolonged and orgasm enhanced. Phenmetrazine prescribed as an anorexiant is the current favorite for this use. With chronic use, however, sexual urges seem to disappear completely.

It is a curious paradox that efforts to regulate the use of drugs by law often lead to the introduction of more dangerous drugs. With the virtual outlawing of amphetamines from legitimate medical practice (based on adverse effects experienced by using doses 2 or 3 orders of magnitude larger than therapeutic doses), cocaine became the substitute. Cocaine may be construed as a highly potent amphetamine ("super-speed") with all of the effects of the latter drug magnified. It is far more likely to lead to dependence than amphetamines, and overdoses leading to death are possible. Cocaine has become the preferred drug of abuse in well-to-do, sophisticated circles. Its expense previously tended to limit its use; however, the drug is no longer used exclusively by the well-to-do but now involves blue-collar workers and students as well.

Two types of administration of cocaine are current. One may "snuff" the drug by sniffing a "line" (a measured amount of drug in a folded piece of paper applied to the nose), or one may smoke "free base." Cocaine is supplied as a hydrochloride salt, and free base is made by alkalinizing the salt and extracting with nonpolar solvents. When free base is smoked, entry through the lungs is almost as fast as by intravenous injection, so that effects are even more accentuated. Intravenous injection is rarely used, as the possibility of overdose is considerable. The purity and potency of cocaine available to users varies widely.

The plasma half-life of cocaine is short, so that effects following a single dose persist only for an hour or two. Consequently, the euphoric experience may be repeated many times during the course of a day or night.

Cocaine may be used sporadically, as at a party, or regularly by those with a self-imposed high level of output, such as rock musicians. It may also be part of the repertoire of the polydrug abuser. A "speedball" is a combination of cocaine and heroin taken intravenously, presumably doubling the "rush" but extinguishing other effects. Patients in methadone maintenance programs who can no longer get much kick from heroin may turn to cocaine, whose euphoriant effects are not altered by methadone.

Besides the paranoid psychosis associated with chronic use of amphetamines, intravenous injection using contaminated syringes leads to the same infectious complications as with heroin. A specific lesion associated with chronic amphetamine use is necrotizing arteritis, which may involve many small and medium-sized arteries and lead to fatal brain hemorrhage or renal failure. Overdoses of amphetamines are rarely fatal; they can be managed by sedating the patient with haloperidol. Overdoses of cocaine are usually rapidly fatal, victims dying within minutes from respiratory depression and seizures. Those who survive for 3 hours usually recover fully. Intravenous administration of diazepam and propranolol may be the best treatment.

Long-Term Treatment

Subjects with residual emotional disorders, either schizophreniform psychosis or mental depression, may require treatment with antipsychotic or antidepressant drugs. Withdrawal from cocaine may be facilitated by treatment with the tricyclic antidepressant, desipramine, which blocks uptake of norepinephrine at noradrenergic synapses. No specific treatment programs have been devised for stimulant users. Those who administer these drugs intravenously have more in common with heroin users than any other group and may be suitable for some of the rehabilitative programs devised for opiate-dependent persons.

HALLUCINOGENS

History

Almost every society, however primitive, has found some bark, skin, leaf, vine, berry, or weed that contains "hallucinogenic" materials. Although the fortuitous discovery of the properties of lysergic acid diethylamide (LSD) occurred in a chemical laboratory 4 decades ago, this was a case in which scientific art was merely imitating nature. Similar compounds have been found in morning glory seeds, and drugs such as mescaline and psilocybin had long been used by North and Central American Indians in the form of cactus buttons or magical mushrooms. Deliriants, such as the alkaloids in *Atropa belladonna* and *Datura stramonium*, were also known in ancient cultures.

Terminology

Although the term "hallucinogen" will be used here, it is not entirely accurate, since hallucinations may be uncommon effects or only part of the overall effects of these drugs. The term "psychotomimetic" is often used to connote the possible action of these drugs in mimicking naturally occurring psychoses. However, the state induced by these agents does not closely resemble that of schizophrenia. The term "psychedelic" was coined to denote a supposed "mind-revealing" aspect of such drug use, but the insights and revelations achieved are not much different from those that have been claimed with many other disinhibiting drugs, most commonly alcohol.

The drugs we here call hallucinogens are taken for many reasons. The one most widely given by users is that the drugs provide new ways of looking at the world and new insights into personal problems. The former claim implies varying degrees of perceptual distortion, while the latter implies changes in mood and increased introspection. LSD has become the prototypical hallucinogenic drug because of the extent of its use; because it represents a family of drugs that are similar; and because it has been most extensively studied.

Chemistry & Pharmacology

The LSD-like group of drugs includes **LSD** and related compounds, **mescaline** and related compounds, and **psilocybin** and related compounds. Although these substances differ chemically, they share some chemical features and even more pharmacologic ones (Fig 30–2). LSD is a semisynthetic chemical not known to occur in nature. It is related to the ergot alkaloids (Chapter 15). The monoethyl—rather than the diethyl—amide is found in hallucinogenic morning glory seeds. Mescaline, a phenethylamine derivative, and psilocybin, an indolethylamine derivative, are found in nature. These drugs also have chemical resemblances to 3 major neurotransmitters: norepinephrine, dopamine, and serotonin.

The mode of action of hallucinogens of the LSD type is uncertain despite much experimental study. Measured electrographically, their effects are to produce a state of hyperarousal of the central nervous system. Neurochemically, LSD seems to work mainly through serotoninergic systems, decreasing activity of this neurotransmitter. It was once thought the drug did this by acting as a false transmitter postsynaptically, replacing the true transmitter. Current opinion is that LSD may act on a presynaptic serotonin receptor, inhibiting the release of serotonin. Decreased turnover of serotonin is manifested by increased brain concentration of serotonin and decreased concentration of its major metabolite, 5-hydroxyindoleacetic acid.

A number of hallucinogenic amphetamine homologs can be synthesized by making various substitutions on the ring portion of the structure. The first of these to become popular as a street drug was 2,5,-dimethoxy-4-methylamephetamine ("STP"), which had a brief vogue in the 1960s. Today's fad drug is 3,4-methylenedioxymethamphetamine ("MDMA," "ecstasy"), which is probably also a hallucinogen of the mescaline type. The amphetamine homolog of this drug ("MDA") was more widely used in the past, and deaths from overdoses have been reported. The extravagant claims of instant insight obtained under the influence of MDMA have a familiar ring.

The deliriant hallucinogens, exemplified by scopolamine (Chapter 7) and some synthetic centrally acting cholinoceptor-blocking agents, are different chemically as well as pharmacologically from the LSD group. Their effects seem to be entirely explainable by blockade of central muscarinic receptors. Similar mental effects may be seen during therapeutic or deliberate overdoses of commonly used medications with antimuscarinic action, such as antiparkinsonism

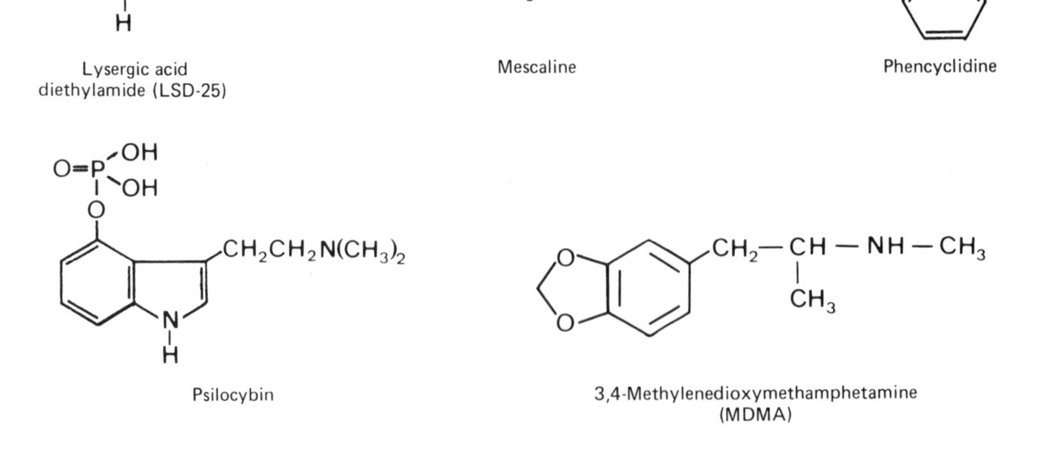

Figure 30–2. Chemical structures of lysergic acid diethylamide (LSD), mescaline, phencyclidine, psilocybin, and "MDMA."

drugs, tricyclic antidepressants, and antispasmodics. Occasional instances of abuse of these therapeutic agents have occurred.

Phencyclidine (PCP, "angel dust," many other names) is a synthetic phenylcyclohexylamine derivative. There is some question about how it should be classified, since it differs in many ways from other hallucinogens, but its primary use is to obtain hallucinogenic effects. The drug was originally introduced as a "dissociative anesthetic" in 1957. Such anesthetics were presumed to work by making patients insensitive to pain by "separating their bodily functions from their minds" without causing loss of consciousness. Hallucinogenic effects were noted in patients emerging from anesthesia. The drug was withdrawn from use in humans but retained in veterinary practice under the name Sernylan. (The veterinary use has given the drug one of its street names—"hog.") **Ketamine**, a homolog, replaced phencyclidine as an anesthetic for use in humans (see Chapter 23). It too produces some emergent hallucinogenic effects. The first street use of PCP was in 1967, when it quickly gained a reputation as a bad drug. Over the next several years, it was mislabeled, being sold as LSD, tetrahydrocannabinol (THC), and other hallucinogens. Since the 1970s PCP has become widely accepted and is now the most used hallucinogenic agent. Phencyclidine may be smoked (by mixing the powder with tobacco), "snorted," taken orally, or injected intravenously. Fortunately, a recent trend toward less frequent use of the drug has been noted.

Some of the early investigators of PCP maintained that it provided a much better model of schizophrenia than LSD, mainly through its action in producing a form of sensory isolation. More recent work, however, indicates that the mode of action of PCP is mainly through dopaminergic mechanisms. Dopaminergic transmission is enhanced as a result of reduced uptake of dopamine. Thus, the schizophreniform psychosis may be mediated in a way postulated for true schizophrenia. The drug is unique among hallucinogens in that animals will self-administer it.

Various harmala alkaloids, especially **harmaline**, have been classified as hallucinogens, but very little recent work has been done with these drugs in humans. The drug has the property of inhibiting monoamine oxidase, which could increase activity of dopamine as well as several other biogenic amine neurotransmitters.

Clinical Effects

LSD produces a series of somatic, perceptual, and psychic effects that overlap each other. Dizziness, weakness, tremors, nausea, and paresthesias are prominent somatic symptoms. Blurring of vision, distortions of perspective, organized visual illusions or "hallucinations," less discriminant hearing, and a change in sense of time are common perceptual abnormalities. Impaired memory, difficulty in thinking, poor judgment, and altered mood are prominent psychic effects. Physiologically, LSD produces signs of overactivity of the sympathetic nervous system and central stimulation, manifested by dilated pupils, increased heart rate, mild elevation of blood pressure, tremor, and alertness. Virtually identical effects are produced by mescaline and psilocybin when they are given in equivalent doses. The onset of effects is fairly rapid, but the duration varies with the dose and is usually measured in hours. Phenomena may vary considerably from one user to another owing to such factors as the personality and expectations of the user and the circumstances under which the drug is taken, but the above effects occur in almost everyone. Waxing and waning of effects is typical.

Usual doses of LSD in humans are approximately 1–2 μg/kg, making it one of the most potent pharmacologic agents known. The drug is equally effective parenterally or orally and consequently is almost always taken by mouth. Psilocybin is usually taken in doses of 250 μg/kg and mescaline in doses of 5–6 mg/kg. Despite these differences in potency, the effects are virtually indistinguishable.

Scopolamine and the "JB" series of antimuscarinic drugs produce a delirium with fluctuating levels of awareness, disorientation, marked difficulty in thinking, marked loss of memory, and bizarre delusions. If doses are large, these impairments may last for more than a day, with some subjects claiming that several days may elapse before they once again feel confident about their memory. Most subjects, at least under experimental conditions, find these drugs to be unpleasant and have little desire to repeat the experience. Some become frightened during the period of drug effect. Others deliberately seek out and use such drugs repeatedly.

PCP produces detachment, disorientation, distortions of body image, and loss of proprioception. Somatic symptoms and signs include numbness, nystagmus, sweating, rapid heart rate, and hypertension. Effects are dose-dependent. Overdosage has been fatal, as contrasted with the absence of known fatalities directly caused by drugs of the LSD group.

Toxicity

Adverse psychologic consequences of hallucinogenic drugs are common. Panic reactions ("bad trips") may be related to excessive doses; they seem to be less common as the doses of street drugs have become more accurate. They are best managed by sedation with a barbiturate or benzodiazepine rather than with a phenothiazine. Simple "talking down" may suffice but is labor-intensive. Acute psychotic or depressive reactions have been precipitated by use of these drugs but usually only in persons with strong predispositions. Acute psychotic reactions are associated with PCP much more commonly than with any of the other hallucinogens. Errors of judgment may lead to reckless acts that threaten life; any person under the influence of one of these drugs should be provided with a non-drugged companion until the effect has dissipated.

Overdoses of the antimuscarinic agents can be treated with infusion of physostigmine (see p 81 for precautions). In mild cases, one may simply allow the patient to sleep off the effects by giving a large dose of a hypnotic drug.

Overdoses of PCP are dangerous but can be managed if recognized promptly. PCP is secreted into the stomach, so that removal may be hastened by continual nasogastric suction. Excretion of this basic drug may be hastened by acidification of the urine to pH 5.5. Diazepam can be given to protect against seizures or to curb excitation; antipsychotics aggravate matters at this point. If a prolonged schizophrenialike illness follows acute intoxication, one may consider antipsychotics on a sustained basis.

Treatment

No systematic program of treatment has been devised for abuse of this class of drugs. Users of hallucinogens are likely to stick to this class of drugs rather than proceed to a pattern of polydrug abuse. Separation of the user from the drug culture is probably the best treatment, but it must be voluntarily accepted.

Therapeutic Uses

No therapeutic indication has yet been accepted for any hallucinogen. LSD was promoted as a cure for alcoholism, but objective evidence of benefit is totally lacking. Facilitation of psychotherapy was another proposed use, again with no substantiation or comparison with other drugs. Although it has been tried in both schizophrenics and depressed individuals, LSD is more likely to precipitate or aggravate these disorders than to alleviate them. Use of the drug in chronic cancer patients was said to diminish the need for opiates, but this work has not been confirmed.

MARIHUANA

History

Use of cannabis has been recorded for thousands of years, especially in Eastern countries such as China and India. It was certainly known to the Greeks at the height of their civilization as well as to Arabic nations somewhat later. It is estimated that about 200–300 million people use cannabis in some form. Thus, it is not only one of the oldest but also one of the most widely used of mind-altering drugs. Since the 1960s, the rise in marihuana use in the USA has been remarkable. Although the drug was known in this country prior to that time, there were only a small number of users, mainly from minority groups. It is estimated now that 30–40 million persons in the USA have used the drug and that a substantial number are regular users. Recent reports suggest that the number of youngsters initiated into use of this drug has declined after a steep rise and an increasingly lower age of first use.

Several species of cannabis (hemp) have been named, but botanists are not agreed that more than one species of plant exists; many morphologic variants occur. Some plants are excellent for fiber, being a source of hemp, and rather poor producers of drug; and the converse also is true. These properties are due to genetic differences. The flowers and small leaves of *Cannabis sativa* supply most of the drug. **Marihuana** is a mixture of ground-up plant materials that resembles grass clippings—thus the street name "grass." Extraction of the resin from the plant provides a more potent product: **hashish**.

Chemistry & Pharmacokinetics of Cannabinoids

Three major cannabinoids have been found in cannabis; cannabidiol (CBD), Δ^9-tetrahydrocannabinol (THC), and cannabinol (CBN). The biosynthetic pathway begins with CBD, proceeds to THC, and ends with CBN (Fig 30–3). Thus, one can deduce from the proportions of these cannabinoids in plant material the age of the plant. Many other variants of these structures have been found in cannabis, but with the exception of THC and its homologs no other cannabinoids have definite psychoactivity. The content of THC varies considerably among plants, so that special genetic lines may produce as much as 4–6% THC content in very selected ("manicured") materials. Most plants have a THC content ranging from trace amounts to 1–2%.

The preferred route of administration in Western countries is by smoking. The high lipid solubility of THC causes it to be readily trapped on the surfactant lining the lungs. Pharmacokinetic studies indicate that smoking is almost equivalent to intravenous administration except that lower peak plasma concentrations of THC are attained. In some Eastern countries, cannabis is taken orally in the form of various confections. The rate of absorption from this route is slow and highly variable, although the duration of action is longer.

THC is extensively metabolized, and new metabolites are still being discovered. One metabolite, 11-hydroxy-THC, is actually more active than the parent compound. However, it is not nearly as abundant, and one must assume that the major part of the activity of cannabis derives from THC itself. The high lipid solubility of the drug leads to extensive sequestration in the lipid compartments of the body, and metabolites may be excreted for as long as a week after a single dose. Whether accumulation of unchanged THC can occur is questionable.

Pharmacodynamics of Cannabinoids

The mechanism of action of THC is not well-defined. Structure-activity relationships indicate that relatively minor changes (such as *cis-trans* isomerization) markedly alter the psychoactivity of THC. One might assume that this would indicate an action on a specific receptor. However, to date none has been discovered. Another potential mode of action of such a lipophilic drug is on the cell membrane itself. It has a variety of pharmacologic effects that suggest actions like those of amphetamines, LSD, alcohol, sedatives,

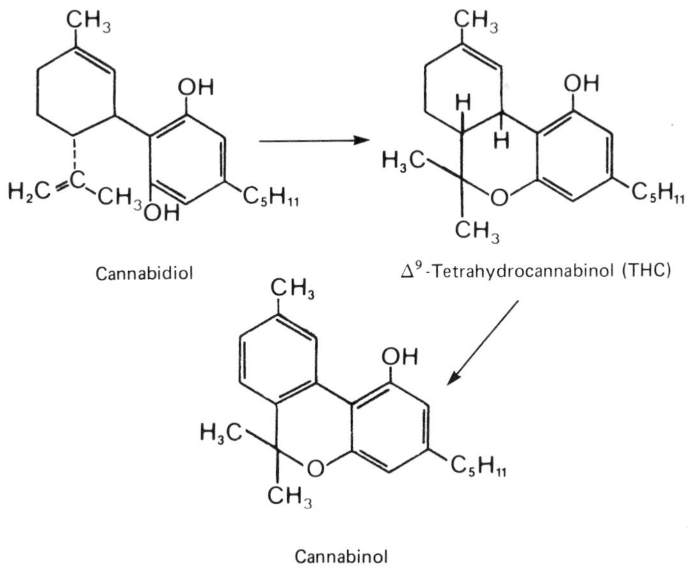

Figure 30–3. Structures of the 3 main cannabinoids in marihuana. Only THC has psychoactivity. C_5H_{11} is *n*-pentyl. Arrows indicate the biosynthetic sequence.

atropine, or morphine. Thus, the drug does not fit traditional pharmacologic classifications and must be considered as a separate class.

Small doses of THC may be associated with a rather definite placebo effect, but large doses are unequivocal in producing the expected range of effects. The expert smoker of marihuana is usually aware of a drug effect after 2 or 3 inhalations. As smoking continues, the effects increase, reaching a maximum about 20 minutes after the smoke has been finished. Most effects of the drug usually have vanished after 3 hours, by which time plasma concentrations are low. Peak effects after oral administration may be delayed until 3–4 hours after drug ingestion but may last for 6–8 hours.

The early stage is one of being "high" and is characterized by euphoria, uncontrollable laughter, alteration of time sense, depersonalization, and sharpened vision. Later the user becomes relaxed and experiences introspective and dreamlike states if not actual sleep. Thinking or concentrating become difficult, although by force of will the subject can attend.

Two characteristic signs of cannabis intoxication are increased pulse rate and reddening of the conjunctiva. The latter correlates well with the presence of detectable plasma concentrations. Pupil size is not changed. The blood pressure may fall, especially in the upright position. An antiemetic effect may be present. Muscle weakness, tremors, unsteadiness, and increased deep tendon reflexes may also be noted.

Virtually any psychologic test shows impairment if the doses are large enough and the test difficult enough. No distinctive biochemical changes have been found in humans.

Tolerance has been demonstrated in virtually every animal species that has been tested. It is apparent in humans only among heavy long-term users of the drug. Different degrees of tolerance develop for different effects of the drug, with tolerance for the tachycardiac effect developing fairly rapidly. A mild withdrawal syndrome has been noted following very high doses.

Health Hazards

Marihuana has raised concern about possible adverse effects on the health of users, probably because so many are very young. The hazards of use are still controversial and ambiguous, and there are many problems with the studies themselves. First, it is difficult to prove or disprove an adverse reaction for humans in an animal model. Second, users thus far have been mostly young people in excellent general health. Third, cannabis is often used in combination with alcohol or tobacco. And fourth, many investigators have biases for or against the drug.

Three epidemiologic studies in developing countries have failed to find definite evidence of impairment among heavy users of cannabis, but field studies may lack sensitivity. Experimental studies in which subjects have smoked heavily for varying periods have shown a lowered serum testosterone level in men and airway narrowing. Effects on immune mechanisms, chromosomes, and cell metabolism are often contradictory. Effects on the fetus are still uncertain.

Heavy smokers of marihuana may be subject to some of the same problems of chronic bronchitis, airway obstruction, and squamous cell metaplasia as smokers of tobacco cigarettes. Angina pectoris may be aggravated by the speeding of the heart rate, orthostatic hypotension, and increased carboxyhemoglobin. Driving ability is likely to be impaired but is not easily demonstrated with usual testing. "Amotivational syndrome," in which promising young people with obvious social advantages lose interest in school and career and enter the drug culture, is a real phenomenon, but one cannot be sure whether drug use is the cause of the problem or simply a matter of personal choice by a disturbed young man or woman. Acute panic reactions, toxic delirium, paranoid states, and frank psychoses are rare. Brain damage has not been confirmed in humans, although some suggestion of ultrastructural damage has been found in animals.

Therapeutic Uses

Cannabis was at one time listed in drug formularies but has not been used medically for some time. Recently, interest in cannabis for therapeutic purposes has revived. A finding of lowered intraocular pressure following oral THC administration has been repeatedly confirmed; it remains to be seen whether preparations of cannabis have any advantages over other forms of treatment for glaucoma. Amelioration of nausea and vomiting associated with cancer chemotherapy appears to be a most promising use. Two homologs, **nabilone (Cesamet)** and **dronabinol (Marinol)**, have recently been approved for this indication. They seem able to reduce nausea and vomiting at doses that are associated with minimal mental effects. **Levonantradol** is another homolog that may have medical use, possibly as an analgesic, as an agent for the relief of muscle spasm, or even as an anticonvulsant. It remains to be proved, however, that any of these homologs have advantages over standard agents.

Treatment

Few users seek treatment, although many who have stopped using the drug have been pleasantly surprised at the increased clarity of their thinking. Although marihuana has been alleged to be a substitute for alcohol, it is more commonly used along with alcohol; alcoholism complicating marihuana use is rare. Marihuana may be used in a pattern of multiple drug use, in which case treatment may be required for the more dangerous drugs being taken.

INHALANTS

History

The modern discovery of the intoxicant effects of inhalants began with Sir Humphry Davy in 1799, who administered nitrous oxide to himself and others. As other anesthetic gases were introduced, such as chloroform and ether, they were also used socially. Such use persists, with occasional instances of halothane inhalation being added to the anesthetic gases previously mentioned. In addition to these agents, 3 other patterns of inhalant use are now prevalent: (1) industrial solvents, including a variety of hydrocarbons, such as toluene; (2) aerosol propellants, such as various fluorocarbons; and (3) organic nitrites, such as amyl or butyl nitrite.

Chemistry & Pharmacology

The structures of some inhalants are shown in Fig 30–4. The mode of action of the inhalant anesthetics has been discussed in Chapter 23.

Clinical Aspects

Nitrous oxide, formerly not easily available, is now sold openly in so-called "head shops." When self-administered, it produces difficulty in concentrating, dreaminess, euphoria, numbness and tingling, unsteadiness, and visual and auditory disturbances. It is usually taken as 35% N_2O mixed with oxygen; administration of 100% nitrous oxide may cause asphyxia and death.

Ether and **chloroform** are readily available through chemical supply houses. Cloths soaked with the material are used for inhalation of the fumes. After an initial period of exhilaration, the person often loses consciousness. Ether is highly flammable. Halothane is usually available only to medical or health care personnel.

A variety of **industrial solvents** used as inhalants are on the market and virtually impossible to control. They include gasoline, paint thinner, glue, rubber cement, acrylic paint sprays, shoe polish, and degreasers. The toxic ingredients may be toluene, heptane, hexane, benzene, trichloroethylene, methylethylketone, and others. Because of their ready availability, this group of inhalants is widely used. Aerosol propellants have also been widely available, though manufacturers of products using propellants have recently changed from fluorocarbons to less hazardous materials.

Motives for use of inhalants include peer influence, low cost, ready availability, convenient packaging, quick intoxication of short duration, and mood enhancement. Boys in their early teen years from lower socioeconomic classes are the principal users. They generally also have worse than average problems at school and at home. Psychologic dependence perpetuates the use of inhalants.

The clinical effects of industrial solvent inhalation are short, lasting only 5–15 minutes. Rags or "toques" are soaked in the solvent and the fumes inhaled. Aerosol propellants are usually inhaled from a plastic bag. Euphoria and a relaxed "drunk" feeling are followed

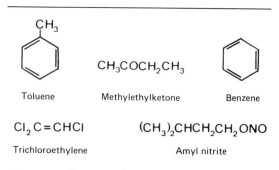

Figure 30–4. Structures of some commonly used inhalants.

by disorientation, slow passage of time, and possibly hallucinations.

Organic nitrites have developed a reputation as a sexual enhancer, a sure avenue to popular acceptance. Amyl nitrite is used medically for angina in the form of fragile glass ampules covered with cloth. When these are broken, they make a popping sound—hence the nickname "poppers." Street forms of bottled isobutyl nitrite (Locker Room, Rush) are readily available in some areas. Inhalation causes dizziness, giddiness, rapid heart rate, lowered blood pressure, "speeding," and flushing of the skin. The effects last only a few minutes and can readily be repeated. The main effect the drug may have on sexual functioning is to diminish inhibition. By reducing the strength of erection, it may prolong sexual intercourse. Except for an occasional instance of methemoglobinemia associated with excessive use of nitrites, few significant adverse effects have been reported despite extensive use of this drug.

Toxicity

Chloroform has been implicated in liver and kidney damage. Industrial solvents have produced a variety of adverse effects: liver and kidney damage, peripheral nerve damage and possibly brain damage in animals, bone marrow suppression, and pulmonary disease. Fluorocarbon inhalation has resulted in sudden deaths, either due to ventricular arrhythmias or asphyxiation. Nitrites have been rather safe but might pose hazards for persons with preexisting cardiovascular problems.

REFERENCES

General

Balster RL, Harris LS: Drugs as reinforcers in animals and humans. (Symposium.) *Fed Proc* 1982;**41:**209.

The Committee on Problems of Drug Dependence: *Testing Drugs for Physical Dependence Potential and Abuse Liability.* JV Brady, SE Lukas (editors). National Institute on Drug Abuse Research Monograph 52, US Government Printing Office, 1984.

Nicholi AM Jr: The nontherapeutic use of psychoactive drugs: A modern epidemic. *N Engl J Med* 1983;**308:**925.

Ray OA: *Drugs, Society and Human Behavior.* Mosby, 1978.

Opiates

Collier HOJ: Physiological basis of opiate dependence. *Drug Alcohol Depend* 1983;**11:**15.

Goldstein A: Heroin addiction: Sequential treatment employing pharmacologic supports. *Arch Gen Psychiatry* 1976; **33:**353.

Sedatives

Cowen PJ, Nutt DJ: Abstinence symptoms after withdrawal of tranquilizing drugs: Is there a common neurochemical mechanism? *Lancet* 1982;**2:**360.

Hollister LE (editor): Valium: A discussion of current issues. *Psychosomatics* 1977;**18:**1.

Stimulants

Kalix P, Braenden O: Pharmacological aspects of the chewing of khat leaves. *Pharmacol Rev* 1985;**37:**149.

Kleber HD, Gawin FH: Cocaine abuse: A review of current and experimental treatments. Page 111 in: *Cocaine: Pharmacology, Effects and Treatment of Abuse.* National Institute on Drug Abuse Research Monograph Series 50, US Government Printing Office, 1984.

Smith DE et al (editors): *Amphetamine Use, Misuse and Abuse.* GK Hall, 1979.

Hallucinogens

Hollister LE: *Chemical Psychoses: LSD and Related Drugs.* Thomas, 1968.

Lewin L: *Phantastics, Narcotic and Stimulating Drugs.* Dutton, 1931.

Martin BR: Pharmacokinetics and mechanism of action of phencyclidine. (Symposium.) *Fed Proc* 1983;**42:**2559.

Cannabis

Maykut MO: *Health Consequences of Acute and Chronic Marihuana Use.* Pergamon Press, 1984.

Milne GM et al (editors): Therapeutic progress in cannabinoid research. *J Clin Pharmacol* 1981;**21(Suppl):**1S.

Nahas GG, Paton WDM (editors): *Marihuana: Biological Effects.* Pergamon, 1979.

Inhalants

Sharp CW, Carroll LT: *Voluntary Inhalation of Industrial Solvents.* DHEW Publication No. (ADM) 79–779, US Government Printing Office, 1979.

31

Agents Used in Anemias: Iron, Vitamin B₁₂, & Folic Acid

Curt A. Ries, MD, & Daniel V. Santi, MD, PhD

Iron, vitamin B$_{12}$, and folic acid are chemically unrelated essential nutrients that are required for normal erythropoiesis. Deficiency of any of these substances results in severe anemia. Iron is required for hemoglobin production; in the absence of adequate iron, small red cells with insufficient hemoglobin are formed, giving rise to microcytic hypochromic anemia. Vitamin B$_{12}$ and folic acid are required for normal DNA synthesis, and deficiency of either of these vitamins results in impaired production and abnormal maturation of erythroid precursor cells, giving rise to the characteristic blood and bone marrow picture known as megaloblastic anemia.

IRON

Basic Pharmacology

Iron forms the nucleus of the iron-porphyrin ring heme, which when combined with appropriate globin chains forms the protein hemoglobin. The structure of hemoglobin allows for reversible binding of oxygen, providing the critical mechanism for oxygen transport from the lungs to other tissues that is essential for humans and other vertebrates. Although iron is also present in other important proteins (myoglobin, cytochromes, etc), the vast majority is normally present in hemoglobin; therefore, anemia is the most prominent clinical feature of iron deficiency.

Pharmacokinetics

Iron is normally available in the diet from a wide variety of foods; dietary iron is usually in the form of heme or iron complexed to various organic compounds. Therapeutic iron, on the other hand, is usually given in the form of iron salts or iron complexed to inorganic substances. These different forms of iron differ widely in the amount of iron available for absorption, as discussed below.

Iron distribution in normal adults is shown in Table 31–1. About 70% of the total body iron content is in the form of hemoglobin in red blood cells, and 10–20% is in the form of storage iron as ferritin and hemosiderin. Women in the reproductive age group usually have less storage iron than men because of iron losses from menstruation and pregnancies. About 10% of the iron is in myoglobin, a heme-containing protein

Table 31–1. Iron distribution in normal adults.*†

	Iron Content (mg)	
	Men	**Women**
Hemoglobin	3050	1700
Myoglobin	430	300
Enzymes	10	8
Transport (transferrin)	8	6
Storage (ferritin and hemosiderin)	750	300
Total	4248	2314

*Adapted, with permission, from Brown EB: Iron deficiency anemia. In: *Cecil Textbook of Medicine,* 16th ed. Wyngaarden JB, Smith LH (editors). Saunders, 1982.
†Values are based on data from various sources and assume "normal" men weigh 80 kg and have a hemoglobin of 16 g/dL and "normal" women weigh 55 kg and have a hemoglobin of 14 g/dL.

in muscle. The remainder (less than 1%) is distributed in trace amounts in cytochromes and other iron-containing enzymes, and as transport iron on transferrin.

Iron is normally absorbed in the duodenum and proximal jejunum, although more distal small bowel sites can absorb iron if necessary. The average American diet contains 10–15 mg of elemental iron daily. A normal non–iron-deficient individual absorbs 5–10% of this iron, or about 0.5–1 mg daily. Iron absorption is increased in response to low iron stores or increased iron requirements. Total iron absorption increases to 1–2 mg/d in normal menstruating women and may be as high as 3–4 mg/d in pregnant women. Infants and adolescents also have increased iron requirements during rapid growth periods.

Iron is available in a wide variety of foods but is especially abundant in meat protein. The iron in meat protein is also more available for absorption and can be more efficiently absorbed, since heme iron in meat hemoglobin and myoglobin can be absorbed intact as hemin (the ferric form of heme) without first having to be broken down into elemental iron. Iron in other foods is often tightly bound to phytates or other complexing agents and may be much less available for absorption. Nonheme iron in foods and iron in inorganic

362

iron salts and complexes must be converted to ferrous ion before it can be absorbed by the intestinal mucosal cells. Such absorption is decreased by the presence of chelators or complexing agents in the intestinal lumen and is increased in the presence of hydrochloric acid and vitamin C. Gastric resection decreases iron absorption by decreasing or eliminating hydrochloric acid production and perhaps even more importantly by removing the site where food is held and digested to make dietary iron more available for absorption by the iron-absorbing areas in the duodenum and proximal jejunum.

Iron is transported across the intestinal mucosal cell by active transport. Absorbed ferrous ion is converted to ferric ion within the mucosal cell, and—together with ferric iron split from hemin—the newly absorbed iron can be made available for immediate transport from the mucosal cell to the plasma via transferrin or can be converted to ferritin and stored in the mucosal cell. In general, when total body iron stores are high and iron requirements by the body are low, newly absorbed iron is diverted into ferritin in the intestinal mucosal cells rather than being transported to other sites. When iron stores are low or iron requirements are high, however, newly absorbed iron is immediately transported from the mucosal cells to the bone marrow for the production of hemoglobin.

Iron is transported in the plasma bound to transferrin, a β-globulin that specifically binds ferric iron. Iron can thus be transported from intestinal mucosal cells or from storage sites in liver or spleen to the developing erythroid cells in bone marrow. Recently, specific receptors for the transferrin–ferric ion complex have been demonstrated on the membranes of maturing erythroid cells (normoblasts) from human bone marrow.

Iron can be stored in 2 forms: ferritin and hemosiderin. Ferritin, the most readily available form of storage iron, is a water-soluble complex consisting of a core crystal of ferric hydroxide covered by a protein shell of apoferritin. Hemosiderin is a particulate substance consisting of aggregates of ferric core crystals partially or completely stripped of apoferritin. Both ferritin and hemosiderin are stored in macrophages in the liver, spleen, and bone marrow; ferritin is also present in intestinal mucosal cells and in plasma. Since the ferritin present in plasma is in equilibrium with storage ferritin in reticuloendothelial tissues, the plasma (or serum) ferritin level can be used to estimate total body iron stores.

There is no mechanism for excretion of iron. Small amounts of iron are lost by exfoliation of intestinal mucosal cells into the stool, and trace amounts are excreted in bile, urine, and sweat. These losses, however, can account for no more than 1 mg of iron per day. Because the body's ability to increase excretion of iron is so limited, regulation of iron balance must be achieved by changing intestinal absorption of iron, depending on the body's needs.

Iron absorption is regulated by the amount of storage iron present, especially the amount of ferritin present in the intestinal mucosal cells, and by the rate of erythropoiesis. Recent studies have shown that increased erythropoiesis is associated with an increase in the number of transferrin receptor sites on developing erythroid cells and that the availability of these receptor sites in some way directly increases the rate of iron absorption. Transferrin and ferritin are both present in intestinal mucosal cells and both appear to regulate iron absorption. Transferrin is increased and ferritin decreased in iron deficiency, promoting increased iron absorption, while transferrin is decreased and ferritin increased in iron overload states, inhibiting further iron absorption.

Clinical Pharmacology of Iron

The only clinical indication for the use of iron preparations is the treatment or prevention of iron deficiency anemia. Iron deficiency is commonly seen in infants, especially premature infants, in children during rapid growth periods, and in pregnant and lactating women. These situations are all associated with increased iron requirements, and individuals in these settings are often routinely supplemented with oral iron to meet the increased need. Iron deficiency also occurs frequently in postgastrectomy states and in patients with severe small bowel disease that results in generalized malabsorption. Iron deficiency in these situations is due to inadequate iron absorption.

The most common cause of iron deficiency in adults, however, is blood loss. Menstruating women lose about 30 mg of iron with each menstrual period; women with heavy or abnormal menstrual bleeding may lose much more. The most common site of unrecognized or occult blood loss is in the gastrointestinal tract. Patients with unexplained iron deficiency anemia must therefore always be evaluated for occult gastrointestinal bleeding, especially to exclude early gastrointestinal cancer, which may present with occult bleeding at a time when the cancer is still surgically curable. Simple nutritional iron deficiency due to inadequate diet is rare in adults and should never be accepted as an explanation of iron deficiency in a patient until a careful search has ruled out occult blood loss and other causes of iron deficiency.

Individuals suspected of being iron-deficient should generally have the diagnosis confirmed before being treated with iron preparations. As iron deficiency develops, storage iron decreases and then disappears; next, serum ferritin decreases; and then serum iron decreases and iron-binding capacity (transferrin) increases, resulting in a decrease in iron-binding (transferrin) saturation. Thereafter, anemia begins to develop. Red cell indices (mean corpuscular volume [MCV]: normal = 80–100 fL; mean corpuscular hemoglobin concentration [MCHC]: normal = 32–36 g/dL) are usually low normal when iron deficiency anemia is mild, but cells become progressively more microcytic and hypochromic as anemia becomes more severe. By the time iron deficiency is diagnosed, serum iron is usually less than 40 μg/dL; total iron-binding capacity (TIBC) is greater than 400

$\mu g/dL$; iron-binding saturation is less than 10%; and serum ferritin is less than 10 $\mu g/L$. One of the most sensitive ways to detect early iron deficiency is to examine bone marrow stained to detect the presence or absence of storage iron.

The treatment of iron deficiency anemia consists of administration of oral or parenteral iron preparations. Oral iron corrects the deficiency just as rapidly and completely as parenteral iron in most cases if iron absorption from the gastrointestinal tract is normal.

A. Oral Iron Therapy: A wide variety of oral iron preparations are available. Since ferrous iron is most efficiently absorbed, only ferrous salts should be used. Ferrous sulfate, ferrous gluconate, and ferrous fumarate are all effective and inexpensive and are recommended for the treatment of most patients. Supplementation with vitamin C and other nutrients is generally not necessary. Sustained-release and enteric-coated iron preparations should not be used, since iron is best absorbed in the duodenum and proximal jejunum.

Different iron salts provide different amounts of elemental iron, as shown in Table 31–2. In an iron-deficient individual, about 50–100 mg of iron can be incorporated into hemoglobin daily, and about 25% of oral iron given as ferrous salt can be absorbed. Therefore, 200–400 mg of elemental iron should be given daily to correct iron deficiency most rapidly. Patients unable to tolerate such large doses of iron can be given lower daily doses of iron, which results in slower—but still complete—correction of iron deficiency.

Treatment with oral iron should be continued for 3–6 months. This will not only correct the anemia but will replenish iron stores. The first measurable response to successful iron therapy can be seen in less than a week, when brisk reticulocytosis occurs, as newly formed hemoglobin-filled red cells from bone marrow enter the bloodstream. The hemoglobin level should increase significantly in 2–4 weeks and should reach normal levels (men = 14–18 g/dL; women = 12–16 g/dL) in 1–3 months. Failure to respond to oral iron therapy may be due to incorrect diagnosis (anemia due to causes other than iron deficiency), continued iron loss (usually secondary to continued blood loss), concurrent chronic inflammation or other illness that suppresses marrow function, or failure of the patient to take or absorb the oral iron.

Common side effects of oral iron therapy include nausea, epigastric discomfort, abdominal cramps, constipation, and diarrhea. These effects are usually dose-related and can often be overcome by lowering the daily dose of iron or by taking the tablets immediately after or with meals. Some patients have less severe gastrointestinal side effects with one iron salt than another and benefit from changing preparations. Patients taking oral iron develop black stools; this itself has no clinical significance but may obscure the diagnosis of continued gastrointestinal blood loss.

B. Parenteral Iron Therapy: Parenteral therapy should be reserved for patients with documented iron deficiency unable to tolerate or absorb oral iron and patients with extensive chronic blood loss who cannot be maintained with oral iron alone. This includes patients with various postgastrectomy states and previous small bowel resections, inflammatory bowel disease involving the proximal small bowel, malabsorption syndromes, and chronic heavy bleeding from nonresectable lesions as may occur in hereditary hemorrhagic telangiectasia.

Iron dextran (many trade names) is a stable complex of ferric hydroxide and low-molecular-weight dextran containing 50 mg of elemental iron per milliliter of solution. It can be given either by deep intramuscular injection (using the "Z track" injection technique to avoid local tissue staining) or by intravenous infusion. Adverse effects of parenteral iron therapy include local pain and tissue staining (brown discoloration of the tissues overlying the injection site), headache, light-headedness, fever, arthralgias, nausea and vomiting, back pain, flushing, urticaria, bronchospasm, and, rarely, anaphylaxis and death.

The total amount of parenteral iron required to correct iron deficiency anemia and to replenish iron stores in a 70-kg adult can be calculated as follows: (normal hemoglobin − patient's hemoglobin) × 0.25 = grams of iron required. Most adults with iron deficiency anemia thus require 1–2 g of replacement iron, or 20–40 mL of iron dextran. Although this amount of parenteral iron can be given as 10–20 daily intramuscular injections, most physicians now prefer to give the entire calculated dose in a single intravenous infusion in several hundred milliliters of normal saline over 1–2 hours. Intravenous administration eliminates the local pain and tissue staining that often occur with the intramuscular route and allows delivery of the entire dose of iron necessary to correct the iron deficiency at one time. There is no clear evidence that any of the adverse effects, including anaphylaxis, are more likely to occur with intravenous than with intramuscular administration.

A small test dose of iron dextran should always be given before full intramuscular or intravenous doses are given. A 0.25–0.5-mL dose can be given by deep intramuscular injection or slow intravenous infusion of very dilute solution 30–60 minutes before proceeding with full therapy. If signs or symptoms of an immediate hypersensitivity reaction occur, additional parenteral iron should not be given, and alternative

Table 31–2. Oral iron preparations.

Preparation	Tablet Size	Elemental Iron Per Tablet	Usual Adult Dose (Tablets Per Day)
Ferrous sulfate, hydrated	320 mg	64 mg	3–6
Ferrous sulfate, dessicated	200 mg	58 mg	3–6
Ferrous gluconate	320 mg	39 mg	5–10
Ferrous fumarate	200 mg	66 mg	3–6
Ferrous fumarate	320 mg	105 mg	2–4

therapy must be considered. Patients with a strong history of allergy and patients who have previously received parenteral iron are more likely to have hypersensitivity reactions following treatment with parenteral iron dextran than those who have not.

Clinical Toxicity

A. Acute Toxicity: Acute iron toxicity is seen almost exclusively in young children who have accidentally ingested iron tablets. Although adults appear to be able to tolerate large doses of oral iron without serious consequences, as few as 10 tablets of any of the commonly available oral iron preparations can be lethal in young children. Oral iron preparations should therefore always be stored in "childproof" containers and kept out of the reach of children.

Large amounts of oral iron cause necrotizing gastroenteritis, with vomiting, abdominal pain, and bloody diarrhea followed by shock, lethargy, and dyspnea. Subsequently, improvement is often noted, but this may be followed by severe metabolic acidosis, coma, and death. Urgent treatment of acute iron toxicity is necessary, especially in young children. Gastric aspiration should be performed, followed by lavage with phosphate or carbonate solutions to form insoluble iron salts. Deferoxamine (Desferal), a potent iron chelating compound, should then be instilled into the stomach to bind any remaining free iron in the gut. Deferoxamine should also be given systemically by intermittent intramuscular injection or by continuous intravenous infusion to bind iron that has already been absorbed and to promote its excretion in urine and feces. Appropriate supportive therapy for gastrointestinal bleeding, metabolic acidosis, and shock must also be provided (see Chapter 62).

B. Chronic Toxicity: Chronic iron toxicity (iron overload), also known as hemochromatosis and hemosiderosis, results when excess iron is deposited in the heart, liver, pancreas, and other organs, leading to organ failure and death. It most commonly occurs in patients with hemochromatosis, an inherited disorder characterized by excessive iron absorption, and in patients who receive many red cell transfusions (each transfusion containing 250 mg of iron) over a long period of time. It is doubtful that clinically significant iron overload can occur in normal individuals who chronically ingest excess iron, because of the protective mechanisms that normally regulate iron absorption and because of the very large amounts of total body iron needed before clinical iron overload becomes apparent. However, continued ingestion of excess iron probably contributes to the development of iron overload in patients who have a higher than normal baseline iron absorption, whether due to inherited factors (subclinical hemochromatosis, etc) or to the presence of non–iron deficiency anemias (anemia of chronic disease, hemolytic anemias, etc).

Chronic iron overload in the absence of anemia is most efficiently treated by intermittent phlebotomy. One unit of blood (containing 250 mg of iron) can be removed every week or so until all of the excess iron is removed. Iron chelation therapy using parenteral deferoxamine is much less efficient as well as more complicated, expensive, and hazardous, but it can be useful for severe iron overload that cannot be managed by phlebotomy.

VITAMIN B$_{12}$ & FOLIC ACID

Basic Pharmacology

Vitamin B$_{12}$ and folic acid are chemically unrelated vitamins essential for normal DNA synthesis. Deficiencies lead to impaired DNA synthesis, inhibition of normal mitosis, and abnormal maturation and function of the cells produced. These changes are most apparent in tissues where cells undergo rapid cell division, such as in bone marrow and the gastrointestinal epithelium, but all dividing cells are affected to some degree. Severe anemia is the chief finding in patients with vitamin B$_{12}$ or folic acid deficiency, but pancytopenia (diminished production of red blood cells, white blood cells, and platelets) may occur, and gastrointestinal symptoms are common. Neurologic abnormalities may also occur in vitamin B$_{12}$ deficiency but not in folic acid deficiency.

Anemias caused by vitamin B$_{12}$ and folic acid deficiency have a characteristic appearance of peripheral blood and bone marrow called megaloblastic anemia. Since the underlying defect in megaloblastic anemias is impaired DNA synthesis, there is diminished cell division in the face of continued RNA and protein synthesis. This leads to production of large (macrocytic) red blood cells that have a high RNA:DNA ratio and are defective in the sense that they are highly susceptible to destruction. Morphologically, the bone marrow is hypercellular, with a marked increase in the number of large abnormal early red cell precursors (megaloblasts) but with very few cells maturing beyond this stage to become circulating red cells. The red cells that do form in the bone marrow characteristically show normal cytoplasmic maturation, including normal hemoglobin formation; it is nuclear maturation and cell division that is impaired in the megaloblastic anemias.

Although megaloblastic anemia can theoretically result from any event that impairs DNA synthesis, in practice almost all cases are due to deficiencies of vitamin B$_{12}$ or folic acid. The biochemical and physiologic bases of these deficiencies are now well understood, and it is possible to describe the mechanisms causing these anemias at the molecular level.

Chemistry

A. Vitamin B$_{12}$: Vitamin B$_{12}$ is made up of a porphyrinlike ring with a central cobalt atom attached to a nucleotide (Fig 31–1). Various ligands may be covalently bound to the cobalt atom, forming different cobalamins. Deoxyadenosylcobalamin and methylcobalamin are the active forms of the vitamin in humans. Cyanocobalamin and hydroxocobalamin (both available for therapeutic use) and other cobalamins

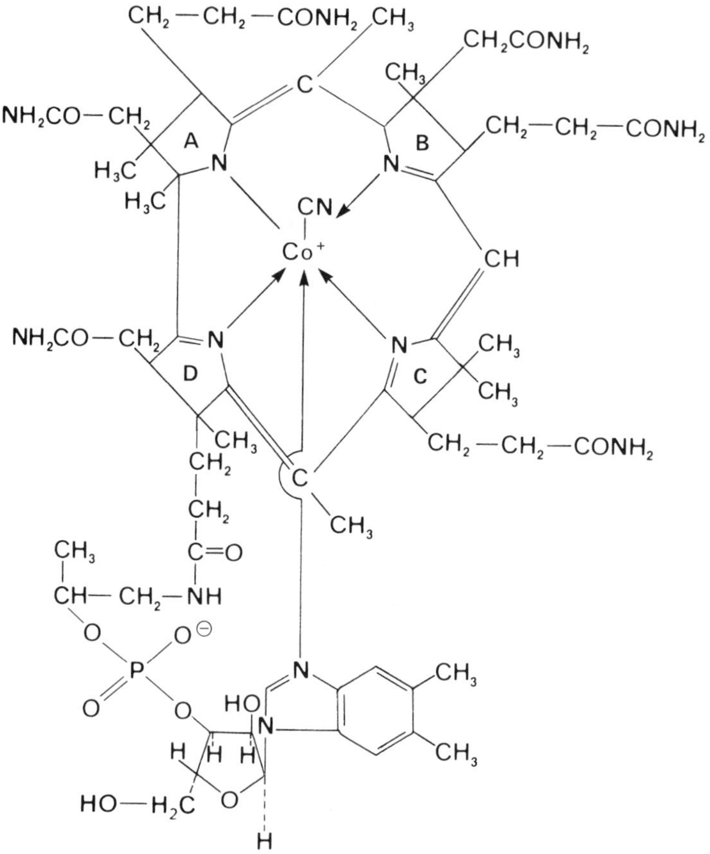

Figure 31–1. Cyanocobalamin; vitamin B_{12} ($C_{63}H_{88}O_{14}N_{14}PCo$). (Reproduced, with permission, from Martin DW Jr et al: *Harper's Review of Biochemistry*, 20th ed. Lange, 1985.)

found in food sources must be converted to the above active forms. The ultimate source of vitamin B_{12} is from microbial synthesis; it is not synthesized by animals or plants. The chief dietary source of vitamin B_{12} is microbially derived vitamin B_{12} in meat (especially liver), eggs, and dairy products. Vitamin B_{12} is sometimes called **extrinsic factor** to differentiate it from intrinsic factor, a substance normally secreted by the stomach.

B. Folic Acid: Folic acid (pteroylglutamic acid) is a compound composed of a pteridine heterocycle, *p*-aminobenzoic acid, and glutamic acid (Fig 31–2). Various numbers of glutamic acid moieties may be attached to the pteroyl portion of the molecule, resulting in monoglutamates, triglutamates, or polyglutamates. The fully oxidized pteridine ring of folic acid can undergo reduction, catalyzed by the enzyme dihydrofolate reductase, to give 7,8-dihydrofolic acid (H_2folate) and then to the fully reduced 5,6,7,8-tetrahydrofolic acid (H_4folate) (Fig 31–3). H_4folate can subsequently be transformed to folate cofactors possessing one-carbon units attached to the 5-nitrogen (5-CH_3–H_4folate and 5-CHO–H_4folate), the 10-nitrogen (10-CHO–H_4folate), or both positions (5,10-CH_2–H_4folate and 5,10-CH^+=H_4folate) (Fig 31–4). The folate cofactors

are interconvertible by various enzymic reactions and serve the important biochemical function of donating one-carbon units at various levels of oxidation. In most instances, H_4folate is regenerated in these reactions and is available for reutilization. Various forms of folic acid are present in a wide variety of plant and animal tissues; the richest sources are yeast, liver, kidney, and green vegetables.

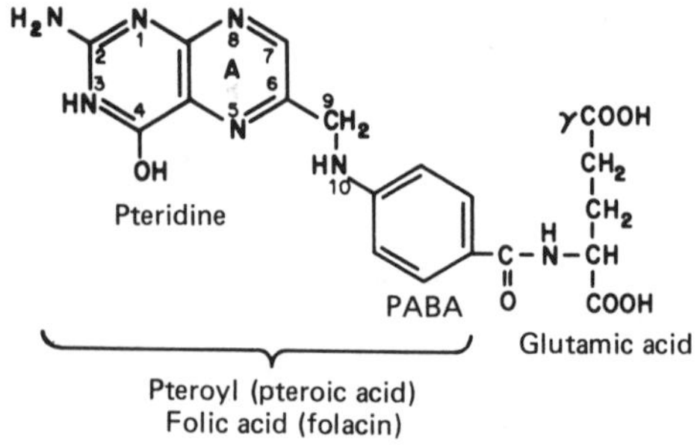

Figure 31–2. The structure and numbering of atoms of folic acid. (Reproduced, with permission, from Martin DW Jr et al: *Harper's Review of Biochemistry*, 20th ed. Lange, 1985.)

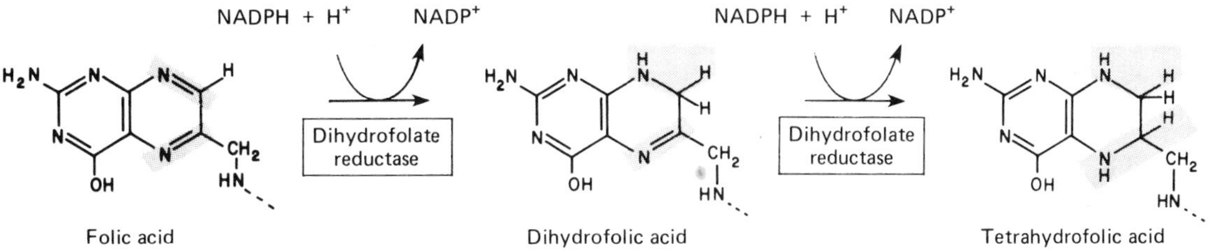

Figure 31–3. The reduction of folic acid to dihydrofolic acid and dihydrofolic acid to tetrahydrofolic acid by the enzyme dihydrofolate reductase. (Reproduced, with permission, from Martin DW Jr et al: *Harper's Review of Biochemistry*, 20th ed. Lange, 1985.)

Pharmacokinetics

A. Vitamin B$_{12}$: The average American diet contains 5–30 μg of vitamin B$_{12}$ daily, 1–5 μg of which is usually absorbed. The vitamin is avidly stored, primarily in the liver, with an average adult having a total vitamin B$_{12}$ storage pool of 3000–5000 μg. Only trace amounts of vitamin B$_{12}$ are normally lost in urine and stool. Since the normal daily requirements of vitamin B$_{12}$ are only about 2 μg, it would take about 5 years for all of the stored vitamin B$_{12}$ to be exhausted and for megaloblastic anemia to develop if B$_{12}$ absorption suddenly or gradually stopped.

Vitamin B$_{12}$ in physiologic amounts is absorbed only after it complexes with intrinsic factor. Intrinsic factor is a glycoprotein with a molecular weight of about 50,000 that is secreted by the parietal cells of the gastric mucosa. Intrinsic factor combines with vitamin

B$_{12}$ liberated from dietary sources in the stomach and duodenum, and the intrinsic factor-vitamin B$_{12}$ complex is subsequently absorbed in the distal ileum by a highly specific receptor-mediated transport system. Vitamin B$_{12}$ deficiency in humans most often results from malabsorption of vitamin B$_{12}$, due either to lack of intrinsic factor or to loss or malfunction of the specific absorptive mechanism in the distal ileum.

Once absorbed, vitamin B$_{12}$ is transported to the various cells of the body bound to a plasma glycoprotein, transcobalamin II. Excess vitamin B$_{12}$ is transported to the liver for storage. Significant amounts of vitamin B$_{12}$ are excreted in the urine only when very large amounts are given parenterally, overcoming the binding capacities of the transcobalamins.

B. Folic Acid: The average American diet contains 500–700 μg of folates daily, 50–200 μg of which

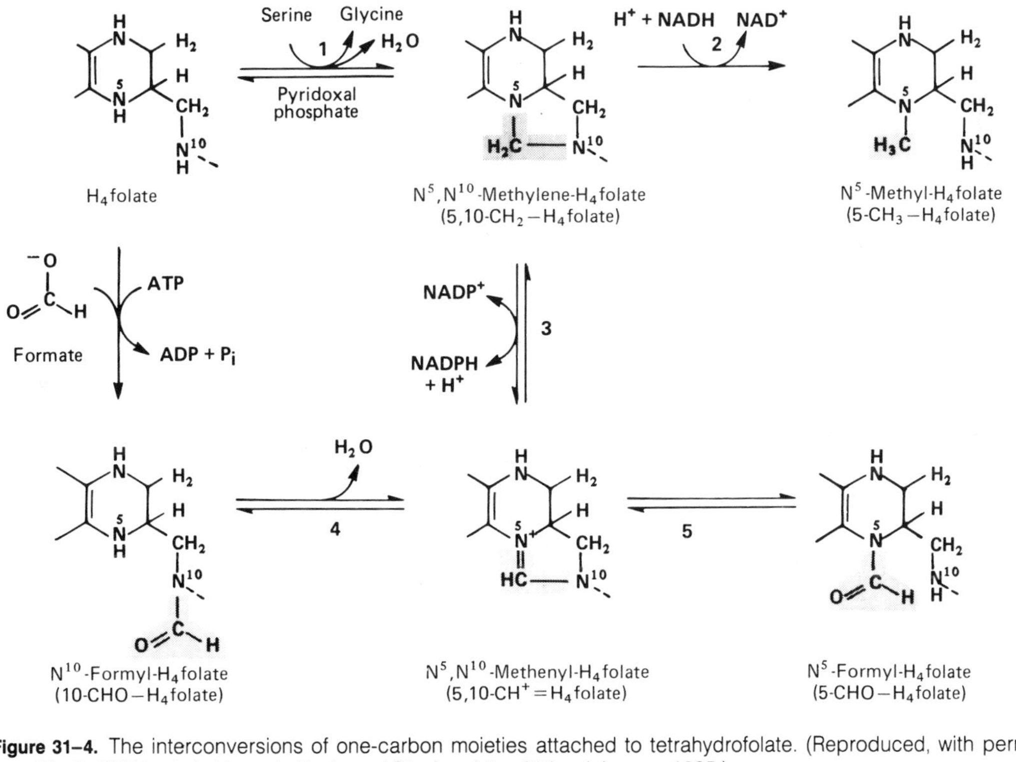

Figure 31–4. The interconversions of one-carbon moieties attached to tetrahydrofolate. (Reproduced, with permission, from Martin DW Jr et al: *Harper's Review of Biochemistry*, 20th ed. Lange, 1985.)

is usually absorbed, depending on metabolic requirements (pregnant women may absorb as much as 300–400 μg of folic acid daily). Normally, 5–20 mg of folates is stored in the liver and other tissues. Folates are excreted in the urine and stool and are also destroyed by catabolism, so serum levels fall within a few days when intake is diminished. Since body stores of folates are relatively low and daily requirements high, folic acid deficiency and megaloblastic anemia can develop within 1–6 months after the intake of folic acid stops, depending on the patient's nutritional status and the rate of folate utilization.

Unaltered folic acid is readily and completely absorbed in the proximal jejunum. Dietary folates, however, consist primarily of polyglutamate forms of 5-CH$_3$–H$_4$folate, with very little unmodified folate present. Before absorption, all but one of the glutamyl residues of the polyglutamates must be hydrolyzed by the enzyme α-L-glutamyl transferase ("conjugase") within the brush border of the intestinal mucosa. The monoglutamate 5-CH$_3$–H$_4$folate is subsequently transported into the bloodstream, both by active and passive transport, and then widely distributed throughout the body.

Pharmacodynamics

A. Vitamin B$_{12}$: There are 2 essential enzymic reactions in humans that require vitamin B$_{12}$ (Fig 31–5). In one reaction, deoxyadenosylcobalamin is a required cofactor in the conversion of methylmalonyl-CoA to succinyl-CoA by the enzyme methylmalonyl-CoA mutase. In the face of vitamin B$_{12}$ deficiency, this conversion cannot take place, and the substrate, methylmalonyl-CoA, accumulates. As a result, aberrant fatty acids are synthesized and incorporated into cell membranes. It is believed that incorporation of such nonphysiologic fatty acids into cell membranes of the central nervous system is responsible for the neurologic manifestations of vitamin B$_{12}$ deficiency.

The other enzymic reaction that requires vitamin B$_{12}$ is conversion of 5-CH$_3$–H$_4$folate and homocysteine to H$_4$folate and methionine by the enzyme 5-CH$_3$–H$_4$folate-homocysteine methyltransferase (Fig 31–5B). In this reaction, cobalamin and methylcobalamin are interconverted, and the vitamin may be considered a true catalyst. When vitamin B$_{12}$ deficiency occurs, conversion of the major dietary and storage folate, 5-CH$_3$–H$_4$folate, to the precursor of folate cofactors, H$_4$folate, cannot occur. As a result, 5-CH$_3$–H$_4$folate accumulates, and a deficiency of folate cofactors necessary for DNA synthesis develops. This accumulation of the body's folate as 5-CH$_3$–H$_4$folate and the associated inability to form folate cofactors in vitamin B$_{12}$ deficiency have been referred to as the "methylfolate trap." This is the biochemical step whereby vitamin B$_{12}$ and folic acid metabolism are linked and explains why the megaloblastic anemia of vitamin B$_{12}$ deficiency (but not the neurologic abnormalities) can be partially corrected by folic acid.

B. Folic Acid: As noted above, the ultimate role of the folates is the formation of folate cofactors essential for one-carbon transfer reactions necessary for DNA synthesis. The de novo synthesis of the purine heterocycle involves 2 enzymic reactions that use folate cofactors. In these, 10-CHO–H$_4$folate and 5,10-CH$^+$=H$_4$folate (Fig 31–4) donate their one-carbon units to ultimately form carbons 2 and 8 of the purine heterocycle. In both of these reactions, H$_4$folate is regenerated and can again accept a one-carbon unit and reenter the H$_4$folate cofactor pool.

Another essential reaction in which a folate cofactor is necessary is the synthesis of thymidylic acid (2'-deoxythymidylate monophosphate, dTMP), an essential precursor of DNA. In this reaction, the enzyme thymidylate synthetase catalyzes the transfer of the one-carbon unit of 5,10-CH$_2$–H$_4$folate to the 5-position of 2'-deoxyuridylate monophosphate (dUMP) to form dTMP (Fig 31–6). Unlike all of the other enzymic reactions that utilize folate cofactors, in this reaction the cofactor is oxidized to H$_2$folate, and for each mole of dTMP produced, 1 mol of H$_4$folate is consumed. In rapidly proliferating tissues, considerable amounts of H$_4$folate can be consumed in this reaction, and continued DNA synthesis requires continued regeneration of H$_4$folate by reduction of H$_2$folate, catalyzed by the enzyme dihydrofolate reductase. The H$_4$folate thus produced can then re-form the cofactor CH$_2$–H$_4$folate by the action of serine transhydroxymethylase and thus allow for the continued synthesis of dTMP. The combined catalytic activities of dTMP synthetase, dihydrofolate reductase, and serine transhydroxymethylase are often referred to as the **dTMP synthesis cycle** (Fig 31–7).

Clinical Pharmacology of Vitamin B$_{12}$ & Folic Acid

Vitamin B$_{12}$ and folic acid should be used specifically to treat or prevent deficiencies of these vita-

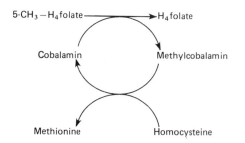

A. Methylmalonyl-CoA mutase

B. 5-CH$_3$–H$_4$folate-homocysteine methyltransferase

Figure 31–5. Enzymic reactions that use vitamin B$_{12}$.

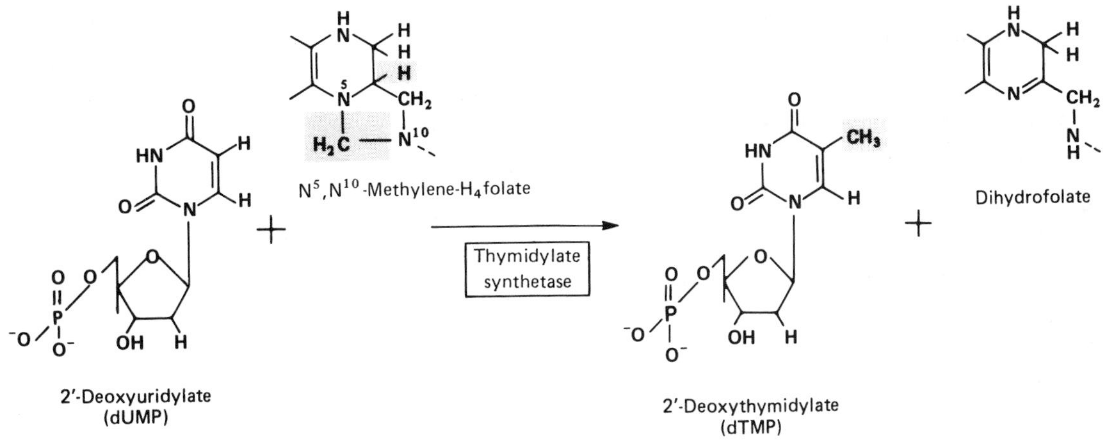

Figure 31–6. The transfer of a methyl moiety from N^5, N^{10}-methylene-H₄folate to deoxyuridylate to generate deoxythymidylate and dihydrofolate (H₂folate). (Reproduced, with permission, from Martin DW Jr et al: *Harper's Review of Biochemistry*, 20th ed. Lange, 1985.)

mins. There is no evidence that vitamin B₁₂ injections have any benefit in persons who do not have vitamin B₁₂ deficiency. Supplemental folic acid, however, may be useful in preventing folic acid deficiency in certain high-risk patients with high folate requirements.

The most characteristic clinical manifestation of vitamin B₁₂ and folic acid deficiency is megaloblastic anemia. Any patient with macrocytosis, with or without anemia, should be evaluated for possible vitamin B₁₂ or folic acid deficiency. Although most patients with neurologic abnormalities caused by vitamin B₁₂ deficiency have full-blown megaloblastic anemia when first seen, occasional patients have few if any hematologic abnormalities, and the diagnosis of vitamin B₁₂ deficiency may at first be obscure. It is particularly important to differentiate vitamin B₁₂ deficiency from other forms of megaloblastic anemia, since treatment with vitamin B₁₂ must be continued for life in most cases and the hematologic abnormalities in vitamin

B₁₂ deficiency may be partially corrected by treatment with large doses of folic acid while the neurologic damage progresses and may become irreversible.

The typical clinical findings in megaloblastic anemia are macrocytic anemia (MCV usually > 120 fL), often with associated mild or moderate leukopenia or thrombocytopenia (or both), and a characteristic hypercellular bone marrow with megaloblastic maturation of erythroid and other precursor cells. Once a diagnosis of megaloblastic anemia is made, it must be determined whether vitamin B₁₂ or folic acid deficiency is the cause. (Other causes of megaloblastic anemia are very rare.) This can usually be accomplished by measuring serum levels of the vitamins, although these measurements occasionally give false-positive or false-negative results. Red blood cell folic acid levels are often of greater diagnostic value than serum levels, since serum folic acid levels tend to be quite labile and do not necessarily reflect tissue levels. The Schilling test, which measures absorption and uri-

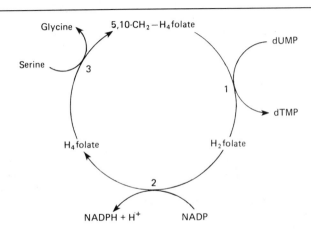

Figure 31–7. dTMP synthesis cycle. (1) dTMP synthetase; (2) H₂folate reductase; (3) serine transhydroxymethylase.

nary excretion of radioactively labeled vitamin B_{12}, can be used to further define the mechanism of vitamin B_{12} malabsorption when this is found to be the cause of the megaloblastic anemia.

A. Vitamin B_{12}: Vitamin B_{12} deficiency is almost always caused by malabsorption of vitamin B_{12}, due either to deficiency of intrinsic factor or to defects in the absorption of the vitamin B_{12}–intrinsic factor complex in the distal ileum. The most common causes of vitamin B_{12} deficiency are pernicious anemia, partial or total gastrectomy, and diseases that affect the distal ileum, such as malabsorption syndromes, inflammatory bowel disease, or small bowel resection. Nutritional deficiency of vitamin B_{12} is rare but may be seen in strict vegetarians after many years without meat, eggs, or dairy products.

Pernicious anemia results from defective secretion of **intrinsic factor** by the gastric mucosal cells. It is most common in older individuals of Northern European extraction, but it may occur at any age and in all races. Patients with pernicious anemia have gastric atrophy and fail to secrete hydrochloric acid (as well as intrinsic factor). The Schilling test shows diminished absorption of radioactively labeled vitamin B_{12}, which is corrected when hog intrinsic factor is administered with radioactive B_{12}, since the vitamin can then be normally absorbed. Pernicious anemia is a lifelong disease, and treatment with vitamin B_{12} injections must be continued indefinitely.

Total or partial gastrectomy removes the parietal cell–containing portion of the stomach that secretes intrinsic factor, resulting in vitamin B_{12} malabsorption similar to that seen in pernicious anemia. Since vitamin B_{12} stores may not be exhausted until as long as 5 years after gastrectomy, megaloblastic anemia will not develop until that time; however, many clinicians routinely start patients on vitamin B_{12} injections after gastrectomy to avoid any chance that vitamin B_{12} deficiency will develop later.

Vitamin B_{12} deficiency also occurs when the region of the distal ileum that absorbs the vitamin B_{12}–intrinsic factor complex is damaged, as when the ileum is involved with inflammatory bowel disease or sprue or when the ileum is surgically resected. In these situations, radioactively labeled vitamin B_{12} is not absorbed in the Schilling test, even when instrinsic factor is added. Other rare causes of vitamin B_{12} deficiency include bacterial overgrowth of the small bowel, blind loop syndrome, fish tapeworm, chronic pancreatitis, and thyroid disease. Rare cases of vitamin B_{12} deficiency in children have been found to be secondary to congenital deficiency of intrinsic factor and congenital selective vitamin B_{12} malabsorption due to defects of the receptor sites in the distal ileum.

Since almost all cases of vitamin B_{12} deficiency are caused by malabsorption of the vitamin, parenteral injections of vitamin B_{12} are required for therapy. For patients with potentially reversible diseases (fish tapeworm, sprue, blind loops), the underlying disease should be treated after initial treatment with parenteral vitamin B_{12}. Most patients, however, do not have cur-

able deficiency syndromes and require lifelong treatment with vitamin B_{12} injections.

Vitamin B_{12} for parenteral injection is available as cyanocobalamin or hydroxocobalamin. Hydroxocobalamin is preferred because it is more highly protein-bound and therefore remains longer in the circulation. Initial therapy should consist of 100–1000 μg of vitamin B_{12} intramuscularly daily or every other day for 1–2 weeks to replenish body stores. Maintenance therapy consists of 100–1000 μg intramuscularly once a month for life. If neurologic abnormalities are present, vitamin B_{12} injections should be given every 1–2 weeks for 6 months before switching to monthly injections. Oral vitamin B_{12}–intrinsic factor mixtures and liver extracts should not be used to treat vitamin B_{12} deficiency; however, oral doses of 1000 μg of vitamin B_{12} daily are usually sufficient to treat patients with pernicious anemia who refuse or cannot tolerate the injections.

The hematologic response to treatment with vitamin B_{12} is rapid. The bone marrow usually returns to normal within 48 hours. Reticulocytosis begins on the second or third day and is usually maximal by the fifth to tenth day. Hemoglobin begins to increase in the first week and returns to normal by 1–2 months. Incomplete correction of the anemia may be due to persistence of other deficiencies (ie, combined vitamin B_{12} and iron deficiency) or the presence of inflammatory disease or other disorders that inhibit erythropoiesis.

B. Folic Acid: Folic acid deficiency, unlike vitamin B_{12} deficiency, is often caused by inadequate dietary intake of folates. Elderly patients, poor patients, and food faddists whose diets lack vegetables, eggs, and meat often develop folic acid deficiency. Prolonged cooking of vegetables destroys folates and can lead to folic acid deficiency if this is the only dietary source of this vitamin. Alcoholics and patients with liver disease develop folic acid deficiency because of poor diet and diminished hepatic storage of folates. There is also evidence that alcohol and liver disease interfere with absorption and metabolism of folates. Pregnant women and patients with hemolytic anemia have increased folate requirements and may become folic acid-deficient, especially if their diets are marginal. Patients with sprue and other malabsorption syndromes also frequently develop folic acid deficiency, perhaps because of a lack of intestinal conjugase. Folic acid deficiency is occasionally associated with cancer, leukemia, myeloproliferative disorders, certain chronic skin disorders, and other chronic debilitating diseases. Patients who require renal dialysis also develop folic acid deficiency, because folates are removed from the plasma each time the patient is dialyzed.

Folic acid deficiency can also be caused by drugs that interfere with folate absorption or metabolism. Phenytoin, some other anticonvulsants, oral contraceptives, and isoniazid can cause folic acid deficiency by interfering with folic acid absorption, possibly by inhibiting intestinal folate conjugases. Other drugs such as methotrexate and, to a lesser extent, trimethoprim and pyrimethamine, inhibit dihydrofolate reductase and may result in a deficiency of folate cofactors and ultimately in megaloblastic anemia.

Folic acid is available as tablets containing 0.1, 0.4, 0.8, and 1 mg of pteroylglutamic acid and as a parenteral solution containing 5 mg per milliliter. Parenteral administration is rarely necessary, since oral folic acid is well absorbed even in patients with malabsorption syndromes. A dose of 1 mg of folic acid orally daily is sufficient to reverse megaloblastic anemia, restore normal serum folate levels, and replenish body stores of folates in almost all patients. Therapy should be continued until the underlying cause of the deficiency is removed or corrected. Therapy may be required indefinitely for patients with malabsorption or dietary inadequacy. Folic acid supplementation to prevent folic acid deficiency should be considered in high-risk patients, including pregnant women, alcoholics, and patients with hemolytic anemia, liver disease, certain skin diseases, and patients on renal dialysis.

The response of patients with folate deficiency to treatment with oral folic acid is rapid and complete and similar to the response of the vitamin B$_{12}$–deficient patient given parenteral vitamin B$_{12}$. The hemoglobin level should begin to rise within the first week, and the anemia should be completely corrected in 1–2 months.

Clinical Toxicology

Vitamin B$_{12}$ and folic acid have no known toxic effects even when administered in very large amounts. Large doses of both vitamins are promptly excreted in urine and to a lesser extent in stool, so that prolonged tissue exposure to very high levels does not occur. There is no evidence that cyanocobalamin, even in huge doses, causes cyanide poisoning.

REFERENCES

Beck WS: Megaloblastic anemias. Chap 103, pp 853–860, in: *Cecil Textbook of Medicine*, 16th ed. Wyngaarden JB, Smith LH (editors). Saunders, 1982.

Brown EB: Iron deficiency anemia. Chap 102.1, pp 844–851, in: *Cecil Textbook of Medicine*, 16th ed. Wyngaarden JB, Smith LH (editors). Saunders, 1982.

Chanarin I: Investigation and management of megaloblastic anemia. *Clin Haematol* 1976;**5**:747.

Chanarin I et al: How vitamin B$_{12}$ acts. *Br J Haematol* 1981; **47**:487.

Dallman PR: Iron deficiency: Diagnosis and treatment. *West J Med* 1981;**134**:496.

Finch CA (editor): Clinical aspects of iron deficiency and excess. *Semin Hematol* 1982;**29**:1. [Entire issue.]

Finch CA, Huebers H: Perspectives in iron metabolism. *N Engl J Med* 1982;**306**:1520.

Reich PR: Hypochromic anemias. Chap 2, pp 35–68, and Megaloblastic anemias. Chap 3, pp 69–107, in: *Hematology: Pathophysiologic Basis for Clinical Practice*, 2nd ed. Little, Brown, 1984.

32

Drugs Used in Disorders of Coagulation

Robert A. O'Reilly, MD

Bleeding and thrombosis are altered states of hemostasis. Inhibition of hemostasis results in spontaneous bleeding; stimulated hemostasis results in thrombus formation. The drugs used to inhibit thrombosis and to arrest bleeding are the subjects of this chapter.

MECHANISMS OF BLOOD COAGULATION

Thrombogenesis

The **platelet** occupies a central position in all thromboembolic disease. Virchow's 19th century triad of hypercoagulability, vessel wall change, and stasis still underlies current theories of thrombogenesis. A **white thrombus** forms initially in high-pressure arteries by adherence of circulating platelets to the arterial wall. These adhered platelets release adenosine diphosphate (ADP), a powerful inducer of platelet aggregation. The growing thrombus of aggregated platelets reduces arterial flow. This localized stasis triggers fibrin formation, and a red thrombus forms around the nidal white thrombus. A **red thrombus** forms in low-pressure veins, especially in their valve pockets, again by adherence of circulating platelets. But venous stasis activates hemostasis so that the bulk of the thrombus forms a long red tail consisting of a fibrin network in which red cells are enmeshed. These tails become detached easily and travel as emboli to the pulmonary arteries. Although all thrombi are mixed, the platelet nidus dominates the arterial thrombus and the fibrin tail the venous thrombus. Arterial thrombi cause serious disease by producing local occlusive ischemia; venous thrombi, by giving rise to distant embolization.

Hemostasis is the spontaneous arrest of bleeding from a damaged blood vessel. The immediate hemostatic response of a damaged vessel is **vasospasm.** Within seconds, platelets stick to the exposed collagen of the vessel (**platelet adhesion**) and to each other (**platelet aggregation**). Platelets then lose their individual membranes and form a gelatinous mass during **viscous metamorphosis.** This platelet plug can quickly arrest bleeding, but it must be reinforced by fibrin for long-term effectiveness. Fibrin reinforcement results from local stimuli to blood coagulation: the exposed collagen of damaged vessels and the membranes and released contents of platelets. The local production of thrombin not only releases more platelet ADP but also stimulates the synthesis of prostaglandins from the arachidonic acid of platelet membranes. These powerful substances are composed of 2 groups of eicosanoids (Chapter 17) that have opposite effects on thrombogenesis. **Thromboxane A$_2$** is synthesized within platelets and induces thrombogenesis. **Prostacyclin** is synthesized within vessel walls and inhibits thrombogenesis.

Blood Coagulation

Blood coagulates by the transformation of soluble fibrinogen into insoluble **fibrin.** More than a dozen circulating proteins (Table 32–1) interact in a cascading series of limited proteolytic reactions (Fig 32–1). At each step, a clotting factor zymogen (eg, factor

Table 32–1. Blood clotting factors and synonyms.*

Factor	Common Synonyms
I	Fibrinogen
I'	Fibrin monomer
I"	Fibrin polymer
II	Prothrombin
III	Tissue thromboplastin
IV	Calcium, Ca^{2+}
V	Proaccelerin
VII	Proconvertin
VIII	Antihemophilic globulin, AHG
IX	Christmas factor; plasma thromboplastin component, PTC
X	Stuart-Prower factor
XI	Plasma thromboplastin antecedent, PTA
XII	Hageman factor
XIII	Fibrin-stabilizing factor
HMW-K	High-molecular-weight kininogen, Fitzgerald factor
Pre-K	Prekallikrein, Fletcher factor
Ka	Kallikrein
PL	Platelet phospholipid

*Modified and reproduced, with permission, from O'Reilly RA: Anticoagulant, antithrombotic, and thrombolytic drugs. Chap 58, pp 1338–1359, in: *Goodman and Gilman's The Pharmacological Basis of Therapeutics,* 7th ed. Gilman AG et al (editors). Macmillan, 1985.

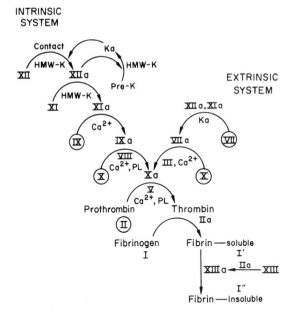

INTRINSIC
SYSTEM

Figure 32–1. Intrinsic and extrinsic systems of blood coagulation. Hageman factor (XII) undergoes contact activation and becomes bound to surfaces. Surface-bound factor XII then undergoes proteolytic activation by kallikrein (Ka) in the presence of high-molecular-weight kininogen (HMW-K). Factor XIIa constitutes an arm of a feedback loop and activates more Ka from prekallikrein (pre-K, or Fletcher factor) in the presence of HMW-K. Factor XIIa in the presence of HMW-K also activates factor XI. Factor XIa in the presence of Ca^{2+} proteolytically activates factor IX to IXa. Factor VIII, factor IXa, Ca^{2+}, and phospholipid micelles (PL) from blood platelets form a lipoprotein complex with factor X and activate it. Factor V, factor Xa, Ca^{2+}, and PL also form a lipoprotein complex with factor II (prothrombin) and activate it to IIa (thrombin). In seconds, thrombin splits 2 pairs of small peptides off the large fibrinogen (I) molecule, followed by rapid noncovalent aggregation of soluble fibrin monomers (I'). Factor XIII, activated by thrombin to XIIIa, cross-links adjacent fibrin monomers (I') covalently to form the insoluble fibrin clot (I"). In the extrinsic system, factor VII undergoes proteolytic activation by factors XIIa, XIa, and Ka from the intrinsic system. Factor VIIa, Ca^{2+}, tissue thromboplastin (III), and factor X form a lipoprotein complex that results in activation of factor X. From this step onward, the extrinsic system is identical to the intrinsic system. Factor Xa is the principal factor that is inhibited by heparin following interaction of heparin with its cofactor, antithrombin III. The circled clotting factors are dependent on vitamin K for their synthesis. (Reproduced, with permission, from O'Reilly RA: Anticoagulant, antithrombotic, and thrombolytic drugs. Chap 58, pp 1338–1359, in: *Goodman and Gilman's, The Pharmacological Basis of Therapeutics*, 7th ed. Gilman AG et al [editors]. Macmillan, 1985.)

XII) undergoes limited proteolysis and becomes an active protease (eg, factor XIIa). This protease activates the next clotting factor (factor XI), until finally a solid fibrin clot is formed. Fibrinogen (factor I), the soluble precursor of fibrin, is the substrate for the enzyme thrombin (factor IIa). This protease is formed during

coagulation by activation of its zymogen prothrombin (factor II). Prothrombin is bound by calcium to a platelet phospholipid (PL) surface, where activated factor X (Xa) in the presence of factor V converts it into circulating thrombin.

Two separate pathways activate factor X. The **intrinsic system** has all the factors necessary for coagulation contained in the circulating blood (Fig 32–1). The **extrinsic system** has an unidentified lipoprotein called tissue thromboplastin (factor III), which is released from damaged tissue into the circulating blood. Tissue thromboplastin in the presence of activated factor VII (VIIa) converts factor X, bound by calcium to phospholipid surfaces, to activated factor X (Xa). In the intrinsic system, factor Xa requires several minutes for formation. In the extrinsic system, factor Xa is formed within seconds, because the early time-consuming reactions are bypassed. Both pathways must be intact for hemostasis to be adequate. The partial thromboplastin time (PTT) is a measure of the function of the intrinsic system. The one-stage prothrombin time measures the extrinsic system.

Regulation of Coagulation & Fibrinolysis

Blood coagulation and thrombus formation must be confined to the smallest possible area to achieve local hemostasis in response to bleeding from trauma or surgery. Two major systems regulate and delimit these processes: **fibrin inhibition** and **fibrinolysis.**

Plasma contains several protease inhibitors that rapidly inactivate the coagulation proteins as they escape from the site of vessel injury. The most important proteins of this system are α_1-antitrypsin, α_2-macroglobulin, α_2-antiplasmin, and antithrombin III. If this system is overwhelmed, generalized intravascular clotting may occur. This process is called **disseminated intravascular coagulation (DIC)** and may follow massive tissue injury, cell lysis in malignant neoplastic disease, obstetric emergencies such as abruptio placentae, or bacterial sepsis.

The central process of fibrinolysis is conversion of inactive plasminogen to the proteolytic enzyme **plasmin.** This process is activated at the onset of blood coagulation by factor XIIa. Injured cells release activators of plasminogen. Plasmin remodels the thrombus and limits the extension of thrombosis by proteolytic digestion of fibrin.

Regulation of the fibrinolytic system is useful in therapeutics. Increased fibrinolysis is effective therapy for thrombotic disease. **Urokinase, streptokinase,** and **tissue plasminogen activator** all activate the fibrinolytic system (Fig 32–2). Conversely, decreased fibrinolysis protects clots from lysis and reduces the bleeding of hemostatic failure. **Aminocaproic acid (Amicar,** EACA) is a clinically useful inhibitor of fibrinolysis. Heparin and the oral anticoagulant drugs do not affect the fibrinolytic mechanism.

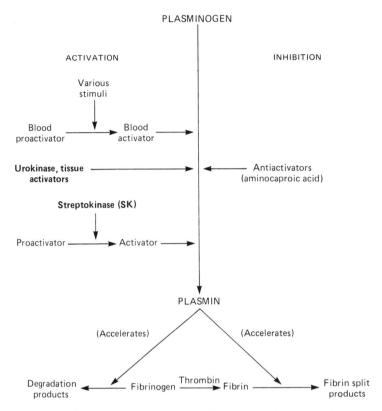

Figure 32–2. Schematic representation of the fibrinolytic system. The sites of action of the activators and the inhibitors of the system are depicted. Urokinase and streptokinase are used clinically, and tissue activators of plasminogen are undergoing clinical trials.

I. BASIC PHARMACOLOGY OF THE ANTICOAGULANT DRUGS

HEPARIN

Chemistry & Mechanism of Action

Heparin is a heterogeneous mixture of sulfated mucopolysaccharides. Its biologic activity is dependent upon the plasma protease inhibitor **antithrombin III,** the cofactor of heparin. Antithrombin inhibits clotting factor proteases by forming equimolar stable complexes with them. In the absence of heparin, these reactions are slow; in the presence of heparin, they are accelerated a thousandfold. Only a third of the molecules in commercial heparin preparations have an accelerating effect and therefore anticoagulant activity. The highly active molecules of heparin bind tightly to antithrombin and cause a conformational change in this inhibitor. This conformational change of antithrombin exposes its active site for rapid interaction with the proteases—the activated clotting factors. Heparin catalyzes the antithrombin-protease reaction without being consumed. Once the antithrombin-protease complex is formed, heparin is released intact for renewed binding to more antithrombin.

The antithrombin-binding region of commercial heparin consists of repeating sulfated disaccharide units composed of D-glucosamine-L-iduronic acid and D-glucosamine-D-glucuronic acid (Fig 32–3). High-molecular-weight fractions of heparin with high affinity for antithrombin markedly inhibit blood coagulation. Low-molecular-weight fractions of heparin inhibit activated factor X but have less effect on antithrombin and on coagulation in general than the high-molecular-weight species. Because commercial heparin consists of a family of molecules of different molecular weights, the correlation between the concentration of a given heparin preparation and its effect on coagulation often is low. Therefore, heparin is standardized as units of activity by bioassay. Heparin sodium USP must contain at least 120 USP units per milligram. Heparin is generally used as the sodium salt, but calcium heparin (Calciparine) is equally effective. Lithium heparin is used in vitro as an anticoagulant for blood samples. Commercial heparin is extracted from porcine intestinal mucosa and bovine lung.

Contraindications

Heparin is contraindicated in patients who are hypersensitive to the drug, are actively bleeding, or have

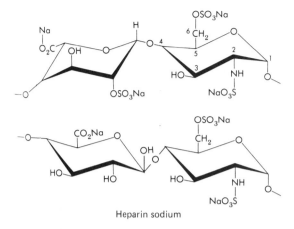

Figure 32–3. Structure of heparin sodium. Commercial heparin consists of polymers containing 8–15 sequences of the 2 disaccharide units depicted here. The upper disaccharide consists of iduronic acid and glucosamine; the lower disaccharide consists of glucuronic acid and glucosamine. The 2 disaccharides occur in varying proportions. Heparin is a strongly acidic molecule because of its high content of anionic sulfate and carboxylic acid. (Modified and reproduced, with permission, from O'Reilly RA: Anticoagulant, antithrombotic, and thrombolytic drugs. Chap 58, pp 1338–1359, in: *Goodman and Gilman's The Pharmacological Basis of Therapeutics*, 7th ed. Gilman AG et al [editors]. Macmillan, 1985.)

hemophilia, thrombocytopenia, purpura, severe hypertension, intracranial hemorrhage, bacterial endocarditis, active tuberculosis, ulcerative lesions of the gastrointestinal tract, threatened abortion, or visceral carcinoma. Heparin should not be given to patients during or after surgery of the brain, spinal cord, or eye or to patients undergoing lumbar puncture or regional anesthetic blocks. Heparin should be used in pregnant women only when clearly indicated despite the apparent lack of placental transfer.

Administration & Dosage

A plasma concentration of heparin of 0.2 unit/mL usually prevents pulmonary emboli in patients with established venous thrombosis. This concentration of heparin will prolong the PTT to 2–2$^{1}/_{2}$ times that of the control value. This degree of anticoagulant effect should be maintained throughout the course of *continuous* intravenous heparin therapy. When *intermittent* heparin administration is used, the PTT should be measured 3–3$^{1}/_{2}$ hours after a heparin dose to adjust the next dose to maintain prolongation of the PTT to 2–2$^{1}/_{2}$ times that of the control value.

The continuous intravenous administration of heparin is accomplished via an infusion pump. After an initial bolus injection of 5000–10,000 units, a continuous infusion of about 900 units/h or 10–15 units/kg/h is required to maintain the PTT at 2–2$^{1}/_{2}$ times that of the control time. Patients with acute pulmonary emboli often require larger doses than these during the first few days because of increased heparin clearance.

With intermittent intravenous administration of heparin, 75–100 units/kg is administered every 4 hours. Subcutaneous administration of heparin, as in low-dose prophylaxis, is achieved with 5000 units every 8 or 12 hours. Heparin must *never* be administered intramuscularly, because of the danger of hematoma formation at the injection site.

Other Heparin Effects

The major adverse effect of heparin is bleeding. This risk can be decreased by scrupulous patient selection, careful control of dosage, and close monitoring of the PTT. Elderly women are particularly prone to hemorrhage. Patients with renal failure often bleed. Heparin is of animal origin and should be used cautiously in patients with allergy. Increased loss of hair and transient reversible alopecia have been reported. Long-term heparin therapy is associated with osteoporosis and spontaneous fractures. Heparin accelerates the clearing of postprandial lipemia by effecting the release of lipoprotein lipase from tissues.

Heparin causes transient thrombocytopenia in 25% of patients and severe thrombocytopenia in 5%. Mild platelet reduction results from heparin-induced aggregation and severe reduction from heparin-induced antiplatelet antibodies. The following points should be considered in all patients receiving heparin: Platelet counts should be performed frequently; thrombocytopenia serious enough to cause bleeding should be considered to be heparin-induced; any new thrombus can be the result of heparin; and thromboembolic disease thought to be heparin-induced should be treated by discontinuation of heparin and administration of an oral anticoagulant if clinically warranted.

Reversal of Heparin Action

Excessive anticoagulant action of heparin is treated by discontinuation of the drug. If bleeding also occurs, administration of a specific antagonist such as protamine sulfate is indicated. Protamine is a highly basic peptide that combines with heparin as an ion pair to form a stable complex devoid of anticoagulant activity. For every 100 units of heparin remaining in the patient, administer 1 mg of protamine sulfate intravenously; the rate of infusion should not exceed 50 mg in any 10-minute period. Excess protamine must be avoided; it also has an anticoagulant effect.

WARFARIN & THE COUMARIN ANTICOAGULANTS

Chemistry & Pharmacokinetics

The clinical use of the coumarin anticoagulants can be traced to the discovery of an anticoagulant substance formed in spoiled sweet clover silage. It produced a deficiency of plasma prothrombin and a consequent hemorrhagic disease in cattle. The toxic agent was identified as bishydroxycoumarin and synthesized as dicumarol. This drug and its congeners, most notably warfarin (Fig 32–4), are widely used as rodenti-

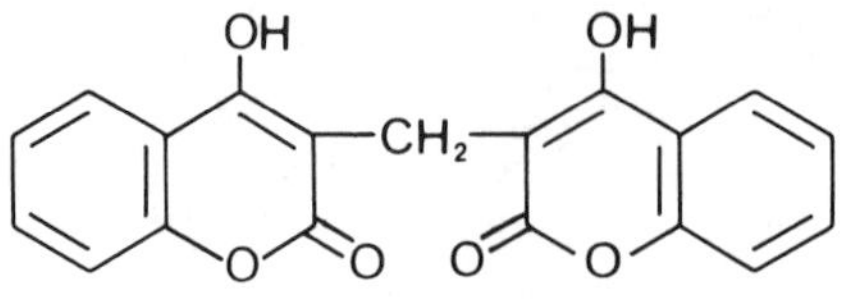

Dicumarol

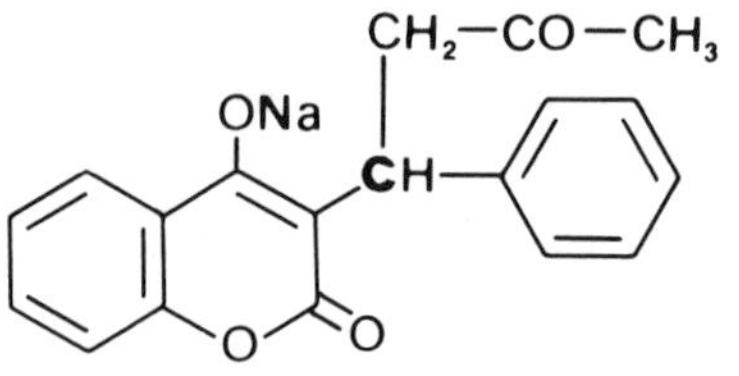

Warfarin sodium

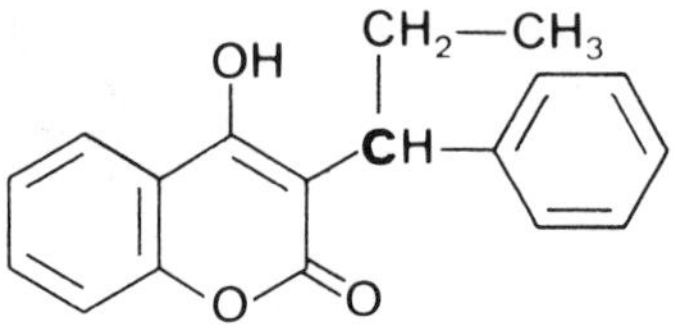

Phenprocoumon

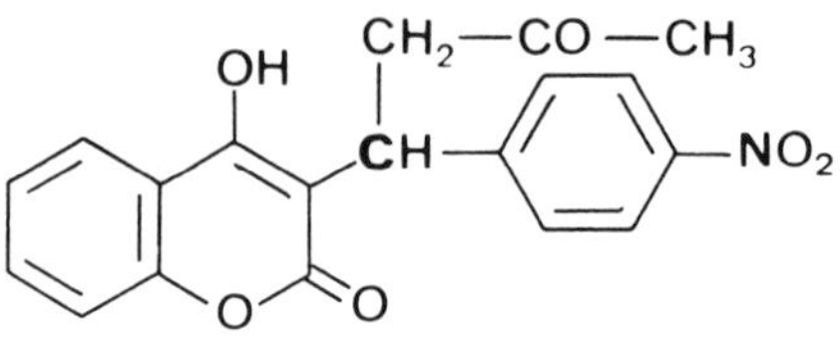

Acenocoumarol

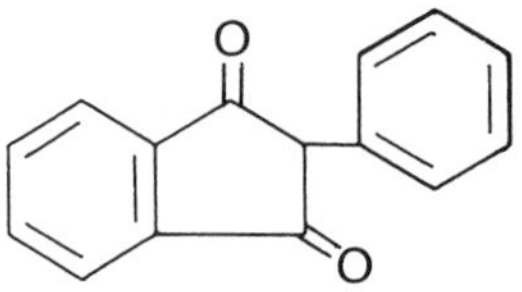

Phenindione

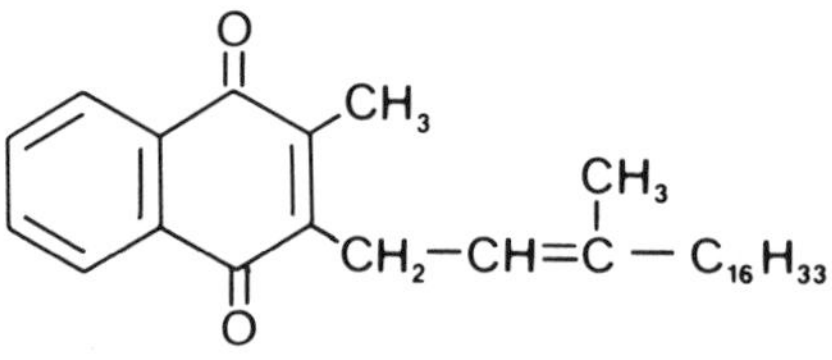

Phytonadione (vitamin K_1)

Figure 32–4. Structural formulas of several oral anticoagulant drugs and of vitamin K. Carbon atoms in bold type are asymmetric centers.

cides in addition to their application as antithrombotic agents in humans. These drugs are often referred to as "oral anticoagulants" because they are administered orally.

Warfarin is generally administered as the sodium salt and has 100% bioavailability. Over 99% of racemic warfarin is bound to plasma albumin, which may contribute to its small volume of distribution (the albumin space), its long half-life in plasma (36 hours), and the lack of urinary excretion of unchanged drug. Warfarin used clinically is a racemic mixture composed of equal amounts of 2 optical isomers. The levorotatory S-warfarin is 4 times more potent than the dextrorotatory R-warfarin. This observation is useful in understanding the stereoselective nature of several drug interactions involving warfarin.

Mechanism of Action

Coumarin anticoagulants block the γ-carboxylation of several glutamate residues in prothrombin and factors VII, IX, and X. The blockade results in incomplete molecules that are biologically inactive in coagulation. This protein carboxylation is physiologically coupled with the oxidative deactivation of vitamin K. The anticoagulant prevents the reductive metabolism of vitamin K epoxide back to its active hydroquinone form (Fig 32–5). Mutational change in the responsible enzyme, vitamin K epoxide reductase, can give rise to genetic resistance to warfarin in humans and in rats.

There is an 8- to 12-hour delay in the action of warfarin. Its anticoagulant effect results from a balance between partially inhibited synthesis and unaltered degradation of the 4 vitamin K-dependent clotting factors. The hypoprothrombinemic effect is dependent on their degradation rate in the circulation. These half-lives are 6, 24, 40, and 60 hours for factors VII, IX, X, and II, respectively. Larger initial doses of warfarin, up to about 0.75 mg/kg, hasten the onset of the anticoagulant effect. Beyond this dosage, the speed of onset is independent of the dose size. The only effect of a larger loading dose is to prolong the time that the plasma concentration of drug remains above that required for suppression of clotting factor synthesis. The 1- to 3-day delay between the peak drug concentration in plasma and its maximum hypoprothrombinemic effect can be described by a model based on the relationship of the plasma concentration of drug and the reduced synthesis of clotting factors. The only difference among oral anticoagulants in producing and maintaining hypoprothrombinemia is the half-life of each drug.

Administration & Dosage

Treatment with warfarin should be initiated with small daily doses of 10–15 mg rather than the large loading doses formerly used. The initial adjustment of the prothrombin time takes about 1 week, which usually results in a maintenance dose of 5–7 mg/d. The prothrombin time should be increased to a level representing 25% of normal activity and maintained there

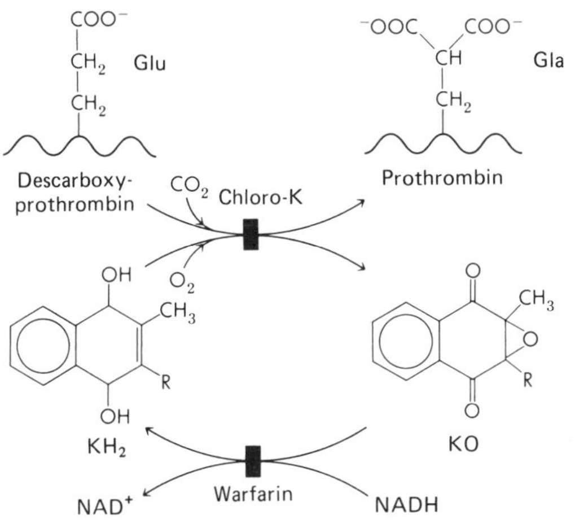

Figure 32–5. Vitamin K cycle—metabolic interconversions of vitamin K associated with the synthesis of vitamin K–dependent clotting factors. Vitamin K_1 or K_2 is reduced to the hydroquinone form (KH_2). Stepwise oxidation to vitamin K epoxide (KO) is coupled to protein carboxylation, wherein descarboxyprothrombin (descarboxy-II) is converted to prothrombin (II) by carboxylation of glutamate residues (Glu) to γ-carboxyglutamate (Gla). Enzymatic reduction of the epoxide with reduced nicotinamide adenine dinucleotide (NADH) as a cofactor regenerates vitamin KH_2. The oxidation of vitamin K is inhibited by the chloro analog of vitamin K (chloro-K), whereas the reduction of vitamin K epoxide is the warfarin-sensitive step (warfarin).The R on the vitamin K molecule represents a 20-carbon phytyl side chain in vitamin K_1 and a 30- to 65-carbon polyprenyl side chain in vitamin K_2. (Artwork reproduced, with permission, from O'Reilly RA: Anticoagulant, antithrombotic, and thrombolytic drugs. Chap 58, pp 1338–1359, in: *Goodman and Gilman's The Pharmacological Basis of Therapeutics,* 7th ed. Gilman AG et al [editors]. Macmillan, 1985.)

for long-term therapy. When the activity is less than 20%, the warfarin dosage should be reduced or omitted until the activity rises above 20%.

Other Effects

Warfarin crosses the placenta readily and can cause a hemorrhagic disorder in the fetus. Furthermore, fetal proteins with γ-carboxyglutamate residues found in bone and blood may be affected by warfarin; the drug

can cause a serious birth defect characterized by abnormal bone formation. Thus, warfarin should never be administered during pregnancy. Cutaneous necrosis unrelated to the degree of anticoagulant effect sometimes occurs during the first weeks of therapy. Rarely, the same process causes frank infarction of breast, fatty tissues, intestine, and extremities. Curiously, the pathologic lesion is venous thrombosis associated with the hemorrhagic infarction.

Drug Interactions

The oral anticoagulants often interact with other drugs and with disease states. These interactions can be broadly divided into pharmacokinetic and pharmacodynamic effects (Appendix I). Pharmacokinetic mechanisms affect the quantity of the administered drug that reaches its receptor site. Pharmacodynamic mechanisms affect the response elicited by the drug at the receptor site. Pharmacokinetic mechanisms for drug interaction with oral anticoagulants are mainly **enzyme induction, enzyme inhibition,** and **reduced plasma protein binding.** Pharmacodynamic mechanisms for interactions with warfarin are **synergism** (impaired hemostasis, reduced clotting factor synthesis, as in hepatic disease), **competitive antagonism** (vitamin K), and **altered physiologic control loop for vitamin K** (hereditary resistance to oral anticoagulants).

The most serious interactions with warfarin are those that increase the anticoagulant effect and the risk of bleeding (Table 32–2). The most dangerous of these interactions are the pharmacokinetic interactions with the pyrazolones phenylbutazone and sulfinpyrazone. These drugs not only augment the hypoprothrombinemia but also inhibit platelet function and may induce peptic ulcer disease (Chapter 34). The mechanisms for their hypoprothrombinemic interaction are a stereoselective inhibition of oxidative metabolic transformation of S-warfarin and displacement of albumin-bound warfarin, increasing the free fraction. Metronidazole, trimethoprim-sulfamethoxazole, and the diuretic ticrynafen also stereoselectively inhibit the metabolic transformation of S-warfarin, whereas disulfiram and cimetidine inhibit metabolism of both enantiomorphs of warfarin. Aspirin, hepatic disease, and hyperthyroidism augment warfarin pharmacodynamically: aspirin by its effect on platelet function and the latter 2

Table 32–2. Pharmacokinetic and pharmacodynamic drug and body interactions with oral anticoagulants.

Increased Prothrombin Time		Decreased Prothrombin Time	
Pharmacokinetic	Pharmacodynamic	Pharmacokinetic	Pharmacodynamic
Cimetidine	**Drugs**	Barbiturates	**Drugs**
Disulfiram	Aspirin (high doses)	Cholestyramine	Diuretics
Metronidazole*	Cephalosporins, third-	Rifampin	Vitamin K
Phenylbutazone*	generation		**Body factors**
Sulfinpyrazone*	Heparin		Hereditary resistance
Ticrynafen*	**Body factors**		Hypothyroidism
Trimethoprim-sulfa-	Hepatic disease		
methoxazole*	Hyperthyroidism		

*Stereoselectively inhibits the oxidative metabolism of the S-warfarin enantiomorph of racemic warfarin.

by increasing the turnover rate of clotting factors. The third-generation cephalosporins apparently eliminate the bacteria in the intestinal tract that produce vitamin K, and, like warfarin, also directly inhibit vitamin K epoxide reductase. Heparin directly prolongs the prothrombin time.

Barbiturates and rifampin both cause a marked decrease of the anticoagulant effect pharmacokinetically by induction of the hepatic enzymes that metabolically transform racemic warfarin. Cholestyramine binds warfarin in the intestine and reduces its absorption and bioavailability. Pharmacodynamic reductions of anticoagulant effect occur with vitamin K (increased synthesis of clotting factors), the diuretics chlorthalidone and spironolactone (clotting factor concentration), hereditary resistance (mutational increase of vitamin K reactivation cycle), and hypothyroidism (decreased turnover rate of clotting factors).

Drugs with *no* significant effect on anticoagulant therapy include ethanol, phenothiazines, benzodiazepines, acetaminophen, narcotics, indomethacin, and most antibiotics.

Reversal of Action

Excessive anticoagulant effect from warfarin can be reversed by stopping the drug and administering large doses of vitamin K_1 (phytonadione) and fresh-frozen plasma or factor IX concentrates such as Konyne and Proplex that also contain large amounts of the prothrombin complex. This disappearance of effect is not correlated with plasma warfarin concentrations but rather with reestablishment of normal activity of the clotting factors. A modest excess of anticoagulant effect without bleeding may require no more than cessation of the drug. Serious bleeding requires large amounts of vitamin K_1 intravenously in 50-mg infusions, factor IX concentrates, and sometimes even transfusion of whole blood.

Analogs & Variants

Vitamin K antagonists other than warfarin are seldom used because they have less favorable pharmacologic properties or greater toxicity. **Dicumarol** is incompletely absorbed and frequently causes gastrointestinal symptoms. **Phenprocoumon (Liquamar** in USA, **Marcumar** or **Marcoumar** in Canada or Europe) has a long half-life of 6 days. The indanedione group, which includes **phenindione** and **diphenadione,** has potentially serious side effects in the kidney and liver and is of little clinical use.

II. BASIC PHARMACOLOGY OF THE FIBRINOLYTIC DRUGS

Fibrinolytic drugs rapidly lyse thrombi by formation of the serine protease **plasmin** (Fig 32–2). These drugs create a generalized lytic state when administered intravenously. Thus, both protective hemostatic thrombi and target thromboemboli are broken down. Two new approaches may reduce these adverse systemic effects. Intra-arterial use of a fibrinolytic drug, as in intracoronary injection, may reduce systemic bleeding. A second generation of prothrombolytic drugs, **tissue plasminogen activators,** can induce thrombolysis without systemic fibrinolysis or fibrinogen breakdown.

STREPTOKINASE & UROKINASE

Pharmacology

Streptokinase is a protein synthesized by streptococci that interacts with the proactivator plasminogen. This enzymatic complex catalyzes the conversion of inactive plasminogen to active plasmin. Urokinase is a human enzyme synthesized by the kidney that directly converts plasminogen to active plasmin. The naturally occurring inhibitors of plasmin in plasma preclude its *direct* use, whereas the absence of inhibitors for urokinase and the streptokinase-proactivator complex permit their use clinically. Plasmin formed inside a thrombus by these activators is protected from plasma antiplasmins, which allows it to lyse the thrombus from within.

Plasminogen can also be activated by endogenous substances called tissue plasminogen activators. These activators preferentially activate plasminogen bound to fibrin, which confines fibrinolysis to the formed thrombus and avoids systemic activation. Recent purification of these activators from cultured human melanoma cells will facilitate clinical trials of these "second-generation" activators.

Indications & Dosage

Use of fibrinolytic drugs intravenously is indicated in cases of multiple pulmonary emboli that are not massive enough to require surgical intervention. Intravenous fibrinolytic drugs are also indicated in cases of central deep venous thrombosis such as the superior vena caval syndrome and ascending thrombophlebitis of the iliofemoral vein. They have also been used intra-arterially, most recently for acute intracoronary thrombosis.

Streptokinase is administered by intravenous infusion of a loading dose of 250,000 units over 30 minutes and a maintenance dose of 100,000 units/h, usually for 24 hours but sometimes longer. Patients with antistreptococcal antibodies can develop fever, allergic reactions, and therapeutic resistance. Urokinase requires a loading dose of 300,000 units given over 10 minutes and a maintenance dose of 300,000 units/h for 12 hours. A course of fibrinolytic drugs is expensive—hundreds of dollars for streptokinase and thousands for urokinase. When therapy is completed, it should be followed by administration of heparin and then warfarin. Thrombolytic treatment with tissue plasminogen activators is still experimental.

Intracoronary administration of streptokinase within the first 6 hours of an acute coronary thrombosis can restore flow in an occluded artery and may reduce the mortality rate. A 10,000-unit bolus of streptokinase followed by 2000 units/min is administered until the vessel is patent, and 2000 units/min is then given for 30–60 minutes more.

DEXTRAN

Dextran is a branched-chain polysaccharide with antithrombotic properties. Although generally used as a plasma volume expander, it has been used to prevent venous thrombosis postoperatively. Dextran interferes with platelet function and fibrin polymerization. The forms of dextran used clinically have molecular weights of 70,000 (**dextran 70**) and 75,000 (**dextran 75**) and are administered by intravenous infusion. Adverse effects include blood volume overload, hemorrhage, and allergic reactions.

III. BASIC PHARMACOLOGY OF ANTITHROMBOTIC DRUGS

Platelet function is regulated by 3 categories of substances. The first group consists of agents generated outside the platelet that interact with platelet membrane receptors, eg, catecholamines, collagen, thrombin, and prostacyclin. The second category contains agents generated within the platelet that interact with the membrane receptors, eg, ADP, prostaglandins D_2 and E_2, and serotonin. The third contains agents generated with the platelet that act within the platelet, eg, prostaglandin endoperoxides and thromboxane A_2, the cyclic nucleotides cAMP and cGMP, and calcium ion. From this list of agents, 2 targets for platelet inhibitory drugs have been identified: inhibition of prostaglandin metabolism and augmentation of platelet cAMP content.

The prostaglandin **thromboxane A_2** is an arachidonate product that causes platelets to change shape, to release their granules, and to aggregate (Fig 32–6). Drugs that antagonize this pathway interfere with platelet aggregation in vitro and prolong the bleeding time. **Aspirin** is the prototype of this class of drugs. Drugs that modulate the intraplatelet concentration of cAMP do not prolong the bleeding time. Dietary therapy can be adjunctive in the prophylaxis of thrombosis. Ingestion of the unsaturated fatty acid **eicosapentaenoic acid**, which is high in the diets of Eskimos, generates prostaglandin I_3, an antiaggregating substance like prostacyclin.

Aspirin inhibits the synthesis of thromboxane A_2 by irreversible acetylation of the enzyme cyclooxygenase (Chapter 17). Because the anuclear platelet cannot synthesize new proteins, it cannot manufacture new enzyme during its 10-day lifetime. Other salicylates and other nonsteroidal anti-inflammatory drugs

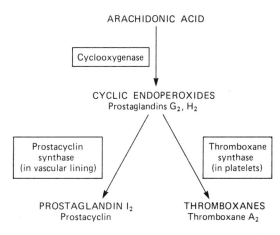

Figure 32–6. Arachidonic acid metabolism in humans. The enzyme cyclooxygenase results in formation of endoperoxides (prostaglandins G_2 and H_2), which are converted in platelets to thromboxane A_2 and in blood vessels to prostacyclin.

have a shorter duration of inhibitory action because they cannot acetylate cyclooxygenase.

Six prospective studies examined the efficacy of aspirin in the secondary prevention of myocardial infarction (see Bouchier-Hayes reference). When these trials were analyzed on the basis of "intention to treat" (all originally assigned patients must be evaluated), the results in favor of aspirin were not statistically significant. However, the previously recommended aspirin dose of 325 mg 3–4 times daily may be too large. This amount of aspirin inhibits production of **prostacyclin** (a potent inhibitor of platelet aggregation) in the vascular epithelium. With lower doses of aspirin, prostacyclin production from endothelial cells recovers more quickly than thromboxane A_2 production from platelets. Thus, low-dose aspirin (less than 350 mg daily) tips the prostaglandin balance in favor of the antithrombotic effect of the drug.

DAZOXIBEN

Dazoxiben, an analog of imidazole, selectively inhibits thromboxane synthase and thereby the formation of the platelet aggregation-facilitating thromboxane A_2. In a recent study, marked inhibition of thromboxane A_2 synthesis by dazoxiben did not prevent arachidonate-induced aggregation unless low-dose aspirin was added to the regimen. The concomitant aspirin reduced the "runoff" of proaggregatory cyclooxygenase products accumulated during blockage of thromboxane A_2 synthesis. Dazoxiben is undergoing clinical study.

SULFINPYRAZONE

The uricosuric drug sulfinpyrazone inhibits cyclooxygenase and reduces platelet consumption but does not prolong the bleeding time. Initial positive reports for sulfinpyrazone in the secondary prophylaxis of myocardial infarction were subsequently criticized for statistical and methodologic reasons. The drug did not receive approval by the United States Food and Drug Administration as an antithrombotic. Dosage is the same as in the treatment of gout (Chapter 34).

BETA-ADRENOCEPTOR–BLOCKING DRUGS

Many clinical trials have been performed with beta-blocking drugs for secondary prophylaxis of myocardial infarction. The Norwegian Multicenter Study of **timolol** was methodologically and statistically sound. Use of timolol resulted in a highly significant reduction of total numbers of deaths and was approved by the FDA for use as a prophylactic agent for myocardial infarction (see Norwegian Multicenter Study reference). It is not certain whether these positive results reflect a direct effect on coagulation, however.

PROSTACYCLIN (Epoprostenol)

Prostacyclin (PGI_2, epoprostenol) has potent platelet inhibitory effects. Its short duration of action (minutes) and vasodepressor action have stimulated a search for nontoxic analogs with more prolonged action. Epoprostenol has been used extensively in hemodialysis and cardiopulmonary bypass machines and is discussed in more detail in Chapter 17.

THIENPYRIDINES

Ticlopidine is a thienpyridine that alters the platelet membrane directly, independently of any inhibition of prostaglandin metabolism. It inhibits platelet aggregation, decreases platelet secretion, decreases platelet and fibrin deposition on artificial surfaces, and prolongs the bleeding time. Ticlopidine has been introduced in Europe but has yet to undergo clinical trial in the USA. It may prove useful in extracorporeal circulation.

DIPYRIDAMOLE

Dipyridamole inhibits platelet adhesion to thrombogenic surfaces but inhibits platelet aggregation in vitro only in high doses. It increases intraplatelet cAMP by inhibiting phosphodiesterase activity. It is effective clinically only when combined with warfarin or aspirin. The usual dose is 400 mg/d.

IV. CLINICAL PHARMACOLOGY OF DRUGS USED TO TREAT THROMBOSIS

The history of pharmacologic treatment of thromboembolism is one of broken promises resulting from the abuse of antithrombotic drugs. Drugs have been used and discarded before being properly evaluated, eg, oral anticoagulants in management of myocardial infarction and hip surgery. Use of prophylactic low-dose heparin during general surgery was undermined by overuse almost as soon as its efficacy had been rigorously established. The antiplatelet drugs are now being widely used despite lack of proof of their efficacy. Their clinical use should not be based on ease of administration, simplicity of monitoring, or infrequency of complications.

VENOUS THROMBOSIS

Antithrombotic Management
A. Prevention: Prevention of venous thrombosis reduces the incidence of and mortality rate from pulmonary emboli. Heparin or dextran is used to prevent venous thrombosis. Platelets have a lesser role in venous than in arterial disease; antiplatelet drugs are not consistently effective in prevention of venous disease. Intermittent administration of low-dose heparin subcutaneously provides effective prophylaxis. Oral anticoagulants are also effective, but the risk of bleeding and the necessity for laboratory monitoring of the prothrombin time limit their use for prophylaxis except in patients with prosthetic heart valves. Early ambulation postoperatively reduces venous stasis. Intermittent external pneumatic compression of the legs also is an effective form of postoperative prophylaxis.

B. Treatment of Established Disease: Established venous thrombosis is treated with maximal dosages of heparin and warfarin. Heparin is used for the first 7–10 days, with a 3–5 day overlap with warfarin. Therapy with warfarin is continued after hospital discharge for 6 weeks (first episode) to 6 months (recurrent episodes). Pulmonary embolism is treated the same way. Small thrombi confined to the calf veins are often managed without anticoagulants. The risk, expense, and inconvenience of unnecessary anticoagulant treatment far exceed those of venography, the definitive diagnostic test. Only a third of patients suspected of having deep venous thrombosis actually have the disease.

Fibrinolytic Therapy
Early treatment with streptokinase or urokinase of a less than massive pulmonary embolus may improve survival and may preserve long-term pulmonary function. The standard course of fibrinolytic therapy should be followed by anticoagulant therapy with hep-

arin and warfarin. Concomitant invasive procedures must be avoided, since bleeding may occur. Therapy is contraindicated after recent surgery or in patients with metastatic cancer, stroke, or underlying hemorrhagic disorders.

Pregnancy

Warfarin readily crosses the placenta. It can cause hemorrhage at any time during pregnancy, as well as developmental defects when administered during the first trimester. Therefore, venous thromboembolic disease in pregnant women should be treated with heparin, best administered by subcutaneous injection. Laboratory monitoring of the anticoagulant effect during pregnancy is mandatory.

ARTERIAL THROMBOSIS

In patients with arterial thrombi, consumption of platelets is excessive. Thus, treatment with platelet-inhibiting drugs (aspirin, dipyridamole, sulfinpyrazone) is indicated. Intracoronary thrombolytic agents are undergoing clinical trials.

DRUGS USED IN BLEEDING DISORDERS

VITAMIN K

Vitamin K confers biologic activity upon prothrombin and factors VII, IX, and X by participating in their postribosomal modification. Severe hepatic failure results in loss of protein synthesis and a hemorrhagic diathesis that is unresponsive to vitamin K.

Vitamin K is a fat-soluble substance found primarily in leafy green vegetables. The dietary requirement is low, because the vitamin is additionally synthesized by bacteria that colonize the human intestine. Two natural forms, vitamins K_1 and K_2, exist. Vitamin K_1 (Fig 32–4) is found in food and is called phytonadione. Vitamin K_2 is found in human tissues, is synthesized by intestinal bacteria, and is called menaquinone.

Vitamins K_1 and K_2 require bile salts for absorption from the intestinal tract. Vitamin K_1 is available clinically in 5-mg tablets and 50-mg ampules. The effect is delayed for 6 hours but is complete by 24 hours when the prothrombin activity is depressed by warfarin excess or vitamin K deficiency. Intravenous administration of vitamin K_1 should be slow, because rapid infusion can produce dyspnea, chest and back pain, and even death. Vitamin K_1 is currently administered to all newborns to prevent the hemorrhagic disease of vitamin K deficiency, which is especially common in pre-

mature infants. Vitamin K deficiency frequently occurs in hospitalized patients because of poor diet, parenteral nutrition, recent surgery, multiple antibiotic therapy, and uremia. The response to vitamin K is prompt and complete.

PLASMA FRACTIONS

Deficiencies in plasma coagulation factors can cause bleeding. Spontaneous bleeding occurs when factor activity is less than 5% of normal. Factor VIII deficiency (classic hemophilia or hemophilia A) and factor IX deficiency (Christmas disease or hemophilia B) account for 95% of the heritable coagulation defects. Concentrated plasma fractions are available for the treatment of these deficiencies. However, the specter of viral hepatitis and of acquired immunodeficiency syndrome (AIDS) is tempering the use of these concentrates in patients with hemophilia. The best use of these therapeutic materials requires diagnostic specificity of the deficient factor and quantitation of its activity in plasma. There are many uncommon inherited and acquired disorders of platelet function.

FACTOR VIII

There are 2 preparations of concentrated human factor VIII. **Cryoprecipitate** is a plasma protein fraction and is obtainable from whole blood. It is used to treat deficiencies of factor VIII in patients with hemophilia and von Willebrand's disease and occasionally to provide fibrinogen. For infusion, the frozen cryoprecipitate unit is thawed and dissolved in a small volume of sterile citrate-saline solution and pooled with other units. Rh-negative women with potential for childbearing should receive only Rh-negative cryoprecipitate because of possible contamination of the product with Rh-positive blood cells. **Lyophilized factor VIII concentrates** are prepared from large pools of plasma. In hemophiliacs with high replacement requirements, concentrates prepared from many donors should be avoided because of the potential exposure to hepatitis and AIDS. Cryoprecipitate prepared from individual donors is probably safer. Treatment of factor VIII concentrates with ultraviolet irradiation may reduce the danger of transmission of AIDS. Commercial freeze-dried concentrates may not suffice for treatment of patients with von Willebrand's disease, because the polymeric structure of factor VIII in the von Willebrand protein that supports platelet adhesion may be lost in the manufacturing process.

An uncomplicated hemorrhage into a joint should be treated with sufficient factor VIII replacement to maintain a level of at least 5% of the normal concentration for 24 hours (Table 32–3). Soft tissue hematomas require a minimum of 10% activity for 7 days. Hematuria requires at least 10% activity for 3 days. Surgery

Table 32–3. Therapeutic products for the treatment of coagulation disorders.*

Factor	Deficiency State	Concentration (Percent) Relative to Normal Plasma Required for Hemostasis†	Half-Life (Days) of Infused Factor	Therapeutic Material
I	Afibrinogenemia, defibrination syndrome.	20	4	Plasma fibrinogen, cryoprecipitate.
II	Prothrombin deficiency.	40	3	Concentrate (factor IX–prothrombin complex).
V	Factor V deficiency.	20	1	Fresh-frozen plasma.
VII	Factor VII deficiency.	Unknown	¼	Concentrate (some preparations of factor IX).
VIII	Hemophilia A (classic).	25	½	Plasma, cryoprecipitate, and other factor VIII concentrates.‡
	von Willebrand's disease.	30	Unknown	
IX	Hemophilia B (Christmas disease).	25	1	Plasma, cryosupernatant, factor IX–prothrombin complex.
X	Stuart-Prower defect.	25	2½	Plasma, concentrate (some preparations of factor IX).
XI	PTA deficiency.	Unknown	3	Fresh-frozen plasma.
XII	Hageman defect.	Not required	Unknown	Treatment not needed.
XIII	Fibrin-stabilizing factor deficiency.	2	6	Fresh-frozen plasma.

*Reproduced, with permission, from Biggs R (editor): *Human Blood Coagulation, Haemostasis, and Thrombosis,* 2nd ed. Blackwell, 1976.
†The immediate postinfusion level may need to be much higher and varied according to the degree of trauma.
‡Highly purified preparations of factor VIII should not be used in the treatment of von Willebrand's disease without specific evidence of their efficacy.

and major trauma require a minimum of 30% activity for 10 days after an initial loading dose of 50 units/kg of body weight to achieve 100% activity of factor VIII. Each unit per kilogram of factor VIII raises its activity in plasma 2%. Replacement should be administered every 12 hours.

Arginine vasopressin (desmopressin acetate, DDAVP) increases the factor VIII activity of patients with mild hemophilia A or von Willebrand's disease. It can be used in preparation for minor surgery such as tooth extraction without any requirement for infusion of clotting factor replacement. **Danazol,** an attenuated androgen that also elevates factor VIII activity, has been used experimentally with success in mild hemophiliacs.

Factor VIII concentrates and cryoprecipitate must not be used to treat deficiencies of vitamin K-dependent factors.

FACTOR IX

Freeze-dried concentrates of plasma containing prothrombin, factors IX and X, and varied amounts factor VII (Proplex and Konyne) are commercially available for treating deficiencies of these factors (Table 32–3). Heparin is often added to inhibit coagulation factors activated by the manufacturing process. Each unit per kilogram of factor IX raises its activity in plasma 1.5%.

Some preparations of factor IX concentrate contain *activated* clotting factors, which has led to their use in treating patients with inhibitors or antibodies to factor VIII or IX. Two new products are available expressly for this purpose: **Autoplex** (with factor VIII correctional activity) and **Feiba** (with factor VIII inhibitor bypassing activity). These products are not uniformly successful in arresting hemorrhage, and the inhibitor titers often rise after treatment with them.

FIBRINOGEN

Fibrinogen may be administered to patients as plasma, cryoprecipitate of factor VIII, or lyophilized concentrates of factor VIII. A single unit of cryoprecipitate contains 300 mg of fibrinogen. Lyophilized concentrates of factor VIII are rich in fibrinogen.

FIBRINOLYTIC INHIBITORS

AMINOCAPROIC ACID

Aminocaproic acid (Amicar, EACA), which is chemically similar to the amino acid lysine, is a synthetic inhibitor of fibrinolysis. It competitively inhibits plasminogen activation (Fig 32–3). It is rapidly absorbed orally and is cleared from the body by the kidney. The usual oral dose of EACA is 6 g 4 times a day. When the drug is administered intravenously, a 5-g loading dose should be infused over 30 minutes to avoid hypotension.

Clinical uses of aminocaproic acid are as adjunctive therapy in hemophilia, as therapy for bleeding from fibrinolytic therapy, and as prophylaxis for rebleeding from intracranial aneurysms. Treatment success has also been reported in patients with postsurgical gastrointestinal bleeding and postprostatectomy bleeding. Side effects of the drug include intravascular thrombosis from inhibition of plasminogen activator, hypotension, myopathy, abdominal discomfort, diarrhea, and nasal stuffiness.

TRANEXAMIC ACID

Tranexamic acid (Amstat) is an analog of aminocaproic acid and an inhibitor of plasminogen activator. It is more potent than EACA, and therefore a lower dosage is needed, which may account for its decreased side effects. It is administered orally with a loading dose of 15 mg/kg and then 30 mg/kg every 6 hours. The indications for tranexamic acid are the same as those for aminocaproic acid.

REFERENCES

Bouchier-Hayes D: Drugs in the treatment of thrombo-embolic disease. (2 parts.) *Ir Med J* 1983;**76**:101, 155.

Buchanan MR et al: Relative importance of thrombin inhibition and factor Xa inhibition of the antithrombotic effects of heparin. *Blood* 1985;**65**:198.

Cowley AJ et al: Effects of dazoxiben, an inhibitor of thromboxane synthetase, on cold-induced forearm vasoconstriction and platelet behavior in different individuals. *Br J Clin Pharmacol* 1985;**19**:1.

Di Minno G et al: Functionally thrombasthenic state in normal platelets following the administration of ticlopidine. *J Clin Invest* 1985;**75**:328.

Eichner ER: Platelets, carotids, and coronaries: Critique on antithrombotic role of antiplatelet agents, exercise, and certain diets. *Am J Med* 1984;**77**:513.

Fareed J: Heparin, its fractions, fragments and derivatives: Some newer aspects. *Semin Thromb Hemost* 1985;**11**:1.

Goldberg RJ et al: Long-term anticoagulant therapy after acute myocardial infarction. *Am Heart J* 1985;**109**:616.

Green D et al: Thrombocytopenia in a prospective, randomized, double-blind trial of bovine and porcine heparin. *Am J Med Sci* 1984;**288**:60.

Gresele P et al: Combining antiplatelet agents: Potentiation between aspirin and dipyridamole. (Correspondence.) *Lancet* 1985;**1**:937.

Hampton JR: Platelets and coronary disease, round three. (Editorial.) *Br Med J* 1985;**290**:414.

Harris WH et al: Prophylaxis of deep-vein thrombosis after total hip replacement: Dextran and external pneumatic compression compared with 1.2 or 0.3 gram of aspirin daily. *J Bone Joint Surg [Am]* 1985;**67**:57.

Hirsh J: Progress review: The relationship between dose of aspirin, side-effects and antithrombotic effectiveness. *Stroke* 1985;**16**:1.

Horrow JC: Protamine: A review of its toxicity. *Anesth Analg* 1985;**64**:348.

Loeliger EA, Van den Besselaar AMHP, Lewis SM: Reliability and clinical impact of the normalization of the prothrombin times in oral anticoagulant control. *Thromb Haemost* 1985;**53**:145.

Mann KG: Biochemistry of coagulation. *Clin Lab Med* 1984;**4**:207.

McCarthy NJ: Factor VIII, factor IX: Prothrombinex. (Correspondence.) *Med J Aust* 1985;**142**:74.

McLeod BC, Scott JP: Use of 'single donor' factor VIII from plasma exchange donation. *JAMA* 1984;**252**:2726.

Motohara K et al: Severe vitamin K deficiency in breast-fed infants. *J Pediatr* 1984;**105**:943.

Multicenter Trial Committee: Dihydroergotamine-heparin prophylaxis of postoperative deep vein thrombosis: A multicenter trial. *JAMA* 1984;**251**:2960.

Norwegian Multicenter Study Group: Timolol-induced reduction in mortality and reinfarction in patients surviving acute myocardial infarction. *N Engl J Med* 1981;**304**:801.

Olson RE: Function and metabolism of vitamin K. *Annu Rev Nutr* 1984;**4**:281.

O'Reilly RA: Complications of anticoagulant therapy. (Editorial.) *West J Med* 1980;**132**:453.

O'Reilly RA: Stereoselective interaction of sulfinpyrazone with racemic warfarin and its separated enantiomorphs in man. *Circulation* 1982;**65**:202.

Rosenberg RD: Role of heparin and heparinlike molecules in thrombosis and atherosclerosis. *Fed Proc* 1985;**44**:404.

Sage JI: Stroke: The use and overuse of heparin in therapeutic trials. (Editorial.) *Arch Neurol* 1985;**42**:315.

Schulman S, Lockner D: Relationship between thromboembolic complications and intensity of treatment during long-term prophylaxis with oral anticoagulants following DVT. *Thromb Haemost* 1985;**53**:137.

Shenkenberg TD, Mackowiak PA, Smith JW: Coagulopathy and hemorrhage associated with cefoperazone therapy in a patient with renal failure. *South Med J* 1985;**78**:488.

TIMI Study Group: Thrombolysis in myocardial infarction (TIMI) trial. (Special report.) *N Engl J Med* 1985;**312**:932.

Vermeulen M et al: Antifibrinolytic treatment in subarachnoid hemorrhage. *N Engl J Med* 1984;**311**:432.

Wessler S, Gitel SN: Warfarin: From bedside to bench. *N Engl J Med* 1984;**311**:645.

33

Agents Used In Hyperlipidemia

Mary J. Malloy, MD, & John P. Kane, MD, PhD

Virtually all of the lipids of human plasma are transported as complexes with proteins. With the exception of fatty acids, which are bound chiefly to albumin, the lipids are carried in special macromolecular complexes termed **lipoproteins.** A number of metabolic disorders that involve elevations in plasma lipoprotein concentrations are thus termed **hyperlipoproteinemias.** The term **hyperlipemia** is restricted to those conditions in which levels of triglycerides in plasma are increased.

The 2 major clinical sequelae of the hyperlipoproteinemias are acute pancreatitis and atherosclerosis. Acute pancreatitis occurs in patients with marked hyperlipemia. In such persons, control of triglyceride levels can prevent recurrent attacks of this life-threatening disease.

Atherosclerosis is the leading cause of death in the USA and other Western countries. Certain plasma lipoproteins are linked to accelerated atherogenesis. The lipoproteins that contain apolipoprotein (apoprotein, apo) B-100 have been identified as the vehicles in which cholesterol is transported into the artery wall. These atherogenic lipoproteins are the low-density **(LDL),** intermediate-density **(IDL),** and very low density **(VLDL)** species. Cholesteryl esters, which are found in the atheroma in cells of smooth muscle origin and in macrophages, also appear in the extracellular matrix and induce collagen production by fibroblasts. Certain other factors also contribute to formation of the atheroma. These include hypertension, which is associated with greater flux of lipoprotein into the subintimal region; low levels of high-density lipoproteins **(HDL),** which appear to be involved in removal of cholesterol from the atheroma; and smoking.

Atherosclerotic disease of both coronary and peripheral arteries appears to be a dynamic process. Evidence from studies both in animals and in humans indicates that progression of atheroma formation can be slowed if elevated serum concentrations of the atherogenic lipoproteins can be reduced. Reversal of atheromas has been demonstrated in animals.

Many of the hyperlipidemic states are associated with the development of xanthomas. These lesions are produced by deposition of lipid in tendons or skin, may be painful or cosmetically unacceptable to the patient and are another reason for treating the associated hyperlipidemia.

An understanding of the biology of the lipoproteins

and the pathophysiology of the various hyperlipidemic states is essential to the rational choice of treatment regimen.

PATHOPHYSIOLOGY OF HYPERLIPOPROTEINEMIA

NORMAL LIPOPROTEIN METABOLISM

Structure

The major lipoproteins of plasma are spherical particles with hydrophobic core regions containing cholesteryl esters and triglycerides. A monolayer of amphiphilic lipids, chiefly unesterified cholesterol and phospholipids, surrounds the core. Specific proteins (apolipoproteins) that bind noncovalently to the lipids are located on the surface. Certain lipoproteins contain very high molecular weight B apoproteins that do not migrate from one particle to another, as do smaller apolipoproteins. There are 2 primary B apoproteins: B-48, found in chylomicrons and their remnants, is formed in the intestine; B-100, found in VLDL, VLDL remnants, and LDL (which are formed from VLDL), arises in the liver.

Smaller apoproteins distribute variably among the lipoproteins. Apo A-I is a cofactor for lecithin:cholesterol acyltransferase (LCAT). Apo C-II is a required cofactor for lipoprotein lipase. Apo D catalyzes the transfer of cholesteryl ester from the HDL subspecies containing LCAT to other lipoproteins. Several isoforms of apo E, based on single amino acid substitutions, are recognized. A normal pattern of these isoforms is required for uptake of lipoprotein remnants by the liver.

The apoprotein contents of various lipoprotein complexes are set forth in Table 33–1.

Synthesis & Catabolism

A. Chylomicrons: Chylomicrons, the largest of the lipoproteins, are formed in the intestine and carry triglycerides of dietary origin (Fig 33–1). Some cholesterol esterified by the acyl-CoA:cholesterol acyltransferase (ACAT) system also appears in the chylomicron core. Phospholipids and free cholesterol, together with newly synthesized apo B-48, A-I, A-II,

Table 33–1. Major lipoproteins of human serum.

	Electrophoretic Mobility in Agarose Gel	Density Interval (g/cm³)	Core Lipids	Diameter (nm)	Apolipoproteins in Order of Quantitative Importance
High-density (HDL)	Alpha	1.063–1.21	Cholesteryl esters	7.5–10.5	A-I, A-II, C, E, D
Low-density (LDL)	Beta	1.019–1.063	Cholesteryl esters	~ 21.5	B-100
Intermediate-density (IDL)	Beta	1.006–1.019	Cholesteryl esters, triglycerides	25–30	B-100, E, C
Very low density (VLDL)	Prebeta, some "slow prebeta"	< 1.006	Triglycerides, some cholesteryl esters	30–100	C species, B-100, E
Chylomicrons	Remain at origin	< 1.006	Triglycerides, some cholesteryl esters	80–500	B-48, C, E, A-I, A-II

and other proteins, form the surface monolayer. The nascent chylomicron enters the extracellular lymph space and travels via the intestinal lymphatics and thoracic duct to the bloodstream.

Triglycerides are removed in extrahepatic tissues through a common pathway with VLDL that involves hydrolysis by the lipoprotein lipase (LPL) system. Heparin and apo C-II are cofactors for this reaction. A progressive decrease in particle diameter occurs as triglycerides in the core are depleted. Surface lipids, apo A-I, apo A-II, and apo C are returned to HDL. The resultant chylomicron "remnants" are taken up by receptor-mediated endocytosis into hepatic parenchymal cells. The cholesteryl esters are hydrolyzed in lysosomes, and cholesterol is then excreted in bile, oxidized and excreted as bile acids, or secreted into plasma in lipoproteins.

B. Very Low Density Lipoproteins (VLDL): VLDL are secreted by liver and are the principal carriers of triglycerides synthesized in liver. VLDL contain apo B-100 but none of the major apoproteins of HDL (Fig 33–2). Some apo C is secreted with the VLDL, and more is acquired from HDL in plasma. Hydrolysis by lipoprotein lipase yields remnant particles that are smaller (25–30 nm in diameter) than those of the chylomicrons (80 nm). Catabolism of a portion of the VLDL remnants results in the formation of LDL, which contain mostly cholesteryl esters in the core regions. The formation of LDL from VLDL explains the clinical phenomenon of the "beta shift," the increase of LDL (β-lipoprotein) in serum as a hypertriglyceridemic state subsides, as in resolving lipemia of diabetes or during treatment with clofibrate. Increased levels of LDL in plasma can thus result from increased

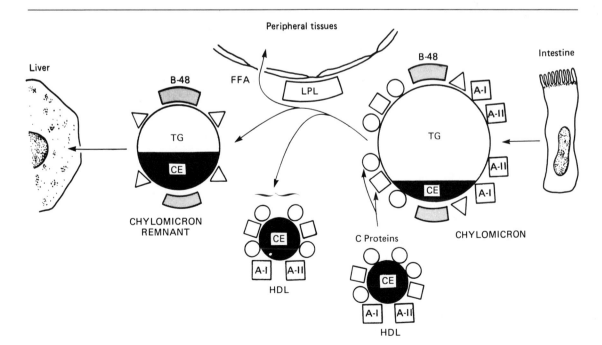

Figure 33–1. Metabolism of chylomicrons. TG = triglyceride; CE = cholesteryl ester.

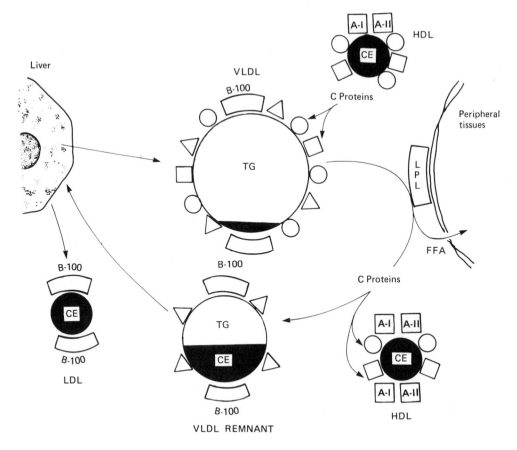

Figure 33–2. Metabolism of very low density lipoproteins. TG = triglyceride; CE = cholesteryl ester.

secretion of its precursor VLDL as well as from decreased LDL catabolism.

C. Low-Density Lipoproteins (LDL): A major pathway by which LDL are catabolized involves high-affinity receptor-mediated adsorptive endocytosis. The apo B binds to the receptor, and an endocytotic vesicle is formed that fuses with a lysosome, and apo B is degraded. Cholesteryl esters from the LDL core are hydrolyzed, and the free cholesterol, some of which is used in synthesis of cell membrane, suppresses the de novo formation of cholesterol and leads to down regulation of the LDL receptors. Excess cholesterol is stored, chiefly as cholesteryl oleate.

D. High-Density Lipoproteins (HDL): HDL are secreted from liver in a nascent bilayer disk form. They are also formed during catabolism of chylomicrons as surface lipids, and apo A-I and apo A-II dissociate from the chylomicron. Phospholipids and cholesterol released from VLDL hydrolysis also contribute to the formation of HDL. In addition to serving as carriers for the various small apoproteins and delivering cholesterol to the adrenal in support of steroidogenesis, HDL play a major role in the transport of surplus cholesterol away from peripheral tissues. Free cholesterol is transferred to a subspecies of HDL with relatively small molecular weight. "Reverse cholesterol transport" is carried further by another subspecies of

HDL, the esterification-transfer particle that contains LCAT. LCAT catalyzes the formation of cholesteryl esters, which are then transferred with the aid of a transfer protein to LDL and triglyceride-rich lipoproteins. Remnants of the latter normally serve to carry the cholesterol to liver. The ways in which HDL are catabolized are not known, but it appears that peripheral tissues are significantly involved, along with the liver.

THE HYPERLIPOPROTEINEMIC STATES

Diagnosis of hyperlipidemia involves a determination that the content of lipids in serum is increased after an overnight fast (cholesterol and triglyceride levels exceeding age- and sex-specific 95th percentile of normal values); differentiation requires identification of the species of lipoproteins that account for the observed increases (Table 33–2). Diagnosis of a specific primary lipoprotein disorder usually necessitates gathering further clinical and genetic data as well as ruling out disorders that can cause secondary hyperlipidemia

Table 33–2. Drug treatment of hyperlipoproteinemia.

	Single Drug*	Drug Combination
Familial hypertriglyceridemia		
Severe	Nicotinic acid.	
Mild	Clofibrate, gemfibrozil, nicotinic acid.	
Familial lipoprotein lipase or cofactor deficiency	(Dietary management.)	
Familial dysbetalipoproteinemia	Clofibrate, gemfibrozil, nicotinic acid.	
Sporadic or unclassified hypertriglyceridemia	Clofibrate, gemfibrozil, nicotinic acid.	
Familial multiple type hyperlipoproteinemia		
VLDL increased	Nicotinic acid.	
LDL increased	Resin, nicotinic acid.	Resin plus nicotinic acid.
VLDL and LDL increased	Nicotinic acid.	Resin plus nicotinic acid.
Familial hypercholesterolemia		
Heterozygous	Resin.	Resin plus nicotinic acid. Neomycin plus nicotinic acid.
Homozygous		Resin plus nicotinic acid.
Polygenic or unclassified hypercholesterolemia	Resin, nicotinic acid, clofibrate, gemfibrozil.	

*Where 2 drugs are listed, the first is the preferred drug. Single-drug therapy should be evaluated before drug combinations are used, except in the case of homozygous familial hypercholesterolemia, where single-drug therapy is known to be ineffective.

Table 33–3. Secondary causes of hyperlipoproteinemia.

Hypertriglyceridemia	Hypercholesterolemia
Diabetes mellitus	Hypothyroidism
Alcohol ingestion	Early nephrosis
Severe nephrosis	Resolving lipemia
Estrogens	Immunoglobulin-lipoprotein complex disorders
Uremia	Anorexia nervosa
Corticosteroid excess	Cholestasis
Hypothyroidism	Hypopituitarism
Glycogen storage disease	Corticosteroid excess
Hypopituitarism	
Acromegaly	
Immunoglobulin-lipoprotein complex disorders	

(Table 33–3). The various patterns of abnormal lipoprotein distribution are described below.

PRIMARY HYPERTRIGLYCERIDEMIA

Although epidemiologic studies have shown only a weak relationship between hypertriglyceridemia and coronary heart disease, atherosclerosis appears to be strongly linked to hypertriglyceridemia in certain kindreds. Therefore, patients in these families should receive drug treatment, whereas such treatment probably need not be given to other patients unless their levels of triglycerides exceed 600–700 mg/dL.

Primary Chylomicronemia

Chylomicrons are not normally present in serum of fasted individuals. The autosomal recessive traits of lipoprotein lipase deficiency and lipoprotein lipase cofactor deficiency are usually associated with severe lipemia (2000–25,000 mg/dL triglycerides), which may, however, go undiagnosed until an attack of acute pancreatitis occurs. Patients may have eruptive xanthomas, hepatosplenomegaly, hypersplenism, and lipid-laden foam cells in bone marrow, liver, and spleen. The lipemia is aggravated by estrogens, since they stimulate VLDL production in the liver, and pregnancy may cause marked increases in triglyceride levels in spite of strict dietary control. Although these patients have a predominant chylomicronemia, they may also have moderately elevated VLDL, presenting with a pattern of mixed lipemia. Lipoprotein lipase deficiency is diagnosed by in vitro assay of lipolytic activity in plasma after intravenous injection of heparin; cofactor deficiency is diagnosed by isoelectric focusing or electrophoresis of the VLDL proteins. A presumptive diagnosis of these disorders is justified by demonstrating a pronounced decrease in levels of plasma triglycerides a few days after sharp restriction of oral fat intake. Marked restriction of the total fat content in the diet provides effective long-term treatment. No drug treatment is indicated.

Mixed Lipemia

A pattern of mixed lipemia (fasting chylomicronemia and elevated VLDL) usually results from impaired removal of triglyceride-rich lipoproteins, although factors that increase VLDL production aggravate the lipemia because VLDL and chylomicrons are competing substrates for lipoprotein lipase. The primary mixed lipemias probably represent a variety of modes of inheritance. Most patients have the hypertrophic form of obesity with impaired effectiveness of insulin. In addition to obesity, other factors that lead to increased rate of secretion of VLDL also aggravate the lipemia. Eruptive xanthomas, lipemia retinalis, epigastric pain, and overt pancreatitis are variably present, depending on the severity of the lipemia. Treatment is primarily dietary, with restriction of total fat, avoidance of alcohol, and weight reduction to ideal levels. Some patients may require treatment with clofibrate, gemfibrozil, or nicotinic acid.

Endogenous Lipemia

Primary increases of VLDL levels probably reflect a number of genetic determinants and are worsened by factors that increase the rate of VLDL secretion from liver, ie, hypertrophic obesity, alcohol ingestion, diabetes, and exogenous estrogens. A major indication for treatment of these patients is the presence of arteriosclerosis. Treatment includes weight reduction to ideal levels, restriction of all types of dietary fat, and avoidance of alcohol. Clofibrate, gemfibrozil, or nicotinic acid usually produces further reduction in triglyceride levels if dietary measures do not reduce them below 600–700 mg/dL.

Multiple Type Hyperlipoproteinemia (Combined Hyperlipidemia)

In kindreds with this disorder, individuals may have elevated levels of VLDL, LDL, or both, and the patterns may change with time. The basic defect is increased production of apo B in VLDL, and factors that increase levels of triglyceride in serum in other disorders do so in this one as well. Elevations of serum cholesterol and triglycerides are usually moderate, and xanthomas do not occur. However, drug treatment is warranted because the risk of coronary atherosclerosis is increased, and diet alone usually does not normalize lipid levels. Patients with elevated VLDL respond to nicotinic acid; those with elevated LDL respond to bile acid resins but often have secondary elevations in VLDL, requiring the addition of nicotinic acid.

Disorders in Which Remnant Particles Accumulate

In familial dysbetalipoproteinemia, normal VLDL of prebeta electrophoretic mobility are present. There are also VLDL with beta mobility and remnant particles of intermediate density (IDL). Levels of LDL are usually decreased. There is a defect in the removal of VLDL and chylomicron remnants from plasma. Because these remnants are rich in cholesteryl esters, the level of serum cholesterol may be as high as that of triglycerides. Diagnosis is confirmed by the virtual absence of the E_3 and E_4 isoforms of apo E detected on isoelectric focusing of the apolipoproteins of VLDL. Patients often develop tuberous or tuberoeruptive xanthomas or characteristic planar xanthomas of the palmar creases. The patients are often obese, and some have impaired glucose tolerance. These factors, together with hypothyroidism, aggravate the lipemia. Coronary and peripheral vascular atherosclerotic disease occurs with increased frequency. A weight reduction diet, together with decreased cholesterol and alcohol ingestion, often is sufficient treatment. Clofibrate, gemfibrozil, or nicotinic acid is needed in some cases. Frequently, low doses are sufficient.

PRIMARY HYPERCHOLESTEROLEMIA

Familial Hypercholesterolemia

This disorder is transmitted as an autosomal dominant trait and, although levels of LDL tend to increase throughout childhood, the diagnosis can often be made at birth on the basis of elevated umbilical cord blood cholesterol level and a family history of affected first-degree relatives. In heterozygous adults, serum cholesterol levels range from about 325 to 500 mg/dL. Triglycerides are usually normal, tendinous xanthomatosis is often present, and arcus corneae and xanthelasma may appear in the third decade. Coronary atherosclerosis tends to occur prematurely, particularly in those who also have HDL deficiencies. Homozygous familial hypercholesterolemia, which can lead to coronary disease in childhood, is characterized by very high levels of cholesterol in serum (often exceeding 1000 mg/dL) and early tuberous and tendinous xanthomatosis. These patients may also develop elevated plaquelike xanthomas of the digital webs, buttocks, and extremities.

The underlying mechanism is genetic deficiency or defects of high-affinity receptors for LDL. Homozygotes have no normal receptors; heterozygotes have about half the usual number; and some individuals apparently have combined heterozygosity.

Treatment of the homozygote is very difficult. Repeated plasmapheresis in conjunction with combined drug therapy is currently the most effective method of management. Levels of LDL in compliant heterozygotes can be normalized with combined drug regimens.

Multiple Type Hyperlipoproteinemia

As described above, some persons in kindreds with this disorder have only an elevation in LDL. Xanthomas are absent, and levels of serum cholesterol usually are less than 350 mg/dL. Premature onset of coronary disease is common. Dietary and drug treatment, usually with a bile acid-binding resin, is indicated. It is frequently necessary to add nicotinic acid to normalize LDL levels or to lower triglycerides which often rise during treatment with the resin.

Other Types of Hypercholesterolemias

Other poorly defined types of hypercholesterolemia occur that are often familial, and usually milder than the disorders described above. At least one of these appears to be polygenic. Individuals in some kindreds who have elevated LDL concentrations have strikingly favorable responses to dietary management.

Some persons have very high levels of Lp(a) lipoprotein, normally only a minor fraction of circulating lipoproteins, which distributes about the ultracentrifugal density that discriminates HDL from LDL. It contains apo B-100 and appears to be atherogenic. The regimen combining resin and nicotinic acid may be useful for these patients.

DEFICIENCY OF HDL

Certain rare genetic disorders are associated with extremely low levels of HDL in serum. More commonly, moderate decreases of HDL levels occur in familial distribution. These patients tend to have premature coronary atherosclerosis and the low HDL levels may be the only identified risk factor. Treatment currently consists only of special attention to avoidance of other risk factors for coronary disease. Nicotinic acid increases HDL cholesterol levels, at least in hyperlipidemic subjects, and may prove to be useful in management of familial hypoalphalipoproteinemia. However, there is no established rationale for such intervention, because there is as yet no evidence that it would modify the risk of vascular disease.

SECONDARY HYPERLIPOPROTEINEMIA

Before the diagnosis of primary hyperlipoproteinemia can be made, secondary causes of the specific phenotype must be considered. The more common conditions that may be associated with hyperlipoproteinemia are summarized in Table 33–3. The lipoprotein abnormality usually resolves with treatment of the underlying disorder.

Certain persons, often with a preexisting mild lipemia, develop severe hypertriglyceridemia when given even small doses of estrogens, such as those in contraceptives. This effect is smaller when the estrogen is used in very low dosage relative to the progestational agent.

Treatment of the hyperlipidemia associated with chronic nephrotic syndrome is probably indicated, since coronary vascular disease is prevalent in these patients. Diet has little effect. Clofibrate and possibly gemfibrozil are contraindicated, because they may precipitate myopathy. Currently, the drugs of choice are bile acid-binding resins combined with nicotinic acid. Tryptophan supplementation ameliorates hypertriglyceridemia in some nephrotic patients who may be deficient in this amino acid.

The hyperlipidemia associated with cholestasis involves abnormal lipoproteins, including LP-X, vesicular particles rich in unesterified cholesterol and phospholipid; LP-Y, which contain large amounts of triglycerides and carry apo B; and LDL containing unusually large amounts of triglycerides. Neuropathy, caused by xanthomatous involvement of nerves, is an indication for treatment of this hyperlipidemia. Although plasmapheresis is most effective, bile acid-binding resins may be of some value. Clofibrate and gemfibrozil are contraindicated, since they can cause an increase in serum cholesterol in these patients.

DIETARY MANAGEMENT OF HYPERLIPOPROTEINEMIA

When the decision is made to treat hyperlipoproteinemia, dietary measures are always initiated first and may obviate the need for drugs. Cholesterol and saturated fats are the principal dietary factors that influence lipoprotein levels in plasma. Dietary cholesterol and saturated fats increase the concentration of LDL independently.

Lipoprotein levels are also affected, but to a lesser extent, by other dietary factors. Transient increases in VLDL occur when carbohydrate intake is acutely increased. Sucrose and other simple sugars may raise VLDL levels in an occasional hypertriglyceridemic patient. Pectin is probably the only form of dietary fiber that reduces LDL levels appreciably. Alcohol can cause significant hypertriglyceridemia by increasing hepatic secretion of VLDL. Synthesis and secretion of VLDL are increased by excess caloric intake. Caloric restriction, especially in obese subjects, reduces VLDL triglycerides and also reduces levels of LDL, particularly in persons with combined hyperlipidemia.

Most patients with hyperlipidemia can be managed appropriately with a diet that is restricted in cholesterol and saturated fat and provides calories to achieve and maintain ideal body weight. Total fat calories should be 20–25%, with saturated fats less than 8% of total calories and cholesterol less than 200 mg/d. Reductions in serum cholesterol range from 20 to 30% on this regimen, except in primary hypercholesterolemias, where the response may be smaller. Increases in complex carbohydrates and fiber are recommended, but large increases in polyunsaturated fats should be avoided. Weight reduction and caloric restriction are especially important for patients with elevated VLDL and IDL. Patients with hypertriglyceridemia should avoid alcohol.

The effect of dietary fats in patients with hypertriglyceridemia is highly dependent upon the disposition of double bonds in the fatty acid carbon chain. Omega-3 (ω-3) fatty acids found in fish oils can induce profound lowering of triglycerides in many patients with endogenous or mixed lipemia. In contrast, the ω-6 fatty acids present in vegetable oils may cause levels of triglycerides to rise in these patients.

Patients with primary chylomicronemia and some individuals with mixed lipemia must consume a diet severely restricted in total fat: 10–15 g/d, of which 5 g should be vegetable oils rich in essential fatty acids. Supplementation of fat-soluble vitamins should be given.

SPECIFIC DRUGS USED IN TREATMENT

Decisions to use drug therapy for hyperlipidemia must be based on the specific physiologic defect and its potential for causing atherosclerosis or pancreatitis. Suggested drug treatments for the principal lipoprotein disorders are presented in Table 33–2. Diet is a necessary adjunct to drug therapy and should be continued for achievement of the full potential of the drug regimen. Drug treatment of hyperlipidemia should be avoided in women who are likely to become pregnant or who are lactating. Children with heterozygous familial hypercholesterolemia may be treated with a bile acid-binding resin, usually after age 7 or 8, when myelination of the central nervous system is essentially complete. Any drug therapy in children is, however, still experimental, and the decision to treat an individual child should be based on the level of plasma LDL, the family history, and the child's age.

NICOTINIC ACID

Nicotinic acid (but not nicotinamide) decreases VLDL and LDL levels in the plasma of patients with a variety of hyperlipidemias.

Chemistry & Pharmacokinetics

Nicotinic acid (niacin) is a water-soluble vitamin with the chemical structure shown below. It is converted in the body to the amide, which is incorporated into nicotinamide adenine dinucleotide (NAD). It is excreted unmodified in the urine and as nicotinamide, N-methyl-2-pyridone-3-carboxamide, N-methyl-2-pyridone-5-carboxamide, and other less abundant metabolites.

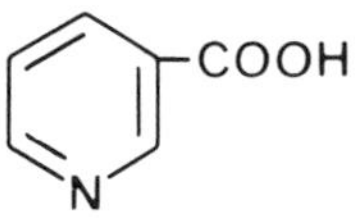

Nicotinic acid

Mechanism of Action

The primary mechanism of action of nicotinic acid probably involves inhibition of VLDL secretion, in turn decreasing production of LDL. Decreased incorporation of amino acids into apo VLDL has been demonstrated. Increased clearance of VLDL via the lipoprotein lipase pathway contributes to the triglyceride-lowering effect of nicotinic acid. The drug has no effect on bile acid production. Excretion of neutral sterols in the stool is increased acutely as cholesterol is mobilized from tissue pools. A new steady state is then reached during chronic administration of the drug. Cholesterogenesis is inhibited, an effect that persists when bile acid-binding resins are given. Decreased synthesis of cholesterol in liver can increase hepatic uptake of LDL in support of increased bile acid synthesis induced by the resin. The catabolic rate for HDL is decreased, with an associated increase in the HDL_2 subfraction and high levels of HDL cholesterol and apo A-1 in plasma. The processes of atherogenesis or thrombosis may be influenced by the substantial reduction of circulating fibrinogen levels produced by nicotinic acid. Increase in levels of tissue plasminogen activator occur and may also be important in preventing occlusive vascular disease. This agent is also a potent inhibitor of the intracellular lipase system of adipose tissue, possibly reducing VLDL production by decreasing the flux of free fatty acids to liver. Sustained inhibition of lipolysis has not been established, however.

Therapeutic Uses & Dosage

In combination with a bile acid-binding resin, nicotinic acid has been found to normalize levels of LDL in patients with heterozygous familial hypercholesterolemia. This drug combination is also indicated in some cases of nephrosis. In severe mixed lipemia that is incompletely responsive to dietary measures, nicotinic acid often produces marked reduction of triglyceride levels in plasma. It is also useful in patients with multiple type hyperlipoproteinemia and in those with familial dysbetalipoproteinemia. It can be used effectively alone or in combination with neomycin to treat hypercholesterolemia.

For combined drug treatment of heterozygous familial hypercholesterolemia, most patients require 6–7.5 g daily orally; more than this should not be given. For other types of hypercholesterolemia and for hypertriglyceridemia, 1.5–3.5 g daily orally is usually sufficient. The drug should be given in divided doses with meals, starting with 100 mg 3 times daily and increasing gradually.

Toxicity

Most persons experience a harmless cutaneous vasodilatation and an uncomfortable sensation of warmth after each dose when the drug is started or the dose is increased. Taking 0.3 g of aspirin about half an hour beforehand blunts this prostaglandin-mediated effect. Tachyphylaxis to this side effect usually occurs within a few days at any dose level. The physician should warn the patient to expect this annoying side effect and should explain why it occurs. Pruritus, rashes, dry skin, and acanthosis nigricans have been reported. Some patients experience nausea and abdominal discomfort. This drug should be avoided in patients with severe peptic disease. Moderate elevations in levels of transaminases or alkaline phosphatase may occur, usually not associated with serious liver toxicity. However, liver function should be monitored regularly. This effect is reversible and is minimized if the daily dose is increased by no more than 2.5 g in a month. Carbohydrate tolerance may be moderately impaired, but this is also reversible. In some patients with latent diabetes, however, this effect may be more evident and incompletely reversible. Nicotinic acid should be used with caution in such persons. Hyperuricemia occurs in about one-fifth of patients receiving nicotinic acid, but it probably becomes symptomatic only in those with preexisting gout. Rarely described conditions associated with the use of nicotinic acid include arrhythmias, mostly atrial, and toxic amblyopia.

CLOFIBRATE

Clofibrate (Atromid-S) decreases levels of VLDL in plasma. Levels of LDL are also decreased in some patients. LDL and HDL levels often increase in hypertriglyceridemic patients during treatment with clofibrate. In some patients with hypertriglyceridemia, there may be marked increases of LDL in plasma as levels of VLDL are reduced. Bile acid-binding resins may be added to control this effect, or nicotinic acid may be substituted for clofibrate.

Chemistry & Pharmacokinetics

Clofibrate is the ethyl ester of chlorphenoxyisobutyric acid. Upon absorption, the ester group is hydrolyzed, by tissue and plasma esterases, and the anion is transported, mostly bound to albumin, in plasma. Although mainly distributed to the extracellular space, some anion is found in tissues (eg, liver). The drug is excreted in urine as the glucuronide. In humans, its plasma half-life is about 12 hours.

Clofibrate

Mechanism of Action

The principal effect of clofibrate is to increase the clearance of triglyceride-rich lipoproteins via an increase in the activity of lipoprotein lipase. Secretion of VLDL from liver is unaffected in hypertriglyceridemic patients and actually appears to be increased in normotriglyceridemic subjects treated with clofibrate. This could explain the lack of significant synergism in most patients with heterozygous familial hypercholesterolemia treated with a combination of bile acid-binding resin and clofibrate. This combination, however, may have some use in persons with mild elevations of LDL. In hypercholesterolemic patients, body cholesterol pools are decreased as fecal and biliary cholesterol excretions are increased. Fecal excretion of bile acids is reduced. Absorption of cholesterol is unaffected. Cholesterol biosynthesis in liver is inhibited, perhaps as a result of changes in VLDL secretion and catabolism. Fatty acid oxidation by liver may be increased. The content of triglycerides in HDL is reduced by clofibrate, whereas total HDL concentration may be slightly increased. These effects appear to be related to the fall in VLDL concentration.

Therapeutic Uses & Dosage

Clofibrate usually produces marked reduction in serum triglycerides and triglyceride-rich lipoproteins in patients with familial dysbetalipoproteinemia. VLDL levels are also reduced in individuals with moderately severe endogenous hypertriglyceridemia. Because its primary effect appears to be stimulation of the lipoprotein lipase mechanism, clofibrate has no effect on the lipemia of patients with primary chylomicronemia due to congenital deficiency of lipoprotein lipase. It has variable effect on severe mixed lipemia and is of no value in treating familial hypercholesterolemia. However, in other disorders where LDL levels are only moderately elevated, it may be of some benefit.

The usual dose of clofibrate (Atromid-S) is 1 g given twice daily; 0.5 g daily may be sufficient in patients with familial dysbetalipoproteinemia.

Toxicity

Nausea and abdominal discomfort are the most common adverse side effects. Myalgia associated with increased plasma levels of creatine phosphokinase has been reported. It occasionally involves the myocardium. Myalgia tends to occur more frequently in patients with low serum albumin levels, and clofibrate should therefore be avoided in nephrotic subjects. It should also be given in reduced dosage (if at all) to patients with azotemia. A weak association with gastrointestinal tract carcinoma has been reported, as has a modest increase in the incidence of cholelithiasis. The hypoglycemic effect of sulfonylureas may be enhanced by clofibrate, and it may also potentiate activities of indandione and coumarin anticoagulants by decreasing platelet reactivity. At least at the onset of clofibrate therapy, dosage of these anticoagulants should be reduced by 30–50%. Dermatitis, hepatic dysfunction, and bone marrow depression are rare toxic effects.

Some men taking clofibrate report decreased libido and breast tenderness. Brittle hair and alopecia have also been reported.

GEMFIBROZIL

Gemfibrozil (Lopid) is a more recently introduced congener of clofibrate that resembles the parent drug pharmacologically.

Chemistry & Pharmacokinetics

The gemfibrozil molecule differs from clofibrate in its aliphatic chain and in the presence of 2 methyl groups rather than a chlorine atom on the phenoxy group. It is supplied as the free carboxylic acid. Gemfibrozil is absorbed quantitatively from the intestine and is tightly bound to plasma proteins. It undergoes enterohepatic circulation and readily passes the placenta. Its plasma half-life is 1½ hours. Seventy percent is eliminated through the kidneys, mostly unmodified. However, the liver modifies some of the drug at the methyl functions to hydroxymethyl or carboxyl derivatives and some of the compound to a quinol.

Mechanism of Action

This agent decreases lipolysis in adipose tissue. There is a decrease in levels of VLDL in plasma. Only modest reductions of LDL levels occur, and HDL

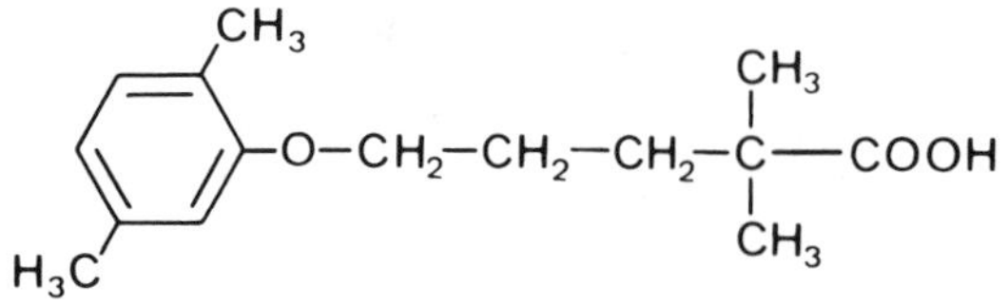

Gemfibrozil

cholesterol levels increase moderately. Whether the latter effect is greater than with clofibrate is not established. Part of the apparent increase of HDL cholesterol levels is a direct consequence of decreasing the content of triglycerides in plasma, with reduction in exchange of triglycerides into HDL in place of cholesteryl esters. Some increase in HDL protein has been reported as well.

Therapeutic Uses & Dosage

The indications for this drug in hypertriglyceridemia are the same as for clofibrate. However, gemfibrozil may be somewhat more effective in reducing triglyceride levels.

The usual dose of gemfibrozil (Lopid) is 600 mg orally twice daily.

Toxicity

Many of the toxic effects associated with clofibrate may be anticipated with this congener also. Skin rashes and gastrointestinal and muscular symptoms have been described. High levels of transaminases or alkaline phosphatase in blood have been reported. A few patients show decreases in white blood count or hematocrit. Gemfibrozil potentiates the action of coumarin or indandione anticoagulants. Doses of these agents must be reduced during therapy with gemfibrozil.

OTHER CONGENERS OF CLOFIBRATE

Several additional congeners of clofibrate are available in Europe. **Fenofibrate (Lipanthyl, Procetofene)** is very similar in action to clofibrate and gemfibrozil, but it may be somewhat more potent in reducing LDL levels. It is hydrolyzed to the anion and is excreted mainly by the kidneys. It is given in doses of 100 mg 3 times a day.

Bezafibrate (Bezalip, Cedur) also resembles clofibrate and gemfibrozil in its effect on VLDL, and, like fenofibrate, it may be somewhat more potent in reducing LDL levels. It is given in doses of 200 mg 3 times daily.

BILE ACID–BINDING RESINS

Colestipol (Colestid) and cholestyramine (Questran) are useful only in hyperlipoproteinemias involving LDL elevations. Patients who have hypertriglyceridemia in addition to elevated LDL may have further increases in levels of VLDL during treatment with the resins.

Chemistry & Pharmacokinetics

Colestipol and cholestyramine are very large polymeric cationic exchange resins that are insoluble in water. They bind bile acids in the intestinal lumen and prevent their reabsorption. Chloride is released from cationic quaternary ammonium binding sites in exchange for bile acids, but the resin itself is not absorbed.

Mechanism of Action

The bile acids, metabolites of cholesterol, are normally reabsorbed in the jejunum with about 95% efficiency. Their excretion is increased up to 10-fold when the resins are given. This results in lower levels of LDL in plasma because, although cholesterol synthesis by both liver and intestine is increased, the fractional catabolic rate of LDL also increases. The increased catabolism of cholesterol reflects its enhanced conversion to bile acids in liver via 7α-hydroxylation, normally controlled by negative feedback by bile acids. The content of cholesteryl esters in LDL decreases somewhat, and body cholesterol pools are decreased during treatment. Increased uptake of LDL from plasma in patients treated with the resins results from increased numbers of high-affinity LDL receptors on cell membranes, particularly in liver. Hence, the resins are without effect in patients with homozygous familial hypercholesterolemia who have no functioning receptors, but they may be useful in patients with receptor-defective combined heterozygosity.

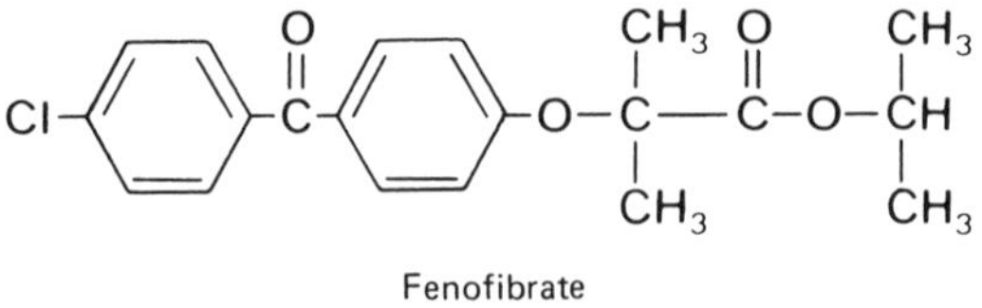

Fenofibrate

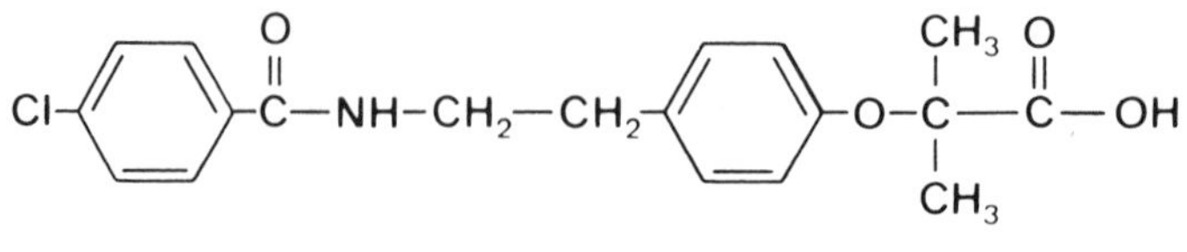

Bezafibrate

Therapeutic Uses & Dosage

The resins are used in treatment of patients with heterozygous familial hypercholesterolemia, producing approximately 20% reduction in LDL cholesterol when used in maximal dosage. Larger reductions at lower dosages may be expected in patients with less severe forms of hypercholesterolemia. If the resins are used to treat LDL elevations in persons with combined hyperlipidemia, they may cause an increase in levels of VLDL that would require the addition of a second agent. The resins are also used in combination with other drugs to achieve further hypocholesterolemic effect (see below). In addition to their use in hyperlipidemia, they may be helpful in relieving itching in patients who have cholestasis and bile salt accumulation. Since they bind digitalis glycosides, the resins may be used to increase the rate of removal of digitalis from the body in severe digitalis toxicity.

Colestipol (Colestid) and cholestyramine (Questran) are granular preparations available in packets of 5 g and 4 g, respectively, or in bulk. The usual starting dose is 20 g orally daily. Total doses of 30–32 g daily may be needed for maximum effect. The usual dose for a child is 15–20 g daily. The resins are mixed with juice or water and allowed to hydrate for 1 minute. They should be taken in 3 doses, preferably with meals.

Toxicity

The most common complaints are constipation and a bloating sensation, easily relieved by eating bran. Heartburn and diarrhea are occasionally reported. In patients who have preexisting bowel disease or cholestasis, steatorrhea may occur. Malabsorption of vitamin K may occur rarely, leading to hypoprothrombinemia. Prothrombin time should be measured frequently in patients who are taking resins and anticoagulants. Malabsorption of folic acid has been reported rarely. Increased formation of gallstones, particularly in obese persons, was an anticipated side effect but has rarely occurred in practice. Another occasional problem is dry flaking skin, which is relieved by application of lanolin. Absorption of certain drugs, including those with neutral or cationic charge as well as anions, may be impaired by the resins. These include digitalis glycosides, chlorothiazide, hydrochlorothiazide, warfarin, tetracycline, vancomycin, thyroxine, iron salts, folic acid, and phenylbutazone. Any additional medication should be given 1 hour before the resin to ensure adequate absorption.

NEOMYCIN

Pharmacokinetics & Mechanism of Action

This poorly absorbed aminoglycoside antibiotic inhibits reabsorption of cholesterol as well as bile acids, producing moderate reductions in levels of LDL. Bile acid excretion is increased, and the total body pool of cholesterol is decreased. It is cleared from plasma by the kidney.

Therapeutic Uses & Dosage

Neomycin is perhaps of greatest value when used in combination with other agents in treating primary hypercholesterolemias (see below). It is of no value in reducing levels of triglycerides.

The total daily dose is 0.5–2 g, usually in 2 divided doses with meals.

Toxicity

The dosage of neomycin is limited by severe side effects. Even at low doses, nausea, abdominal cramps, diarrhea, and malabsorption have been reported. Overgrowth of resistant microorganisms may lead to enterocolitis. In patients with bowel disease, absorption of the drug may be enhanced, so that otic, hepatic, and hematopoietic toxicity will occur with greater frequency. In patients with normal bowel function, these effects are unusual at doses under 2 g daily. Neomycin also impairs absorption of digitalis glycosides. It should not be given to patients with renal disease.

COMPETITIVE INHIBITORS OF HMG-CoA REDUCTASE

Two fungal inhibitors of cholesterol biosynthesis, **compactin** and **mevinolin,** are now under investigation for treatment of hypercholesterolemia. These agents are structural analogs of the substrate for HMG-CoA reductase, a rate-limiting enzyme in synthesis of sterols and other isoprenoid compounds. LDL levels are reduced about 40% in patients with familial hypercholesterolemia taking a daily dose of 40 mg of mevinolin. This is chiefly the result of induction of increased numbers of high-affinity membrane receptors for LDL, which increases LDL uptake. However, increased numbers of receptors in the liver could also decrease LDL production by removing VLDL remnants from plasma.

Though dolichol, ubiquinone, and isopentenyl adenine are synthesized via HMG-CoA, they appear to be less affected than cholesterol, probably owing to the high affinity of enzymes in these pathways for the product of HMG-CoA reductase, mevalonic acid. Ubiquinone levels in blood have been shown to be unaffected by therapeutic doses of compactin. Few significant side effects have been reported to date. If their safety is established, compactin and mevinolin are likely to become highly important in the treatment of hypercholesterolemia.

OTHER DRUGS

DEXTROTHYROXINE

L-Thyroxine increases neutral sterol excretion and oxidation of cholesterol to bile acids and induces LDL receptors on cell membranes. Dextrothyroxine

(Choloxin) is a synthetic analog that appears to retain these effects with some reduction in calorigenic activity. Sufficient calorigenic and adrenergic effect remains, however, to cause increased angina and serious arrhythmias in some patients. Because of the presence of covert coronary disease in many patients with hyperlipidemia, there is little justification for the use of this agent.

PROBUCOL

Probucol (Lorelco) does not resemble in chemical structure any of the other agents used to lower lipoprotein levels. Its mechanisms of action are unclear, but it may inhibit sterol biosynthesis. Increased uptake of LDL into cells by low-affinity processes may be an important effect. Probucol is lipophilic, distributes into adipose tissue, and thus persists in tissues for a long time. An average of 20% of peak blood levels persist 6 months following cessation of treatment. Serious toxicity has been demonstrated in animals (arrhythmias, prolonged QT interval). Substantial reduction of HDL cholesterol and apo A-I levels in plasma occur. If it affects subspecies of HDL that play a protective role against atherosclerosis, it is doubtful that treatment with this drug would have a net beneficial effect. It usually produces only a very limited reduction in LDL cholesterol levels in most patients. Some individuals with mildly elevated levels of LDL may show a moderate effect. The usual dose is 500 mg twice daily.

Probucol

TREATMENT WITH DRUG COMBINATIONS

Combined drug therapy is useful in the following instances (1) when VLDL levels are significantly increased during treatment of hypercholesterolemia with a bile acid-binding resin; (2) when LDL and VLDL levels are both elevated initially; and (3) when LDL levels are not normalized with a single agent.

CLOFIBRATE/ BILE ACID–BINDING RESIN

In familial hypercholesterolemia, this combination produces some decrease in VLDL levels in plasma but

offers no advantage over the resins alone in lowering LDL levels. Although clofibrate is said to inhibit cholesterol biosynthesis, it apparently cannot overcome the massively increased cholesterogenesis induced by the resin. There is a theoretical risk of further increasing stone formation in bile with this drug combination.

NEOMYCIN COMBINATIONS

Combination of neomycin with bile acid-binding resins may be more effective than either agent alone in treating some patients with hypercholesterolemia. This is presumably due to the ability of neomycin to block the absorption of cholesterol as well as bile acids. Neomycin and nicotinic acid appear to be highly complementary in hypercholesterolemic patients and may be considered for patients who tolerate the resins poorly.

HMG-CoA REDUCTASE INHIBITORS/BILE ACID– BINDING RESIN

Highly synergistic effects in lowering LDL cholesterol levels in animals and in humans have been reported with these combinations. However, these combinations probably increase HDL levels to a lesser degree than the combination of bile acid sequestrants and nicotinic acid (see below).

NICOTINIC ACID/ BILE ACID–BINDING RESIN

This combination is effective both in controlling VLDL levels (during treatment with resins or in treating disorders in which VLDL and LDL levels are both increased) and in normalizing levels of LDL in patients with familial hypercholesterolemia.

Nicotinic acid, when used alone, has a marked effect on levels of VLDL and chylomicrons and usually normalizes triglyceride levels if they increase when the patient is given a bile acid-binding resin. When VLDL and LDL levels are both increased initially, the doses of nicotinic acid required for treatment in combination with a resin may be as low as 1.5–3 g daily.

The nicotinic acid-colestipol combination is highly effective for treating heterozygous familial hypercholesterolemia. This probably reflects the summation of (1) increased catabolism of LDL due to the resin, (2) decreased synthesis of its precursor VLDL attributable to nicotinic acid, and perhaps also (3) the ability of nicotinic acid to inhibit cholesterol biosynthesis in the liver. The nicotinic acid also produces significant elevation in levels of HDL cholesterol.

Diameters of tendinous xanthomas in patients with heterozygous familial hypercholesterolemia are significantly reduced during treatment with this regimen, indicating that it is capable of mobilizing cholesterol from tissue sites. Effects on lipoprotein levels are sustained (some patients have now been treated as long as 10 years), and no additional toxicity or side effect beyond those encountered when the drugs are used singly has developed. In fact, because the resin has acid-neutralizing properties, the gastric irritation produced by the nicotinic acid in some persons is relieved when they take the drugs in combination. The drugs may be taken together, because it has been shown that although nicotinic acid is an anion, it does not bind to the resins, so that its absorption from the intestine is not impeded. Complete normalization of levels of LDL in heterozygous familial hypercholesterolemia is usually attained with daily doses of 6.5 g of nicotinic acid in conjunction with 24–30 g of resin.

Some patients with homozygous familial hypercholesterolemia have a modest decrease in LDL levels when taking this drug combination, but most have had no change. This combination does potentiate the effect of plasmapheresis in such patients, however.

REFERENCES

Differentiation of Hyperlipidemias

Goldstein JL, Brown MS: Familial hypercholesterolemia. Chap 33, pp 672–712, in: *The Metabolic Basis of Inherited Disease,* 5th ed. Stanbury JB et al (editors). McGraw-Hill, 1983.

Havel RJ: Familial dysbetalipoproteinemia: New aspects of pathogenesis and diagnosis. *Med Clin North Am* 1982; **66**:441.

Havel RJ (editor): Approach to the patient with hyperlipidemia. *Med Clin North Am* 1982;**66**:319.

Havel RJ, Goldstein JL, Brown MS: Lipoproteins and lipid transport. Pages 393–494 in: *Metabolic Control and Disease,* 8th ed. Bondy PK, Rosenberg LE (editors). Saunders, 1980.

Dietary Treatment

Connor WE, Connor SL: The dietary treatment of hyperlipidemia. *Med Clin North Am* 1982;**66**:485.

Phillipson BE et al: Reduction of plasma lipids, lipoproteins, and apoproteins by dietary fish oils in patients with hypertriglyceridemia. *N Engl J Med* 1985;**312**:1210.

Drug Treatment

AHA Special Report: Recommendations for the treatment of hyperlipidemia in adults. *Circulation* 1984;**69**:443A.

Bilhemier DW et al: Mevinolin and colestipol stimulate receptor-mediated clearance of low density lipoprotein from plasma in familial hypercholesterolemia heterozygotes. *Proc Natl Acad Sci USA* 1983;**80**:4124.

Brensike JF et al: Effects of therapy with cholestyramine on progression of coronary arteriosclerosis: Results of the NHLBI type II coronary intervention study. *Circulation* 1984;**69**:313.

Grundy SM: Hypertriglyceridemia: Mechanisms, clinical significance, and treatment. *Med Clin North Am* 1982; **66**:519.

Hoeg JM et al: Normalization of plasma lipoprotein concentrations in patients with type II hyperlipoproteinemia by combined use of neomycin and niacin. *Circulation* 1984;**70**:1004.

Illingworth DR: Mevinolin plus colestipol in therapy for severe familial hypercholesterolemia. *Ann Intern Med* 1984;**101**:598.

Kane JP, Havel RJ: Treatment of hypercholesterolemia. *Annu Rev Med* 1986;**37**:427.

Kane JP, Malloy MJ: Treatment of hypercholesterolemia. *Med Clin North Am* 1982;**66**:537.

Kane JP et al: Normalization of low-density lipoprotein levels in heterozygous familial hypercholesterolemia with a combined drug regimen. *N Engl J Med* 1981;**304**:251.

The Lipid Research Clinics Coronary Primary Prevention Trial Results. *JAMA* 1984;**251**:351.

Mabuchi H et al: Reduction of serum cholesterol in heterozygous patients with familial hypercholesterolemia: Additive effects of compactin and cholestyramine. *N Engl J Med* 1983;**308**:609.

Tobert JA et al: Cholesterol-lowering effect of mevinolin, an inhibitor of 3-hydroxy-3-methylglutaryl-coenzyme A reductase, in healthy volunteers. *J Clin Invest* 1982;**69**:313.

34

Nonsteroidal Anti-inflammatory Agents; Nonopiate Analgesics; Drugs Used in Gout

Martin A. Shearn, MD

THE INFLAMMATORY RESPONSE

Inflammation is an important mechanism for protection of the body from attack by invading organisms. However, inflammation is also the cause of the disability that accompanies a variety of disorders. In arthritis, perpetuation of the inflammatory reaction can lead to limitation of joint function and destruction of bone and of cartilage and other articular structures.

The inflammatory response is usually initiated by antigens, eg, viral, bacterial, protozoal, or fungal, or by trauma. The cell damage associated with inflammation causes release of lysosomal enzymes from leukocytes through action on cell membranes; arachidonic acid is then liberated from precursor compounds by phospholipases (Chapter 17). The enzyme cyclooxygenase converts arachidonic acid to endoperoxides, which are biologically active and short-lived. These compounds are rapidly converted to prostaglandins and thromboxane. Lipoxygenases are enzymes that convert arachidonic acid to leukotrienes. Leukotrienes have a powerful chemotactic effect on eosinophils, neutrophils, and macrophages and promote bronchoconstriction and vascular permeability. Kinins and histamines are also released at the site of tissue injury, as are complement components and other products of leukocytes and platelets. Stimulation of the neutrophil membranes produces oxygen-derived free radicals. Superoxide anion is formed by the reduction of molecular oxygen, which may stimulate the production of other reactive molecules such as hydrogen peroxide and hydroxyl radicals. The interaction of these substances with arachidonic acid results in the generation of chemotactic substances, thus perpetuating the inflammatory process.

I. NONSTEROIDAL ANTI-INFLAMMATORY AGENTS

Salicylates and other agents used to treat rheumatic disease share the capacity to suppress the signs and symptoms of inflammation. Some of the drugs also exert antipyretic and analgesic effects, but it is their anti-inflammatory properties that make them useful in management of disorders in which pain is related to the intensity of the inflammatory process. Drugs employed for their anti-inflammatory properties are heterogeneous in chemical structure and diverse in mechanism of action.

ASPIRIN

Aspirin and the newer nonsteroidal anti-inflammatory drugs (NSAIDs) (ibuprofen, naproxen, etc) are related chemically in that they are weak organic acids; in addition, they share the important property of inhibiting prostaglandin biosynthesis. They may also decrease the production of free radicals and of superoxide and may interact with adenylate cyclase to alter the cellular concentration of cAMP. Although these drugs effectively inhibit inflammation, there is no evidence that—in contrast to drugs such as gold and penicillamine—they alter the course of an arthritic disorder. Aspirin's long history of use and availability without prescription diminish its glamour compared to that of the newer NSAIDs. However, because of its low cost (Table 34–1) and long history of safety, aspirin remains the drug of initial choice for treating the majority of articular and musculoskeletal disorders. Aspirin is also the standard against which all anti-inflammatory agents are measured, and it should not be abandoned unless specific contraindication exists or another NSAID offers a clearly demonstrable advantage.

History
Quinine from cinchona bark is one of the oldest remedies for relief of mild pain and fever. Willow bark was used in folk medicine for years for similar indications. In 1763, Reverend Edmund Stone, in a letter to the president of the Royal Society, described his success in treating fever with a powdered form of the bark of the willow. He had noted that the bitterness of willow bark was reminiscent of the taste of cinchona bark, the source of quinine. The active ingredient of

Table 34–1. Comparison of aspirin and newer nonsteroidal anti-inflammatory drugs.

	Total Daily Dose for Rheumatoid Arthritis (mg)	Recommended Number of Divided Daily Doses	Plasma Half-Life (hours)	Approximate Cost to Patient for 100-Day Supply
Aspirin, generic	4000	3	12	$ 10.00
Diflunisal (Dolobid)	1000	2	10	112.00
Fenoprofen (Nalfon)	2400	4	2	130.00
Ibuprofen* (Motrin)	2400	4	2	67.00
Indomethacin (Indocin)	150	3	5	87.00
Meclofenamate (Meclomen)	400	4	2	159.00
Naproxen (Naprosyn)	750	2	13	105.00
Piroxicam (Feldene)	20	1	45	103.00
Sulindac (Clinoril)	400	2	16	107.00
Tolmetin (Tolectin)	1600	4	1	159.00

*Also available over the counter as Advil or Nuprin.

willow bark, salicin, which on hydrolysis yields salicylic acid, was later found in other natural sources. Acetylsalicylic acid was synthesized in 1853, but the drug was not used until 1899, when it was found to be effective in arthritis and well tolerated. The name aspirin was coined from the German word for the compound, *a*cetyl*spir*säure (*Spirea*, the genus of plants from which it was obtained, and *Säure*, the German word for acid). Because of its greater efficacy and lower cost, aspirin rapidly replaced the natural products then in use and has remained one of the most widely employed remedies for over 80 years.

Chemistry & Pharmacokinetics

Salicylic acid is a simple organic acid with a pK_a of 3. Aspirin (acetylsalicylic acid) has a pK_a of 3.5 (Table 1–1). It is about 50% more potent than sodium salicylate, although the latter compound causes less gastric irritation.

The salicylates (Fig 34–1) are rapidly absorbed from the stomach and upper small intestine, yielding a peak plasma salicylate level within 1–2 hours. The acid medium in the stomach keeps a large fraction of the salicylate in the nonionized form, promoting absorption. However, when high concentrations of salicylate enter the mucosal cell, the drug may damage the mucosal barrier. If the gastric pH is raised by a suitable buffer to 3.5 or higher, gastric irritation is minimized.

Aspirin is absorbed as such and is hydrolyzed to acetic acid and salicylate by esterases in tissue and blood. Salicylate is bound to albumin, but, as the serum concentration of salicylate increases, a greater fraction remains unbound and available to tissues. Ingested salicylate and that generated by the hydrolysis of aspirin may be excreted unchanged, but most is converted to water-soluble conjugates that are rapidly cleared by the kidney (Fig 34–1). When this pathway becomes saturated, a small increase in aspirin dose re-sults in a large increase in plasma levels. Alkalinization of the urine increases the rate of excretion of free salicylate. When aspirin is used in low doses (600 mg), elimination is in accordance with first-order kinetics and the serum half-life is 3–5 hours. With higher dosage, zero-order kinetics prevail; at anti-inflammatory dosage (≥ 4 g/d), the half-life increases to 15 hours or more. This effect occurs in about a week and is related to saturation of hepatic enzymes that catalyze the formation of salicylate conversion compounds, salicylphenylglucuronide and salicyluric acid.

Pharmacodynamics

A. Anti-inflammatory Effects: The effectiveness of aspirin is largely due to its capacity to inhibit prostaglandin biosynthesis (see Chapter 17). It does this by irreversibly blocking the enzyme cyclooxygenase (prostaglandin synthase), which catalyzes the reaction of arachidonic acid to endoperoxide compounds; in high doses, the drug decreases the formation of both the prostaglandins and thromboxane A_2 (Fig 34–2). Aspirin also interferes with the chemical mediators of the kallikrein system (Chapter 16). Aspirin inhibits granulocyte adherence to damaged vasculature, stabilizes lysosomes, and inhibits the migration of polymorphonuclear leukocytes and macrophages into the site of inflammation.

B. Analgesic Effect: Aspirin is most effective in reducing pain of mild to moderate intensity. It alleviates pain of varying causes, such as that of muscular, vascular, and dental origin, postpartum states, arthritis, and bursitis. Aspirin acts peripherally through its effects on inflammation but probably also depresses pain stimuli at a subcortical site.

C. Antipyretic Effect: Aspirin reduces elevated temperature, whereas normal body temperature is only slightly affected. The fall in temperature is related to

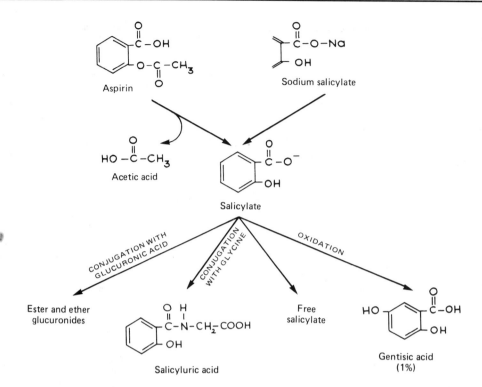

Figure 34–1. Structure and metabolism of the salicylates. (Modified and reproduced, with permission, from Meyers FH, Jawetz E, Goldfien A: *Review of Medical Pharmacology*, 7th ed. Lange, 1980.)

increased dissipation of heat caused by dilatation of superficial blood vessels. The antipyresis may be accompanied by profuse sweating.

The fever associated with infection is thought to result from the production of prostaglandins in the central nervous system in response to bacterial pyrogens. Aspirin, by blocking this effect, may reset the "temperature control" in the hypothalamus and thereby facilitate heat dissipation by vasodilatation.

D. Platelet Effects: Aspirin affects hemostasis. Single doses of aspirin produce a slightly prolonged bleeding time, which doubles if administration is continued for a week. The change is explained by the inhibition of platelet aggregation secondary to inhibition of thromboxane synthesis (Chapter 32). Because thromboxane accelerates platelet aggregation, aspirin inhibits platelet aggregation for up to 8 days—ie, until new platelets are formed.

Aspirin has a longer duration of effect than the many other compounds that inhibit platelet aggregation—clofibrate, phenylbutazone, dipyridamole, tranquilizers, antidepressants, etc. There is no relationship between the platelet dysfunction and gastrointestinal bleeding, nor is the hazard of surgery increased in a patient taking aspirin.

Therapeutic Uses

A. Analgesia and Anti-inflammatory Effects: Aspirin is one of the most frequently employed drugs for reducing mild to moderate pain of varied origin. Aspirin is often combined with other mild analgesics,

and over 200 such products may be purchased without prescription. These more costly combinations have never been shown to be more effective or less toxic than aspirin alone, and treating poisoning due to overdoses of such combinations is more difficult. Furthermore, the phenacetin contained in many such compounds may cause interstitial nephritis with serious renal impairment. Aspirin is not effective in the treatment of visceral pain such as that associated with acute abdomen, renal colic, pericarditis, or myocardial infarction.

The anti-inflammatory properties of salicylates in high doses are responsible for their recommendation as initial therapy for rheumatoid arthritis, rheumatic fever, and other inflammatory joint conditions. In mild arthritis, many patients can be managed using salicylates as their sole medication.

B. Other Indications:

1. Antipyresis–Except for a few diseases (eg, neurosyphilis, chronic brucellosis), there is no evidence that elevation of body temperature is a useful defense mechanism. Aspirin is the best available drug for reducing fever when doing so is desirable.

2. Inhibition of platelet aggregation–Aspirin has been shown to decrease the incidence of transient ischemic attacks and unstable angina in men and has been used as a prophylactic agent in these conditions. It may also be effective in reducing the incidence of thrombosis in coronary artery bypass grafts. Its efficacy in reducing the incidence of coronary artery thrombosis has not been proved.

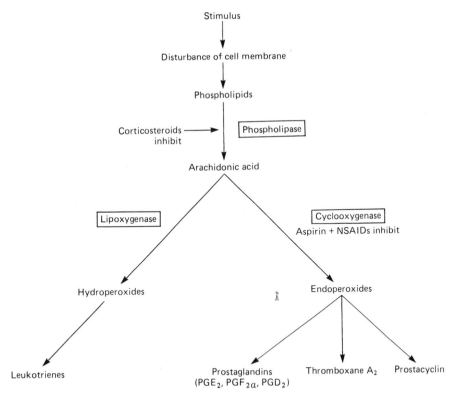

Figure 34–2. Scheme for prostaglandin biosynthesis.

3. Cataract—Preliminary studies suggest that aspirin may reduce cataract formation.

Dosage

The optimal analgesic or antipyretic dose of aspirin is less than the 0.6-g oral dose commonly used. Larger doses may prolong the effect. The usual dose may be repeated every 4 hours and smaller doses (0.3 g) every 3 hours. The dose for children is 50–75 mg/kg/d in divided doses.

The average anti-inflammatory dose of 4 g daily can be tolerated by most adults. For children, 50–75 mg/kg/d usually produces adequate blood levels. Blood levels of 15–30 mg/dL are associated with anti-inflammatory effects. A simple reliable method for determining salicylate blood levels is available, and the drug can thus be titrated to the proper level. Because of the long half-lives (about 12 hours) of aspirin and its metabolites, frequent dosing is not necessary when daily doses of 4 g or more are required. A convenient method is to give the total amount divided into 3 doses taken after meals.

The relationship of salicylate blood levels to therapeutic effect and toxicity is illustrated in Fig 34–3.

Preparations Available

Aspirin is available from many different manufacturers, and although it may vary in texture and appearance, the content of aspirin is constant. A disintegration test is part of the official standard, and there is little evidence that differences among tablets have clinical significance. The most popular buffered aspirin does not contain sufficient alkali to modify gastric irritation, and there is no evidence that these more expensive preparations are associated with higher blood levels, greater clinical effectiveness, or a lower incidence of side effects. Enteric-coated aspirin (many trade names) may be suitable for patients in whom buffering fails to control gastritis, since the coating prevents the tablet from dissolving in the stomach and the drug is absorbed in the alkaline medium of the small intestine. Therapeutic blood levels with this preparation may be similar to those achieved with the same doses of regular aspirin. Enteric coating increases the cost of aspirin, but these products are still less costly than the newer NSAIDs. The use of cimetidine to counteract gastric acidity increases the cost considerably and adds another drug with potential side effects.

Adverse Effects

A. Gastrointestinal Effects: At the usual dosage, the main adverse effect is gastric intolerance. This effect can be minimized with suitable buffering (taking aspirin with meals followed by a glass of water or antacids). The gastritis that occurs with aspirin may be due to irritation of the gastric mucosa by the undissolved tablet, to absorption in the stomach of nonionized salicylate, or to inhibition of protective prostaglandins. In animals, administration of prostaglandins

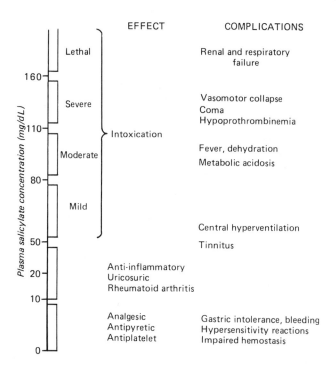

Figure 34–3. Approximate relationships of plasma salicylate levels to pharmacodynamics and complications. (Modified and reproduced, with permission, from Hollander J, McCarty D Jr: *Arthritis and Allied Conditions*. Lea & Febiger, 1972.)

has prevented gastric erosions, suggesting that the absence of a prostaglandin may make the gastric mucosa more vulnerable.

Vomiting may occur as a result of central nervous system stimulation after absorption of large doses. Upper gastrointestinal bleeding is usually related to erosive gastritis. A small increase in fecal blood loss is routinely associated with aspirin administration; about 1 mL of blood normally lost in the stool daily increases to about 4 mL daily in persons using ordinary aspirin doses and more for higher doses.

Aspirin has never been shown to cause peptic ulcers in humans, and with appropriate therapy, ulcers have been shown to heal while aspirin was taken concomitantly. Nevertheless, because of its irritant properties, aspirin should be avoided or taken with effective buffers by individuals with peptic disease.

B. Central Nervous System Effects: With higher doses, patients may experience "salicylism"—tinnitus, decreased hearing, and vertigo—reversible by reducing the dosage. Still larger doses of salicylates cause hyperpnea through a direct effect on the medulla. At low toxic salicylate levels, respiratory alkalosis may occur as a result of the increased ventilation. Later, acidosis supervenes from accumulation of salicylic acid derivatives and depression of the respiratory center.

C. Other Adverse Effects: Aspirin in a daily dose of 2 g or less usually increases serum uric acid levels, whereas doses exceeding 4 g daily decrease urate levels below 2.5 mg/dL. (See Drugs Used in Gout, below.)

Aspirin may cause mild, usually asymptomatic hepatitis, especially in patients with underlying disorders such as systemic lupus erythematosus and juvenile and adult rheumatoid arthritis.

Salicylates may cause reversible decrease of glomerular filtration rate in patients with underlying renal disease, but this may also occur (though rarely) in normal persons.

Aspirin in usual doses has a negligible effect on glucose tolerance. Toxic amounts affect the cardiovascular system directly and may depress cardiac function and dilate peripheral blood vessels. Large doses directly affect smooth muscles.

Hypersensitivity reactions may occur in patients with asthma and nasal polyps and may be associated with bronchoconstriction and shock. These reactions are mediated by leukotrienes.

Aspirin is contraindicated in patients with hemophilia. Aspirin is not recommended for pregnant women. Although a relationship to peptic ulcer disease has not been proved, aspirin is best avoided in patients with active peptic ulcer.

Use of aspirin during an antecedent viral infection has been associated with an increase in the incidence of Reye's syndrome (see Hurwitz reference).

Overdosage Toxicity

Aspirin is such a common household drug that it is a frequent cause of poisoning in young children. Serious intoxication results when the amount ingested exceeds 150–175 mg/kg of body weight.

Most aspirin is sold and used without prescription.

The drug must be kept out of reach of children and in the child-resistant container in which it is dispensed. Colorful, flavored, and liquid preparations should be kept in locked cabinets.

When overdosing occurs, either accidentally or with suicidal intent, gastric lavage is advised (Chapter 62). Hyperthermia may be treated with alcohol sponges or ice packs. It is important to maintain a high urine volume and to treat acid-base abnormalities. In severe toxic reactions, ventilatory assistance may be required. Sodium bicarbonate infusions may be employed to alkalinize the urine, which will increase the amount of salicylate excreted.

Drug Interactions

Drugs that enhance salicylate intoxication include acetazolamide and ammonium chloride. Alcohol increases gastrointestinal bleeding produced by salicylates. Aspirin displaces a number of drugs from protein binding sites in the blood. These include tolbutamide, chlorpropamide, nonsteroidal anti-inflammatory agents, methotrexate, phenytoin, and probenecid. Corticosteroids may decrease salicylate concentration. Aspirin reduces the pharmacologic activity of spironolactone, antagonizes the effect of heparin, competes with penicillin G for renal tubular secretion, and inhibits the uricosuric effect of sulfinpyrazone and probenecid.

NEWER NONSTEROIDAL ANTI-INFLAMMATORY DRUGS

The side effects of aspirin—especially the gastric irritation that occurs when large doses are employed—have led to the search for alternative compounds. Starting with ibuprofen in 1974, several drugs with aspirinlike properties (designated nonsteroidal anti-inflammatory drugs, NSAIDs) have been approved for use in the USA for the treatment of rheumatoid arthritis or osteoarthritis (Table 34–1). In addition to their use in joint disease, ibuprofen, naproxen, and mefenamic acid have been approved for use in primary dysmenorrhea. Over 50 drug applications for NSAIDs are on file with the FDA. Although aspirin is an NSAID, this term has come into use to designate the newer aspirin substitutes.

Chemistry

The NSAIDs (Fig 34–4) are grouped in 7 major classes: (1) propionic acid derivatives, (2) indole derivatives, (3) fenamates, (4) pyrrolealkanoic acids, (5) pyrazolone derivatives, (6) oxicams, and (7) salicylic acids. This chemical diversity yields such a broad range of pharmacokinetic characteristics that these properties are best discussed in connection with the individual agents.

Pharmacodynamics

The anti-inflammatory activity of the NSAIDs is similar in mechanism to that of aspirin and is mediated chiefly through inhibition of biosynthesis of prostaglandins. Inflammation is reduced by decreasing the release of mediators from granulocytes, basophils, and mast cells. The NSAIDs decrease the sensitivity of vessels to bradykinin and histamine, affect lymphokine production from T lymphocytes, and reverse vasodilatation. To varying degrees, all are inhibitors of prothrombin synthesis; all are analgesic, anti-inflammatory, and antipyretic; and all inhibit platelet aggregation. They are all gastric irritants as well, although as a group they tend to cause less gastric irritation than aspirin. Nephrotoxicity has increasingly been observed for all of the drugs for which extensive experience has been reported.

IBUPROFEN

Ibuprofen (Motrin, Rufen) is a simple derivative of phenylpropionic acid. In doses of about 2400 mg daily, ibuprofen is equivalent to 4 g of aspirin in anti-inflammatory effect. It is available over the counter in lower dosage as Advil or Nuprin. The drug is usually prescribed in lower doses, at which it is analgesic but inferior as an anti-inflammatory agent. The half-life is 2 hours. Ibuprofen is metabolized in the liver, and less than 10% is excreted unchanged. Gastrointestinal irritation and bleeding occur, although less frequently than with aspirin. The use of ibuprofen concomitantly with aspirin may decrease the total anti-inflammatory effect. The drug is contraindicated in individuals with nasal polyps, angioedema, and bronchospastic reactivity to aspirin. In addition to the gastrointestinal symptoms (which can be modified by ingestion with meals), rash, pruritus, tinnitus, dizziness, headache, anxiety, aseptic meningitis, and fluid retention have been reported. Interaction with anticoagulants is uncommon. Serious hematologic effects include agranulocytosis and aplastic anemia; effects on the kidney include acute renal failure, interstitial nephritis, and nephrotic syndrome.

NAPROXEN & FENOPROFEN

Naproxen (Anaprox, Naprosyn) is a naphthylpropionic acid that binds to plasma protein and has a long half-life (13 hours). Antacids delay its absorption. Naproxen is excreted in the urine as an inactive glucuronide metabolite. Like ibuprofen, naproxen competes with aspirin for plasma protein binding sites. It also prolongs prothrombin time. The average dose for inflammatory arthritis is 375 mg twice daily.

Fenoprofen (Nalfon), another propionic acid derivative, has a short half-life (2 hours) so that multiple dosing is required. The dose for inflammatory arthritis is 600–800 mg 4 times daily.

Side effects and drug interactions of naproxen and fenoprofen are similar to those of ibuprofen, ie, nephrotoxicity, jaundice, nausea, dyspepsia, periph-

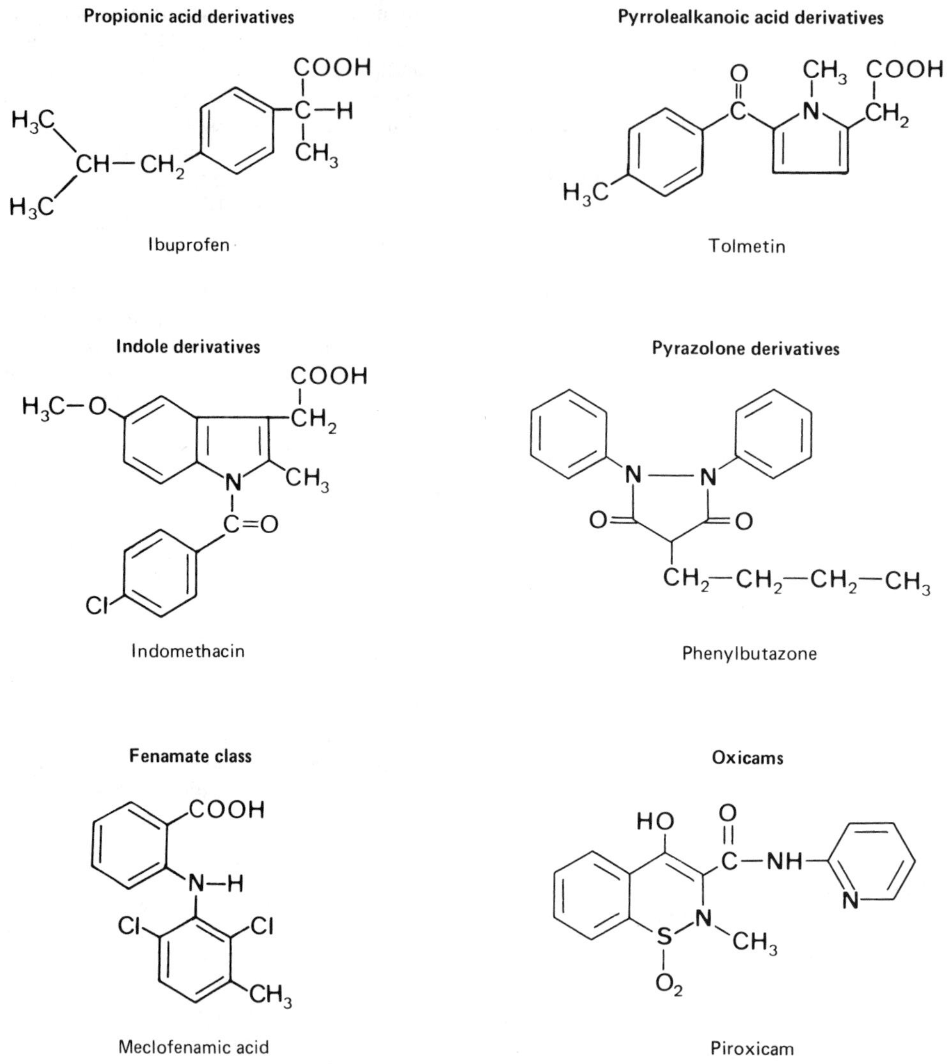

Propionic acid derivatives

Ibuprofen

Pyrrolealkanoic acid derivatives

Tolmetin

Indole derivatives

Indomethacin

Pyrazolone derivatives

Phenylbutazone

Fenamate class

Meclofenamic acid

Oxicams

Piroxicam

Figure 34–4. Chemical structures of some NSAIDs.

eral edema, rash, pruritus, central nervous system and cardiovascular effects, and tinnitus.

INDOMETHACIN

Indomethacin (Indocin), introduced in 1963, is an indole derivative. It is more toxic but in certain circumstances more effective than aspirin or any of the other NSAIDs (Fig 34–4). In the laboratory, it is the most potent of the inhibitors of prostaglandin synthesis. Indomethacin is well absorbed after oral administration and highly bound to plasma proteins. Metabolism occurs in the liver, and unchanged drug and inactive metabolites are excreted in bile and urine. The serum half-life is 2 hours.

Clinical Uses

Indomethacin is not suggested for general use as an analgesic. Except for the treatment of patent ductus arteriosus (discussed below), it should not be used in children. It is useful in special situations, including acute gouty arthritis, ankylosing spondylitis, and osteoarthritis of the hip and has also been effective in extra-articular inflammatory conditions such as pericarditis and pleurisy and in Bartter's syndrome. In acute gout, indomethacin has virtually replaced colchicine as the initial medication (see section on gout).

A special investigational application of indomethacin is in the management of patent ductus arteriosus in premature infants.

Adverse Reactions

Indomethacin produces a high incidence of dose-related toxic effects. At higher dosage levels, at least a third of patients have reactions requiring discontinuance of the medication. The gastrointestinal effects may include abdominal pain, diarrhea, gastrointestinal hemorrhage, and pancreatitis. Severe headache is experienced by 20–25% of patients and may be associated with dizziness, confusion, and depression. Rarely, psychosis with hallucinations has been reported. Hepatic abnormalities are rare. Serious hematologic reactions have been noted, including thrombocytopenia and aplastic anemia. Coronary vasoconstriction has been demonstrated. Hyperkalemia has been reported and is related to inhibition of the effect of prostaglandins on the kidney. A number of interactions with other drugs have been reported (see Appendix I). Use of indomethacin should be avoided in patients with nasal polyps or angioedema, in whom asthma may be precipitated. The drug is contraindicated in pregnancy and should be used with caution in persons with psychiatric disorders or peptic disease.

SULINDAC

Sulindac (Clinoril), a sulfoxide, is a pro-drug, closely related to indomethacin. The drug is effective only after it is converted by liver enzymes to a sulfide, which is excreted in bile and then reabsorbed from the intestine. The enterohepatic cycling prolongs the duration of action to about 16 hours.

The indications and adverse reactions are similar to those of other NSAIDs. Stevens-Johnson epidermal necrolysis syndrome, thrombocytopenia, agranulocytosis, and nephrotic syndrome have all been observed. The average dose for inflammatory arthritis is 200 mg twice daily.

MECLOFENAMATE

Meclofenamate (Meclomen), a fenamate agent, reaches a peak plasma level in 30–60 minutes, with a half-life of 2 hours. It is excreted in the urine, largely as the glucuronide conjugates. Although long-term experience is lacking, meclofenamate appears to have adverse effects similar to those of related agents and to have no advantage over them. This drug enhances the effect of oral anticoagulants.

Meclofenamate is contraindicated in pregnancy; its efficacy and safety have not been established for young children.

In inflammatory arthritis, the recommended dosage is 200–400 mg daily divided into 4 equal doses.

MEFENAMIC ACID

Mefenamic acid (Ponstel), another fenamate, possesses analgesic properties but is probably less effective than aspirin as an anti-inflammatory agent and is clearly more toxic. It should not be used for longer than 1 week and never in children.

TOLMETIN

Tolmetin (Tolectin), a pyrrolealkanoic acid agent, is similar to aspirin in effectiveness in juvenile and adult rheumatoid arthritis and osteoarthritis. The drug

has a short half-life (60 minutes), which means that it must be given repeatedly. The average adult dose is 400 mg 4 times daily.

PHENYLBUTAZONE

Phenylbutazone (Butazolidin), a pyrazolone derivative, rapidly gained favor after its introduction in 1949 for the treatment of rheumatoid arthritis, ankylosing spondylitis, acute gouty arthritis, and various musculoskeletal disorders. It has potent anti-inflammatory properties and is thus still commonly prescribed, even though aspirin and newer NSAIDs are superior in most applications.

The package insert lists a panoply of adverse effects. The most serious are agranulocytosis and aplastic anemia, which have led to a number of deaths. Phenylbutazone has also caused hemolytic anemia, nephrotic syndrome, optic neuritis, deafness, serious allergic reactions, exfoliative dermatitis, and hepatic and renal tubular necrosis. The main indications for phenylbutazone are for the short-term therapy of such painful conditions as acute gouty arthritis and superficial thrombophlebitis.

PIROXICAM

Piroxicam (Feldene), an oxicam, is an NSAID of novel structure (Fig 34–4). It has a half-life of 45 hours, permitting once-daily dosing, which should favor compliance. It is rapidly absorbed in the stomach and reaches 80% of its peak plasma concentration in 1 hour. It is excreted as the glucuronide conjugate and to a small extent unchanged.

Gastrointestinal symptoms are encountered in 20% of patients. Other adverse reactions include dizziness, tinnitus, headache, and rash. The drug may be used in the treatment of rheumatoid arthritis, ankylosing spondylitis, and osteoarthritis. The average daily dose is 20 mg.

DIFLUNISAL

Diflunisal (Dolobid) is a difluorophenyl derivative of salicylic acid. The drug has a plasma half-life of 8–12 hours, reaching a steady state after several days. Like aspirin, it has analgesic and anti-inflammatory effects; unlike aspirin, it has little antipyretic activity.

The indications for use of diflunisal include pain and osteoarthritis. It is not yet approved for rheumatoid arthritis. Adverse reactions are similar to those of other NSAIDs.

CLINICAL PHARMACOLOGY OF THE NSAIDs

Most patients with inflammatory joint disorders benefit from aspirin when administered in sufficient doses (4 g or more) and when special attention is given to lessening gastric irritation by proper buffering. About 15% of patients develop troublesome side effects from aspirin; it is primarily for these patients that NSAIDs are indicated. As a group, these newer agents tend to cause less gastric irritation, and the dosing schedule of some is simpler (one tablet once or twice daily). In choosing an agent, it is worth remembering that the cost to the patient is $67–159 for a 100-day supply of the newer agents compared to about $10 for generic over-the-counter aspirin (Table 34–1). In addition, a reliable method for determining salicylate blood levels is available to establish therapeutic range, which is not true for the newer drugs. These advantages must be weighed against easier dosage schedules, better compliance, and lower incidence of gastric irritation with some of the newer agents. Surveys show that most patients with inflammatory arthritis receive NSAIDs without an adequate trial of salicylates, yet none of these newer drugs have proved more effective than aspirin in controlled studies. Moreover, although less gastrointestinal irritation has been shown for most of them, some are proving more toxic in other ways.

The NSAIDs have been responsible for many instances of acute renal failure and nephrotic syndrome, which develops insidiously and is neither dose-dependent nor related to duration of drug use. Patients rarely have symptoms suggestive of a hypersensitivity reaction, so the condition may go undetected until advanced.

If the decision is made to use an NSAID, it is important to consider adverse effects, cost, and dosing schedules. It is not possible to know which patient will respond in a specific way to which NSAID, for some patients derive benefit from one and not from another. How much of this variability of response is related to the agent per se, to individual differences in metabolism of the drug, or to a placebo effect is difficult to evaluate. When compliance is a problem, drugs such as piroxicam, sulindac, and naproxen are useful because only one or 2 doses are required daily. If a patient is taking a hypoglycemic agent or warfarin, ibuprofen or tolmetin might be considered, since, unlike sulindac, they do not potentiate the effect of the hypoglycemic drugs or warfarin. Hypersensitivity to one of the phenylalkanoic acids, however, should preclude use of the others in that group. Dosing schedules listed for the drugs are those recommended by the manufacturer, but it is becoming clear that some patients require and may tolerate higher doses. Until blood level assays become available, it is probably safest to use the dosages as listed.

SLOW-ACTING ANTI-INFLAMMATORY AGENTS

ANTIMALARIAL DRUGS (Chloroquine, Hydroxychloroquine)

The pharmacology of the 4-aminoquinoline derivatives is fully discussed in Chapter 56. Chloroquine (Aralen) and hydroxychloroquine (Plaquenil) have been used in the treatment of rheumatoid arthritis and systemic lupus erythematosus since the 1950s, and their efficacy in inducing remission has been confirmed in carefully controlled studies. Rheumatoid factor declines after prolonged chloroquine use; however, there is no evidence that chloroquine decreases the progression of erosive bone lesions as is observed with gold.

The mechanism of anti-inflammatory action of chloroquine and hydroxychloroquine in rheumatic disorders is unclear. They suppress the responsiveness of T lymphocytes to mitogens, interfere with the replication of viruses, decrease leukocyte chemotaxis, stabilize lysosomal membranes, inhibit DNA and RNA synthesis, and trap free radicals. The action of chloroquine is not apparent until after a latent period of 4–12 weeks. The drug is often useful as an adjunct to treatment with NSAIDs and has no adverse interaction with other antirheumatic agents.

Indications

Antimalarials are often administered to patients with rheumatoid arthritis who have not responded optimally to salicylates and NSAIDs. In addition to their use in rheumatoid arthritis, antimalarials have been used successfully for their anti-inflammatory effect in juvenile chronic arthritis, Sjögren's syndrome, and systemic lupus erythematosus (in which they have a beneficial effect on both joint and skin findings). The antimalarial drugs should not be used in psoriatic arthritis because of the possible development of exfoliative dermatitis.

Adverse Effects

These are described in Chapter 56.

Dosage

Hydroxychloroquine sulfate, available in tablets of 200 mg (155 mg of base), is the preferred drug. Initial dosage is 2 tablets orally daily. Once clinical improvement is established, the dose can often be decreased to one tablet daily.

GOLD

Gold compounds were introduced for treatment of rheumatoid arthritis in the 1920s, but it was not until 1960, following a report of a large double-blind trial, that the efficacy of gold salts in the management of rheumatoid arthritis was clearly established. Subsequent controlled studies have confirmed the value of the drug and have demonstrated that these agents *retard the progression of bone and articular destruction* determined roentgenographically. In this regard, gold salts have special value in treating rheumatoid arthritis. Further impetus to the popularity of gold salts has been the demonstration that the drug may be continued for years, allaying earlier fears of toxicity from accumulation.

Chemistry

The 2 most commonly administered gold preparations are gold sodium thiomalate (Myochrysine) and aurothioglucose (Solganal). Both are administered intramuscularly as water-soluble gold salts containing 50% elemental gold. Auranofin (Ridaura) is a newly released oral gold preparation. Its superiority over parenteral forms has not been established.

Pharmacokinetics

Gold salts are approximately 95% bound to plasma protein during transport by the blood. Although they tend to concentrate in synovial membranes, gold salts are also concentrated in the liver, kidney, spleen, adrenal glands, lymph nodes, and bone marrow. After oral administration, only about 25% is absorbed. Following intramuscular injection, peak levels are reached in 2–6 hours; 40% is excreted within a week, about two-thirds in the urine and one-third in the feces. One month after intramuscular injection of 50 mg, 75–80% of the drug has been eliminated. Certain tissue compartments such as the epithelial cells of the renal tubules, which have a particular affinity for gold, show its presence many years after therapy has ceased. Most studies have failed to show a correlation between serum gold concentration and either therapeutic effect or toxicity.

Pharmacodynamics

The precise manner in which gold salts produce their beneficial effects in patients with rheumatoid arthritis and allied disorders is unknown. Gold alters the morphologic and functional capabilities of human macrophages; this may be its major mode of action. Other effects ascribed to gold include inhibition of lysosomal enzyme activity, reduction of histamine release from mast cells, inactivation of the first component of complement, suppression of phagocytic activity of the polymorphonuclear leukocytes, and inhibition of the Shwartzman phenomenon.

Indications

Gold therapy is indicated for active rheumatoid arthritis in patients who have been given an adequate trial of therapy with NSAIDs for a period of 3–4 months and continue to show active synovitis. Patients who later in the course of their disease show active inflammation and erosive changes are also candidates for gold. Patients with rheumatoid arthritis in the pres-

ence of Sjögren's syndrome and those with juvenile rheumatoid arthritis may also be considered, whereas the usefulness of gold in the treatment of psoriatic arthritis is less clear.

The major contraindications to gold are a confirmed history of previous toxicity from the drug, pregnancy, serious impairment of liver or renal function, and blood dyscrasias. Gold is not given in conjunction with penicillamine, because this chelator will remove much of the administered gold.

Adverse Effects

Approximately one-third of patients receiving gold salts experience some form of toxicity. Dermatitis, which is usually pruritic, is the most common side effect, occurring in 15–20% of patients. Eosinophilia may precede or be associated with cutaneous lesions. Hematologic abnormalities, including thrombocytopenia, leukopenia, and pancytopenia, occur in 1–10% of patients. Aplastic anemia, although rare, may be fatal. About 8–10% of patients develop proteinuria that may progress to nephrotic syndrome in a few cases. Other side effects include stomatitis, a metallic taste in the mouth, skin pigmentation, enterocolitis, cholestatic jaundice, peripheral neuropathy, pulmonary infiltrates, and corneal deposition of gold. Nitritoid reactions (sweating, faintness, flushing, and headaches) may occur, especially with gold thiomalate, and are presumably due to the vehicle rather than the gold salts themselves. Transient aggravation of arthritic symptoms may occur after injections of gold. Gastrointestinal disturbances (especially diarrhea) and dermatitis are the most common side effects of oral gold therapy.

Method of Administration

Parenteral gold is usually given as a 50-mg dose intramuscularly weekly until a total of 1000 mg has been injected (unless there is no response by the time 600–700 mg has been given, in which case the drug can be stopped). If 1 g is given without serious adverse effects and a favorable response is observed, the drug can be continued indefinitely in lengthening intervals of 2, 3, then 4 weeks. Oral gold is given as a 6-mg dose daily, increasing to 9 mg/d if a response is not seen after 3 months. Clinical response usually requires a few months to become evident and may be delayed for as long as 4 months. Urinalysis and blood and platelet counts should be performed every other week and liver function tests less frequently. Patients should avoid strong light and be warned to promptly report any skin or mucous membrane lesions. Gold should be stopped if dermatitis occurs but may be reintroduced cautiously if the skin lesions clear. Nephrosis, thrombocytopenia, leukopenia, and exfoliative dermatitis require cessation of gold therapy, and reintroduction of the drug is contraindicated. Penicillamine and dimercaprol have been used to treat toxicity with varying success. Improvement may be expected in 60–70% of patients who tolerate the drug.

PENICILLAMINE

Penicillamine, a metabolite of penicillin, is an analog of the amino acid cysteine. The drug can be resolved into D and L isomers; it is the D form that is used clinically.

$$HS-\underset{\underset{CH_3}{|}}{\overset{\overset{CH_3}{|}}{C}}-\underset{\underset{NH_2}{|}}{\overset{\overset{H}{|}}{C}}-COOH$$

Penicillamine

Pharmacokinetics

Radiolabeling studies indicate that about half of orally administered penicillamine is absorbed. Peak serum concentrations occur in 1–2 hours; 80% of the plasma penicillamine is protein-bound. Absorption is enhanced if the drug is administered 1½ hours after meals. Free penicillamine and its metabolites may be found in urine and feces. About 60% of the drug is excreted in 24 hours. No satisfactory method is available for determining blood levels.

Pharmacodynamics

Penicillamine suppresses arthropathy in experimental animal models and has been shown to interact with lymphocyte membrane receptors. It may interfere with the synthesis of DNA, collagen, and mucopolysaccharides. Rheumatoid factor titer falls following administration of drug, probably reflecting disruption of disulfide bonds of macroglobulins but perhaps also reflecting a basic action of the drug on the immune system. The mechanism of penicillamine's action in rheumatoid arthritis is unclear.

Indications

Penicillamine is similar to gold in its latency period (3–4 months) and in its anti-inflammatory properties. Like gold, it may retard the progression of bone and articular destruction. About 70% of patients who tolerate the drug are improved, and complete remissions have been observed. Penicillamine is reserved for patients with active, progressive erosive rheumatoid disease not controlled by conservative therapy. Penicillamine is usually prescribed for patients who have not responded to gold therapy. Penicillamine is not useful in seronegative arthropathies. Caution is required when administering other drugs simultaneously, because penicillamine impedes absorption of many drugs and prevents them from reaching therapeutic levels.

Adverse Effects

The side effects of penicillamine limit its usefulness. Animal studies have shown inhibition of wound healing and evidence of muscle and blood vessel damage. In humans, side effects are reduced by giving lower doses and by slow progression to maintenance dosages. Proteinuria is encountered in 20% of patients. Immune complex nephritis has been seen in 4% of patients; it is often reversible when the drug is withdrawn. Leukopenia and thrombocytopenia may occur at any time and may herald aplastic anemia. Most deaths related to penicillamine are due to aplastic anemia. Skin and mucous membrane reactions, the most common side effects, may occur at any time during therapy and may respond to lowering the dose. Drug fever, which may be seen as an early response to penicillamine, is often associated with cutaneous eruptions.

Loss of taste perception or a metallic taste may develop. The blunting of taste perception relates to zinc chelation. Anorexia, nausea, and vomiting occur.

A variety of autoimmune diseases, including myasthenia gravis, Goodpasture's syndrome, lupus erythematosus, hemolytic anemia, and thyroiditis may be seen. The drug must be discontinued permanently when any of these conditions is encountered.

Mammary hyperplasia, alopecia, and psychologic changes have also been observed.

Penicillamine is contraindicated in pregnancy and in the presence of renal insufficiency and should not be given in combination with gold, cytotoxic drugs, or phenylbutazone.

Side effects necessitating cessation of the drug occur in about 40% of patients. Blood counts (including platelet count) and urinalysis are performed twice a month for 4–6 months, then monthly. The drug should be stopped if the platelet count falls below 100,000/μL or the white count below 3000/μL. A history of penicillin allergy is not a contraindication to penicillamine. Patients who develop renal involvement, drug fever, autoimmune syndromes, and hematologic problems should not be rechallenged with the drug.

Dosage

Penicillamine (Cuprimine, Depen) is taken orally 1½ hours after meals. If clinical benefits are to occur, they should be apparent by 6 months. Treatment begins with 125 mg or 250 mg daily for 1–3 months; if no side effects are seen and improvement does not occur, the dose is doubled. If therapeutic effects are absent after 3–4 months, the dose is increased at monthly intervals up to 750 mg daily (250 mg 3 times daily), which it is rarely necessary to exceed. When therapy is discontinued after improvement, most patients relapse within 6 months.

EXPERIMENTAL ANTIRHEUMATIC AGENTS

LEVAMISOLE

Levamisole (Ketrax), a drug employed for the treatment of helminthic infections (especially *Ascaris lumbricoides*), was found to have immunostimulant properties that led to its trial in rheumatic diseases, in which immune *enhancement* was considered (paradoxically) to be of potential benefit. Levamisole restored impaired cellular immune responses in arthritis induced by adjuvant injection in rats. The drug increases chemotaxis and phagocytosis of macrophages and polymorphonuclear leukocytes and appears to enhance T lymphocyte function, especially in situations where delayed hypersensitivity is impaired.

Pharmacokinetics

Levamisole is administered orally and is rapidly absorbed, reaching peak blood levels at 2 hours. The plasma half-life is about 4 hours; the drug is metabolized by the liver and excreted mainly in urine and to a lesser degree in feces.

Indications

Levamisole has proved in randomized double-blind studies to be effective in rheumatoid arthritis. It decreases inflammatory changes while simultaneously lowering the erythrocyte sedimentation rate and the titer of rheumatoid factor.

Adverse Effects

Reactions occur in up to 20% of patients. Rash is the most common side effect, but more toxic reactions include leukopenia, agranulocytosis, and thrombocytopenia. Influenzalike illnesses, mouth ulcers, and nausea and vomiting also occur. Reversible immune complex glomerulonephritis has been reported.

Dosage

The usual dosage schedule for levamisole is 40–50 mg orally daily for the first week, increased to 80–100 mg daily for the second week and 120–150 mg daily thereafter. Administering 150 mg on 3 consecutive days and none the rest of the week has proved as effective as daily dosing. Like gold and penicillamine, there is a latent period of 3–4 months before clinical improvement is observed. The FDA has not yet approved levamisole for treatment of rheumatic diseases in the USA.

IMMUNOSUPPRESSIVE DRUGS

The immunosuppressive agents (see Chapter 59) have been employed for over 4 decades in the therapy of rheumatic diseases. The drugs are considered experimental, and their current use is largely restricted to certain life-threatening disorders or seriously crippling diseases with reversible lesions after conventional therapy has failed. Because of their toxic potential, they should be employed only by physicians completely familiar with their actions. Reliable methods of selecting one drug instead of another are not available, and acceptable controlled studies demonstrating efficacy in humans are lacking for most of the drugs.

Drugs for which there is adequate experience include the alkylators mechlorethamine, cyclophos-phamide, and chlorambucil; the purine antagonist aza-thioprine, which is FDA-approved for treatment in rheumatoid arthritis; and the folate antagonist meth-otrexate.

Immunosuppressive agents have been shown to be effective in some patients, especially those with vasculitis syndromes, such as Wegener's granulomatosis and panarteritis. They are useful in lupus nephritis, in seropositive progressive rheumatoid arthritis, and occasionally in patients with other rheumatic diseases. Because of the severity of side effects—especially the oncogenic effects and bone marrow depression—immunosuppressive drugs should be given only after safer agents have been tried.

GLUCOCORTICOID AGENTS

The pharmacology of corticosteroids and their effect on inflammation are discussed in Chapter 38. The indications for management of rheumatic disease are briefly discussed here.

Rheumatoid Arthritis

The effect of prednisone on rheumatoid arthritis is prompt and dramatic. However, the prolonged use of the drug leads to serious, disabling side effects. Corticosteroids do not alter the course of the disease, and bone and cartilage destruction continues while inflammation is decreased. Corticosteroids may be administered for certain serious extra-articular manifestations such as pericarditis or eye involvement or during periods of exacerbation. When prednisone is required for long-term therapy, the dosage should not exceed 10 mg daily, and gradual reduction of the dose should be encouraged. Alternate-day corticosteroid therapy is unsuccessful in arthritis: patients become symptomatic on the day they do not take the drug.

Intra-articular corticosteroids are often helpful to alleviate painful symptoms and, when successful, are preferable to increasing the dosage of systemic medication.

Cranial Arteritis & Polymyalgia Rheumatica

Patients with headache, jaw claudication, and other symptoms of cranial arteritis should be started on prednisone, 60 mg daily. The dose is maintained for about a month, then decreased to the lowest level compatible with normal erythrocyte sedimentation rate. In polymyalgia rheumatica without cranial artery symptoms and negative temporal artery biopsy, 15 mg daily often suffices.

Necrotizing Vasculitis

Prednisone, 60 mg daily, is indicated, although cyclophosphamide appears to be of equal or possibly greater effectiveness.

Systemic Lupus Erythematosus

Prednisone is used for complications such as hemolytic anemia, thrombocytopenic purpura, and involvement of lung, brain, heart, and kidney. Articular symptoms may respond to more conservative therapy.

Polymyositis-Dermatomyositis

Corticosteroids are usually effective in doses of 60 mg daily, which are tapered in accordance with improvement and reduction of muscle enzymes.

Mixed Connective Tissue Disease

Lower doses are usually required than in lupus erythematosus and depend on the site and degree of involvement.

Scleroderma

Corticosteroids are usually of little benefit.

Wegener's Granulomatosis

Although corticosteroids may be used, cyclophosphamide is the preferred agent.

II. NONOPIOID ANALGESIC AGENTS

For the treatment of mild to moderate pain when an anti-inflammatory effect is not necessary, the drugs discussed below have been used.

PHENACETIN

Phenacetin can no longer be prescribed in the USA and has been removed from many over-the-counter analgesic combinations such as Anacin and Empirin Compound. However, it is still present in a number of proprietary analgesics in this country and is in common use in many other parts of the world. The association between the excessive use of analgesic combinations—especially those that contain phenacetin—and the development of renal failure has been recognized for almost 30 years. Estimates of the percentage of patients with end-stage renal disease resulting from this kind of analgesic abuse range from 5 to 15%. After prohibition of the use of phenacetin in proprietary analgesics in Finland, Scotland, and Canada, the number of new cases of analgesic nephropathies in those countries decreased significantly.

ACETAMINOPHEN

Acetaminophen (Tempra, Tylenol, etc) is the active metabolite of phenacetin responsible for its analgesic effect. It is a weak prostaglandin inhibitor and possesses no significant anti-inflammatory effects.

Phenacetin
(acetophenetidin)

N-acetyl-*p*-amino-
phenol (acetaminophen)

Pharmacokinetics

Acetaminophen is administered orally. Absorption is related to the rate of gastric emptying, and peak blood concentrations are usually reached in 30–60 minutes. Acetaminophen is slightly bound to plasma proteins and is partially metabolized by hepatic microsomal enzymes and converted to acetaminophen sulfate and glucuronide, which are pharmacologically inactive (Fig 3–10). Less than 5% is excreted unchanged. A minor but highly active metabolite (N-acetyl-*p*-benzoquinone) is important in large doses because of its toxicity to both liver and kidney. The half-life of acetaminophen is 2–3 hours and is relatively unaffected by renal function. With toxic quantities or liver disease, the half-life may be increased 2-fold or more.

Indications

Although equivalent to aspirin as an effective analgesic and antipyretic agent, acetaminophen differs by its lack of anti-inflammatory properties. It does not affect uric acid levels and lacks platelet-inhibiting properties. The drug is useful in mild to moderate pain such as headache, myalgia, postpartum pain, and other circumstances in which aspirin is an effective analgesic. Acetaminophen alone is inadequate therapy for inflammatory conditions such as rheumatoid arthritis, although it may be used as an analgesic adjunct to anti-inflammatory therapy. For mild analgesia, acetaminophen is the preferred drug in patients allergic to aspirin or when salicylates are poorly tolerated. It is preferable to aspirin in patients with hemophilia or a history of peptic ulcer and in those in whom bronchospasm is precipitated by aspirin. Unlike aspirin, acetaminophen does not antagonize the effects of uricosuric agents; it may be used concomitantly with probenecid in the treatment of gout. Concomitant use with aspirin may increase blood levels of the latter drug.

Adverse Effects

In therapeutic doses, a mild increase in hepatic enzymes may occasionally occur in the absence of jaundice: this is reversible when the drug is withdrawn. With larger doses, dizziness, excitement, and disorientation are seen. Ingestion of 15 g of acetaminophen may be fatal, death being caused by severe hepatotoxicity with central lobular necrosis, sometimes associated with acute renal tubular necrosis (Chapter 62).

Early symptoms of hepatic damage include nausea, vomiting, diarrhea, and abdominal pain. Therapy is much less satisfactory than for aspirin overdose. In addition to supportive therapy, measures that have proved extremely useful are the provision of sulfhydryl groups to neutralize the toxic metabolites. Acetylcysteine (Mucomyst) has been used for this purpose (see also Chapter 3, Part II).

Hemolytic anemia and methemoglobinemia, reported with the use of phenacetin, have rarely been noted with acetaminophen. Interstitial nephritis and papillary necrosis, serious complications of phenacetin, although anticipated with widespread chronic use of acetaminophen, have not occurred despite the fact that about 80% of phenacetin is rapidly metabolized to acetaminophen. Gastrointestinal bleeding does not occur. Caution should be exercised in patients with liver disease.

Dosage

Acute pain and fever may be managed by 325–500 mg 4 times daily and proportionately less for children. Steady-state conditions are attained within a day.

III. DRUGS USED IN GOUT

Gout is a familial metabolic disease characterized by recurrent episodes of acute arthritis due to deposits of monosodium urate in joints and cartilage. Formation of uric acid calculi in the kidneys may also occur. Gout is associated with high serum levels of uric acid, a poorly soluble substance that is the major end product of purine metabolism. In most mammals, uricase converts uric acid to the more soluble allantoin; this enzyme is absent in humans.

The treatment of gout is aimed at relieving the acute gouty attack and preventing recurrent gouty episodes and urate lithiasis. Before therapy for gout is started, patients in whom hyperuricemia is associated with gout and urate lithiasis must be clearly distinguished from those who have only hyperuricemia. In an asymptomatic person with hyperuricemia, the efficacy of long-term drug treatment is unproved. Uric acid levels may be elevated up to 2 standard deviations above the mean for a lifetime without adverse consequences in some individuals.

COLCHICINE

Colchicine is an alkaloid isolated from the autumn crocus, *Colchicum autumnale*. Its structure is shown in Fig 34–5.

Pharmacokinetics

Colchicine is absorbed readily after oral administration and reaches peak plasma levels within 2 hours.

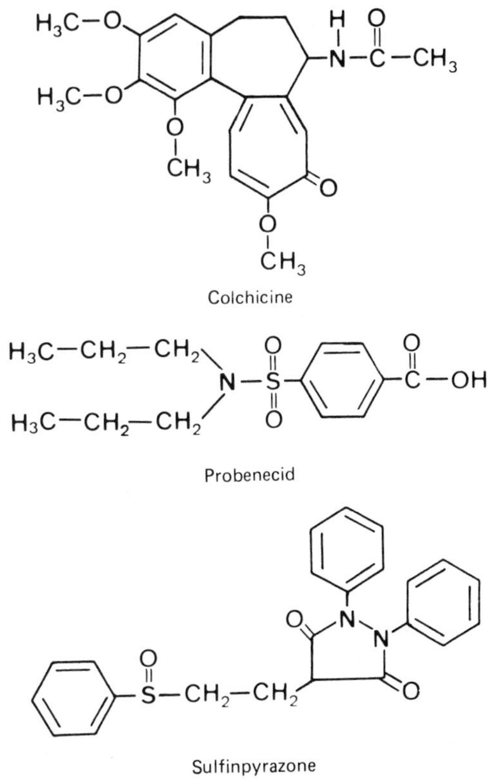

Figure 34–5. Colchicine and uricosuric drugs.

Metabolites of the drug are excreted in the intestinal tract and urine.

Pharmacodynamics

Colchicine dramatically relieves the pain and inflammation of gouty arthritis in 12–24 hours without altering the metabolism or excretion of urates and without other analgesic effects. Colchicine is effective in this disorder by means of its anti-inflammatory properties. Gouty arthritis is produced by the deposition of urate crystals in synovial tissue. An inflammatory process results through activation of the kallikrein-kinin system, plasminogen, and complement. Phagocytosis of crystals by polymorphonuclear leukocytes and discharge of proteolytic enzymes result in decreased pH, which further increases urate deposition and intensifies inflammation. Recent evidence indicates that monosodium urate activates the lipoxygenase pathway, leading to the formation of leukotriene B_4. Colchicine apparently exerts its anti-inflammatory effects through binding to the microtubular protein tubulin, preventing its polymerization and leading to inhibition of leukocyte migration and phagocytosis. It also inhibits the formation of leukotriene B_4.

Indications

Colchicine has been the traditional drug used for alleviating the inflammation of acute gouty arthritis. Although colchicine is more specific in gout than the NSAIDs, other agents (eg, indomethacin) are often employed because of the troublesome diarrhea associated with colchicine therapy. Colchicine is preferred for the prophylaxis of recurrent episodes of gouty arthritis, is effective in preventing attacks of acute Mediterranean fever, and may have a mild beneficial effect in sarcoid arthritis.

Adverse Effects

Colchicine may occasionally cause nausea, vomiting, and abdominal pain. Colchicine may rarely cause hair loss and bone marrow depression as well as peripheral neuritis and myopathy.

Acute intoxication after ingestion of large (nontherapeutic) doses of the alkaloid is characterized by burning throat pain, bloody diarrhea, shock, hematuria, and oliguria. Fatal ascending central nervous system depression has been reported. Treatment is supportive.

Dosage

For terminating an attack of gout, the initial dose of colchicine is usually 0.5 or 1 mg, followed by 0.5 mg every 2 hours until pain is relieved or nausea and diarrhea appear. The total dose can be given intravenously, if necessary, but it should be remembered that as little as 8 mg in 24 hours may be fatal.

The prophylactic dose of colchicine is 0.5 mg 1–3 times daily.

NSAIDs IN GOUT

Indomethacin may be used as initial treatment of gout or as an alternative drug when colchicine is unsuccessful or causes too much discomfort. Indomethacin is the agent most often used today to treat acute gout. Three to 4 doses of 50 mg every 6 hours are given; when a response occurs the dosage is reduced to 25 mg 3 or 4 times daily for about 5 days.

Phenylbutazone also is effective in the treatment of acute attacks of gout. Because the drug is used for a few days only, the serious side effects of phenylbutazone are rarely a problem in this application. The usual initial dose is 400 mg followed by 200 mg every 6 hours until the attack subsides. Phenylbutazone should not be continued after 3 days.

The newer NSAIDs are also being used with success in the acute episode. Ibuprofen in doses of 2400 mg daily has alleviated attacks. These agents appear to be as effective and safe as the older drugs.

URICOSURIC AGENTS

Probenecid (Benemid) and sulfinpyrazone (Anturane) are uricosuric drugs employed to decrease the body pool of urate in patients with tophaceous gout or in those with increasingly frequent gouty attacks. In a patient who excretes large amounts of uric acid, the uricosuric agents should be avoided so as not to precipitate the formation of uric acid calculi.

Chemistry

Uricosuric drugs are organic acids (Fig 34–5) and, as such, act at the anionic transport sites of the renal tubule (Chapter 14). Sulfinpyrazone is a metabolite of an analog of phenylbutazone.

Pharmacokinetics

Probenecid is completely reabsorbed by the renal tubules and is metabolized very slowly. Sulfinpyrazone or its active hydroxylated derivative is rapidly excreted by the kidneys. Even so, the duration of its effect after oral administration is almost as long as that of probenecid.

Pharmacodynamics

Uric acid is freely filtered at the glomerulus (Fig 34–6, site 1). Like many other weak acids, uric acid is then completely reabsorbed in the proximal convoluted tubule (site 2). Uricosuric drugs—sulfinpyrazone, probenecid, and large doses of aspirin—act at this site to decrease reabsorption. Small amounts of both aspirin and uricosuric drugs reduce urate secretion at site 3. Finally, most of the urate is reabsorbed in the postsecretory segment (site 4). Because aspirin in small doses causes net retention of uric acid, it should not be used for analgesia in patients with gout. The secretion of other organic acids—eg, penicillin—is reduced by uricosuric agents. Probenecid was originally developed as an agent to prolong penicillin blood levels.

As the urinary excretion of uric acid increases, the plasma level may not be greatly reduced, but the size of the urate pool decreases. In patients who respond favorably, tophaceous deposits of urate will be reabsorbed, with relief of arthritis and remineralization of bone. With the ensuing increase in uric acid excretion, a predisposition to the formation of renal stones is augmented rather than decreased; therefore, the urine volume should be maintained at a high level and—at least early in treatment—the urine pH kept above 6.0 by the administration of alkali.

Indications

Uricosuric therapy should be initiated if several acute attacks of gouty arthritis have occurred, when evidence of tophi appears, or when plasma levels of uric acid in patients with gout are so high that tissue damage is almost inevitable. Therapy should not be started until 2–3 weeks after an acute attack.

Sulfinpyrazone has also been suggested for preventing sudden death after myocardial infarction, but questions have been raised about the methodology of the study.

Adverse Effects

Side effects do not provide a basis for preferring one or the other of the uricosuric agents. Both of these organic acids cause gastrointestinal irritation, but

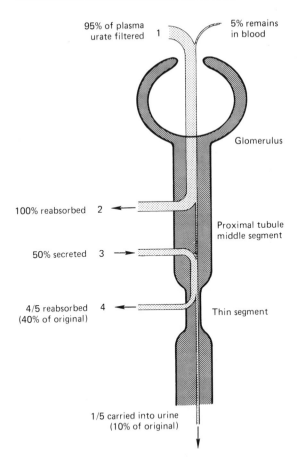

Figure 34–6. Renal handling of uric acid. Ninety-five percent of plasma urate is filtered by the glomerulus (site 1). Urate is completely reabsorbed in the middle segment of the proximal tubule (site 2), but 50% of this is secreted by the weak acid carrier in the same portion of the nephron (site 3). Finally, of the secreted uric acid, four-fifths (40% of original) is reabsorbed at a downstream site (site 4). (Modified and reproduced, with permission, from Meyers FH, Jawetz E, Goldfien A: *Review of Medical Pharmacology,* 7th ed. Lange, 1980.)

sulfinpyrazone is more active in this regard. Probenecid is more likely to cause allergic dermatitis, but a rash may appear after the use of either compound. Nephrotic syndrome has resulted from the use of probenecid. Both sulfinpyrazone and probenecid may (though rarely) cause aplastic anemia.

Contraindications & Cautions
It is essential to maintain a large urine volume to minimize the possibility of stone formation.

Dosage
Probenecid is usually started at a dosage of 0.5 g orally daily in divided doses, progressing to 1 g daily after 1 week. Sulfinpyrazone is started at a dosage of 200 mg orally daily, progressing to 400–800 mg daily. It should be given in divided doses with food to reduce gastrointestinal side effects.

ALLOPURINOL

An alternative to increasing uric acid excretion in the treatment of gout is to reduce its synthesis by inhibiting xanthine oxidase with allopurinol (Zyloprim).

Chemistry
The structure of allopurinol, an isomer of hypoxanthine is shown in Fig 34–7.

Pharmacokinetics
Allopurinol is approximately 80% absorbed after oral administration. Like uric acid, allopurinol is itself metabolized by xanthine oxidase. The resulting compound, alloxanthine, retains the capacity to inhibit xanthine oxidase and has a long enough duration of action so that allopurinol need be given once a day only.

Pharmacodynamics
Dietary purines are not an important source of uric acid. The quantitatively important amounts of purines are formed from amino acids, formate, and carbon dioxide in the body. Those purine ribonucleotides not incorporated into nucleic acids and those derived from the degradation of nucleic acids are converted to xanthine or hypoxanthine and oxidized to uric acid (Fig 34–7). When this last step is inhibited by allopurinol, there is a fall in the plasma urate level and a decrease in the size of the urate pool with a concurrent rise in the more soluble xanthine and hypoxanthine.

Indications
Treatment of gout with allopurinol, as with uricosuric agents, is begun with the expectation that it will be continued for years if not for life. Allopurinol for the treatment of gout is indicated in the following circumstances: (1) in chronic tophaceous gout, in which reabsorption of tophi is more rapid than with uricosuric agents; (2) in patients with gout whose 24-hour urinary uric acid on purine-free diet exceeds 1.1 g; (3) when probenecid or sulfinpyrazone cannot be used because of side effects or allergic reactions, or when they are providing less than optimal therapeutic effect; (4) for recurrent renal stones; (5) in patients with renal functional impairment; or (6) when serum urate levels are grossly elevated. One should attempt to lower urate levels to less than 6.5 mg/dL. Aside from gout, allopurinol is indicated to prevent the massive uricosuria following therapy of blood dyscrasias that could otherwise lead to renal calculi.

Adverse Effects
Acute attacks of gouty arthritis occur early in treatment with allopurinol when urate crystals are being withdrawn from the tissues and plasma levels are below normal. To prevent acute attacks, colchicine should be given during the initial period of therapy with allopurinol unless allopurinol is being used in combination with probenecid or sulfinpyrazone. Gastrointestinal intolerance, including nausea and vomiting and diarrhea, may occur. Peripheral neuritis and

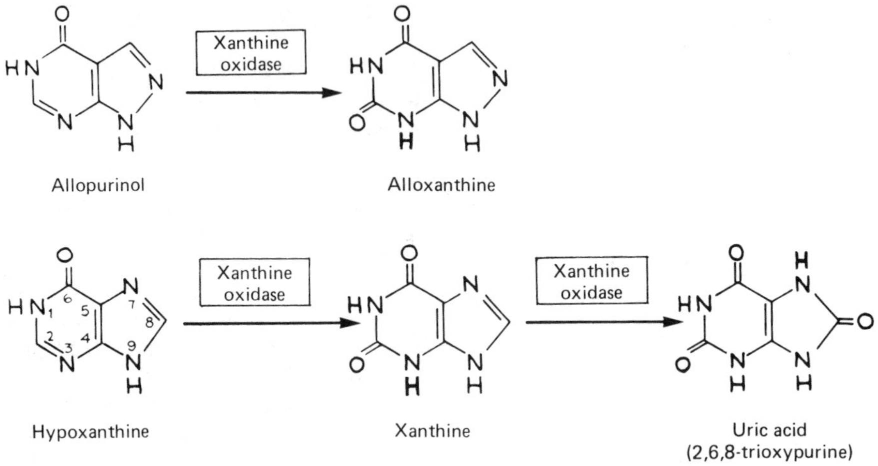

Figure 34–7. Inhibition of uric acid synthesis by allopurinol. (Modified and reproduced, with permission, from Meyers FH, Jawetz E, Goldfien A: *Review of Medical Pharmacology,* 7th ed. Lange, 1980.)

necrotizing vasculitis, depression of bone marrow elements, and, rarely, aplastic anemia may also occur. Hepatic toxicity and interstitial nephritis have been reported. An allergic skin reaction characterized by pruritic maculopapular lesions develops in 3% of patients. Isolated cases of exfoliative dermatitis have been reported. Allopurinol may become bound to the lens, resulting in cataracts.

Interactions & Contraindications

When chemotherapeutic mercaptopurines are being given concomitantly, their dose must be reduced to about 25%. Allopurinol may also increase the effect of cyclophosphamide. Allopurinol inhibits the metabolism of probenecid and oral anticoagulants and may increase hepatic iron concentration. Safety in children and during pregnancy has not been established.

Dosage

The initial dose of allopurinol is 100 mg daily. A daily dose of 300 mg is reached in 3 weeks and is adequate for most patients.

Colchicine, 0.5 mg twice daily, should be given during the first weeks of allopurinol therapy to prevent the gouty arthritis episodes that sometimes occur.

REFERENCES

General

Lasagna L, McMahon FG (editors): New perspectives on aspirin therapy: Proceedings of a symposium co-sponsored by the Aspirin Foundation of America and Tulane University Medical Center. *Am J Med* 1983;**74**:1. [Entire issue.]

Lorenzen I: Treatment of severe rheumatoid arthritis: Pharmacotherapy, immunoregulation, present state, and perspectives. *Ann Clin Res* 1983;**15**:80.

Settipane GA (editor): National symposium on aspirin and endogenous mediators of disease. *N Eng Soc Allergy Proc* 1981;**2**:54.

Shearn MA: Arthritis and muscular skeletal disorders. Chapter 14 in: *Current Medical Diagnosis & Treatment 1986.* Krupp MA, Chatton MJ, Tierney LM Jr (editors). Lange, 1986.

Salicylates

Bradlow BA, Chetty N: Dosage frequency for suppression of platelet function by low dose aspirin therapy. *Thromb Res* 1982;**27**:99.

Cotlier E, Sharma YR: Aspirin and senile cataracts in rheumatoid arthritis. (Letter.) *Lancet* 1981;**1**:338.

Gordon IJ et al: Algorithm for modified alkaline diuresis in salicylate poisoning. *Br Med J* 1984;**289**:1039.

Henry J, Volans G: ABC of poisoning. Analgesic poisoning:

I—Salicylates. *Br Med J* 1984;**289**:820.

Hurwitz ES et al: Public Health Service study on Reye's syndrome and medications. *N Engl J Med* 1985;**313**:849.

Mehta J: Platelets and prostaglandins in coronary artery disease: Rationale for use of platelet-suppressive drugs. *JAMA* 1983;**249**:2818.

Pedersen AK, Fitzgerald GA: Dose-related kinetics of aspirin: Presystemic acetylation of platelet cyclooxygenase. *N Engl J Med* 1984;**311**:1206.

Snyderman R: Pharmacologic manipulation of leukocyte chemotaxis: Present knowledge and future trends. *Am J Med* 1983;(**75–No. 4B**):10.

Tubwell P et al: Controlled trial of clinical utility of serum salicylate monitoring in rheumatoid arthritis. *J Rheumatol* 1984;**11**:457.

Waldman RJ et al: Aspirin as a risk factor in Reye's syndrome. *JAMA* 1982;**247**:3089.

White RL et al: Salicylate removal during plasma exchange in normal volunteers. *Clin Pharm* 1984;**3**:396.

Other Nonsteroidal Drugs (NSAIDs)

Chan WY: Prostaglandins and nonsteriodal anti-inflammatory drugs in dysmenorrhea. *Annu Rev Pharmacol Toxicol* 1983;**23**:131.

Clive DM, Stoff JS: Renal syndromes associated with nonsteroidal antiinflammatory drugs. *N Engl J Med* 1984; **310**:563.

Coles LS et al: From experiment to experience: Side effects of nonsteroidal anti-inflammatory drugs. *Am J Med* 1983; **74**:820.

Forre O et al: Non-steroidal anti-inflammatory drugs in rheumatoid arthritis: Effects on clinical parameters and cellular immunity. *Inflammation* 1984;**8**:S109.

Garella S, Matarese RA: Renal effects of prostaglandins and clinical adverse effects of nonsteroidal anti-inflammatory agents. *Medicine* 1984;**63**:165.

Indomethacin for patent ductus arteriosus. *Med Lett Drugs Ther* (Oct 30) 1981;**23**:39.

Nuki G: Non-steroidal analgesic and anti-inflammatory agents. *Br Med J* 1983;**287**:39.

Percy JS: Gastric mucosa, epigastric distress and anti-inflammatory agents. (Editorial.) *J Rheumatol* 1982;**9**:351.

Verbeeck RK, Blackburn JL, Loewen GR: Clinical pharmacokinetics of non-steroidal anti-inflammatory drugs. *Clin Pharmacokinet* 1983;**8**:297.

Slow-Acting Anti-Inflammatory Drugs (Remission-Inducing Drugs)

Blodgett RC: Auranofin: Experience to date. *Am J Med* 1983; **75**:86.

Delamere JP et al: Penicillamine-induced myasthenia in rheumatoid arthritis: Its clinical and genetic features. *Ann Rheum Dis* 1983;**42**:500.

Iannuzzi L et al: Does drug therapy slow radiographic deterioration in rheumatoid arthritis? *N Engl J Med* 1983; **309**:1023.

Lipsky PE: Remission-inducing therapy in rheumatoid arthritis. *Am J Med* 1983;(**75**–No. 4B):40.

Sharp JT, Lidsky MD, Duffy J: Clinical responses during gold therapy for rheumatoid arthritis: Changes in synovial, radiologically detectable erosive lesions, serum proteins, and serologic abnormalities. *Arthritis Rheum* 1982;**25**:540.

Weinblatt ME et al: Efficacy of low-dose methotrexate in rheumatoid arthritis. *N Engl J Med* 1985;**312**:818.

Williams HJ et al: Low-dose D-penicillamine therapy in rheumatoid arthritis: A controlled, double-blind clinical trial. *Arthritis Rheum* 1983;**26**:581.

Miscellaneous Antirheumatic Drugs

Drugs for rheumatoid arthritis. *Med Lett Drugs Ther* 1985; **27**:25.

Gutierrez-Rodriguez O: Thalidomide: A promising new treatment for rheumatoid arthritis. *Arthritis Rheum* 1984; **27**:1118.

Scherbel AL: Use of synthetic antimalarial drugs and other agents for rheumatoid arthritis: Historic and therapeutic perspectives. *Am J Med* 1983;**75**:1.

Shearn MA, Tu WH: Proliferative glomerulonephritis associated with levamisole therapy of rheumatoid arthritis. *J Rheumatol* 1981;**8**:55.

Veys EM et al: Levamisole as basic treatment of rheumatoid arthritis: Longterm evaluation. *J Rheumatol* 1981;**8**:45.

Nonopiate Analgesic Drugs

Black M: Acetaminophen hepatotoxicity. *Annu Rev Med* 1984;**35**:577.

Dietz AJ Jr et al: Effects of alcoholism on acetaminophen pharmacokinetics in man. *J Clin Pharmacol* 1984;**24**:205.

Dubach UC, Rosner B, Pfister E: Epidemiologic study of abuse of analgesics containing phenacetin: Renal morbidity and mortality (1968–1979). *N Engl J Med* 1983;**308**:357.

Gonwa TA, Hamilton RW, Buckalew VM Jr: Chronic renal failure and end-stage renal disease in northwest North Carolina. *Arch Intern Med* 1981;**141**:462.

Linden CH, Rumack BH: Acetaminophen overdose. *Emerg Med Clin North Am* 1984;**2**:103.

Drugs Used In Gout

Dieppe PA: Crystal deposition and inflammation. *Q J Med* 1984;**53**:309.

Emmerson BT: Therapeutics of hyperuricaemia and gout. *Med J Aust* 1984;**141**:31.

Ferraccioli G, Spisni A, Ambanelli U: Hypouricemic action of diflunisal in gouty patients: In vitro and in vivo studies. *J Rheumatol* 1984;**11**:330.

Griffing WL, O'Duffy JD: Oxipurinol in allopurinol-allergic patients. *Clin Res* 1983;**31**:803A.

Hande KR, Noone RM, Stone WJ: Severe allopurinol toxicity: Description and guidelines for prevention in patients with renal insufficiency. *Am J Med* 1984;**76**:47.

Lerman S, Megaw JM, Gardner K: Allopurinol therapy and cataract progenesis in humans. *Am J Ophthalmol* 1982; **94**:141.

Levinson DJ, Decker DE, Sorensen LB: Renal handling of uric acid in man. *Ann Clin Lab Sci* 1982;**12**:73.

Palella TD, Kelley WN: An approach to hyperuricemia and gout. *Geriatrics* 1984;**39**:89.

Widmark PH: Piroxicam: Its safety and efficacy in the treatment of acute gout. *Am J Med* 1982;**72**:63.

35

Introduction to Endocrine Pharmacology

Henry R. Bourne, MD

Endocrine drugs, like many other drugs, act by mimicking or interfering with chemical signals that mediate normal biologic regulation. Because hormones are synthesized in discrete anatomic sites and circulate in the blood, these chemical signals are particularly amenable to experimental manipulation and chemical analysis. As a result, the physiologic and even molecular mechanisms of many endocrine drugs have been specifically identifed. This chapter will describe the cellular mechanisms involved in endocrine regulation in an idealized system, as a basis for understanding the actions and uses of drugs described in later chapters.

THERAPEUTIC USES & SITES OF ACTION OF ENDOCRINE DRUGS

The clinical uses of endocrine drugs can be summarized as follows:

(1) To repair a deficiency of a specific hormone (or of its normal effect): The first triumphs of clinical endocrinology came from observations that extracts of certain glands—eg, adrenal, thyroid, and pancreatic islet cells—could restore normal physiologic function in animals from which the glands had been surgically removed. Administration of hormones to treat specific deficiencies still constitutes one of the most gratifying and effective modes of drug therapy in modern clinical medicine.

(2) To compensate for excess or inappropriate effect of a specific hormone: When surgical removal of a hyperfunctioning gland is not possible or must be delayed, drugs can often be used to decrease the secretion or effects of the excess hormone.

(3) To alter (or test) the functional integration of an endocrine system: Many endocrine responses are controlled by feedback loops (see below). By stimulation or pharmacologic blockade of one component in the loop, it is often possible to alter the hormonal response of a second component. Oral contraceptives employ this principle in preventing ovulation. Diagnostically, the same principle may be used to identify the site of a pathologic lesion, eg, in determining whether excess endogenous cortisol is due to a tumor in the pituitary or adrenal gland.

(4) Treatment of nonendocrine disease by stimulation or blockade of normally functioning endocrine responses: With the exception of diabetes mellitus, most classic endocrine diseases are relatively rare. Accordingly, endocrine drugs are most commonly used in treatment of nonendocrine disorders—as in therapy of asthma with glucocorticoids, breast cancer with sex steroids, or hypertension with mineralocorticoid antagonists. Subsequent chapters describe many additional examples of each of these uses of endocrine drugs.

In order to understand how endocrine drugs work, it is useful first to review the basic mechanism of endocrine regulation and the 3 general sites of drug action in an idealized endocrine system: hormone-producing cells, the circulating hormone itself, and the target cells or tissue on which the hormone acts (Fig 35–1).

HORMONE-PRODUCING CELLS

These specialized cells may be localized in a discrete gland or dispersed (like pancreatic islet cells) throughout a larger organ. Such cells may synthesize a peptide hormone, eg, insulin or parathyroid hormone, from larger precursor polypeptides and store the hormone in intracellular granules for release on demand. Alternatively, they may respond to stimulation by increasing synthesis of a hormone that is immediately secreted, as in the case of steroid hormones. Hormone secretion may be regulated by another hormone (eg, corticotropin and cortisol); by neural influences (cholinergic stimulation of catecholamine release from the adrenal medulla); by the concentration of a circulating ion or metabolite (ionized calcium and parathyroid hormone, glucose and glucagon); or by all 3 kinds of regulation (as is the case with the insulin-secreting beta cells of pancreatic islets).

In most cases, synthesis or secretion of a hormone is negatively regulated by one or more mechanisms that sense an effect of the hormone produced. Such negative feedback loops may be relatively simple (elevated blood glucose → increased insulin secretion → reduction of blood glucose → decreased insulin secretion) or may involve multiple interacting pathways in different organs (as exemplified by relations between renin, angiotensin, aldosterone, and blood volume and concentration of Na^+ and K^+).

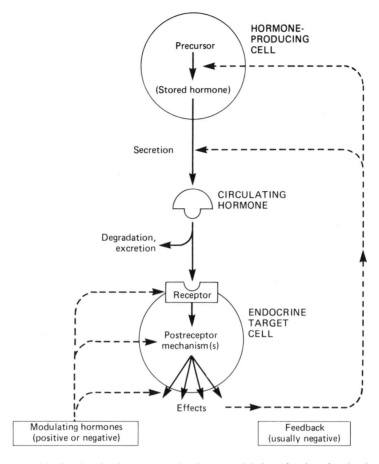

Figure 35–1. An idealized endocrine system, showing potential sites of action of endocrine drugs.

CIRCULATING HORMONE

As is the case with all drugs, the chemical structure of a hormone determines its distribution among tissues, its susceptibility to enzymatic degradation, and its excretion from the body. In addition, certain hormones (eg, cortisol, sex steroids) are transported in blood by specific carrier proteins. Any of these processes may alter the concentration of a hormone in blood and its accessibility to the target cell and thereby alter its effects.

ENDOCRINE TARGET CELLS

Each target cell possesses its own complement of specific hormone receptors capable of discriminating between the appropriate hormone and other circulating molecules. Binding of the hormone to cell receptors initiates a sequence of postreceptor events that results in the characteristic hormonal response of that cell— lipolysis, thermogenesis, production of a second hormone, etc. In addition, the cell's responsiveness to one hormone in many cases can be modified by additional hormones, which may act by altering the receptors for the first hormone or the enzymes involved in

postreceptor mediation of the hormonal effect. Thus, for example, glucocorticoids can regulate responsiveness of many tissues to insulin, and thyroid hormones can alter responsiveness of the cardiovascular system to catecholamines.

The 3 components of this idealized endocrine system present a multitude of potential sites of drug action. The remainder of this chapter surveys these sites in order to introduce concepts that underlie the actions of currently useful endocrine drugs and to suggest opportunities for development of new drugs.

DRUG ACTIONS ON HORMONE-PRODUCING CELLS

Table 35–1 lists drugs that are clinically useful because of their primary actions on hormone-producing cells. These drugs are divided into 2 groups depending on whether they act via hormone receptors or not.

The drugs listed in group A in Table 35–1 are used as *hormones* to produce effects normally produced by endogenous hormones. Thus, corticotropin and thyrotropin are used to test the ability of their target glands

Table 35–1. Drugs used for their primary action on hormone-producing cells.

Drug	Action	Clinical Use
Group A: Drugs that act via hormone receptors.		
Growth hormone	Increases somatomedin release.	Pituitary dwarfism.
Corticotropin	Increases cortisol release.	Test adrenal responsiveness.
Thyrotropin	Increases production of T_4 and T_3.	Test thyroid responsiveness.
Oral contraceptives	Decrease gonadotropin production.	Prevent ovulation.
T_3	Decreases thyrotropin production.	Test integrity of pituitary-thyroid axis.
Dexamethasone	Decreases corticotropin production.	Test integrity of pituitary-thyroid axis.
Bromocriptine	Decreases prolactin secretion.	Prolactinoma.
Group B: Drugs that do not act via hormone receptors.		
Iodide, thionamides	Decrease production of T_4 and T_3.	Thyrotoxicosis.
Sulfonylureas	Increase insulin production.	Diabetes mellitus.
Metyrapone	Decreases cortisol production.	Test integrity of pituitary-adrenal axis.
Aminoglutethimide	Decreases cortisol production.	Cushing's syndrome.
Mitotane (o,p'-DDD)	Destroys adrenocortical cells.	Adrenal carcinoma.
Streptozocin	Destroys pancreatic islet cells.	Pancreatic islet cell carcinoma.

to produce cortisol and thyroid hormones, respectively. Conversely, triiodothyronine (T_3) or dexamethasone (a potent synthetic analog of cortisol) is used to determine whether the pituitary's stimulation of thyroid or adrenocortical hormone production can be appropriately suppressed by the hormonal product of the target gland. These negative feedback loops are described in more detail in Chapters 37 and 38. (*Note:* In addition to their use in endocrine tests, T_3 and dexamethasone are used clinically for their direct effects on tissues.)

The other 3 drugs in group A are used in therapy rather than in tests of endocrine function. Estrogens and progestins act as contraceptives by suppressing pituitary production of gonadotropins, which are necessary for induction of ovulation. These effects of oral contraceptives take advantage of the negative feedback regulation normally exerted by sex steroids on the pituitary. The efficacy of these contraceptives results from altering the timing and extent of normal pituitary suppression (see Chapter 39). Growth hormone promotes growth, in part, by stimulating hepatic production of somatomedins (Chapter 36) and is used in replacement therapy for pituitary dwarfism. Bro-

mocriptine acts as a dopamine agonist to prevent pituitary release of prolactin. Although this drug is used to prevent pathologic galactorrhea (eg, caused by pituitary cells that autonomously secrete prolactin), it acts by augmenting a normal regulatory pathway that is mediated by dopamine.

Thus, all the drugs in group A act via hormone receptors that are essential control points in normal regulatory pathways. These drugs were discovered by the classic method of endocrinology: surgical extirpation of a gland and demonstration that an extract of the gland can restore a normal endocrine function, followed eventually by isolation of the pure hormone and, in some cases, by synthesis of a congener of the hormone.

In contrast, none of the drugs in group B act via normal hormone receptors, and most of them were discovered serendipitously, as a result of investigations not directed toward understanding endocrine regulation. For example, the sulfonylureas—now widely used in treating non–insulin-dependent diabetes (Chapter 40)—were developed because of the clinical observation that a sulfonamide caused hypoglycemia in the course of treatment of typhoid fever. Similarly, goiters in rabbits fed a diet composed largely of cabbage led to discovery of the thionamides. Prototypes of this class of drug—now extremely useful in suppressing thyrotoxicosis—were isolated from cabbage seeds (Chapter 37).

Such fortuitous advances suggest that hormone-producing cells contain many potential sites at which synthesis or secretion of hormones can be specifically altered by drugs. Even when the specific drug is already available, it is not always easy to determine exactly where these sites are. Thus, despite considerable research, it is still not clear, at a molecular level, how sulfonylureas stimulate insulin release or precisely how the thionamides block incorporation of iodine into thyroid hormones (see Chapters 37 and 40). Similarly, although mitotane and streptozocin are cytotoxic to many cell types, they show considerable specificity in killing tumors derived from adrenal cortex and pancreatic islets, respectively. This specificity must indicate quite specific molecular targets in the 2 cell types, although the molecules involved are unknown.

The molecular sites of action of aminoglutethimide and metyrapone are well established. These drugs inhibit specific enzymatic steps in the biosynthesis of cortisol (Chapter 38). Pharmacologic inhibition of cortisol production provides additional probes for testing the integrity of the pituitary-adrenal axis and may also be useful in preventing or decreasing the deleterious effects of excess cortisol in some patients (eg, when Cushing's syndrome is caused by ectopic corticotropin in an inoperable lung carcinoma).

None of the agents in group B specifically affect the endocrine function of cells that produce peptide hormones such as parathyroid hormone, growth hormone, calcitonin, or the pituitary trophic hormones. Such drugs will eventually be developed as a result of continuing advances in understanding the molecular mechanisms involved in synthesis, storage, and release of these hormones.

We have contrasted drugs that alter hormone production by acting on hormone receptors (group A) with those that act on other components of the hormone-producing cell (group B). Development of agents in the first group directly followed characterization of normal hormones, which provided chemical structures to be copied or modified. Consequently, these drugs possess the advantage of biologic specificity, selected by evolution.

Drugs in the second group have exactly the opposite potential advantage: Because they do *not* act through hormone receptors, their potential actions are not confined to those of endogenous hormones. Thus, in spite of the fact that no known hormone directly inhibits production of thyroid hormones, it was possible to develop drugs like the thionamide propylthiouracil that have precisely this effect.

A survey of endocrine diseases reveals obvious clinical needs for new agents that might be added to the list in group B. For example, a new drug (analogous to mitotane) that selectively kills parathyroid cells or a drug (analogous to aminoglutethimide) that specifically inhibits synthesis of parathyroid hormone would rapidly find a place in the therapy of parathyroid tumors or primary or secondary hyperparathyroidism, respectively. Similarly, a drug that specifically inhibits synthesis of gonadotropins without producing the potentially undesirable effects of sex steroids would be an obvious candidate for use as an oral contraceptive in both men and women.

PHARMACOLOGIC IMPORTANCE OF THE METABOLISM, DISTRIBUTION, & EXCRETION OF HORMONES

In principle, the effect of a natural hormone could be regulated by varying its rate of production, its rate of degradation, or the sensitivity of its target cell. With few exceptions, nature appears to have concentrated on the first and last of these mechanisms. In most endocrine systems, investigation has failed to uncover physiologically meaningful regulation of the rate of clearance of a hormone from the compartment in which it acts.* Nonetheless, the rate of clearance of a hormone or hormone congener from the bloodstream can be of crucial clinical importance, because it helps to determine the rate of onset and the duration of action of exogenously administered hormones.

Thyroid hormones exemplify this principle. Thus, the maximal effect of a given daily dose of T_3 (plasma half-life less than 2 days) occurs much sooner than does the maximal effect of thyroxine (plasma half-life more than 7 days). Correspondingly, the effects dissipate much more rapidly upon withdrawal of T_3 than when thyroxine administration is stopped. The clinical implications of these differences are examined in Chapter 37.

The very much shorter plasma half-lives of most peptide hormones create a different set of therapeutic problems. Thus, hormone replacement therapy with insulin (plasma half-life 9 minutes) would be impossible if insulin could not be injected in forms that release active hormone into the bloodstream over several hours. The therapeutic challenge posed by varying metabolic requirements for insulin over the course of a day—depending upon ingestion of carbohydrate, exercise, etc—has stimulated development of short-, intermediate-, and long-acting insulin preparations. The specific characteristics of these preparations must be thoroughly understood by both the physician and the diabetic patient (see Chapter 40).

As a therapeutic strategy, deliberate manipulation of the metabolism and distribution of endogenous hormones and endocrine drugs is just beginning to be explored. The pharmacology of catecholamines, refined over more than 4 decades, provides many examples of such a strategy (see Chapters 8–10). These include the following: (1) specific enzyme inhibitors that increase the concentration of endogenous neurohormone (monoamine oxidase inhibitors); (2) structural modification of catecholamine congeners to bypass metabolizing enzymes (eg, terbutaline, which is not a substrate for catechol-O-methyltransferase); (3) structural modifications that enhance gastrointestinal absorption or distribution to specific sites such as the brain (eg, amphetamine); (4) administration of a precursor of specific neurohormone or congener (methyldopa, levodopa); and (5) coadministration of an enzyme inhibitor (carbidopa) with a catecholamine precursor (levodopa) to reduce accumulation of the active drug (dopamine) at receptors where an effect is not desired.

This general strategy can be more easily pursued with chemically simple hormones—biogenic amines, steroids, etc—than with the peptide hormones, for obvious reasons. Thus, development of peptide hormone congeners that can be administered orally presents a difficult challenge. Similarly, it will be difficult to design congeners of insulin, parathyroid hormone, or gonadotropins that are simultaneously resistant to biodegradation, nonantigenic, and effective at appropriate receptor sites. The development of captopril, a specific inhibitor of the protease that generates angiotensin II and degrades bradykinin (see Chapters 10 and 16), suggests that it should be possible to develop specific inhibitors of the proteolytic synthesis or degradation of other peptide hormones.

---

*Norepinephrine, the sympathetic neurotransmitter, is a possible exception in that presynaptic reuptake of the transmitter is regulated by norepinephrine itself. This reuptake process is a determinant of the extent and duration of stimulation of postsynaptic receptors, as described in Chapter 5.

DRUGS THAT ACT ON ENDOCRINE TARGET CELLS

Most endocrine drugs act directly on endocrine target cells by binding to receptors for endogenous hormones. The mechanisms of action and therapeutic uses of these drugs vary greatly in complexity. In the simplest case, the drug substitutes for a deficient hormone and may indeed be chemically identical to the hormone. The therapeutic strategies followed in administering most endocrine drugs are more complex. These include administration of supraphysiologic doses of hormones, use of hormone congeners with enhanced receptor specificity (greater than observed with the normal hormone), and use of hormone antagonists. In addition, hormones and hormone antagonists that bind to one class of receptor can be used to modulate the effects of hormones that act through a different class of receptor. After a review of the postreceptor mechanisms by which different classes of receptors produce their effects, the pharmacologic and therapeutic principles that underlie all these strategies will be considered, proceeding from the simplest case to the most complex.

POSTRECEPTOR MECHANISMS OF HORMONE ACTION

The mechanisms of action of hormones fall into 2 general groups: **Gene-active hormones** promote synthesis of specific messenger RNA (mRNA) and thus increase synthesis of key proteins whose activities produce the effects seen in the target cell. **Membrane-active hormones** employ several mechanisms to change the activities of enzymes and proteins that have already been synthesized.

Gene-Active Hormones

The steroid hormones (glucocorticoids, mineralocorticoids, sex steroids, and vitamin D metabolites) all act by a common general mechanism, as depicted in Fig 35–2. The hormone enters the cytoplasm, where it binds to a specific receptor. The steroid-receptor complex then undergoes an activation process that enables it to enter the nucleus, where it binds to sites on chromatin and regulates transcription of specific gene sequences into RNA. The RNA molecules are processed to form mRNAs, which leave the nucleus and bind to ribosomes where their nucleotide sequences are translated into the corresponding amino acid sequences of specific enzymes and proteins. Note that the specificity of action of a steroid hormone thus depends upon the type of steroid receptor involved. Once it has formed a complex with hormone, each type of steroid receptor is able to activate the transcription of a limited number of specific genes. Thus, although a cell may possess both glucocorticoid and sex steroid receptors,

the 2 different classes of hormone will induce synthesis of different sets of mRNAs and proteins.

Thyroid hormones act by a similar mechanism. The sequence of events differs from that shown for steroid hormones in that the thyroid hormones bind to receptors that are already present in the nucleus, so that the cytoplasmic binding and receptor activation steps are omitted. Thyroid hormones also bind with some specificity to sites in the plasma membrane, cytoplasm, and mitochondria. Because some experimentally observed effects of these hormones do not require de novo protein synthesis, these effects may be mediated by extranuclear receptors via mechanisms that do not alter gene expression.

Two important therapeutic implications follow from the mechanisms of action of the gene-active hormones: (1) As a class, all of these hormones produce their effects after a characteristic lag period of 30 minutes to several hours—a period that is required for synthesis of new proteins. An increase in blood concentration of these hormones will produce an increased effect after a similar lag period. This means that the gene-active hormones cannot be expected to alter a pathologic state within minutes—eg, glucocorticoids will not immediately relieve the symptoms of acute bronchial asthma. (2) When tissues are exposed for a brief period to increased concentrations of these hormones in plasma, the effects characteristically persist for hours or days. This may be due in part to high affinity of hormone for receptor (which means that the agonist dissociates slowly from the receptor once it has been bound). The persistence of effect is also due to the relatively slow turnover of most enzymes and proteins, which can remain active in cells for hours or even days after they have been synthesized. In this way, a cell or tissue can "remember" that it came in contact with a gene-active hormone at an earlier time. Therapeutically, this means that the beneficial (or toxic) effects of a gene-active hormone will usually decrease slowly when the administration of the hormone is discontinued and that there will not be a simple temporal correlation between plasma concentration of the hormone and its effects.

Membrane-Active Hormones

Many hormones—including most peptide hormones, the biogenic amines, and the prostaglandins—combine with receptors in the plasma membrane. These hormones produce their effects on target cells by a diverse set of mechanisms. The best-established mechanism involves synthesis of an intracellular "second messenger," cyclic $3',5'$-adenosine monophosphate (cyclic AMP, cAMP) (Fig 35–3). The hormone-receptor complex interacts with a guanine nucleotide-binding membrane protein, which in turn stimulates conversion of intracellular ATP to cAMP by a third membrane-bound protein, the enzyme adenylate cyclase. Within the cell, cAMP relays the hormonal message by combining with its own receptor, cAMP-dependent protein kinase. Activated by cAMP, the protein kinase catalyzes phosphorylation

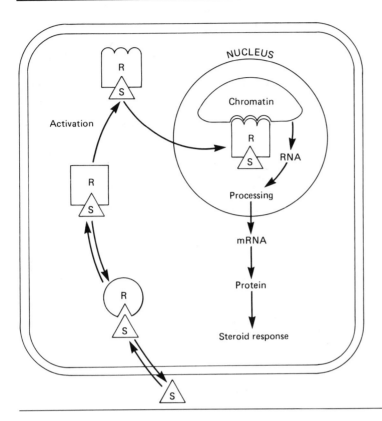

Figure 35–2. Mechanism of action of steroid hormones in mammalian cells. The steroid hormone (S) binds reversibly to a cytoplasmic receptor (R), and the steroid-receptor complex undergoes an irreversible activation step that allows it to enter the nucleus, where it activates transcription of specific genes into RNA. After processing in the nucleus, the corresponding mRNAs code for ribosomal synthesis of the specific proteins that mediate the steroid response.

of specific enzymes, thus stimulating or inhibiting their activities. Either directly or through a series of subsequent metabolic steps, altered activities of these enzymes produce the characteristic effect of a hormone on its target cell.

The cAMP-dependent phosphorylation mechanism produces very rapid responses to hormone (ie, within seconds), because it only requires activation of enzymes already present in the cell. Similarly, disappearance of the hormone is rapidly followed by disappearance of its effect, owing to degradation of intracellular cAMP by cyclic nucleotide phosphodiesterases and dephosphorylation of kinase substrates by phosphatases. This quick-on, quick-off mechanism is well suited for moment-to-moment regulation of physiologic responses to rapid changes in the environment—as in the "fight-or-flight" sympathetic response, which involves several cAMP-mediated processes (cardioacceleration, glycogenolysis, lipolysis, etc).

Table 35–2 lists the membrane-active hormones that are thought to act by stimulating cAMP synthesis and an additional group of hormones that are not. (Note that some hormones, such as the catecholamines, appear in both groups, because some of their actions are clearly mediated by cAMP, while others are not.)

Actions of the membrane-active hormones that do not exert their effects by elevating cAMP are not understood in detail. For this group, however, 3 potential mechanisms are beginning to emerge: (1) Some hor-

mones *reduce* adenylate cyclase activity in membranes of their target tissues, via a GTP-binding inhibitory coupling protein analogous to the stimulatory coupling protein that mediates activation of the same enzyme by other ligands. This group includes α_2-adrenoceptor agonists in platelets, prostaglandin E_1 in adipose tissue, and muscarinic agonists and somatostatin in other tissues. (2) Other neurotransmitters and hormones (eg, α_1-adrenoceptor agonists, vasopressin, and gonadotropin-releasing hormone) appear to produce some of their effects by stimulating the metabolism of membrane phosphoinositides to produce 2 intracellular messengers, inositoltrisphosphate (which elevates cytosolic calcium) and diacylglycerol (which stimulates the activity of protein kinase C). Steps in the actions of these hormones distal to calcium elevation and protein kinase C activation are poorly understood. (3) Still other hormones (eg, insulin and epidermal growth factor) stimulate an intrinsic enzymatic activity of their receptors—tyrosine-specific protein phosphorylation. Because physiologically relevant substrates phosphorylated by these receptors have not yet been identified, it is not clear how (or even whether) the kinase activity mediates cellular regulation by these hormones.

Although the biochemical mechanisms of hormone action are the subject of intensive investigation, relatively few drugs act to block or enhance the actions of hormones at sites distal to the hormone receptor. The methylxanthines caffeine and theophylline inhibit cyclic nucleotide phosphodiesterases and may produce some of their effects, such as bronchodilatation, by blocking intracellular degradation of cAMP.

Despite the lack of drugs that act specifically on postreceptor mechanisms, the multiplicity of these mechanisms has important therapeutic implications. Many important homeostatic functions are regulated by more than one hormone and often by both gene-active and membrane-active hormones. When excess or deficiency of one of these hormones is difficult to treat directly, indirect therapy based on the actions of a second hormone can often be effective. The therapeutic uses of such hormone-hormone interactions are discussed in a later section of this chapter.

THERAPY BASED ON RECEPTOR SPECIFICITY OF THE TARGET CELL

Whatever their ultimate mechanism of action on the target cell, hormones and hormone analogs derive their therapeutic usefulness from specific interactions with hormone receptors. Receptor specificity allows direct replacement of a missing hormone, use of hormone analogs with greater potency or specificity than the natural hormone, and use of hormone antagonists.

Hormone Replacement Therapy

Conceptually, treatment of endocrine deficiency disorders appears quite straightforward, now that the chemical structures of most hormones are well established and they are available in pure form. Clinically, however, effective therapy is not always simple.

In order to design an effective replacement regimen, the physician must first understand the hormone's role in normal regulation. What is the hormone's normal plasma concentration? What is the normal rate of its secretion? What are the environmental and physiologic stresses that require increased secretion of the hormone in a normal person? What additional problems in a sick patient may modify either end organ responsiveness to the hormone or its metabolism and thus alter the effectiveness or toxicity of the exogenously administered agent?

Right or wrong answers to these questions may dramatically affect the outcome of insulin replacement therapy in diabetes—determining the frequency of life-threatening ketoacidosis or hypoglycemic coma and perhaps influencing the incidence and severity of vascular complications of this disease (Chapter 40). In a more subtle fashion, knowing that the normal adrenal produces 10–20 times more cortisol under conditions of severe stress may avert disaster when a patient with adrenal insufficiency is subjected to major surgery or develops pneumonia (Chapter 38). Many similar examples are presented in subsequent chapters.

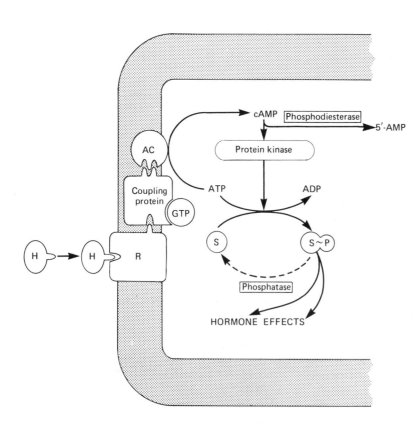

Figure 35–3. Cyclic AMP (cAMP) as an intracellular second messenger for hormones. The diagram depicts an idealized cell containing the enzymes involved in mediating the actions of hormones that work via cAMP. Hormone (H) binds to its membrane receptor (R), triggering the guanosine triphosphate (GTP)–dependent activation of adenylate cyclase (AC) by a membrane-bound coupling protein. cAMP synthesized by adenylate cyclase diffuses through the cytoplasm and activates cAMP-dependent protein kinase, which in turn catalyzes the phosphorylation of specific substrate proteins (S), usually enzymes. Altered activity of the phosphorylated substrates, denoted S~P, produces the characteristic effects of cAMP (and therefore of the hormone) in a particular cell. The stimulatory action of hormones is opposed by cyclic nucleotide phosphodiesterase, which degrades cAMP, and by phosphatases, which dephosphorylate substrates of cAMP-dependent protein kinase.

Table 35–2. Postreceptor mechanisms of action of membrane-active hormones.*

cAMP as "Second Messenger"	Other Mechanisms
Adrenocorticotropic hormone (ACTH)	Angiotensin
Calcitonin	Catecholamines (α)
Catecholamines (β)	Chorionic somatomammotropin (placental lactogen, PL)
Chorionic gonadotropin (hCG)	Epidermal growth factor (EGF)
Follicle-stimulating hormone (FSH)	Fibroblast growth factor (FGF)
Glucagon	Gonadotropin-releasing hormone (GNRH)
Histamine (H_2)	Growth hormone
Luteinizing hormone (LH)	Histamine (H_1)
Melanocyte-stimulating hormone (MSH)	Insulin
Prostacyclin (epoprostenol), prostaglandin E_1	Nerve growth factor (NGF)
Thyrotropin-releasing hormone (TRH)	Oxytocin
Thyroid-stimulating hormone (TSH)	Prolactin
Vasopressin (ADH)	Prostaglandin $F_{2\alpha}$
	Somatomedin
	Somatostatin
	Vasopressin (ADH)

*Modified and reproduced, with permission, from Baxter JD, McLeod KM: Molecular basis for hormone action. In: *Duncan's Diseases of Metabolism.* Bondy PK, Rosenberg LE (editors). Saunders, 1980.

Enhanced Specificity of Hormonal Agonists

Some endocrine drugs are used in an "extraphysiologic" fashion to produce an effect not usually observed in a normally regulated endocrine system rather than to replace a missing hormone. In this more complex situation, the physician often seeks to induce an intense pharmacologic effect in certain tissues and risks producing toxic effects in other target tissues. A cardinal example is the use of glucocorticoids for their anti-inflammatory, immunosuppressive, or lympholytic actions. The glucocorticoids may be lifesaving, but they also can produce a host of dangerous toxicities that include acute psychosis, increased catabolism of protein, arrested growth (in children), hyperglycemia, cataracts, retention of salt and water, etc (see Chapter 38).

To avoid or minimize such toxic effects, 2 therapeutic strategies may be used. The first of these—simple to describe, often difficult to use in practice—is to administer the hormonal agonist (eg, the glucocorticoid) in the lowest dose and for the shortest period possible. In every case, the drug dosage should be reduced or discontinued as soon as the disorder—bronchial asthma, Crohn's disease, thrombocytopenic purpura, etc—is amenable to less dangerous treatment.

The second strategy takes advantage of the fact that a single hormone or hormone analog may interact with more than one kind of receptor. If one of these receptors mediates the desired therapeutic effect while a second receptor is responsible for a toxic effect, the chemist may be able to design a synthetic agonist that selectively binds to the first receptor. Thus, in comparison to the natural hormone cortisol, synthetic steroids such as prednisone and dexamethasone have much greater affinity for glucocorticoid receptors. This "improvement on nature" can reduce or eliminate one of the toxic effects of adrenal steroids—retention of salt and water.

Exploitation of this kind of receptor selectivity has been most successful with chemically simple hormones such as the adrenal steroids and catecholamines. The diversity of receptors for many other hormones—including histamine, dopamine, endogenous opioids, vasopressin, and even insulin—is just beginning to be explored.

Hormone Antagonists

Disorders of hormone excess present obvious potential opportunities for use of specific hormone antagonists. Here again, the chemically simple hormones have been exploited most successfully, as with the use of α- and β-adrenoceptor antagonists in treatment of pheochromocytoma. In treating more common diseases, hormone antagonists are used to block regulatory pathways that may be physiologically normal but are nonetheless deleterious to the patient suffering from a nonendocrine disorder—eg, propranolol for hypertension, cimetidine for peptic ulcer, tamoxifen to block estrogen actions that may support growth of breast cancer, or spironolactone to block the sodium-retaining effects of aldosterone in congestive heart failure.

Useful antagonists to most of the peptide hormones have proved more difficult to synthesize, probably owing to their chemical complexity. Saralasin, an angiotensin II antagonist, is finding restricted use in the diagnosis of some kinds of hypertension (Chapter 10). Antagonists (or partial agonists) to corticotropin, luteinizing hormone–releasing hormone, glucagon, oxytocin, and parathyroid hormone have been used experimentally in animals or isolated cells but not yet in humans. Obstacles to development of such antagonist drugs include chemical complexity, the fact that they often turn out to be partial agonists (like tamoxifen and saralasin), and—especially with peptides—the difficulty of finding a drug that is effective when administered orally.

Hormone-Hormone Interactions

Virtually every important homeostatic function is regulated by more than one control system. In most cases, as with regulation of arterial blood pressure or the concentration of plasma glucose, it is possible to delineate a finely tuned network of multiple synergistic and antagonistic controls, mediated by autonomic nerves and hormones. In pathologic states where the therapeutic strategies discussed above prove inadequate, it is often possible to take advantage of these redundant regulatory mechanisms by administering hormones or hormone antagonists.

The cardiovascular and metabolic effects of excess thyroid hormone, for example, can produce a medical emergency that is difficult to treat. No specific receptor antagonist to thyroid hormone is available; drugs that suppress synthesis and release of thyroid hormone act too slowly to provide the immediate relief that may be necessary; and thyroid surgery in the thyrotoxic state is extremely dangerous. In such a situation, propranolol, a β-adrenoceptor antagonist, can swiftly reduce many of the signs and symptoms caused by excess thyroid hormone and allow time for other therapy to take effect. The physiologic basis of this therapy is fairly well understood: Thyroid hormones and β-agonist catecholamines normally regulate many functions, such as heart rate, in the same direction; in addition, thyroid hormones increase the sensitivity of the heart to β-agonists (see Chapters 9 and 37).

In the other direction, synergistic actions of hormones can sometimes be used to treat a hormone defi-

ciency when direct replacement of the hormone is difficult or impossible. Examples include the use of mineralocorticoids to maintain blood pressure in patients with autonomic insufficiency and the use of vitamin D metabolites to elevate serum calcium in hypoparathyroidism.

Note that each of these examples involves a physiologic synergism between a gene-active and a membrane-active hormonal signal (thyroid hormone and catecholamines, mineralocorticoids and catecholamines, vitamin D and parathyroid hormone). The existence of multiple hormonal controls, acting through distinct postreceptor mechanisms, allows the physician to treat disorders that are not yet amenable to more "specific" therapy.

REFERENCES

Baxter JD, McLeod KM: Molecular basis for hormone action. Chap 4, pp 104–160, in: *Duncan's Diseases of Metabolism.* Bondy PK, Rosenberg LE (editors). Saunders, 1980.

Berridge MJ, Irvine RF: Inositoltrisphosphate, a novel second messenger in signal transduction. *Nature* 1984;**312**:315.

Gilman AG: G proteins and dual control of adenylate cyclase. *Cell* 1984;**36**:577.

Roth J, Grunfeld C: Endocrine systems: Mechanisms of disease, target cells, and receptors. Chap 2, pp 15–72, in: *Textbook of Endocrinology.* Williams RH (editor). Saunders, 1981.

Sutherland EW: Studies on the mechanism of hormone action. *Science* 1972;**177**:401.

Williams RH: *Textbook of Endocrinology,* 6th ed. Saunders, 1981.

Hypothalamic & Pituitary Hormones

36

David C. Klonoff, MD, & John H. Karam, MD

Neuroendocrine control of metabolism, growth, and certain aspects of reproduction is mediated by a combination of neural and endocrine systems located in the hypothalamus and pituitary gland. The pituitary gland weighs an average of about 0.6 g and rests in the bony sella turcica under a layer of dura mater. It is connected to overlying brain by a stalk from the hypothalamus containing neurosecretory fibers surrounded by a complex of blood vessels, including a portal venous system that drains the hypothalamus and perfuses the anterior pituitary.

The pituitary gland consists of an anterior lobe (adenohypophysis), intermediate lobe, and posterior lobe (neurohypophysis), which under hypothalamic influence release a number of hormones that either control the secretion of other endocrine glands or affect metabolic actions of target tissues directly.

The secretion of anterior lobe hormones is regulated by hormones formed in the median eminence of the hypothalamus and carried to the adenohypophysis by the hypothalamic-hypophyseal portal venous system (Fig 36–1). These hormones are small peptides that function as releasing or inhibiting hormones. The structures of several of these peptides have been determined, thus permitting the synthesis of the natural hormones as well as of experimentally modified forms.

The posterior lobe hormones are synthesized in the hypothalamus and transported via the neurosecretory fibers in the stalk of the pituitary to the posterior lobe, from which they are released into the circulation.

The hormones of the intermediate lobe have melanocyte-stimulating properties that are important in animals that utilize skin color changes as adaptive mechanisms. They have not been identified as discrete hormones in humans and therefore have no role at present in clinical pharmacology.

Therapeutic preparations of pituitary and hypothalamic peptide hormones are usually synthetic; a few are purified from human sources. Their applications lie in 3 areas: (1) as replacement therapy for hormone deficiency states; (2) as drug therapy for a variety of disorders using pharmacologic doses to elicit a hormonal effect that is not present at physiologic blood levels; and (3) as diagnostic tools for performing stimulation tests to diagnose hypo- or hyperfunctional endocrine states.

HYPOTHALAMIC & ANTERIOR PITUITARY HORMONES

Hypothalamic regulatory hormones that have been identified and (in most cases) synthesized include growth hormone–releasing hormone (GRH), a growth hormone–inhibiting hormone (somatostatin), thyrotropin-releasing hormone (TRH), corticotropin-releasing hormone (CRH), gonadotropin-releasing hormone (GnRH, LHRH), and prolactin-inhibiting hormone (PIH, now believed to be dopamine).

Six anterior pituitary hormones are recognized: growth hormone (GH), thyrotropin (TSH), adrenocorticotropin (ACTH), follicle-stimulating hormone (FSH), luteinizing hormone (LH), and prolactin. Another polypeptide, β-lipotropin (β-LPH), is derived from the same prohormone, pro-opiomelanocortin, as adrenocorticotropin. β-Lipotropin is secreted from the pituitary along with adrenocorticotropin, but its hormonal function is unknown. It is a precursor of the opioid polypeptide, β-endorphin (Chapter 29).

It also appears that certain hormones from the thyroid, adrenal cortex, and gonads inhibit hypophyseal-pituitary release of their respective tropic hormones, while neurotransmitters such as serotonin, norepinephrine, and dopamine directly influence the secretion of the hypothalamic hormones by the peptidergic neurons of the median eminence.

In the discussion below, the hypothalamic control peptides are paired with their pituitary target hormones in the order in which they are listed above.

GROWTH HORMONE–RELEASING HORMONE (GRH)

The precise structure of human growth hormone–releasing hormone (GRH; tentatively called somatocrinin) has not been determined; however, 2 factors with growth hormone–releasing activity have been isolated from pancreatic islet cell tumors in patients with clinical evidence of acromegaly associated with hyperplasia of their pituitary somatotrophs (cells that synthesize somatotropin). Structural analysis has

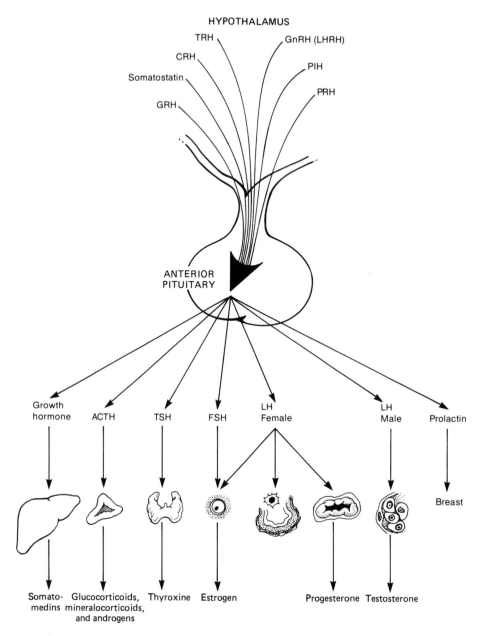

Figure 36–1. Hypothalamic releasing hormones and actions of anterior pituitary hormones. GRH, growth hormone–releasing hormone; TRH, thyrotropin-releasing hormone; CRH, corticotropin-releasing hormone; GnRH (LHRH), gonadotropin-releasing hormone, luteinizing hormone–releasing hormone; PIH, prolactin-inhibiting hormone (dopamine); and PRH, prolactin-releasing hormone.

disclosed a linear peptide with identical amino acid sequences for the first 40 amino acids in both factors. An additional 4 amino acids at the carboxy terminal end of the molecule were present in one of the factors. While GRH has yet to be isolated from human hypothalamus, there is evidence of its presence in the median eminence in human, primate, and rat hypothalamus.

Clinical Pharmacology

Both GRH$_{40}$ and GRH$_{44}$ are effective in rapidly elevating growth hormone in normal subjects as well as in

patients with idiopathic growth hormone deficiency. Doses as low as 0.5 μg/kg of body weight given intravenously rapidly elevate growth hormone levels within minutes and achieve peak responses at 1 hour. It has been found that stimulation of growth hormone release can be produced in humans after intranasal application of GRH. The effect of GRH on pituitary somatotrophs appears to be quite specific, and no other anterior pituitary hormones are secreted following GRH administration.

Except for mild facial flushing and a feeling of

warmth over the head, neck, and chest in about 60% of subjects, there were no toxic effects from acute administration of GRH to humans.

Somatostatin and somatomedin C noncompetitively inhibit the secretion of growth hormone induced by GRH at the level of the pituitary.

Diagnostic & Therapeutic Uses

GRH will be available for diagnostic evaluation of patients with idiopathic growth hormone deficiency in order to characterize anterior pituitary responsiveness. In patients whose pituitary somatotrophs are responsive to GRH and whose bone age is amenable to further growth, a therapeutic trial with GRH administration would deserve consideration, particularly if the convenience of nasal administration is substantiated by further trials of effectiveness without significant toxicity.

Preparations & Dosage

Preparations of GRH$_{44}$ are available from Bachem Inc., Torrance, California, for investigational use. An intravenous bolus of 0.5 μg/kg is effective for diagnostic purposes in humans. A therapeutic dose of 3 μg/kg of GRH$_{40}$ given subcutaneously over 1 minute every 3 hours by infusion pump produced acceleration of growth in growth hormone–deficient children.

SOMATOSTATIN
(Growth Hormone–Inhibiting Hormone, GIH, Somatotropin Release–Inhibiting Hormone)

Somatostatin, a tetradecapeptide, has been isolated from the hypothalamus and other parts of the central nervous system. It has been sequenced (Fig 36–2) and synthesized. This substance has been shown to inhibit growth hormone release in response to a wide variety of stimuli in normal individuals. It produces a decrease in circulating insulin levels and interferes with the ability of thyrotropin-releasing hormone to cause thyrotropin release. Somatostatin has also been identified in the pancreas and other sites in the gastrointestinal tract. It has been shown to inhibit the release of glucagon, insulin, and gastrin.

Exogenously administered somatostatin is rapidly cleared from the circulation, with an initial half-life of 1–3 minutes. The kidney appears to play an important role in its metabolism and excretion.

Somatostatin can effectively inhibit growth hormone release in patients with acromegaly. However, it is of no use in the treatment of this disorder because of its lack of specificity and short duration of action.

Peptides have been synthesized that partially separate the various properties of somatostatin, and a 7-aminoheptanoic acid derivative containing only 4 of the 14 amino acids of somatostatin has been found to block the effect of somatostatin.

A 28-amino-acid peptide called prosomatostatin isolated from intestine and hypothalamus is believed to be the precursor of somatostatin. It is 10 times more potent than somatostatin in inhibiting insulin secretion in rats, but its effect on glucagon secretion is only twice that of somatostatin. Its greater potency and prolonged action make prosomatostatin more useful than somatostatin in testing hormonal control mechanisms.

GROWTH HORMONE
(Somatotropin, GH)

Growth hormone is a peptide hormone produced by the anterior pituitary. Growth hormone has direct metabolic effects on lipolysis in adipose tissue and on insulin action and indirect anabolic effects mediated through another class of factors known as somatomedins.

Chemistry & Pharmacokinetics

A. Structure: Growth hormone is a 191-amino-acid peptide with 2 sulfhydryl bridges. Its structure closely resembles that of prolactin and the placental hormone human chorionic somatomammotropin. Growth hormone for pharmacologic use is presently extracted from human cadaver pituitaries.

B. Absorption, Metabolism, and Excretion: Circulating endogenous growth hormone has a half-life of 20–25 minutes and is predominantly cleared by the liver. Human growth hormone can be dissolved in a 15% w/v gelatin solution and administered intramuscularly, with peak levels occurring in 2–4 hours and active blood levels persisting for 36 hours.

Pharmacodynamics

Growth hormone has both metabolic and anabolic effects. The metabolic consequence of a pharmacologic dose of growth hormone is an initial insulinlike effect with increased tissue uptake of both glucose and amino acids and decreased lipolysis. Within a few hours there is a peripheral insulin-antagonistic effect with impaired glucose uptake and increased lipolysis.

The major anabolic consequence of a pharmacologic dose of growth hormone is longitudinal growth. The anabolic effects of growth hormone are mediated indirectly via another class of peptide hormones, the somatomedins, or insulinlike growth factors. Growth hormone stimulates synthesis of somatomedins (predominantly in the liver); somatomedins promote uptake of sulfate into cartilage and are probably the actual mediators of the cellular processes associated with bone growth. This growth can be traced back to the molecular level, where increased incorporation of

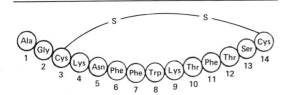

Figure 36–2. Amino acid sequence of somatostatin.

thymidine into DNA and uridine into RNA occur (indicating cellular proliferation) along with increased conversion of proline to hydroxyproline (indicating cartilage synthesis).

It has long been recognized that growth hormone deficiency leads to inadequate somatomedin production and dwarfism. There are also states of dwarfism in which elevated plasma growth hormone levels fail to induce adequate production of somatomedins.

Clinical Pharmacology

Timely growth hormone replacement therapy will permit achievement of full predicted adult height in children with growth hormone deficiency. Criteria for diagnosis of growth hormone deficiency usually include (1) stature more than 2 SD below the mean for age and sex, (2) growth velocity (measured over 1 year) below the 25th percentile for age, and (3) impaired growth hormone secretion during an insulin tolerance test. The prevalence of congenital growth hormone deficiency is approximately one in 4000. Congenital growth hormone deficiency can result from lesions affecting the hypophyseal-pituitary region such as craniopharyngiomas but is most often due to lack of hypothalamic growth hormone–releasing factors, resulting in pituitary dwarfism. In the newborn, hypoglycemia and even seizures can occur in the absence of growth hormone.

In addition to isolated growth hormone deficiency, congenital deficiencies of multiple pituitary hormones occur with approximately equal frequency. Affected children will respond with normal growth to administration of growth hormone plus other appropriate pituitary replacement preparations. Acquired growth hormone deficiency, which is often accompanied by multiple hormone deficiencies, may also respond well to growth hormone plus other hormone replacements as needed provided the underlying disease process can be controlled.

Short-term growth hormone therapy has been reported to increase growth in some young children whose short stature and delayed bone age have *not* been associated with low levels of somatomedin C or with impaired responsiveness of growth hormone to intense combined stimuli. However, until long-term studies have documented that growth hormone therapy will increase final height of these short "normal" children without producing adverse effects, use of human growth hormone should be limited to therapy of those children with short stature due to growth hormone deficiency.

Preparations & Dosage

Animal preparations of growth hormone are ineffective in humans. Treatment of children with human growth hormone has been limited by the scarcity of the hormone as well as its expense.

In the past, all commercially available growth hormone (somatropin) was freeze-extracted from human pituitaries. It was available in vials containing 4 IU (Crescormon) or 2 or 10 IU (Asellacrin). Specific activity of these preparations is approximately 21 IU per milligram of protein. Biosynthetic growth hormone has replaced these human-derived preparations (see below).

Stimulated by the great need for a larger supply of growth hormone, a massive research effort has been successful in producing a biosynthetic human growth hormone through recombinant DNA technology. The expressed product contains the same amino acid sequence as human growth hormone, except for the addition of a methionyl residue at the N-terminal end. By all of the indices measured in short-term studies, synthetic methionyl human growth hormone (somatrem, Protropin) is equipotent with pituitary human growth hormone and justifies current optimism that adequate supplies of growth hormone will soon be available to meet clinical needs. The recommended dosage of somatrem is 0.1 mg/kg (0.2 IU/kg) intramuscularly, given 3 times per week.

Toxicity & Contraindications

In 1985, the National Hormone and Pituitary Program halted distribution of human pituitary–derived growth hormone in the USA after it received reports that 3 patients had died of Creutzfeldt-Jakob disease 5, 6, and 7 years after cessation of therapy with growth hormone. Because Creutzfeldt-Jakob disease is extremely rare in young adults (the patients were 20, 22, and 24 years old), it was considered possible that they had been infected with the neurotropic virus in the growth hormone preparations. One similar case has been reported in the UK.

Antibody formation may occur in 10–20% of patients treated with pituitary growth hormone and in over half of patients treated with synthetic methionyl hormone. These antibodies rarely interfere with the activity of this hormone.

Growth hormone is contraindicated in a patient with closed epiphyses or an expanding intracranial mass. Patients receiving growth hormone should be screened regularly for diabetes. If growth slows in the absence of rising antibody titers, hypopituitarism should be ruled out. Untreated hypothyroidism or excessive glucocorticoid replacement therapy can impair growth.

THYROTROPIN-RELEASING HORMONE (TRH)

Thyrotropin-releasing hormone, or protirelin, is a tripeptide hormone found in the hypothalamus as well as in other parts of the brain. TRH is secreted into the portal venous system and stimulates the pituitary to produce thyrotropin, which in turn stimulates the thyroid to produce thyroxine (T_4). TRH stimulation of thyrotropin is blocked by thyroxine and stimulated by lack of thyroxine such that the extent of thyrotropin response to TRH stimulation forms the basis for using TRH as a diagnostic agent in the evaluation of hyperthyroid and hypothyroid states.

Chemistry & Pharmacokinetics

A. Structure: TRH is (pyro)Glu-His-Pro-NH$_2$.

Thyrotropin-releasing hormone
(protirelin)

B. Absorption, Metabolism, and Excretion: TRH is usually administered intravenously. Rapid plasma inactivation occurs, with a half-life of 4–5 minutes.

Pharmacodynamics

TRH stimulates pituitary production of thyrotropin, possibly through stimulation of adenylate cyclase. TRH stimulation of thyrotropin may be blocked by pretreatment with thyroxine, corticosteroids, and somatostatin. TRH stimulation of prolactin production is not blocked.

Peak serum thyrotropin levels occur 20–30 minutes after an intravenous TRH injection in healthy individuals. In hyperthyroidism, high serum thyroxine levels blunt the thyrotropin response to TRH. In primary hypothyroidism, thyrotropin levels start high, and the pituitary response to TRH may be quite large, with a particularly brisk outpouring of additional thyrotropin. In secondary (pituitary) hypothyroidism, serum thyrotropin levels start low and fail to rise after TRH administration. In tertiary (hypothalamic) hypothyroidism, the baseline serum thyrotropin level may be low or normal, and the thyrotropin response to TRH may be delayed.

TRH infusion leads to stimulation of prolactin release by the pituitary in healthy individuals but has no effect on cells producing growth hormone or ACTH. In certain types of pituitary tumors, however, the neoplastic cells may respond abnormally to TRH by releasing growth hormone (in acromegaly), by releasing ACTH (in Cushing's disease), or by failing to release prolactin (in prolactinoma). Timely high-dose TRH infusion may improve the outcome of spinal cord injuries. This property of TRH is currently being investigated. The mechanism is unknown.

Clinical Pharmacology

TRH is used only for diagnostic purposes. A TRH infusion test is the most sensitive method for diagnosing mild hyperthyroidism and mild hypothyroidism in the minimally symptomatic patient with equivocal serum thyroxine or thyrotropin levels. In spite of overlap in the responses between various hyper- and hypothyroid states and normals, the test is quite valuable in some patients.

A blunted thyrotropin response to TRH occurs in approximately half of euthyroid patients with Graves' exophthalmopathy, whereas orbital mass lesions are associated with a normal thyrotropin response.

TRH infusion has also been suggested as a diagnostic test for differentiating unipolar and bipolar depressions. However, a blunted thyrotropin response can occur in many psychiatric disorders, making such a test useless.

Preparations & Dosage

TRH is available as protirelin (Relefact TRH, Thypinone) in ampules for intravenous injection. The dosage is 500 μg for adults and 7 μg/kg for children age 6 or older but not to exceed the adult dose. A baseline thyrotropin level should be obtained, followed by 3 further determinations at 15, 30, and 60 minutes postinfusion.

Toxicity

Up to 50% of patients tested may note side effects lasting for a few minutes: nausea, an urge to urinate, light-headedness, a metallic taste, or abdominal discomfort. Transient hypertension may occur.

THYROID-STIMULATING HORMONE (Thyrotropin, TSH)

Thyrotropin is an anterior pituitary hormone that regulates thyroid function by stimulating production of thyroxine. Diagnostic use of thyrotropin in various states of borderline thyroid function has been largely supplanted by measurement of the baseline thyrotropin concentration and its response to TRH as well as by sensitive radionuclide scanning methods. Therapeutic use of thyrotropin in conjunction with ^{131}I ablation is established in selected cases of thyroid carcinoma to enhance thyroid radioiodine uptake.

Chemistry & Pharmacokinetics

A. Structure: Thyrotropin consists of 2 peptides (α and β), each containing branched carbohydrate side chains. Therapeutic thyrotropin is prepared from bovine anterior pituitaries. There is 70% homology between human and bovine TSH-α subunits and 90% homology between human and bovine TSH-β subunits. The TSH-α subunit sequence in humans is virtually identical to that of the α subunit of FSH, LH, and hCG.

B. Absorption, Metabolism, and Excretion: Thyrotropin is administered intramuscularly or subcutaneously. Its half-life is approximately 1 hour, with degradation occurring in the kidneys. However, unlike gonadotropins, little thyrotropin appears in the urine.

Pharmacodynamics

Thyrotropin stimulates thyroid cell adenylate cyclase activity. Increased cAMP production causes increased iodine uptake and, ultimately, increased production of thyroid hormones. Increased thyroid size and vascularity follow thyrotropin administration.

Clinical Pharmacology

A. Diagnostic Uses: Radioiodine uptake following thyrotropin uptake has been used to distinguish primary and secondary hypothyroidism from the euthyroid state. This method has been largely replaced by TRH stimulation of thyrotropin production, which is quicker, less expensive, and easier to interpret.

B. Therapeutic Uses: Thyrotropin has a role in the therapy of metastatic thyroid carcinoma. Following a tumoricidal dose of ^{131}I, the patient is maintained on triiodothyronine for 10 weeks and then taken off hormone replacement for 3 weeks. Finally, the patient is given thyrotropin, 5–10 units subcutaneously daily for 3–7 days, in an attempt to elicit iodine uptake by remaining metastatic tissue. Additional ^{131}I is then administered if needed.

Preparations & Dosage

Thyrotropin (Thytropar) is derived from beef pituitaries and is intended for intramuscular or subcutaneous administration. A dose of 5 units per day for 3 days is used for diagnostic purposes; 5–10 units per day for 3–7 days is used in conjunction with ^{131}I for ablation of thyroid carcinoma.

Toxicity

Local soreness at the injection site is common. Nausea, vomiting, thyroid tenderness, allergic symptoms, and symptoms of hyperthyroidism may occur. This drug should be used cautiously in the presence of heart disease or adrenocortical insufficiency.

CORTICOTROPIN-RELEASING HORMONE (CRH)

This hypothalamic peptide contains 41 amino acids. It has been chemically synthesized and proved to have corticotropin-releasing action on cultured pituitary cells. This effect is associated with cAMP generation. The hormone-releasing action of CRH is specific for corticotrophs (cells that synthesize corticotropin), since only ACTH and β-endorphin release occurs, with no observed effect on growth hormone, gonadotropin prolactin, or thyrotropin secretion.

Clinical Pharmacology

Glucocorticoids prevent the release of ACTH by cultured pituitary corticotrophs in response to CRH. However, in patients with Cushing's disease, CRH can elevate plasma ACTH levels despite supranormal plasma cortisol values. This contrasts with the failure of TRH to stimulate TSH release when circulating thyroxine levels are supranormal. The corticotroph response to CRH is dose-dependent, and sensitivity to CRH is the same regardless of whether it is administered in the evening or early morning. Vasopressin

clearly potentiates the ACTH-releasing effects of submaximal doses of CRH.

Diagnostic Uses

CRH has been administered in a variety of hypothalamic-pituitary-adrenal disorders in attempts to differentiate hypothalamic versus pituitary causes of ACTH deficiency or excess. Plasma ACTH responses in Cushing's disease are variable but generally show a stimulation of plasma ACTH. Peak levels achieved may exceed those of normals, but the incremental increase above baseline is generally less than that seen in normals receiving CRH. Patients with Addison's disease and Nelson's syndrome show an exaggerated response of plasma ACTH, while patients with Sheehan's syndrome—or with Cushing's syndrome due to a primary tumor of the adrenal—do not show a rise in plasma ACTH after receiving CRH.

The availability of CRH should permit the development of specific radioimmunoassays to elucidate its physiologic role and to determine whether it contributes to the pathogenesis of Cushing's disease.

Toxicity

Intravenous bolus doses of 1 $\mu g/kg$ of body weight or higher result in flushing of the head and chest. Bolus doses of 3 $\mu g/kg$ or more often cause shortness of breath, tightness of the chest, and a transient slight fall in blood pressure. At doses less than 1 $\mu g/kg$, these side effects do not occur.

ADRENOCORTICOTROPIN (Corticotropin, ACTH)

Adrenocorticotropin is a peptide hormone produced in the anterior pituitary. Its primary endocrine function is to stimulate synthesis and release of adrenocortical hormones. Pharmacologic administration of corticotropin results in increased production not only of cortisol but of adrenal androgens and mineralocorticoids as well. Corticotropin can be used therapeutically, but its primary usefulness is in the assessment of adrenocortical responsiveness. A substandard adrenocortical response to exogenous corticotropin administration indicates adrenocortical insufficiency.

Chemistry & Pharmacokinetics

A. Structure: Human ACTH is a single polypeptide chain of 39 amino acids (Fig 36–3). The N-terminal portion containing amino acids 1–24 is necessary for full biologic activity. The remaining amino acids (25–39) confer species specificity. Therapeutic ACTH preparations are derived from porcine pituitaries and differ in structure from human ACTH only in the nonessential 25–39 region. Synthetic human $ACTH_{1-24}$ is known as cosyntropin (Cortrosyn). The N-terminal amino acids 1–13 are identical to melanocyte-stimulating hormone (α-MSH), which has been found in animals but not in humans. In states of

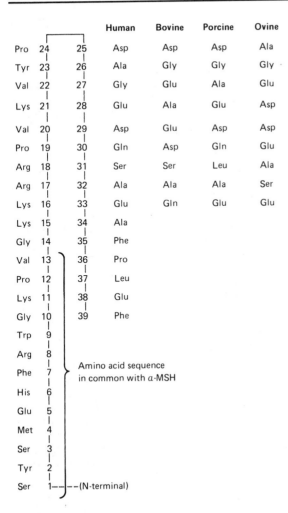

			Human	Bovine	Porcine	Ovine
Pro	24	25	Asp	Asp	Asp	Ala
Tyr	23	26	Ala	Gly	Gly	Gly
Val	22	27	Gly	Glu	Ala	Glu
Lys	21	28	Glu	Ala	Glu	Asp
Val	20	29	Asp	Glu	Asp	Asp
Pro	19	30	Gln	Asp	Gln	Glu
Arg	18	31	Ser	Ser	Leu	Ala
Arg	17	32	Ala	Ala	Ala	Ser
Lys	16	33	Glu	Gln	Glu	Glu
Lys	15	34	Ala			
Gly	14	35	Phe			
Val	13	36	Pro			
Pro	12	37	Leu			
Lys	11	38	Glu			
Gly	10	39	Phe			
Trp	9					
Arg	8					
Phe	7	} Amino acid sequence in common with α-MSH				
His	6					
Glu	5					
Met	4					
Ser	3					
Tyr	2					
Ser	1	(N-terminal)				

Figure 36–3. Amino acid sequences of human, bovine, porcine, and ovine adrenocorticotropin.

excessive pituitary ACTH secretion, hyperpigmentation, due to the α-MSH activity intrinsic to ACTH, may be noted.

ACTH from animal sources is assayed biologically by measuring the depletion of adrenocortical ascorbic acid that follows subcutaneous administration of the ACTH. Synthetic ACTH can be assayed by weight. The steroidogenic activity of 1 unit of porcine ACTH is approximately equal to that of 10 μg of cosyntropin.

B. Absorption, Metabolism, and Excretion: Both porcine and synthetic corticotropin are well absorbed by the intramuscular route. Corticotropin cannot be administered orally because of gastrointestinal proteolysis.

The biologic half-lives of $ACTH_{1-39}$ and $ACTH_{1-24}$ are under 20 minutes. Tissue uptake occurs in the liver and kidneys. $ACTH_{1-39}$ is transformed into a biologically inactive substance with a structure similar to that of $ACTH_{1-39}$, probably by modification of a side chain. ACTH is not excreted in the urine in significant amounts.

The effects of a long-acting repository form of porcine corticotropin persist for up to 18 hours with an ACTH-gelatin complex, and up to several days with an ACTH-zinc hydroxide complex.

Pharmacodynamics

ACTH stimulates the adrenal cortex to produce glucocorticoids, mineralocorticoids, and androgens. ACTH increases the activity of cholesterol esterase, the enzyme that catalyzes the rate-limiting step of steroid hormone production: cholesterol → pregnenolone. ACTH also stimulates adrenal hypertrophy and hyperplasia. In pharmacologic doses, corticotropin may cause adipose tissue lipolysis and increased skin pigmentation.

Clinical Pharmacology

A. Therapeutic Uses: Corticotropin may be prescribed for patients with normal adrenal function when increased glucocorticoid concentrations are desired. In choosing between ACTH and glucocorticoids, side effects should be considered, since their effectiveness is similar. On balance, the disadvantages of ACTH appear to outweigh its advantages, making glucocorticoids the drugs of choice in chronic conditions where anti-inflammatory or immunosuppressive therapy is warranted.

B. Diagnostic Uses: ACTH stimulation of the adrenals will fail to elicit an appropriate response in states of adrenal insufficiency. A rapid test for ruling out adrenal insufficiency employs cosyntropin (see below). Plasma cortisol levels are measured before and either 30 or 60 minutes following an intramuscular or intravenous injection of 0.25 mg of cosyntropin. A normal plasma cortisol response is a stimulated increment exceeding 7 μg/dL and a peak level exceeding 18 μg/dL. A subnormal response indicates primary or secondary adrenocortical insufficiency that can be differentiated using plasma ACTH levels (which are increased in primary adrenal insufficiency and decreased in the secondary form). An incremental rise in plasma aldosterone generally occurs in secondary but not primary adrenal insufficiency after cosyntropin stimulation.

The plasma 17-hydroxyprogesterone level rises in response to rapid ACTH infusion in patients with classic congenital adrenal hyperplasia due to 21-hydroxylase deficiency. Detection of the carrier state for this gene may be possible using this method, since heterozygotes also show enhanced production of 17-hydroxyprogesterone with ACTH infusion.

A milder type of 21-hydroxylase deficiency "acquired" as teenager or adult can be biochemically distinguished from classic "congenital" 21-hydroxylase deficiency by prolonged ACTH stimulation. A normal cortisol response occurs in the nonclassic type, whereas the response is subnormal in the classic type.

Preparations & Dosage

Porcine corticotropin is available in vials containing 25, 40, and 80 units per milliliter for parenteral use. Repository preparations containing gelatin for intramuscular or subcutaneous use or zinc hydroxide for intramuscular use only are available in vials containing 40 or 80 units/mL. Cosyntropin (Cortrosyn) (synthetic human $ACTH_{1-24}$) is available in vials of 0.25 mg for intravenous or intramuscular use. ACTH may be used therapeutically in doses of 10–20 units 4 times daily. Repository ACTH, 40–80 units, may be administered every 24–72 hours. Cosyntropin, 0.25 mg (= 25 units), is used for diagnostic studies.

Toxicity & Contraindications

The toxicity of ACTH resembles that of the glucocorticoids. The occasional development of antibodies to animal ACTH or to depot cosyntropin (a preparation not currently available in the USA) has produced anaphylactic reactions or refractoriness to ACTH therapy in a few individuals. Painful swelling occurs at the injection site more often with the zinc hydroxide depot preparation than with the gelatin preparation.

Contraindications are similar to those of glucocorticoids. Use of ACTH during pregnancy should be minimized. When immediate effects are desired, glucocorticoids are preferable.

GONADOTROPIN-RELEASING HORMONE (GnRH; Luteinizing Hormone–Releasing Hormone [LHRH])

Gonadotropin-releasing hormone is a decapeptide that controls release of the gonadotropins FSH and LH.

Chemistry & Pharmacokinetics

A. Structure: GnRH is a decapeptide found in all mammals. Pharmaceutical GnRH is synthetic.

PGlu-His-Trp-Ser-Tyr-Gly-Leu-Arg-Pro-Gly-NH$_2$
  1   2   3   4   5   6   7   8 9 10

Gonadotropin-releasing hormone (GnRH)

PGlu-His-Trp-Ser-Tyr-D-Leu-Leu-Arg-Pro-NHCH$_2$CH$_3$
  1   2   3   4   5   6   7   8 9

Leuprolide

B. Absorption, Metabolism, and Excretion: GnRH may be administered intravenously or subcutaneously. Long-acting analogs of GnRH may eventually be administered by nasal spray or vaginal pessary. Intravenous GnRH has a half-life of 5–27 minutes and is almost completely degraded in the blood except for 2%, which is excreted in the urine.

Pharmacodynamics

GnRH binds to receptors on pituitary gonadotropes. When administered intermittently, it stimulates FSH and LH secretion. Prolonged GnRH administration blocks gonadotropin release.

Clinical Pharmacology

A. Diagnostic Uses: GnRH is currently approved only for diagnostic use. It is of limited benefit in evaluating selected cases of suspected hypogonadism. Following intravenous or subcutaneous administration of a 100-μg bolus of GnRH, serum LH levels are measured sequentially. An appropriate LH surge indicates the presence of functional pituitary gonadotropes but does not predict pituitary gonadotropic reserve. A flat LH curve does not distinguish pituitary from hypothalamic disease, however.

B. Therapeutic Uses: There is promising experimental evidence that pulsatile administration of GnRH causing pituitary stimulation can induce ovulation in women with hypothalamic amenorrhea and spermatogenesis in men with hypogonadotropic hypogonadism. Experimental data also demonstrate that administration of long-acting GnRH analogs which cause pituitary suppression can be effective for treating polycystic ovary syndrome, endometriosis, premenstrual syndrome, and precocious puberty. One GnRH analog, **leuprolide** (shown above), offers promise in the treatment of prostatic cancer.

Preparations & Dosage

GnRH is available as gonadorelin hydrochloride (Factrel) in 100-μg and 500-μg vials. Dosage is described above under diagnostic uses. In women, the test should be performed during the first 7 days of the menstrual cycle.

Toxicity

Systemic complaints such as headache, abdominal discomfort, and flushing are reported rarely. Subcutaneous administration can cause a rash.

FOLLICLE-STIMULATING HORMONE (FSH)

Follicle-stimulating hormone is a glycoprotein hormone produced in the anterior pituitary that, along with LH, regulates gonadal function. It is composed of 2 peptide chains. The principal function of FSH is to stimulate gametogenesis and follicular development in women and spermatogenesis in men.

A naturally modified form of FSH is available for therapeutic use. The urine of postmenopausal women contains a substance with FSH-like properties but with 4% of the potency and a different dose-response curve. There is also an LH-like substance in such urine. The use of these excreted menotropins (postmenopausal gonadotropins) is discussed below.

FSH acts on the immature follicular cells of the ovary and induces development of the mature follicle and oocyte. In the testes, FSH acts on the Sertoli cells and stimulates their production of androgen-binding protein.

LUTEINIZING HORMONE
(LH)

Luteinizing hormone is a glycoprotein hormone consisting of 2 chains and, like FSH, is produced by the anterior pituitary. LH is primarily responsible for regulation of gonadal steroid hormone production. No LH preparation is presently available for clinical use. Human chorionic gonadotropin—with an almost identical structure—is available and can be used as a luteinizing hormone substitute in many gonadotropin-deficient states.

LH acts on testicular Leydig cells to stimulate testosterone production. In the ovary, LH acts in concert with FSH to stimulate follicular development. LH acts on the mature follicle to induce ovulation, and it stimulates the corpus luteum in the luteal phase of the menstrual cycle to produce progesterone and androgens.

HUMAN MENOPAUSAL GONADOTROPINS
(hMG)

Human menopausal gonadotropins are a mixture of partially catabolized human FSH and LH extracted from the urine of postmenopausal women. The commercial preparation of hMG, or menotropins (Pergonal), is biologically standardized for FSH and LH content. It is used in states of infertility to stimulate ovarian follicle development in women and spermatogenesis in men. In both sexes, it must be used in conjunction with a luteinizing hormone, ie, human chorionic gonadotropin (hCG), to permit ovulation and implantation in women and testosterone production and full masculinization in men.

Pharmacokinetics

Over a 14-day course of daily hMG administration intended to mimic the follicular phase of the ovarian cycle in women with hypothalamic amenorrhea, FSH levels gradually rise to twice their baseline level, and LH levels increase to 1½ times the baseline.

Pharmacodynamics

Ovarian follicular growth and maturation will occur during hMG treatment of gonadotropin-deficient women. Ovulation requires administration of chorionic gonadotropin when adequate follicular maturation has occurred.

In men with gonadotropin deficiencies, pretreatment with chorionic gonadotropin produces external sexual maturation; addition of a course of hMG will stimulate spermatogenesis and lead to fertility.

Clinical Pharmacology

Human menopausal gonadotropin is indicated for pituitary or hypothalamic hypogonadism with infertility. Anovulatory women with the following conditions may benefit from hMG: primary amenorrhea, secondary amenorrhea, polycystic ovary syndrome, and anovulatory cycles.

Over 50% of men with hypogonadotropic hypogonadism become fertile after hMG administration.

Preparations & Dosage

An ampule of menotropins (Pergonal) contains 75 IU of FSH and 75 IU of LH. By bioassay, 1 IU of LH is approximately equivalent to 0.5 IU of hCG. Human menopausal gonadotropin is administered intramuscularly.

A. Women: One ampule is administered daily for 9–12 days until evidence of adequate follicular maturation is present. Serum estradiol levels and a cervical examination should be performed daily. When appropriate follicular maturation has occurred, hMG is discontinued; the following day, hCG, 10,000 IU, is administered intramuscularly to induce ovulation.

B. Men: Following pretreatment with 4000–5000 IU of hCG 3 times weekly for up to 6 months in order to achieve masculinization, menotropins is administered as one ampule weekly in combination with hCG, 2000 IU twice weekly. At least 4 months of combined treatment are usually necessary before spermatozoa appear in the ejaculate.

Toxicity & Contraindications

Overstimulation of the ovary can lead to uncomplicated ovarian enlargement in approximately 20% of patients. This usually resolves spontaneously. The "hyperstimulation syndrome" occurs in 0.5–4% of patients. It is characterized by hMG-induced ovarian enlargement, ascites, hydrothorax, and hypovolemia, sometimes to the point of shock. Hemoperitoneum (from a ruptured ovarian cyst), fever, or arterial thromboembolism can occur. The frequency of multiple births is approximately 20%. A reported 25% incidence of spontaneous abortions may be due to earlier diagnosis of pregnancy in treated than in untreated patients, with recognition of very early abortion. There may, however, be abnormal development and premature degeneration of corpus luteum in some treated patients. Gynecomastia occasionally occurs in men.

Human menopausal gonadotropin should be administered only by a physician experienced in treating infertility. Before treatment of women, a thorough gynecologic evaluation must be performed to rule out uterine, tubal, or ovarian disease as well as pregnancy. In cases of irregular bleeding, uterine cancer should be ruled out.

HUMAN CHORIONIC GONADOTROPIN
(hCG)

Human chorionic gonadotropin is a hormone produced by the human placenta and excreted into the urine, whence it can be extracted and purified. The function of hCG is to stimulate the ovarian corpus luteum to produce progesterone and maintain the placenta. It is very similar to LH in structure and is used to treat both men and women with LH deficiency.

Human chorionic gonadotropin is a glycoprotein consisting of an alpha chain virtually identical to that of FSH, LH, and TSH and a beta chain of 147 amino acids that resembles that of LH except for the presence of a carboxy terminal sequence of 30 amino acids not present in LH.

Pharmacokinetics

Human chorionic gonadotropin is well absorbed after intramuscular administration and has a biologic half-life of 8 hours, compared to 30 minutes for LH. The difference may lie in the high sialic acid content of hCG compared to LH. It is apparently modified in the body prior to urinary excretion, because the half-life measured by immunoassay far exceeds that measured by bioassay.

Pharmacodynamics

Human chorionic gonadotropin stimulates production of gonadal steroid hormones. The interstitial and corpus luteal cells of the female produce progesterone, and the Leydig cells of the male produce testosterone. It can be used to mimic a midcycle LH surge and trigger ovulation in a hypogonadotropic woman.

Human chorionic gonadotropin has no established effect on fat mobilization, fat distribution, or appetite. It has been advocated without justification as an adjunct to dietary management in obese patients.

Clinical Pharmacology

A. Diagnostic Uses: In prepubertal boys with undescended gonads, a truly retained (cryptorchid) testis can be distinguished from a retracted (pseudocryptorchid) one using hCG. Testicular descent during a course of hCG administration usually foretells permanent testicular descent at puberty, when circulating LH levels rise. Lack of descent usually means that orchiopexy will be necessary at puberty to preserve spermatogenesis.

Patients with constitutional delay in onset of puberty can be distinguished from those with hypogonadotropic hypogonadism using repeated hCG stimulation. Serum testosterone and estradiol levels rise in the former but not in the latter group.

B. Therapeutic Uses: As described above, hCG can be used in combination with human menotropins to induce ovulation in women with secondary hypogonadism or to induce spermatogenesis in men with secondary hypogonadism.

Preparations & Dosage

Lyophilized powder preparations are available. The dosages for female and male infertility are described under hMG dosage. For prepubertal cryptorchidism, a dosage of 500–4000 units 3 times weekly for up to 6 weeks has been advocated.

Toxicity & Contraindications

Reported side effects include headache, depression, edema, precocious puberty, gynecomastia, or (rarely) production of antibodies to hCG.

Human chorionic gonadotropin should be administered for infertility only by a physician with experience in this field. Androgen-dependent neoplasia and precocious puberty are contraindications to its use.

PROLACTIN

Prolactin is a glycoprotein hormone produced in the anterior pituitary whose structure resembles that of growth hormone. Prolactin is the principal hormone responsible for lactation. Milk production is stimulated by prolactin when appropriate circulating levels of estrogens, progestins, corticosteroids, and insulin are present. Deficiency of prolactin—which can occur in states of pituitary deficiency—is manifested only by failure to lactate. In hypothalamic destruction, prolactin levels may be elevated as a result of impaired transport of prolactin-inhibiting hormone (dopamine) to the pituitary. Hyperprolactinemia can produce galactorrhea and hypogonadism and may be associated with symptoms of a pituitary mass. No preparation is available for use in prolactin-deficient patients. For patients with symptomatic hyperprolactinemia, inhibition of prolactin secretion can be achieved with bromocriptine, a dopamine agonist (see below), or with pergolide, an experimental dopamine agonist related to bromocriptine.

BROMOCRIPTINE

Although bromocriptine is not a hormone, it has important inhibitory effects on the pituitary that warrant its discussion here.

Bromocriptine is an ergot derivative with dopamine agonist properties that lowers circulating prolactin levels. Its chemical structure and pharmacokinetic features are presented in Chapter 15.

Bromocriptine decreases pituitary prolactin secretion through dopaminemimetic action on the pituitary at 2 central nervous system loci: (1) It decreases dopamine turnover in the tuberoinfundibular neurons of the arcuate nucleus, generating increased hypothalamic dopamine; and (2) it acts directly on pituitary dopamine receptors to inhibit spontaneous prolactin release and that evoked by thyrotropin-releasing hormone. Bromocriptine stimulates pituitary growth hormone release in normal subjects and—paradoxically, and for unknown reasons—suppresses growth hormone release in acromegalics.

Clinical Pharmacology

A. Amenorrhea/Galactorrhea: Bromocriptine is approved in the USA for short-term treatment of amenorrhea/galactorrhea associated with various hyperprolactinemic states other than pituitary tumors. Idiopathic hyperprolactinemia responds well to bromocriptine. Upon cessation of therapy, hyperprolactinemia and galactorrhea generally recur.

B. Physiologic Lactation: Bromocriptine suppresses the prolactin secretion that occurs after parturition or abortion and is used to prevent breast engorgement when breast feeding is not desired.

C. Prolactin-Secreting Adenomas: Although not yet approved in the USA for this purpose, bromocriptine is gaining wide acceptance as initial treatment for prolactinomas. Significant reduction in both tumor size and serum prolactin levels can be demonstrated with bromocriptine treatment. For definitive therapy of such tumors, eventual surgical excision with or without radiation therapy probably remains necessary, because the effects of long-term bromocriptine therapy are not known, and expansion of these tumors may occur if bromocriptine is discontinued.

D. Acromegaly: Although not approved for this indication in the USA, bromocriptine has also been used for acromegaly. Acromegalic patients demonstrate improvement of symptoms less frequently than those with prolactinomas and rarely achieve clinical remissions. There may also be dissociation between clinical improvement and plasma growth hormone levels, which may fall but rarely to normal. The role of bromocriptine in acromegaly remains to be determined.

E. Parkinson's Disease: The use of bromocriptine in Parkinson's disease is discussed in Chapter 26.

Preparations & Dosage

Bromocriptine (Parlodel) is supplied as 2.5-mg tablets and 5-mg capsules (as the mesylate). For amenorrhea/galactorrhea or prevention of physiologic lactation, 2.5–10 mg in divided doses taken with meals is used, and this dose is generally adequate to treat prolactin microadenomas. For larger prolactinomas, daily doses up to 20 mg may be needed, and even higher doses are required in acromegaly. Doses should be increased by no more than 2.5–5 mg/d.

Toxicity & Contraindications

Doses up to 10 mg daily may cause nausea, lightheadedness, orthostatic hypotension, or constipation. Doses above 10 mg daily may cause cold-induced peripheral digital vasospasms, neuropsychiatric symptoms, or, rarely, peptic ulcer.

Although bromocriptine therapy during the first 3 weeks of pregnancy has not been associated with an increased risk of spontaneous abortion or congenital malformations, there are few data on the safety of bromocriptine if used throughout gestation. Therefore, bromocriptine should not be used in a woman known to be pregnant. A woman receiving bromocriptine therapy whose period is late should be tested for pregnancy.

POSTERIOR PITUITARY HORMONES

Two posterior pituitary hormones are known: vasopressin and oxytocin. Their structures are very similar (Fig 36–4), and they probably have a common phylogenetic precursor. Secretion of posterior pituitary hormones is not regulated by hypothalamic releasing hormones, as is the case with anterior pituitary hormones. Posterior pituitary hormones are synthesized in the hypothalamus and then transported intracellularly to the posterior pituitary, from which they are released into the circulation.

OXYTOCIN

Oxytocin is a peptide secreted by the posterior pituitary that elicits milk ejection in lactating women. In therapeutic doses, oxytocin can be used to induce uterine contractions and maintain labor; however, at physiologic blood levels, the contribution of this hormone to parturition is probably small.

Chemistry & Pharmacokinetics

A. Structure: Oxytocin is a 9-amino-acid peptide composed of a 6-amino-acid disulfide ring and a 3-membered tail containing the carboxy terminus. Oxytocin and vasopressin differ by only one amino acid residue each from vasotocin, which is the only posterior pituitary hormone found in nonmammalian vertebrates.

B. Absorption, Metabolism, and Excretion: Oxytocin is usually administered intravenously for stimulation of labor, although buccal absorption is possible. Oxytocin is inactive if swallowed, because it is destroyed in the stomach and intestine. Oxytocin is not bound to plasma proteins and is catabolized by the

Cys-Tyr-Phe-Gln-Asn-Cys-Pro-Arg-Gly-NH$_2$
1   2   3   4   5   6   7   8   9

Arginine vasopressin

Cys-Tyr-Ile-Gln-Asn-Cys-Pro-Leu-Gly-NH$_2$
1   2   3   4   5   6   7   8   9

Oxytocin

Figure 36–4. Arginine vasopressin and oxytocin. In some species, lysine is substituted for arginine in position 8 of the vasopressin molecule. (Reproduced, with permission, from Ganong WF: *Review of Medical Physiology,* 12th ed. Lange, 1985.)

kidneys and liver, with a circulating half-life of 5 minutes.

Pharmacodynamics

Oxytocin alters transmembrane ionic currents in myometrial smooth muscle cells to produce sustained uterine contraction. The sensitivity of the uterus to oxytocin increases during pregnancy. Oxytocin-induced myometrial contractions can be inhibited by β-adrenoceptor agonists, magnesium sulfate, or inhalation anesthetics. Oxytocin also causes contraction of myoepithelial cells surrounding mammary alveoli, which leads to milk ejection. Without oxytocin-induced contraction, normal lactation cannot occur. Oxytocin is a weak antidiuretic acting at the same renal tubular location as vasopressin.

Clinical Pharmacology

A. Therapeutic Uses: Oxytocin is used for induction and reinforcement of labor in women with mild preeclampsia near term, uterine inertia, and incomplete abortion. The drug should not be used for elective induction of labor in the absence of these indications. Oxytocin can also be used for control of postpartum uterine hemorrhage. Impaired milk ejection may respond to oxytocin.

B. Diagnostic Uses: Oxytocin infusion near term will produce uterine contractions that decrease the fetal blood supply. The fetal heart rate response to a standardized oxytocin challenge test provides information about placental circulatory reserve. An abnormal response suggests intrauterine growth retardation and may warrant immediate cesarean delivery.

Preparations & Dosage

Oxytocin is available in vials (Pitocin, Syntocinon) for parenteral use and as oxytocin nasal spray (Syntocinon). Intravenous oxytocin should be administered via an infusion pump with appropriate fetal monitoring. For induction of labor, an initial infusion rate of 1 mU/min is gradually increased up to 5–20 mU/min until a physiologic contraction pattern is established. For postpartum uterine bleeding, 10–40 units is added to 1 L of 5% dextrose, and the infusion rate is titrated to control uterine atony. Alternatively, 10 units can be given intramuscularly after delivery of the placenta. To induce lactation, one puff is sprayed into each nostril in the sitting position 2–3 minutes before nursing.

Toxicity & Contraindications

Among the reported adverse reactions to oxytocin administration are maternal deaths due to hypertensive episodes, uterine rupture, and water intoxication and fetal deaths. Afibrinogenemia has been reported.

Contraindications include fetal distress, prematurity, abnormal fetal presentation, cephalopelvic disproportion, and other predispositions for uterine rupture. Sympathomimetic agents should not be used with oxytocin.

VASOPRESSIN
(Antidiuretic Hormone, ADH)

Vasopressin is a peptide hormone released by the posterior pituitary in response to rising plasma tonicity or falling blood pressure. Vasopressin possesses antidiuretic and vasopressor properties. A deficiency of this hormone results in diabetes insipidus (Chapters 14 and 16).

Chemistry & Pharmacokinetics

A. Structure: Vasopressin is a nonapeptide with a 6-amino-acid ring and a 3-amino-acid side chain. The residue at position 8 is arginine in humans and most other mammals except pigs and related species, whose vasopressin contains lysine at position 8 (Fig 36–4).

B. Absorption, Metabolism, and Excretion: Vasopressin must be administered parenterally. Intravenous, intramuscular, or inhalational routes of administration may be selected. The half-life of circulating ADH is approximately 20 minutes, with renal and hepatic catabolism via reduction of the disulfide bond and peptide cleavage. A small amount of vasopressin is excreted as such in the urine, but urinary clearance is less than 5% of that of creatinine and does not reflect plasma levels.

Pharmacodynamics

The antidiuretic effect of vasopressin is mediated through activation of cAMP in renal collecting duct cells, leading to an increase in permeability and increased resorption of water from the collecting tubule. Vasopressin is a vasoconstrictor of splanchnic vessels, which makes it useful in certain types of gastrointestinal bleeding. Unfortunately, vasopressin may also cause coronary artery vasoconstriction and can result in myocardial depression.

Clinical Pharmacology

Vasopressin is the treatment of choice for pituitary diabetes insipidus (Chapter 14). Vasopressin infusion is also effective in some cases of esophageal variceal bleeding and of colonic diverticular bleeding. It is much less effective in bleeding caused by gastric or small intestine mucosal damage.

Synthetic vasopressin antagonists are being investigated for use in states of vasopressin-induced water retention.

Preparations & Dosage

Four preparations are in common use.

A. Aqueous Vasopressin: Aqueous vasopressin (Pitressin Synthetic) is a short-acting preparation for intramuscular, subcutaneous, or intravenous administration. The dose is 5–10 units subcutaneously or intramuscularly every 3–6 hours for transient diabetes insipidus; 0.1–0.5 unit/min intravenously for gastrointestinal bleeding.

B. Vasopressin Tannate in Oil: Vasopressin (Pitressin) tannate in oil is a long-acting form for intramuscular injection. The dosage is 2.5–5 units every 24–72 hours.

C. Lysine Vasopressin: Lypressin (Diapid) is a short-acting nasal spray. The dosage is 10–20 units sprayed deeply into one or both nostrils every 4–6 hours.

D. Desmopressin Acetate: Desmopressin acetate (DDAVP)—1-desamino-8-D-arginine vasopressin—is a long-acting synthetic analog of vasopressin. It is usually the preferred form for chronic therapy of diabetes insipidus, although it is the most expensive. The dosage is 10–40 μg/d (0.1–0.4 mL) in 2 or 3 divided doses, usually as 0.1 mL (10 μg) inhaled deeply through a flexible graduated plastic nasal tube into a single nostril once at bedtime and once during the day. Ten micrograms of desmopressin is equivalent to 40 IU of vasopressin. Injectable desmopressin

(DDAVP), 4 μg/mL, may be administered intravenously or subcutaneously, 0.5–1 mL every 8–12 hours as needed.

Desmopressin is now approved for the treatment of coagulopathy in hemophilia A and von Willebrand's disease (see Chapter 32).

Toxicity & Contraindications

Headache, nausea, abdominal cramps, and allergic reactions have been reported. Overdosage can result in hyponatremia.

Vasopressin should be used cautiously in patients with coronary artery disease. Drugs known to potentiate the effects of vasopressin include chlorpropamide, clofibrate, and carbamazepine. Inhalation of vasopressin may be ineffective when nasal congestion is present.

REFERENCES

Hypothalamic Releasing Hormones

Bouchard P et al: Gonadotropin-releasing hormone pulsatile administration restores luteinizing hormone pulsatility and normal testosterone levels in males with hyperprolactinemia. *J Clin Endocrinol Metab* 1985;**60**:258.

Chrousos GP et al: Clinical applications of corticotropin-releasing factor. *Ann Intern Med* 1985;**102**:344.

Cutler GB Jr et al: Therapeutic applications of luteinizing hormone–releasing hormone and its analogs. *Ann Intern Med* 1985;**102**:643.

Faden AI et al: Thyrotropin-releasing hormone in experimental spinal injury: Dose response and late treatment. *Neurology* 1984;**34**:1280.

Gelato MC et al: Effects of growth hormone–releasing factor on growth hormone secretion in acromegaly. *J Clin Endocrinol Metab* 1985;**60**:251.

Jackson IMD: Thyrotropin-releasing hormone. *N Engl J Med* 1982;**306**:145.

The Leuprolide Study Group: Leuprolide versus diethylstilbestrol for metastatic prostate cancer. *N Engl J Med* 1984; **311**:1281.

Plewe G et al: Long acting and selective suppression of growth hormone secretion by somatostatin analogue SMS 201–995 in acromegaly. *Lancet* 1984;**2**:782.

Sheldon WR et al: Rapid sequential intravenous administration of four hypothalamic releasing hormones as a combined anterior pituitary function test in normal subjects. *J Clin Endocrinol Metab* 1985;**60**:623.

Thorner MO et al: Acceleration of growth in two children treated with human growth hormone–releasing factor. *N Engl J Med* 1985;**312**:4.

Ziporyn T: LHRH: Clinical applications growing. *JAMA* 1985;**253**:469.

Anterior Pituitary Hormones

Beck-Peccoz P et al: Decreased receptor binding of biologically inactive thyrotropin in central hypothyroidism: Effect of treatment with thyrotropin-releasing hormone. *N Engl J Med* 1985;**312**:1085.

Cunningham SK et al: Normal cortisol response to corticotropin in patients with secondary adrenal failure. *Arch Intern Med* 1983;**143**:2276.

D'Agata RD et al: hCG-induced maturation of the seminiferous epithelium in hypogonadotropic men. *Horm Res* 1984;**19**:23.

Donald RA: ACTH and related peptides. *Clin Endocrinol (Oxf)* 1980;**12**:491.

Dunkel L et al: Single versus repeated dose human chorionic gonadotropin stimulation in the differential diagnosis of hypogonadotropic hypogonadism. *J Clin Endocrinol Metab* 1985;**60**:333.

Kater CE et al: Effects of continued adrenocorticotropin stimulation on the mineralocorticoid hormones in classical and nonclassical simple virilizing types of 21-hydroxylase deficiency. *J Clin Endocrinol Metab* 1985;**60**:1057.

Malone DNS, Strong JA: The present status of corticotropin therapy. *Practitioner* 1972;**208**:329.

March CM: The use of Pergonal for the induction of ovulation. *Clin Obstetrics Gynaecol* 1984;**27**:966.

Martin TL et al: The natural history of idiopathic hyperprolactinemia. *J Clin Endocrinol Metab* 1985;**60**:855.

Molitch ME: Pregnancy and the hyperprolactinemic woman. *N Engl J Med* 1985;**312**:1364.

Raiti S: Human growth hormone and Creutzfelt-Jakob disease. *Ann Intern Med* 1985;**103**:288.

Underwood LE: Report of the conference on uses and possible abuses of biosynthetic human growth hormone. *N Engl J Med* 1984;**311**:606.

Vance ML et al: Bromocriptine. *Ann Intern Med* 1985; **60**:855.

Posterior Pituitary Hormones

Horenstein JM, Phelan JP: Previous cesarean section: The risks and benefits of oxytocin usage in a trial of labor. *Am J Obstet Gynecol* 1985;**151**:564.

Richardson DW, Robinson AG: Desmopressin. *Ann Intern Med* 1985;**103**:228.

Schrier RW: Treatment of hyponatremia. *N Engl J Med* 1985;**312**:1121.

Seitchik J et al: Oxytocin augmentation of dysfunctional labor. 5. An alternative oxytocin regimen. *Am J Obstet Gynecol* 1985;**151**:757.

37

Thyroid & Antithyroid Drugs

Francis S. Greenspan, MD, & Betty J. Dong, PharmD

Because of its anatomic prominence, the thyroid was one of the first of the endocrine glands to be correctly associated with the clinical conditions caused by its malfunction. However, the fact that this gland releases 2 very different types of hormones was not appreciated until recently. This chapter discusses the pharmacology of the thyroid hormones essential for growth and development and for regulation of energy metabolism: thyroxine and triiodothyronine. The second type of thyroid hormone, calcitonin, is important in the regulation of calcium metabolism and is discussed in Chapter 41.

THYROID PHYSIOLOGY

The normal thyroid gland secretes sufficient amounts of the thyroid hormones—triiodothyronine (T_3) and tetraiodothyronine (T_4, thyroxine)—to maintain normal growth and development, normal body temperature, and normal energy levels. These hormones contain 59% and 65% (respectively) of iodine as an essential part of the molecule.

Iodide Metabolism

Nearly all of the iodide (I^-)* intake is via the gastrointestinal tract from food, water, or medication. The recommended daily adult intake is 150 μg. This ingested iodide is rapidly absorbed and enters an extracellular fluid pool. The thyroid gland removes about 75 μg a day from this pool for hormone secretion, and the balance is excreted in the urine. If iodide intake is increased, the fractional iodine uptake by the thyroid is diminished.

Biosynthesis of Thyroid Hormones

Once taken up by the thyroid gland, iodide undergoes a series of enzymatic reactions that convert it into active thyroid hormone (Fig 37–1). The first step is the transport of iodide into the thyroid gland, called **iodide trapping.** This can be inhibited by such anions as SCN^-, BF_4^-, NO_3^-, and ClO_4^-. Iodide is then oxidized to iodine, in which form it rapidly iodinates tyrosine residues within the thyroglobulin molecule to form monoiodotyrosine (MIT) and diiodotyrosine (DIT).

*In this chapter, "iodine" is used to refer to all forms of the element. Iodide refers only to the ionic form, I^-.

This process is called **iodide organification.** Two molecules of DIT combine within the thyroglobulin molecule to form L-thyroxine (T_4). One molecule of MIT and one molecule of DIT will combine to form T_3. In addition to thyroglobulin, other proteins within the gland may be iodinated, but these iodoproteins do not have hormonal activity. Thyroid hormones are released from thyroglobulin by pinocytosis and proteolysis of thyroglobulin at the apical colloid border. The colloid droplets of thyroglobulin merge with lysosomes containing proteolytic enzymes, which hydrolyze thyroglobulin and release T_4, T_3, MIT, and DIT. The MIT and DIT are deiodinated, and the iodine is reutilized. The ratio of T_4 to T_3 within thyroglobulin is approximately 5:1, so that most of the hormone released is thyroxine. Most of the T_3 circulating in the blood is derived from peripheral metabolism of thyroxine (see below).

Transport of Thyroid Hormones

T_4 and T_3 in plasma are reversibly bound to protein, primarily thyroxine-binding globulin (TBG). About 0.04% of total T_4 and 0.4% of T_3 exist in the free form.

Many physiologic and pathologic states and drugs affect T_4, T_3, and thyroid transport. However, the actual levels of free hormone generally remain normal, reflecting feedback control.

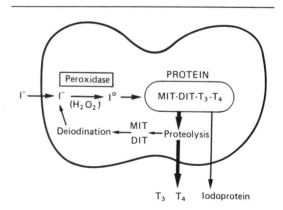

Figure 37–1. Hormone synthesis in the thyroid gland. I^-, iodide ion; I°, oxidized iodine; MIT, monoiodotyrosine; DIT, diiodotyrosine; T_3, triiodothyronine; and T_4, thyroxine. (Modified and reproduced, with permission, from Greenspan FS. In: *Gynecologic Endocrinology*, 3rd ed. Gold JJ, Josimovich JB [editors]. Harper & Row, 1980.)

Peripheral Metabolism of Thyroid Hormones

A small amount of thyroxine is biologically inactivated by deamination, decarboxylation, or conjugation and excretion as a glucuronide or sulfate. The primary pathway for the peripheral metabolism of thyroxine, however, is deiodination. Deiodination of T_4 may occur by monodeiodination of the outer ring, producing 3,5,3'-triiodothyronine (T_3), which is 3–4 times more potent than T_4. Alternatively, deiodination may occur in the inner ring, producing 3,3',5'-triiodothyronine (reverse T_3, or rT_3), which is metabolically inactive (Fig 37–2).

Fig 37–3 shows the amounts of thyroid hormone produced and metabolized per day in normal adults. Normal levels of thyroid hormone in the serum are listed in Table 37–1. The low serum levels of T_3 (Table 37–1) and rT_3 in normal individuals are due to the high metabolic clearances of these 2 compounds.

Control of Thyroid Function

The tests used to evaluate thyroid function are listed in Table 37–2.

A. Thyroid-Pituitary Relationships: Control of thyroid function via the thyroid-pituitary feedback is discussed in Chapter 36. Briefly, hypothalamic cells secrete thyrotropin-releasing hormone (TRH). TRH is secreted into capillaries of the pituitary portal venous system, and in the pituitary gland TRH stimulates the synthesis and release of thyroid-stimulating hormone (TSH). TSH in turn stimulates an adenylate cyclase mechanism in the thyroid cell to increase the synthesis and release of T_4 and T_3. These thyroid hormones, in a negative feedback fashion, act in the pituitary to block the action of TRH and in the hypothalamus to inhibit the synthesis and secretion of TRH. Other hormones or drugs may also affect the release of TRH or TSH.

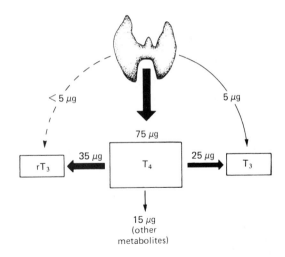

Figure 37–3. Quantitative aspects (per day) of thyroid hormone production and metabolism in normal adults.

B. Autoregulation of the Thyroid Gland: The thyroid gland also regulates its uptake of iodide and thyroid hormone synthesis by intrathyroidal mechanisms that are independent of TSH. These mechanisms are primarily related to the level of iodine in the blood. Large doses of iodine inhibit iodide organification. In certain disease states, this can result in inhibition of thyroglobulin iodination and thyroid hormone synthesis.

C. Abnormal Thyroid Stimulators: In Graves' disease (see below), lymphocytes secrete a thyroid-stimulating immunoglobulin (TSI). This immunoglobulin is probably bound to the TSH receptor site and turns on the gland in exactly the same fashion as TSH itself. The duration of the effect, however, is much longer than that of TSH.

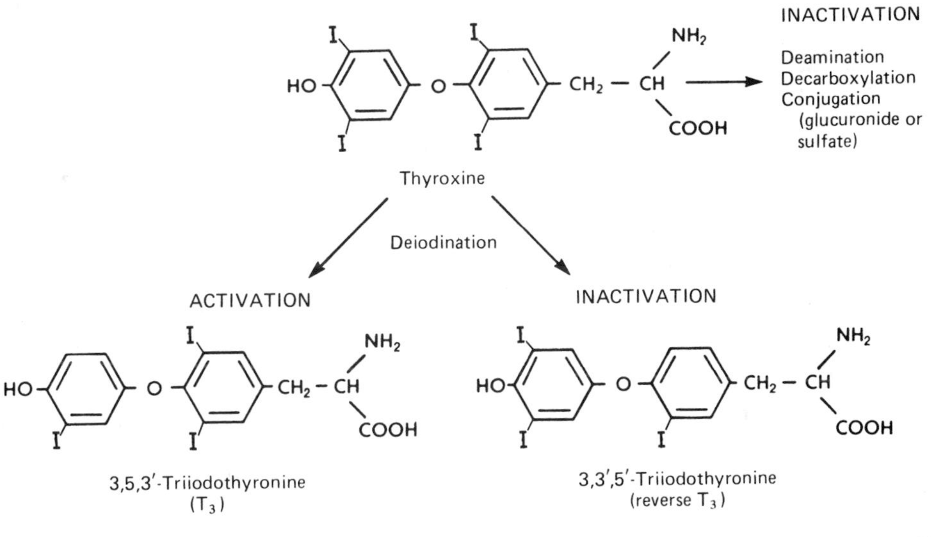

Figure 37–2. Peripheral metabolism of thyroxine. (Modified and reproduced, with permission, from Greenspan FS. In: *Gynecologic Endocrinology,* 3rd ed. Gold JJ, Josimovich JB [editors]. Harper & Row, 1980.)

Table 37–1. Summary of thyroid hormone kinetics.

Kinetic Variable	T_4	T_3
Volume of distribution	10 L	40 L
Extrathyroidal pool	800 μg	54 μg
Daily production	80 μg	30 μg
Fractional turnover per day	10%	60%
Metabolic clearance per day	1.1 L	24 L
Half-life (biologic)	7 days	1 day
Serum levels	5–12 μg/dL	80–180 ng/dL
Amount bound	99.96%	99.6%
Amount free	0.04%	0.4%
Biologic potency	1	4
Oral absorption	65%	95%

I. BASIC PHARMACOLOGY OF THYROID & ANTITHYROID DRUGS

THYROID HORMONES

Chemistry

The structural formulas of thyroxine (T_4) and triiodothyronine (T_3) as well as reverse triiodothyronine (rT_3) are shown in Figure 37–2. All of these naturally occurring molecules are levo (L) isomers. The synthetic dextro (D) isomer of thyroxine, dextrothyroxine, has approximately 4% of the biologic activity of the L isomer as evidenced by its ability to suppress TSH secretion and correct hypothyroidism.

Mechanism of Action

The precise mechanism of action of thyroid hormone is still controversial. The detection of high-affinity binding sites for T_3 and T_4 in the nucleus, mitochondria, and plasma membranes suggests multiple sites of action rather than a single site.

Large numbers of receptors are found in the most hormone-responsive tissues (pituitary, liver, kidney, heart, skeletal muscle, lung, and intestine), while few receptor sites occur in hormone-unresponsive tissues (spleen, testes). The brain, which lacks an anabolic response to T_3, contains an intermediate number of receptors. In agreement with their biologic potencies, the affinity of the receptor site for T_4 is about 10 times lower than that for T_3. The number of nuclear receptors may be altered to preserve body homeostasis. For example, starvation lowers both circulating T_3 and T_3 receptors.

A model for the 3 sites of thyroid hormone action is depicted in Fig 37–4. In this model, thyroid hormone T_3 binds to a receptor protein in the cell membrane and increases the uptake of glucose and amino acid into the cell. T_3 can also enter the cell by diffusion. Once within the cell, T_3 binds to cytosol-binding protein (CBP), which exists in equilibrium with free T_3. In the cell, free T_3 may bind to receptors in the inner mitochondrial membrane or to receptors in the nuclear chromatin.

The responses that follow these hormone-receptor interactions are quite diverse. In the nucleus, an increase in RNA polymerase activity and transcription

Table 37–2. Normal values for thyroid function tests.

Name	Normal Value	Results in Hypothyroidism	Results in Hyperthyroidism
Total thyroxine by RIA (T_4 [RIA])	5–12 μg/dL	Low	High
Total triiodothyronine by RIA (T_3 [RIA])	80–180 ng/dL	Normal or low	High
Resin T_3 uptake (RT_3U)	25–35%	Low	High
Free thyroxine index (FT_4I)	1.3–4.2	Low	High
Free T_3 index (FT_3I)	20–63	Normal or low	High
Free T_4 (FT_4)	0.8–2.4 ng/dL	Low	High
Thyrotropic hormone (TSH)	0.4–4.8 μU/mL	High	Low
^{123}I uptake at 24 hours	5–35%	Low	High
Antithyroglobulin antibodies (Atg-ab)	Not detectable	Often present	Usually present
Antimicrosomal antibodies (Am-ab)	Titer less than 1:100	Often present	Usually present
Thyrotropin-releasing hormone test (TRH)	Three- to 5-fold rise in serum TSH 15–30 minutes after injection	Exaggerated rise	No response
Isotope scan with ^{123}I or ^{99m}TcO$_4$	Normal pattern	Not done	Diffusely enlarged gland
Thin needle aspiration biopsy (TNA)	Normal pattern	Not done	Not done
Serum thyroglobulin	< 50 ng/mL*	Low	High
Serum calcitonin	< 200 pg/mL*	Not done	Not done

*Results may vary with different laboratories.

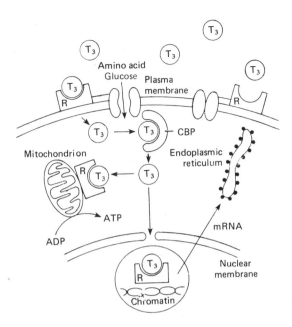

Figure 37–4. Proposed mechanism of thyroid hormone action. Thyroid hormone (in this case triiodothyronine or T₃) binds to receptor proteins (R) on the cell surface and increases the uptake of glucose and amino acids. T₃ also enters the cell where it reacts with cytoplasmic binding proteins (CBP) and receptors on chromatin and mitochondria. In the nucleus, the T₃-receptor complex leads to the synthesis of new protein. (Courtesy of JA Williams.)

of DNA into RNA results in increased mRNA synthesis, leading to stimulation of protein synthesis and subsequent enzyme and cell activity. Interactions with the mitochondrial receptor may affect regulation of energy metabolism directly and protein synthesis indirectly. Thyroid hormones directly stimulate membrane Na^+,K^+-ATPase, increasing Na^+ and K^+ transport (the sodium pump) and oxygen utilization. In addition, interaction with the cell membrane receptor results in increased uptake of amino acids and glucose independent of protein synthesis.

Most of the effects of thyroid on metabolic processes appear to be mediated by activation of nuclear receptors that lead to increased formation of RNA and subsequent protein synthesis. For example, increased formation of the protein Na^+,K^+-ATPase and the consequent increase in ATP turnover and oxygen consumption are responsible for some of the calorigenic effects of thyroid hormones. This is consistent with the observation that the action of thyroid is manifested in vivo after a time lag of hours or days after its administration.

Effects of Thyroid Hormones

The thyroid hormones are responsible for optimal growth, development, function, and maintenance of all body tissues (Table 37–3). Since T₃ and T₄ are qualitatively similar, they may be considered as one hormone in the discussion that follows.

Thyroid hormone is critical for nervous, skeletal, and reproductive tissues. Its effects depend upon protein synthesis as well as potentiation of the secretion and action of growth hormone. Thyroid deprivation in early life results in irreversible mental retardation and dwarfism—symptoms typical of congenital cretinism.

Effects on growth and calorigenesis are accompanied by a pervasive influence on metabolism of drugs as well as carbohydrates, fats, proteins, and vitamins. Many of these changes are dependent upon or modified by activity of other hormones. Conversely, the secretion and degradation rates of virtually all other hormones, including catecholamines, cortisol, estrogens, testosterone, and insulin, are affected by thyroid status.

Many of the manifestations of thyroid hyperactivity resemble sympathetic nervous system overactivity, although catecholamine levels are not increased. Possible explanations have included an increased number of beta-receptor sites or enhanced amplification of the beta-receptor signal without an increase in the number of receptor sites. Changes in catecholamine-stimulated adenylate cyclase activity as measured by cAMP are found with changes in thyroid activity. The most dramatic effects of this catecholamine hyperactivity are seen in the cardiovascular system. Other clinical symptoms reminiscent of excessive epinephrine activity and partially alleviated by adrenoceptor antagonists include lid lag and retraction, tremor, excessive sweating, anxiety, nervousness, and muscle weakness. The opposite constellation of symptoms is seen in hypothyroidism (Table 37–3).

Pharmacokinetics

Data on oral absorption of thyroid hormones are derived from administration of exogenous hormones. T₄ is absorbed best in the ileum and colon and is modified by intraluminal contents such as plasma proteins, food, and intestinal flora. Oral absorption in humans ranges from 35 to 80% (average, 65%; see Table 37–1). In contrast, T₃ is almost completely absorbed (95%) and minimally interfered with by intraluminal binding proteins. T₄ and T₃ absorption appears not to be affected by mild hypothyroidism but may be impaired in severe myxedema with ileus. These factors are important in switching from oral to parenteral therapy. For parenteral use, the intravenous route is preferred for both hormones (even though no commercial intravenous preparation of T₃ is available).

In patients with hyperthyroidism, the metabolic clearance rates of T₄ and T₃ are increased and the half-life decreased; the opposite is true in patients with hypothyroidism. Drugs such as phenobarbital that induce hepatic microsomal enzymes increase the metabolism of both T₄ and T₃. However, despite this change, the normal hormone concentration is maintained in euthyroid patients as a result of compensatory hyperfunction of the thyroid. A similar compensation occurs if binding sites are altered. If TBG sites are increased by pregnancy, estrogens, or oral contraceptives, there is an initial shift of hormone from the free to the bound

Table 37–3. Summary of thyroid hormone effects.

System	Thyrotoxicosis	Hypothyroidism
Skin and appendages	Warm, moist skin; sweating; heat intolerance; fine, thin hair; Plummer's nails.	Pale, cool, puffy skin; dry and brittle hair; brittle nails.
Eyes, face	Retraction of upper lid with wide stare; periorbital edema; exophthalmos; diplopia.	Drooping of eyelids; periorbital edema; loss of temporal aspects of eyebrows; puffy, nonpitting facies; large tongue.
Cardiovascular system	Increased peripheral vascular resistance, heart rate, stroke volume, cardiac output, pulse pressure; high-output congestive heart failure; increased inotropic/chronotropic effects; arrhythmias; angina.	Decreased peripheral vascular resistance, heart rate, stroke volume, cardiac output, pulse pressure; low-output congestive heart failure; ECG: bradycardia, prolonged PR interval, flat T wave, low voltage; pericardial effusion.
Respiratory system	Dyspnea; decreased vital capacity.	Pleural effusions; hypoventilation and CO_2 retention.
Gastrointestinal system	Increased appetite; increased frequency of bowel movements; hypoproteinemia.	Decreased appetite; decreased frequency of bowel movements; ascites.
Central nervous system	Nervousness; hyperkinesia; emotional lability.	Lethargy; general slowing of mental processes; neuropathies.
Musculoskeletal system	Weakness and muscle fatigue; increased deep tendon reflexes; hypercalcemia; osteoporosis.	Stiffness and muscle fatigue; decreased deep tendon reflexes; increased alkaline phosphatase, LDH, SGOT.
Renal system	Mild polyuria; increased renal blood flow; increased glomerular filtration rate.	Impaired water excretion; decreased renal blood flow; decreased glomerular filtration rate.
Hematopoietic system	Increased erythropoiesis; anemia.	Decreased erythropoiesis; anemia.
Reproductive system	Menstrual irregularities; decreased fertility; increased gonadal steroid metabolism.	Hypermenorrhea; infertility; decreased libido; impotence; oligospermia; decreased gonadal steroid metabolism.
Metabolic system	Increased basal metabolic rate; negative nitrogen balance; hyperglycemia; increased free fatty acids; decreased cholesterol and triglycerides; increased hormone degradation; increased requirements for fat- and water-soluble vitamins; increased drug detoxification.	Decreased basal metabolic rate; slight positive nitrogen balance; delayed degradation of insulin, with increased sensitivity; increased cholesterol and triglycerides; decreased hormone degradation; decreased requirements for fat- and water-soluble vitamins; decreased drug detoxification.

state and a decrease in its metabolic clearance until the normal hormone concentration is reached. Thus, the concentration of total and bound hormone will increase, but the concentration of free hormone and the steady-state clearance will remain normal. The reverse occurs when thyroid binding sites are decreased.

Thyroid Preparations

Available preparations can be classified as either synthetic (levothyroxine, liothyronine, liotrix) or of animal origin (desiccated thyroid, thyroglobulin).

Thyroid USP is derived primarily from pork thyroid glands, although beef and sheep are also used. Because the FDA requires only that desiccated thyroid contain between 0.17% and 0.23% organic iodine by weight and says nothing about the appropriate $T_4:T_3$ ratio, potency may vary from one lot to the next. The disadvantages of thyroid USP outweigh the advantage of low cost and include protein antigenicity, product instability, and difficulty in laboratory monitoring. Thyroglobulin (Proloid) is a purified extract of hog gland, standardized biologically to give a $T_4:T_3$ ratio of 2.5:1. It offers no advantages over desiccated thyroid and is more expensive. Sixty-five milligrams (1 gr) of thyroglobulin is equivalent to 65 mg of desiccated thyroid.

Levothyroxine sodium (Levothroid, Synthroid, etc) is the drug of choice for replacement and suppression therapy. Advantages include stability, uniform potency, low cost, lack of allergenic foreign protein, easy interpretation of laboratory values, and a half-life of 7 days, so that once-daily administration is feasible. Absorption is variable (approximately 65%) and is increased by fasting. Generic preparations should probably not be used until problems of erratic bioavailability are corrected. T_4 for intravenous use is available when indicated. Sixty-five milligrams (1 gr) of desiccated thyroid is approximately equivalent to 60 μg of levothyroxine.

Liothyronine (Cytomel) is often used as a diagnostic agent in the T_3 suppression test and when short-term suppression of TSH is necessary. Although it is 3–4 times more active than T_4, it is not recommended for routine replacement because of its shorter half-life ($1^1/_2$ days) and higher cost and the difficulty of using conventional laboratory tests to monitor adequacy of replacement. Serum TSH is the only laboratory index that can be used to monitor T_3 replacement. T_3 should not be used for replacement therapy in patients with cardiac disease, since therapy is so difficult to monitor and the potential for cardiotoxicity so great. T_3 for intravenous use is not commercially available but can be prepared by dissolving crystalline liothyronine in a few drops of 0.1 N sodium hydroxide. The solution is then diluted with about 5 mL of sterile 1% human serum albumin in 0.85% saline, mixed by swirling, and then sterilized by passage through a Millipore filter.

Liotrix (Euthroid, Thyrolar) is a combination of synthetic T_4 and T_3 in a standard ratio of 4:1. It is an expensive form of thyroid medication but is stable, has predictable potency, lacks antigenicity, and is easily monitored. Furthermore, since a significant amount of T_4 is peripherally converted to T_3, the rationale that it is better because it mimics normal secretion is not valid. It is also important to note that Euthroid is 20% more potent than Thyrolar when corresponding milligram equivalents are compared.

The shelf life of the synthetic hormone preparations is excellent, particularly if they are stored in a dark bottle to minimize spontaneous deiodination. If desiccated thyroid is kept dry and free from moisture, potency is better preserved.

ANTITHYROID AGENTS

Reduction of thyroid activity and hormone effects can be accomplished by agents that interfere with the production of thyroid hormones; by agents that modify the tissue response to thyroid hormones; or by glandular destruction with radiation or surgery. "Goitrogens" are agents that suppress secretion of T_3 and T_4 to subnormal levels and thereby increase TSH to produce goiter. The antithyroid compounds used clinically include the thionamides, iodides, and radioactive iodine, which will be discussed later.

THIONAMIDES

The thionamides—propylthiouracil and methimazole (Tapazole)—are major drugs for treatment of thyrotoxicosis. In the United Kingdom, carbimazole, which is converted to methimazole in vivo, is widely used. Methimazole is about 10 times more active than propylthiouracil.

The chemical structures of these compounds are shown in Fig 37–5. The thiocarbamide group (see below) is essential for antithyroid activity.

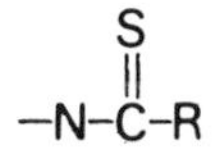

$$\begin{array}{c} S \\ \parallel \\ -N-C-R \end{array}$$

Pharmacokinetics

Propylthiouracil is rapidly absorbed, reaching peak serum levels after 1 hour. The bioavailability of 50–80% may be due to incomplete absorption or a large first-pass effect in the liver. The volume of distribution approximates total body water with accumula-

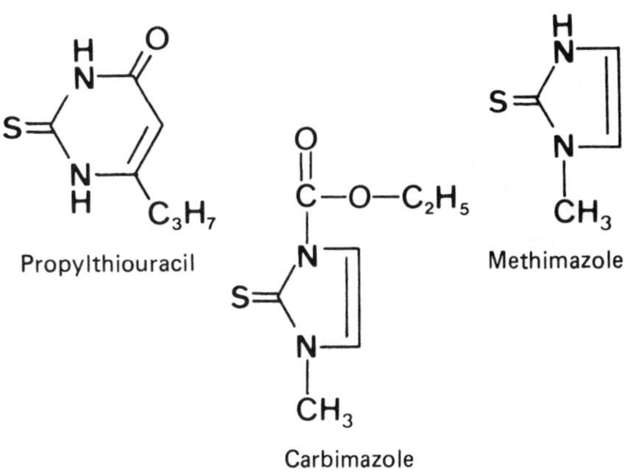

Figure 37–5. Structure of thionamides.

tion in the thyroid gland. Most of an ingested dose of propylthiouracil is excreted by the kidney as the inactive glucuronide within 24 hours.

In contrast, methimazole is completely absorbed but at variable rates. It is readily accumulated by the thyroid gland and has a volume of distribution similar to that of propylthiouracil. Excretion is slower than with propylthiouracil; 65–70% of a dose is recovered in the urine in 48 hours.

The short plasma half-life of these agents ($1^1/_2$ hours for propylthiouracil and 6 hours for methimazole) has little bearing on the duration of the antithyroid action or the dosing interval, since both agents are accumulated by the thyroid gland. For propylthiouracil, giving the drug every 6 hours is reasonable since a single 100-mg dose can inhibit 60% of iodine organification for 7 hours. Likewise, for methimazole, giving the drug every 8 hours is reasonable since a single 10-mg dose of methimazole inhibits over 90% of iodine organification for 8 hours. Since a single 30-mg dose of methimazole exerts an antithyroid effect for longer than 24 hours, a single daily dose may be effective in the management of mild to moderate hyperthyroidism.

Both thionamides cross the placental barrier and are concentrated by the fetal thyroid, so that caution must be employed while using these drugs in pregnancy. Methimazole appears to cross the placenta more readily than propylthiouracil. Recent data suggest that propylthiouracil is not secreted in sufficient quantity in breast milk to preclude breast feeding.

Pharmacodynamics

The thionamides act by multiple mechanisms. The major action is to prevent hormone synthesis by inhibiting the thyroid peroxidase-catalyzed reactions to block iodine organification. In addition, they block coupling of the iodotyrosines—primarily the formation of DIT. They do not block uptake of iodide by the gland. Propylthiouracil and (to a much lesser extent) methimazole inhibit the peripheral deiodination of T_4 and T_3. An immunosuppressive action has also been suggested. Since the synthesis rather than the release of hormones is affected, the onset of these agents is slow, often requiring 3–4 weeks before stores of T_4 are depleted.

Preparations

Propylthiouracil is available in 50-mg tablets and methimazole (Tapazole) in 5- and 10-mg tablets for oral administration. Since methimazole is water-soluble, both oral liquid and intravenous preparations can be prepared. In contrast, propylthiouracil is very insoluble and not suitable for intravenous use. A suspension of propylthiouracil can be compounded by dissolving tablets in carboxymethylcellulose flavored with cherry syrup.

Toxicity

Adverse reactions to the thionamides occur in about 3–12% of treated patients. Most reactions occur early. The most common side effect is a maculopapular pruritic rash, at times accompanied by systemic signs such as fever. Rare adverse effects include an urticarial rash, vasculitis, arthralgia, a lupuslike reaction, cholestatic jaundice, lymphadenopathy, hypoprothrombinemia, and polyserositis. Leukopenia, which is dose-dependent, should be differentiated from that occurring in Graves' disease. The most dangerous complication is agranulocytosis, an infrequent but potentially fatal adverse reaction. It occurs in about 0.3–0.6% of patients taking thionamides, but the risk is increased in older patients and in those receiving high-dose methimazole therapy (over 40 mg/d). The reaction is usually rapidly reversible when the drug is discontinued, but antibiotic therapy may be necessary for complicating infections. The cross-sensitivity between propylthiouracil and methimazole is not clear.

ANION INHIBITORS

Monovalent anions such as perchlorate (ClO_4), pertechnetate (TcO_4), and thiocyanate (SCN^-) can block uptake of iodide by the gland through competitive inhibition of the iodide transport mechanism. Since these effects can be overcome by large doses of iodides, their effectiveness is somewhat unpredictable.

Most of these agents, because of their toxicity, are used clinically only for diagnostic purposes. Potassium perchlorate was used clinically in the treatment of thyrotoxicosis until it was shown to cause aplastic anemia.

IODIDES

Iodides have been known since the 1920s to have multiple effects on the thyroid gland. Prior to the introduction of the thionamides in the 1940s, iodides were the major antithyroid agents; today they are rarely used as sole therapy.

Pharmacodynamics

Iodides have several actions on the thyroid. They inhibit organification (see physiology section), inhibit hormone release, and decrease the size and vascularity of the hyperplastic gland. In susceptible individuals, iodides can induce hyperthyroidism (jodbasedow) or precipitate hypothyroidism.

In pharmacologic doses (> 6 mg daily), the major action of iodides is to inhibit hormone release, possibly through inhibition of thyroglobulin proteolysis. Rapid improvement in thyrotoxic symptoms occurs within 2–7 days—hence the value of iodide therapy in thyroid storm. In addition, iodides decrease the vascularity, size, and fragility of a hyperplastic gland, making the drugs valuable as preoperative preparation for surgery.

Preparations

Stable iodine is available either as Lugol's solution (5% iodine and 10% potassium iodide) containing 8 mg of iodide per drop or as the more palatable saturated solution of potassium iodide (SSKI), containing 50 mg of iodide per drop. Parenteral preparations of sodium iodide, 1 and 2 g/10 mL, are also available. Disadvantages of iodide therapy include an increase in intraglandular stores of iodine, which may delay onset of thionamide therapy or prevent use of radioactive iodine therapy for several weeks. Thus, iodides should be initiated after onset of thionamide therapy and avoided if treatment with radioactive iodine seems likely. Iodide should not be used alone, since its withdrawal may produce severe exacerbation of thyrotoxicosis in an iodine-enriched gland. Chronic use of iodides in pregnancy should be avoided, since they cross the placenta and can cause fetal goiter.

Toxicity

Adverse reactions to iodine (iodism) are uncommon and in most cases reversible upon discontinuation. They include acneiform rash (similar to that of bromism), swollen salivary glands, mucous membrane ulcerations, conjunctivitis, rhinorrhea, drug fever, metallic taste, bleeding disorders, and, rarely, anaphylactoid reactions.

IPODATE

A most promising agent (now investigational) in the clinical treatment of hyperthyroidism is ipodate sodium (Oragrafin), an iodinated contrast medium that contains 61.4% iodine and can inhibit conversion of T_4 to T_3 in the liver, kidney, pituitary, and brain. When it is administered in a dose of 3 g orally every third day to thyrotoxic patients, improvement occurs in both subjective and objective symptoms, ie, decreased pulse rate and increased weight. The prolonged effect of suppressing T_4 as well as T_3 levels suggests that inhibition of hormone release due to the iodine released from ipodate may be an additional mechanism of action.

Since ipodate is relatively nontoxic, it may prove to be useful in the treatment of thyrotoxicosis.

RADIOACTIVE IODINE

^{131}I is the only isotope used for treatment of thyrotoxicosis. Administered orally in solution as sodium ^{131}I, it is rapidly absorbed, concentrated by the thyroid, and incorporated into storage follicles. Its therapeutic effect depends on emission of beta rays with an effective half-life of 5 days and a penetration range of 400–2000 μm. Within a few weeks after treatment, destruction of the thyroid parenchyma occurs as evidenced by epithelial swelling and necrosis, follicular disruption, edema, and leukocyte infiltration. Advantages of radioiodine include easy administration, effectiveness, low expense, and absence of pain. Fears of radiation-induced genetic damage, leukemia, and neoplasia have caused some clinics to restrict the use of radioiodine in the treatment of hyperthyroidism to adults over some specified age such as 35 years. However, after more than 30 years of clinical experience with radioiodine, these fears have not been realized. Radioactive iodine should not be administered to pregnant women or nursing mothers, since it crosses the placenta and is excreted in breast milk.

ADRENOCEPTOR-BLOCKING AGENTS

Since many of the symptoms of thyrotoxicosis mimic those associated with sympathetic stimulation, agents that deplete catecholamines such as guanethidine—or agents such as beta blockers that impair the tissue response at the receptor site—are useful therapeutic adjuncts. Beta-adrenoceptor–blocking drugs are the agents of choice because they are effective in patients refractory to guanethidine and reserpine. Propranolol has been the drug in this group most widely used and studied in the therapy of thyrotoxicosis. For a more complete discussion of this important class of drugs, see Chapter 9.

DIET-INDUCED THYROID DISEASE

Naturally occurring goitrogens of the Brassicaceae family include cabbage, turnips, rutabagas, and mustards. Thiocyanate is present in cabbage, and the others contain progoitrins that become goitrogenic when acted upon by enzymes present in the plant or in intestinal bacteria. These agents rarely produce goiter or hypothyroidism unless consumed raw in large quantities by susceptible individuals.

II. CLINICAL PHARMACOLOGY OF THYROID & ANTITHYROID DRUGS

HYPOTHYROIDISM

Hypothyroidism is a syndrome resulting from deficiency of thyroid hormones manifested by a general slowing of almost all body functions. In infants and children, there is striking retardation of growth and development, with resulting dwarfism and irreversible mental retardation. In adults, hypothyroidism is manifested largely by reversible slowing down of all body functions (Table 37–3).

The etiology and pathogenesis of hypothyroidism are outlined in Table 37–4. Hypothyroidism can occur with or without thyroid enlargement (goiter). The most common cause of hypothyroidism in the USA at this time is probably Hashimoto's thyroiditis, an immunologic disorder in genetically predisposed individuals. There is evidence of humoral immunity in the presence of antithyroid antibodies (see above) and lymphocyte sensitization to thyroid antigens. The laboratory diagnosis of hypothyroidism in the adult is easily made by the combination of a low free thyroxine (or low free thyroxine index) and elevated serum TSH (Table 37–2). Antithyroid antibodies are often positive, indicating underlying thyroiditis.

Table 37–4. Etiology and pathogenesis of hypothyroidism.

Cause	Pathogenesis	Goiter	Degree of Hypothyroidism
Hashimoto's thyroiditis	Autoimmune destruction of thyroid.	Present early, absent later	Mild to severe
Drug-induced*	Blocked hormone formation.	Present	Mild to moderate
Dyshormonogenesis	Impaired synthesis of T$_4$ due to enzyme deficiency.	Present	Mild to severe
Radiation, ^{131}I, x-ray	Destruction of gland.	Absent	Severe
Congenital (cretinism)	Athyreosis or ectopic thyroid, iodine deficiency.	Absent or present	Severe
Secondary (TSH deficit)	Pituitary or hypothalamic disease.	Absent	Mild

*Iodides, lithium, fluoride, thionamides, aminosalicylic acid, phenylbutazone, amiodarone, etc.

Management of Hypothyroidism

Except for hypothyroidism caused by drugs (Table 37–4), which can be treated by simply removing the depressant agent, the general strategy of replacement therapy is appropriate. The most satisfactory preparation is levothyroxine (Levothroid, Synthroid). Infants and children require somewhat more T_4 per kilogram of body weight than adults. The average dose for an infant 1–6 months of age is about 10 μg/kg, whereas the average dose for an adult is about 2.25 μg/kg (1 μg/lb). There is some variability in the absorption of thyroxine, so this dosage may vary from patient to patient. Because of the long half-life of thyroxine, the dose need be given only once daily. Children should be monitored for normal growth and development. Serum TSH and free thyroxine levels should be measured at regular intervals and maintained within a normal range. It takes about 6–8 weeks after starting a given dose of thyroxine to reach steady-state levels in the bloodstream. Thus, dosage changes should be made slowly.

In long-standing hypothyroidism, in older patients, and in patients with underlying cardiac disease, it is imperative to start treatment with reduced dosage. In such adult patients, levothyroxine is given in a dose of 0.0125–0.025 mg/d for 2 weeks, increasing by 0.025 mg every 2 weeks until euthyroidism or drug toxicity is observed. In older patients, the heart is very sensitive to the level of circulating thyroxine, and if angina pectoris or cardiac arrhythmia develops, it is essential to reduce the dose of thyroxine immediately. In younger patients or those with very mild disease, full replacement therapy may be started immediately.

The toxicity of thyroxine is directly related to the hormone level. In children, restlessness, insomnia, and accelerated bone maturation and growth may be signs of thyroxine toxicity. In adults, increased nervousness, heat intolerance, episodes of palpitation and tachycardia, or unexplained weight loss may be the presenting symptoms of thyroid toxicity. If these symptoms are present, it is important to monitor free thyroxine (Table 37–2), which will determine whether the symptoms are due to excess thyroxinemia.

Special Problems in Management of Hypothyroidism

A. Myxedema and Coronary Artery Disease: Since myxedema frequently occurs in older persons, it is often associated with underlying coronary artery disease. In this situation, the low levels of circulating thyroid hormone actually protect the heart against increasing demands that could result in angina pectoris or myocardial infarction. Correction of myxedema must be done cautiously to avoid provoking arrhythmia, angina, or acute myocardial infarction. Restoration of euthyroid state may not be possible in patients with severe coronary artery disease unless bypass coronary artery surgery restores a more normal coronary circulation.

B. Myxedema Coma: Myxedema coma is an end state of untreated hypothyroidism. It is associated with progressive weakness, stupor, hypothermia, hypoventilation, hypoglycemia, hyponatremia, water intoxication, shock, and death. Symptoms usually develop quite slowly, with a gradual onset of lethargy, progressing to stupor or coma.

The pathophysiology of myxedema coma involves 3 major aspects: (1) CO_2 retention and hypoxia associated with decreased sensitivity of the respiratory center; (2) fluid and electrolyte imbalance with hyponatremia; and (3) marked hypothermia, with body temperatures as low as 24 °C (75 °F). Serum tests are consistent with severe hypothyroidism (see above).

Management of myxedema coma is an acute medical emergency. The patient should be treated in the intensive care unit, since intubation and mechanical ventilation may be required. Associated illnesses such as infection or heart failure must be treated by appropriate therapy. Patients with myxedema coma absorb drugs poorly. It is therefore important to give all preparations intravenously. Intravenous fluids should be administered with caution to avoid excessive water intake. These patients have large pools of free T_3 and T_4 binding sites in their sera that must be filled before there is adequate free thyroxine to affect tissue metabolism. Accordingly, the treatment of choice in myxedema coma is to give a loading dose of levothyroxine intravenously—usually 300–400 μg initially, followed by 50 μg daily. Intravenous hydrocortisone is indicated if the patient has associated adrenal or pituitary insufficiency but is probably not necessary in most patients with primary myxedema. Narcotics and sedatives must be used with extreme caution.

Clinically, improvement is evidenced by an increase in body temperature and arousal from the comatose state. Once the patient is able to breathe normally, assisted mechanical ventilation can be removed, and steady improvement will ensue.

C. Hypothyroidism and Pregnancy: Hypothyroid females frequently have anovulatory cycles and are therefore relatively infertile until restoration of the euthyroid state. This has led to the widespread use of thyroid hormone for infertility, although there is no evidence for its usefulness in this situation unless the patient is clearly hypothyroid. In a pregnant hypothyroid patient receiving thyroxine, it is extremely important that the daily dose of thyroxine be maintained. In most cases, the dose in the nonpregnant state is the same as that in the pregnant state, and no change in dose is required. Because of the elevated maternal TBG, the free thyroxine index (FT_4I) or free thyroxine (FT_4) (Table 37–2) must be used to monitor maternal thyroxine dosages.

HYPERTHYROIDISM

Hyperthyroidism, or thyrotoxicosis, is the clinical syndrome that results when tissues are exposed to high levels of thyroid hormone.

GRAVES' DISEASE

The most common form of hyperthyroidism is Graves' disease, or diffuse toxic goiter. The presenting signs and symptoms of Graves' disease are set forth in Table 37–3.

Pathophysiology

Graves' disease is considered to be an autoimmune disorder in which there is a genetic defect in suppressor T lymphocytes, and helper T lymphocytes stimulate B lymphocytes to synthesize antibodies to thyroidal antigens. One such antibody (thyroid-stimulating immunoglobulin, or TSI) is directed against the TSH receptor site in the thyroid cell membrane and has the capacity to stimulate the thyroid cell.

Laboratory Diagnosis

In most patients, T_3, T_4, RT_3U, FT_4, and FT_4I will all be elevated (Table 37–2). Radioiodine uptake is usually markedly elevated as well. Antithyroglobulin antibodies, antimicrosomal antibodies, and TSI are also present.

Management of Graves' Disease

The 3 primary methods for controlling hyperthyroidism are antithyroid drug therapy, surgical thyroidectomy, and destruction of the gland with radioactive iodine.

A. Antithyroid Drug Therapy: Drug therapy is most useful in young patients with small glands and mild disease. Either propylthiouracil or methimazole is administered until the disease undergoes spontaneous remission, which may take from 1 year to 15 years. This is the only therapy that leaves an intact thyroid gland, but it does require a long period of treatment and observation (1–2 years), and there is a 60–70% incidence of relapse.

Antithyroid drug therapy is usually begun with large divided doses, shifting to single-dose maintenance therapy when the patient becomes clinically euthyroid. Therapy is frequently started with propylthiouracil, 100–150 mg every 6 hours, and then, after 4–8 weeks, gradual reduction of the dose to maintenance therapy of 50–150 mg once daily. Propylthiouracil inhibits the conversion of T_4 to T_3, so it brings the level of activated thyroid hormone down more quickly than does methimazole. However, methimazole has a longer duration of action and is more useful if one is striving to achieve a single daily dose regimen. The best clinical guide to remission is reduction in the size of the goiter. Laboratory tests most useful in monitoring the course of therapy are serum T_3 by RIA, FT_4 or FT_4I, and serum TSH (Table 37–2).

Reactions to antithyroid drugs have been described above. A minor rash can often be controlled by antihistamine therapy. The more severe reaction of agranulocytosis is heralded by a sore throat or high fever. Thus, all patients receiving antithyroid drugs are instructed that if they develop sore throat or fever they must immediately discontinue the drug and seek a physician, who should obtain a throat culture and white blood cell and differential counts and then institute appropriate antibiotic therapy. Cholestatic jaundice, hepatocellular toxicity, exfoliative dermatitis, and acute arthralgia are rare adverse reactions to antithyroid drugs also requiring cessation of drug therapy.

B. Thyroidectomy: Subtotal thyroidectomy is the treatment of choice for patients with very large glands or multinodular goiters. Patients are treated with antithyroid drugs until euthyroid (about 6 weeks). In addition, for 2 weeks prior to surgery, they receive saturated solution of potassium iodide, 5 drops twice daily, to diminish vascularity of the gland and simplify surgery. About 50–60% of patients will require thyroid supplementation following subtotal thyroidectomy.

C. Radioactive Iodine: Radioiodine therapy utilizing ^{131}I is the preferred treatment for most patients over 21 years of age. In patients without heart disease, the therapeutic dose may be given immediately in a range of 80–100 $\mu Ci/g$ of estimated thyroid weight corrected for uptake. In patients with underlying heart disease or relatively large glands, it is desirable to treat with antithyroid drugs until euthyroid before giving ^{131}I. The medication is then stopped for 5–7 days; radioiodine uptake is determined; and a dose of 120–150 $\mu Ci/g$ of estimated thyroid weight is administered. Iodides should be avoided to assure maximal ^{131}I uptake. Six to 12 weeks following the administration of radioiodine, the gland will shrink in size and the patient will usually become euthyroid. A second dose may be required in some patients. The major complication of radioiodine therapy is hypothyroidism, which occurs in about 80% of patients. Serum FT_4 and TSH levels should be monitored. When hypothyroidism develops, prompt replacement with levothyroxine, 0.15–0.2 mg orally daily, is instituted.

D. Adjuncts to Antithyroid Therapy: During the acute phase of thyrotoxicosis, beta-adrenoceptor–blocking agents are extremely helpful. Propranolol, 10–40 mg orally every 6 hours, will control tachycardia, hypertension, and atrial fibrillation. Propranolol is gradually withdrawn as serum thyroxine levels return to normal. Adequate nutrition and vitamin supplements are essential. Barbiturates accelerate T_4 breakdown (by hepatic enzyme induction) and may be helpful both as a sedative and to lower T_4 levels.

TOXIC UNINODULAR GOITER & TOXIC MULTINODULAR GOITER

These forms of hyperthyroidism occur often in older women with nodular goiters. FT_4 is moderately elevated or occasionally normal, but T_3 by RIA is strikingly elevated. Single toxic adenomas can be managed with either surgical excision of the adenoma or with radioiodine therapy. Toxic multinodular goiter is usually associated with a large goiter and best treated by preparation with propylthiouracil followed by subtotal thyroidectomy.

SUBACUTE THYROIDITIS

During the acute phase of viral infection of the thyroid gland, thyroid hormones are produced that result in transient thyrotoxicosis. This syndrome has been called "spontaneously resolving hyperthyroidism." Supportive therapy is usually all that is necessary, such as propranolol for tachycardia and aspirin to control local pain and fever.

THYROTOXICOSIS FACTITIA

This is due to excessive ingestion of thyroid hormones, either accidentally or purposely. Treatment consists of supportive therapy and discontinuing excessive medication.

SPECIAL PROBLEMS

Thyroid Storm

Thyroid storm, or thyrotoxic crisis, is sudden acute exacerbation of all of the symptoms of thyrotoxicosis, presenting as a life-threatening syndrome. The clinical manifestations are variable in intensity but reflect hypermetabolism and excessive adrenergic activity. Fever is present, often associated with flushing and sweating. Tachycardia is common, often with atrial fibrillation, high pulse pressure, and occasionally heart failure. Central nervous system symptoms include marked agitation, restlessness, delirium, and coma. Gastrointestinal symptoms include nausea, vomiting, diarrhea, and jaundice. Death may occur from heart failure and shock.

Vigorous management is mandatory. Propranolol, 1–2 mg slowly intravenously or 40–80 mg orally every 6 hours, is helpful to control the severe cardiovascular manifestations. If propranolol is contraindicated by the presence of severe heart failure or asthma, reserpine, 1 mg orally, intramuscularly, or intravenously every 6–12 hours, or guanethidine, 1–2 mg/kg orally in divided doses, may help control hypertension and tachycardia. Release of thyroid hormones from the gland is retarded by the administration of sodium iodide, 1 g intravenously over a 24-hour period, or saturated solution of potassium iodide, 10 drops orally daily. Hormone synthesis is blocked by the administration of propylthiouracil, 250 mg orally every 6 hours. If the patient is unable to take propylthiouracil by mouth, methimazole may be prepared for intravenous administration in a dose of 25 mg every 6 hours. Hydrocortisone, 50 mg intravenously every 6 hours, will protect the patient against shock and will block the conversion of T_4 to T_3, bringing down the level of thyroactive material in the blood quickly.

Supportive therapy is essential to control fever, heart failure, and any underlying disease process that may have precipitated the acute storm. In rare situations, where the above methods are not adequate to control the problem, plasmapheresis or peritoneal dialysis has been used to lower the levels of circulating thyroxine.

Ophthalmopathy

Although severe ophthalmopathy is rare, it is difficult to treat. Management requires effective treatment of the thyroid disease, usually by total surgical excision or ^{131}I ablation of the gland. In addition, local therapy may be necessary, eg, elevation of the head to diminish periorbital edema and artificial tears to relieve corneal drying. For the severe, acute inflammatory reaction, a short course of prednisone, 100 mg orally daily for about a week and then 100 mg every other day, tapering the dose over a period of 6–12 weeks, may be effective. If steroid therapy fails or is contraindicated, irradiation of the posterior orbit, using well-collimated high-energy x-ray therapy, will frequently result in marked improvement of the acute process. Threatened loss of vision is an indication for surgical decompression of the orbit. Eyelid or eye muscle surgery may be necessary to correct residual problems after the acute process has subsided.

Dermopathy

Dermopathy or pretibial myxedema will often respond to topical corticosteroids applied to the involved area and covered with an occlusive dressing.

Thyrotoxicosis During Pregnancy

Ideally, women in the childbearing period with severe disease should have definitive therapy with ^{131}I or subtotal thyroidectomy prior to pregnancy in order to avoid an acute exacerbation of the disease during pregnancy or following delivery. If thyrotoxicosis does develop during pregnancy, radioiodine is contraindicated because it crosses the placenta and may injure the fetal thyroid. In the first trimester, the patient can be prepared with propylthiouracil and a subtotal thyroidectomy performed safely during the middle trimester. It is essential to give the patient a thyroid supplement during the balance of the pregnancy. Alternatively, the patient can be treated with propylthiouracil during the pregnancy, and the decision regarding long-term management can be made after delivery. The dosage of propylthiouracil must be kept to the minimum necessary for control of the disease, because it may affect the function of the fetal thyroid gland. Methimazole is not recommended, because of the risk of fetal scalp defects.

Neonatal Graves' Disease

Graves' disease may occur in the newborn infant, either due to passage of TSI through the placenta, stimulating the thyroid gland of the neonate, or to genetic transmission of the trait to the fetus. Laboratory studies reveal an elevated free thyroxine, a markedly elevated T_3, and a *low* TSH, in contrast to the normal infant, in whom TSH is *elevated* at birth. TSI is usually found in the serum of both the child and the mother.

If caused by maternal TSI, the disease is usually self-limited and subsides over a period of 4–12 weeks, coinciding with the fall in the infant's TSI level. However, treatment is necessary because of the severe metabolic stress the infant is subjected to. Therapy includes propylthiouracil in a dose of 5–10 mg/kg/d in divided doses at 8-hour intervals; Lugol's solution (8 mg of iodide per drop), 1 drop every 8 hours; and propranolol, 2 mg/kg/d in divided doses. Careful supportive therapy is essential. If the infant is very ill, prednisone, 2 mg/kg/d orally in divided doses, will help block conversion of T_4 to T_3. These medications are gradually reduced as the clinical picture improves and can be discontinued by 6–12 weeks.

NONTOXIC GOITER

Nontoxic goiter is a syndrome of thyroid enlargement without excessive thyroid hormone production. Enlargement of the thyroid gland is usually due to TSH stimulation from inadequate thyroid hormone synthesis. The most common cause of nontoxic goiter worldwide is iodide deficiency, but in the USA it is Hashimoto's thyroiditis. Less common causes include dietary goitrogens, dyshormonogenesis, and neoplasms (see below).

Goiter due to iodide deficiency is best managed by prophylactic administration of iodide. The optimal daily iodide intake is 150–300 μg. Iodized salt and iodate used as preservatives in flour and bread are excellent sources of iodine in the diet. In areas where it is difficult to introduce iodized salt or iodate preservatives, a solution of iodized poppyseed oil has been administered intramuscularly to provide a long-term source of inorganic iodine.

Goiter due to ingestion of goitrogens in the diet is managed by elimination of the goitrogen or by adding sufficient thyroxine to shut off TSH stimulation. Similarly, in Hashimoto's thyroiditis and dyshormonogenesis, adequate thyroxine therapy—0.15–0.2 mg/d orally—will suppress pituitary TSH and result in slow regression of the goiter as well as correction of hypothyroidism.

THYROID NEOPLASMS

Neoplasms of the thyroid gland may be benign (adenomas) or malignant. Thin needle aspiration biopsy has proved effective for differentiation of benign from malignant disease. Some adenomas will regress following thyroxine therapy; those that do not should be rebiopsied or surgically removed. Management of thyroid carcinoma requires a near-total thyroidectomy, postoperative radioiodine therapy in selected instances, and lifetime replacement with levothyroxine.

REFERENCES

Physiology & Pharmacology

Brennan MD: Series on pharmacology in practice. 5. Thyroid hormones. *Mayo Clin Proc* 1980;**55**:33.

Hershman JM, Bray GA (editors): *The Thyroid: Physiology and Treatment of Disease*. Pergamon, 1979.

Larsen PR: Thyroid pituitary interaction: Feedback regulation of thyrotropin secretion by thyroid hormones. *N Engl J Med* 1982;**306**:23.

Marchant B, Lees JFH, Alexander WD: Antithyroid drugs. *Pharmacol Ther [B]* 1978;**3**:305.

Miller LJ, Gorman CA, Go VLW: Gut-thyroid interrelationships. *Gastroenterology* 1978;**75**:901.

Oppenheimer JH: Thyroid hormone action at the nuclear level. *Ann Intern Med* 1985;**102**:374.

Shenfield GM: Influence of thyroid dysfunction on drug pharmacokinetics. *Clin Pharmacokinet* 1981;**6**:275.

Hypothyroidism

Evered D, Hall R (editors): *Hypothyroidism and Goitre*. Vol 8 of: *Clinics in Endocrinology and Metabolism*. Saunders, 1979.

Fisher DA et al: Results of screening one million North American infants. *J Pediatr* 1979;**94**:700.

Hennessey JV, Burman KD, Wartofsky L: The equivalency of two L-thyroxine preparations. *Ann Intern Med* 1985;**102**:770.

Maeda M et al: Changes in serum triiodothyronine, thyroxine and thyrotropin during treatment with thyroxine in severe primary hypothyroidism. *J Clin Endocrinol Metab* 1976;**43**:10.

Odell WD, Fisher DA: Treatment of hypothyroidism. Pages 92–110 in: *Diagnosis and Treatment of Common Thyroid Diseases*. Selenkow HA, Hoffman F (editors). Excerpta Medica International Congress Series No. 227, 1971.

Urbanic RC, Mazzaferri EL: Thyrotoxic crisis and myxedema coma. *Heart Lung* 1978;**7**:435.

Hyperthyroidism

Bierwaltes WH: The treatment of hyperthyroidism with iodine-131. *Semin Nucl Med* 1978;**8**:95.

Burman KD, Baker JR Jr: Immune mechanisms on Graves' disease. *Endocr Rev* 1985;**6**:183.

Burrow GN: Hyperthyroidism during pregnancy. *N Engl J Med* 1978;**298**:150.

Cooper DS: Antithyroid drugs. *N Engl J Med* 1984;**311**:1353.

Dobyns BM: Prevention and management of hyperthyroid storm. *World J Surg* 1978;**2**:293.

Dunn JT: Choice of therapy in young adults with hyperthyroidism of Graves' disease: A brief, case-directed poll of fifty-four thyroidologists. *Ann Intern Med* 1984;**100**:891.

Rapoport B: The ophthalmopathy of Graves' disease. (Medical Staff Conference, University of California, San Francisco.) *West J Med* 1985;**142**:532.

Nontoxic Goiter, Nodules, & Cancer

Clark OH: Thyroid nodules and thyroid cancer: Surgical aspects. *West J Med* 1980;**133:**1.

Miller JM, Hamburger JI, Kim S: Diagnosis of thyroid nodules: Use of fine needle aspiration and needle biopsy. *JAMA* 1979;**241:**481.

Papapetrou PD et al: Long-term treatment of Hashimoto's thyroiditis with thyroxine. *Lancet* 1972;**2:**1045.

Stanbury JB: Familial goiter. Page 206 in: *The Metabolic Basis of Inherited Disease,* 4th ed. Stanbury JB, Wyngaarden JB, Frederickson DS (editors). McGraw-Hill, 1978.

Adrenocorticosteroids & Adrenocortical Antagonists

38

Alan Goldfien, MD

The natural adrenocortical hormones are steroid molecules produced and released by the adrenal cortex. Both natural and synthetic corticosteroids are used for diagnosis and treatment of disorders of adrenal function. They are also used—in much larger quantities—for treatment of a variety of inflammatory and immunologic disorders.

Secretion of adrenocortical steroids is controlled by the pituitary release of corticotropin (ACTH). Secretion of the salt-retaining hormone aldosterone is also under the influence of angiotensin. Corticotropin has some actions that do not depend upon its effect on adrenocortical secretion. However, its pharmacologic value as an anti-inflammatory agent and its use in testing adrenal function depend on its trophic action. Its pharmacology was discussed in Chapter 36 and will be reviewed with the adrenocortical hormones.

Antagonists of the synthesis or action of ACTH and the adrenocortical steroids are important in the treatment of several tumors. These agents are described at the end of this chapter.

I. ADRENOCORTICOSTEROIDS

The adrenal cortex releases a large number of steroids into the circulation. Some have minimal biologic activity and function primarily as precursors, and there are some for which no function has been established. The hormonal steroids may be classified as those having important effects on intermediary metabolism (glucocorticoids), those having principally salt-retaining activity (mineralocorticoids), and those having androgenic or estrogenic activity (see Chapter 39). In humans, the major glucocorticoid is cortisol and the most important mineralocorticoid is aldosterone. Quantitatively, dehydroepiandrosterone (DHEA) is the major androgen, since about 20 mg is secreted daily, partly as the sulfate. However, both DHEA and androstenedione are very weak androgens. A small amount of testosterone is secreted by the adrenal and may be of greater importance as an androgen. Little is known about the estrogens secreted by the adrenal. However, it has been shown that the

adrenal androgens such as testosterone and androstenedione can be converted to estrone in small amounts by nonendocrine tissues and that they constitute the major endogenous source of estrogen in women after menopause and in some patients in whom ovarian function is abnormal.

THE NATURALLY OCCURRING GLUCOCORTICOIDS; CORTISOL (Hydrocortisone)

Pharmacokinetics

The major glucocorticoid in humans is cortisol. It is synthesized from cholesterol (as shown in Fig 38–1) by the cells of the zona fasciculata and zona reticularis and released into the circulation under the influence of ACTH. The mechanisms controlling its secretion are discussed in Chapter 36.

In the normal adult in the absence of stress, about 20 mg of cortisol is secreted daily. The rate of secretion changes in a circadian rhythm (Fig 38–2). In plasma, cortisol is bound to plasma proteins. Corticosteroid-binding globulin (CBG), an α_2-globulin synthesized by the liver, binds 95% of the circulating hormone under normal circumstances. The remainder is free or loosely bound to albumin and is available to exert its effect on target cells. When plasma cortisol levels exceed 20–30 μg/dL, CBG is saturated and most of the excess is loosely bound to albumin.

The half-life of cortisol in the circulation is normally about 90–110 minutes; it may be increased when large amounts are present or in hypothyroidism. Cortisol is removed from the circulation in the liver, where it is reduced and conjugated to form water-soluble compounds that are excreted into the urine (Fig 38–3). The side chain (C20 and C21) is removed from about 5–10% of the cortisol, and the resulting compounds are further metabolized and excreted into the urine as 11-oxy 17-ketosteroids.

In some species (eg, the rat), corticosterone is the major glucocorticoid. It is less firmly bound to protein and therefore metabolized more rapidly. The pathways of its degradation are similar to those of cortisol.

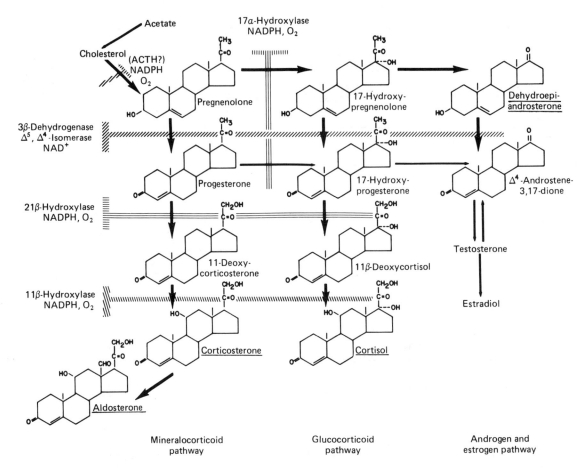

Figure 38–1. Outline of major pathways in adrenocortical hormone biosynthesis. The major secretory products are under-lined. Pregnenolone is the major precursor of corticosterone and aldosterone, and 17-hydroxypregnenolone is the major precursor of cortisol. The enzymes and cofactors for the reactions progressing down each column are shown on the left and from the first to the second column at the top of the figure. When a particular enzyme is deficient, hormone production is blocked at the points indicated by the shaded bars. (Modified after Welikey et al; reproduced, with permission, from Ganong WF: *Review of Medical Physiology*, 12th ed. Lange, 1985.)

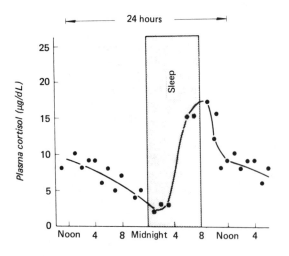

Figure 38–2. Circadian rhythm of plasma cortisol (free and protein-bound). (After Liddle, 1966).

Pharmacodynamics

A. Mechanism of Action: Natural and synthetic glucocorticoids and anti-inflammatory steroids bind to specific intracellular receptors upon entering target tis-sues as described in Chapter 35. The macromolecular complex thus formed is transported into the nucleus, where it interacts with chromosomal constituents to al-ter gene expression. These hormones alter the regula-tion of many cellular processes, including enzyme synthesis and activity, membrane permeability, trans-port processes, and structure.

B. Physiologic Effects: The glucocorticoids have widespread effects because they influence the function of most cells in the body. The major met-abolic consequences of glucocorticoid secretion or ad-ministration are due to direct actions of these hor-mones in the cell. However, some important effects are the result of homeostatic responses by insulin and glucagon. Although many of the effects are dose-re-lated and become magnified when large amounts are administered for therapeutic purposes, there are also

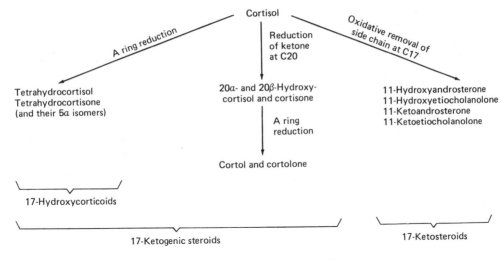

Figure 38–3. Primary excretion products of cortisol.

"permissive" effects. In other words, many normal reactions that take place at a significant rate only in the presence of corticoids are not further stimulated in the presence of larger amounts of corticoids. For example, the response of vascular and bronchial muscle to catecholamines is diminished in the absence of cortisol and restored by physiologic amounts of this glucocorticoid. The lipolytic responses of fat cells to catecholamines, ACTH, and growth hormone are also attenuated in the absence of glucocorticoid. The mechanism of these effects has not been determined.

C. Metabolic Effects: The glucocorticoids have important dose-related effects on carbohydrate, protein, and fat metabolism. The same effects are responsible for some of the serious adverse effects associated with their use in therapeutic doses. Glucocorticoids stimulate—and are required for—gluconeogenesis in the fasted state and in diabetes. Glucocorticoids also increase amino acid uptake by the liver and kidney and increase the activity of enzymes required for gluconeogenesis.

Glucocorticoids increase liver glycogen deposition by stimulating glycogen synthase activity and increasing glucose production from protein. The increase in glucose levels also stimulates insulin release.

Glucocorticoids inhibit the uptake of glucose by fat cells, leading to increased lipolysis. However, the increased insulin secretion described above stimulates lipogenesis, leading to a net increase in fat deposition.

The net results of these actions are most apparent in the fasting state, when the supply of glucose from gluconeogenesis, the release of amino acids from muscle catabolism, the inhibition of peripheral glucose uptake, and the stimulation of lipolysis all contribute to the maintenance of an adequate glucose supply to the brain.

D. Catabolic Effects: Although glucocorticoids stimulate protein and RNA synthesis in the liver, they have catabolic effects in lymphoid and connective tissue, muscle, fat, and skin. Supraphysiologic amounts of glucocorticoids lead to decreased muscle mass and weakness. Catabolic effects on bone are the cause of osteoporosis in Cushing's syndrome and constitute a major limitation in the long-term therapeutic use of glucocorticoids. In children, the catabolic effects of excessive amounts of glucocorticoid reduce growth. This effect is not prevented by growth hormone.

E. Anti-inflammatory and Immunosuppressive Effects: Glucocorticoids have the capacity to dramatically reduce the manifestations of inflammation. This is due largely to their profound effects on the concentration, distribution, and function of peripheral leukocytes. After a single dose of a short-acting glucocorticoid, the concentration of neutrophils increases while the lymphocytes (T and B cells), monocytes, eosinophils, and basophils decrease in number. The changes are maximal at 6 hours and are dissipated in 24 hours. The increase in neutrophils is due both to the increased influx from the bone marrow and decreased migration from the blood vessels, leading to a reduction in the number of cells at the site of inflammation. The reduction in circulating lymphocytes, monocytes, eosinophils, and basophils is the result of their movement from the vascular bed to lymphoid tissue. Glucocorticoids inhibit the functions of leukocytes and tissue macrophages. The ability of these cells to respond to antigens and mitogens is reduced. The effect on macrophages is particularly marked and limits their ability to phagocytize and kill microorganisms and to produce pyrogen, collagenase, elastase, and plasminogen activator. Although the evidence is conflicting, large doses of glucocorticoids have also been reported to stabilize lysosomal membranes, thereby reducing the concentration of proteolytic enzymes at the site of inflammation.

In addition to their effects on leukocyte function, glucocorticoids may influence the inflammatory response by their vascular effects. They cause vasoconstriction when applied directly to vessels. They decrease capillary permeability by inhibiting the activity of kinins and bacterial endotoxins and by reducing the amount of histamine released by basophils.

The anti-immune effect of glucocorticoids is largely due to the effects described above. In humans, complement activation is unaltered, but its effects are inhibited. Antibody production can be reduced by large doses of steroids, although it is unaffected by moderate doses (eg, 20 mg/d of prednisone). However, inhibition of the production and effects of interleukin-2 and blocking the effects of migration inhibition factor and macrophage inhibition factor impair delayed hypersensitivity reactions. The use of these steroids in the control of homograft rejection is augmented by their ability to reduce antigen release from the grafted tissue, delay revascularization, and interfere with the sensitization of antibody-forming cells.

The anti-inflammatory (and immunosuppressive) effects of these agents are widely useful therapeutically but are also responsible for some of their most serious adverse effects (see below).

F. Other Effects: Glucocorticoids have important effects on the nervous system. Adrenal insufficiency causes marked slowing of the alpha rhythm of the EEG. Increased amounts lower the threshold for electrically induced convulsions in rats and often produce behavioral disturbances in humans. Increased intracranial pressure (pseudotumor cerebri) occurs rarely.

Glucocorticoids suppress the pituitary release of ACTH and β-lipotropin but do not decrease circulating levels of β-endorphin (Chapter 36).

Large doses of glucocorticoids stimulate excessive production of acid and pepsin in the stomach and may cause peptic ulcer. They facilitate fat absorption and appear to antagonize the effect of vitamin D on calcium absorption. The glucocorticoids also have important effects on the hematopoietic system. In addition to their effects on leukocytes described above, they increase the number of platelets and red blood cells.

In the absence of physiologic amounts of cortisol, renal function (particularly glomerular filtration) is impaired and there is an inability to excrete a water load.

Glucocorticoids also have some effects on the development of the fetus. The structural and functional changes near term, including the production of pulmonary surface-active material required for air breathing, are stimulated by glucocorticoids.

SYNTHETIC ADRENOCORTICOSTEROIDS

ACTH and steroids having glucocorticoid activity have become important agents for use in the treatment of many inflammatory and allergic disorders. This has stimulated the search for and development of many steroids with anti-inflammatory activity.

Pharmacokinetics

A. Source: Although the natural corticosteroids can be obtained from animal adrenals, they are usually synthesized from cholic acid (obtained from cattle) or steroid sapogenins, diosgenin in particular, found in plants of the Liliaceae and Dioscoreaceae families. Further modifications of these steroids have led to the marketing of a large group of synthetic steroids with special characteristics that are pharmacologically and therapeutically important (Table 38–1).

B. Metabolism: The metabolism of the naturally occurring adrenal steroids has been discussed above. The synthetic corticosteroids for oral use (Table 38–1) are in most cases rapidly and completely absorbed when given by mouth. Although they are transported and metabolized in a fashion similar to the endogenous steroids, important differences exist.

Alterations in the molecule influence the degree of protein binding, side chain stability, rate of reduction, and end products. Halogenation at the 9 position, unsaturation of the Δ1-2 bond of the A ring, and methylation at the 2 or 16 position will prolong the half-life by more than 50%. The 11-hydroxyl group also appears to inhibit destruction, since the half-life of 11-deoxycortisol is half that of cortisol. The Δ1 compounds are excreted in the free form.

Pharmacodynamics

The actions of the synthetic steroids are similar to those of cortisol (see above). They bind to the specific intracellular receptor proteins and produce the same effects with different ratios of glucocorticoid to mineralocorticoid potency (Table 38–1).

Clinical Pharmacology

A. Diagnosis and Treatment of Disturbed Adrenal Function:

1. Adrenocortical insufficiency–

a. Chronic (Addison's disease)–Chronic adrenocortical insufficiency is characterized by hyperpigmentation, weakness, fatigue, weight loss, hypotension, and inability to maintain the blood glucose level with fasting. In such individuals, minor noxious, traumatic, or infectious stimuli may produce acute adrenal insufficiency with shock and finally death.

In adrenal insufficiency, whether primary or following adrenalectomy, about 20–30 mg of cortisol must be given daily, with increased amounts during periods of stress. This must be supplemented by an appropriate amount of salt-retaining hormone such as desoxycorticosterone (DOC) or fludrocortisone. It is for this reason that glucocorticoids devoid of salt-retaining activity are not indicated for these patients.

b. Acute–When acute adrenocortical insufficiency is suspected, treatment must be instituted immediately. In addition to large amounts of parenteral cortisol, therapy includes correction of fluid and electrolyte abnormalities and treatment of precipitating factors.

Cortisol hemisuccinate or phosphate in doses of 100 mg intravenously is given every 6–8 hours until the patient is stable. The dose is then gradually reduced, achieving maintenance dosage in 5 days. The

Table 38–1. Some commonly used natural and synthetic corticosteroids for general use.

Agent	Activity*			Equivalent Oral Dose (mg)	Forms Available
	Anti-inflammatory	Topical	Salt-Retaining		
Short-acting glucocorticoids					
Hydrocortisone (cortisol) (various trade names)	1	1	1	20	Oral, injectable, topical.
Cortisone (various trade names)	0.8	0	0.8	25	Oral, injectable, topical.
Prednisone (various trade names)	4	0	0.3	5	Oral.
Prednisolone (various trade names)	5	4	0.3	5	Oral, injectable, topical.
Fluocortolone[†]				5	Oral, topical.
Methylprednisolone (Medrol, etc)	5	5	0	4	Oral, injectable, topical.
Meprednisone (Betapar, etc)	5		0	4	Oral, injectable.[†]
Intermediate-acting glucocorticoids					
Triamcinolone (Aristocort, Kenalog, etc)	5	5[‡]	0	4	Oral, injectable, topical.
Paramethasone (Haldrone, etc)	10		0	2	Oral, injectable.[†]
Fluprednisolone (Alphadrol)	15	7	0	1.5	Oral.
Long-acting glucocorticoids					
Betamethasone (Celestone)	25–40	10	0	0.6	Oral, injectable, topical.
Dexamethasone (Decadron, etc)	30	10	0	0.75	Oral, injectable, topical.
Mineralocorticoids					
Fludrocortisone (Florinef, etc)	10	10	250	2	Oral, injectable, topical.
Desoxycorticosterone (various trade names)	0	0	20		Injectable.

*Potency relative to hydrocortisone.
[†]Outside USA.
[‡]Acetonide: Up to 100.

administration of salt-retaining hormone is resumed when the total cortisol dosage has been reduced to 50 mg/d.

2. Adrenocortical hyperfunction–

a. Congenital adrenal hyperplasia–This group of disorders is characterized by specific defects in the synthesis of cortisol. The most common is a decrease in or lack of 21-hydroxylase activity. As can be seen in Fig 38–1, this would lead to a reduction in cortisol synthesis and produce a compensatory increase in ACTH release. If sufficient enzyme activity is present, a normal amount of cortisol will be produced in response to the increased level of ACTH, but the gland will become hyperplastic and produce abnormally large amounts of precursors such as 17-hydroxyprogesterone that can be diverted to the androgen pathway, leading to virilization. Metabolism of this compound in the liver leads to pregnanetriol, which is characteristically excreted into the urine in large amounts in this disorder.

If the defect is in 11-hydroxylation, hypertension is prominent. When 17-hydroxylation is defective in the adrenals and gonads, hypogonadism will be present. However, increased amounts of 11-deoxycorticosterone (DOC) (see below) are formed and the signs and symptoms associated with mineralocorticoid excess—such as hypertension and hypokalemia—are found.

Cortisol and cortisone have been used in the treatment of congenital adrenal hyperplasia. Since ACTH suppression is an important objective of therapy, slowly absorbed parenteral preparations can be given in smaller amounts than the oral preparations, which are rapidly absorbed and metabolized and must be given in divided doses. When treating these patients, larger doses of cortisone (25–100 mg daily intramuscularly, depending upon age) can be given for 5–10 days to achieve adequate suppression of adrenal secretion. The dose is then reduced to 4–6 mg/d and adjusted to maintain a low urinary ketosteroid excretion. Treatment with orally administered hydrocortisone in a dose of 18 mg/d/m² of body surface or less in 3 divided doses can be used as the basis of therapy. Undesirable effects are minimized by giving a larger part of the dose in the morning. The dose must also be adjusted over the long course of therapy to permit normal growth, since excessive amounts of glucocorticoids inhibit linear growth in children. In some infants, salt-retaining hormone therapy is also required.

b. Cushing's syndrome–Cushing's syndrome is usually the result of bilateral adrenal hyperplasia secondary to a pituitary adenoma but occasionally is due to tumors of the adrenal gland or ectopic production of ACTH by other tumors. The manifestations are those associated with the presence of excessive glucocorticoids. When changes are marked, a rounded, plethoric face and trunk obesity are striking in appearance. In general, the manifestations of protein loss are severe and include muscle wasting, thinning of the skin, striae, easy bruisability, poor wound healing, and osteoporosis. Other serious disturbances include mental disorders, hypertension, and diabetes. This disorder is treated by surgical removal of the tumor producing the hormone, irradiation or removal of a pituitary microadenoma producing ACTH, or resection of hyperplastic adrenals. These patients must receive large doses of cortisol during and following the surgical procedure. Doses of 300 mg of soluble hydrocortisone are given as a continuous intravenous infusion on the day of surgery. The dose must be reduced slowly to normal replacement levels, since rapid reduction in dose may produce symptoms including fever and joint pain. If adrenalectomy has been performed, long-term maintenance is similar to that outlined above for adrenal insufficiency.

c. Hyperaldosteronism–Primary hyperaldosteronism usually results from the excessive production of aldosterone by an adrenal adenoma (Conn's syndrome). It may result from abnormal secretion of hyperplastic glands or from a malignant tumor. The clinical findings of hypertension, polyuria, polydipsia, weakness, and tetany are related to the continued renal loss of potassium, which leads to hypokalemia, alkalosis, and hypernatremia. This syndrome can be produced by excessive secretion of desoxycorticosterone, corticosterone, or 18-hydroxycorticosterone.

In contrast to patients with secondary hyperaldosteronism (see below), these patients have low (suppressed) levels of plasma renin activity and angiotensin II. When treated with desoxycorticosterone acetate (20 mg intramuscularly daily for 3 days) or fludrocortisone (0.2 mg twice daily orally for 3 days), they fail to retain sodium and their secretion of aldosterone is not significantly reduced. They are generally improved when treated with spironolactone, and their response to this agent is of diagnostic value.

3. Use of glucocorticoids for diagnostic purposes–It is sometimes necessary to suppress the production of ACTH in order to identify the source of a particular hormone or to establish whether or not its production is influenced by the secretion of ACTH. In these circumstances, it is advantageous to employ a very potent substance such as dexamethasone or betamethasone. Although these preparations are no more effective, the use of small quantities reduces the possibility of confusion in the interpretation of hormone assays in blood or urine. For example, if complete suppression is achieved by the use of 50 mg of cortisol, the urinary 17-hydroxycorticoids will be 15–18 mg/24 h, since one-third of the dose is recovered in urine as 17-hydroxycorticoid. If 1.5 mg of dexamethasone is employed, the excretion will be only 0.5 mg/24 h.

The **dexamethasone suppression test** is useful for the diagnosis of Cushing's syndrome and has also been used in the differential diagnosis of depressive states. Dexamethasone, 1 mg, is given orally at 11 PM, and a plasma sample is obtained in the morning. In normal individuals, the cortisol concentration is usually less than 5 μg/dL (Fig 38–2), whereas in Cushing's syndrome the level is usually greater than 10 μg/

dL. The results are less reliable in the presence of depression, anxiety, illness, and other stressful conditions.

Suppression of the adrenal with glucocorticoids and of the ovary with estrogens can be useful in locating the source of androgen production in a hirsute woman if the effect on testosterone levels in blood can be measured before and during hormone administration.

B. Adrenocorticosteroids and Stimulation of Lung Maturation in the Fetus: Lung maturation in the fetus is regulated by the fetal secretion of cortisol. Treatment of the mother with large doses of glucocorticoid reduces the incidence of respiratory distress syndrome in infants delivered prematurely. When delivery is anticipated before 34 weeks of gestation, betamethasone, 12 mg, followed by an additional dose of 12 mg 18–24 hours later, is commonly used. Protein binding of this corticosteroid is less than that of cortisol, allowing increased transfer across the placenta to the fetus. Corticosteroid levels achieved in the fetus are equivalent to those observed when the fetus is stressed. The safety of this treatment in patients with severe preeclampsia or hypertension—or diabetes with renal complications—has not been established.

C. Adrenocorticosteroids and Nonadrenal Disorders: Cortisol and its synthetic analogs have been found to be useful in the treatment of a diverse group of diseases unrelated to any known disturbance of adrenal function. The usefulness of corticosteroids in these disorders is a function of their ability to suppress inflammatory and immune responses as described above. In disorders in which host response is the cause of the major manifestations of the disease, these agents are useful. In instances where the inflammatory or immune response is important in controlling the pathologic process, therapy with corticosteroids may be dangerous but justified, if used in conjunction with specific therapy for the disease process, to prevent irreparable damage from an inflammatory response.

Since the corticosteroids are not usually curative, the pathologic process may progress while clinical manifestations are suppressed. Therefore, chronic therapy with these drugs should be undertaken with great care and only when the seriousness of the disorder warrants their use and less hazardous measures have been exhausted.

In general, attempts should be made to bring the disease process under control using short-acting glucocorticoids as well as all ancillary measures possible to keep the dose low. Where possible, alternate-day therapy should be utilized (see below). Therapy should not be decreased or stopped abruptly. When prolonged therapy is anticipated, it is helpful to obtain chest films and a tuberculin test. The presence of diabetes, peptic ulcer, osteoporosis, and psychologic disturbances should be excluded, and cardiovascular function should be assessed.

The following supplemental measures should be considered: The diet should be rich in potassium and low in sodium to prevent electrolyte disturbances. Caloric management to prevent obesity should be instituted. High protein intake is required to compensate for the loss due to the increased breakdown of protein from gluconeogenesis. Antacids should be used 3–4 times daily in patients prone to epigastric distress. Where osteoporosis is of concern, the use of physical therapy, fluorides, androgens, and vitamin D (with careful monitoring of serum calcium levels) has been recommended.

1. Some therapeutic indications for glucocorticoids in nonadrenal disorders–

Allergic disorders (angioneurotic edema, asthma, bee stings, contact dermatitis, drug reactions, allergic rhinitis, hay fever, serum sickness, urticaria)

Arthritis, bursitis, and tenosynovitis

Cerebral edema

Collagen vascular disorders (giant cell arteritis, lupus erythematosus, mixed connective tissue syndromes, polymyositis, polymyalgia rheumatica, rheumatoid arthritis, temporal arteritis)

Eye diseases (acute uveitis, allergic conjunctivitis, choroiditis, optic neuritis)

Gastrointestinal diseases (inflammatory bowel disease, nontropical sprue, regional enteritis, subacute hepatic necrosis, ulcerative colitis)

Hematologic disorders (acquired hemolytic anemia, acute allergic purpura, leukemia, autoimmune hemolytic anemia, idiopathic thrombocytopenic purpura, lymphoblastic leukemia, multiple myeloma)

Hypercalcemia (immunosuppression [transplants], carcinoma, sarcoidosis)

Infection (gram-negative septicemia, shock; occasionally helpful to suppress excessive inflammation)

Malignant exophthalmos and subacute thyroiditis

Neurologic diseases

Pulmonary diseases (aspiration pneumonia, bronchial asthma, prevention of infant respiratory distress syndrome, sarcoidosis)

Renal diseases (certain nephrotic syndromes)

Skin disorders (atopic dermatitis, dermatoses [see above], lichen simplex chronicus [localized neurodermatitis], mycosis fungoides, pemphigus, seborrheic dermatitis, xerosis)

Toxicity

The benefits obtained from the use of these compounds vary considerably. They must be carefully weighed in each patient against the widespread effects on every part of the organism. The major undesirable effects of the glucocorticoids are predictable exaggerations of their hormonal actions (see above) and lead to the clinical picture of iatrogenic Cushing's syndrome.

When the glucocorticoids are used for short periods (less than 1 week), it is unusual to see serious side effects even with moderately large doses. However, behavioral changes and acute peptic ulcers are occasionally observed.

A. Adrenal Suppression: When corticosteroids are administered for a period of months or years, adrenal suppression occurs and the patient should be given supplementary therapy at times of severe stress such as accidental trauma or surgery. With very rare exceptions, recovery occurs when the drug is withdrawn. Treatment with ACTH does not significantly reduce the suppression of pituitary-adrenal function.

B. Metabolic Effects: Most patients who are given daily doses of 100 mg of cortisol or more (or the equivalent amount of synthetic steroid) for longer than 2 weeks undergo a series of changes that have been termed iatrogenic Cushing's syndrome. The rate of development is a function of the dose. The appearance of the face is altered by rounding, puffiness, and plethora. Fat tends to be redistributed from the extremities to the trunk and face. There is an increased growth of fine hair over the thighs and trunk and sometimes the face. Acne may increase or appear, and insomnia and increased appetite are noted. In the treatment of dangerous or disabling disorders, these changes may not require cessation of therapy. However, the underlying metabolic changes accompanying them can be very serious by the time they become obvious. The continuing breakdown of protein and diversion of amino acids to glucose production increase the need for insulin and over a period of time result in **weight gain;** fat deposition; muscle wasting; thinning of the skin, with striae and bruising; hyperglycemia; and eventually the development of **osteoporosis** and **diabetes.** When diabetes occurs, it is treated by diet and insulin. These patients are often resistant to insulin but rarely develop ketoacidosis. In general, patients treated with corticosteroids should be on high-protein diets, and increased potassium and anabolic steroids should be used when required.

C. Other Complications: Other serious complications include the development of **peptic ulcers** and their complications. The clinical findings associated with other disorders, particularly bacterial and mycotic infections, may be masked by the corticosteroids, and patients must be carefully watched to avoid serious mishap when large doses are used. Some patients develop a myopathy the nature of which is unknown. The frequency of myopathy is greater in patients treated with triamcinolone. The administration of this drug as well as of methylprednisolone has been associated with nausea, dizziness, and weight loss in some patients. It is treated by changing drugs, reducing dosage, and increasing the potassium and protein intake.

Psychosis may occur, particularly in patients receiving large doses of corticosteroids. Long-term therapy is associated with the development of posterior subcapsular **cataracts.** Increased intraocular pressure is common, and **glaucoma** may be induced. **Benign intracranial hypertension** also occurs. In doses of 45 mg/m^2/d or more, **growth retardation** occurs in children.

When given in greater than physiologic amounts, steroids such as cortisone and hydrocortisone, which have mineralocorticoid effects in addition to glucocorticoid effects, cause some sodium and fluid retention and loss of potassium. In patients with normal cardiovascular and renal function, this leads to a **hypokalemic, hypochloremic alkalosis** and eventually a rise in blood pressure. In patients with hypoproteinemia, renal disease, or liver disease, edema may also occur. In patients with heart disease, even small degrees of sodium retention may lead to congestive heart failure. These effects can be minimized by sodium restriction and judicious use of potassium supplements.

Children with asthma treated for prolonged periods with these steroids have been reported to develop cataracts with increased frequency. Periodic slit lamp examination is indicated in such patients.

Contraindications & Cautions

A. Special Precautions: Patients receiving these drugs must be observed carefully for the development of hyperglycemia, glycosuria, sodium retention with edema or hypertension, hypokalemia, peptic ulcer, osteoporosis, and hidden infections.

The dosage should be kept as low as possible and intermittent dosage (eg, alternate-day) employed when satisfactory therapeutic results can be obtained on this schedule. In patients being maintained on relatively low doses of corticosteroids, supplementary therapy may be required at times of stress such as when surgical procedures are performed or accidents occur.

B. Contraindications: These agents must be used with the greatest of caution in patients with peptic ulcer, heart disease or hypertension with congestive heart failure, infections, psychoses, diabetes, osteoporosis, glaucoma, or herpes simplex infection.

Selection of Drug & Dosage Schedule

Since these preparations differ with respect to relative anti-inflammatory and mineralocorticoid effect (Table 38–1), duration of action, cost, and dosage forms available, these factors should be taken into account in selecting the drug to be used.

A. ACTH Versus Adrenocortical Steroids: In patients with normal adrenals, ACTH has been used to induce the endogenous production of cortisol to obtain similar effects. However, except when the increase in androgens is desirable, the use of ACTH as a therapeutic agent is probably unjustified. Instances in which ACTH has been claimed to be more effective than glucocorticoids are probably due to the administration of smaller amounts of corticoids than were produced by the dosage of ACTH.

B. Dosage: In determining the dose to be used, the physician must consider the seriousness of the disease, the amount of drug likely to be required to obtain the desired effect, and the duration of therapy. In some diseases, the amount required for maintenance of the desired therapeutic effect is less than the dose needed to obtain the initial effect, and the lowest possible dose for the needed effect should be determined by gradually lowering the dose until an increase in signs or symptoms is noted.

Many types of dosage schedules have been used in administering glucocorticoids. When it is necessary to maintain continuously elevated plasma corticosteroid levels in order to suppress ACTH, a slowly absorbed parenteral preparation or small doses at frequent intervals are required. The opposite situation exists with respect to the use of corticosteroids in the treatment of inflammatory and allergic disorders. The same total quantity given in a few doses may be more effective than when given in many smaller doses or in a slowly absorbed parenteral form. Severe autoimmune conditions involving vital organs must be treated aggressively, and under-treatment is as dangerous as overtreatment. In order to minimize the deposition of immune complexes and the influx of leukocytes and macrophages, 1 mg/kg/d of prednisone in divided doses is required initially. This dose is maintained until the serious manifestations respond. The dose can then be gradually reduced. When large doses are required for prolonged periods of time, **alternate-day** administration of the compound may be tried. When used in this manner, very large amounts (eg, 100 mg prednisone) can sometimes be administered with only minimal side effects because there is a recovery period between each dose. The transition to an alternate-day schedule can be made after the disease process is under control. It should be done gradually and with additional supportive measures between doses. A typical schedule for a patient maintained on 50 mg of prednisone daily would be as follows:

Day 1: 50 mg	Day 7: 75 mg
2: 40 mg	8: 5 mg
3: 60 mg	9: 70 mg
4: 30 mg	10: 5 mg
5: 70 mg	11: 65 mg
6: 10 mg	12: 5 mg, etc

When selecting a drug for use in large doses, a shorter-acting synthetic steroid with little mineralocorticoid effect is advisable. If possible, it should be given as a single morning dose.

Methylprednisolone in doses of 1 g given intravenously over 30–60 minutes at monthly intervals has been reported to be useful in treatment of rheumatoid arthritis in a few cases. The indications for this mode of therapy are not established.

C. Special Dosage Forms: The use of local therapy such as topical preparations for skin disease, ophthalmic forms for eye disease, intra-articular injections for joint disease, and hydrocortisone enemas for ulcerative colitis provides a means of delivering large amounts of steroid to the diseased tissue with reduced systemic effects.

For example, beclomethasone dipropionate administered as an aerosol in doses of 400 μg daily has been found to be effective in the treatment of asthma. In this dose, endogenous adrenal function is not significantly depressed in adults, and systemic effects are minimal. This agent and its metabolites are excreted mainly in feces. The switch from therapy with systemic glucocorticoids to aerosol therapy with beclomethasone must be undertaken with caution, since adrenal insufficiency will occur if adrenal function is suppressed. In such patients, a slow, graded reduction of systemic therapy and monitoring of endogenous adrenal function should accompany the institution of aerosol administration.

Beclomethasone dipropionate and flunisolide are available as nasal sprays for the treatment of allergic rhinitis. They are effective at doses that in most patients result in plasma levels too low to influence adrenal function. Beclomethasone is administered as a powder delivered as an aerosol; flunisolide is provided as 0.025% solution sprayed by a hand-activated pump. The dose of beclomethasone is 200–400 μg daily; of flunisolide, 200 μg daily. Both are given in divided doses 2–4 times daily.

TOPICAL CORTICOSTEROIDS

Corticosteroids incorporated into ointments, creams, lotions, and sprays are used for the treatment of atopic dermatitis, eczema, psoriasis, and some localized forms of vulvitis. These preparations are discussed in more detail in Chapter 65.

MINERALOCORTICOIDS (Aldosterone, Desoxycorticosterone, Fludrocortisone)

The most important mineralocorticoid in humans is aldosterone. However, small amounts of desoxycorticosterone (DOC) are also formed and released. Although the amounts are normally insignificant, DOC is of some importance therapeutically. Its actions, effects, and metabolism are similar to those described below for aldosterone. Fludrocortisone, a synthetic corticosteroid, is the most commonly used salt-retaining hormone.

ALDOSTERONE

Aldosterone is synthesized mainly in the zona glomerulosa of the adrenal cortex. Its structure and synthesis are illustrated in Fig 38–1.

The rate of aldosterone secretion is subject to several influences. ACTH produces a moderate stimulation of its release, but this effect is not sustained for more than a few days in the normal individual. Although aldosterone is no less than one-third as effective as cortisol in suppressing ACTH, the minute quantities of aldosterone produced by the adrenal cortex prevent it from participating in any feedback relationship in the control of ACTH secretion.

After hypophysectomy, aldosterone secretion gradually falls to about half the normal rate, which means that other factors are able to maintain and perhaps regulate its secretion. Independent variations between cortisol and aldosterone secretion can also be demonstrated by means of lesions in the nervous system such as decerebration, which decreases the secretion of hydrocortisone while increasing the secretion of aldosterone.

One of the important stimuli of aldosterone secretion is a reduction in blood volume, whether due to hemorrhage, dietary sodium restriction, or sodium loss following administration of diuretics. These stimuli lead to a decrease in mean renal arterial pressure that is associated with an increase in the release of renin by the cells of the juxtaglomerular apparatus. The enzyme renin then acts upon a circulating α_2-globulin (renin substrate), releasing angiotensin I, which is then converted to angiotensin II. Angiotensin is a powerful stimulant of aldosterone production, only a few micrograms being required to show an effect in humans (Chapter 16). A metabolite of angiotensin II, the heptapeptide formed by the removal of asparagine from the N-terminus, is also a potent stimulator of aldosterone production.

Physiologic & Pharmacologic Effects

Aldosterone and other steroids with mineralocorticoid properties induce the reabsorption of sodium from urine by the distal renal tubules, loosely coupled to the secretion of potassium and hydrogen ion. Sodium reabsorption in the sweat and salivary glands, gastrointestinal mucosa, and across cell membranes in general is also increased. Excessive levels of aldosterone produced by tumors or overdosage with other mineralocorticoids lead to hypernatremia, hypokalemia, metabolic alkalosis, increased plasma volume, and hypertension.

Aldosterone has a delayed action on sodium transport. Its action is dependent upon the synthesis of an enzyme required by the transport mechanism.

Metabolism

Aldosterone is secreted at the rate of 100–200 μg/d in normal individuals with a moderate dietary salt intake. The plasma level in males (resting supine) is about 0.007 μg/dL. The half-life of aldosterone injected in tracer quantities is 15–20 minutes, and it does not appear to be firmly bound to serum proteins.

The metabolism of aldosterone is similar to that of cortisol, about 50 μg/24 h appearing in the urine as conjugated tetrahydroaldosterone. Approximately 5–15 μg/24 h is excreted free or as the 3-oxo glucuronide.

DESOXYCORTICOSTERONE (DOC)

DOC, which also serves as a precursor of aldosterone (Fig 38–1), is normally secreted in amounts of about 200 μg/d. Its half-life when injected into the human circulation is about 70 minutes. Preliminary estimates of its concentration in plasma are approximately 0.03 μg/dL. The control of its secretion differs from that of aldosterone in that the secretion of DOC is primarily under the control of ACTH. Although the response to ACTH is enhanced by dietary sodium restriction, a low-salt diet does not increase DOC asecretion.

FLUDROCORTISONE

This compound, a potent glucocorticoid and mineralocorticoid, has become the most widely used mineralocorticoid. Doses of 0.1 mg 2–7 times weekly have potent salt-retaining activity and are used in the treatment of adrenocortical insufficiency but are too small to have important anti-inflammatory effects.

The clinical uses of fludrocortisone are discussed in the section on adrenocortical insufficiency. The available preparations are listed in Table 38–1.

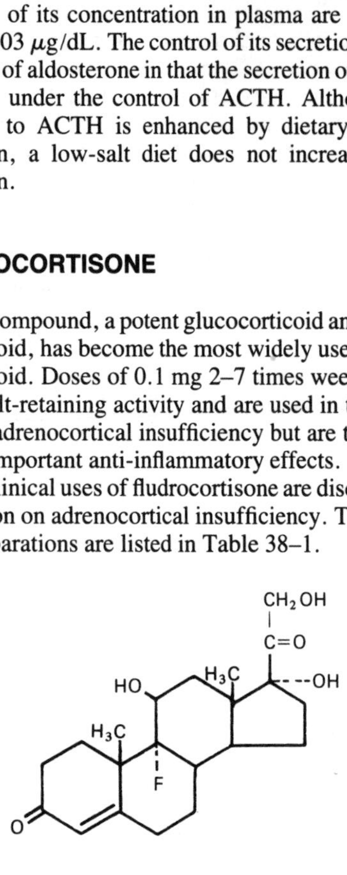

Fludrocortisone

ALDOSTERONE ANTAGONISTS

In addition to agents that interfere with aldosterone synthesis such as amphenone B (see below), there are steroids that compete with aldosterone for binding sites and decrease its effect peripherally. Progesterone is mildly active in this respect. However, it has been found that substitution of a 17-spironolactone group for the C20–C21 side chain of desoxycorticosterone results in a compound capable of blocking the sodium-retaining effect of aldosterone.

Spironolactone (Aldactone) is a 7α-acetylthiospironolactone. Little is known about its metabolism. The onset of activity is slow, and the effects last for 2–3 days after the drug is discontinued. It is used in the treatment of primary hyperaldosteronism in doses of 50–100 mg/d in divided doses. This agent will reverse many of the findings of hyperaldosteronism. It has been useful in establishing the diagnosis in some patients and in ameliorating the signs and symptoms when surgical removal of an adenoma is delayed. When used diagnostically for the detection of hyperaldosteronism in hypokalemic patients with hyperten-

sion, doses of 400–500 mg/d for 4–8 days—with an adequate intake of sodium and potassium—will restore potassium levels to or toward normal. This agent is also useful in preparing these patients for surgery. Doses of 300–400 mg/d for 2 weeks are used for this purpose and may reduce the incidence of cardiac arrhythmias.

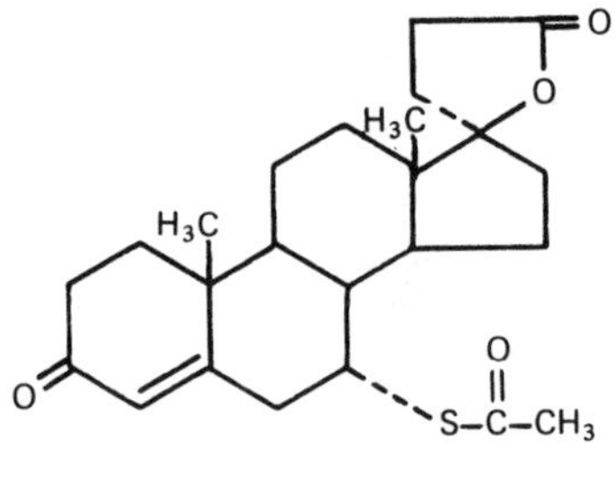

Spironolactone

Spironolactone is also used in treatment of hirsutism in women. Doses of 50–200 mg/d cause a reduction in the density, diameter, and rate of growth of facial hair in patients with idiopathic hirsutism or hirsutism secondary to androgen excess. The effect can usually be seen in 2 months and becomes maximal in about 6 months. It may be due to inhibition of androgen production and action at the hair follicle.

Spironolactone has limited usefulness as a diuretic (Chapter 14).

Side effects reported for spironolactone include hyperkalemia, menstrual abnormalities, gynecomastia, sedation, headache, gastrointestinal disturbances, and skin rashes.

II. ANTAGONISTS OF ADRENOCORTICAL AGENTS

MITOTANE

Mitotane (o,p'-DDD, Lysodren) produces adrenal atrophy in dogs and will interfere with biosynthetic pathways (Fig 38–4). Doses of up to 10 g daily have been administered to patients with carcinoma of the adrenal. The production of corticosteroids was reduced, and in a few patients some reduction in tumor size was noted. However, severe toxic effects, including central nervous system depression, tremors, and skin and gastrointestinal disturbances, limit the effective use of this experimental compound.

AMPHENONE B

Amphenone B is a more potent inhibitor of synthesis than mitotane, blocking hydroxylation at the 11, 17, and 21 positions (Fig 38–4). It does not have a de-

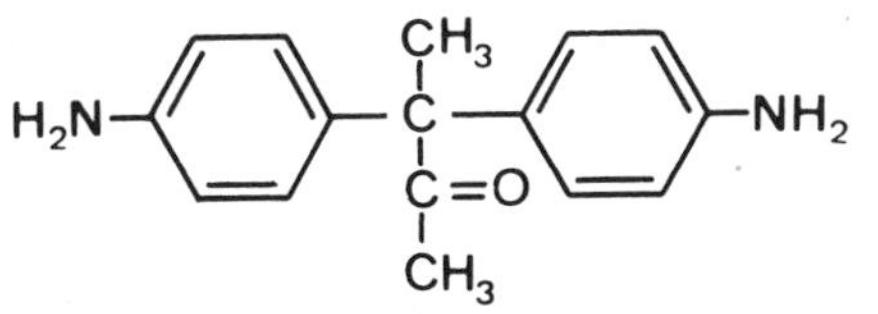

Amphenone B

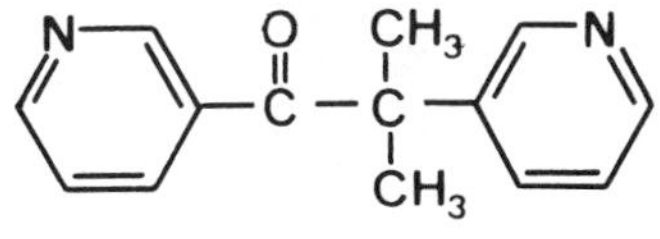

Metyrapone (Su 4885)

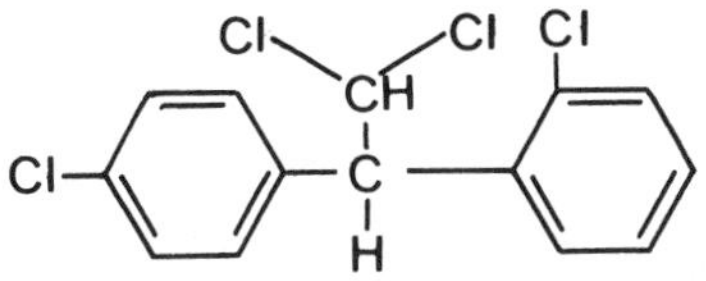

Mitotane (*o,p'*-DDD; dichloro-diphenyldichloroethane)

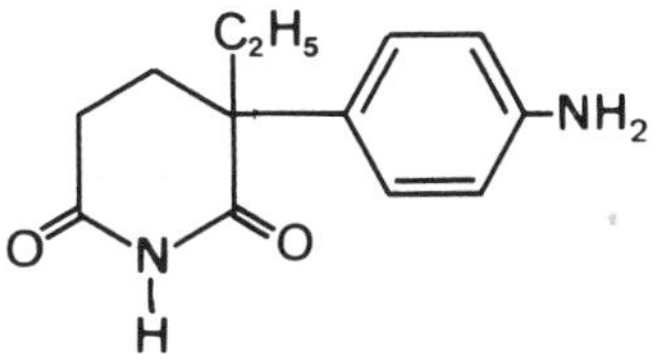

Aminoglutethimide

Figure 38–4. Adrenocortical antagonists.

structive effect on the tissue, and the synthetic block leads to increased production of ACTH and hyperplasia of the gland. It is considered too toxic for use in humans. Amphenone causes central nervous system depression and gastrointestinal tract and skin disorders, and impairs liver and thyroid function.

METYRAPONE

Metyrapone (Metopirone) (Fig 38–4) has a more selective effect at low doses than either mitotane or amphenone B. It inhibits 11-hydroxylation, interfering with cortisol and corticosterone synthesis and leading to secretion of 11-deoxycortisol. In the presence of a normal pituitary gland, there is a compensatory increase in 11-deoxycortisol production. This response is a measure of the capacity of the anterior pituitary to produce ACTH and has been adapted for clinical use as a diagnostic test. Although the toxicity of metyrapone is much lower than that of the above agents, it does produce transient dizziness and gastrointestinal disturbances. This agent has not been widely used for the treatment of Cushing's syndrome. However, in doses of 0.25 g twice daily to 1 g 4 times daily, metyrapone can reduce cortisol production to normal levels in some patients with adrenal tumors, ectopic ACTH syndromes, and hyperplasia. It may be useful in the management of severe manifestations of cortisol excess while the cause is being determined or in conjunction with radiation or surgical treatment. The major side effects observed are salt and water retention and hirsutism resulting from diversion of precursor to DOC and androgen synthesis.

Metyrapone is most commonly used in tests of adrenal function. The blood levels of 11-deoxycortisol and the urinary excretion of 17-hydroxycorticoids are measured before and after administration of the compound. Normally, there is a 2-fold or greater increase in the urinary 17-hydroxycorticoid excretion. A dosage of 300–500 mg every 4 hours for 6 doses is commonly used, and urine collections are made on the day before and the day after treatment. In patients with Cushing's syndrome, a normal response to metyrapone indicates that the cortisol excess is not the result of adrenal carcinoma or autonomous adenoma, since secretion by such tumors produces suppression of ACTH and atrophy of normal adrenal cortex.

Adrenal function may also be tested by administering metyrapone, 2–3 g orally at midnight, and measuring the level of ACTH or 11-deoxycortisol in blood drawn at 8:00 AM, or by comparing the excretion of 17-hydroxycorticosteroids in the urine during the 24-hour periods preceding and following administration of the drug.

In patients with suspected or known lesions of the pituitary, this procedure is a means of estimating the ability of the gland to produce ACTH.

AMINOGLUTETHIMIDE

Aminoglutethimide (Cytadren) (Fig 38–4) blocks the conversion of cholesterol to pregnenolone and causes a reduction in the synthesis of all hormonally active steroids (Fig 38–1). It has been used in conjunction with dexamethasone to reduce or eliminate estrogen and androgen production in patients with carcinoma of the breast. In doses of 1 g daily it was well tolerated; however, with higher doses, lethargy was a common effect. This drug may prove to be useful in reducing steroid secretion in patients with adrenocortical malignancy. It has been shown to enhance the metabolism of dexamethasone. During treatment, the half-life of ^{3}H-dexamethasone was reduced from 264 to 120 minutes.

REFERENCES

Adinoff AD, Hollister RJ: Steroid-induced fractures and bone loss in patients with asthma. *N Engl J Med* 1983;**309**:265.

Axelrod L: Glucocorticoid therapy. *Medicine* 1976;**55**:39.

Bartter FC (editor): *The Clinical Use of Aldosterone Antagonists*. Thomas, 1960.

Baxter JD, Rousseau GG (editors): *Glucocorticoid Action*. Monographs on Endocrinology. Vol 12. Springer-Verlag, 1979.

Bethune JE: *The Adrenal Cortex*. A Scope Monograph. Upjohn, 1974.

Bongiovanni AM, Root AW: The adrenogenital syndrome. (3 parts.) *N Engl J Med* 1963;**268**:1283, 1342, 1391.

Brook CGD et al: Experience with long-term therapy in congenital adrenal hyperplasia. *J Pediatr* 1974;**85**:12.

Burdick KH, Poulsen B, Place VA: Extemporaneous formulation of corticosteroids for topical usage. *JAMA* 1970;**11**:462.

Byyny RL: Withdrawal from glucocorticoid therapy. *N Engl J Med* 1976;**295**:30.

Cope CL: *Adrenal Steroids and Disease*. Lippincott, 1972.

Cumming DC et al: Treatment of hirsutism with spironolactone. *JAMA* 1982;**247**:1295.

Cupps TR, Fauci AS: Corticosteroid-mediated immunoregulation in man. *Immunol Rev* 1982;**65**:133.

Davis JO, Freeman RH: Mechanisms regulating renin release. *Physiol Rev* 1976;**56**:1.

Edelman IS, Fimognari GM: On the biochemical mechanism of action of aldosterone. *Recent Prog Horm Res* 1968;**24**:1.

Fauci AS, Dale DC, Balow JE: Glucocorticosteroid therapy: Mechanisms of action and clinical considerations. *Ann Intern Med* 1976;**84**:304.

Ferriss JB et al: Treatment of low-renin ("primary") hyperaldosteronism. *Am Heart J* 1978;**96**:97.

Graber AL et al: Natural history of pituitary-adrenal recovery following long-term suppression with corticosteroids. *J Clin Endocrinol Metab* 1965;**25**:11.

Hahn TJ: Corticosteroid-induced osteopenia. *Arch Intern Med* 1978;**138**:882.

Hutter AM Jr, Kayhoe DE: Adrenal cortical carcinoma: Results of treatment with o,p′DDD in 138 patients. *Am J Med* 1966;**41**:581.

Jeffcoate WJ et al: Metyrapone in long-term management of Cushing's disease. *Br Med J* 1977;**2**:215.

Jubiz W et al: Plasma metyrapone, adrenocorticotropic hormone, cortisol, and deoxycortisol levels: Sequential changes during oral and intravenous metyrapone administration. *Arch Intern Med* 1970;**125**:468.

Kaplan NM: Assessment of pituitary ACTH secretory capacity with Metopirone [metyrapone]. *J Clin Endocrinol Metab* 1963;**23**:945.

Morimoto Y, Yagura T, Yamamura Y: The effect of prolonged administration of beclomethasone dipropionate inhaler on adrenocortical functions in bronchial asthma. *J Med* 1977; **8**:1.

Myles AB, Daly JR: *Corticosteroid and ACTH Treatment*. Williams & Wilkins, 1974.

A new topical corticosteroid. *Med Lett Drugs Ther* (Nov 26) 1982;**24**:103.

Reid IA, Ganong WF: Control of aldosterone secretion. Pages 265–292 in: *Hypertension*. Genest J, Koiw E, Kuchel O (editors). McGraw-Hill, 1976.

Santen RJ, Lipton A, Kendall J: Successful medical adrenalectomy with amino-glutethimide. *JAMA* 1974;**230**:1661.

Scoggins RB, Kliman B: Percutaneous absorption of corticosteroids: Systemic effects. *N Engl J Med* 1965;**273**:831.

Slaunwhite W Jr, Sandberg A: Transcortin: A corticosteroid-binding protein of plasma. *J Clin Invest* 1959;**38**:384.

Thompson DG, Mason AS, Goodwin FJ: Mineralocorticoid replacement in Addison's disease. *Clin Endocrinol* 1979; **10**:499.

Thorn GW: Clinical considerations in the use of corticosteroids. *N Engl J Med* 1966;**274**:775.

Thorn GW, Lauler DP: Clinical therapeutics of adrenal disorders. *Am J Med* 1972;**53**:673.

Weinberger M et al: Primary aldosteronism: Diagnosis, localization, and treatment. *Ann Intern Med* 1979;**90**:386.

Zachmann M et al: Effect of aminoglutethimide on urinary cortisol and cortisol metabolites in adolescents with Cushing's syndrome. *Clin Endocrinol* 1977;**7**:63.

The Gonadal Hormones & Inhibitors

39

Alan Goldfien, MD

I. THE OVARY (Estrogens, Progestins, Other Ovarian Hormones, Oral Contraceptives, Antiestrogens, & Ovulation-Inducing Agents)

The ovary has important gametogenic functions that are integrated with its hormonal activity. In the human female, the gonad is relatively quiescent during the period of rapid growth and maturation. At puberty, the ovary begins a 30- to 40-year period of cyclic function called the menstrual cycle because of the regular episodes of bleeding that are its most obvious manifestation. It then fails to respond to gonadotropins secreted by the anterior pituitary gland, and the cessation of cyclic bleeding that occurs is called the menopause.

The mechanism responsible for the onset of ovarian function at the time of puberty is thought to be neural in origin, because the immature gonad can be stimulated by gonadotropins already present in the hypothalamus and because the pituitary is responsive to hypothalamic gonadotropin-releasing hormones. The maturation of centers such as the amygdala in the brain may release an inhibition of the cells in the median eminence of the hypothalamus, allowing them to produce gonadotropin-releasing hormone (GnRH, LHRH), which stimulates the release of follicle-stimulating hormone (FSH) and luteinizing hormone (LH) (see Chapter 36). At first, small amounts of these latter 2 hormones are released, and the limited quantities of estrogen ssecreted in response to FSH cause breast development, alterations in fat distribution, and a growth spurt associated with epiphyseal closure in the long bones. The small amounts of androgens produced by the ovary and adrenal may contribute to the appearance of axillary and pubic hair at this time.

After a year or 2, sufficient estrogen is produced to induce endometrial changes and periodic bleeding. After the first few cycles, which may be anovulatory, normal cyclic function is established (Fig 39–1).

At the beginning of each cycle, a variable number of follicles (vesicular follicles), each containing an ovum, begin to enlarge in response to FSH. After 5 or 6 days, one of the follicles begins to develop more rapidly. The granulosa cells of this follicle multiply and, under the influence of LH, synthesize estrogens and release them at an increasing rate. The estrogens appear to inhibit FSH release, which may lead to regression of the smaller, less mature follicles and produces local stimulation of the maturing follicle. The ovarian follicle consists of an ovum surrounded by a fluid-filled antrum lined by granulosa and theca cells. The estrogen secretion reaches a peak just before midcycle and stimulates the brief surge in LH and FSH release that precedes (and causes) ovulation. At the time of ovulation, the granulosa cells are beginning to secrete progesterone. When the follicle ruptures, the ovum is released into the abdominal cavity near the uterine tube.

Following the above events, the cavity of the ruptured follicle fills with blood (corpus hemorrhagicum), and the luteinized theca and granulosa cells proliferate and replace the blood to form the corpus luteum. The cells of this structure produce estrogens and progesterone for the remainder of the cycle, or longer if pregnancy occurs.

If pregnancy does not occur, the corpus luteum begins to degenerate and ceases hormone production, eventually becoming a corpus albicans. The cause of luteolysis is unknown. Most other hormonal events occurring during the normal ovarian cycle can be explained on the basis of feedback regulation. The endometrium, which proliferated during the follicular phase and developed its glandular structure during the

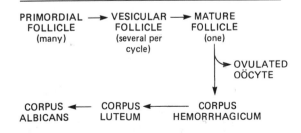

Figure 39–1. Sequence of follicular development and regression during a normal menstrual cycle. The mature follicle produces estrogen, while the corpus luteum produces both estrogen and progesterone.

luteal phase, is shed in the process of menstruation. These events are summarized in Fig 39–2.

The ovary normally ceases its gametogenic and endocrine function with time. This change is accompanied by a cessation in uterine bleeding (menopause) and occurs at a mean age of 52 years in the USA. Although the ovary ceases to secrete estrogen, significant levels of estrogen persist in many women as a result of conversion of adrenal steroids such as androstenedione to estrone and estradiol in nonendocrine tissues.

Disturbances in Ovarian Function

Disturbances of cyclic function are common even during the peak years of reproduction. A minority of these result from inflammatory or neoplastic processes that destroy the uterus, ovaries, or pituitary, but the causes of most menstrual problems are poorly understood. Many of the minor disturbances leading to periods of amenorrhea or anovulatory cycles are self-limited. They are often associated with emotional or environmental changes and are thought to represent temporary disorders in the centers in the brain that control the secretion of the hypothalamic releasing factors. Normal ovarian function can be modified by androgens produced by the adrenal cortex or tumors arising from it. The ovary also gives rise to androgen-producing neoplasms such as arrhenoblastomas and Leydig cell tumors and estrogen-producing granulosa cell tumors.

THE ESTROGENS

Estrogenic activity is shared by a large number of chemical substances. In addition to the variety of steroidal estrogens derived from animal sources, nonsteroidal estrogens have been synthesized. Many phenols are estrogenic, and estrogenic activity has been identified in such diverse forms of life as those found in the sediments of the seas and certain species of clover.

The Natural Estrogens

The major estrogens produced by women are estradiol, estrone, and estriol (Fig 39–3). Estradiol appears to be the major secretory product of the ovary. Although some estrone is produced in the ovary, most of it (and estriol) is formed in the liver from estradiol or formed in peripheral tissues from androstenedione and other androgens. As noted above, during the first part of the menstrual cycle estrogens are produced in the ovarian follicle by the theca cells. After ovulation, the estrogens as well as progesterone are synthesized by the granulosa cells of the corpus luteum, and the pathways of biosynthesis are slightly different.

During pregnancy, a large amount of estrogen is synthesized by the fetoplacental unit. The estriol synthesized by the fetoplacental unit is released into the maternal circulation and excreted into the urine. Repeated assay of maternal urinary estriol excretion has been useful in the assessment of fetal well-being.

One of the most prolific natural sources of estrogenic substances is the stallion, which liberates more of this hormone than the pregnant mare or pregnant woman. The equine estrogens—equilenin and equilin—and their congeners are unsaturated in the B as well as the A ring and are excreted in large quantities in urine, from which they can be recovered and used for medicinal purposes.

In normal women, estradiol is produced at a rate that varies during the cycle. Plasma levels of estradiol vary during the menstrual cycle (Fig 39–2) from a low of 50 pg/mL to as high as 350–850 pg/mL at the time of the preovulatory peak. When released into the circulation, estradiol binds strongly to an α_2-globulin (sex hormone–binding globulin [SHBG]) and to albumin with less affinity. Estradiol is converted by the liver and other tissues to estrone and estriol and their 2-hydroxylated derivatives and other metabolites (Fig 39–3). The catechol estrogens compete for catechol-O-methyltransferase and in high concentration inhibit

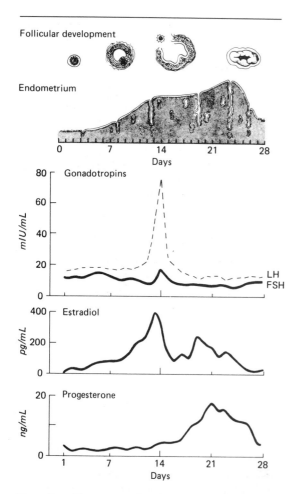

Figure 39–2. The menstrual cycle, showing plasma levels of pituitary and ovarian hormones and histologic changes.

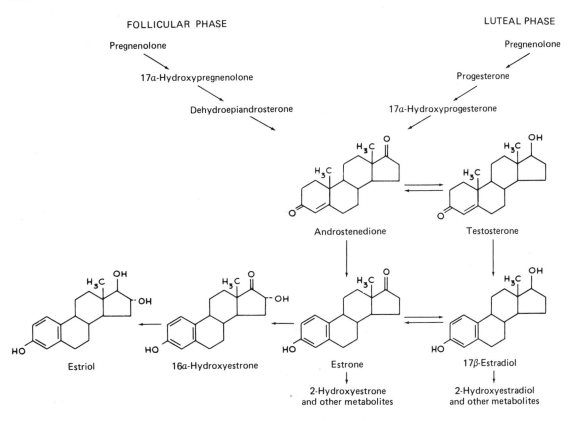

Figure 39–3. Biosynthesis and metabolism of estrogens.

the inactivation of catecholamines by the enzyme. Estrogens are also excreted in small amounts in the breast milk of nursing mothers.

Synthetic Estrogens

A variety of chemical alterations have been produced in the natural estrogens. The most important effect of these alterations has been to increase the effectiveness of the estrogens when administered orally. Some structures are shown in Fig 39–4. Those with therapeutic uses as listed in Table 39–1.

In addition to the steroidal estrogens, a variety of nonsteroidal compounds with estrogenic activity have been synthesized and used clinically. These include dienestrol, benzestrol, hexestrol, methestrol, methallenoestril, and chlorotrianisene (Fig 39–4).

Physiologic Effects

The estrogens are required for the normal maturation of the female. They stimulate the development of the vagina, uterus, and uterine tubes as well as the secondary sex characteristics. They stimulate stromal development and ductal growth in the breast and are responsible for the accelerated growth phase and the closing of the epiphyses of the long bones that occur at puberty. They contribute to the growth of the axillary and pubic hair and alter the distribution of body fat so as to produce typical female body contours. Larger quantities also stimulate development of pigmentation in the skin, most prominent in the region of the nipples and areolas and in the genital region.

In addition to its growth effects on the uterine muscle, estrogen also plays an important role in the development of the endometrial lining. Continuous exposure to estrogens for prolonged periods leads to an abnormal hyperplasia of the endometrium that is usually associated with abnormal bleeding patterns. When the estrogen production is properly coordinated with the production of progesterone during the normal human menstrual cycle, regular periodic bleeding and shedding of the endometrial lining occur.

Estrogens have a number of important metabolic effects. They seem to be partially responsible for the maintenance of the normal structure of the skin and blood vessels in women. Estrogens decrease the rate of resorption of bone by antagonizing the effect of parathyroid hormone on bone but do not stimulate bone formation. Estrogens may have important effects on intestinal absorption because they reduce the motility of the bowel. In addition to stimulating the synthesis of enzymes leading to uterine growth, they alter the production and activity of many other enzymes in the body. In the liver, metabolism of α_2-globulin is altered, so that there is a higher circulating level of this group of proteins (Table 39–2). This results in an increase in proteins responsible for the transport of thyroxine, estrogen, testosterone, iron, copper, and other substances.

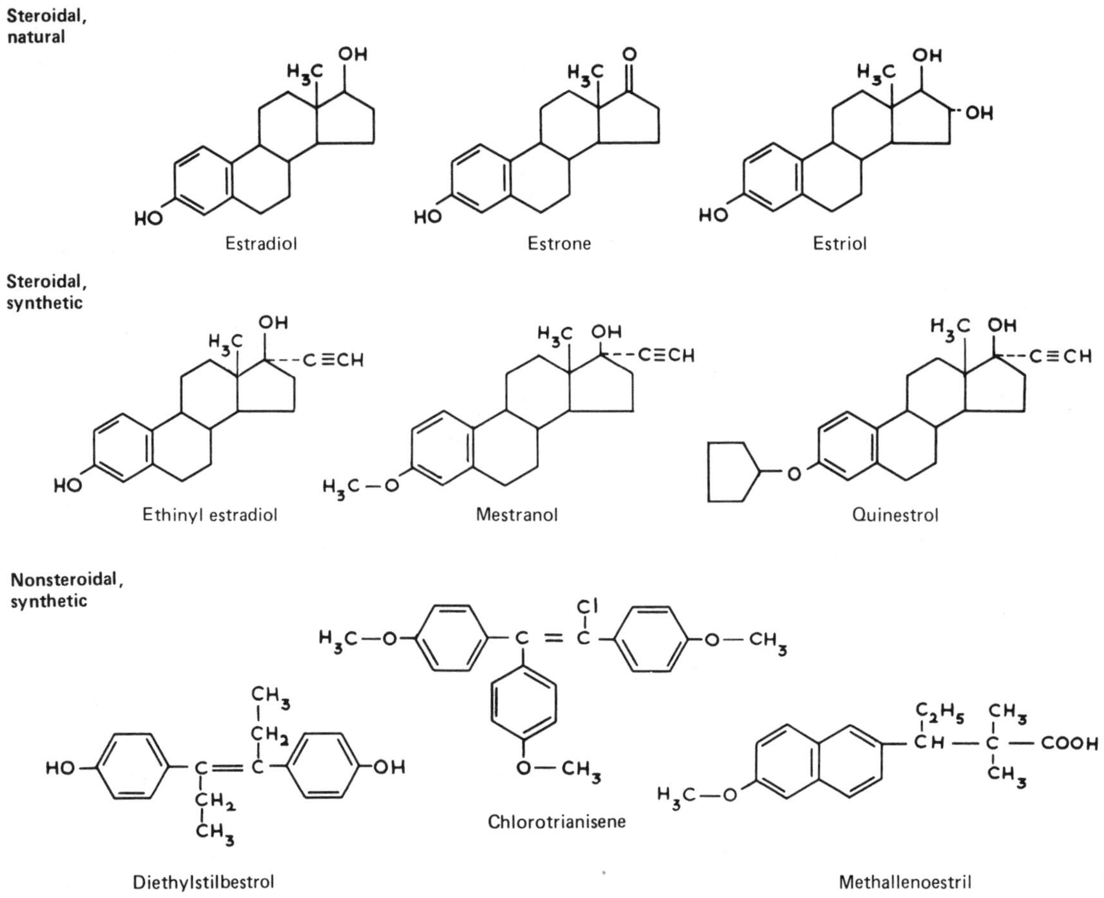

Figure 39–4. Compounds with estrogenic activity.

Estrogens enhance the coagulability of blood. Many changes in factors influencing coagulation have been reported, including increased circulating levels of factors II, VII, IX, and X. Increased plasminogen levels and decreased platelet adhesiveness have also been found (see section on oral contraceptives).

Alterations in the composition of the plasma lipids caused by estrogens are characterized by an increase in the alpha lipoproteins, a slight reduction in the beta lipoproteins, and a reduction in plasma cholesterol levels. Plasma triglyceride levels are increased.

Estrogens have many other effects. They are responsible for estrous behavior in animals and influence libido in humans. They facilitate the loss of intravascular fluid into the extracellular space, producing edema. The resulting decrease in plasma volume causes a compensatory retention of sodium and water by the kidney. Estrogens also modulate sympathetic nervous system control of smooth muscle function.

Clinical Uses

A. Primary Hypogonadism: Estrogens have been used extensively for replacement therapy in estrogen-deficient patients. The estrogen deficiency may be due to primary failure of development of the ovaries, castration, or menopause.

Treatment of primary hypogonadism is usually begun at 11–13 years of age in order to stimulate the development of secondary sex characteristics and menses, to stimulate optimal growth, and to avoid the psychologic consequences of delayed puberty. Treatment consists mainly of the administration of estrogens and progestins and should be done by a specialist.

Table 39–1. Commonly used estrogens.

	Average Replacement Dose
Ethinyl estradiol	0.005–0.02 mg/d
Micronized estradiol	1–2 mg/d
Estradiol cypionate	2–5 mg every 3–4 weeks
Estradiol valerate	2–20 mg every other week
Estropipate (Ogen)	1.25–2.5 mg/d
Conjugated, esterified, or mixed estrogenic substances:	
Oral	0.3–1.25 mg/d
Injectable	0.2–2 mg/d
Topical	. . .
Diethylstilbestrol	0.1–0.5 mg/d
Quinestrol (Estrovis)	0.1–0.2 mg/week
Dienestrol (Synestrol)	. . .
Chlorotrianisene (Tace)	12–25 mg/d
Methallenoestril	3–9 mg/d

Table 39–2. The effects of testosterone, progesterone, estradiol, and pregnancy on plasma proteins. [*][†]

Measurement	Testosterone	Progesterone	Estradiol	Pregnancy
Serum proteins	–	–	↓	↓
TBPA[‡]	↑	–	↓	↓
Albumin	–	–	↓	↓
Orosomucoid	. . .	–	↓	↓
TBG[§]	↓	–	↑	↑
Trypsin inhibitor	–	–	↑	↑
CBG[**]	↓	–	↑	↑
Transferrin	↓	–	–	↑
Ceruloplasmin	–	–	↑	↑
Haptoglobin	–	–	↓	–
Immunoglobulins	–	–	–	–
Plasminogen	–	–	↑	↑
Fibrinogen	↓	–	↑	↑
Renin substrate	. . .	–	↑	↑
Plasma amino acids	↑	↓	↑	. . .

*Modified and reproduced, with permission, from Salhanick HA, Kipnis DM, Vande Wiele RL (editors): *Metabolic Effects of Gonadal Hormones and Contraceptive Steroids.* Plenum Press, 1969.

† ↑ = increased, ↓ = decreased, – = unchanged.

‡Thyroxine-binding prealbumin.

§Thyroxine-binding globulin.

**Corticosteroid-binding globulin.

B. Hormonal Therapy in Postmenopausal Women:

Estrogens are widely used after the menopause. The need for and response to estrogen are quite variable, and many symptoms and disorders in menopausal women are probably unrelated to its deficiency. Hot flushes, sweating, and atrophic vaginitis are generally relieved by estrogens, and many patients experience some increased sense of well-being, but depression and other psychopathologic states are seldom improved.

The role of estrogens in the prevention and treatment of osteoporosis has been carefully studied. The amount of bone present is maximal in the young active adult and begins to decline in middle age in men and women. The development of osteoporosis depends on the amount of bone present at the start of this process as well as activity. Since estrogen opposes the resorption caused by parathyroid hormone, bone loss is accelerated at the time of the menopause (artificial or natural). Estrogen therapy has been shown to reduce this loss. However, estrogens cannot repair the process by increasing bone formation. Factors other than change in estrogen secretion are important in the development of osteoporosis. In these patients and others, calcium supplements are useful in bringing the total daily calcium intake up to 1500 mg. Fluoride in adequate amounts can increase bone density, but the effects on bone strength have not been assessed. Vitamin D therapy can be useful when calcium intake is less than optimal. Adequate protein intake and exercise are also useful.

The major indications for hormonal therapy in menopausal women are hot flushes, atrophic vaginitis, and a high risk of osteoporosis. The risk of osteoporosis is highest in smokers who are thin, Caucasian, and inactive and have a low calcium intake and a strong family history of osteoporosis. Estrogens should be used in the smallest dose consistent with relief of symptoms. In women who have not undergone hysterectomy, it is most convenient to prescribe estrogen on the first 21–25 days of each month. Studies indicate that 10 mg/d of medroxyprogesterone for the last 10–14 days of estrogen administration markedly reduces the risk of endometrial carcinoma in these patients. The recommended dosages of estrogen are 0.3–1.25 mg/d of conjugated estrogen or 0.01–0.02 mg/d of ethinyl estradiol. Doses in the middle of this range have been shown to be maximally effective in preventing the decrease in bone density occurring at menopause. From this point of view, it is important to begin therapy as soon as possible after the menopause for maximum effect.

Patients at low risk of developing osteoporosis who manifest only mild atrophic vaginitis can be treated with topical preparations. This route of application is also useful in the treatment of urinary tract symptoms in these patients. It is important to realize, however, that locally administered estrogens are almost completely absorbed into the circulation, and these preparations should be given cyclically.

In patients in whom estrogen replacement therapy is contraindicated, such as those with estrogen-sensitive tumors, relief of vasomotor symptoms can be obtained by the use of progestational agents.

C. Other Uses: Estrogens combined with progestins can be used to suppress ovulation in patients with intractable dysmenorrhea or when suppression of ovarian function is used in the treatment of hirsutism and amenorrhea due to excessive secretion of androgens by the ovary. Under these circumstances, marked suppression is needed, and oral contraceptives containing 80–100 μg of estrogen may be required (Table 39–4).

Estrogens have been used to stop excessive uterine bleeding due to endometrial hyperplasia. Repeated doses of 20 μg of ethinyl estradiol every few hours or the administration of 20 mg of conjugated estrogens intravenously has been useful in arresting blood loss temporarily.

Adverse Effects

Adverse effects of variable severity have been reported with the therapeutic use of estrogens. Many other effects reported in conjunction with hormonal contraceptives may be related to their estrogen content. These are discussed on pp 470–473.

Estrogen therapy has now become the major cause of **postmenopausal bleeding.** Unfortunately, vaginal bleeding at this time of life may also be due to carcinoma of the endometrium. In order to avoid this complication, patients should be treated with the smallest amount of estrogen possible. It should be given cyclically so that bleeding, when it occurs, will be more likely to occur during the withdrawal period. As noted above, endometrial hyperplasia can be prevented by administration of a progestational agent with estrogen in each cycle.

Nausea and **breast tenderness** are common and can be minimized by using the smallest effective dose of estrogen. **Hyperpigmentation** also occurs. Estrogen therapy is associated with an increase in frequency of **migraine headaches** as well as **cholestasis, hypertension,** and **gallbladder disease.**

The relationship of estrogen therapy to **cancer** continues to be the subject of intensive investigation. Although it has not been possible to establish that there is an increased risk in the incidence of breast cancer, it is not clear that it is safe to use these agents in patients considered to be at high risk for this tumor. Many studies have been published showing an increased risk of endometrial carcinoma in patients taking estrogens. The risk seems to vary with the dose and duration of treatment: 15 times as great in patients taking large doses of estrogen for 5 or more years, in contrast with 2–4 times greater in patients receiving lower doses for short periods. Several recent studies indicate that the concomitant use of a progestin not only prevents this increased risk but actually reduces the incidence of endometrial cancer below that in the general population.

A number of papers have appeared reporting the occurrence of adenocarcinoma of the vagina in young women whose mothers were treated with large doses of diethylstilbestrol early in pregnancy. These cancers are most common in young women (ages 14–44). Studies indicate that the incidence is less than one per 1000 women exposed. The risks for infertility, ectopic pregnancy, and premature delivery are also increased. It is now recognized that there is no indication for its use at that time, and it should be avoided. It is not known whether other estrogens have a similar effect or whether this is peculiar to diethylstilbestrol. This agent should be limited to use in the treatment of cancer (eg, prostate) or to use as a "morning after" contraceptive (see p 475).

Contraindications

Estrogens should not be used in patients with estrogen-dependent neoplasms such as carcinoma of the endometrium or in patients with known or suspected carcinoma of the breast. They should be avoided in patients with undiagnosed genital bleeding, liver disease, or a history of thromboembolic disorder.

Preparations & Dosages

The commonly used natural and synthetic preparations and equivalent dosages are given in Table 39–1. Although estrogens have both metabolic and gonadal effects, the intensity of these effects is not identical. For example, diethylstilbestrol and ethinyl estradiol have a greater effect on hepatic production of the steroid-binding globulins than on suppression of FSH.

THE PROGESTINS

PROGESTERONE

Progesterone is the most important progestin in humans. In addition to having important hormonal effects, it serves as a precursor to the estrogens, androgens, and adrenocortical steroids. It is synthesized in the ovary, testis, and adrenal from acetate, cholesterol, and pregnenolone, as shown in Fig 39–5. Large amounts are also synthesized and released by the placenta during pregnancy.

In the ovary, progesterone is produced primarily by the corpus luteum. Normal males appear to secrete 1–5 mg of progesterone daily, resulting in plasma levels of about 0.03 μg/dL. The level is only slightly higher in the female during the follicular phase of the cycle, when only a few milligrams per day of progesterone are secreted. During the luteal phase, plasma levels range from 0.5 to more than 2 μg/dL (Fig 39–2).

Progesterone is rapidly absorbed following administration by any route. Its half-life in the plasma is approximately 5 minutes, and small amounts are stored temporarily in body fat. It is almost completely metab-

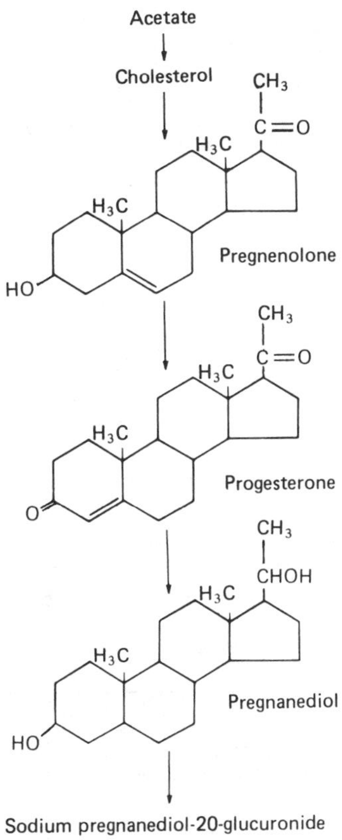

Figure 39–5. Biosynthesis of progesterone and major pathway for its metabolism. Other metabolites are also formed. (Reproduced, with permission, from Ganong WF: *Review of Medical Physiology*, 12th ed. Lange, 1985.)

motes glycogen storage, possibly by facilitating the effect of insulin. Progesterone also promotes ketogenesis.

Progesterone can compete with aldosterone at the renal tubule, causing a decrease in Na^+ reabsorption. This leads to an increased secretion of aldosterone by the adrenal cortex (eg, in pregnancy). Progesterone increases the body temperature in humans. The mechanism of this effect is not known, but an alteration of the temperature-regulating centers in the hypothalamus has been suggested. Progesterone also alters the function of the respiratory centers. The ventilatory response to CO_2 is increased (synthetic progestins with an ethinyl group do not have respiratory effects). This leads to a measurable reduction in arterial and alveolar P_{CO_2} during pregnancy and in the luteal phase of the menstrual cycle. Progesterone and related steroids also have depressant and hypnotic effects on the brain.

Progesterone is responsible for the alveolobular development of the secretory apparatus in the breast. It also causes the maturation and secretory changes in the endometrium that are seen following ovulation (Fig 39–2).

Progesterone decreases the plasma levels of many amino acids and leads to increased urinary nitrogen excretion. It has been found to induce changes in the smooth endoplasmic reticulum and its functions in experimental animals.

Other effects are noted in the section on oral contraceptives, below.

SYNTHETIC PROGESTATIONAL AGENTS

A variety of progestational compounds have now been synthesized. Some of these are active when given by mouth. They are not a uniform group of compounds, and all of them differ from progesterone in one or more respects. Table 39–3 lists some of these compounds.

In general, the compounds chemically related to progesterone (21-carbon) can produce a secretory endometrium and maintain pregnancy in animals. They antagonize aldosterone-induced sodium retention (see above) and have no androgenic or estrogenic effects. The remaining compounds (19-carbon) produce a decidual change in the endometrial stroma, do not support pregnancy in test animals, are more effective gonadotropin inhibitors, and may have minimal estrogenic and androgenic or anabolic activity. They are sometimes referred to as "impeded androgens."

Therapeutic Uses

The major use of progestational hormones is for hormonal contraception (see below). However, they are useful in producing long-term ovarian suppression for other purposes. When used alone in large doses parenterally (eg, medroxyprogesterone acetate, 150 mg intramuscularly every 90 days), prolonged anovulation and amenorrhea are produced. This procedure

olized in one passage through the liver, and for that reason it is quite ineffective when administered orally.

In the liver, progesterone is metabolized to pregnanediol and conjugated with glucuronic acid. It is excreted into the urine as pregnanediol glucuronide (Fig 39–5). The amount of pregnanediol in the urine has been used as an index of progesterone secretion. It has been very useful in spite of the fact that the proportion of secreted progesterone converted to this compound varies from day to day and from individual to individual.

In addition to progesterone, 20α- and 20β-hydroxyprogesterone (20α- or 20β-hydroxy-4-pregnene-3-one) are also found. These compounds have about one-fifth the progestational activity of progesterone in humans and other species. Little is known of the role of these compounds, but 20α-hydroxyprogesterone is produced in large amounts in some species and may be of some importance biologically.

Progesterone has little effect on protein metabolism (Table 39–2). It stimulates lipoprotein lipase activity and seems to favor fat deposition. The effects on carbohydrate metabolism are more marked. Progesterone increases basal insulin levels and the insulin response to glucose. There is usually no manifest change in carbohydrate tolerance. In the liver, progesterone pro-

Table 39–3. Activities of progestational agents.

	Activities*						
	Duration of Action	Estro-genic	Andro-genic	Anti-estrogenic	Anti-androgenic	Anabolic	Preparations Available
Progesterone and derivatives							
Progesterone (various trade names)	1 d	−	−	+	−	−	Aqueous suspension: 25 and 50 mg/mL. In oil: 25 and 50 mg/mL. Suppository: 25–200 mg.†
Hydroxyprogesterone caproate (Delalutin)	8–14 d	sl	sl	−	−	−	Injection: 125 and 250 mg/mL.
Medroxyprogesterone acetate (Amen, Provera)	Tablets: 1–3 d Injection: 4–12 weeks	−	+	+	−	−	Tablet: 2.5 and 10 mg. Injection: 50 and 100 mg/mL.
Megestrol acetate (Megace)	1–3 d	−	−	+	+	−	Tablet: 20 and 40 mg.
17α-Ethinyl testosterone derivatives **Testosterone derivatives** Dimethisterone	1–3 d	−	−	sl	−	−	
19-Nortestosterone derivatives Norethynodrel‡ (Enovid)	1–3 d	+	−	−	−	−	
Lynestrenol (not available in USA)	1–3 d	+	+	−	−	+	
Norethindrone‡ (Micronor, etc)	1–3 d	sl	+	+	−	+	Tablet: 5 mg.
Norethindrone acetate‡ (Norlutate, etc)	1–3 d	sl	+	+	−	+	Tablet: 5 mg.
Ethynodiol diacetate‡ (Demulen)	1–3 d	sl	+	+	−	−	
dl-Norgestrel‡ (Ovrette)	1–3 d	−	+	+	−	+	
L-Norgestrel‡	1–3 d	−	+	+	−	+	

*Interpretation: + = active; − = inactive; sl = slight activity. Activities have been reported in various species using various end points and may not apply to humans.
†Formulated by prescription.
‡See Table 39–4.

has been employed in the treatment of dysmenorrhea, endometriosis, hirsutism, and bleeding disorders when estrogens are contraindicated. The major problem with this regimen is the prolonged time required for ovulatory function to return after cessation of therapy in some patients. It should not be used for patients planning a pregnancy in the near future.

Progestins do not appear to have any place in the therapy of threatened or habitual abortion. Early reports of the usefulness of these agents resulted from the unwarranted assumption that after several abortions the likelihood of repeated abortions was over 90%. When progestational agents were administered to patients with previous abortions, a salvage rate of 80% was obtained. It is now recognized that similar patients abort only 20% of the time even when untreated.

Progesterone and progestational agents administered early in pregnancy have been incriminated in the masculinization of the external genitalia in the female fetus. Prolonged postpartum bleeding has been reported in some patients treated with repository me-droxyprogesterone or hydroxyprogesterone caproate.

Progesterone and medroxyprogesterone have been used in the treatment of women who have difficulty in conceiving and who demonstrate a slow rise in basal body temperature. There is no convincing evidence that this treatment is effective.

Preparations of progesterone and medroxyprogesterone have been used to treat premenstrual syndrome. Controlled studies have not confirmed the effectiveness of such therapy. However, the placebo effect is substantial.

Diagnostic Uses

Progesterone can also be used as a test of estrogen secretion. The administration of progesterone, 150 mg/d, or medroxyprogesterone, 10 mg/d for 5–7 days, is followed by withdrawal bleeding in amenorrheic patients only when the endometrium has been stimulated by estrogens. A combination of estrogen and progestin can be given to test the responsiveness of the endometrium in patients with amenorrhea.

Contraindications, Cautions, & Adverse Effects

Recent studies with progestational compounds and with combination oral contraceptives indicate that the progestin in these agents may increase blood pressure in some patients. The more potent progestins also reduce plasma high-density lipoprotein levels in women. Lower HDL levels are associated with an increased incidence of arterial disease. See also Hormonal Contraception, below.

Preparations & Dosages

See Table 39–3.

DANAZOL

Danazol (Danocrine), an isoxazole derivative of ethisterone (17α-ethinyl testosterone) with weak progestational and androgenic activities, is used to suppress ovarian function. Danazol inhibits the midcycle surge of LH and FSH and can prevent the compensatory increase in LH and FSH following castration in animals, but it does not significantly lower or suppress basal LH or FSH levels in normal women. Danazol binds to androgen, progesterone, and glucocorticoid receptors and can translocate the androgen receptor into the nucleus to initiate androgen-specific RNA synthesis. It does not bind to intracellular estrogen receptors, but it does bind to sex hormone–binding globulin (SHBG) and corticosteroid-binding globulins (CBG). It inhibits the cholesterol-cleaving enzyme, 3-β-hydroxysteroid dehydrogenase, 17-α-hydroxysteroid dehydrogenase, 17,21-lyase, 17α-hydroxylase, 11β-hydroxylase, and 21-hydroxylase, but it does not inhibit aromatase. It increases the mean clearance rate of progesterone, probably by displacing the hormone from binding proteins, and may have similar effects on other active steroid hormones. Ethisterone, a major metabolite, has both progestational and mild androgenic effects.

Danazol is slowly metabolized in humans, having a half-life of over 15 hours. This results in stable circulating levels when the drug is administered twice daily. It has been found to be highly concentrated in the liver, adrenals, and kidneys and is excreted in both feces and urine.

Danazol has been employed as an inhibitor of gonadal function and has found its major use in the treatment of endometriosis. For this purpose, it can be given in a dose of 600 mg/d. The dose is reduced to 400 mg/d after 1 month and to 200 mg/d in 2 months. About 85% of patients show marked improvement in 3–12 months.

Danazol has also been used for the treatment of fibrocystic disease of the breast. It has been effective in some patients for the relief of severe cyclic breast pain and tenderness but should be reserved for use in patients in whom analgesics and other drugs have failed.

Preliminary studies indicate that danazol may be useful in the treatment of patients with hematologic disorders, including hemophilia, Christmas disease, and idiopathic thrombocytopenic purpura.

The major side effects are weight gain, edema, decreased breast size, acne and oily skin, increased hair growth, deepening of the voice, headache, hot flushes, changes in libido, and muscle cramps. Although mild side effects are very common, it is seldom necessary to discontinue the drug because of them.

Danazol should be used with great caution in patients with hepatic dysfunction, since it has been reported to produce mild to moderate hepatocellular damage in some patients, as evidenced by enzyme changes. It is also contraindicated during pregnancy and breast feeding, as it may produce urogenital abnormalities in the offspring. Therefore, women taking the drug should be advised to use an effective form of contraception.

OTHER OVARIAN HORMONES

The normal ovary produces small amounts of androgens, including testosterone, androstenedione, and dehydroepiandrosterone. Only testosterone has a significant amount of biologic activity, although androstenedione can be converted to estrone in peripheral tissues. The normal woman produces a total of less than 200 μg of testosterone in 24 hours, and about one-third of this is probably formed in the ovary directly. The physiologic significance of these small amounts of androgens is not established, but they may be partly responsible for normal hair growth at puberty and may have other important metabolic effects. The androgen production by the ovary may be markedly increased in some abnormal states, usually in association with hirsutism and amenorrhea as noted above.

The ovary also produces one or more substances similar to the inhibin produced by the testis that decreases the pituitary release of FSH.

RELAXIN

Relaxin is a polypeptide that has been extracted from the ovary. The 3-dimensional structure of relaxin is related to that of the growth-promoting polypeptides and similar to that of insulin. Although the amino acid sequence differs from that of insulin, it consists of 2 chains linked by disulfide bonds, cleaved from a prohormone. It is found in the ovary, placenta, uterus, and blood. Relaxin synthesis has been demonstrated in luteinized granulosa cells of the corpus luteum. It has been shown to increase glycogen synthesis and water uptake by the myometrium and decreases uterine contractility. In some species it changes the mechanical properties of the cervix and pubic ligaments, facilitating delivery.

In women, relaxin has been measured by immunoassay. Levels were highest immediately after the LH surge and during menstruation. A physiologic role for this hormone has not been established.

Clinical trials with relaxin have been carried out in patients with dysmenorrhea. Relaxin has also been administered to patients in premature labor and during prolonged labor. The therapeutic value of this hormone has not been established.

HORMONAL CONTRACEPTION
(Oral Contraceptives)

A large number of oral contraceptives containing estrogens or progestins (or both) are now available for clinical use (Table 39–4). These preparations vary chemically and, as might be expected, have many properties in common, but they exhibit definite differences. Experience with some of the drugs has been much greater than with others, and more differences may emerge as further experience accumulates.

Two types of preparations are used for oral contraception: (1) combinations of estrogens and progestins and (2) continuous progestin therapy without concomitant administration of estrogens.

The preparations for oral use are all well absorbed, and the metabolism of the drugs is not known to be profoundly altered by simultaneous administration. Little information is available concerning the turnover time and excretion of some of these compounds.

Pharmacologic Effects
A. Mechanism of Contraceptive Action: The combinations of estrogens and progestins exert their effect largely through inhibition of ovulation. The combination agents also produce a change in the cervical mucus, in the uterine endometrium, and in the motility and secretion in the fallopian tubes, all of which decrease the likelihood of conception and implantation. The continuous use of progestins alone does not always inhibit ovulation. The other factors mentioned, therefore, play a major role in the prevention of pregnancy when these agents are used.

B. Effects on the Ovary: ′Chronic use of combination agents depresses ovarian function. The gross appearance of the ovary is that of relative inactivity; there is a minimum of follicular development; and corpora lutea, larger follicles, stromal edema, and other morphologic features normally seen in ovulating women are absent. In general, the amounts of the endogenous estrogens excreted in the urine are less than those observed in normal menstruating women, and pregnanediol excretion is not usually increased in the latter phase of the cycle. Although cystic follicles have been described in patients being treated with oral contraceptives, the ovaries usually become smaller even when enlarged before therapy.

The great majority of patients return to normal menstrual patterns when these drugs are terminated. About 75% will ovulate in the first posttreatment cycle, and 97% by the third posttreatment cycle. Patients with a history of irregular cycles seem more liable to the development of amenorrhea following cessation of therapy.

About 2% of patients remain amenorrheic for periods of up to several years after therapy has been concluded, and the prevalence of amenorrhea, often with galactorrhea, is higher in women who have used this form of contraception.

These preparations have important effects on the genital tract. The cytologic findings on vaginal smears vary depending on the preparation used. However, with almost all of the combined drugs, a low maturation index is found because of the presence of progestational agents.

C. Effects on the Uterus: After prolonged use, the cervix may show some hypertrophy and polyp formation. There are also important effects on the cervical mucus, making it more like postovulation mucus, ie, thick and less copious.

The endometrial changes vary with the preparation. Agents containing both estrogens and progestins produce a stromal deciduation toward the end of the cycle. The agents containing the 19-nor compounds—particularly those with the smaller amounts of estrogen—tend to produce more glandular atrophy and usually less bleeding, whereas combination agents containing progestins that produce more physiologic changes in the endometrium (eg, medroxyprogesterone) are associated with spotting between periods and more bleeding at the time of menses.

Although studies in rodents suggest that the development of the blastocyst and the endometrium must be very precisely matched for implantation to occur, pregnancies occur in some patients who omit a few tablets or when the medication was begun too late in a given cycle to prevent ovulation.

Although studies in humans are not available, animal experiments indicate that transport of the gamete through the fallopian tube is altered by estrogens and progestins. The effect on transport is thought by some to be an important mechanism for the impairment of fertility, particularly with the use of low-dosage continuous progestin therapy as noted above.

D. Effects on the Breast: Stimulation of the breasts occurs in most patients receiving estrogen-containing agents. Some enlargement is generally noted. The administration of estrogens and combinations of estrogens and progestins tends to suppress lactation. When the doses are small, the effects on breast feeding are not appreciable. Preliminary studies of the transport of the oral contraceptives into the breast milk suggest that only small amounts of these compounds are found, and they have not been considered to be of importance.

E. Other Effects of the Oral Contraceptives:
1. Central nervous system effects–The central nervous system effects of the oral contraceptives have not been well studied in humans. A variety of effects

Table 39–4. Oral contraceptive agents in use. The estrogen-containing compounds are arranged in order of increasing content of estrogen (ethinyl estradiol and mestranol have similar potencies). The relative progestational potencies are shown in the last column.

	Estrogen (mg)	Progestin (mg)	PP*
Monophasic combination tablets			
Loestrin 1/20	Ethinyl estradiol 0.02	Norethindrone acetate 1.0	4
Loestrin 1.5/30	Ethinyl estradiol 0.03	Norethindrone acetate 1.5	6
Lo/Ovral	Ethinyl estradiol 0.03	dl-Norgestrel 0.3	18
Nordette	Ethinyl estradiol 0.03	L-Norgestrel 0.15	18
Brevicon Modicon	Ethinyl estradiol 0.035	Norethindrone 0.5	1
Demulen 1/35	Ethinyl estradiol 0.035	Ethynodiol diacetate 1.0	30
Norinyl 1/35 Ortho-Novum 1/35	Ethinyl estradiol 0.035	Norethindrone 1.0	2
Ovcon 35	Ethinyl estradiol 0.035	Norethindrone 0.4	0.8
Demulen 1/50	Ethinyl estradiol 0.05	Ethynodiol diacetate 1.0	30
Norlestrin 1/50	Ethinyl estradiol 0.05	Norethindrone acetate 1.0	4
Norlestrin 2.5/50	Ethinyl estradiol 0.05	Norethindrone acetate 2.5	10
Ovcon 50	Ethinyl estradiol 0.05	Norethindrone 1.0	2
Ovral	Ethinyl estradiol 0.05	dl-Norgestrel 0.5	30
Norinyl 1/50 Ortho-Novum 1/50	Mestranol 0.05	Norethindrone 1.0	2
Enovid 5	Mestranol 0.075	Norethynodrel 5.0	11
Norinyl 1/80 Ortho-Novum 1/80	Mestranol 0.08	Norethindrone 1.0	2
Enovid E	Mestranol 0.1	Norethynodrel 2.5	6
Norinyl-2 Ortho-Novum-2	Mestranol 0.1	Norethindrone 2.0	4
Ovulen	Mestranol 0.1	Ethynodiol diacetate 1.0	30
Biphasic combination tablets Ortho-Novum 10/11			
Days 1–10	Ethinyl estradiol 0.035	Norethindrone 0.5	1
Days 11–21	Ethinyl estradiol 0.035	Norethindrone 1.0	2
Triphasic combination tablets Triphasil			
Days 1–6	Ethinyl estradiol 0.03	L-Norgestrel 0.05	2
Days 7–11	Ethinyl estradiol 0.04	L-Norgestrel 0.075	3
Days 12–21	Ethinyl estradiol 0.03	L-Norgestrel 0.125	5
Ortho-Novum 7/7/7			
Days 1–7	Ethinyl estradiol 0.035	Norethindrone 0.5	1
Days 8–14	Ethinyl estradiol 0.035	Norethindrone 0.75	1.5
Days 15–21	Ethinyl estradiol 0.035	Norethindrone 1.0	2
Tri-Norinyl			
Days 1–7	Ethinyl estradiol 0.035	Norethindrone 0.5	1
Days 8–16	Ethinyl estradiol 0.035	Norethindrone 1.0	2
Days 17–21	Ethinyl estradiol 0.035	Norethindrone 0.5	1
Daily progestin tablets			
Micronor	. . .	Norethindrone 0.35	0.7
Nor-QD	. . .	Norethindrone 0.35	0.7
Ovrette	. . .	dl-Norgestrel 0.075	3

*Progestational potency.

of estrogen and progesterone have been noted in animals. Estrogens tend to increase excitability in the brain, whereas progesterone tends to decrease it. The thermogenic action of progesterone and some of the synthetic progestins is also thought to be in the central nervous system. The suppression of ovarian function that results from inhibition of gonadotropin secretion is also thought to be due to an influence on the hypothalamus or other parts of the nervous system.

It is very difficult to evaluate any behavioral or emotional effects of these compounds. Although the incidence of pronounced changes in mood, affect, and behavior reported in most studies is low, milder changes are common. These changes are variable and therefore difficult to evaluate in relation to the pharmacologic effects of the drug. They may be psychologically induced by the act of using contraception or the circumstances surrounding it. However, it is possible that the changes in neuronal activity produced by these drugs may lead to behavioral changes which are conditioned by other factors.

2. Effects on endocrine function–The inhibition of pituitary gonadotropin secretion has been mentioned. Estrogens are known to alter adrenal structure and function. Estrogens increase the plasma concentration of the α_2-globulin that binds hydrocortisone (cortisol-binding globulin). This does not appear to lead to any chronic alteration in the rate of secretion of cortisol, but plasma concentrations may be more than double the levels found in untreated individuals. It has also been observed that the ACTH response to the administration of metyrapone (see Chapter 36) is attenuated by estrogens and the oral contraceptives.

These preparations cause alterations in the angiotensin-aldosterone system. Plasma renin activity has been found to increase, and there is an increase in aldosterone secretion. The relationship between these alterations and the hypertension that occurs in some patients taking oral contraceptives is not clear.

Thyroxine-binding globulin is increased. As a result, plasma thyroxine (T_4) levels are increased to those commonly seen during pregnancy. Since more of the thyroxine is bound, the free thyroxine level in these patients is normal.

3. Hematologic effects–Serious thromboembolic phenomena occurring in women taking oral contraceptives have stimulated a great many studies of the effects of these compounds on blood coagulation. A clear picture of such effects has not yet emerged. The oral contraceptives do not consistently alter bleeding or clotting time. Preliminary indications are that the changes observed are similar to those reported in pregnancy. There is an increase in factors VII, VIII, IX, and X. Increased amounts of coumarin derivatives are required to produce a reduction in prothrombin time in patients taking oral contraceptives.

In addition to the changes in clotting factors, there are important changes in serum proteins. There is an increase in the α_2-globulins that affects the concentrations of hormones and other serum constitutents that are protein-bound (Table 39–2). There is an increase

in serum iron and total iron-binding capacity similar to that reported in patients with hepatitis.

Significant alterations in the cellular components of blood have not been reported with any consistency. A number of patients have been reported to develop folic acid deficiency anemias.

4. Hepatic effects–The liver plays an important role in the inactivation and conversion to water-soluble conjugates of the estrogens and progestins used in oral contraceptives. These hormones also have profound effects on the function of the liver. Some of these effects are deleterious and will be considered below under Adverse Reactions.

The effects on serum proteins noted above result from the effects of the estrogens on the synthesis of the various α_2-globulins and fibrinogen. Serum haptoglobins that also arise from the liver are depressed rather than increased by estrogen.

Some of the effects on carbohydrate and lipid metabolism are probably influenced by changes in liver metabolism (see below).

Important alterations in drug excretion and metabolism also occur in the liver. Estrogens in the amounts seen during pregnancy or used in oral contraceptive agents delay the clearance of sulfobromophthalein and reduce the flow of bile. These alterations result from impairment of the transfer of cholephilic substances from hepatic cells into the bile. These agents increase the saturation of cholesterol in bile. The proportion of cholic acid in bile acids is increased while the proportion of chenodeoxycholic acid is decreased. These changes may cause the observed increase in cholelithiasis associated with the use of these agents.

5. Effects on lipid metabolism–The available studies indicate that estrogens increase serum triglycerides and free and esterified cholesterol. Phospholipids are also increased, as are high-density lipoproteins. Low-density lipoproteins usually decrease. Although the effects are marked with doses of 100 μg of mestranol or ethinyl estradiol, doses of 50 μg or less have minimal effects. The progestins (particularly the 19-nortestosterone derivatives) tend to antagonize the effects of estrogen. Preparations containing small amounts of estrogen and a progestin may slightly decrease triglycerides and high-density lipoproteins.

6. Effects on carbohydrate metabolism–The administration of oral contraceptives produces alterations in carbohydrate metabolism similar to those observed in pregnancy. There is a reduction in the rate of absorption of carbohydrates from the gastrointestinal tract. Progesterone increases basal insulin levels and the insulin rise induced by carbohydrate ingestion. Preparations with more potent progestins such as norgestrel may cause progressive decreases in carbohydrate tolerance over the years. However, the changes in glucose tolerance are reversible on discontinuing medication.

7. Cardiovascular effects–These agents cause small increases in cardiac output associated with higher systolic and diastolic blood pressure and heart rate. Pathologic increases in blood pressure have been reported in a small number of patients. The pressure returns to normal when treatment is terminated. Although the magnitude of the pressure change is small in many patients, it is marked in others. It is important that blood pressure be followed in each patient. An increase in blood pressure has been reported to occur in few postmenopausal women treated with estrogens alone.

8. Effects on the skin–The oral contraceptives have been noted to increase pigmentation of the skin of patients (chloasma). This effect seems to be enhanced in women who have dark complexions and by exposure to ultraviolet light. Some of the androgenlike progestins may increase the production of sebum. The sequential oral contraceptive preparations as well as estrogens often decrease sebum production. This may be due to suppression of the ovarian production of androgens. Estrogens also decrease pore size and lead to acne in some patients.

Clinical Uses

The most important use of the estrogens and progestins is for oral contraception. A large number of preparations are available for this specific purpose, some of which are listed in Table 39–4. They are specially packaged to provide for ease of administration. In general, they are very effective; when these agents are taken according to directions, the risk of conception is extremely small. The pregnancy rate is estimated to be about 0.5–1 per 100 woman years at risk with combination agents. Contraceptive failure has been observed in some patients taking phenytoin or antibiotics or when one or more doses are missed.

Progestins and estrogens are also useful in the treatment of endometriosis. When severe dysmenorrhea is the major symptom, the suppression of ovulation with estrogen may be followed by painless periods. However, in most patients this approach to therapy is inadequate. The long-term administration of large doses of progestins or combinations of progestins and estrogens prevents the periodic breakdown of the endometrial tissue and in some cases will lead to endometrial fibrosis and prevent the reactivation of implants for prolonged periods.

As is true with most hormonal preparations, many of the side effects are physiologic or pharmacologic effects that are objectionable only because they are not pertinent to the situation for which they are being used. Therefore, the product containing the smallest effective amounts of hormones should be selected for use.

Adverse Reactions

The incidence of serious known side effects associated with the use of these drugs is low. There are a number of reversible changes in intermediary metabolism. However, the long-term effects of such changes as an increase in plasma triglycerides or decrease in glucose tolerance cannot be assessed as yet. Minor side effects are frequent, but most are mild and many are transient. Although it is not often necessary to discontinue medication for these, as many as one-third of all patients started on oral contraception with combined or sequential agents discontinue therapy for reasons other than a desire to become pregnant.

Common minor problems may respond to simple changes in pill formulation. A brief summary of some symptoms and suggested changes is as follows:

(1) Nausea, breast tenderness, edema, chloasma: Decrease estrogen content.

(2) Early and midcycle spotting, decreased flow or amenorrhea: Increase estrogen content or decrease progestin content (or both).

(3) Weight gain, hair growth, depression, tiredness: Decrease progestin content.

(4) Excessive bleeding, late cycle spotting: Increase progestin content or decrease estrogen content (or both).

A. Mild Side Effects:

1. Nausea, mastalgia, breakthrough bleeding, and edema are related to the amount of estrogen in the preparation. They were more common with the sequential preparations because of the larger amounts of estrogen present and can often be alleviated by a shift to a preparation containing smaller amounts of estrogen or to agents containing progestational compounds with androgenlike effects.

2. Changes in serum proteins and other effects on endocrine function (see above) must be taken into account when thyroid, adrenal, or pituitary function is being evaluated. Increases in sedimentation rate are thought to be due to increased levels of fibrinogen.

3. Psychologic changes are often transient and are not predictable with any of the preparations. In general, most patients "feel better" because they are relieved of anxiety about becoming pregnant. Some patients experience premenstrual-like symptoms of irritability and depression throughout the cycle.

4. Headache is mild and often transient. Migraine is often made worse and has been reported to be associated with an increased frequency of cerebrovascular accidents. When this occurs, or when migraine has its onset during therapy with these agents, treatment should be discontinued.

5. Libido is increased or decreased in a few patients and unchanged in the majority. Similar changes have been observed with placebo therapy.

6. Withdrawal bleeding sometimes fails to occur—most often with combination preparations—and may cause confusion with regard to pregnancy. If this is disturbing to the patient, a different preparation may be tried or other methods of contraception used.

B. More Annoying Side Effects: Any of the following may require discontinuation of oral contraceptives:

1. Breakthrough bleeding is the most common problem in using progestational agents alone for contraception. It occurs in as many as 25% of patients. It is more frequently encountered in patients taking low-dose preparations than in those taking combination pills with higher levels of progestin and estrogen. The

recently introduced biphasic and triphasic oral contraceptives (Table 39–4) decrease breakthrough bleeding without increasing the total hormone content.

2. Weight gain is more common with the combination agents containing androgenlike progestins. It can usually be controlled by shifting to preparations with less progestin effect or by dieting.

3. Increased skin pigmentation may be distressing in dark-skinned women. It tends to increase with time, the incidence being about 5% at the end of the first year and about 40% after 8 years. It is thought to be exacerbated by vitamin B deficiency. It is often reversible upon discontinuance of medication, but in occasional cases the pigmentation disappears very slowly.

4. Acne may be exacerbated by agents containing androgenlike progestins, whereas agents containing large amounts of estrogen frequently cause marked improvement in acne.

5. Hirsutism may also be aggravated by the 19-nortestosterone derivatives, and the combination containing nonandrogenic progestins is preferred.

6. Ureteral dilatation similar to that observed in pregnancy has been reported, and bacteriuria is more frequent.

7. Vaginal infections are more common and more difficult to treat in patients who are receiving oral contraceptives.

8. Amenorrhea after discontinuation–Following cessation of administration of oral contraceptives, 95% of patients with normal menstrual histories resume normal periods and all but a few resume normal cycles during the next few months. However, some patients remain amenorrheic for several years. Many of these patients also have galactorrhea. Patients who have had menstrual irregularities before taking oral contraceptives are particularly susceptible to prolonged amenorrhea when the agents are discontinued.

C. Severe Side Effects:

1. Vascular disorders–Thromboembolism was one of the earliest of the serious unanticipated effects to be reported and has been the most thoroughly studied.

a. Venous thromboembolic disease–Epidemiologic studies indicate that about one patient per 1000 woman years not using oral contraceptives will develop superficial or deep thromboembolic disease. The overall incidence of these disorders in patients taking low-dose oral contraceptives is about 3 per 1000 woman years. The risk for this disorder is increased during the first month of contraceptive use and remains constant for several years or more. The risk returns to normal within a month when use is discontinued. The risk of venous thrombosis or pulmonary embolism among women with predisposing conditions may be higher than that in normal women.

The incidence of this complication is related to the estrogen but not the progestin content of oral contraceptives. The risk of superficial or deep thromboembolic disease in patients treated with oral contraceptives is not related to age, parity, mild obesity, or cigarette smoking. However, some studies indicate a genetic susceptibility to this disorder and suggest that oral contraceptives multiply the effect. Decreased venous blood flow, endothelial proliferation in veins and arteries, and increased coagulability of blood resulting from changes in platelet coagulation and fibrinolytic systems contribute to the increased incidence of thrombosis. The major plasma inhibitor of thrombin, antithrombin III, is substantially decreased during oral contraceptive use. This change occurs in the first month of treatment and lasts as long as treatment persists, reversing within a month thereafter.

b. Myocardial infarction–The use of oral contraceptives is associated with a slightly higher risk of myocardial infarction in women who are obese, have a history of preeclampsia or hypertension, or have hyperlipoproteinemia or diabetes. There is a much higher risk in women who smoke. Since 40% of women 20–50 years of age smoke 15 or more cigarettes a day, this risk factor is very important. The risk attributable to oral contraceptives in women 30–39 years of age who do not smoke is about 4 cases per 100,000 users per year, as compared to 185 cases per 100,000 among women 40–44 who smoke heavily. The association with myocardial infarction is thought to involve acceleration of atherogenesis because of decreased glucose tolerance, decreased levels of high-density lipoproteins, increased levels of low-density lipoproteins, and increased platelet aggregation. However, facilitation of coronary arterial spasm may also play a role in some of these patients. The progestational component of oral contraceptives decreases high-density lipoprotein cholesterol, although the estrogenic component has also been found to increase it. The net difference, therefore, will depend on the specific composition of the pill used and the patient's susceptibility to the particular effects. Recent studies suggest that risk of infarction is not increased in past users who used these agents for less than 5 years.

c. Cerebrovascular disease–The risk of strokes is concentrated in women over 35. It is increased in current users of oral contraceptives but not in past users. However, subarachnoid hemorrhages have been found to be increased among both current and past users and may increase with time. The risk of thrombotic or hemorrhagic stroke attributable to oral contraceptives is about 37 cases per 100,000 users per year. Ten percent of these strokes were fatal, and most of the fatal ones were due to subarachnoid hemorrhage. Insufficient data are available on which to base an assessment of the effects of smoking and other risk factors. However, it is thought that the pattern of risk is similar to that seen for myocardial infarction.

Elevations in blood pressure may also increase the risk, since there is a 3- to 6-fold increase in the incidence of overt hypertension in women taking oral contraceptives.

In summary, available data indicate that oral contraceptives increase the risk of various cardiovascular disorders at all ages and among both smokers and nonsmokers. However, this risk appears to be concentrated in women 35 years of age or older who are heavy smokers. It is clear that the presence of these risk factors must be considered in each individual patient for whom oral contraceptives are considered.

2. Gastrointestinal disorders–Many cases of cholestatic jaundice have been reported in patients taking progestin-containing drugs. The differences in incidence of these disorders from one population to another suggest that genetic factors may be involved.

The jaundice caused by these agents is similar to that produced by other 17-alkyl-substituted steroids. It is most often observed in the first 3 cycles and is particularly common in women with a history of cholestatic jaundice during pregnancy. Liver biopsies taken from such women show bile thrombi in the canaliculi and occasional focal necrosis. Serum alkaline phosphatase and SGPT are increased. Sulfobromophthalein retention and serum enzyme changes observed in some patients may indicate liver damage.

Jaundice and pruritus disappear 1–8 weeks after the drug is discontinued.

These agents have also been found to increase the incidence of symptomatic gallbladder disease, including cholecystitis and cholangitis. This is probably the result of the alterations in bile described above.

It also appears that the incidence of hepatic adenomas is increased in women taking oral contraceptives. Ischemic bowel disease secondary to thrombosis of the celiac and superior and inferior mesenteric arteries and veins has also been reported in women using these drugs.

3. Depression–Depression of sufficient degree to require cessation of therapy occurs in about 6% of patients treated with some preparations.

4. Cancer–The occurrence of malignant tumors in patients taking oral contraceptives has been studied extensively. It is now clear that these compounds *reduce* the risk of endometrial and ovarian cancer. One recent study suggests that in young women using compounds with high progestin content for 6 years or longer before the age of 25, there is an increased risk for breast cancer. No such increase was found in older women or in those using combination oral contraceptives with low progestin content. However, another study failed to confirm even this limited increase in breast cancer risk.

In addition to the above effects, a number of other adverse reactions have been reported for which a causal relationship has not been established. These include alopecia, erythema multiforme, erythema nodosum, and other skin disorders.

Contraindications & Cautions

These drugs are contraindicated in patients with thrombophlebitis, thromboembolic phenomena, and cerebrovascular disorders or a past history of these conditions. They should not be used to treat vaginal bleeding when the cause is unknown. They should be avoided in patients with known or suspected tumor of the breast or other estrogen-dependent neoplasm.

Since these preparations have caused aggravation of preexisting disorders, they should be avoided or used with caution in patients with liver disease, asthma, eczema, migraine, diabetes, hypertension, optic neuritis, retrobulbar neuritis, or convulsive disorders.

The oral contraceptives may produce edema, and for that reason they should be used with great caution in patients in congestive failure or in whom edema is otherwise undesirable or dangerous.

Estrogens may increase the rate of growth of fibroids. Therefore, for women with these tumors, agents with the smallest amounts of estrogen and the most androgenic progestins should be selected. The use of progestational agents alone for contraception might be especially useful in such patients (see below).

At present, these agents are contraindicated in adolescents in whom epiphyseal closure has not yet been completed.

Since the introduction of oral contraceptives and the recognition of serious adverse effects, the trend has been toward reduction of first the estrogen content and more recently the progestin content. Recent reports showing a reduction in adverse effects probably reflect changes in the selection of patients as well as the effects of dose reduction. However, it seems prudent to utilize the smallest effective doses of estrogen and progestin compatible with the patient's needs.

Contraception with progestins alone. Small doses of progestins administered orally can be used for contraception. They are particularly suited for use in patients for whom estrogen administration is undesirable. They are about as effective as intrauterine devices or combination pills containing 20–30 μg of ethinyl estradiol. There is a high incidence of abnormal bleeding. The use of infrequent injections of long-acting progestins (see above) such as medroxyprogesterone acetate has also found limited usefulness. The use of large doses of oral progestins at the time of intercourse is under study.

A new method of hormonal contraception is presently undergoing clinical trials. This method utilizes the subcutaneous implantation of capsules containing a progestin such as levonorgestrel. These capsules release one-fifth to one-third as much steroid as oral agents, are extremely effective, and last for 5–6 years. The low levels of hormone have little effect on lipoprotein and carbohydrate metabolism or blood pressure. The disadvantages include the need for surgical insertion and removal of capsules and some irregular bleeding rather than predictable menses.

Postcoital contraceptives. Pregnancy can be prevented following coitus by the administration of estrogens alone or in combination with progestins ("morning after" contraception). When treatment is begun within 72 hours, it is effective 99% of the time. The effective schedules are shown in Table 39–5. The hormones are often administered with antiemetics, since 40% of patients have nausea or vomiting. Other side effects include headache, dizziness, breast tenderness, and abdominal and leg cramps.

Table 39–5. Schedules for use of postcoital contraceptives.

Conjugated estrogens: 10 mg 3 times daily for 5 days
Ethinyl estradiol: 2.5 mg twice daily for 5 days
Diethylstilbestrol: 50 mg daily for 5 days
Norgestrel, 0.5 mg, with ethinyl estradiol, 0.05 mg: 2 tablets and
    2 in 12 hours

Health Benefits of Hormonal Contraceptives

It has become apparent during the last decade that reduction in the dose of the constituents of oral contraceptives has markedly reduced mild and severe adverse effects, providing a relatively safe and convenient contraceptive for many young women. Treatment with oral contraceptives has now been shown to be associated with many benefits unrelated to contraception. These include a reduced risk of ovarian cysts, ovarian and endometrial cancer, and benign breast disease. There is a lower incidence of pelvic inflammatory disease and ectopic pregnancy. Iron deficiency, duodenal ulcer, and rheumatoid arthritis are less common, and premenstrual symptoms, dysmenorrhea, and endometriosis are ameliorated with their use.

ANTIESTROGENS

TAMOXIFEN

Tamoxifen (Nolvadex) is a competitive inhibitor of estradiol at the receptor and is being used in the palliative treatment of advanced breast cancer in postmenopausal women. It is a nonsteroidal agent that is given orally. Peak plasma levels are reached in a few hours. It has an initial half-life of 7–14 hours in the circulation and is predominantly excreted by the liver. It is dispensed as the citrate in the form of tablets containing the equivalent of 10 mg tamoxifen. It is used in doses of 10–20 mg twice daily. Hot flashes and nausea and vomiting occur in 25% of patients, and many other adverse effects are observed.

CLOMIPHENE

Clomiphene citrate (Clomid) is a weak estrogen that also acts as a competitive inhibitor of endogenous estrogens. It has found use as an ovulation-inducing agent (see below).

GONADOTROPIN-RELEASING HORMONE (GnRH) ANALOGS

As noted below, GnRH administered in pulses will stimulate ovarian function and induce ovulation in women with amenorrhea. However, continuous administration suppresses ovarian function by down regulation of the receptor and desensitization. The development of potent polypeptide analogs such as nafarelin and buserelin has made it possible to produce ovarian suppression by daily subcutaneous or intranasal administration of these agents. The marked suppression produced by large doses has found use in the treatment of precocious puberty and gonadal hormone-dependent tumors. Smaller doses have been found to be effective in the treatment of endometriosis.

OVULATION-INDUCING AGENTS

CLOMIPHENE

Interest in antiestrogenic compounds has been stimulated by the increasing need for antifertility compounds. Several of the synthetic estrogens have been shown to have significant antiestrogen or partial agonist properties. They are able to successfully compete for binding sites, yet have weaker hormonal properties. Clomiphene citrate (Clomid) is one such compound. It is closely related to other pharmacologically active compounds such as the estrogen chlorotrianisene (Fig 39–4) and the cholesterol inhibitor triparanol.

$(C_2H_5)_2$—N—CH_2—CH_2—O—⟨⟩—C=C⟨⟩Cl

Clomiphene

This compound is active when taken orally, since it is readily absorbed. Very little is known about its metabolism, but about half of the compound is excreted into the stools within 5 days after administration. It has been suggested that clomiphene is slowly excreted from an enterohepatic pool.

Pharmacologic Effects

A. Mechanisms of Action: Clomiphene is a partial agonist estrogen. The estrogenic effects are best demonstrated in animals with marked gonadal deficiency. Clomiphene has also been shown to effectively inhibit the action of stronger estrogens. In humans it leads to an increase in the secretion of gonadotropins and estrogens.

B. Effects: The pharmacologic importance of this compound rests on its ability to stimulate ovulation in women with amenorrhea and other ovulatory disorders. The mechanism by which ovulation is produced is not known. It has been suggested that it blocks an inhibitory influence of estrogens on the hypothalamus and increases the production of gonadotropins.

Clinical Uses

Clomiphene is used for the treatment of disorders of ovulation in patients wishing to become pregnant. In general, a single ovulation is induced by a single course of therapy, and the patient must be treated repeatedly until pregnancy is achieved, since normal ovulatory function does not usually resume. The compound is of no use in patients with ovarian or pituitary failure.

When clomiphene is administered in doses of 100 mg daily for 5 days, a rise in plasma LH and FSH is observed several days after starting. In patients who ovulate, the initial rise is followed by a second rise of gonadotropin levels just prior to ovulation.

Adverse Reactions

The most common side effects in patients treated with this drug are hot flushes, which resemble those experienced by menopausal patients. They tend to be mild and disappear when the drug is discontinued. There have been occasional reports of eye symptoms due to intensification and prolongation of after-images. These are generally of short duration. Headache, constipation, allergic skin reactions, and reversible hair loss have been reported occasionally.

The effective use of clomiphene is associated with some stimulation of the ovaries and usually with ovarian enlargement. The degree of enlargement tends to be greater and its incidence higher in patients who have enlarged ovaries at the beginning of therapy.

A variety of other symptoms such as nausea and vomiting, increased nervous tension, depression, fatigue, breast soreness, weight gain, urinary frequency, and heavy menses have also been reported. However, these appear to be due to the hormonal changes associated with an ovulatory menstrual cycle rather than a result of the medication. The incidence of multiple pregnancy is approximately 10%.

Clomiphene has not been shown to have an adverse effect in human pregnancy. However, since the only current indication for clomiphene therapy is to achieve pregnancy, existing pregnancy is a contraindication to its use.

Contraindications & Cautions

Special precautions should be observed in patients with enlarged ovaries. These women are thought to be more sensitive to this drug and should receive small doses. Any patient who complains of abdominal symptoms should be carefully examined. The maximum ovarian enlargement occurs after the 5-day course has been completed, and many patients can be shown to have a palpable increase in ovarian size by the seventh to tenth days.

Special precautions must also be taken in patients who have visual symptoms associated with clomiphene therapy, since these symptoms may make activities such as driving more hazardous.

Dosages

The recommended dose of clomiphene citrate (Clomid) at the beginning of therapy is 50 mg/d for 5 days. If ovulation occurs, this same course may be repeated until pregnancy is achieved. If ovulation does not occur, the dose is doubled to 100 mg/d for 5 days. If ovulation and menses occur, the next course can be started on the fifth day of the cycle. Experience to date suggests that patients who do not ovulate after 3 courses of 100 mg/d of clomiphene are not likely to respond to continued therapy.

About 80% of patients with anovulatory disorders or amenorrhea can be expected to respond by having ovulatory cycles. Approximately half of these patients will become pregnant.

BROMOCRIPTINE

In some amenorrheic women, an elevated level of prolactin appears to be the causative factor. These patients may have prolactin-secreting tumors or "empty sella" syndrome, which should be excluded before treatment is begun. The criteria for selecting medical, surgical, and radiation therapy for prolactinomas have not been firmly established.

Bromocriptine (Parlodel), an ergot alkaloid (Chapter 15), acts by binding to dopamine receptors in the pituitary and inhibits prolactin secretion. In 90% or more of patients, treatment leads to the onset of menses in 3–5 weeks. The usual dose required is 2.5 mg 2 or 3 times a day. Prolactin levels should be depressed to normal if treatment is adequate.

HUMAN MENOPAUSAL GONADOTROPIN (hMG, Menotropins)

Human menopausal gonadotropin—in conjunction with human chorionic gonadotropin (hCG), see p 431—is used to stimulate ovulation in patients who do not ovulate but have potentially functional ovarian tissue. It has been successful in the induction of ovulation in patients with hypopituitarism and other defects in gonadotropin secretion. It has also been used in patients with amenorrhea or anovulatory cycles and in patients in whom ovulatory disturbances are associated with galactorrhea or hirsutism.

Preparations of human menopausal gonadotropin can stimulate spermatogenesis in males with isolated gonadotropin deficiency. Using hMG in conjunction with hCG (see Chapter 36), endocrine and gametogenic function can be restored in some of these patients.

The pulsatile administration of GnRH is an effective means of inducing ovulation in patients with hypothalamic amenorrhea. It is cumbersome in that it requires the use of a peristaltic pump which delivers a pulse of 1–10 μg of this hypothalamic hormone every 60–120 minutes. It has the advantage of maintaining the normal processes for the control of follicular development, thus avoiding the complications seen with menotropins.

II. THE TESTIS
(Androgens & Anabolic Steroids, Antiandrogens, & Male Contraception)

The testis, like the ovary, has both gametogenic and endocrine functions. The gametogenic function of the testes is controlled largely by the secretion of FSH by the pituitary. High concentrations of androgens locally are also required for sperm production in the seminiferous tubules. The Sertoli cells in the seminiferous tubules may be the source of the estradiol produced in the testes. The androgens are produced in the interstitial or Leydig cells found in the spaces between the seminiferous tubules.

In humans the most important androgen secreted by the testis is testosterone. The pathways of synthesis of testosterone in the testes are similar to those previously described for the adrenal and ovary (Figs 38–1 and 39–3).

In the male, approximately 8 mg of testosterone is produced daily. About 95% is produced by the Leydig cells and only 5% by the adrenal. The testis also secretes small amounts of another potent androgen, dihydrotestosterone, as well as androstenedione and dehydroepiandrosterone, which are weak androgens. Pregnenolone and progesterone and their 17-hydroxylated derivatives are also released in small amounts.

Plasma levels of testosterone in males are about 0.6 μg/dL after puberty and do not appear to vary significantly with age. Testosterone is also present in the plasma of women in concentrations of approximately 0.03 μg/dL and is derived in approximately equal parts from the ovaries, the adrenals, and by the peripheral conversion of other hormones.

About 65% of circulating testosterone is bound to sex hormone–binding globulin (SHBG), a specific protein produced by the liver. This protein is increased in plasma by estrogen, by thyroid hormone, and in patients with cirrhosis of the liver. It is decreased by androgen and growth hormone and is lower in obese individuals. Most of the remaining testosterone is bound to albumin. However, approximately 2% remains free and available to enter cells and bind to intracellular receptors.

Metabolism

In many target tissues, testosterone is converted to dihydrotestosterone by the enzyme 5α-reductase. In these tissues, dihydrotestosterone is the major androgen. The conversion of testosterone to estradiol also occurs in some tissues, including the hypothalamus, and may be of importance in regulating gonadal function.

The major pathway for the degradation of testosterone in humans is illustrated in Fig 39–6. In the liver, the reduction of the double bond and ketone in the A ring, as is seen in other steroids with a Δ^4-ketone configuration in the A ring, leads to the production of inactive substances such as androsterone and etiocholanolone that are then conjugated and excreted into the urine.

Androstenedione and dehydroepiandrosterone are also produced in significant amounts in humans, although largely in the adrenal rather than in the testes.

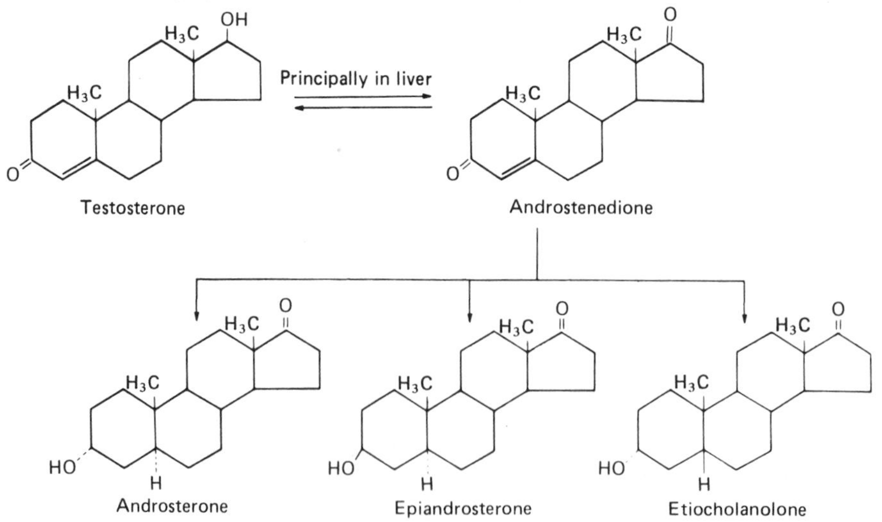

Figure 39–6. Metabolism of testosterone. (Reproduced, with permission, from Ganong WF: *Review of Medical Physiology,* 8th ed. Lange, 1977.)

These compounds do not have significant androgenic activity, but they are to a large extent metabolized in the same fashion as testosterone. Both compounds—but particularly androstenedione—can be converted by peripheral tissues to estrone in very small amounts (1–5%).

Physiologic Effects

In the normal male, testosterone is responsible for the many changes that occur in puberty. In addition to the general growth-promoting properties of androgens on the body tissues, these hormones are responsible for penile and scrotal growth. Changes in the skin include the appearance of pubic hair, axillary hair, and beard hair. The sebaceous glands become more active, and the skin tends to become thicker and oilier. The larynx grows and the vocal cords become thicker, leading to a lower pitched voice. Skeletal growth is stimulated and epiphyseal closure accelerated. Other effects include growth of the prostate and seminal vesicles, darkening of the skin, and increased skin circulation. Psychologic and behavioral changes also occur.

Synthetic Steroids With Androgenic & Anabolic Action

Testosterone, when administered by mouth, is rapidly absorbed. However, it is largely converted to inactive metabolites, and only about one-sixth of the dose administered is available in active form. Testosterone can be administered parenterally, but it has a more prolonged absorption time and greater activity when esterified. Methyltestosterone and fluoxymesterone are active when given by mouth.

Testosterone and its derivatives have been used for their anabolic effects as well as for the replacement of testosterone deficiency. Although testosterone and other known active steroids can be isolated in pure form and measured by weight, biologic assays are still used in the investigation of new compounds. In some of these studies in animals, the anabolic effects of the compound—as measured by trophic effects on muscles or the reduction of nitrogen excretion—may be dissociated from the other androgenic effects. This has led to the marketing of a substantial group of compounds that are supposed to have marked anabolic activity associated with only weak androgenic effects. This dissociation does not appear to be complete, and in humans it is less marked than in the animals used for testing (Table 39–6).

Pharmacologic Effects

A. Mechanisms of Action: Testosterone acts intracellularly in target cells. In skin, prostate, seminal vesicles, and epididymis, it is converted to 5α-dihydrotestosterone by the enzyme 5α-reductase. In these tissues, dihydrotestosterone is the dominant androgen. The distribution of this enzyme in the fetus is different and has important developmental implications.

Testosterone and dihydrotestosterone bind to the

Table 39–6. Androgens: Preparations available and relative androgen/anabolic activity in animals.

	Androgenic/Anabolic Activity
Testosterone	1:1
Testosterone cypionate	1:1
Testosterone enanthate	1:1
Testosterone propionate	1:1
Methyltestosterone	1:1
Fluoxymesterone	1:2
Methandrostenolone (metandienone)	1:3
Oxymetholone	1:3
Ethylestrenol	1:4–1:8
Oxandrolone	1:3–1:13
Nandrolone phenpropionate	1:3–1:6
Nandrolone decanoate	1:2.5–1:4
Stanozolol	1:3–1:6
Dromostanolone propionate	1:3–1:4

5α-Dihydrotestosterone
(androstanolone, stanolone, DHT)

cytosol androgen receptor, initiating a series of events leading to growth, differentiation, and synthesis of a variety of enzymes and other functional proteins (Chapter 35).

B. Effects: In the male at puberty, androgens cause development of the secondary sex characteristics (see above). In the adult male, large doses of testosterone or its derivatives suppress the secretion of gonadotropins and result in some atrophy of the interstitial tissue and the tubules of the testes. Since fairly large doses of androgens are required to suppress gonadotropic secretion, it has been postulated that estrogens produced in the testis (either in combination with androgens or instead of androgens) are responsible for the feedback control of secretion. In women, androgens are capable of producing changes similar to those observed in the prepubertal male. These include growth of facial hair and body hair, deepening of the voice, enlargement of the clitoris, frontal baldness, and prominent musculature. The natural androgens stimulate erythrocyte production.

The administration of androgens reduces the excretion of nitrogen into the urine, indicating an increase in protein synthesis or decrease in protein breakdown within the body. This effect is much more pronounced in women and children than in normal men.

Clinical Uses

A. Androgen Replacement Therapy in Men: Androgens are used to replace or augment endogenous androgen secretion in hypogonadal men (Table 39–7). Even in the presence of hypogonadotropism, androgens are used rather than gonadotropin except when normal spermatogenesis is to be achieved. When androgen deficiency occurs prior to completion of sexual maturation, large doses of androgens are required, and orally administered androgens are not sufficiently efficacious. In these patients, therapy should begin using testosterone enanthate or cypionate in doses of 200 mg intramuscularly every 1–2 weeks until maturation is complete. The dose can then be reduced to 200 mg at 2- to 3-week intervals. Testosterone propionate, though potent, is not practical for long-term use. The development of polycythemia or hypertension may require some reduction in dose.

In patients with hypopituitarism, androgens are not added to the treatment regimen until puberty, at which time they are instituted in gradually increasing doses to achieve the growth spurt and the development of secondary sex characteristics.

B. Gynecologic Disorders: Androgens are used occasionally in the treatment of certain gynecologic disorders, but the undesirable effects in women are such that they must be used with great caution. Androgens have been used to reduce breast engorgement during the postpartum period, usually in conjunction with estrogens.

Androgens are sometimes given in combination with estrogens for replacement therapy in the postmenopausal period in an attempt to eliminate the endometrial bleeding that may occur when only estrogens are used. They are also used for the chemotherapy of breast tumors in premenopausal women.

C. Use as Protein Anabolic Agents: Androgens and anabolic steroids have been used in conjunc-

tion with dietary measures and exercises in an attempt to reverse protein loss after trauma, surgery, or prolonged immobilization and in patients with debilitating diseases.

D. Anemia: Large doses of androgens have been employed in the treatment of refractory anemias and have resulted in some increase in reticulocytosis and hemoglobin levels. The large amounts required prevent this from being a useful method of therapy in women.

E. Osteoporosis: Androgens and anabolic agents have been used in the treatment of osteoporosis, either alone or in conjunction with estrogens.

F. Use as Metabolic Stimulators: These agents have been used to stimulate growth in prepubertal boys. If the drugs are used carefully, these children will probably achieve their expected adult height (and sooner than normal). If treatment is too vigorous, the patient may grow rapidly at first but will not achieve full stature because of the accelerated epiphyseal closure that occurs. It is difficult to control this type of therapy adequately even with frequent x-ray examination of the epiphyses, since the action of the hormones on epiphyseal centers may continue for many months after therapy is discontinued.

Adverse Reactions

The adverse effects of these compounds are due largely to their masculinizing actions and are most noticeable in women and prepubertal children. In women, the administration of more than 200–300 mg of testosterone per month is usually associated with hirsutism, acne, depression of menses, clitoral enlargement, and deepening of the voice. These effects may occur with even smaller doses in some women. Some of the androgenic steroids exert progestational activity leading to endometrial bleeding. These hormones also alter serum lipids and could conceivably increase susceptibility to atherosclerotic disease in women. Except under the most unusual circumstances, androgens should not be used in infants. Recent studies in animals suggest that administration of androgens in early life may have profound effects on maturation of central nervous system centers governing sexual development, particularly in the female. Administration of these drugs to pregnant females may lead to masculinization of the external genitalia in the infant. Although the above-mentioned effects may be less marked with the anabolic agents, they do occur.

Sodium retention and edema are not common but must be carefully watched for in patients with heart and kidney disease.

Most of the synthetic androgens and anabolic agents are 17-alkyl-substituted steroids. Administration of drugs with this structure is associated with increase in sulfobromophthalein retention and SGOT levels. Alkaline phosphatase values are also elevated. These changes usually occur early in the course of treatment, and the degree is proportionate to the dose. Bilirubin levels occasionally increase until clinical

Table 39–7. Androgen preparations for replacement therapy.

	Route of Administration	Dose
Methyltestosterone (Metandren, etc)	Oral	25–50 mg/d
	Sublingual (buccal)	5–10 mg/d
Fluoxymesterone (Halotestin, etc)	Oral	2–10 mg/d
Testosterone propionate (Synandrol, etc)	Sublingual (buccal)	5–20 mg/d
	Intramuscular	10–50 mg 3 times weekly
Testosterone enanthate (Delatestryl, etc)	Intramuscular	200 mg every 1–2 weeks until maturation is complete, then every 2–3 weeks for maintenance.
Testosterone cypionate (Depovirin, etc)	Intramuscular	
Testosterone pellets	Subcutaneous	450 mg every 4–6 months

jaundice is apparent. The cholestatic jaundice is reversible upon cessation of therapy, and permanent changes do not occur. In older males, prostatic hyperplasia may develop, causing urinary obstruction.

Contraindications & Cautions

The use of androgenic steroids is contraindicated in pregnant women or women who may become pregnant during the course of therapy.

Androgens should not be administered to male patients with carcinoma of the prostate or breast.

Until more is known about the effects of these hormones on the central nervous system in developing children, they should be avoided in infants and young children.

Special caution is required in giving these drugs to children to produce a growth spurt.

Care should be exercised in the administration of these drugs to patients with renal or cardiac disease predisposed to edema. If sodium and water retention occurs, it will respond to diuretic therapy.

Methyltestosterone therapy is associated with creatinuria, but the significance of this finding is not known.

Caution: Several cases of hepatocellular carcinoma have been reported in patients with aplastic anemia treated with androgen anabolic therapy.

ANTIANDROGENS

The potential usefulness of antiandrogens for the treatment of patients producing excessive amounts of testosterone has led to the search for effective drugs that can be used for this purpose. Two approaches to the problem have met with limited success.

Several compounds have been developed that inhibit the 17-hydroxylation of progesterone or pregnenolone, thereby preventing the action of the side chain–splitting enzyme and the further transformation of these steroid precursors to active androgens. A few of these compounds have been tested clinically but have been too toxic for prolonged use.

Another approach has been the development of steroids that are chemically similar and act as competitive inhibitors. A few of these have been tried in patients on a limited basis. Cyproterone and cyproterone acetate are effective antiandrogens that inhibit the action of the androgens at the target organ. The acetate form has a marked progestational effect that suppresses the feedback enhancement of LH and FSH leading to a more effective antiandrogen effect. These compounds have been used in women for the treatment of hirsutism and in men to decrease excessive sexual drive and are being studied in other conditions in which the reduction of androgenic effects would be useful. **Cyproterone acetate** in doses of 2 mg/d administered concurrently with an estrogen is used in the treatment of hirsutism in women, but it is not available for use in the USA.

Spironolactone, a competitive inhibitor of aldosterone (see Chapter 14), competes with dihydrotestosterone for the androgen receptors in target tissues. It also reduces 17α-hydroxylase activity, lowering plasma levels of testosterone and androstenedione. It is used in doses of 50–200 mg/d for the treatment of hirsutism in women.

Flutamide (2-methyl-N-[4-nitro-3-(trifluoromethyl)phenyl]-propanamide), a substituted anilide, is a potent antiandrogen that has been used in the treatment of prostatic carcinoma. It behaves like a competitive antagonist at the androgen receptor. It is rapidly metabolized in humans. It frequently causes mild gynecomastia (probably by increasing testicular estrogen production) and occasionally causes mild reversible hepatic toxicity. Administration of this compound causes some improvement in most patients who have not had prior endocrine therapy.

ANDROGEN SUPPRESSION

The treatment of advanced prostatic carcinoma often requires orchiectomy or large doses of estrogens to reduce available androgen. The psychologic effects of the former and gynecomastia produced by the latter make these approaches undesirable. As noted above, the gonadotropin-releasing hormone analogs such as nafarelin, buserelin, and leuprolide acetate produce gonadal suppression when given daily intranasally or by injection. **Leuprolide acetate,** the only preparation currently available for use, is injected subcutaneously daily in doses of 1 mg for the treatment of prostatic carcinoma. Although testosterone levels fall to 10% of their initial values after a month, they increase significantly in the beginning. This increase is usually associated with a flare of tumor activity and an increase in symptoms. Recent studies suggest that the combination of a GnRH agonist and flutamide can prevent the initial stimulation and provide a more effective inhibition of androgenic activity.

HORMONAL CONTRACEPTION IN THE MALE

A large number of studies conducted over the past few decades have been unsuccessful in identifying an effective oral contraceptive for men. Various androgens, including testosterone and testosterone enanthate, in doses of 400 mg per month, will produce azoospermia in less than half of the men treated. Minor adverse reactions, including gynecomastia and acne, were encountered. Testosterone in combination with danazol was well tolerated but no more effective than testosterone alone. Androgens in combination with a progestin such as depomedroxyprogesterone acetate were no more effective. Cyproterone acetate, a very potent progestin, will also produce oligospermia but has not produced reliable contraception. Potent analogs of GnRH are also under study.

GOSSYPOL

Extensive trials of this cottonseed derivative are being conducted in China. This compound destroys elements of the seminiferous epithelium but does not alter the endocrine function of the testis.

Large numbers of men have been treated with 20 mg/d of gossypol or gossypol acetic acid for 2 months, followed by a maintenance dose of 60 mg a week. On this regimen, 99% of men developed sperm counts below 4 million per milliliter. Preliminary data indicate that recovery (return of normal sperm count) following discontinuation of gossypol administration is more apt to occur in men whose counts do not fall to extremely low levels and when administration is not continued for over 2 years. Hypokalemia is the major side effect and may lead to transient paralysis.

Gossypol

REFERENCES

General

Belchetz PE et al: Hypophyseal responses to continuous and intermittent delivery of hypothalamic gonadotropin-releasing hormone. *Science* 1978;**202**:631.

Hertz R: Physiologic effects of androgens and estrogens in man. *Am J Med* 1956;**21**:671.

Rosemberg E (editor): *Gonadotropin Therapy in Female Infertility.* International Congress Series No. 266. Excerpta Medica, 1973.

Salhanick HA, Kipnis DM, Vande Wiele RL (editors): *Metabolic Effects of Gonadal Hormones and Contraceptive Steroids.* Plenum Press, 1969.

Wise AJ, Gross MA, Schalch DS: Quantitative relationships of the pituitary-gonadal axis in postmenopausal women. *J Lab Clin Med* 1973;**81**:28.

Estrogens & Progestins

Ahn YS et al: Danazol for the treatment of idiopathic thrombocytopenic purpura. *N Engl J Med* 1983;**308**:1396.

Antunes CMF et al: Endometrial cancer and estrogen use. *N Engl J Med* 1979;**300**:9.

Barbieri RL, Ryan KJ: Danazol: Endocrine pharmacology and therapeutic applications. *Am J Obstet Gynecol* 1981;**141**:453.

Bibbo M et al: Follow-up study of male and female offspring of DES-exposed mothers. *Obstet Gynecol* 1977;**49**:1.

Cann CE et al: Spinal mineral loss by quantitative computed tomography in oophorectomized women. *JAMA* 1980;**244**:2056.

Christiansen C et al: Prevention of early postmenopausal bone loss. *Eur J Clin Invest* 1980;**10**:273.

Conte FA, Grumbach MM: Estrogen use in children and adolescents: A survey. *Pediatrics* 1978;**62(6–Part 2)**:1091.

Dmowski WP: Endocrine properties and clinical application of danazol. *Fertil Steril* 1979;**31**:237.

Goldzieher JW, Dozier TS, de la Pena A: Plasma levels and pharmacokinetics of ethynyl estrogens in various populations. 1. Ethynylestradiol. *Contraception* 1980;**21**:1.

Gralnick HR, Rick ME: Danazol increases factor VIII and factor IX in classic hemophilia and Christmas disease. *N Engl J Med* 1983;**308**:1393.

Gusberg SB: Current concepts in cancer: The changing nature of endometrial cancer. *N Engl J Med* 1980;**302**:729.

Hahn HB Jr, Hayles AB, Albert A: Medroxyprogesterone [Provera] and constitutional precocious puberty. *Mayo Clin Proc* 1964;**39**:182.

Hammond CS et al: Effects of long-term estrogen replacement therapy. *Am J Obstet Gynecol* 1979;**133**:525.

Heaney RP, Recker RR, Saville PD: Menopausal changes in calcium balance performance. *J Lab Clin Med* 1978;**92**:953.

Herbst AL: Diethylstilbestrol exposure 1984. *N Engl J Med* 1984;**311**:1433.

Horsman A et al: The effect of estrogen dose on postmenopausal bone loss. *N Engl J Med* 1983;**309**:1405.

Jewelewicz R: Management of infertility resulting from anovulation. *Am J Obstet Gynecol* 1975;**122**:909.

Kalkhoff RK: Metabolic effects of progesterone. *Am J Obstet Gynecol* 1982;**142**:735.

Kase NG: Progestin therapy for perimenopausal women. *J Reprod Med* 1982;**27**:522.

Mandanes AE, Farber M: Danazol. *Ann Intern Med* 1982;**96**:625.

Mandel FP et al: Biologic effects of various doses of ethinyl estradiol in postmenopausal women. *Obstet Gynecol* 1982;**59**:673.

Mann JI: Progestogens in cardiovascular disease: An introduction to the epidemiologic data. *Am J Obstet Gynecol* 1982;**142**:752.

Mashchak AC et al: Comparison of pharmacodynamic properties of various estrogen formulations. *Am J Obstet Gynecol* 1982;**144**:511.

Meema S, Bunker ML, Meema HE: Preventive effect of estrogen on postmenopausal bone loss. *Arch Intern Med* 1975;**135**:1436.

Nachtigall LE et al: Estrogen replacement therapy. 1. A ten

year prospective study in the relationship to osteoporosis. *Obstet Gynecol* 1979;**53**:277.

Riggs LB et al: Effect of the fluoride/calcium regimen on vertebral fracture occurrence in postmenopausal osteoporosis. *N Engl J Med* 1982;**306**:446.

Robboy SJ, Bradley R: Changing trends and prognostic features in endometrial cancer associated with exogenous estrogen therapy. *Obstet Gynecol* 1979;**54**:269.

Sampson GA: Premenstrual syndrome: A double blind controlled trial of progesterone and placebo. *Br J Psychiatry* 1979;**135**:209.

Spellacy WN, Buhi WC, Birk SA: Effect of estrogen treatment for one year on carbohydrate and lipid metabolism in women with normal and abnormal glucose tolerance test results. *Am J Obstet Gynecol* 1978;**131**:87.

Weiss G et al: Distribution of relaxin in women during pregnancy. *Obstet Gynecol* 1978;**52**:569.

Yen SSC et al: Circulating estradiol, estrone and gonadotropin levels following the administration of orally active 17α-estradiol in postmenopausal women. *J Clin Endocrinol Metab* 1975;**40**:518.

Yuzpe AA: Postcoital hormonal contraception: Uses, risks and abuses. *Int J Gynaecol Obstet* 1977;**133**:136.

Oral Contraceptives

Bradley BD et al: Serum high-density-lipoprotein cholesterol in women using oral contraceptives, estrogen and progestins. *N Engl J Med* 1978;**299**:17.

Centers for Disease Control Cancer and Steroid Hormone Study: Long-term oral contraceptive use and the risk of breast cancer. *JAMA* 1983;**249**:1591.

Centers for Disease Control Cancer and Steroid Hormone Study: Oral contraceptive use and the risk of endometrial cancer. *JAMA* 1983;**249**:1600.

Centers for Disease Control Cancer and Steroid Hormone Study: Oral contraceptive use and the risk of ovarian cancer. *JAMA* 1983;**249**:1596.

Gambrell RD, Maier RC, Sanders BI: Decreased incidence of breast cancer in postmenopausal estrogen-progestogen users. *Obstet Gynecol* 1983;**62**:435.

Garattini S, Berendes HW: *Pharmacology of Steroid Contraceptive Drugs.* Raven Press, 1977.

Goldzieher JW (editor): Advances in oral contraception: An international review of levonorgestrel and ethinyl estradiol. *J Reprod Med* 1983;**28(1–Suppl)**:53.

Huggins GR, Guintoli RL: Oral contraceptives and neoplasia. *Fertil Steril* 1979;**32**:1.

Jeppsson S, Johansson EDB: Medroxyprogesterone acetate, estradiol, FSH and LH in peripheral blood after intramuscular administration of Depo-Provera to women. *Contraception* 1976;**14**:461.

Jick H, Dinan B, Rothman KJ: Oral contraceptives and nonfatal myocardial infarction. *JAMA* 1979;**239**:1403.

Jick H et al: Myocardial infarction and other vascular diseases in young women: Role of estrogens and other factors. *JAMA* 1978;**240**:2548.

Larsson-Cohn U et al: Lipoprotein changes may be minimized by proper composition of a combined oral contraceptive. *Fertil Steril* 1981;**35**:172.

Mishell DR Jr: Noncontraceptive health benefits of oral contraceptives. *Am J Obstet Gynecol* 1982;**142**:809.

Nora JJ et al: Exogenous progestogen and estrogen implicated in birth defects. *JAMA* 1978;**240**:837.

Pike MC et al: Breast cancer in young women and use of oral contraceptives: Possible modifying effect of formulation and age at use. *Lancet* 1983;**2**:926.

Shapiro S et al: Oral-contraceptive use in relation to myocardial infarction. *Lancet* 1979;**1**:743.

Stadel BV: Oral contraceptives and cardiovascular disease. (2 parts.) *N Engl J Med* 1981;**305**:612, 672.

Wahl P et al: Effect of estrogen/progestin potency on lipid/lipoprotein cholesterol. *N Engl J Med* 1983;**308**:862.

Weiss NS, Sayvetz TA: Incidence of endometrial cancer in relation to the use of oral contraceptives. *N Engl J Med* 1980; **302**:551.

Wynn V: Cardiovascular effects and progestins in oral contraceptives. *Am J Obstet Gynecol* 1982;**142(6–Part 2)**:718.

Wynn V: Effect of duration of low-dose oral contraceptive administration on carbohydrate metabolism. *Am J Obstet Gynecol* 1982;**142(6–Part 2)**:739.

Androgens

Androgens II and antiandrogens. Vol 35, part 2, in: *Handbook of Experimental Pharmacology.* (New series.) Springer, 1974.

Franchimont P et al: Effects of oral testosterone undecanoate in hypogonadal male patients. *Clin Endocrinol* 1978; **9**:313.

Griffin JE, Wilson JD: The syndromes of androgen resistance. *N Engl J Med* 1980;**302**:198.

Johnson FL et al: Association of androgenic-anabolic steroid therapy with development of hepatocellular carcinoma. *Lancet* 1972;**2**:1273.

Labrie F et al: Long term treatment with luteinising hormone releasing hormone agonists and maintenance of serum testosterone to castration concentrations. *Br Med J* 1985; **291**:369.

Linde R et al: Reversible inhibition of testicular steroidogenesis and spermatogenesis by a potent gonadotropin-releasing hormone agonist in normal men. *N Engl J Med* 1981; **305**:663.

Neumann F: Pharmacology and potential use of cyproterone acetate. *Horm Metab Res* 1977;**9**:1.

Nieschlag E, Wickings EJ, Breuer H: Chemical methods for male fertility control. *Contraception* 1981;**23**:1.

Rigberg SV, Brodsky I: Potential roles of androgens and the anabolic steroids in the treatment of cancer: A review. *J Med* 1975;**6**:271.

Sogani PC, Vagaiwala MR, Whitmore WF: Experience with flutamide in patients with advanced prostatic cancer without prior endocrine therapy. *Cancer* 1984;**54**:744.

Wolstenholme GEW, O'Connor M (editors): Endocrinology of the testis. *Ciba Found Colloq Endocrinol* 1967;**16**:1.

Pancreatic Hormones & Antidiabetic Drugs

John H. Karam, MD

THE ENDOCRINE PANCREAS

The endocrine pancreas in the adult human consists of approximately 1 million islets of Langerhans interspersed throughout the pancreatic gland. Within the islets, at least 4 hormone-producing cells have been identified (Table 40–1). Their hormone products include **insulin,** the storage and anabolic hormone of the body; **glucagon,** the hyperglycemic factor that mobilizes glycogen stores; **somatostatin,** a universal inhibitor of secretory cells; and **pancreatic polypeptide,** a small protein that facilitates digestive processes by a mechanism not yet clarified.

Diabetes mellitus is the most important disease involving the endocrine pancreas. Its major manifestations include disordered metabolism and inappropriate hyperglycemia. A "therapeutic" classification presently recommended by the American Diabetes Association includes 2 major types: insulin-dependent (IDDM) and non–insulin-dependent (NIDDM) diabetes mellitus. An estimated 5.5 million people in the USA are known to have diabetes, and 440,000 have the insulin-dependent type.

Type I diabetes (IDDM) is a severe form associated with ketosis in the untreated state. It occurs most commonly in juveniles but occasionally in adults, especially the nonobese and those who are elderly when hyperglycemia first appears. It is a catabolic disorder in which circulating insulin is virtually absent, plasma glucagon is elevated, and the pancreatic B cells fail to respond to all insulinogenic stimuli. Exogenous insulin is therefore required to reverse the catabolic state, prevent ketosis, and reduce the hyperglucagonemia and the elevated blood glucose level.

Because of certain immune characteristics, type I diabetes is felt to result from an infectious or toxic environmental insult to pancreatic B cells such as coxsackievirus B4, or from chemical agents. An underlying genetic defect on chromosome 6 relating to B cell replication or function may predispose to development of B cell failure after viral infection; alternatively, specific HLA genes may increase susceptibility to a diabetogenic virus or may be linked to certain immune response genes that predispose patients to a destructive autoimmune response against their own islet cells (auto-aggression).

Type II diabetes (NIDDM) represents a heterogeneous group comprising milder forms of diabetes that occur predominantly in adults but occasionally in juveniles. Circulating endogenous insulin is sufficient to prevent ketoacidosis but is often either subnormal or relatively inadequate because of tissue insensitivity. Obesity, which generally results in impaired insulin action, is a common risk factor for this type of diabetes, and most patients with NIDDM are obese.

In addition to tissue insensitivity to insulin, which has been noted in most NIDDM patients irrespective of weight, there is an accompanying deficiency of the pancreatic B cell's response to glucose. Both the tissue resistance to insulin and the impaired B cell response to glucose appear to be further aggravated by increased hyperglycemia, and both of these defects are ameliorated by therapeutic maneuvers that reduce the hyperglycemia.

When dietary treatment and attempts at weight reduction of obesity fail to correct hyperglycemia, sulfonylurea drugs are usually prescribed. Insulin therapy may be required to achieve satisfactory glycemic control even though it is not needed to prevent ketoacidosis in patients with NIDDM.

Table 40–1. Pancreatic islet cells and their secretory products.

Cell Types	Approximate Percent of Islet Mass	Secretory Products
A cell (alpha)	20	Glucagon, proglucagon.
B cell (beta)	75	Insulin, C-peptide, proinsulin.
D cell (delta)	3–5	Somatostatin.
F cell (PP cell)*	< 2	Pancreatic polypeptide (PP).

*Within pancreatic polypeptide–rich lobules of adult islets, located only in the posterior portion of the head of the human pancreas, glucagon cells are scarce (less than 0.5%), and F cells make up as much as 80% of the cells.

INSULIN

Chemistry

Insulin is a small protein with a molecular weight in humans of 5808. It contains 51 amino acids arranged in 2 chains (A and B) linked by disulfide bridges; there are species differences in the amino acids of both chains. Within the B cell, insulin precursor is produced by DNA/RNA-directed synthesis. Initially, proinsulin, a long single-chain protein molecule, is processed within the Golgi apparatus and packaged into granules, where it is hydrolyzed into insulin and a residual connecting segment called the C-peptide by removal of 4 amino acids (shown in dashed lines in Fig 40–1). Insulin and C-peptide are secreted in equimolar amounts in response to all insulin secretogogues; a small quantity of unprocessed or partially hydrolyzed proinsulin is released as well. Neither proinsulin nor C-peptide is known to have any physiologic function. Granules within the B cell store the insulin in the form of crystals consisting of 2 atoms of zinc and 6 molecules of insulin. The entire human pancreas contains up to 8 mg of insulin, representing approximately 200 biologic "units." Originally, the unit was defined on the basis of the hypoglycemic activity of insulin in rabbits. With improved purification techniques, the unit is presently defined on the basis of weight, and present insulin standards used for assay purposes are 28 units per milligram.

Insulin Degradation

The liver and kidney are the 2 main organs that remove insulin from the circulation, presumably by hydrolysis of the disulfide connections between the A and B chains through the action of glutathione insulin transhydrogenase (insulinase). After this reductive cleavage, further degradation by proteolysis occurs. The liver normally clears the blood of approximately 60% of the insulin released from the pancreas by virtue of its location as the terminal site of portal vein blood flow, with the kidney removing 35–40% of the endogenous hormone. However, in insulin-treated diabetics receiving subcutaneous insulin injections, this

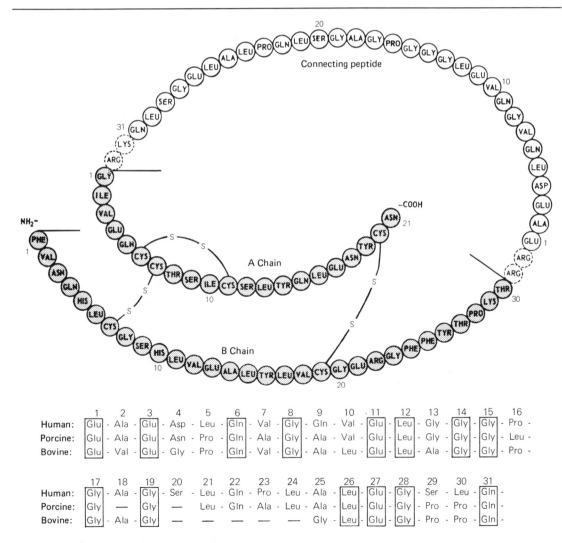

	1	2	3	4	5	6	7	8	9	10	11	12	13	14	15	16
Human:	Glu	Ala	Glu	Asp	Leu	Gln	Val	Gly	Gln	Val	Glu	Leu	Gly	Gly	Gly	Pro
Porcine:	Glu	Ala	Glu	Asn	Pro	Gln	Ala	Gly	Ala	Val	Glu	Leu	Gly	Gly	Gly	Leu
Bovine:	Glu	Val	Glu	Gly	Pro	Gln	Val	Gly	Ala	Leu	Glu	Leu	Ala	Gly	Gly	Pro

	17	18	19	20	21	22	23	24	25	26	27	28	29	30	31
Human:	Gly	Ala	Gly		Ser	Leu	Gln	Pro	Leu	Ala	Leu	Glu	Gly	Ser	Leu	Gln
Porcine:| Gly	—	Gly		—	Leu	Gln	Ala	Leu	Ala	Leu	Glu	Gly	Pro	Pro	Gln
Bovine:	Gly	Ala	Gly		—	—	—	—	—	Gly	Leu	Glu	Gly	Pro	Pro	Gln

Figure 40–1. Structure of human proinsulin. Comparisons of human, porcine, and bovine C-peptides are shown in the accompanying diagram. Identical residues are shown in boxes. Insulin is shown as the shaded polypeptide chains.

ratio is reversed, with as much as 60% of exogenous insulin being cleared by the kidney and the liver removing no more than 30–40%. The half-life of circulating insulin is 3–5 minutes.

Measurement of Circulating Insulin

The radioimmunoassay of insulin permits detection of insulin in picogram quantities, which is below the capabilities of ordinary chemical methods of peptide analysis. The assay is based on antibodies developed in guinea pigs against bovine or pork insulin. Because of the similarities between these 2 insulins and human insulin, the assay successfully measures the human hormone.

With this assay, basal insulin values of 5–15 μU/mL are found in normal humans, with a peak rise to 60–90 μU/mL during meals. Similar assays for measuring all of the known hormones of the endocrine pancreas (including C-peptide and proinsulin) have been developed.

Biologic Effect of Insulin

Insulin promotes the storage of fat as well as glucose (both sources of energy) within specialized target cells (Fig 40–2) and influences cell growth and the metabolic functions of a wide variety of tissues. Once insulin has entered the circulation, it is taken up by specialized receptors that have been found on the membranes of most tissues. However, the biologic responses promoted by these insulin-receptor complexes have been identified in only a few target tissues, eg, liver, muscle, and adipose tissue. The receptors bind insulin with high specificity and affinity in the picomolar range. Various hormonal agents (eg, hydrocortisone) lower the affinity of insulin receptors to insulin; growth hormone in excess increases this affinity slightly. The concentration of these specific receptor molecules as well as their affinity for binding insulin seems to be affected by the concentration of insulin molecules to which they are exposed. In clinical situations associated with elevated blood levels of circulating insulin, such as obesity or insulinoma, the concentration of insulin receptors is reduced. This phenomenon of "down regulation" of insulin receptors seems to provide an intrinsic mechanism whereby target cells limit their response to excessive hormone concentrations.

Traditionally, it had been thought that a "second messenger" was generated by the combination of insulin with its membrane receptor to initiate both rapid (transport) effects of insulin and more sustained (anabolic) effects. However, recent evidence suggests that the insulin receptor is a tyrosine protein kinase. After binding insulin at the outside surface of the cell,

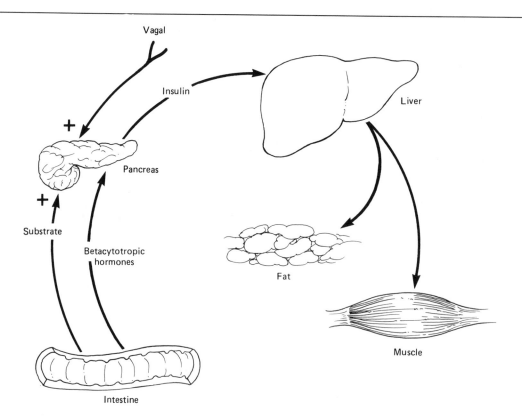

Figure 40–2. Insulin promotes synthesis (from circulating nutrients) and storage of glycogen, triglycerides, and protein in its major target tissues: liver, fat, and muscle. The release of insulin from the pancreas is stimulated by increased blood glucose, vagal nerve stimulation, and other factors (see text).

the insulin-receptor complex is internalized, and kinase activity results in phosphorylation of the receptor protein as well as other proteins within the cell. This cascade of phosphorylation may represent the "second message." However, it remains controversial whether internalization contributes to further action of insulin or is merely a means of limiting further effects of insulin by removing insulin and its receptor within scavenger lysosomes.

Effects of Insulin on Its Target Cells (Table 40–2)

A. Action of Insulin on Liver: The first major organ endogenous insulin reaches via the portal circulation is the liver, where it acts to increase storage of glucose as glycogen and to reset the liver to the fed state by reversing a number of catabolic mechanisms associated with the postabsorptive state: glycogenolysis, ketogenesis, and gluconeogenesis. These effects are brought about in part through the induction, by insulin, of increased synthesis of pyruvate kinase, phosphofructokinase, and glucokinase, and in part through the repression of gluconeogenic enzymes, including pyruvate carboxylase, phosphoenolpyruvate carboxykinase, fructose bisphosphatase, and glucose 6-phosphatase. In addition, insulin decreases urea production, protein catabolism, and cAMP in the liver and increases potassium and phosphate uptake by the organ.

B. Effect of Insulin on Muscle: Insulin promotes protein synthesis by increasing amino acid transport and by stimulating ribosomal activity. It also promotes glycogen synthesis to replace glycogen stores expended by muscle activity. This is accomplished by increasing glucose transport into the muscle

Table 40–2. Endocrine effects of insulin.

Effect on liver:
  Reversal of catabolic features of insulin deficiency
    Inhibits glycogenolysis.
    Inhibits conversion of fatty acids and amino acids to keto acids.
    Inhibits conversion of amino acids to glucose.
  Anabolic action
    Promotes glucose storage as glycogen (induces glucokinase and glycogen synthase, inhibits phosphorylase).
    Increases triglyceride synthesis and very low density lipoprotein formation.
Effect on muscle:
  Increased protein synthesis
    Increases amino acid transport.
    Increases ribosomal protein synthesis.
  Increased glycogen synthesis
    Increases glucose transport.
    Induces glycogen synthase and inhibits phosphorylase.
Effect on adipose tissue:
  Increased triglyceride storage
    Lipoprotein lipase is induced and activated by insulin to hydrolyze triglycerides from lipoproteins.
    Glucose transport into cell provides glycerol phosphate to permit esterification of fatty acids supplied by lipoprotein transport.
    Intracellular lipase is inhibited by insulin.

cell, inducing glycogen synthase, and inhibiting phosphorylase. Approximately 500–600 g of glycogen is stored in muscle tissue of a 70-kg male.

C. Effect of Insulin on Adipose Tissue: The most efficient means of storing energy is in the form of triglyceride depots. This provides 9 kcal per gram of stored substrate and, unlike glycogen, does not require water to maintain it within cells. A normal 70-kg man has 12–14 kg of fat in storage, chiefly in adipose tissue.

Insulin acts to reduce circulating free fatty acids and to promote triglyceride storage in adipocytes by 3 primary mechanisms: (1) induction of lipoprotein lipase, which actively hydrolyzes triglycerides from circulating lipoproteins; (2) glucose transport into cells to generate glycerophosphate as a metabolic product, which permits esterification of fatty acids supplied by lipoprotein hydrolysis; and (3) reduction of intracellular lipolysis of stored triglyceride by a direct inhibition of intracellular lipase. These effects appear to involve suppression of cAMP production and dephosphorylation of the lipases in the fat cell.

Characteristics of Available Insulin Preparations

Commercial insulin preparations differ in a number of ways, including differences in the animal species from which they are obtained; their purity, concentration, and solubility; and the time of onset and duration of their biologic action. In the past few years, a number of additional preparations have been added to the list of available insulins. As a result, in 1985, at least 47 different insulin formulations were available for purchase in the USA. As the use of human insulin increases, the number of available insulins from animal sources should decline.

A. Principal Types and Duration of Action of Insulin Preparations: Three principal types of insulins are available: (1) short-acting, with rapid onset of action; (2) intermediate-acting; and (3) long-acting, with slow onset of action (Fig 40–3) (Table 40–3). Short-acting insulin is a crystalline zinc-insulin complex provided in soluble form and dispensed as a clear solution at neutral pH. All other commercial insulins have been modified to provide prolonged action and are dispensed as turbid suspensions at neutral pH with either protamine in phosphate buffer (protamine zinc and NPH insulin) or varying concentrations of zinc in acetate buffer (ultralente, lente, and semilente insulins). Treatment with protamine zinc insulin or semilente preparations is currently decreasing, and almost no clinical indications for their use exist. Conventional subcutaneous insulin therapy presently consists of split-dose injections of mixtures of short-acting and intermediate-acting insulins (NPH or lente) or multiple doses of short-acting insulin preprandially in association with any of 3 insulin suspensions (NPH, lente, or ultralente) whose prolonged duration of action provides overnight basal insulin levels.

1. Short-acting insulin–Regular insulin is a short-acting soluble crystalline zinc insulin whose ef-

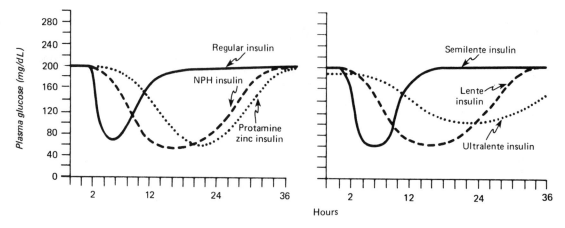

Figure 40–3. Extent and duration of action of various types of insulin (in a fasting diabetic).

fect appears within 15 minutes of subcutaneous injection and lasts 5–7 hours. It is the only type of insulin that can be administered intravenously or by infusion pumps. Short-acting soluble insulin is particularly useful for intravenous therapy in the management of diabetic ketoacidosis and when the insulin requirement is changing rapidly, such as after surgery or during acute infections.

2. Lente and ultralente insulin–Lente insulin is a mixture of 30% semilente (an amorphous precipitate of insulin with zinc ions in acetate buffer that has a relatively rapid onset of action) with 70% ultralente insulin (a poorly soluble crystal of zinc and beef insulin that has a delayed onset and prolonged duration of action). These 2 components provide a combination of relatively rapid absorption, with sustained long action making lente insulin a useful therapeutic agent. While

both beef and pork insulin can readily form zinc crystals in acetate buffer under the conditions employed, only the beef insulin has the proper hydrophobic alignment within the crystal to provide the delayed, sustained release of insulin characteristic of ultralente. Zinc crystals of pork insulin dissolve more rapidly, and while the appearance of the crystals is virtually identical to that of zinc crystals of beef insulin, the onset of action is earlier and the duration shorter. Accordingly, there is no ultralente insulin made of porcine insulin alone. Until data become available on onset and duration of action of the more recently developed pure pork or human forms of lentelike insulin (Monotard or Novolin-L, from Squibb-Novo; and Pork Lente Iletin II or Humulin-L, from Lilly), one must assume that their time course may be less sustained than that of lente insulin containing beef crystals of ultralente.

Lente insulin is the most widely used of the lente series of insulins, particularly in combination with regular insulin, which has a more rapid onset of action than the semilente component. Ultralente has a very slow onset of action with a prolonged duration, and its administration once or twice daily has been advocated to provide a basal level of insulin comparable to that achieved by basal endogenous insulin secretion or the overnight infusion rate programmed into insulin pumps. There has recently been a resurgence of use of ultralente insulin in combination with multiple injections of regular insulin as a means of attempting optimal control in patients with insulin-dependent diabetes.

3. NPH (neutral protamine Hagedorn, or isophane) insulin–NPH insulin is an intermediate-acting insulin wherein the onset of action is delayed by combining appropriate amounts of insulin and protamine so that neither is present in an uncomplexed form ("isophane"). Protamine isolated from the sperm of rainbow trout is a mixture of 6 major and some minor compounds of similar structure. They appear to be arginine-rich peptides with an average molecular weight of approximately 4400. To form an isophane

Table 40–3. Commercial insulin: Sources and activity.

Type of Preparations	Source	Activity (hours)	
		Peak	Duration*
Rapid-acting			
Insulin injection USP (regular, crystalline zinc)	Human, beef, pork, or mixture	½–3	5–7
Insulin zinc suspension USP (prompt, semilente)	Beef, pork, or mixture	1–4	12–16
Intermediate-acting			
Isophane insulin suspension USP (NPH insulin)	Human, beef, pork, or mixture	8–12	18–24
Insulin zinc suspension USP (lente)	Human, beef, pork, or mixture	8–12	18–24
Long-acting			
Protamine zinc insulin suspension USP (PZI)	Beef, pork, or mixture	8–16	24–36
Insulin zinc suspension extended USP (ultralente)	Beef or mixture	8–16	24–36

*The duration of action is increased with increasing doses.

complex (one in which neither component retains any free binding sites), approximately a 1:10 ratio by weight of protamine to insulin is required—eg, 0.3–0.4 mg of protamine to 4 mg of insulin (100 units). This represents approximately 6 molecules of insulin per molecule of protamine. In the complex, asparagine (the terminal amino acid on insulin's A chain) combines with an arginine-binding site on protamine. After subcutaneous injection, proteolytic enzymes degrade the protamine to permit absorption of insulin.

The onset and duration of action of NPH insulin is comparable to that of lente insulin (Table 40–3); it is usually mixed with regular insulin and given at least twice daily for insulin replacement in patients with insulin-dependent diabetes.

4. Mixtures of insulins–Since intermediate-acting insulins require several hours to reach adequate therapeutic levels, their use in insulin-dependent diabetic patients requires supplements of regular insulin preprandially. For convenience, these may be mixed together in the same syringe and injected subcutaneously in split dosage before breakfast and supper.

Recent reports warn that insulin mixtures containing increased portions of lente or NPH to regular insulin may retard the rapid action of admixed regular insulin, particularly if not injected immediately after mixing. The excess zinc in lente insulin and the protamine contained in NPH insulin can precipitate some of the soluble regular insulin when mixed in vitro (even at equal proportions), which may explain the slight retardation of regular insulin's absorption and biologic effect when mixed in ratios of 2 parts or greater of intermediate insulin to 1 part regular insulin.

B. Species of Insulin: Most commercial insulin in the USA contains beef insulin as its chief component. Beef insulin differs by 3 amino acids from human insulin, whereas only a single amino acid distinguishes pork and human insulins (Fig 40–1). The beef hormone is slightly more antigenic in humans than is pork insulin. The most commonly prescribed preparations in the USA are standard mixtures containing 70% beef and 30% pork insulin. However, supplies of "monospecies" pork or beef insulin are commercially available and are particularly useful in patients with conditions in which pure monospecies insulin may be indicated, such as insulin allergy or insulin resistance (see below). Recent advances in the mass production of human insulin by recombinant DNA techniques are quite promising, and biosynthetic **human insulin** has been prepared by inserting synthetic nucleotides, which separately transcribe both the human insulin A and B chains, into *Escherichia coli* and combining the extracted purified chains to form the human insulin molecule. A semisynthetic human insulin has also been produced by chemical modification of pork insulin, in which the carboxy terminal alanine of the B chain has been replaced by threonine.

Human insulin prepared by the recombinant DNA method is available for clinical use as Humulin (Lilly) and dispensed as either regular, NPH, or lente Humulin. Human insulin prepared by enzymatic conversion of pork insulin is marketed by Squibb-Novo as human insulin injection (Novolin R), Monotard Human Insulin (Novolin L), and an isophane suspension of human insulin (Novolin N). The postscripts R, L, and N refer to the formulations: regular, lente, and NPH, respectively. The Nordisk Company also produces a semisynthetic human insulin marketed as Velosulin (regular) and Insulatard (NPH) human insulins. Since human insulin tends to be slightly more hydrophilic than beef insulin, it has not yet been possible to produce an ultralente formulation of human insulin with the required degree of insolubility characteristic of beef insulin products. They appear to be as safe and effective as conventional animal insulins, and human insulin appears to be considerably less immunogenic in diabetic patients than beef-pork insulins and slightly less immunogenic than pork insulin.

C. Purity of Insulin: Recent improvements in purification techniques (using gel columns) have greatly reduced contaminating proteins with molecular weights greater than that of insulin. These include proinsulin and partially cleaved proinsulins that are metabolically inactive yet capable of inducing anti-insulin antibodies. Further purification with chromatography can virtually eliminate these larger proteins and markedly lower the concentration of smaller peptide contaminants. Conventional formulations of insulin contain less than 50 ppm of proinsulin. When proinsulin content is less than 10 ppm, manufacturers are entitled by FDA regulations in the USA to label the insulin as "purified."

D. Concentration: Currently, all insulins are available in a concentration of 100 units/mL (U100), and are dispensed in 10-mL vials. To accommodate children and occasional adults who may require small quantities, U40 insulin continues to be produced. For use in rare cases of severe insulin resistance in which large quantities of insulin are required, a limited supply of U500 regular porcine insulin is available.

E. Human Proinsulin: Human proinsulin is now available from recombinant DNA synthesis and shows biologic activity in humans which is 8–12% that of human insulin. Since it has a circulating half-life 4–6 times that of human insulin, it is undergoing clinical trials as an alternative form of longer-acting insulin. It would have certain advantages over NPH and lente formulations of human insulin in that it could provide prolonged insulin action without need for fish protamine additives or large concentrations of zinc acetate to precipitate the insulin.

Insulin Delivery Systems

A. Closed Loop Systems: Automated administration of soluble insulin by "closed loop" systems (blood glucose-controlled insulin infusion systems) has recently been successful in acute situations such as management of diabetic ketoacidosis or maintaining insulin balance of diabetics undergoing surgery. Chronic use of such systems is prevented by the need for uninterrupted aspiration of blood to reach an external glucose sensor and by the size of the computerized insulin pump system used on present models.

B. Open Loop Systems: Research into smaller "open loop" methods of insulin delivery (insulin reservoir and pump programmed to deliver regular insulin at a calculated rate without a glucose sensor) has resulted in readily portable pumps for subcutaneous, intravenous, or intraperitoneal infusion. As methods for self-monitoring of blood glucose are increasingly accepted by patients, these pump systems are becoming less "open loop" and therefore potentially more useful for managing insulin-dependent diabetics. However, at present, intensive therapy using conventional daily administration of multiple subcutaneous injections of soluble, rapid-acting insulin and a single daily injection of long-acting insulin appears to provide blood glucose control as effective as either type of loop system for most patients.

C. Nasal Insulin Delivery: When insulin is combined with a detergent and administered as an aerosol to the nasal mucosa, effective circulating levels of insulin can be achieved almost as rapidly as when an intravenous bolus of insulin is administered. If this route can be shown to produce reliable and reproducible absorption over the long term without toxicity to the nasal mucosa, it may improve insulin delivery to the circulation while reducing the need for injections.

Treatment With Insulin

The current classification of diabetes mellitus identifies a group of patients who have virtually no insulin secretion and whose survival is dependent on administration of exogenous insulin. This "insulin-dependent" group (type I) represents only about 8% of the diabetic population in the USA. Most type II diabetics do not require exogenous insulin for survival but may need exogenous supplementation of their endogenous secretion to achieve optimum health.

Complications of Insulin Therapy

A. Hypoglycemia:

1. Mechanisms and diagnosis–Hypoglycemic reactions are the most common complication of insulin therapy. They may result from a delay in taking a meal, unusual physical exertion, or a dose of insulin that is too large for immediate needs. With more patients attempting "tight" control without frequent capillary blood glucose home monitoring, hypoglycemia is likely to become an even more frequent complication.

In older diabetics and those taking longer-acting insulins, autonomic warning signals of hypoglycemia are less frequent, and the manifestations of insulin excess are mainly those of impaired function of the central nervous system, ie, mental confusion, bizarre behavior, and ultimately coma. More rapid development of hypoglycemia from the effects of regular insulin causes signs of autonomic hyperactivity, both sympathetic (tachycardia, palpitations, sweating, tremulousness) and parasympathetic (nausea, hunger), that may progress to convulsions and coma.

An identification bracelet, necklace, or card in the wallet or purse should be carried by every diabetic who may require hypoglycemic drug therapy.

2. Treatment–All of the manifestations of hypoglycemia are rapidly relieved by glucose administration. In a case of mild hypoglycemia in a patient who is conscious and able to swallow, orange juice, glucose, or any sugar-containing beverage or food may be given. If more severe hypoglycemia has produced unconsciousness or stupor, the treatment of choice is to give 20–50 mL of 50% glucose solution by intravenous infusion over a period of 2–3 minutes. If intravenous therapy is not available, 1 mg of glucagon injected either subcutaneously or intramuscularly will usually restore consciousness within 15 minutes to permit ingestion of sugar. Family members or others in the household should be taught how to give glucagon when the need arises. If the patient is stuporous and glucagon is not available, small amounts of honey or syrup can be inserted within the buccal pouch. In general, however, oral feeding is contraindicated in unconscious patients.

B. Immunopathology of Insulin Therapy: At least 5 molecular classes of insulin antibodies may be produced during the course of insulin therapy in diabetes: IgA, IgD, IgE, IgG, and IgM. There are 2 major types of immune disorders in these patients:

1. Insulin allergy–Insulin allergy, an immediate type hypersensitivity, is a rare condition in which local or systemic urticaria is due to histamine release from tissue mast cells sensitized by anti-insulin IgE antibodies. In severe cases, anaphylaxis results. A subcutaneous nodule appearing several hours later at the site of insulin injection and lasting for up to 24 hours has been attributed to an IgG-mediated complement-binding Arthus reaction. Because sensitivity is often to noninsulin protein contaminants, the new highly purified insulins have markedly reduced the incidence of insulin allergy, especially local reactions. When allergy to beef insulin is present, a species change (eg, to pure pork or human insulin) may correct the problem. Antihistamines, corticosteroids, and even desensitization may be required, especially for systemic hypersensitivity.

2. Immune insulin resistance–All insulin-treated patients develop a low titer of circulating IgG anti-insulin antibodies that neutralize the action of insulin to a small extent. In some diabetic patients, principally those with some degree of tissue insensitivity to insulin (such as occurs in obese diabetics) and a history of interrupted insulin therapy with preparations of beef insulin, a high titer of circulating IgG anti-insulin antibodies develops. This results in extremely high insulin requirements—often more than 200 units daily. This is often a self-limited condition and may clear spontaneously after several months. However, in cases where the circulating antibody is specifically more reactive with beef insulin—a more potent antigen in humans than pork insulin—switching to a less antigenic (pork or human) insulin may make possible a dramatic reduction in insulin dosage or may at least shorten the duration of immune resistance. Other forms of therapy include sulfated beef insulin (a chemically modified form of beef insulin containing an average of 6 sulfate groups per molecule) and immunosuppression with corticosteroids. In some adults, the foreign insulin can be completely discontinued and the patient maintained on diet alone with oral sulfonylureas. This is possible only when the circulating antibodies do not effectively neutralize the patient's own insulin.

C. Lipodystrophy at Injection Sites: Atrophy of subcutaneous fatty tissue may occur at the site of injection. This complication has become rare since the development of highly concentrated, pure insulin preparations of neutral pH. Injection of these preparations directly into the atrophic area often results in restoration of normal contours. Hypertrophy of subcutaneous fatty tissue remains a problem, even with the purified insulins, if injected repeatedly at the same site.

ORAL HYPOGLYCEMIC AGENTS

A large number of substances are capable of modifying insulin release (Table 40–4), including drugs that are useful in the treatment of diabetes. In the USA, the only oral medications available for treating hyperglycemia in non–insulin-dependent diabetics are the class of compounds known as sulfonylureas, which increase the release of endogenous insulin as well as improve its peripheral effectiveness. In other countries, a much wider choice of preparations is available, including a second class of compounds, the biguanides, that reduce blood glucose even in the absence of pancreatic B cell function. Biguanides were

Table 40–4. Regulation of insulin release in humans.*

Stimulants of insulin release
Glucose, mannose
Leucine
Vagal stimulation
Sulfonylureas
Amplifiers of glucose-induced insulin release
1. Enteric hormones:
   Gastrin inhibitory polypeptide
   Cholecystokinin
   Secretin, gastrin
2. Neural amplifiers:
   β-Adrenoceptor stimulation
3. Amino acids:
   Arginine
Inhibitors of insulin release
Neural: α-Sympathomimetic effect of catecholamines
Humoral: Somatostatin
Drugs: Diazoxide, phenytoin, vinblastine, colchicine

*Modified and reproduced, with permission, from Greenspan FS, Forsham PH (editors): *Basic & Clinical Endocrinology*, 2nd ed. Lange, 1986.

removed from the market in the USA in 1977, because the use of phenformin was reported to be associated with a relatively high incidence of lactic acidosis.

SULFONYLUREAS

In 1955, sulfonylurea drugs became widely available for treatment of non–insulin-dependent diabetics. The compounds are arylsulfonylureas with substitutions on the benzene and urea groups. Table 40–5 depicts the chemical structures of the 6 sulfonylureas used in the USA, including 2 "second-generation" preparations of higher potency that were introduced in 1984.

Mechanism of Action

At least 3 mechanisms of sulfonylurea action have been proposed: (1) release of insulin from B cells, (2) reduction of serum glucagon levels, and (3) an extrapancreatic effect to increase the number of insulin receptors.

A. Insulin Release From Pancreatic B Cells: When therapy is started, release of preformed insulin is stimulated by sulfonylureas by an unknown mechanism. Insulin synthesis is not stimulated and may even be reduced. Release of insulin in response to the major physiologic stimulus—glucose—is enhanced. There is some evidence, however, that after prolonged sulfonylurea therapy, serum insulin levels are no longer increased by the drug and may even be decreased. This observation is complicated by the fact that most such data are obtained from oral glucose tolerance testing—an unphysiologic measure of pancreatic response. After mixed meals containing protein as well as carbohydrate, the beneficial effect of chronic sulfonylurea treatment is generally associated with increased levels of serum insulin.

B. Reduction of Serum Glucagon Concentrations: It is now established that chronic administration of sulfonylureas to non–insulin-dependent diabetics reduces serum glucagon levels. This could contribute to the hypoglycemic effect of the drugs. The mechanism for this suppressive effect of sulfonylureas on glucagon levels is unclear but may involve a direct inhibition of pancreatic A cell secretion or an indirect inhibition due to enhanced release of both insulin and somatostatin, which inhibit A cell secretion.

C. Increase in Numbers of Insulin Receptors: There is evidence that increased binding of insulin to tissue receptors occurs during in vivo (but not in vitro) sulfonylurea administration. As shown in Fig 2–6, an increase in receptor number can increase the effect achieved with a given concentration of agonist; such an action by the sulfonylureas would potentiate the effect of the patient's low levels of insulin as well as that of exogenous insulin. However, in insulin-dependent diabetics with no endogenous insulin secretion, therapy with sulfonylureas has yet to be shown to improve blood glucose control, enhance sensitivity to

Table 40–5. Sulfonylureas.

Sulfonylurea	Chemical Structure	Daily Dose	Duration of Action (hours)
Tolbutamide (Orinase)	H_3C—⟨⟩—SO_2—NH—C(=O)—NH—$(CH_2)_3$—CH_3	0.5–2 g in divided doses	6–12
Tolazamide (Tolinase)	H_3C—⟨⟩—SO_2—NH—C(=O)—NH—N⟨⟩	0.1–1 g as single dose or in divided doses	10–14
Acetohexamide (Dymelor)	H_3C—C(=O)—⟨⟩—SO_2—NH—C(=O)—NH—⟨⟩	0.25–1.5 g as single dose or in divided doses	12–24
Chlorpropamide (Diabinese)	Cl—⟨⟩—SO_2—NH—C(=O)—NH—$(CH_2)_2$—CH_3	0.1–0.5 g as single dose	Up to 60
Glyburide [Glibenclamide*] (DiaBeta, Micronase)	Cl, OCH_3 ring—C(=O)—NH—$(CH_2)_2$—⟨⟩—SO_2—NH—C(=O)—NH—⟨⟩	0.0025–0.02 g	10–24
Glipizide [Glydiazinamide*] (Glucotrol)	H_3C—pyrazine—C(=O)—NH—$(CH_2)_2$—⟨⟩—SO_2—NH—C(=O)—NH—⟨⟩	0.0025–0.02 g	10–24[†]

*Outside USA.
[†]Elimination half-life considerably shorter (see text).

administered insulin, or increase receptor binding of insulin.

Efficacy & Safety of the Sulfonylureas

In 1970, the University Group Diabetes Program (UGDP) reported that the number of deaths due to cardiovascular disease in diabetic patients treated with tolbutamide was excessive compared to either insulin-treated patients or those receiving placebos. Controversy persists about the validity of the conclusions reached by the UGDP, because of the heterogeneity of the population studied and certain features of the experimental design such as the use of a fixed dose of tolbutamide. However, in 1984 a package insert warning of a possible increased risk of death due to cardiovascular disease was placed in all sulfonylureas by order of the FDA.

TOLBUTAMIDE

Tolbutamide (Orinase) is well absorbed but rapidly oxidized in the liver. Its duration of effect is relatively short (6–10 hours). Tolbutamide is best administered in divided doses (eg, 500 mg before each meal and at bedtime); however, some patients require only 1 or 2 tablets daily. Acute toxic reactions are rare; skin rash occurs infrequently. Prolonged hypoglycemia has been reported rarely, mostly in elderly people or in pa-

tients receiving certain drugs (eg, dicumarol, phenylbutazone, or some of the sulfonamides). These drugs apparently compete for oxidative enzymes in the liver, resulting in higher levels of unmetabolized, active tolbutamide in the circulation.

CHLORPROPAMIDE

Chlorpropamide (Diabinese) has a half-life of 32 hours and is slowly metabolized; approximately 20–30% is excreted unchanged in the urine. Chlorpropamide also interacts with the drugs mentioned above that depend on hepatic oxidative catabolism, and it is contraindicated in patients with hepatic or renal insufficiency. The average maintenance dose is 250 mg daily, given as a single dose in the morning. Prolonged hypoglycemic reactions are more common than with tolbutamide, particularly in elderly patients, in whom chlorpropamide therapy should be monitored with special care. Doses in excess of 500 mg daily increase the risk of jaundice, which is uncommon at lower doses. Patients with a genetic predisposition who are taking chlorpropamide may experience a hyperemic flush when alcohol is ingested. Dilutional hyponatremia has been recognized as a complication of chlorpropamide therapy in some patients. This appears to result from both a stimulation of vasopressin secretion and a potentiation of its action at the renal tubule by chlorpropamide. The antidiuretic effect of chlorpropamide appears to be independent of the sulfonylurea part of its structure, since 3 other sulfonylureas (acetohexamide, tolazamide, and glyburide) have diuretic effects in humans. Hematologic toxicity (transient leukopenia, thrombocytopenia) occurs in less than 1% of patients.

TOLAZAMIDE

Tolazamide (Tolinase) is comparable to chlorpropamide in potency but has a shorter duration of action, similar to that of acetohexamide. Tolazamide is more slowly absorbed than the other sulfonylureas, and its effect on blood glucose does not appear for several hours. Its half-life is about 7 hours. Tolazamide is metabolized to several compounds that retain hypoglycemic effects. If more than 500 mg per day is required, the dose should be divided and given twice daily. Doses larger than 1000 mg daily do not further improve the degree of blood glucose control.

ACETOHEXAMIDE

Acetohexamide (Dymelor) has a duration of action of 10–16 hours—intermediate between tolbutamide and chlorpropamide. Therapeutic doses consist of 0.25–1.5 g daily in one or 2 doses. Liver metabolism is rapid, but the metabolite produced remains active. Side effects are similar to those of the other sulfonylurea drugs.

SECOND-GENERATION SULFONYLUREAS

In April 1984, the FDA approved 2 potent sulfonylurea compounds: glyburide and glipizide. Initial use of these drugs in other countries (glyburide in 1969, glipizide in 1971) was associated with a high rate of severe hypoglycemic reactions and even some deaths, due probably to lack of familiarity with their potent effects. These drugs should be used with caution in patients with cardiovascular disease or in elderly patients, in whom hypoglycemia would be especially dangerous.

Diabetes patients who have not responded to tolbutamide or tolazamide may respond to the more potent first-generation sulfonylurea chlorpropamide or to either of the second-generation sulfonylureas. It has not been established that the second-generation agents are more efficacious than chlorpropamide.

Glyburide (Glibenclamide; DiaBeta, Micronase) is metabolized in the liver into products with such low hypoglycemic activity that they are considered clinically unimportant. Although assays specific for the unmetabolized compound suggest a short plasma half-life, the biologic effects of glyburide are clearly persistent 24 hours after a single morning dose in diabetic patients. The usual starting dose is 2.5 mg/d, and the average maintenance dose is 5–10 mg/d given as a single morning dose; maintenance doses higher than 20 mg/d are not recommended.

Glyburide has few adverse effects other than its potential for causing hypoglycemia. Flushing has rarely been reported after ethanol ingestion. It does not cause water retention, as chlorpropamide does, but slightly enhances free water clearance. Glyburide is particularly contraindicated in the presence of hepatic impairment and probably should not be used in patients with renal insufficiency.

Glipizide (Glucotrol) has the shortest half-life of the more efficacious agents (2–4 hours). For maximum effect in reducing postprandial hyperglycemia, this agent should be ingested 30 minutes before breakfast, since rapid absorption is delayed when the drug is taken with food. The recommended starting dose is 5 mg/d, with up to 15 mg/d given as a single daily dose. When higher daily doses are required, they should be divided and given before meals. The maximum recommended dose is 40 mg/d.

At least 90% of glipizide is metabolized in the liver to inactive products, and 10% is excreted unchanged in the urine. Glipizide therapy is therefore contraindicated in patients with hepatic or renal impairment, who would therefore be at high risk for hypoglycemia.

COMBINED THERAPY WITH SULFONYLUREAS & INSULIN

Since sulfonylurea drugs not only increase the pancreatic B cell secretion of insulin but also restore peripheral tissue sensitivity to insulin, their use in combination with insulin has been advocated to reduce the total insulin dose required to control hyperglycemia. Currently, however, there are no data from prospective clinical trials with appropriate controls and crossover studies to justify the expense of prescribing both insulin and sulfonylureas to treat NIDDM.

BIGUANIDES

The structure of biguanides is shown in Table 40–6.

Phenformin was discontinued in the USA because of its association with lactic acidosis and because there was no documentation of any long-term benefit from its use. Metformin, buformin, and phenformin continue to be used elsewhere, although in some areas the indications for biguanide therapy are being reevaluated.

Mechanism of Action

An explanation of the mechanism of action of biguanides remains elusive. Their blood glucose–lowering action does not depend on the presence of functioning pancreatic B cells. Glucose is not lowered in normal subjects after an overnight fast, but postprandial blood glucose levels are considerably lower dur-

Table 40–6. Biguanides.

Biguanide $H_2N-C \overset{\overset{H}{\underset{|}{N}}}{\underset{\underset{NH}{\|}}{}} C \overset{}{\underset{\underset{NH}{\|}}{}}-R$		Daily Dose	Duration of Action (hours)
Phenformin (DBI, Meltrol-50)	$-NH-(CH_2)_2-$ ⬡	0.025–0.10 g as single dose or in divided doses	4–6 8–14
Buformin*	$-NH-(CH_2)_3-CH_3$	0.05–0.3 g in divided doses	...
Metformin*	$-N-(CH_3)_2$	1–3 g in divided doses	...

*In clinical use outside USA.

ing phenformin administration. Patients with non–insulin-dependent diabetes have considerably less fasting hyperglycemia as well as postprandial hyperglycemia after biguanides; however, hypoglycemia during biguanide therapy is essentially unknown. These agents might therefore be more appropriately termed "euglycemic" rather than hypoglycemic agents. Currently proposed mechanisms of action include (1) direct stimulation of glycolysis in peripheral tissues, with increased glucose removal from blood; (2) reduced hepatic gluconeogenesis; (3) slowing of glucose absorption from the gastrointestinal tract; (4) inhibition of plasma glucagon levels; and (5) increased insulin binding to insulin receptors.

Metabolism & Excretion

Phenformin is bound to plasma protein, and therapeutic dose levels range from 100 to 250 ng/mL. The half-life is approximately 11 hours. Phenformin is about one-third metabolized by hydroxylation of its benzene ring and thereby rendered biologically inactive; the remainder is excreted in the active unmetabolized form. In patients with renal insufficiency, unmetabolized phenformin accumulates in high concentration and thereby increases the risk of lactic acidosis, which appears to be a dose-related complication. Metformin is not metabolized and is excreted by the kidneys as the active compound. Lactic acidosis occurs with less frequency in patients treated with metformin compared to those treated with phenformin.

Clinical Use of Biguanides

Biguanides have been most often prescribed for patients with refractory obesity whose hyperglycemia is due to ineffective insulin action. Another indication for their use is in certain nonobese non–insulin-dependent diabetics in whom sulfonylurea therapy alone is less effective than when combined with phenformin.

Phenformin is contraindicated in patients with renal disease, alcoholism, hepatic disease, or conditions predisposing to tissue anoxia, such as chronic cardiopulmonary dysfunction, because of an increased risk of lactic acidosis induced by this drug in the presence of these diseases.

In the UGDP study, phenformin given in a dosage of 100 mg daily showed no therapeutic advantages in comparison with a control group of placebo-treated patients. A slight increase in heart rate and blood pressure was noted in the phenformin-treated diabetics, and an increased risk of cardiovascular mortality was reported.

GLUCAGON

Chemistry & Metabolism

Glucagon is synthesized in the A cells of the pancreatic islets of Langerhans (Table 40–1). Glucagon is a polypeptide—identical in all mammals—consisting of a single chain of 29 amino acids (Fig 40–4), with a molecular weight of 3485. Selective proteolytic cleavage converts a large precursor molecule of approximately MW 18,000 to glucagon. One of the precursor intermediates consists of a 100-amino-acid polypeptide called **glicentin,** which contains the glucagon sequence interposed between peptide extensions.

Glucagon is extensively degraded in the liver and kidney as well as in plasma, and at its tissue receptor sites. Because of its rapid deactivation by plasma, chilling of the collecting tubes and addition of antiproteolytic enzymes such as aprotinin are necessary when samples of blood are collected for immunoassay of circulating glucagon. Its half-life in plasma is between 3 and 6 minutes, which is similar to that of insulin.

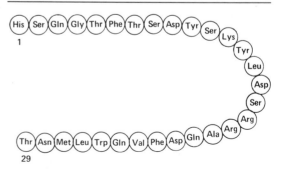

Figure 40–4. Amino acid sequence of glucagon polypeptide.

"Gut Glucagon"

Glicentin immunoreactivity has been found in cells of the small intestine as well as in pancreatic A cells and in effluents of perfused pancreas. The intestinal cells secrete **enteroglucagon,** a family of glucagon-like polypeptides, of which glicentin is a member. Unlike the pancreatic A cell, these intestinal cells lack the enzymes to convert glucagon precursors to true glucagon by removing the carboxy terminal extension from the molecule. Accordingly, the enteroglucagons do not react with antibody directed against the carboxy terminus of glucagon.

The function of the enteroglucagons has not been clarified, although smaller precursors can bind hepatic glucagon receptors where they exert partial activity.

Pharmacologic Effects of Glucagon

A. Metabolic Effects: The first 6 amino acids at the N-terminus of the glucagon molecule bind to specific receptors on liver cells. This leads to an increase in production of cAMP, which facilitates catabolism of stored glycogen and increases gluconeogenesis and ketogenesis. The immediate pharmacologic result of glucagon infusion is to raise blood glucose at the expense of stored hepatic glycogen. There is no effect on skeletal muscle glycogen, presumably because of the lack of glucagon receptors on skeletal muscle. Pharmacologic amounts of glucagon cause release of insulin from normal pancreatic B cells, catecholamines from pheochromocytoma, and calcitonin from medullary carcinoma cells.

B. Cardiac Effects: Glucagon has been shown to have an inotropic and chronotropic effect on the heart. However, it has not proved to be clinically useful in the management of cardiac failure.

C. Effects on Smooth Muscle: Glucagon has also been used extensively in radiology as an aid to x-ray visualization of the bowel, because large doses produce a profound relaxation of the intestine.

Clinical Uses

A. Severe Hypoglycemia: The major use of glucagon is for emergency treatment of severe hypoglycemic reactions in insulin-dependent patients when unconsciousness prohibits oral feedings (see p 490). Nasal sprays have been developed for this purpose and are presently undergoing clinical trials.

B. Endocrine Diagnosis: Several diagnostic tests use glucagon to diagnose endocrine pathophysiologic processes. In patients with insulin-dependent diabetes mellitus, a standard test of pancreatic B cell secretory reserve utilizes 1 mg of glucagon administered as an intravenous bolus. Since insulin-treated patients develop circulating anti-insulin antibodies that interfere with radioimmunoassays of insulin, measurements of C-peptide are used to indicate B cell secretion. Normal persons achieve a standard serum concentration of pancreatic C-peptide within 10 minutes of the injection, and in insulin-treated diabetics various degrees of B cell insufficiency can be quantitated. Most long-standing insulin-dependent diabetics show no C-peptide response to glucagon.

In patients with suspected endocrine tumors such as insulinoma, pheochromocytoma, or medullary carcinoma of the thyroid, a bolus of 0.5–1 mg of glucagon intravenously is occasionally effective in discharging hormonal products from a tumor, although negative tests may not rule out the diagnosis.

Adverse Reactions

Transient nausea and occasional vomiting can result from glucagon administration. These are generally mild, and glucagon is relatively free of severe adverse reactions.

REFERENCES

Berger M et al: Absorption kinetics and biologic effects of subcutaneously injected insulin preparations. *Diabetes Care* 1982;**5**:77.

Binder C et al: Insulin pharmacokinetics. *Diabetes Care* 1984;**7**:188.

Galloway JA et al: Factors influencing the absorption, serum insulin concentration, and blood glucose response, after injections of regular insulin and various insulin mixtures. *Diabetes Care* 1981;**4**:366.

Garvey WT et al: The effect of insulin treatment on insulin secretion and insulin action in type II diabetes mellitus. *Diabetes* 1985;**34**:222.

Grodsky GM et al: Pancreatic action of the sulfonylureas. *Fed Proc* 1977;**36**:2714.

Heine R-J et al: Absorption kinetics and action profiles of mixtures of short- and intermediate-acting insulins. *Diabetologia* 1984;**27**:558.

Herman WH et al: An epidemiological model for diabetes mellitus: Incidence, prevalence, and mortality. *Diabetes Care* 1984;**7**:367.

Howell SL: The mechanism of insulin secretion. *Diabetologia* 1984;**26**:319.

Jacobs S, Cuatrecasas P: Insulin receptors. *Annu Rev Pharmacol Toxicol* 1983;**23**:461.

Kadowaki T et al: Chlorpropamide-induced hyponatremia: Incidence and risk factors. *Diabetes Care* 1983;**6**:468.

Karam JH, Etzwiler DD (editors): International symposium on human insulin. *Diabetes Care* 1983;**6(Suppl 1)**:1.

Karam JH, Matin SB, Forsham PH: Antidiabetic drugs after the University Group Diabetes Program. *Annu Rev Pharmacol* 1975;**15**:351.

Kreisberg RA: The second-generation sulfonylureas: Change or progress? *Ann Intern Med* 1985;**102**:126.

Lebovitz HE, Feinglos MN: Mechanism of action of the second-generation sulfonylurea glipizide. *Am J Med* 1983;**75(Suppl 5B)**:46.

Lockwood DH, Gerich JE, Goldfine I (editors): Symposium on effects of oral hypoglycemic agents on receptor and postreceptor actions of insulin. *Diabetes Care* 1984;**7(Suppl 1)**:1.

Lord JM et al: Effect of metformin on insulin receptor binding and glycemic control in type II diabetes. *Br Med J* 1983;**286**:830.

Marliss EB et al: Present and future expectations regarding insulin infusion systems. *Diabetes Care* 1981;**4**:325.

Melander A, Wahlen-Bohl E: Clinical pharmacology of glipizide. *Am J Med* 1983;**75(Suppl 5B):**41.

Muhlhauser I, Koch J, Berger M: Pharmacokinetics and bioavailability of injected glucagon: Differences between intramuscular, subcutaneous, and intravenous administration. *Diabetes Care* 1985;**8:**39.

Nolte MS et al: Reduced solubility of short-acting soluble insulins when mixed with longer-acting insulins. *Diabetes* 1983;**32:**1177.

Peden N, Newton RW, Feely J: Oral hypoglycemic agents. *Br Med J* 1983;**286:**1564.

Peterson CM (editor): Symposium on optimal insulin delivery. *Diabetes Care* 1982;**5(Suppl 1):**1.

Pfeifer MA et al: Acute and chronic effects of sulfonylurea drugs on pancreatic islet function in man. *Diabetes Care* 1984; **7(Suppl 1):**25.

Pontiroli AE, Alberetto M, Pozza G: Intranasal glucagon raises blood glucose concentrations in healthy volunteers. *Br Med J* 1983;**287:**462.

Raskin P: Treatment of insulin-dependent diabetes mellitus with portable insulin infusion devices. *Med Clin North Am* 1982; **66:**1269.

Revers RR et al: The effects of biosynthetic human proinsulin on carbohydrate metabolism. *Diabetes* 1984;**33:**762.

Roth RA, Cassell DJ: Insulin receptor: Evidence that it is a protein kinase. *Science* 1983;**219:**299.

Salzman R et al: Intranasal aerosolized insulin: Mixed-meal studies and long term use in type I diabetes. *N Engl J Med* 1985;**312:**1078.

Seltzer HS: Efficacy and safety of oral hypoglycemic agents. *Annu Rev Med* 1980;**31:**261.

Skyler JS (editor): Symposium on human insulin of recombinant DNA origin. *Diabetes Care* 1982;**5(Suppl 2):**186.

Tattersal RB, Gale EAM: Patient self-monitoring of blood glucose and refinements of conventional insulin treatment. *Am J Med* 1981;**70:**177.

Unger RH: Meticulous control of diabetes: Benefits, risks, and precautions. *Diabetes* 1982;**31:**479.

Agents That Affect Bone Mineral Homeostasis

41

Daniel D. Bikle, MD, PhD

I. BASIC PHARMACOLOGY

Calcium and phosphate, the major mineral constituents of bone, are also 2 of the most important minerals for general cellular function. Accordingly, the body has evolved a complex set of mechanisms by which calcium and phosphate homeostasis is carefully maintained. Approximately 98% of the 1–2 kg of calcium and 85% of the 1 kg of phosphorus in the human adult is found in bone, the principal reservoir for these minerals. This function is dynamic, with constant remodeling of bone and ready exchange of bone mineral with that in the extracellular fluid. Bone also serves as the principal structural support for the body and provides the space for hematopoiesis. Thus, abnormalities in bone mineral homeostasis can lead not only to a wide variety of cellular dysfunction (eg, tetany, coma, muscle weakness) but also to disturbances in structural support of the body (eg, osteoporosis with fractures) and loss of hematopoietic capacity (eg, infantile osteopetrosis).

Calcium and phosphate enter the body from the intestine. The average American diet provides 600–1000 mg of calcium per day, of which approximately 100–250 mg is absorbed. This figure represents net absorption, since both absorption (principally in the duodenum and upper jejunum) and secretion (principally in the ileum) occur. The amount of phosphorus in the American diet is about the same as that of calcium. However, the efficiency of absorption (principally in the jejunum) is greater, ranging from 70 to 90% depending on intake. In the steady state, renal excretion of calcium and phosphate balances intestinal absorption. In general, over 95% of filtered calcium and 85% of filtered phosphate is reabsorbed by the kidney. The movement of calcium and phosphate across the intestinal and renal epithelia is closely regulated. Intrinsic disease of intestine (eg, nontropical sprue) or kidney (eg, chronic renal failure) disrupts bone mineral homeostasis.

Two hormones serve as the principal regulators of calcium and phosphate homeostasis: the polypeptide parathyroid hormone (PTH) and the steroid vitamin D. Vitamin D is a prohormone, rather than a true hormone, since it must be further metabolized to gain bio-logic activity. Other hormones—calcitonin, prolactin, growth hormone, insulin, thyroid hormone, glucocorticoids, and sex steroids—influence calcium and phosphate homeostasis under certain physiologic circumstances and can be considered secondary regulators. Deficiency or excess of these secondary regulators within a physiologic range does not produce the disturbance of calcium and phosphate homeostasis observed in situations of deficiency or excess PTH and vitamin D. However, certain of these secondary regulators—especially calcitonin, glucocorticoids, and estrogens—are useful therapeutically and will be discussed in subsequent sections.

In addition to these hormonal regulators, calcium and phosphate themselves, other ions such as sodium and fluoride, and a variety of drugs (diphosphonates, mithramycin, and thiazides) also alter calcium and phosphate homeostasis. This chapter is concerned with the pharmacology of these agents.

PRINCIPAL HORMONAL REGULATORS OF BONE MINERAL HOMEOSTASIS

PARATHYROID HORMONE

Parathyroid hormone (PTH) is a single-chain polypeptide hormone composed of 84 amino acids. It is produced in the parathyroid gland in a precursor form of 115 amino acids, the remaining 31 N-terminal amino acids being cleaved off prior to secretion. Within the gland is a calcium-sensitive protease capable of cleaving the intact hormone into fragments. Biologic activity resides in the N-terminal region such that synthetic 1–34 PTH is fully active. Loss of the first 2 N-terminal amino acids eliminates most biologic activity.

The metabolic clearance rate of intact PTH in dogs has been estimated to be 20 mL/min/kg, with a half-time of disappearance measured in minutes. Most of the clearance occurs in the liver and kidney. The biologically inactive C-terminal fragments produced during metabolism of the intact hormone have a much lower clearance rate, especially in renal failure. This accounts, in part, for the very high PTH values often observed in patients with renal failure when measured by radioimmunoassays directed against the C-terminal region of the molecule. The appearance of N-terminal fragments of PTH in the blood is difficult to demonstrate, consistent with the observations that only small amounts of such fragments are released into the blood and that their clearance is high.

PTH regulates calcium and phosphate flux across cellular membranes in bone and kidney, resulting in increased serum calcium and decreased serum phosphate. In bone, PTH increases the activity and number of osteoclasts, the cells responsible for bone resorption. However, it appears that this stimulation of osteoclasts is not a direct effect. This action increases bone turnover or bone remodeling, a specific sequence of cellular events initiated by osteoclastic bone resorption and followed by osteoblastic bone formation. Although both bone resorption and bone formation are enhanced by PTH, the net effect of excess PTH is to increase bone resorption. PTH in low doses may actually increase bone formation without first stimulating bone resorption. Although cAMP is involved in the action of PTH on bone cells, other mediators (including calcium) probably play a role.

In the kidney, PTH increases the ability of the nephron to reabsorb calcium and magnesium but reduces its ability to reabsorb phosphate, amino acids, bicarbonate, sodium, chloride, and sulfate. Although PTH markedly stimulates the renal production and excretion of cAMP and cAMP reproduces a number of the renal actions of PTH, cAMP may not be the sole mediator of PTH action on the kidney. Another important action of PTH on the kidney is its stimulation of 1,25-dihydroxyvitamin D (1,25[OH]$_2$D) production.

Recent evidence has called attention to vasoactive and cardiotropic actions of PTH. These observations may explain the ability of PTH to increase the glomerular filtration rate acutely. Whether such actions are involved in the apparent association of hyperparathyroidism and hypertension remains to be determined.

VITAMIN D

Vitamin D is a secosteroid produced in the skin from 7-dehydrocholesterol under the influence of ultraviolet irradiation. Vitamin D is also found in certain foods and is used to supplement dairy products. Both the natural form (vitamin D$_3$, cholecalciferol) and the plant-derived form (vitamin D$_2$, ergocalciferol) are present in the diet. These forms differ in that ergocalciferol contains a double bond (C22–23) and an additional methyl group in the side chain. This difference in humans apparently is of little physiologic consequence, and the following comments apply equally well to both forms of Vitamin D.

Vitamin D, which is a prohormone, serves as precursor to a number of biologically active metabolites (Fig 41–1). Vitamin D is first hydroxylated in the liver to form 25-hydroxyvitamin D (25[OH]D). This metabolite is further converted in the kidney to a number of other forms the best-studied of which are 1,25-dihydroxyvitamin D (1,25[OH]$_2$D), 24,25-dihydroxyvitamin D (24,25[OH]$_2$D), 25,26-dihydroxyvitamin D (25,26[OH]$_2$D), 1,24,25-trihydroxyvitamin D (1,24,25[OH]$_3$D), 1,25,26-trihydroxyvitamin D (1,25,26[OH]$_3$D), and the 25(OH)D-26,23-lactone. Only vitamin D, 25(OH)D (as calcifediol), and 1,25(OH)$_2$D (as calcitriol), are available for clinical use (see Table 41–1), although clinical studies with 24,25(OH)$_2$D are under way. The regulation of vitamin D metabolism is complex, involving calcium, phosphate, and a variety of hormones the most important of which is PTH.

Vitamin D and its metabolites circulate in plasma tightly bound to a carrier protein, the vitamin D-binding protein. This α-globulin binds 25(OH)D and 24,25(OH)$_2$D with comparable high affinity and vitamin D and 1,25(OH)$_2$D with lower affinity. In normal subjects, the terminal half-life of injected calcifediol is 23 days, whereas in anephric subjects it is longer (42 days). The half-life of 24,25(OH)$_2$D is probably similar. Tracer studies with vitamin D have shown a rapid clearance from the blood. The liver appears to be the principal organ for clearance. Excess vitamin D is stored in adipose tissue. The metabolic clearance rate of calcitriol in humans indicates a rapid turnover, with a terminal half-life measured in hours.

The mechanism of action of the vitamin D metabolites remains under active investigation. However, calcitriol is well established as the most potent agent with respect to stimulation of intestinal calcium and phosphate transport and bone resorption. Calcitriol appears to act on the intestine both by induction of new

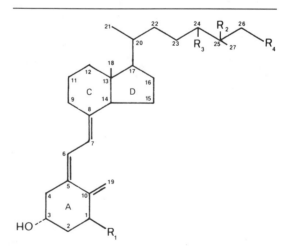

Figure 41–1. The structure of vitamin D$_3$. R$_1$–R$_4$ represent the sites of principal hydroxylation by which vitamin D$_3$ is converted to biologically active metabolites. R$_1$ = 1α-(OH); R$_2$ = 25(OH); R$_3$ = 24(OH); R$_4$ = 26(OH). The letters in the rings (A, C, D) and the carbon numbering are derived from the steroid nucleus of 7-dehydrocholesterol.

Table 41–1. Vitamin D and its clinically available metabolites and analogs.

Chemical Name	Abbreviation	Generic Name
Vitamin D$_3$	D$_3$	Cholecalciferol
Vitamin D$_2$	D$_2$	Ergocalciferol
25-Hydroxyvitamin D$_3$	25(OH)D$_3$	Calcifediol
1,25-Dihydroxyvitamin D$_3$	1,25(OH)$_2$D$_3$	Calcitriol
Dihydrotachysterol	DHT	Dihydrotachysterol

Table 41–2. Actions of PTH and vitamin D on gut, bone, and kidney.

	PTH	Vitamin D
Intestine	Increased calcium and phosphate absorption (by increased 1,25[OH]$_2$D production).	Increased calcium and phosphate absorption (by 1,25[OH]$_2$D).
Kidney	Decreased calcium excretion, increased phosphate excretion.	Calcium and phosphate excretion may be decreased by 25(OH)D and 1,25(OH)$_2$D.
Bone	Calcium and phosphate resorption increased by high doses. Low doses may increase bone formation.	Increased calcium and phosphate resorption by 1,25(OH)$_2$D. Bone formation may be increased by 24,25(OH)$_2$D.
Net effect on serum levels	Serum calcium increased, serum phosphate decreased.	Serum calcium and phosphate both increased.

proteins (eg, calcium-binding protein) and by modulation of calcium flux across the brush border and mitochondrial membranes by a means that does not require new protein synthesis. The molecular action of calcitriol on bone has received less attention. The metabolites 25(OH)D and 24,25(OH)$_2$D are far less potent stimulators of intestinal calcium and phosphate transport or bone resorption. However, 25(OH)D appears to be more potent than 1,25(OH)$_2$D in stimulating renal reabsorption of calcium and phosphate and may be the major metabolite regulating calcium flux and contractility in muscle. Recent evidence suggests that 24,25(OH)$_2$D stimulates bone formation. Specific receptors for 1,25(OH)$_2$D exist in target tissues. However, the role and even the existence of receptors for 25(OH)D and 24,25(OH)$_2$D remain controversial.

INTERACTION OF PTH & VITAMIN D

A summary of the principal actions of PTH and vitamin D on the 3 main target tissues—intestine, kidney, and bone—is presented in Table 41–2. The net effect of PTH is to raise serum calcium and reduce serum phosphate; the net effect of vitamin D is to raise both. Regulation of calcium and phosphate homeostasis is achieved through a variety of feedback loops. Calcium is the principal regulator of PTH secretion; as serum calcium levels rise, PTH secretion falls. Phosphate regulates PTH secretion indirectly, by forming complexes with calcium in the serum. Since it is the ionized concentration of calcium that is detected by the parathyroid gland, increases in serum phosphate levels reduce the ionized calcium and lead to stimulation of PTH secretion. Such feedback regulation is appropriate to the net effect of PTH to raise serum calcium and reduce serum phosphate levels. Likewise, both calcium and phosphate at high levels reduce the amount of 1,25(OH)$_2$D produced by the kidney and increase the amount of 24,25(OH)$_2$D produced. Since 1,25(OH)$_2$D raises serum calcium and phosphate, whereas 24,25(OH)$_2$D has less effect, such feedback regulation is again appropriate.

A different type of interaction is observed between PTH secretion and vitamin D metabolism. PTH stimulates 1,25(OH)$_2$D production and may reduce 24,25(OH)$_2$D production by the kidney. Conversely, 24,25(OH)$_2$D appears to suppress PTH secretion, whereas 1,25(OH)$_2$D may not if serum calcium is fixed. These interactions suggest a feed-forward or amplification interaction between PTH secretion and 1,25(OH)$_2$D production such that these hormone levels can rise or fall together if required to maintain normal serum calcium levels.

SECONDARY HORMONAL REGULATORS OF BONE MINERAL HOMEOSTASIS

A number of hormones modulate the actions of PTH and vitamin D in regulating bone mineral homeostasis. Compared to PTH and vitamin D, the physiologic impact of such secondary regulation on bone mineral homeostasis is minor. However, in pharmacologic amounts, a number of these hormones have actions on the bone mineral homeostatic mechanisms that can be exploited therapeutically.

CALCITONIN

The calcitonin secreted by the parafollicular cells of the mammalian thyroid (and by piscine ultimobranchial bodies) is a single-chain polypeptide hormone with 32 amino acids and a molecular weight of 3600. A disulfide bond between positions 1 and 7 is essential for biologic activity. Calcitonin is produced in these glands from a precursor with MW 15,000. The circulating forms of calcitonin are multiple, ranging in size from the monomer (MW 3600) to forms with an apparent molecular weight of 60,000. Whether such heterogeneity includes precursor forms or covalently linked oligomers is not known. Because of its heterogeneity, calcitonin is standardized by bioassay in rats. Activity is compared to a standard maintained by the

British Medical Research Council (MRC) and expressed as MRC units.

Human calcitonin monomer has a half-life of about 10 minutes with a metabolic clearance rate of 8–9 mL/kg/min. Salmon calcitonin has a longer half-life and a reduced metabolic clearance rate (3 mL/kg/min). Much of the clearance occurs in the kidney, although little intact calcitonin appears in the urine.

The principal effects of calcitonin are to lower serum calcium and phosphate by actions on bone and kidney. Calcitonin inhibits osteoclastic bone resorption. Although bone formation is not impaired at first after calcitonin administration, with time both formation and resorption of bone are reduced. Thus, the early hope that calcitonin would prove useful in restoring bone mass has not been realized. In the kidney, calcitonin reduces both calcium and phosphate reabsorption as well as reabsorption of other ions, including sodium, potassium, and magnesium. Although calcitonin stimulates cAMP formation in both bone and kidney, a requirement for cAMP in mediating these actions is not established. PTH also stimulates cAMP accumulation in these tissues, yet the effects of PTH and calcitonin are generally antagonistic. Tissues other than bone and kidney are affected by calcitonin. Calcitonin in pharmacologic amounts decreases gastrin secretion and reduces gastric acid output while increasing secretion of sodium, potassium, chloride, and water in the gut. Pentagastrin is a potent stimulator of calcitonin secretion (as is hypercalcemia), suggesting a possible physiologic relationship between gastrin and calcitonin. In the adult human, no readily demonstrable problem develops in cases of calcitonin deficiency (thyroidectomy) or excess (medullary carcinoma of the thyroid). However, the ability of calcitonin to block bone resorption and lower serum calcium makes it a useful drug for the treatment of Paget's disease, hypercalcemia, and osteoporosis.

GLUCOCORTICOIDS

Glucocorticoid hormones alter bone mineral homeostasis by antagonizing vitamin D–stimulated intestinal calcium transport, by blocking bone collagen synthesis, and by increasing PTH-stimulated bone resorption (although this last action is not universally accepted). Although these observations underscore the negative impact of glucocorticoids on bone mineral homeostasis, these hormones have proved useful in 2 situations involving bone mineral homeostasis: in the intermediate term treatment of hypercalcemia and as a diagnostic test of the cause of hypercalcemia.

ESTROGENS

Estrogens can prevent accelerated bone loss during the immediate postmenopausal period. Estrogens probably do not restore bone in the patient who already has osteoporosis. The prevailing hypothesis to explain these observations is that estrogens reduce the bone-resorbing action of PTH. The renal response to PTH may also be altered by estrogens. Estrogen administration leads to an increased $1,25(OH)_2D$ level in blood, but estrogens have no direct effect on $1,25(OH)_2D$ production in vitro. Conceivably, most—if not all—of the observed increase in $1,25(OH)_2D$ levels with estrogen therapy reflects the increase in vitamin D–binding protein and may not be associated with increased $1,25(OH)_2D$ production or free $1,25(OH)_2D$ levels. The principal therapeutic application for estrogen administration in disorders of bone mineral homeostasis is the treatment or prevention of postmenopausal osteoporosis.

NONHORMONAL AGENTS AFFECTING BONE MINERAL HOMEOSTASIS

DIPHOSPHONATES

The diphosphonates are analogs of pyrophosphate in which the P–O–P bond has been replaced with a nonhydrolyzable P–C–P bond (Fig 41–2). Only ethane-1-hydroxy-1,1-diphosphonate (EHDP, etidronate) is available for clinical use, although other forms are undergoing clinical trials. The diphosphonates owe their clinical usefulness and toxicity to their abil-

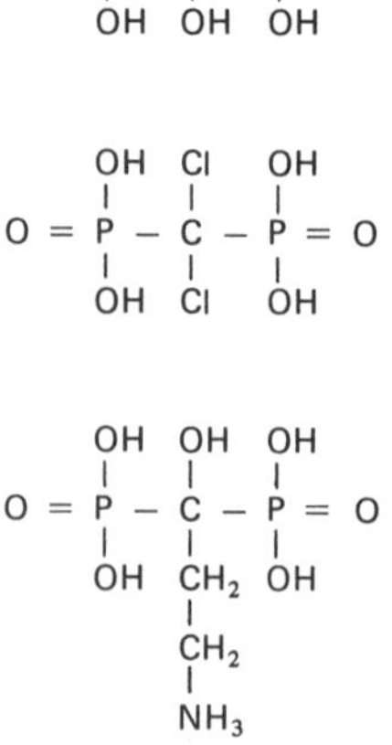

Inorganic pyrophosphoric acid

Ethane-1-hydroxy-1,1-diphosphonic acid (EHDP)

Dichloromethane diphosphonic acid (Cl_2MDP)

3-Amino-1-hydroxy-propane-1,1-diphosphonic acid (AHPDP)

Figure 41–2. The structure of pyrophosphate and the 3 diphosphonates that have been most studied: EHDP (etidronate), Cl_2MDP, and AHPDP.

ity to retard formation and dissolution of hydroxyapatite crystals within and without the skeletal system.

The results from animal studies indicate that 1–10% of an oral dose of etidronate is absorbed. Nearly half of the absorbed drug accumulates in bone; the remainder is excreted unchanged in the urine. That portion bound to bone is retained for weeks, depending on the turnover of bone itself.

Etidronate and the other diphosphonates exert a variety of effects on bone mineral homeostasis. Their physicochemical properties of reducing hydroxyapatite formation and dissolution make them clinically useful. However, the diphosphonates exert a variety of other cellular effects, including inhibition of 1,25(OH)$_2$D production, inhibition of intestinal calcium transport, metabolic changes in bone cells such as inhibition of glycolysis, inhibition of cell growth, and changes in acid and alkaline phosphatase. These effects vary depending on the diphosphonate being studied and may account for some of the clinical differences observed in the effects of the various diphosphonates on bone mineral homeostasis.

MITHRAMYCIN

Mithramycin is a cytotoxic antibiotic (see Chapter 58) that has been used clinically for 2 disorders of bone mineral metabolism: Paget's disease and hypercalcemia. The cytotoxic properties of the drug appear to involve its binding to DNA and interruption of DNA-directed RNA synthesis. The reasons for its usefulness in the treatment of Paget's disease and hypercalcemia are unclear but may relate to the need for protein synthesis to sustain bone resorption. The doses required to treat Paget's disease and hypercalcemia are about one-tenth the amounts required to achieve cytotoxic effects.

THIAZIDES

The chemistry and pharmacology of this family of drugs are covered in Chapter 14. The principal application of thiazides in the treatment of bone mineral disorders is in reducing renal calcium excretion. Thiazides may increase the effectiveness of parathyroid hormone in stimulating reabsorption of calcium by the renal tubules or may act on calcium reabsorption secondarily by increasing sodium reabsorption in the proximal tubule, thus reducing sodium delivery to the distal tubule. Thiazides have proved to be quite useful in reducing the hypercalciuria and incidence of stone formation in subjects with idiopathic hypercalciuria. Part of their efficacy in reducing stone formation may also lie in their ability to decrease urine oxalate excretion and increase urine magnesium and zinc levels (both of which inhibit calcium oxalate stone formation).

FLUORIDE

Fluoride is well established as effective for the prophylaxis of dental caries and is currently under investigation for the treatment of osteoporosis. Both therapeutic applications originated from epidemiologic observations that subjects living in areas with naturally fluoridated water (1–2 ppm) had less dental caries and fewer vertebral compression fractures than subjects living in nonfluoridated water areas. Fluoride is accumulated by bones and teeth, where it may act by stabilizing the hydroxyapatite crystal. Such a mechanism may explain the effectiveness of fluoride in increasing the resistance of teeth to dental caries, but it does not explain new bone growth.

Fluoride in drinking water appears to be most effective in preventing dental caries if consumed prior to the eruption of the permanent teeth. The optimum concentration in drinking water supplies is 0.5–1 ppm. Topical application is most effective if administered just as the teeth erupt. There is little further benefit to giving fluoride after the permanent teeth are fully formed. Excess fluoride in the drinking water leads to mottling of the enamel proportionate to the concentration above 1 ppm.

Because of the general lack of effectiveness of other agents in stimulating new bone growth in patients with osteoporosis, interest in the use of fluoride for this disorder has been renewed. Results of earlier studies indicated that fluoride alone without adequate calcium supplementation produced osteomalacia. More recent studies, in which calcium supplementation has been adequate, have demonstrated an improvement in calcium balance, an increase in bone mineral, an increase in trabecular bone volume, and a reduction in fracture incidence. The doses required range from 40 to 100 mg/d, maintaining serum fluoride levels between 5 and 10 μmol/L. Side effects observed include nausea and vomiting, gastrointestinal blood loss, arthralgias, and arthritis in a substantial proportion of patients. Such side effects are usually responsive to reducing the dose or giving fluoride with meals (or both). At present, fluoride is not approved by the Food and Drug Administration for use in osteoporosis. The most readily available formulation is a 2.2-mg pediatric tablet, so that at least 20 tablets per day are required for adequate therapy.

Acute toxicity, generally due to ingestion of fluoride-containing rat poisons, includes gastrointestinal symptoms and neurologic signs of hypocalcemia presumably related to the calcium-binding properties of fluoride. Fluoride in acutely toxic doses may also cause cardiovascular collapse or respiratory failure. Chronic exposure to very high levels of fluoride dust in the inspired air results in **crippling fluorosis,** characterized by thickening of the cortex of long bones and bony exostoses, especially in the vertebrae.

II. CLINICAL PHARMACOLOGY

Disorders of bone mineral homeostasis generally present with abnormalities in serum or urine calcium levels (or both), often accompanied by abnormal serum phosphate levels. These abnormal mineral concentrations may themselves cause symptoms requiring immediate treatment (eg, malignant hypercalcemia or tetany). More commonly, they serve as clues to an underlying disorder in hormonal regulators (eg, primary hyperparathyroidism), target tissue response (eg, chronic renal failure), or drug abuse (eg, vitamin D intoxication). In such cases, treatment of the underlying disorder is of prime importance.

Since bone and kidney play central roles in bone mineral homeostasis, conditions that alter bone mineral homeostasis usually affect either or both of these tissues secondarily. Effects on bone can result in osteoporosis (abnormal loss of bone; remaining bone histologically normal), osteomalacia (abnormal bone formation due to inadequate mineralization), or osteitis fibrosa (excessive bone resorption with fibrotic replacement of resorption cavities). Biochemical markers of skeletal involvement include changes in serum levels of the skeletal isoenzyme of alkaline phosphatase (reflecting osteoblastic activity) and urine levels of hydroxyproline (reflecting osteoclastic activity). The kidney becomes involved when the calcium-times-phosphate product in serum exceeds the point at which ectopic calcification occurs (often in renal parenchyma) or when the calcium-times-oxalate (or phosphate) product in urine exceeds saturation, leading to nephrocalcinosis and nephrolithiasis. Subtle early indicators of such renal involvement include polyuria, nocturia, and hyposthenuria. Radiologic evidence of nephrocalcinosis and stones is not generally observed until later. The degree of the ensuing renal failure is best followed by monitoring the decline in creatinine clearance.

ABNORMAL SERUM CALCIUM & PHOSPHATE LEVELS

HYPERCALCEMIA

Hypercalcemia is potentially lethal. Its major causes (other than thiazide therapy) are hyperparathyroidism and cancer with or without bone metastases. Less common causes are hypervitaminosis D, sarcoidosis, thyrotoxicosis, milk-alkali syndrome, adrenal insufficiency, and immobilization. With the possible exception of hypervitaminosis D, these latter disorders seldom require emergency lowering of serum calcium. A number of approaches are used to manage the hypercalcemic crisis.

SALINE DIURESIS

In hypercalcemia of sufficient severity to produce symptoms, rapid reduction of serum calcium is required. The first steps include rehydration with saline and diuresis with furosemide. Most patients presenting with severe hypercalcemia have a substantial component of prerenal azotemia owing to dehydration, which prevents the kidney from compensating for the rise in serum calcium by excreting more calcium in the urine. Therefore, the initial infusion of 500–1000 mL/h of saline to reverse the dehydration and restore urine flow can by itself substantially lower serum calcium. The addition of a loop diuretic such as furosemide (Chapter 14) not only enhances urine flow but floods the distal tubule with sodium, which competes with calcium for reabsorption at this site. Monitoring central venous pressure is important to forestall the development of congestive heart failure and pulmonary edema in predisposed subjects. In many subjects, saline diuresis will suffice to reduce serum calcium levels to a point at which more definitive diagnosis and treatment of the underlying condition can be achieved. If this is not the case or if more prolonged medical treatment of hypercalcemia is required, the following agents are available (discussed in order of preference).

CALCITONIN

Calcitonin has proved useful as ancillary treatment in a large number of patients. Calcitonin by itself seldom restores serum calcium to normal, and refractoriness frequently develops. However, its lack of toxicity permits frequent administration at high doses (200 MRC units or more). An effect on serum calcium is observed within 4–6 hours and lasts for 6–10 hours. Calcimar (salmon calcitonin) is available for parenteral administration only.

MITHRAMYCIN

Because of its toxicity, mithramycin is not the drug of first choice for the treatment of hypercalcemia. However, when other forms of therapy fail, 25–50 μg/kg given intravenously usually lowers serum calcium substantially within 24–48 hours. This effect can last for several days. This dose can be repeated as necessary. The most feared toxic effect is sudden thrombocytopenia followed by hemorrhage. Hepatic and renal toxicity can also occur. Hypocalcemia, nausea, and vomiting may limit therapy. Use of this drug must be accompanied by careful monitoring of platelet counts, liver and kidney function, and serum calcium levels.

PHOSPHATE

Giving intravenous phosphate is probably the fastest and surest way to reduce serum calcium, but it is a hazardous procedure if not done properly. Intravenous phosphate should be used only after other methods of treatment (calcitonin, saline diuresis with furosemide, and mithramycin) have failed to control symptomatic hypercalcemia. Phosphate must be given slowly (50 mmol or 1.5 g elemental phosphorus over 6–8 hours) and the patient switched to oral phosphate (1–2 g elemental phosphorus daily) as soon as symptoms of hypercalcemia have cleared. The risks of intravenous phosphate therapy include sudden hypocalcemia, ectopic calcification, acute renal failure, and hypotension. Oral phosphate can also lead to ectopic calcification and renal failure if serum calcium and phosphate levels are not carefully monitored, but the risk is less and the time of onset much longer. Phosphate is available in oral and intravenous forms as the sodium or potassium salt. Amounts required to provide 1 g of elemental phosphorus are as follows:

Intravenous:
  In-Phos: 40 mL
  Hyper-Phos-K: 15 mL
Oral:
  Fleet's Phospho-Soda: 6.2 mL
  Neutra-Phos: 300 mL
  Phos-Tab: 6 tablets

GLUCOCORTICOIDS

Glucocorticoids have no clear role in the acute treatment of hypercalcemia. However, the chronic hypercalcemia of sarcoidosis, vitamin D intoxication, and certain cancers (particularly multiple myeloma and related lymphoproliferative diseases) may respond within several days to glucocorticoid therapy. Prednisone in doses of 30–60 mg orally daily is generally used, although equivalent doses of other glucocorticoids are effective. The rationale for the use of glucocorticoids in these diseases differs, however. The hypercalcemia of sarcoidosis appears to be secondary to increased production of $1,25(OH)_2D$, possibly by the sarcoid tissue itself. Glucocorticoid therapy directed at the reduction of sarcoid tissue results in restoration of normal serum calcium and $1,25(OH)_2D$ levels. The treatment of hypervitaminosis D with glucocorticoids probably does not alter vitamin D metabolism significantly but is thought to reduce vitamin D–mediated intestinal calcium transport. An action of glucocorticoids to reduce vitamin D–mediated bone resorption has not been excluded, however. The effect of glucocorticoids on the hypercalcemia for cancer is probably 2-fold. The malignancies responding best to glucocorticoids (ie, multiple myeloma and related lymphoproliferative diseases) are sensitive to the lytic action of glucocorticoids, so part of the effect may be related to decreased tumor mass and activity. Glucocorticoids have also been shown to inhibit the effectiveness of osteoclast activating factor, a humoral substance elaborated by multiple myeloma and related cancers that stimulates osteoclastic bone resorption.

Other causes of hypercalcemia—particularly primary hyperparathyroidism—do not respond to glucocorticoid therapy.

This difference in response of the various forms of hypercalcemia to glucocorticoids forms the basis for the glucocorticoid suppression test, in which the response of serum calcium to a 10-day course of prednisone, 60 mg orally daily, helps differentiate the hypercalcemia of primary hyperparathyroidism from other causes such as sarcoidosis, vitamin D intoxication, and certain cancers. This test may be misleading and should not be used as a substitute for more specific tests for primary hyperparathyroidism such as serum immunoreactive PTH determinations.

HYPOCALCEMIA

The main features of hypocalcemia are neuromuscular—tetany, paresthesias, laryngospasm, muscle cramps, and convulsions. The major causes of hypocalcemia in the adult are hypoparathyroidism, vitamin D deficiency, renal failure, and malabsorption. Neonatal hypocalcemia is a common disorder that usually resolves without therapy. The roles of PTH, vitamin D, and calcitonin in the neonatal syndrome are under active investigation. Large infusions of citrated blood can produce hypocalcemia by the formation of citrate-calcium complexes. Calcium and vitamin D (or its metabolites) form the mainstay of treatment of hypocalcemia.

CALCIUM

A number of calcium preparations are available for intravenous, intramuscular, and oral use. Calcium gluceptate (0.9 meq calcium/mL), calcium gluconate (0.45 meq calcium/mL), and calcium chloride (0.68–1.36 meq calcium/mL) are available for intravenous therapy. Calcium gluconate is the preferred form because it is less irritating to veins. Oral preparations include calcium carbonate (40% calcium), calcium lactate (13% calcium), calcium phosphate (25% calcium), and calcium chloride (27% calcium). Calcium carbonate is often the preparation of choice because of its high percentage of calcium, ready availability (eg, Tums), low cost, and antacid properties. In achlorhydric patients, calcium carbonate should be given with meals to increase absorption. Combinations of vitamin D and calcium are available, but treatment must be tailored to the individual patient and individual disease, a flexibility lost by fixed-dosage combinations. Treatment of severe symptomatic hypocalcemia can be accomplished with slow infusion of 5–20 mL of 10% calcium gluconate. Rapid infusion can lead to cardiac arrhythmias. Less severe hypocalcemia is best treated with oral forms sufficient to provide approximately 400–800 mg of elemental calcium (1–2 g calcium carbonate per day). Dosage must be adjusted to avoid hypercalcemia and hypercalciuria.

VITAMIN D

When rapidity of action is required, $1,25(OH)_2D_3$ (calcitriol), $0.25–1 \mu g$ daily, is the vitamin D metabolite of choice, since it is capable of raising serum calcium within 24–48 hours. Calcitriol also raises serum phosphate, although this action is usually not observed early in treatment. The combined effects of calcitriol and all other vitamin D metabolites and analogs on both calcium and phosphate make careful monitoring of these mineral levels especially important to avoid ectopic calcification secondary to an abnormally high serum calcium-times-phosphate product. Since the choice of the appropriate vitamin D metabolite or analog for long-term treatment of hypocalcemia depends on the nature of the underlying disease, further discussion of vitamin D treatment will be found under the headings of the specific diseases.

HYPERPHOSPHATEMIA

Hyperphosphatemia is a frequent complication of renal failure but is also found in all types of hypoparathyroidism (idiopathic, surgical, and pseudo), vitamin D intoxication, and the rare syndrome of tumoral calcinosis. Emergency treatment of hyperphosphatemia is seldom necessary but can be achieved by dialysis or glucose and insulin infusions. In general, control of hyperphosphatemia involves restriction of dietary phosphate plus the use of phosphate binding gels such as $Al(OH)_3$-containing antacids.

HYPOPHOSPHATEMIA

A variety of conditions are associated with hypophosphatemia, including primary hyperparathyroidism, vitamin D deficiency, idiopathic hypercalcemia, vitamin D-resistant rickets, various other forms of renal phosphate wasting (eg, Fanconi's syndrome), overzealous use of $Al(OH)_3$-containing antacids, and parenteral nutrition with inadequate phosphate content. Acute hypophosphatemia may lead to a reduction in the intracellular levels of high-energy organic phosphates (eg, ATP), interfere with normal hemoglobin-to-tissue oxygen transfer by decreasing red cell 2,3-diphosphoglycerate levels, and lead to rhabdomyolysis. However, clinically significant acute effects of hypophosphatemia are seldom seen, and emergency treatment is generally not indicated. The long-term effects of hypophosphatemia include proximal muscle weakness and abnormal bone mineralization (osteomalacia). Therefore, hypophosphatemia should be avoided during other forms of therapy and treated in conditions such as vitamin D–resistant rickets of which it is a cardinal feature. Oral forms of phosphate available for use are listed above in the section on hypercalcemia.

SPECIFIC DISORDERS INVOLVING THE BONE MINERAL REGULATING HORMONES

PRIMARY HYPERPARATHYROIDISM

This rather common disease, if associated with symptoms and significant hypercalcemia, is best treated surgically. Oral phosphate has been tried but cannot be recommended.

HYPOPARATHYROIDISM

In the absence of PTH (idiopathic or surgical hypoparathyroidism) or a normal target tissue response to PTH (pseudohypoparathyroidism), serum calcium falls and serum phosphate rises. In such patients, $1,25(OH)_2D$ levels are usually low, presumably reflecting the lack of stimulation by PTH of $1,25(OH)_2D$ production. The skeletons of patients with idiopathic or surgical hypoparathyroidism are normal except for a slow turnover rate. A number of patients with pseudohypoparathyroidism appear to have osteitis fibrosa, suggesting that the normal or high PTH levels found in such patients are capable of acting on bone but not on the kidney. The distinction between pseudohypoparathyroidism and idiopathic hypoparathyroidism is made on the basis of normal or high PTH levels but deficient renal response (ie, diminished excretion of cAMP or phosphate) in patients with pseudohypoparathyroidism.

The principal therapeutic concern is to restore normocalcemia and normophosphatemia. Under most circumstances, vitamin D (25,000–100,000 units 3 times per week) and dietary calcium supplements suffice. More rapid increments in serum calcium can be achieved with calcitriol, although it is not clear that this metabolite offers a substantial advantage over vitamin D itself for long-term therapy. Many patients treated with vitamin D develop episodes of hypercalcemia. This complication is more rapidly reversible with cessation of therapy using calcitriol rather than vitamin D. This would be of importance to the patient in whom such hypercalcemic crises are common. Dihydrotachysterol and 25(OH)D have not received much study as therapy for hypoparathyroidism, although both should be effective. Whether they offer advantages over vitamin D sufficient to justify their added expense remains to be seen.

NUTRITIONAL RICKETS

Vitamin D deficiency, once thought to be rare in this country, is being recognized more often, especially in the pediatric and geriatric populations on vegetarian diets and with reduced sunlight exposure. This problem can be avoided by daily intake of 400 units of vitamin D and treated by somewhat higher doses (4000 units per day). No other metabolite is indicated. The diet should also contain adequate amounts of calcium and phosphate.

CHRONIC RENAL FAILURE

The major problems of chronic renal failure that impact on bone mineral homeostasis are the loss of $1,25(OH)_2D$ and $24,25(OH)_2D$ production, the retention of phosphate that reduces ionized calcium levels, and the secondary hyperparathyroidism that results. With the loss of $1,25(OH)_2D$ production, less calcium is absorbed from the intestine and less bone is resorbed under the influence of PTH. As a result hypocalcemia usually develops, furthering the development of hyperparathyroidism. The bones show a mixture of osteomalacia and osteitis fibrosa. Some patients may become hypercalcemic from 2 causes other than overzealous treatment with calcium supplements and high dialysate calcium levels. The most common cause of hypercalcemia is the development of severe secondary (sometimes referred to as tertiary) hyperparathyroidism. In such cases, the PTH level in blood is very high. Serum alkaline phosphatase levels also tend to be high. Treatment often requires parathyroidectomy. A less common circumstance leading to hypercalcemia is development of a form of osteomalacia characterized by a profound decrease in bone cell activity and loss of the calcium buffering action of bone. In the absence of kidney function, any calcium absorbed from the intestine accumulates in the blood. Therefore, such patients are very sensitive to the hypercalcemic action of $1,25(OH)_2D$. These individuals generally have a high serum calcium but nearly normal alkaline phosphatase and PTH levels. Recent evidence suggests that bone in such patients has a high aluminum content, especially in the mineralization front, which may block normal bone mineralization. These patients do not respond favorably to parathyroidectomy. Deferoxamine, an agent used to chelate iron (Chapter 61), also binds aluminum and is undergoing clinical trials as therapy for this disorder.

The choice of vitamin D preparation to be used in the setting of chronic renal failure in the dialysis patient depends on the type and extent of bone disease and hyperparathyroidism. No consensus has been reached regarding the advisability of using any vitamin D metabolite in the predialysis patient. $1,25(OH)_2D_3$ (calcitriol) will rapidly correct hypocalcemia and at least partially reverse the secondary hyperparathyroidism and osteitis fibrosa. Many patients with muscle weakness and bone pain gain an improved sense of well-being. Dihydrotachysterol, an analog of $1,25(OH)_2D$, is also available for clinical use. Dihydrotachysterol appears to be as effective as calcitriol, differing principally in its time course of action; calcitriol increases serum calcium in 1–2 days, whereas dihydrotachysterol requires 1–2 weeks. For an equipotent dose (0.2 mg dihydrotachysterol versus 0.5 μg calcitriol), dihydrotachysterol costs about one-fourth as much as calcitriol. A disadvantage of dihydrotachysterol is the inability to measure it in serum. Neither dihydrotachysterol nor calcitriol corrects the osteomalacic component of renal osteodystrophy in the majority of patients, and neither should be used in patients with hypercalcemia, especially if the bone disease is primarily osteomalacic. Calcifediol $(25[OH]D_3)$ may also be used to advantage. Calcifediol is less effective than calcitriol in stimulating intestinal calcium transport, so that hypercalcemia is less of a problem with calcifediol. Like dihydrotachysterol, calcifediol requires several weeks to restore normocalcemia in hypocalcemic individuals with chronic renal failure. Presumably because of the reduced ability of the diseased kidney to metabolize calcifediol to more active metabolites, high doses (50–100 μg daily) must be given to achieve the supraphysiologic serum levels required for therapeutic effectiveness.

Vitamin D has been used in treating renal osteodystrophy. However, patients with a substantial degree of renal failure who are thus unable to convert vitamin D to its active metabolites usually are refractory to vitamin D. Its use is decreasing as more effective alternatives become available. Regardless of the drug employed, careful attention to serum calcium and phosphate levels is required. Calcium supplements (dietary and in the dialysate) and phosphate restriction (dietary and with oral ingestion of phosphate binders) should be employed along with the use of vitamin D metabolites. Monitoring serum PTH and alkaline phosphatase levels is useful in determining whether therapy is correcting or preventing secondary hyperparathyroidism. Although not generally available, percutaneous bone biopsies for quantitative histomorphometry are becoming increasingly important in choosing appropriate therapy and following the effectiveness of such therapy. Unlike the rapid changes in serum values, changes in bone morphology require months to years. Monitoring serum levels of the vitamin D metabolites is useful to determine compliance, absorption, and metabolism.

INTESTINAL OSTEODYSTROPHY

A number of gastrointestinal and hepatic diseases result in disordered calcium and phosphate homeostasis that ultimately leads to bone disease. The bones in such patients show a combination of osteoporosis and osteomalacia. Osteitis fibrosa does not occur (as it does in renal osteodystrophy). The common features that appear to be important in this group of diseases are malabsorption of calcium and vitamin D. Liver disease may, in addition, reduce the production of $25(OH)D$ from vitamin D, although the importance of this in all but patients with terminal liver failure remains in dispute. The malabsorption of vitamin D is probably not limited to exogenous vitamin D. The liver secretes into bile a substantial number of vitamin

D metabolites and conjugates that are reabsorbed in (presumably) the distal jejunum and ileum. Interference with this process could deplete the body of endogenous vitamin D metabolites as well as limit absorption of dietary vitamin D.

In mild forms of malabsorption, vitamin D (25,000–50,000 units 3 times per week) should suffice to raise serum levels of 25(OH)D into the normal range. Many patients with severe disease do not respond to vitamin D. Clinical experience with the other metabolites is limited, but both calcitriol and calcifediol have been used successfully in doses similar to those recommended for treatment of renal osteodystrophy. Theoretically, calcifediol should be the drug of choice under these conditions, since no impairment of the renal metabolism of 25(OH)D to 1,25(OH)$_2$D and 24,25(OH)$_2$D exists in these patients. Both calcitriol and calcifediol may be of importance in reversing the bone disease. As in the other diseases discussed, treatment of intestinal osteodystrophy with vitamin D and its metabolites should be accompanied by appropriate dietary calcium supplementation and monitoring of serum calcium and phosphate levels.

OSTEOPOROSIS

Osteoporosis is defined as abnormal loss of bone predisposing to fractures. It is most common in postmenopausal women but may occur in older men also. It may occur as a side effect of chronic administration of glucocorticoids or other drugs; as a manifestation of endocrine disease such as thyrotoxicosis or hyperparathyroidism; as a feature of malabsorption syndrome; as a consequence of alcohol abuse; or without obvious cause (idiopathic). The postmenopausal form of osteoporosis is accompanied by lower 1,25(OH)$_2$D levels and reduced intestinal calcium transport. This form of osteoporosis appears to be due to estrogen deficiency and is best treated with cyclic doses of estrogen. It is important to note that the most rapid loss of bone occurs within the first 5 years after menopause and that administration of estrogens after this time may be less effective. Furthermore, if estrogen therapy is discontinued, a period of accelerated bone loss may occur. Thus, treatment with estrogens should be started prior to the onset of osteoporosis (ie, in the perimenopausal period) and may need to be continued for life. Since continuous estrogen therapy is associated with increased risk of endometrial carcinoma, among other complications, the recommendation to treat all postmenopausal women with estrogens has not been universally accepted. With the advent of sensitive means of measuring vertebral bone mineral content (CT scan, dual photon absorptiometry), estrogen therapy may be reserved for women wth reduced bone mineral content at the time of menopause or those who lose bone rapidly in the first year after menopause. Recent evidence, however, indicates that cyclic estrogen therapy in combination with a progestational agent reduces or eliminates this added risk of cancer. There-

fore, estrogens should be administered for 21 of 28 days in the lowest effective dose (eg, 0.625 mg of conjugated estrogens or 25–50 μg of ethinyl estradiol), with addition of a progestational agent on days 14–21 (eg, 10 mg of medroxyprogesterone acetate). This may reinitiate menstrual bleeding, so the patient must be advised of this in advance. Other complications of estrogen therapy such as hypertension and thrombophlebitis must also be kept in mind when such treatment is initiated.

To counter the reduced intestinal calcium transport, vitamin D therapy is often employed in addition to dietary calcium supplementation. There is no clear evidence that pharmacologic doses of vitamin D are of much additional benefit beyond cyclic estrogens and calcium supplementation. Studies are under way in which calcitriol and calcifediol are being tried in an effort to restore bone or to prevent further bone loss, but definitive results are not yet available.

A recent large study from the Mayo Clinic (see Riggs reference) indicated that fluoride furthered the efficacy of estrogen therapy and calcium in preventing vertebral compression fractures. High doses of fluoride must be used (40–100 mg/d). A significant number of patients receiving fluoride therapy develop gastrointestinal or rheumatic symptoms. Currently, fluoride has not been approved by the Food and Drug Administration for the treatment of osteoporosis, so that its use in this condition remains investigational (see p 501).

Calcitonin has recently been approved for use in the treatment of postmenopausal osteoporosis. Whether this agent, which reduces bone resorption acutely, will have a long-term effect on bone mass remains uncertain. It has few side effects.

The cause of idiopathic osteoporosis in men is not known. Treatment usually consists of giving vitamin D and dietary calcium supplements, but little information is available about its efficacy. It is important to exclude more treatable forms of osteoporosis such as that accompanying corticosteroid therapy, alcohol abuse, hyperparathyroidism, thyrotoxicosis, malabsorption, or occult nutritional osteomalacia.

VITAMIN D–RESISTANT RICKETS

This X-linked recessive disorder is manifested by the appearance of rickets and hypophosphatemia in children. The disease can present in adulthood, presumably reflecting either less severe disease or a missed diagnosis in childhood. The main defect appears to be an abnormality in renal phosphate reabsorption. Phosphate is critical to normal bone mineralization; when phosphate stores are deficient, a clinical and pathologic picture resembling vitamin D–deficient rickets develops. However, such children fail to respond to the usual doses of vitamin D employed in the treatment of nutritional rickets. A defect in 1,25(OH)$_2$D production by the kidney has also been suggested by some investigators, because the serum

1,25(OH)₂D levels tend to be low relative to the degree of hypophosphatemia observed. This combination of low serum phosphate and low or low-normal serum 1,25(OH)₂D provides the rationale for treating such patients with oral phosphate (1–3 g daily) and large doses of vitamin D (25,000–100,000 units daily). Recently, some groups have used calcitriol with good effect (0.25–1 μg daily). Reports of such combination therapy are encouraging in this otherwise debilitating disease.

VITAMIN D–DEPENDENT RICKETS

This entity actually represents 2 different diseases (types I and II). Both present as childhood rickets that does not respond to conventional doses of vitamin D. Type I vitamin D–dependent rickets is due to an isolated deficiency of 1,25(OH)₂D production. This condition can be treated with vitamin D (4000 units daily) or calcitriol (0.25–0.5 μg daily). Type II vitamin D–dependent rickets is caused by a target tissue defect in response to 1,25(OH)₂D. The serum levels of 1,25(OH)₂D are very high in type II but not in type I. Treatment with large doses of calcitriol has been claimed to be effective in restoring normocalcemia. Such patients are totally refractory to vitamin D. One recent report indicates a reversal of resistance to calcitriol when 24,25(OH)₂D was given. These diseases are rare.

NEPHROTIC SYNDROME

Patients with nephrotic syndrome can lose vitamin D metabolites into their urine, presumably by loss of the vitamin D–binding protein. Such patients may have very low 25(OH)D levels. At least some of them develop bone disease. It is not yet clear what value vitamin D therapy has in such patients, since this complication of the nephrotic syndrome has only recently been recognized, and therapeutic trials with vitamin D (or any other vitamin D metabolite) have not yet been carried out. Since the problem is not related to vitamin D metabolism, one would not anticipate any advantage in using the more expensive vitamin D metabolites in place of vitamin D itself.

IDIOPATHIC HYPERCALCIURIA

This syndrome, characterized by hypercalciuria and nephrolithiasis with normal serum calcium and PTH levels, has been subdivided into 3 groups of patients: (1) hyperabsorbers, patients with increased intestinal absorption of calcium, resulting in high-normal serum calcium, low-normal PTH, and a secondary increase in urine calcium; (2) renal calcium leakers, patients with a primary decrease in renal reabsorption of filtered calcium, leading to low-normal serum calcium and high-normal serum PTH; and (3) renal

phosphate leakers, patients with a primary decrease in renal reabsorption of phosphate, leading to stimulation of 1,25(OH)₂D production, increased intestinal calcium absorption, increased ionized serum calcium, low-normal PTH levels, and a secondary increase in urine calcium. There is some disagreement about this classification, and in many cases patients are not readily categorized. Many such patients present with mild hypophosphatemia, and oral phosphate has been used with some success to reduce stone formation. However, a clear role for phosphate in the treatment of this disorder has not been established. Therapy with hydrochlorothiazide, 50 mg twice daily, is recommended, although equivalent doses of other thiazide diuretics work as well. Loop diuretics such as furosemide and ethacrynic acid should not be used, since they increase urinary calcium excretion. The major toxicity of thiazide diuretics, besides hypokalemia and hyperglycemia, is hypercalcemia. This is seldom more than a biochemical observation unless the patient has a disease such as hyperparathyroidism in which bone turnover is accelerated. Accordingly, one should screen patients for such disorders before starting thiazide therapy and monitor serum and urine calcium when therapy has begun. An alternative to thiazides is allopurinol. Some studies indicate that hyperuricosuria is associated with idiopathic hypercalcemia and that a small nidus of urate crystals could lead to the calcium oxalate stone formation characteristic of idiopathic hypercalciuria. Allopurinol, 300 mg daily, may reduce stone formation by reducing uric acid excretion.

OTHER DISORDERS OF BONE MINERAL HOMEOSTASIS

PAGET'S DISEASE OF BONE

Paget's disease is a localized bone disease characterized by uncontrolled osteoclastic bone resorption with secondary increases in bone formation. This new bone is poorly organized, however. The cause of Paget's disease is obscure, although recent studies suggest that a slow virus may be involved. The disease is fairly common, although symptomatic bone disease is less common. The biochemical parameters of elevated serum alkaline phosphatase and urinary hydroxyproline are useful for diagnosis. Along with the characteristic radiologic and bone scan findings, these biochemical determinations provide good markers by which to follow therapy. The goal of treatment is to reduce bone pain and stabilize or prevent other problems such as progressive deformity, hearing loss, high-output cardiac failure, and immobilization hypercalcemia. Calcitonin can be used as sole treatment or in combination with diphosphonates for this disease. Treatment failures may respond to mithramycin. Calcitonin is administered subcutaneously or intramuscularly in doses of 50–100 MRC units every day or every other day. Higher or more frequent doses have been advocated when this initial regimen is ineffective. Improvement in bone pain and reduction in serum alkaline phosphatase and urine hydroxyproline levels require weeks to months. Often a patient who responds well initially will lose the response to calcitonin. This refractoriness is not correlated with the development of antibodies.

Sodium etidronate is the only diphosphonate currently available for clinical use. The recommended dosage is 5 mg/kg of the sodium salt daily by oral administration. Long-term (months to years) remission may be expected in patients who respond to etidronate. Treatment should not exceed 6 months per course but can be repeated after 3 months if necessary. The principal toxicity of etidronate is the development of osteomalacia and increased incidence of fractures when the dose is raised substantially above 5 mg/kg. Other diphosphonates such as dichloromethane diphosphonate or aminohydroxypropane diphosphonate are less toxic in this regard. Some patients treated with etidronate develop bone pain similar in nature to the bone pain of osteomalacia. This subsides after stopping the drug.

The use of a potentially lethal cytotoxic drug such as mithramycin in a generally benign disorder like Paget's disease is recommended only when other less toxic agents (calcitonin, etidronate) have failed and the symptoms are debilitating. Insufficient clinical data on long-term use of mithramycin are available to determine its usefulness for extended therapy. However, short courses involving 15–25 μg/kg intravenously for 5–10 days followed by 15 μg/kg intravenously each week have been used to control the disease.

ENTERIC OXALURIA

Patients with short bowel syndromes associated with fat malabsorption can present with renal stones composed of calcium and oxalate. Such patients characteristically have normal or low urine calcium levels but elevated urine oxalate levels. The major reasons for the development of oxaluria in such patients are thought to be decreased availability of luminal calcium (which is bound to fat) to bind to oxalate to prevent its absorption and increased production of oxalate by enteric flora acting on the increased supply of nutrients reaching the colon. Although one would ordinarily avoid treating a patient with calcium oxalate stones with calcium supplementation, this is precisely what is done in patients with enteric oxaluria. One to 2 g of calcium carbonate can be given daily in divided doses, with careful monitoring of urinary calcium and oxalate to be certain that urinary oxalate falls without a dangerous increase in urinary calcium.

REFERENCES

Austin LA, Heath HH III: Calcitonin: Physiology and pathophysiology. *N Engl J Med* 1981;**304:**269.

Bikle DD: The vitamin D endocrine system. *Adv Intern Med* 1982;**27:**45.

Bikle DD et al: Bone disease in alcohol abuse. *Ann Intern Med* 1985;**103:**42.

Coburn JW, Massry SG (editors): Uses and actions of 1,25 dihydroxyvitamin D$_3$ in uremia. *Contrib Nephrol* 1980;**18:**1.

Dambacher MD, Binswanger U, Fischer JA: Diagnosis and treatment of primary hyperparathyroidism. *Urol Res* 1979;**7:**171.

Ettinger B, Genant HK, Cann CE: Long-term estrogen replacement therapy prevents bone loss and fractures. *Ann Intern Med* 1985;**102:**319.

Forscher BK, Arnaud CD (editors): The Third F. Raymond Keating, Jr., Memorial Symposium: Parathyroid hormone, calcitonin and vitamin D. *Am J Med* 1974;**56:**743 and **57:**1.

Lei DBM, Zawada ET, Kleeman CR: The pathophysiology and clinical aspects of hypercalcemic disorders. *West J Med* 1978;**129:**278.

Long RG: Hepatic osteodystrophy: Outlook good but some problems unsolved. *Gastroenterology* 1980;**78:**644.

Malluche HH et al: The use of deferoxamine in the management of aluminum accumulation in bone in patients with renal failure. *N Engl J Med* 1984;**311:**140.

Pak CYC (editor): Symposium on urolithiasis. *Kidney Int* 1978;**13:**341.

Riggs BL et al: Changes in bone mineral density of the proximal femur and spine with aging: Differences between the postmenopausal and senile osteoporosis syndromes. *J Clin Invest* 1982;**70:**716.

Riggs BL et al: Effect of the fluoride/calcium regimen on vertebral fracture occurrence in postmenopausal osteoporosis. *N Engl J Med* 1982;**306:**446.

Wallach S: Treatment of Paget's disease. *Adv Intern Med* 1982;**27:**1.

Principles of Antimicrobial Drug Action

42

Ernest Jawetz, MD, PhD

An ideal antimicrobial drug exhibits **selective toxicity.** This term implies that the drug is harmful to a parasite without being harmful to the host. In many instances, selective toxicity is relative rather than absolute, meaning that a drug may damage a parasite in a concentration that can be tolerated by the host.

Selective toxicity may be a function of a specific receptor required for drug attachment, or it may depend on the inhibition of biochemical events that exist in or are essential to the parasite but not the host. For a majority of antimicrobial drugs, the mechanism of action is not completely understood. However, for purposes of discussion, it is convenient to present antimicrobial mechanisms under 4 distinct headings:

(1) Inhibition of cell wall synthesis.

(2) Alteration in the permeability of cell membrane or active transport across cell membrane.

(3) Inhibition of protein synthesis (ie, inhibition of translation and transcription of genetic material).

(4) Inhibition of nucleic acid synthesis.

ANTIMICROBIAL ACTION THROUGH INHIBITION OF CELL WALL SYNTHESIS (Bacitracin, Cephalosporins, Cycloserine, Penicillins, Ristocetin, Vancomycin)

In contrast to animal cells, bacteria possess a rigid outer layer, the cell wall. It maintains the shape of microorganisms and "corsets" the bacterial cell, which possesses an unusually high internal osmotic pressure.

The internal pressure is 3–5 times greater in gram-positive than in gram-negative bacteria. Injury to the cell wall (eg, by lysozyme) or inhibition of its formation may lead to lysis of the cell. In a hypertonic environment (eg, 20% sucrose), damaged cell wall formation leads to formation of spherical bacterial "protoplasts" from gram-positive organisms or "spheroplasts" from gram-negative organisms, which are limited by the fragile cytoplasmic membrane. If such flexible cells are placed in an environment of ordinary tonicity, they take up fluid rapidly and may explode.

The cell wall contains a chemically distinct complex polymer "mucopeptide" ("murein," "peptidoglycan") consisting of polysaccharides and a highly cross-linked polypeptide. The polysaccharides regularly contain the amino sugars N-acetylglucosamine and acetylmuramic acid. The latter is found only in bacteria. To the amino sugars are attached short peptide chains. The final rigidity of the cell wall is imparted by cross-linking of the peptide chains (eg, through pentaglycine bonds) as a result of "transpeptidation" reactions carried out by several enzymes (Fig 42–1). The peptidoglycan layer is much thicker in the cell wall of gram-positive bacteria than in the cell wall of gram-negative bacteria.

All penicillins and all cephalosporins (β-lactam antibiotics) are selective inhibitors of bacterial cell wall synthesis. While this is only one of many different activities of these drugs, it is perhaps the best understood. The initial step in drug action consists of binding of the drug to cell receptors. These "penicillin-binding proteins" (PBP) number 3–6 (MW 40,000–120,000) on many bacteria, and some are transpeptidation enzymes. Different receptors (PBP) may possess different affinity for a drug, and each may mediate a different mode of action. For example, attachment of penicillin to one PBP may result chiefly in abnormal elongation of the cell, whereas attachment to another may lead to a cell wall defect at the periphery with resulting cell lysis. After a β-lactam antibiotic has attached to the receptor, the transpeptidation reaction is inhibited and peptidoglycan synthesis is blocked. The next step probably involves the removal or inactivation of an inhibitor of autolytic enzymes in the cell wall. This activates the lytic enzyme in some microorganisms and may result in lysis in an isotonic environment. In a hypertonic environment (eg, 20% sucrose), the microbes may change to protoplasts or spheroplasts covered only by the fragile cell membrane. In such cells, synthesis of proteins and nucleic acids may continue for some time.

Inhibition of the transpeptidation enzymes by the penicillins and cephalosporins may be due to a structural similarity of these drugs to acyl-D-alanyl-D-alanine. The transpeptidation reaction involves the loss of a D-alanine from the pentapeptide (Fig 42–1).

The remarkable lack of toxicity of β-lactam antibiotics to mammalian cells must be attributed to the absence of a bacterial type cell wall, with its peptidoglycan, in animal cells. The differences in susceptibility of gram-positive and gram-negative bacteria to various penicillins or cephalosporins probably depends on structural differences in their cell walls (eg, amount of peptidoglycan, presence of receptors and lipids, na-

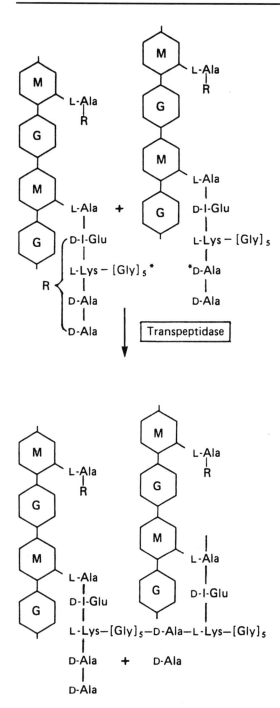

Figure 42–1. The transpeptidation reaction in *Staphylococcus aureus* that is inhibited by β-lactam antibiotics. The cell wall of gram-positive bacteria is made up of long peptidoglycan polymer chains consisting of the alternating aminohexoses N-acetylglucosamine (G) and N-acetylmuramic acid (M) with pentapeptide side chains linked (in *S aureus*) by pentaglycine bridges. The exact composition of the side chains varies between species. The diagram illustrates small segments of 2 such polymer chains and their amino acid side chains. These linear polymers must be cross-linked by transpeptidation of the side chains at the points indicated by asterisks to achieve the strength necessary for cell viability. D-I-Glu, D-isoglutamine.

ture of cross-linking, activity of autolytic enzymes) that determine penetration, binding, and activity of the drugs.

Susceptibility of bacteria to β-lactam antibiotics depends on various structural and functional characteristics. In order to reach receptors, the drugs must permeate the outer layers of the cell envelope. In gram-negative bacteria, there is an outer phospholipid membrane that may hinder passage of these drugs. Hydrophilic molecules (eg, ampicillin, amoxicillin) may pass more readily than penicillin G. In gram-positive bacteria, the phospholipid membrane is lacking and its barrier function is absent.

The number and type of receptor proteins (PBP) vary in different species. They are under chromosomal control, and mutation may alter their number or their affinity for β-lactam drugs.

Amdinocillin is an amidinopenicillanic acid derivative that binds *only* to PBP 2 and is more active against gram-negative than against gram-positive bacteria. Amdinocillin can act synergistically with other β-lactam drugs that attach to other PBPs.

Some bacteria may be inhibited by β-lactam drugs as peptidoglycan formation is inhibited, but they may fail to lyse. This "tolerance" may be due to a lack of activation of autolytic enzymes (hydrolases) in the cell wall. This in turn may be a function of the presence or absence of precursors or of the nature of the enzyme inhibitor.

The most important clinically encountered mechanism of insusceptibility to β-lactam drugs is the production by the bacteria of β-lactamases. These enzymes break the β-lactam ring and nullify the biologic effect of the drug.

There are many types of β-lactamases, most of them under the genetic control of plasmids. Such gene-bearing plasmids are widespread among staphylococci and enteric gram-negative rods. Some β-lactamases can be firmly bound by compounds such as clavulanic acid and can thus be prevented from attacking hydrolyzable penicillins (eg, amoxicillin). A mixture of amoxicillin and clavulanic acid is used to treat β-lactamase–producing *Haemophilus* sp infections. Certain β-lactam antibiotics are resistant to β-lactamases because their β-lactam ring is protected by steric hindrance by methoxy or other groups (eg, methicillin, cefoxitin). Such antibiotics can attack β-lactamase–producing bacteria, inhibit their transpeptidation, or lyse them. The basis for resistance of some bacteria to the latter type of drug (eg, methicillin-resistant staphylococci) is not well understood. It may depend on varying affinity of receptors for the drug or on the lack of required PBP.

Several other drugs, including bacitracin, vancomycin, and ristocetin, inhibit early steps in the biosynthesis of the peptidoglycan (Fig 42–2). Since the early stages of synthesis take place inside the cytoplasmic membrane, these drugs must penetrate the membrane to be effective. For these drugs, the inhibition of peptidoglycan synthesis is not the sole mode of antibacterial action.

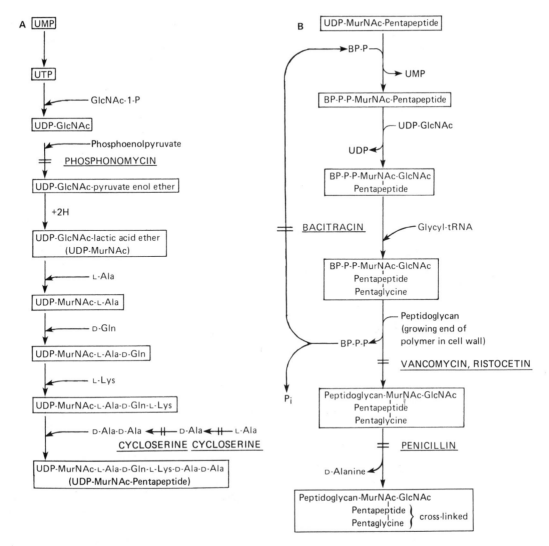

Figure 42–2. The biosynthesis of cell wall peptidoglycan, showing the sites of action of 6 antibiotics. BP, bactoprenol; Mur-NAc, N-acetylmuramic acid; GLcNAc, N-acetylglucosamine. *(A)* Synthesis of UDP–acetylmuramic acid–pentapeptide. *(B)* Synthesis of peptidoglycan from UDP–acetylmuramic acid–pentapeptide, UDP–N-acetylglucosamine, and glycyl residues. (Modified and reproduced, with permission, from Jawetz E et al: *Review of Medical Microbiology,* 17th ed. Lange, 1987.)

Cycloserine, an analog of D-alanine, also interferes with peptidoglycan synthesis. This drug blocks the action of alanine racemase, an essential enzyme in the incorporation of D-alanine in the pentapeptide of peptidoglycan. Phosphonopeptides also inhibit enzymes needed for early steps in the synthesis of peptidoglycans.

ANTIMICROBIAL ACTION THROUGH INHIBITION OF CELL MEMBRANE FUNCTION (Amphotericin B, Colistin, Imidazoles, Nystatin, Polymyxins)

The cytoplasm of all living cells is bounded by the cytoplasmic membrane, which serves as a selective permeability barrier, carries out active transport functions, and thus controls the internal composition of the cell. If the functional integrity of the cytoplasmic membrane is disrupted, macromolecules and ions escape from the cell, and cell damage or death ensues. The cytoplasmic membrane of certain bacteria and fungi can be more readily disrupted by certain agents than can the membranes of animal cells. Consequently, selective chemotherapeutic activity is possible.

Good examples of this mechanism are the polymyxins acting on gram-negative bacteria (polymyxins selectively act on membranes rich in phosphatidyl ethanolamine and act like cationic detergent) and the polyene antibiotics acting on fungi. However, polymyxins are inactive against fungi, and polyenes are inactive against bacteria. This is because ergosterol is present in the fungal cell membrane and absent in the bacterial cell membrane. Polyenes require ergosterol as a receptor in the fungal cell membrane, prior to exerting their effect. Bacterial cell membranes do not contain that sterol and (presumably for this reason) are resistant to polyene action—a good example of cell individuality and of selective toxicity. Fungi that are resistant to polyenes exhibit a decrease in membrane ergosterol or a modification in its structure, so that it combines less well with the drug. The antifungal imidazoles (miconazole, clotrimazole, ketoconazole) impair the integrity of fungal cell membranes by inhibiting the biosynthesis of membrane lipids.

ANTIMICROBIAL ACTION THROUGH INHIBITION OF PROTEIN SYNTHESIS (Chloramphenicol, Erythromycins, Lincomycins, Tetracyclines; Aminoglycosides: Amikacin, Gentamicin, Kanamycin, Neomycin, Streptomycin, Tobramycin, Etc)

It is established that aminoglycosides, tetracyclines, chloramphenicol, erythromycins, and lincomycins can inhibit protein synthesis through an action on ribosomes in bacteria. Puromycin is an inhibitor of protein synthesis in animal and other cells. The concepts of protein synthesis are undergoing rapid change, and the precise mechanism of action is not fully established for these drugs.

Bacteria have 70S ribosomes, whereas mammalian cells have 80S ribosomes. The subunits of each type of ribosome, their chemical composition, and their functional specificities are sufficiently different to explain why antimicrobial drugs can inhibit protein synthesis in bacterial ribosomes without having a major effect on mammalian ribosomes.

In normal microbial protein synthesis, the mRNA message is simultaneously "read" by several ribosomes that are strung out along the mRNA strand. These are called polysomes.

Aminoglycosides

The mode of action of streptomycin has been studied far more than that of other aminoglycosides (kanamycin, neomycin, gentamicin, tobramycin, amikacin, etc), but probably all act similarly. The first step is the attachment of the aminoglycoside to a specific receptor protein (P 12 in the case of streptomycin) on the 30S subunit of the microbial 70S ribosome. Second, the aminoglycoside blocks the normal activity of the "initiation complex" of peptide formation (mRNA + formyl methionine + tRNA). Third, the mRNA message is misread on the "recognition region" of the ribosome, and, as a result, the wrong amino acid is inserted into the peptide, resulting in a nonfunctional protein. Fourth, aminoglycoside attach-

ment results in the breakup of polysomes and their separation into "monosomes" incapable of protein synthesis. These activities occur more or less simultaneously, and the overall effect is usually an irreversible event—killing of the cell.

Chromosomal resistance of microbes to aminoglycosides depends principally on the lack of a specific protein receptor on the 30S subunit of the ribosome. Plasmid-dependent resistance to aminoglycosides depends on the production by the microorganism of adenylylating, phosphorylating, or acetylating enzymes that destroy the drugs. A third type of resistance consists of a "permeability defect," an outer membrane change that reduces active transport of the aminoglycoside into the cell with the result that the drug cannot reach the ribosome. This is—at least sometimes—plasmid-mediated. The active transport of aminoglycosides into the cell is an energy-dependent, oxygen-dependent process. Therefore, strict anaerobes are relatively insusceptible to aminoglycosides.

Tetracyclines

Tetracyclines bind to the 30S subunit of microbial ribosomes. They inhibit protein synthesis by blocking the attachment of charged aminoacyl-tRNA. Thus, they prevent introduction of new amino acids into the nascent peptide chain. The action is usually bacteriostatic and reversible upon withdrawal of the drug. Resistance to tetracyclines results from changes in permeability of the microbial cell envelope. In susceptible cells, the drug is concentrated from the environment by an energy-dependent process of active transport and does not readily leave the cell. In resistant cells, the drug either is not actively transported into the cell or leaves it so rapidly that inhibitory concentrations are not maintained. This is often plasmid-controlled. Mammalian cells do not actively concentrate tetracyclines.

Chloramphenicol

Chloramphenicol attaches to the 50S subunit of the ribosome. It interferes with the binding of new amino acids to the nascent peptide chain, largely because chloramphenicol inhibits peptidyl transferase. Chloramphenicol is mainly bacteriostatic, and growth of microorganisms resumes (ie, drug action is reversible) when the drug is withdrawn. Microorganisms resistant to chloramphenicol produce the enzyme chloramphenicol acetyl transferase, which destroys drug activity. The production of this enzyme is usually under control of a plasmid.

Macrolides (Erythromycins)

These drugs bind to the 50S subunit of the ribosome and can compete with lincomycins for binding sites (a 23S rRNA). Macrolides may interfere with formation of initiation complexes for peptide chain synthesis or may interfere with aminoacyl translocation reactions. Some macrolide-resistant bacteria lack the proper receptor on the ribosome (through methylation of the rRNA); this may be under plasmid or chromosomal control.

Lincomycins (Clindamycin)

Lincomycins bind to the 50S subunit of the microbial ribosome and resemble macrolides in binding site, antibacterial activity, and mode of action. There may be mutual interference between these drugs, presumably because they share the same receptor. Chromosomal mutants are resistant by virtue of lacking the proper binding site on the 50S subunit.

ANTIMICROBIAL ACTION THROUGH INHIBITION OF NUCLEIC ACID SYNTHESIS (Nalidixic Acid, Novobiocin, Pyrimethamine, Rifampin, Sulfonamides, Trimethoprim)

Drugs such as the actinomycins are effective inhibitors of DNA synthesis. Actually, they form complexes with DNA by binding to the deoxyguanosine residues. The DNA-actinomycin complex inhibits the DNA-dependent RNA polymerase and blocks mRNA formation. Actinomycin also inhibits DNA virus replication. Mitomycins result in the firm cross-linking of complementary strands of DNA and subsequently block DNA replication. Both actinomycins and mitomycin inhibit bacterial as well as animal cells but are not sufficiently selective to be employed in antibacterial chemotherapy.

Rifampin inhibits bacterial growth by binding strongly to the DNA-dependent RNA polymerase of bacteria. Thus, it inhibits bacterial RNA synthesis. Rifampin resistance develops as a chromosomal mutation of high frequency that results in a change in RNA polymerase.

Nalidixic acid and oxolinic acid, used mainly as urinary antiseptics, are potent inhibitors of DNA synthesis. They block DNA gyrase action. However, it is not known whether their antibacterial action depends solely on this effect.

For many microorganisms, p-aminobenzoic acid (PABA) is an essential metabolite. It is used by them as a precursor in the synthesis of folic acid in the pathway leading to the synthesis of nucleic acids. The specific mode of action of PABA probably involves an adenosine triphosphate (ATP)–dependent condensation of a pteridine with PABA to yield dihydropteroic acid, which is subsequently converted to folic acid. Sulfonamides are structural analogs of PABA and inhibit dihydropteroate synthetase.

Sulfonamides can enter into the reaction in place of PABA and compete for the active center of the enzyme. As a result, nonfunctional analogs of folic acid are formed, preventing further growth of the bacterial cell. The inhibiting action of sulfonamides on bacterial growth can be counteracted by an excess of PABA in the environment (competitive inhibition). Animal cells cannot synthesize folic acid and must depend upon exogenous sources. Some bacteria, like animal cells, are not inhibited by sulfonamides. Many other bacteria, however, synthesize folic acid as mentioned above and consequently are susceptible to inhibition by sulfonamides.

Tubercle bacilli are not inhibited markedly by sulfonamides, but their growth is inhibited by PAS (p-aminosalicylic acid). Conversely, most sulfonamide-susceptible bacteria are resistant to PAS. This suggests that the receptor site for PABA differs in different types of organisms.

Trimethoprim (3,4,5-trimethoxybenzyl pyrimidine) inhibits the dihydrofolic acid reductase of bacteria 50,000 times more efficiently than the same enzyme of mammalian cells. This enzyme reduces dihydrofolic to tetrahydrofolic acid, a stage in the sequence leading to the synthesis of purines and ultimately of DNA. Sulfonamides and trimethoprim produce sequential blocking of this pathway, resulting in marked enhancement (synergism) of activity. Such sulfonamide (5 parts) + trimethoprim (1 part) mixtures have been used in a variety of parasitic (eg, malaria, *Pneumocystis*) and bacterial (eg, *Shigella*, *Salmonella*, coliform) infections.

Pyrimethamine (Daraprim) also inhibits dihydrofolate reductase, but it is more active against the mammalian cell enzyme and therefore more toxic than trimethoprim. Pyrimethamine plus sulfonamides is the current treatment of choice in toxoplasmosis and some other protozoal infections.

Many different chemicals that can interfere with the synthesis of viral nucleic acids have been employed for chemoprophylaxis and chemotherapy of viral infections. These are discussed in some detail in Chapter 49, and their mechanism of action is presented there.

RESISTANCE TO ANTIMICROBIAL DRUGS

There are many different mechanisms by which microorganisms might exhibit resistance to drugs. The following are fairly well supported by evidence:

(1) Microorganisms produce enzymes that destroy the active drug. *Examples:* Staphylococci resistant to penicillin G produce a β-lactamase that destroys the drug. Other β-lactamases are produced by gram-negative rods. Gram-negative bacteria resistant to aminoglycosides (usually mediated by a plasmid) produce adenylylating, phosphorylating, or acetylating enzymes that destroy the drug. Gram-negative bacteria may be resistant to chloramphenicol if they produce a chloramphenicol acetyl transferase.

(2) Microorganisms change their permeability to the drug. *Examples:* Tetracyclines accumulate in susceptible bacteria through active transport through the cell membrane. Resistant bacteria lack this mechanism. Resistance to polymyxins is probably associated with a change in permeability to the drugs. Streptococci have a natural permeability barrier to aminogly-

cosides. This can be partly overcome by the simultaneous presence of a cell wall–active drug, eg, a penicillin. Resistance to amikacin and some other aminoglycosides may depend on a lack of permeability to the drugs, apparently due to an outer membrane change that impairs active transport into the cell.

(3) Microorganisms develop an altered structural target for the drug (see also ¶ [5]). *Examples:* Chromosomal resistance to aminoglycosides is associated with the loss (or alteration) of a specific protein on the 30S subunit of the bacterial ribosome that serves as a receptor in susceptible organisms. Erythromycin-resistant organisms have an altered receptor site on the 50S subunit of the bacterial ribosome, resulting from methylation of a 23S ribosomal RNA. Resistance to some penicillins may be a function of the loss or alteration of PBP.

(4) Microorganisms develop an altered metabolic pathway that bypasses the reaction inhibited by the drug. *Example:* Some sulfonamide-resistant bacteria do not require extracellular PABA but, like mammalian cells, can utilize preformed folic acid.

(5) Microorganisms develop an altered enzyme that can still perform its metabolic function but is much less affected by the drug than the enzyme in the susceptible organism. *Example:* In some sulfonamide-susceptible bacteria, dihydropteroate synthetase has a much higher affinity for sulfonamide than for PABA. In sulfonamide-resistant mutants, the opposite is the case.

Origin of Drug Resistance

The origin of drug resistance may be genetic or nongenetic.

A. Nongenetic Origin: Active replication of bacteria is usually required for most antibacterial drug actions. Consequently, microorganisms that are metabolically inactive (nonmultiplying) may be resistant to drugs. However, their offspring are fully susceptible. *Example:* Mycobacteria often survive in tissues for many years after infection yet are restrained by the host's defenses and do not multiply. Such "persisting" organisms are resistant to treatment and cannot be eradicated by drugs. However, if they start to multiply (eg, following corticosteroid treatment of the patient), they are fully susceptible to the same drug.

Microorganisms may lose the specific target structure for a drug for several generations and thus be resistant. *Example:* Penicillin-susceptible organisms may change to L forms (protoplasts) during penicillin administration. Lacking most cell wall, they are then resistant to cell wall–inhibitor drugs (penicillins, cephalosporins) and may remain so for several generations as "persisters." When these organisms revert to their bacterial parent forms by resuming cell wall production, they are again fully susceptible to penicillin.

B. Genetic Origin: The vast majority of drug-resistant microbes have emerged as a result of genetic changes and subsequent selection processes. Genetic changes may be chromosomal or extrachromosomal.

Bacteria contain chromosomes made of a double-stranded circular molecule of DNA. These chromosomes are supercoiled and folded within the cell to allow for orderly segregation into the daughter cells. Bacterial chromosomes replicate semiconservatively and sequentially. In some bacteria, replication is known to proceed bidirectionally.

1. Chromosomal resistance–This develops as a result of spontaneous mutation in a locus that controls susceptibility to a given antimicrobial. The presence of the drug serves as a selecting mechanism to suppress susceptibles and promote the growth of drug-resistant mutants. Spontaneous mutation occurs with a frequency of 10^{-12} to 10^{-7} and thus is an infrequent cause for the emergence of clinical drug resistance within a given patient. However, chromosomal mutants for resistance to rifampin occur in many bacteria with a high frequency (10^{-7}–10^{-5}). Consequently, treatment of bacterial infections with rifampin as the sole drug generally fails.

Chromosomal mutants are commonly resistant by virtue of a change in a structural receptor for a drug. Thus, the P 12 protein on the 30S subunit of the bacterial ribosome serves as a receptor for streptomycin attachment. Mutation in the gene that controls that structural protein results in streptomycin resistance. A narrow region of the bacterial chromosome contains structural genes that code for a number of drug receptors, including those for erythromycin, tetracycline, lincomycin, aminoglycosides, etc. Mutation may also result in a loss of penicillin receptors in some microbial species, making the mutant penicillin-resistant.

2. Extrachromosomal resistance–Bacteria also contain extrachromosomal genetic elements called **plasmids.** Plasmids are circular DNA molecules, have 1–3% of the weight of the bacterial chromosome, may exist free in the bacterial cytoplasm, or may be integrated into the bacterial chromosome. Some carry their own genes for replication and transfer. Others rely on genes in other plasmids.

R factors are a class of plasmids that carry genes for resistance to one—and often several—antimicrobial drugs and heavy metals. Plasmid genes for antimicrobial resistance often control the formation of enzymes capable of destroying antimicrobial drugs. Thus, plasmids determine resistance to penicillins and cephalosporins by carrying genes for the formation of β-lactamases. Plasmids code for enzymes that destroy chloramphenicol (acetyl transferase); enzymes that acetylate, adenylylate, or phosphorylate various aminoglycosides; enzymes that determine the permeability of the cell envelope to tetracyclines; and others.

Genetic material and plasmids can be transferred by the following mechanisms:

a. Transduction–Plasmid DNA is enclosed in a bacterial virus and transferred by the virus to another bacterium of the same species. *Example:* The plasmid carrying the gene for β-lactamase production can be transferred from a penicillin-resistant to a susceptible staphylococcus if carried by a suitable bacteriophage. Similar transduction occurs in salmonellae.

b. Transformation–Naked DNA passes from one cell of a species to another cell, thus altering the genotype of the latter. This can occur through laboratory manipulation, such as in recombinant DNA technology, and perhaps spontaneously.

c. Bacterial conjugation–A unilateral transfer of genetic material between bacteria of the same or different genera occurs during a mating (conjugation) process. This is mediated by a fertility (F) factor that results in the extension of sex pili from the donor (F^+) cell to the recipient. Plasmid or other DNA is transferred through these protein tubules from the donor to the recipient cell. A series of closely linked genes, each determining resistance to one drug, may thus be transferred from a resistant to a susceptible bacterium. Such a resistance transfer factor (RTF) is the commonest method of spread of multidrug resistance among various genera of gram-negative bacteria and also among some gram-positive cocci.

d. Translocation or transposition–An exchange of short DNA sequences (transposons) occurs between one plasmid and another or between a plasmid and a portion of the bacterial chromosome within a bacterial cell.

Cross-Resistance

Microorganisms resistant to a certain drug may also be resistant to other drugs that share a mechanism of action or attachment. Such relationships exist mainly between agents that are closely related chemically (eg, polymyxin B–colistin; erythromycin-oleandomycin; neomycin-kanamycin), but they may also exist between unrelated chemicals (erythromycin-lincomycin). In certain classes of drugs, the active nucleus of the chemical is so similar among many congeners (eg, tetracyclines) that full cross-resistance is to be expected.

REFERENCES

Beeuwkes H, Rutgers VH: A combination of amoxicillin and clavulanic acid in the treatment of respiratory tract infections caused by amoxicillin-resistant *Haemophilus influenzae*. *Infection* 1981;**9**:244.

Buchanan CE, Strominger JL: Altered penicillin-binding components in penicillin-resistant mutants of *Bacillus subtilis*. *Proc Natl Acad Sci USA* 1976;**73**:1816.

Datta N (editor): Antibiotic resistance in bacteria. *Br Med Bull* 1984;**40**:1.

Falkow S: *Infectious Multiple Drug Resistance*. Pion Ltd, 1975.

Finland M: Emergence of antibiotic resistance in hospitals 1935–75. *Rev Infect Dis* 1979;**1**:4.

Gale EF et al: *The Molecular Basis of Antibiotic Action*, 2nd ed. Wiley, 1981.

Jacobs MR et al: Emergence of multiply resistant pneumococci. *N Engl J Med* 1978;**299**:735.

Jawetz E: Antimicrobial drugs: Mechanisms and factors influencing their action. Chap 1, pp 3–10, in: *Antimicrobial Therapy*, 3rd ed. Kagan BM (editor). Saunders, 1980.

Mandell GL, Douglas RG, Bennett JE (editors): *Principles and Practice of Infectious Diseases*, 2nd ed. Wiley, 1985.

McDonnell RW et al: Conjugational transfer of gentamicin resistance plasmids intra- and interspecifically in *Staphylococcus aureus* and *Staphylococcus epidermidis*. *Antimicrob Agents Chemother* 1983;**23**:151.

Moellering RC Jr, Nelson JD, Neu HC (editors): An international review of amdinocillin. (Symposium.) *Am J Med* 1983;**75**:1.

Neu HC: Changing mechanisms of bacterial resistance. *Am J Med* 1984;**77**:11.

Reynolds PE: Resistance of the antibiotic target site. *Br Med Bull* 1984;**40**:3.

Sanders CC, Sanders WE: Microbial resistance to newer generation β-lactam antibiotics. *J Infect Dis* 1985;**151**:399.

Tipper DJ: Mode of action of beta-lactam antibiotics. *Rev Infect Dis* 1979;**1**:39.

Tomasz A: From penicillin-binding proteins to the lysis and death of bacteria: A 1979 view. *Rev Infect Dis* 1979;**1**:434.

Zighelboim S, Tomasz A: Multiple antibiotic resistance in South African strains of *Streptococcus pneumoniae:* Mechanism of resistance to bɛ a lactam antibiotics. *Rev Infect Dis* 1981; **3**:267.

43

Penicillins & Cephalosporins

Ernest Jawetz, MD, PhD

PENICILLINS

In 1929, Fleming reported his observation that colonies of staphylococci lysed on a plate that had become contaminated with a *Penicillium* mold. His efforts to extract the bacteriolytic substance failed, but in 1940 Chain, Florey, and their associates succeeded in producing significant quantities of the first penicillins from cultures of *Penicillium notatum*. Fermentation methods improved rapidly, so that by 1949 virtually unlimited quantities of penicillin were available for clinical use. Of the several fermentation products, penicillin G proved to be the best.

The 2 principal limitations of penicillin G were its susceptibility to destruction by β-lactamase (penicillinase) and its relative inactivity against most gram-negative bacteria. A research assault on these problems organized by Chain, Rolinson, and Batchelor led, in 1957, to the isolation of 6-aminopenicillanic acid in bulk amounts. Thus began the development of a long series of semisynthetic penicillins. This resulted in the selective design of drugs resistant to β-lactamase, stable to acid pH, and active against both gram-positive and gram-negative bacteria.

Penicillins and cephalosporins are large groups of drugs that share features of chemistry, mechanism of action, pharmacologic and clinical effects, and immunologic characteristics. These drugs are referred to as β-lactam drugs or cell wall inhibitors.

Chemistry

All penicillins share the basic structure shown in Fig 43–1 (top). There is a thiazolidine ring (A) attached to a β-lactam ring (B) that carries a secondary amino group (R–NH–). Acidic radicals (R, shown in Fig 43–2) can be attached to the amino group and can be separated from the amino group by bacterial and other amidases. Similar basic structures incorporating the β-lactam ring provide the cephalosporin and monobactam families, as shown in Fig 43–1. The structural integrity of the 6-aminopenicillanic acid nucleus is essential to the biologic activity of the molecules. If the β-lactam ring is enzymatically cleaved by bacterial β-lactamases (penicillinases), the resulting product, penicilloic acid, is devoid of antibacterial activity. However, it carries an antigenic determinant of the penicillins, acts as a sensitizing structure when attached to host proteins, and can be used as

skin testing material when attached to peptide chains. Products of alkaline hydrolysis of the penicillins also contribute to sensitization.

The attachment of different radicals (R) to the amino group of 6-aminopenicillanic acid determines the essential pharmacologic properties of the resulting molecules. Clinically important penicillins available in 1986 fall into several groups: (1) Highest activity against gram-positive organisms but susceptible to hydrolysis by β-lactamases, eg, penicillin G. (2) Relatively resistant to staphylococcal β-lactamases but of lower activity against gram-positive organisms and inactive against gram-negatives, eg, nafcillin, methicillin. (3) Relatively high activity against both gram-negative and gram-positive organisms but destroyed by β-lactamases, eg, carbenicillin, ticarcillin (*extended-spectrum* agents). (4) Relatively stable to gastric acid and suitable for oral administration, eg, penicillin V, ampicillin, cloxacillin.

Some representatives of each group are shown in Fig 43–2, with a few distinguishing characteristics. Amdinocillin (mecillinam) is an amidinopenicillanic acid derivative that binds only to penicillin-binding protein (PBP) 2 (below) and is more active against gram-negative than against gram-positive bacteria. Its antibacterial mechanism is different from that of β-lactam drugs. It may act synergistically with them.

Most penicillins are dispensed as the sodium or potassium salt of the free acid. Potassium penicillin G contains about 1.7 meq of K^+ per million units of penicillin (2.8 meq/g). Nafcillin contains Na^+, 2.8 meq/g. Procaine salts (procaine penicillin) and benzathine salts (benzathine penicillin; Bicillin) are employed to provide repository forms for intramuscular injection.

In dry crystalline form, penicillin salts are stable for long periods (eg, for years at 4°C). Solutions lose their activity rapidly (eg, 24 hours at 20°C) and must be prepared fresh for administration.

Antimicrobial Activity of Beta-Lactam Drugs

Beta-lactam agents share general mechanisms of antibacterial action that involve damage to the cell wall of bacteria. These complex mechanisms are incompletely understood and may not be the same for all drugs. Only a simplified outline is presented here. (See also Chapter 42.)

The initial step in penicillin action consists of bind-

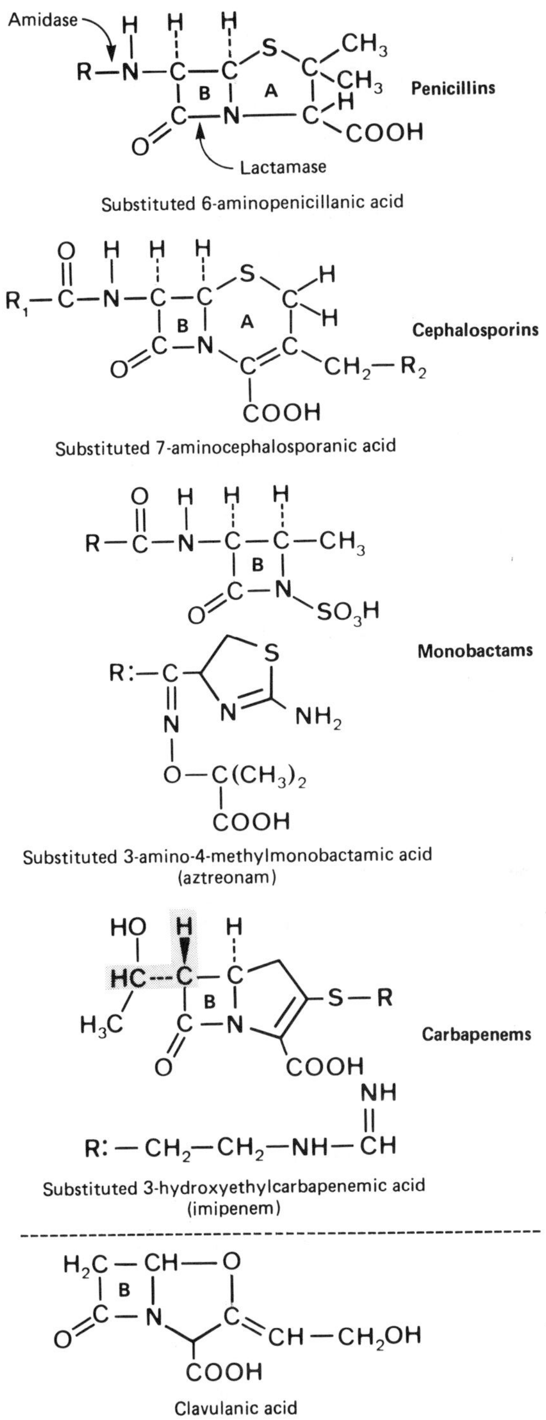

Substituted 6-aminopenicillanic acid

Substituted 7-aminocephalosporanic acid

Substituted 3-amino-4-methylmonobactamic acid
(aztreonam)

Substituted 3-hydroxyethylcarbapenemic acid
(imipenem)

Clavulanic acid

Figure 43–1. Core structures of 4 β-lactam antibiotic families and of clavulanic acid. The ring marked B in each structure is the β-lactam ring. The penicillins are susceptible to bacterial metabolism and inactivation by amidases and lactamases at the points shown. Note that the carbapenems have a different stereochemical configuration in the lactam ring (shaded bonds) that apparently imparts resistance to β-lactamases. Substituents for the penicillin and cephalosporin families are shown in Figs 43–2 and 43–3, respectively.

ing of the drug to cell receptors. These penicillin-binding proteins (PBP) are 3–6 in number, and some of them are transpeptidation enzymes. Different receptors have different affinities for a given drug, and each may mediate a different effect, eg, abnormal cell elongation versus cell wall defect in the periphery. After attachment, the penicillins and cephalosporins inhibit the activity of various transpeptidation enzymes, and transpeptidation reactions are blocked. As a result, the synthesis of cell wall peptidoglycan remains incomplete. The next step in the action of these drugs probably involves removal or inactivation of an inhibitor of autolytic enzymes in the cell wall. This activates the lytic enzymes and may result in lysis of the organism if the environment is isotonic. In a markedly hypertonic environment (eg, 20% sucrose), the cells change to protoplasts or spheroplasts, covered only by the fragile cell membrane. In such forms, the synthesis of proteins and nucleic acids may continue for some time.

Penicillins and cephalosporins can be bactericidal only if active peptidoglycan synthesis takes place. Metabolically inactive cells are unaffected.

Different penicillins possess different quantitative activity against certain organisms. Whereas 0.002–0.5 μg/mL of penicillin G is lethal for a majority of susceptible gram-positive bacteria, nafcillin and other β-lactamase–resistant penicillins are 10–100 times less active against the same organisms. While ampicillin, 0.01–0.5 μg/mL, is active against most organisms susceptible to penicillin G, it is also active against gram-negative non–β-lactamase–producing organisms in similar concentrations. The susceptibility of microorganisms is in part a function of the genus and in part a characteristic of individual strains. The difference in susceptibility of gram-positive and gram-negative organisms must depend in part on the frequency and avidity of drug receptors; on the relative amount of peptidoglycan present (gram-positive organisms usually possess far more); on the amount of lipids in the cell wall; and on other chemical differences that determine binding, penetration, and resistance to lysis or rupture. The gram-negative neisseriae are as susceptible to penicillin G as many gram-positive organisms.

The activity of penicillin G was originally defined in units. Crystalline sodium penicillin G contains approximately 1600 units/mg (1 unit = 0.6 μg; 1 million units of penicillin = 0.6 g). Most semisynthetic penicillins are prescribed by weight rather than units.

Resistance

Resistance to penicillins falls into several distinct categories.

A. Certain bacteria (eg, many *Staphylococcus aureus*, some *Haemophilus influenzae* and gonococci, most gram-negative enteric rods) produce β-lactamases (penicillinases), enzymes that inactivate some penicillins by breaking the β-lactam ring. The genetic control of β-lactamase production—there are about 50 different such enzymes—resides in transmissible plas-

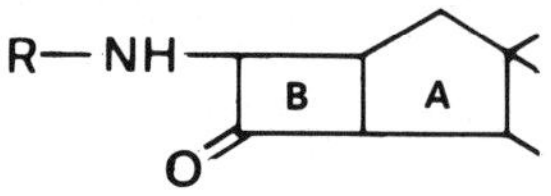

6-Aminopenicillanic acid nucleus, simplified from Fig 43–1. The following structures can each be substituted at R to produce a new penicillin.

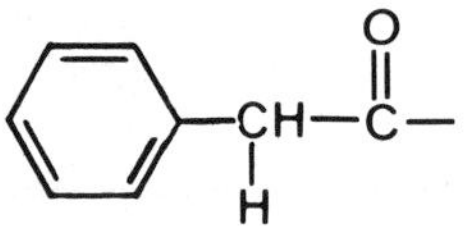

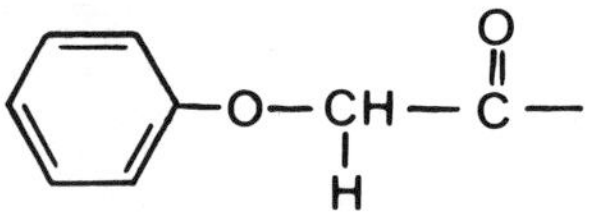

Penicillin V (phenoxymethylpenicillin):
Similar to penicillin G but relatively acid-resistant and can be taken orally.

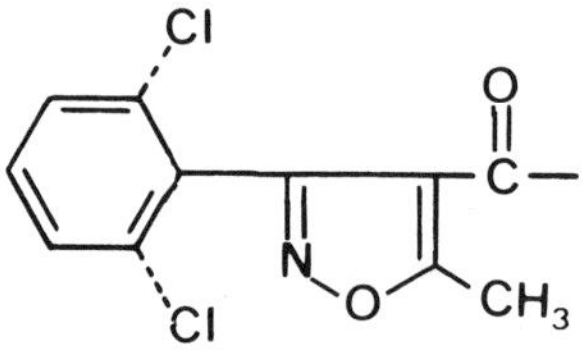

Penicillin G (benzylpenicillin):
High activity against gram-positive bacteria. Low activity against gram-negative bacteria. Acid-labile. Destroyed by β-lactamase. 60% protein-bound.

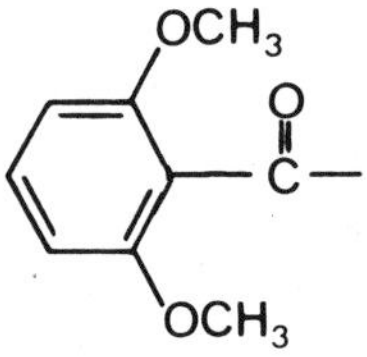

Oxacillin (no Cl atoms); cloxacillin (one Cl in structure); dicloxacillin (2 Cls in structure); flucloxacillin (one Cl and one F in structure) (isoxazolyl penicillins):
Similar to methicillin in β-lactamase resistance, but acid-stable. Can be taken orally. Highly protein-bound (95–98%).

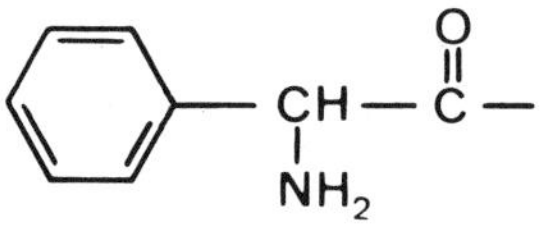

Methicillin (dimethoxyphenylpenicillin):
Lower activity than penicillin G but resistant to β-lactamase. Acid-labile. 40% protein-bound.

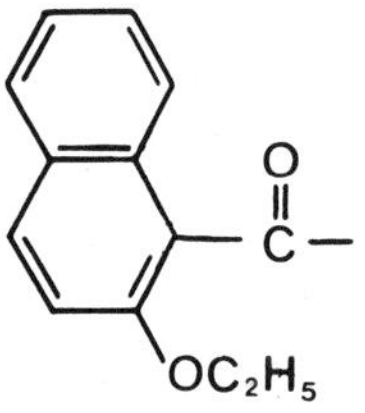

Ampicillin (alpha-aminobenzylpenicillin):
Similar to penicillin G (destroyed by β-lactamase) but acid-stable and more active against gram-negative bacteria. Carbenicillin has —COONa instead of —NH$_2$ group.

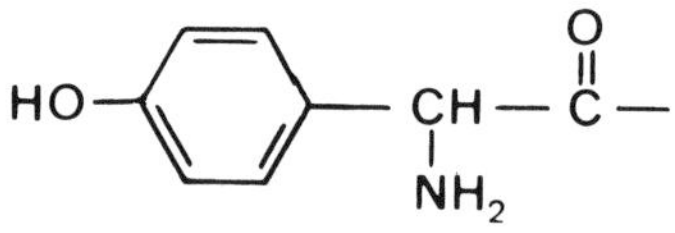

Nafcillin (ethoxynaphthamidopenicillin):
Similar to isoxazolyl penicillins. Less strongly protein-bound (90%). Can be given by mouth or by vein. Resistant to staphylococcal β-lactamase.

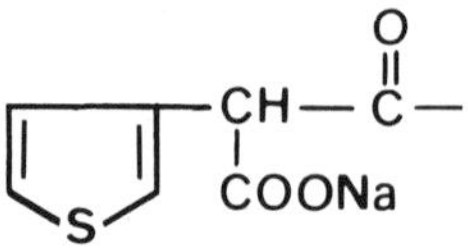

Amoxicillin:
Similar to ampicillin but better absorbed, gives higher blood levels.

Ticarcillin
Similar to carbenicillin but gives higher blood levels. Piperacillin, azlocillin, and mezlocillin resemble ticarcillin in action against gram-negative aerobes.

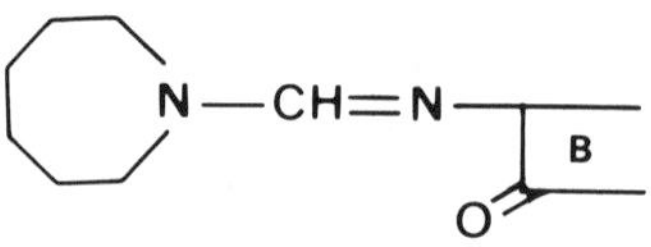

Amdinocillin:
An *amidino* substituent, not amino. Enhanced activity against gram-negative organisms.

Figure 43–2. Structures of some penicillins.

mids (see Chapter 42). Other penicillins (eg, nafcillin) and cephalosporins are β-lactamase–resistant because the β-lactam ring is protected by parts of the R side chain. Such penicillins are active against β-lactamase–producing organisms.

B. Other bacteria do not produce β-lactamases but are resistant to the action of penicillins either because they lack specific receptors or because of lack of permeability of outer layers, so that the drug cannot reach the receptors.

C. Some bacteria may be insusceptible to the killing action of penicillins because the autolytic enzymes in the cell wall are not activated. Such "tolerant" organisms (eg, certain staphylococci, streptococci, *Listeria*) are inhibited but not killed.

D. Organisms that lack cell walls (*Mycoplasma*, L forms) or are metabolically inactive are insusceptible to penicillins and other cell wall inhibitors because they do not synthesize peptidoglycans.

E. Some bacteria (eg, *Staphylococcus* sp) may be resistant to the action of β-lactamase-resistant penicillins, eg, methicillin. The mechanism of this resistance appears to depend on a deficiency or inaccessibility of PBP receptors; it is independent of any β-lactamase production, and its frequency varies greatly with time and place.

Absorption, Metabolism, & Excretion

After parenteral administration, absorption of most penicillins is complete and rapid. Because of the irritation and consequent local pain produced by the intramuscular injection of large doses, administration by the intravenous route (intermittent bolus addition to a continuous drip) is often preferred. After oral administration, absorption differs greatly for different penicillins, depending in part on their acid stability and protein binding. In order to minimize binding to foods, oral penicillins should not be preceded or followed by food for at least 1 hour.

After absorption, penicillins are widely distributed in body fluids and tissues. Penicillins are lipid-insoluble and do not enter living cells well. With parenteral doses of 3–6 g (5–10 million units) of penicillin G, injected in divided doses into a continuous infusion or by intramuscular injections, average serum levels of the drug reach 1–10 units (0.6–6 μg)/mL. A rough relationship of 6 g given parenterally per day yielding serum levels of 1–6 μg/mL also applies to other penicillins. Highly protein-bound penicillins (eg, oxacillin, dicloxacillin) tend to produce lower levels of free drug in serum than less protein-bound penicillins (eg, penicillin G, ampicillin). However, the relevance of protein binding to clinical efficacy of drug is not fully understood.

Special dosage forms of penicillin have been designed for delayed absorption to yield low blood and tissue levels for long periods. The outstanding example is benzathine penicillin G. After a single intramuscular injection of 0.75 g (1.2 million units), serum levels in excess of 0.03 unit/mL are maintained for

10 days and levels in excess of 0.005 unit/mL for 3 weeks. The latter is sufficient to protect against β-hemolytic streptococcal infection; the former to treat an established infection with these organisms. Procaine penicillin also has delayed absorption, yielding useful levels for 24 hours after a single intramuscular injection.

In many tissues, penicillin concentrations are equal to those in serum. Lower levels are found in the eye, the prostate, and the central nervous system. However, with active inflammation of the meninges, as in bacterial meningitis, penicillin levels in the cerebrospinal fluid exceed 0.2 μg/mL with a daily parenteral dose of 12 g. Thus, pneumococcal and meningococcal meningitis may be treated with systemic penicillin and there is no need for intrathecal injection. It is probable that high levels of penicillins in the cerebrospinal fluid in meningitis are due to (1) increased permeability of meninges, (2) inhibition of the normal active transport of penicillin out of the cerebrospinal fluid, or (3) some binding of penicillin to cerebrospinal fluid proteins. Absorbed penicillins also reach pleural, pericardial, and joint fluids well, so that local injection is rarely warranted.

Most of the absorbed penicillin is rapidly excreted by the kidneys into the urine; small amounts are excreted by other channels. About 10% of renal excretion is by glomerular filtration and 90% by tubular secretion, to a maximum of about 2 g/h in an adult. The normal half-life of penicillin G is ½–1 hour; in renal failure, it may be up to 10 hours. Ampicillin is secreted more slowly than penicillin G. Nafcillin is excreted 80% into the biliary tract and only 20% by tubular secretion; therefore, it is little affected by renal failure. Tubular secretion can be partially blocked by probenecid (Benemid) to achieve higher systemic and cerebrospinal fluid levels. Because renal clearance is less efficient in the newborn, proportionately smaller doses result in higher systemic levels that are maintained longer than in the adult.

Renal excretion of penicillin results in very high levels in the urine. Thus, systemic daily doses of 6 g of penicillin may yield urine levels of 500–3000 μg/mL—enough to suppress not only gram-positive but also many gram-negative bacteria in the urine (provided they produce little β-lactamase).

Penicillin is also excreted into sputum and milk to levels of 3–15% of those present in the serum. This is the case in both humans and cattle. The presence of penicillin in the milk of cows treated for mastitis presents a problem in human allergy.

Clinical Uses

Penicillins are by far the most widely effective and the most extensively used antibiotics. All oral penicillins should be given at other than mealtimes (1 hour before or 1–2 hours after), to reduce binding and acid inactivation. Oxacillin is most strongly bound to food (ie, protein-bound), dicloxacillin somewhat less so. Blood levels of all penicillins can be raised by simultaneous administration of probenecid, 0.5 g every 6 hours orally (10 mg/kg every 6 hours), which impairs tubular secretion.

A. Penicillin G is the drug of choice for infections caused by pneumococci, streptococci, meningococci, non–β-lactamase–producing staphylococci and gonococci, *Treponema pallidum* and many other spirochetes, *Bacillus anthracis* and other gram-positive rods, clostridia, *Actinomyces, Listeria*, and *Bacteroides* (except *Bacteroides fragilis*). Most of these infections respond to daily doses of penicillin G, 0.6–5 million units (0.36–3 g). Intermittent intramuscular injection is the usual method of administration. Much larger amounts (6–50 g daily) can be given by injection during a 20-minute period every 4–6 hours into an intravenous infusion. Such a procedure is useful in serious or complicated infections due to these organisms. Oral administration of **penicillin V** is indicated only in minor infections—eg, of the respiratory tract or its associated structures, especially in children (pharyngitis, otitis, sinusitis)—in a daily dose of 1–4 g. Oral administration is subject to such variable efficacy that it should not be relied upon in seriously ill patients. Many non–β-lactamase–producing gonococci have developed partial resistance to penicillin, requiring 1–3 units/mL for inhibition. Treatment of such gonorrhea now requires procaine penicillin, 4.8 million units once, with probenecid, 1 g orally. In gonococcal prostatitis, arthritis, salpingitis, or other closed lesions, 10 million units must be given daily for 4–14 days, combined with drainage when needed. When β-lactamase–producing gonococci are present, alternative drugs, eg, spectinomycin, cefoxitin, or tetracycline, must be used.

Penicillin G is inhibitory for enterococci *(Streptococcus faecalis)*, but the simultaneous administration of an aminoglycoside is often necessary for bactericidal effects, eg, in enterococcal endocarditis. In urinary tract infections, large doses of penicillin G (eg, 1–10 million units intramuscularly) may provide sufficiently high levels in the urine to inhibit some gram-negative coliform bacteria and, in particular, *Proteus mirabilis*. However, such treatment is likely to fail in the presence of large numbers of bacteria producing large amounts of β-lactamase.

B. Benzathine penicillin G is a salt of very low water solubility for intramuscular injection that yields low but prolonged drug levels. A single injection of 1.2 million units intramuscularly is satisfactory for treatment of beta-hemolytic streptococcal pharyngitis. A similar injection given intramuscularly once every 3–4 weeks provides satisfactory prophylaxis against reinfection with beta-hemolytic streptococci. Benzathine penicillin G (2.4 million units intramuscularly once a week for 1–3 weeks) is effective in the treatment of early or latent syphilis. This drug should never be given by mouth.

C. Ampicillin, Amoxicillin, Carbenicillin, Ticarcillin, Piperacillin, Mezlocillin, Azlocillin: These drugs differ from penicillin G in having greater activity against gram-negative bacteria. Carbenicillin, ticarcillin, piperacillin, mezlocillin, and azlocillin have good activity against *Pseudomonas* and are often referred to as **extended-spectrum** penicillins, but they are inactivated by β-lactamases.

Ampicillin, 500 mg orally every 6–8 hours, is used to treat common urinary tract infections with gram-negative coliform bacteria or mixed secondary bacterial infections of the respiratory tract (sinusitis, otitis, bronchitis). Ampicillin is also sometimes given for infections in which penicillin G is the drug of choice but oral therapy is preferred (eg, in acute uncomplicated gonorrhea, 3.5 g once, with probenecid). Ampicillin, 300 mg/kg/d intravenously, is a current choice for bacterial meningitis in children, especially if the disease is caused by *H influenzae*. However, in some locations, β-lactamase–producing *H influenzae* are emerging. Therefore, chloramphenicol or cefuroxime must be used.

Ampicillin is ineffective against *Enterobacter, Pseudomonas*, and indole-positive *Proteus* infections. In invasive *Salmonella* infections (eg, typhoid), ampicillin, 6–12 g/d intravenously, can suppress signs and symptoms and eliminate organisms from some carriers. In typhoid and paratyphoid fevers, ampicillin is an alternative to chloramphenicol or trimethoprim-sulfamethoxazole. However, it is not beneficial in noninvasive *Salmonella* gastroenteritis and may even prolong carriage and shedding. An exception may be salmonellosis in severely malnourished children. In enterococcal sepsis or endocarditis, ampicillin may be more active than penicillin G when combined with an aminoglycoside.

Amoxicillin is similar to ampicillin but is somewhat better absorbed from the gut. The same applies to the esters pivampicillin and bacampicillin. These 3 drugs are comparable in spectrum, activity, and side effects to ampicillin but can be given somewhat less frequently (eg, amoxicillin, 500 mg 3 times daily, instead of ampicillin, 500 mg 4 times daily).

Carbenicillin resembles ampicillin but has more activity against *Pseudomonas* and *Proteus* organisms, although *Klebsiella* are usually resistant. In susceptible populations of *Pseudomonas*, resistance to carbenicillin may emerge rapidly. Therefore, in *Pseudomonas* sepsis (eg, burns, immunosuppressed patients), carbenicillin, 12–30 g/d intravenously (300–500 mg/kg/d), is usually combined with an aminoglycoside, eg, gentamicin, 5–7 mg/kg/d intramuscularly, to delay emergence of resistance and perhaps to obtain synergistic effects. Carbenicillin contains Na^+, 4.7 meq/g. Carbenicillin indanyl sodium is acid-stable and can be given orally in urinary tract infections.

Ticarcillin resembles carbenicillin in single and combined activity, but the dose may be lower, eg, 200–300 mg/kg/d intravenously. Hetacillin is converted to ampicillin and should not be used. Piperacillin, mezlocillin, azlocillin, and others resemble ticarcillin and claim special effectiveness against gram-negative aerobic rods, including *Pseudomonas* sp. However, in serious *Pseudomonas* infections, they should probably be used in combination with an aminoglycoside.

Ampicillin, amoxicillin, ticarcillin, and others in this group can be protected from destruction by β-lactamases if they are administered together with lactamase inhibitors such as clavulanic acid or sulbactam. Such mixtures have been employed against lactamase-producing *Haemophilus influenzae* or coliform organisms. The possible advantages of such mixtures over appropriate cephalosporins are not fully evident.

D. Penicillins Resistant to Beta-Lactamases: These are relatively resistant to destruction by staphylococcal β-lactamases. The sole indication for their use is infection by β-lactamase–producing staphylococci.

Oxacillin, cloxacillin, dicloxacillin, or nafcillin, 0.25–0.5 g every 4–6 hours by mouth, is suitable for treatment of mild localized staphylococcal infections (50–100 mg/kg/d for children). All of these drugs are relatively acid-stable and reasonably well absorbed from the gut. They are all highly protein-bound (95–98%). Food interferes with their absorption, and the drugs must be administered 1 hour away from meals.

For serious systemic staphylococcal infections, nafcillin, 8–12 g/d, is administered intravenously, usually by introducing 1–2 g during 20–30 minutes every 2–4 hours into a continuous infusion of 5% dextrose in water. The dose for children is 50–100 mg/kg/d. Methicillin has similar indications, but it appears to be more nephrotoxic than nafcillin and is therefore employed less often.

Adverse Reactions

The penicillins undoubtedly possess less direct toxicity than any other antibiotics. Most of the serious side effects are due to hypersensitivity.

A. Allergy: All penicillins are cross-sensitizing and cross-reacting. Any preparation containing penicillin may induce sensitization, including foods or cosmetics. In general, sensitization occurs in direct proportion to the duration and total dose of penicillin received in the past. The responsible antigenic determinants appear to be degradation products of penicillins, particularly penicilloic acid and products of alkaline hydrolysis bound to host protein. Skin tests with penicilloylpolylysine, with alkaline hydrolysis products, and with undegraded penicillin will identify many hypersensitive individuals. Among positive reactors to skin tests, the incidence of subsequent penicillin reactions is high and is associated with cell-bound IgE antibodies. Although many persons develop IgG antibodies to antigenic determinants of penicillin, the presence of such antibodies does not appear to be correlated with allergic reactivity (except rare hemolytic anemia), and serologic tests have little predictive value. A history of a penicillin reaction in the past is not reliable; about 5–8% of people claim such a history in the USA. However, in such cases, penicillin should be administered with caution or a substitute drug given.

About 10–15% of persons with a past history of a penicillin reaction have an allergic reaction when given penicillin again. Less than 1% of persons who previously received penicillin without incident will have an allergic reaction when given penicillin again. The incidence of allergic reactions in small children is negligible.

Allergic reactions may occur as typical anaphylactic shock (very rare—0.05% of recipients), typical serum sickness type reactions (now rare—urticaria, fever, joint swelling, angioneurotic edema, intense pruritus, and respiratory embarrassment occurring 7–12 days after exposure), and a variety of skin rashes, oral lesions, fever, interstitial nephritis (an autoimmune reaction to a penicillin-protein complex), eosinophilia, hemolytic anemia and other hematologic disturbances, and vasculitis.

At times, individuals known to be hypersensitive to penicillin can tolerate the drug during corticosteroid administration. "Desensitization" with gradually increasing doses of penicillin is rarely indicated. Most patients allergic to penicillins can be treated with alternative drugs. Anaphylactic reactions are less common after oral penicillin administration than after parenteral administration.

B. Toxicity: Since the action of penicillin is directed against a unique bacterial structure, the cell wall, it is virtually without effect on most animal cells. The toxic effects of penicillin G are due to the direct irritation caused by intramuscular or intravenous injection of exceedingly high concentrations (eg, 1 g/mL). Such concentrations may cause local pain, induration, thrombophlebitis, or degeneration of an accidentally injected nerve. All penicillins are irritating to the central nervous system and greatly increase the excitability of neurons. For that reason, no more than 20,000 units can be given intrathecally on any one day, but there is little indication for intrathecal administration at present. In rare cases, a patient receiving high doses (eg, more than 20 million units of penicillin G daily) has exhibited signs of cerebrocortical irritation as a result of the passage of unusually large amounts of penicillin into the central nervous system. With doses of this magnitude, direct cation toxicity (Na^+, K^+) can also occur (see Chemistry, above), particularly in patients with renal failure.

Large doses of penicillins given orally may lead to gastrointestinal upset, particularly nausea, vomiting, and diarrhea. This is more pronounced with the broad-spectrum forms (ampicillin, amoxicillin) than with other penicillins. Oral therapy may also be accompanied by luxuriant overgrowth of staphylococci, *Pseudomonas, Proteus,* or yeasts, which may occasionally cause enteritis. Superinfections in other organ systems may occur with penicillins as with any antibiotic therapy. Methicillin, nafcillin, and other penicillins have occasionally caused granulocytopenia, especially in children. Methicillin causes nephritis more commonly than does nafcillin: The tubular basement membrane protein serves to bind penicillin, and antibody to the carrier-hapten antigen forms a complex, with binding of complement. Carbenicillin can cause hypokalemic alkalosis and transaminase elevation in serum. It can also induce hemostatic defects leading to bleeding tendency. Ampicillin frequently causes skin rashes, some of which are not allergic in nature.

Problems Relating to the Use of the Penicillins

The penicillins are by far the most widely used antibiotics. Several thousand tons of these drugs have been administered to humans during the past 40 years. Therefore, penicillins have been responsible for some of the most drastic consequences of antibiotic misuse.

A significant proportion (perhaps 1–5%) of the population of many countries has become hypersensitive. In many cases, there is no doubt that sensitization has occurred when penicillin was administered without proper indication. It would be desirable to have penicillin-hypersensitive individuals definitely identified, but hypersensitivity may be temporary.

The saturation of certain environments (eg, hospitals) with penicillin has produced a selection pressure against penicillin-sensitive microorganisms and resulted in greater numbers of penicillin-resistant organisms. In the 1950s, hospitals were an important site for the proliferation and selection of β-lactamase–producing staphylococci; subsequently, there were outbreaks of sepsis in newborn nurseries and surgical units. Now β-lactamase–producing staphylococci prevail everywhere; they cause about 80% of community-acquired staphylococcal infections.

The suppression of normal flora creates a partial void that is regularly filled with drug-resistant, prevalent organisms. Penicillins are administered to a high proportion of patients in hospitals. These patients are made selectively susceptible to superinfections with microorganisms derived from the hospital environment (*Proteus, Pseudomonas, Enterobacter, Serratia*, yeasts, staphylococci, etc). Such organisms become established in organ systems where the normal flora has been suppressed (eg, the respiratory tract, gut, skin) and can cause disease processes there.

Plasmids that control β-lactamase production are being distributed with increasing frequency among different genera of microorganisms. *Neisseria gonorrhoea* has recently acquired such plasmids, probably from *Haemophilus* sp. In West Africa and in the Philippines, outbreaks of β-lactamase–producing gonococci are seen. Local endemic foci have also been found in the USA (eg, Los Angeles), presenting problems for their control.

Although pneumococci have long been considered an example of total and regular susceptibility to penicillins, this is no longer entirely true. In New Guinea and South Africa, outbreaks of relatively penicillin-resistant pneumococci have been observed, causing pneumonia and meningitis. The pneumococci do not produce β-lactamase, but up to 6 μg/mL of penicillin G may be necessary to kill them. Such concentrations of penicillin cannot be obtained in the central nervous system, and the mortality rate has consequently been high. Sporadic cases of similar resistance have been observed in the USA.

CEPHALOSPORINS

Fungi of *Cephalosporium* sp yielded several antibiotics that resembled penicillins but were resistant to β-lactamase and were active against both gram-positive and gram-negative bacteria. Methods were eventually developed for the large-scale production of the common nucleus, 7-aminocephalosporanic acid. This made possible the synthesis of many derivatives, the cephalosporins. A bewildering array of semisynthetic cephalosporins has been developed. In addition to the synthetics derived from cephalosporanic acid, the cephamycins (fermentation products of *Streptomyces*) have very similar properties, as do totally synthetic new drugs such as moxalactam.

Chemistry

The nucleus of the cephalosporins, 7-aminocephalosporanic acid, bears a close resemblance to 6-aminopenicillanic acid (Fig 43–1) and also to the nucleus of the cephamycin antibiotics. The intrinsic antimicrobial activity of natural cephalosporins is low, but the attachment of various R_1 and R_2 groups has yielded drugs of good therapeutic activity and low toxicity (Fig 43–3).

The cephalosporins have molecular weights of 400–450. They are soluble in water and relatively stable to pH and temperature changes. They vary in resistance to β-lactamases. The sodium salt of cephalothin contains 2.4 meq Na^+ per gram.

Antimicrobial Activity

The antimicrobial spectrum of cephalosporins varies with "generations" of the drugs. The "first-generation" cephalosporins are highly active against gram-positive organisms (with the exception of enterococci, methicillin-resistant staphylococci, and penicillin-resistant pneumococci) but only moderately active against gram-negative bacteria. The "second-generation" cephalosporins are somewhat more active against gram-negative bacteria and fairly active against gram-positives. The "third-generation" cephalosporins are much more active against gram-negative bacteria, including Enterobacteriaceae and—at times—*Pseudomonas*, but generally much less active against gram-positives. There is much variation between different drugs of the same "generation," especially in their effect on anaerobes and the likelihood of superinfection with gram-positive cocci.

Many cephalosporins are active against coliforms such as *Escherichia coli, Klebsiella*, and some strains of *Proteus* and *Enterobacter*, while *Serratia* and *Pseudomonas* are often insusceptible. Superinfections with enterococci and staphylococci are not rare. A group of the newer drugs (eg, cefotaxime, cefuroxime, ceftazidime, moxalactam, cefoperazone) stand out because they reach therapeutic concentrations in the central nervous system and are often active against hospital-borne enteric gram-negative aerobic bacteria.

The mechanism of action of cephalosporins is analogous to that described for penicillins. The recep-

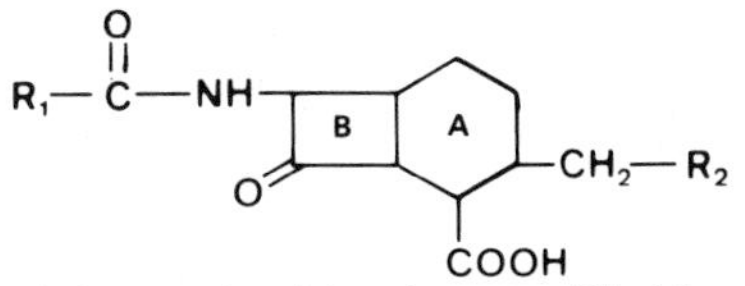

7-Aminocephalosporanic acid nucleus, simplified from Fig 43–1. The following structures can each be substituted at R_1 and R_2 to produce the named derivatives.

R_1		R_2

"First generation"

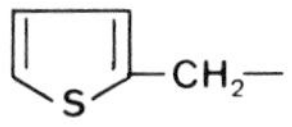

Cephalothin

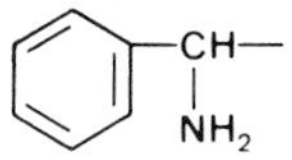

Cephalexin

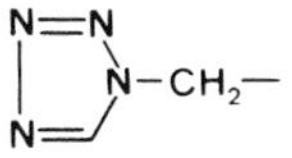

Cefazolin

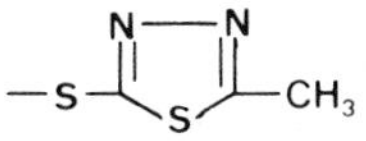

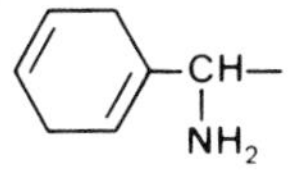

Cephradine

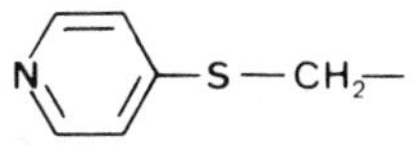

Cephapirin

"Second generation"

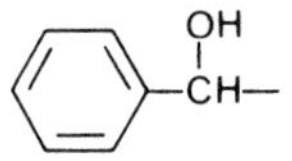

Cefamandole

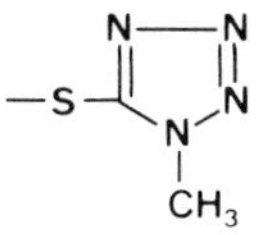

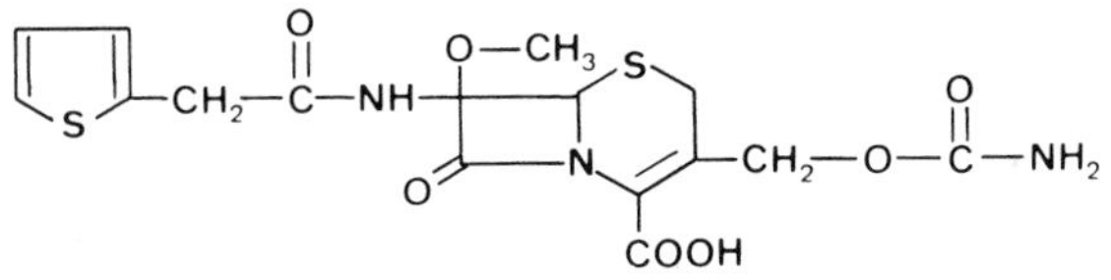

Cefoxitin (a cephamycin)

"Third generation"

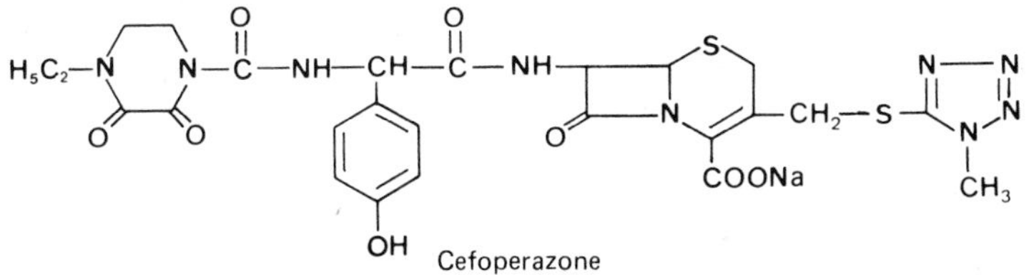

Cefoperazone

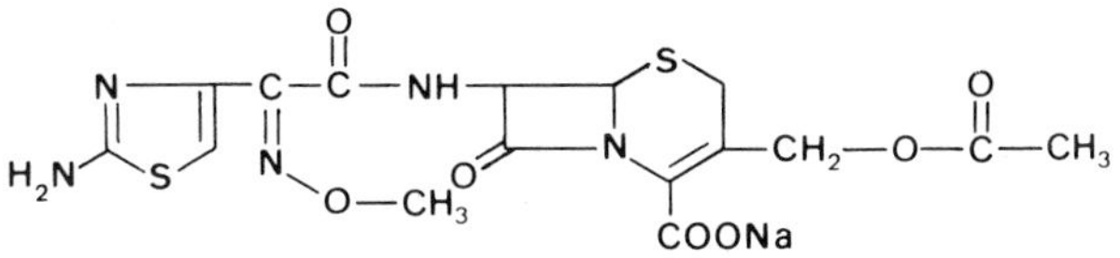

Cefotaxime

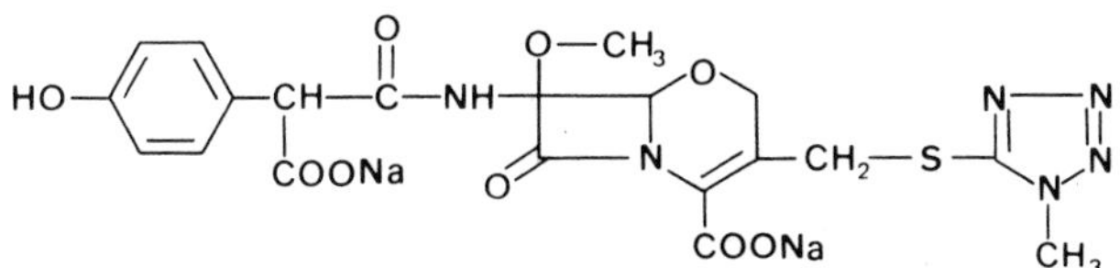

Moxalactam

Figure 43–3. Structures of some cephalosporins.

tors are similar or identical proteins, but different drugs may bind to different receptors. Transpeptidation enzymes are inhibited, resulting in blockage of terminal cross-linking of bacterial cell wall peptidoglycan. Autolytic enzymes in the cell wall may be activated. It appears that the mechanism is not identical for every drug and for every bacterial species.

Resistance to cephalosporins can be associated with (1) lack of outer membrane permeability to the drug in a particular microbial strain; (2) lack of a proper receptor on the bacterium, most receptors appearing to be analogous or identical to penicillin-binding proteins (PBP); and (3) production by the bacterium of a β-lactamase capable of splitting the β-lactam ring of cephalosporins (cephalosporinase). Many such enzymes exist. Among *Enterobacter, Serratia*, and *Pseudomonas* strains and others, resistance to "third-generation" cephalosporins has been observed, associated with the induction of special β-lactamases during exposure to these drugs. Some instances of bacterial tolerance have been observed when strains were inhibited but not killed by cephalosporins. This has been attributed to a deficiency (or lack of activation) of autolytic enzymes in the cell wall.

Absorption, Distribution, & Excretion

Of the more than 30 cephalosporins available in the USA in 1985, only 4 (cephalexin, cephradine, cefaclor, cefadroxil) are sufficiently well absorbed after oral intake to give systemic levels or urine levels suitable for treatment. The other drugs in this class are usually given intravenously because intramuscular injection is too painful. Commonly, a bolus of 0.5–2 g is added 4–8 times daily to an intravenous drip, resulting in serum levels ranging from 10 to 40 μg/mL. The serum half-life typically ranges from 30 to 90 minutes. There are significant variations between individual drugs.

Cephalosporins are distributed widely into tissues and body fluids, including pleural, pericardial, and synovial fluids. The earlier cephalosporins failed to penetrate the central nervous system and were singularly unsuccessful in the treatment of meningitis. However, cefotaxime, cefuroxime, ceftriaxone, moxalactam, cefoperazone, and others do enter the central nervous system and reach therapeutic concentrations there, sufficient for the treatment of meningitis caused by aerobic gram-negative bacteria. Conversely, these same drugs may particularly favor superinfection by enterococci and other resistant gram-positive organisms.

Cephalosporins are excreted mainly by glomerular filtration and tubular secretion into the urine, where levels may reach 200–2000 μg/mL. Tubular blocking agents (eg, probenecid) may increase serum levels substantially. Those cephalosporins containing acetyl groups in the R_2 position (cephalothin, cephapirin) are deacetylated in the liver, the metabolic product is less biologically active. In renal failure, the dose must be reduced, since the excretion of cephalosporins may be markedly impaired, and high fluid and tissue levels may exert toxic effects. Levels of cephalosporins in bile are similar to those in serum. Cefoperazone is primarily excreted into the bile, and its serum level is not greatly influenced by renal failure.

Clinical Uses

Cephalosporins can be considered for the following major applications:

(1) Suspected bacteremia due to an unknown organism (most likely *Klebsiella*, coliform bacteria, *Proteus*, or *Pseudomonas*), especially in debilitated or immunosuppressed patients. Such infections are often nosocomial and can be managed with a "third-generation" cephalosporin, often given together with an aminoglycoside.

(2) Selected "surgical prophylaxis." A cephalosporin is given parenterally for 2–6 hours before and 12–24 hours after a surgical procedure that has more than a 5% risk of infection. Drugs with a long half-life, high tissue levels, and low cost (eg, cefazolin) are often preferred.

(3) Mixed infections, especially those including anaerobes, involving chest, abdomen, or pelvis. Cefoxitin and several "third-generation" drugs are particularly effective against anaerobes, including *Bacteroides* sp.

(4) Penicillinase-producing *N gonorrhoeae* and other special infections. An alternative choice in urinary tract infections.

(5) Gram-negative rod bacterial meningitis may be treated by choice with cefuroxime, cefoperazone, cefotaxime, or other cephalosporins that reach the central nervous system.

A. Oral Administration: Cephalexin and cephradine seem virtually identical in terms of absorption, levels in blood (10 μg/mL after 0.5 g every 6 hours), protein binding (20%), antimicrobial activity, and excretion in urine. Use is limited to infections of the urinary tract (levels in urine may reach 500 μg/mL) or to minor infections of the respiratory tract (otitis, sinusitis, tracheobronchitis) caused by susceptible organisms. Cefadroxil (1 g every 12 hours) has similar indications. Cefaclor is similar to these drugs but is also active against β-lactamase–producing *H influenzae*. It is given 3–4 times daily in a dose of 15–30 mg/kg/d (up to 1 g/d for children).

B. Parenteral Administration:

1. Intramuscular–Cefazolin, cefamandole, cefoxitin, cefotaxime, and others may be given by this route in the same dose as intravenously. However, pain on injection may be a major objection to this route of administration.

2. Intravenous–Typically, a portion of the daily dose (below) is added as a bolus every 4–8 hours to an intravenous infusion. Cefazolin, 4 g/d (50–200 mg/kg/d), has been used for surgical prophylaxis because it gives unusually high and prolonged levels. Cephalothin, 6–12 g/d (50–200 mg/kg/d), yields somewhat lower serum levels, but it is highly resistant to staphylococcal β-lactamase. Cephapirin is similar.

Cefamandole, 6–12 g/d (75–200 mg/kg/d), is often active against *Klebsiella, Enterobacter, Proteus*, and anaerobes but is probably a poor choice in *H influenzae* infections. Cefoxitin may be preferred in *B fragilis* and mixed anaerobic infections. It and ceftriaxone are alternative drugs for penicillinase-producing *N gonorrhoeae*. With all of these drugs, individual strains may exhibit resistance.

Laboratory tests for susceptibility of a given isolate may occasionally be helpful. Cefotaxime (4–12 g/d [50–200 mg/kg/d]), moxalactam (4–12 g/d), and cefoperazone (6–12 g/d), are given every 4–8 hours as a bolus into an intravenous infusion. Ceforanide (2–4 g/d) and ceftriaxone (2–4 g/d) can be given at 12-hour intervals, and it is claimed that cefonicid (2–3 g/d) is effective when given as a single daily dose. These are competing in the USA, claiming broader spectrum, enhanced activity, greater β-lactamase resistance, and greater clinical efficacy. Cefotaxime, cefuroxime, ceftriaxone, moxalactam, cefoperazone, and some others can be used for treatment of gram-negative bacterial meningitis but are very expensive and should not be used for surgical prophylaxis. The experience available in 1985 does not justify any definite preference for one of the newer cephalosporins. They have been overused, and resistance to them is appearing among gram-negative enteric organisms.

Adverse Reactions

A. Toxicity: Local irritation can produce severe pain after intramuscular injection and thrombophlebitis after repeated intravenous injection. Other toxic reactions include anaphylaxis, urticaria, skin rashes, fever, eosinophilia, granulocytopenia, and hemolytic anemia. Some of these are probably hypersensitivity reactions (see below). Renal toxicity producing tubular necrosis has been demonstrated for several cephalosporins. Interstitial nephritis has occurred in elderly patients. For this reason, cephaloridine has been abandoned.

The oral cephalosporins also can produce diarrhea, nausea, vomiting, and SGOT elevation.

Some of the newest cephalosporins can have a disulfiramlike effect if combined with alcohol. They may also induce hypoprothrombinemia and a bleeding tendency, so that supplemental vitamin K is indicated. Moxalactam can produce severe bleeding disorders. Induced platelet defects have been observed to contribute to coagulopathy at times.

B. Allergy: Cephalosporins can be sensitizing, and specific hypersensitivity reactions, including anaphylaxis, can occur. Because of the difference in the chemical structure of the drug nucleus, the antigenicity of cephalosporins differs from that of penicillins. Consequently, many individuals who are hypersensitive to penicillins can tolerate cephalosporins. The degree of cross-allergenicity between penicillins and cephalosporins remains controversial (6–16%). Some cross-antigenicity can be demonstrated both in vitro and in humans.

MISCELLANEOUS AGENTS

Monocyclic Beta-Lactams

Certain gram-negative bacteria produce monocyclic β-lactam agents (monobactams) with weak antimicrobial activity. Extensive structural manipulation of the naturally occurring drugs has led to the development of drugs with enhanced activity and lactamase resistance. The first of these agents to become available for clinical investigation is **aztreonam** (Fig 43–1). It has high activity against gram-negative organisms, including *Pseudomonas, Serratia*, and *E coli*, but is inactive against gram-positives. Its clinical efficacy remains to be determined.

Carbapenems

A novel class of β-lactam antibiotics isolated from various *Streptomyces* spp has been given the name carbapenems. The first agent from this group to be extensively studied in humans is the semisynthetic **imipenem** (Fig 43–1). It has high resistance against bacterial β-lactamases and activity against a variety of both gram-positive and gram-negative organisms. Its major mechanism appears to be inhibition of cell wall transpeptidation—like that of other β-lactams. A major disadvantage is extensive metabolism in renal tubular cells, resulting in low urinary concentrations and significant renal toxicity in experimental animals. Therefore, an inhibitor of renal dehydropeptidase, cilastatin, is coadministered with imipenem to reduce intrarenal inactivation. This drug combination has recently been released in the USA as Primaxin.

Clavulanic Acid

Clavulanic acid (Fig 43–1) was originally isolated from cultures of *Streptomyces clavuligerus*. Although a β-lactam molecule, it has little inhibitory effect on the transpeptidase enzymes of the bacterial cell wall. However, it is a powerful inhibitor of many β-lactamase enzymes formed by gram-negative and gram-positive organisms and can therefore potentiate the effects of β-lactam agents that are normally inactivated by the enzyme. It has recently been released for clinical use in combination with amoxicillin and ticarcillin.

REFERENCES

Aronoff GR et al: Interactions of moxalactam and tobramycin in normal volunteers and in patients with impaired renal function. *J Infect Dis* 1984;**149**:9.

Barza M: Antimicrobial spectrum, pharmacology and therapeutic use of penicillins. *Am J Hosp Pharm* 1977;**34**:57.

Birnbaum J et al: Carbapenems, a new class of beta-lactam antibiotics. *Am J Med* 1985;**78(Suppl 6A)**:3.

Border WA et al: Antitubular basement membrane antibodies in methicillin-associated interstitial nephritis. *N Engl J Med* 1974;**291**:381.

Brown CH et al: The hemostatic defect produced by carbenicillin. *N Engl J Med* 1974;**291**:265.

Buchanan CE, Strominger JL: Altered penicillin-binding components in penicillin-resistant mutants of *Bacillus subtilis*. *Proc Natl Acad Sci USA* 1976;**73**:1816.

Eliopoulous GM, Moellering RC: Azlocillin, mezlocillin and piperacillin: New broad-spectrum penicillins. *Ann Intern Med* 1982;**79**:755.

Erffmeyer JE: Adverse reactions to penicillin. *Ann Allergy* 1981;**47**:288.

Finegold SM et al: Comparative trial of bacampicillin and amoxicillin in bacterial infections of the lower respiratory tract. *Rev Infect Dis* 1981;**3**:150.

Hartman B, Tomasz A: Altered penicillin-binding proteins in methicillin-resistant strains of *Staphylococcus aureus*. *Antimicrob Agents Chemother* 1981;**19**:726.

Heseltine PN et al: Cefoxitin: Clinical evaluation in thirty-eight patients. *Antimicrob Agents Chemother* 1977;**11**:427.

Kancir LM et al: Adverse reactions to methicillin and nafcillin during treatment of serious *Staphylococcus aureus* infections. *Arch Intern Med* 1978;**138**:909.

Kitzing W et al: Comparative toxicities of methicillin and nafcillin. *Am J Dis Child* 1981;**135**:52.

Landesman SH et al: Gram-negative bacillary meningitis: New therapy and changing concepts. *Arch Intern Med* 1982;**142**:939.

Love LJ et al: Randomized trial of empiric antibiotic therapy with ticarcillin in combination with gentamicin, amikacin, or netilmicin in febrile patients with granulocytopenia and cancer. *Am J Med* 1979;**66**:603.

Mangi RJ et al: Development of meningitis during cephalothin therapy. *Ann Intern Med* 1973;**78**:347.

Murray BE, Mederskisamajoj B: Transferable beta-lactamase: A new mechanism for in vitro penicillin resistance in *Streptococcus faecalis*. *J Clin Invest* 1983;**72**:1168.

Murray BE, Moellering RC Jr: Cephalosporins. *Annu Rev Med* 1981;**32**:559.

Neu HC: The emergence of bacterial resistance and its influence on empiric therapy. *Rev Infect Dis* 1983;**5**:S9.

Neu HC: The new beta-lactamase–stable cephalosporins. *Ann Intern Med* 1982;**97**:408.

Pacter RL et al: Coagulopathy associated with the use of moxalactam. *JAMA* 1982;**248**:1100.

Parker CW: Drug allergy. (3 parts.) *N Engl J Med* 1975; **292**:511, 732, 957.

Petz LD: Immunologic cross reactivity between penicillins and cephalosporins: A review. *J Infect Dis* 1978;**137(Suppl)**:S74.

Phillips JA et al: Ampicillin-associated diarrhea. *Pediatrics* 1976;**58**:869.

Rahal JJ: Moxalactam therapy for gram-negative bacillary meningitis. *Rev Infect Dis* 1982;**4**:606.

Reyes MP et al: Granulocytopenia associated with carbenicillin. *Am J Med* 1973;**54**:413.

Rolinson GN: 6-APA and the development of the beta-lactam antibiotics. *J Antimicrob Chemother* 1979;**5**:7.

Rudolph AH, Price EV: Penicillin reactions among patients in venereal disease clinics. *JAMA* 1973;**223**:499.

Sanders CC: Novel resistance selected by the new expanded-spectrum cephalosporins: A concern. *J Infect Dis* 1983; **147**:585.

Scheifele DW et al: Evaluation of rapid β-lactamase test for detecting ampicillin-resistant strains of *Hemophilus influenzae* type b. *Pediatrics* 1976;**58**:382.

Spector R, Lorenzo AV: Inhibition of penicillin transport from the cerebrospinal fluid after intracisternal inoculation of bacteria. *J Clin Invest* 1974;**54**:316.

Sykes RB: The classification and terminology of enzymes that hydrolyze β-lactam antibiotics. *J Infect Dis* 1982;**145**:762.

Tipper DJ: Mode of action of beta-lactam antibiotics. *Rev Infect Dis* 1979;**1**:39.

Ward TT, Amon MB, Krause LK: Combination amdinocillin and cefoxitin therapy of multiply-resistant *Serratia marcescens* urinary tract infections. *Am J Med* 1983;**75(2A)**:85.

Wendel GD et al: Penicillin allergy and desensitization in serious infections during pregnancy. *N Engl J Med* 1985; **312**:1229.

Chloramphenicol & Tetracyclines

44

Ernest Jawetz, MD, PhD

CHLORAMPHENICOL

Chloramphenicol was first isolated from cultures of *Streptomyces venezuelae* in 1947 and was synthesized in 1949, the first completely synthetic antibiotic of importance to be produced commercially. It is the only available representative of its chemical type.

Chemistry

Crystalline chloramphenicol is a neutral, stable compound with the following structure:

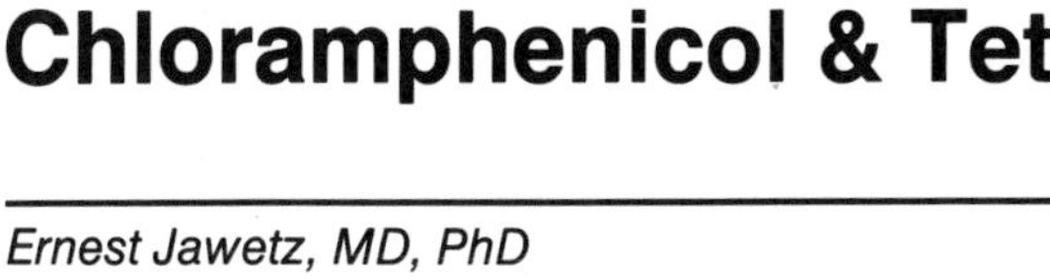

Chloramphenicol

It consists of colorless crystals with an intensely bitter taste. It is highly soluble in alcohol and poorly soluble in water. Saturated aqueous solutions (0.25%) keep their activity for many months at refrigerator or room temperature if protected from light. Chloramphenicol succinate is highly soluble in water and is hydrolyzed in tissues with the liberation of free chloramphenicol; it is used for parenteral injection.

Antimicrobial Activity

Chloramphenicol is a potent inhibitor of microbial protein synthesis and has little effect on other microbial metabolic functions. Chloramphenicol binds reversibly to a receptor site on the 50S subunit of the bacterial ribosome. There it interferes markedly with the incorporation of amino acids into newly formed peptides by blocking the action of peptidyl transferase (see Chapter 42). Chloramphenicol also inhibits mitochondrial protein synthesis of mammalian bone marrow cells but does not greatly affect other intact cells.

Chloramphenicol is bacteriostatic for many bacteria and for rickettsiae but is clinically ineffective against chlamydiae. Its action is reversible by removal of the drug. Most gram-positive bacteria are inhibited by chloramphenicol in concentrations of 1–10 μg/mL, and many gram-negative bacteria are inhibited by concentrations of 0.2–5 μg/mL. *Haemophilus influenzae*, *Neisseria meningitidis*, and some strains of *Bacteroides* are highly susceptible, and for them chloramphenicol may be bactericidal. Some salmonellae are

susceptible, but plasmid-mediated resistance to chloramphenicol has appeared with increasing frequency.

Resistance

In most bacterial species, large populations of chloramphenicol-susceptible cells contain occasional resistant mutants that are less permeable to the drug. These mutants are usually only 2–4 times more resistant than the parent populations; consequently, they emerge slowly in treated individuals. There is no cross-resistance between chloramphenicol and other drugs, but plasmids (resistance transfer factors, RTF) may transmit multiple drug resistance (chloramphenicol, tetracycline, streptomycin, etc) from one bacterium to another by conjugation (see Chapter 42). Such plasmid-mediated resistance to chloramphenicol results from the production of chloramphenicol acetyl transferase, a bacterial enzyme that destroys the drug. Consequently, the resistance of such plasmid-containing microorganisms is of high order.

Absorption, Metabolism, & Excretion

After oral administration, crystalline chloramphenicol is rapidly and completely absorbed. With daily doses of 2 g orally, blood levels usually reach 8 μg/mL. Chloramphenicol palmitate, administered to children in doses up to 50 mg/kg/d orally, is hydrolyzed in the intestine to yield free chloramphenicol, but the usual blood levels rarely exceed 10 μg/mL. For parenteral injection, chloramphenicol succinate, 25–50 mg/kg/d intravenously, yields free chloramphenicol by hydrolysis, giving blood levels somewhat lower than those achieved with the orally administered drug.

After absorption, chloramphenicol is widely distributed to virtually all tissues and body fluids, including the central nervous system and cerebrospinal fluid. In fact, the concentration of chloramphenicol in brain tissue may be equal to that in serum—a unique property for the treatment of central nervous system infections.

Circulating chloramphenicol is about 30% protein-bound. The drug penetrates cell membranes readily. Most of the drug is inactivated in the body either by conjugation with glucuronic acid (principally in the liver) or by reduction to inactive aryl amines. Excretion of active chloramphenicol (about 10% of the total dose administered) and of inactive degradation products (about 90% of the total) occurs by way of the urine. It may be that the active drug is cleared mainly by glomerular filtration and the inactive products mainly by tubular secretion. Only small amounts of active drug are excreted into bile or feces.

The systemic dosage of chloramphenicol need not be altered in renal insufficiency, but it must be reduced markedly in hepatic failure.

Clinical Uses

Chloramphenicol is a possible drug of choice in only a few types of infections: (1) Symptomatic *Salmonella* infection, eg, typhoid fever (some strains in Central and South America are now resistant). (2) *H influenzae* meningitis, laryngotracheitis, or pneumonia caused by β-lactamase-producing strains. (3) Meningococcal infections in patients hypersensitive to penicillin. (4) Anaerobic or mixed infections in the central nervous system, eg, brain abscess. (5) Severe rickettsial infections.

Chloramphenicol is occasionally used topically in the treatment of eye infections because of its wide antibacterial spectrum and its penetration of ocular tissues and the aqueous humor. However, it is not effective in chlamydial eye infections.

A. Salmonellosis: For *Salmonella* infections (eg, typhoid or paratyphoid fever), adults should receive chloramphenicol, 2–3 g daily orally for 14–21 days, and children 30–50 mg/kg/d orally for 14–21 days. Prolonged treatment tends to reduce the frequency of relapses. A similar program may be followed in severe rickettsial infections (eg, scrub typhus or Rocky Mountain spotted fever).

B. Haemophilus: For *H influenzae* meningitis or laryngotracheitis (in small children) or pneumonia (in the elderly), chloramphenicol, 50–100 mg/kg/d orally or intravenously, has been given for 8–14 days, depending upon clinical response and cerebrospinal fluid changes. However, ampicillin is the drug of first choice at present unless ampicillin-resistant *Haemophilus* strains have been encountered in the community. Up to 20% of *H influenzae* type b strains in the USA may now be β-lactamase producers. Initial treatment for *Haemophilus* meningitis should consist of both chloramphenicol and ampicillin until it can be shown that the organism does not produce β-lactamase. On the other hand, chloramphenicol-resistant *Haemophilus* strains have also appeared. Cefuroxime, cefotaxime, and ceftizoxime are alternative drugs.

C. Other Uses: In life-threatening sepsis probably originating in the lower bowel, chloramphenicol, 2 g/d, is sometimes combined with an aminoglycoside (eg, amikacin, 15 mg/kg/d). Because of the excellent penetration by chloramphenicol of all parts of the central nervous system, it is sometimes used in cerebritis, brain abscess, or meningitis of ill-defined origin. Sepsis caused by some species of *Bacteroides* and severe melioidosis may respond to chloramphenicol.

Adverse Reactions

A. Gastrointestinal Disturbances: Adults taking chloramphenicol, 1.5–2.5 g daily, occasionally develop nausea, vomiting, and diarrhea in 2–5 days.

This is rare in children. After 5–10 days, the results of microbial flora alteration may become apparent, with prominent candidiasis of mucous membranes (especially of the mouth and vagina).

B. Bone Marrow Disturbances: Adults taking chloramphenicol in excess of 50 mg/kg/d regularly exhibit disturbances in red cell maturation after 1–2 weeks of blood levels above 25–30 μg/mL. These are characterized by the appearance of markedly vacuolated nucleated red cells in the marrow, anemia, and reticulocytopenia. These anomalies usually disappear when chloramphenicol is discontinued. The disturbance appears to be a maturation arrest associated with a rise in serum iron concentration and a depression of serum phenylalanine levels and is not related to the rare occurrence of aplastic anemia.

Aplastic anemia is a rare consequence of chloramphenicol administration by any route. It probably represents a specific genetically determined idiosyncrasy of the individual. It is not related to dose or time of intake but is seen more frequently with prolonged use. It tends to be irreversible and fatal. The precise incidence of fatal aplastic anemia as a toxic reaction to chloramphenicol administration is not known, but the disease is estimated to occur 13 times more frequently after the use of the drug than it does spontaneously. Aplastic anemia probably develops once in 24,000–40,000 patients who have taken chloramphenicol. Leukemia may follow the development of hypoplastic anemia.

C. Toxicity for Newborn Infants: Newborn infants lack an effective glucuronic acid conjugation mechanism for the degradation and detoxification of chloramphenicol. Consequently, when infants are given doses of 75 mg/kg/d or more, the drug may accumulate, resulting in the "gray syndrome," with vomiting, flaccidity, hypothermia, gray color, shock, and collapse. To avoid this toxic effect, chloramphenicol should be used with caution in infants and the dosage should be limited to 50 mg/kg/d or less in full-term infants and 30 mg/kg/d or less in prematures.

D. Interaction With Other Drugs: Chloramphenicol may prolong the half-life and raise the blood concentration of phenytoin, tolbutamide, chlorpropamide, and coumadin. This is attributable to inhibition of liver microsomal enzymes by chloramphenicol. It may precipitate a variety of other drugs from solutions. Like other bacteriostatic inhibitors of microbial protein synthesis, chloramphenicol can antagonize the bactericidal action of penicillins or aminoglycosides (see Chapter 52).

Medical & Social Implications of Overuse

Because of its "broad spectrum" and its apparent lack of toxicity, chloramphenicol was used indiscriminately between 1948 and 1951 without specific indications. It has been estimated that more than 8 million people received the drug for minor complaints, respiratory (usually viral) illnesses, etc. This inappropriate use was followed by a wave of cases of aplastic anemia, which, in turn, almost resulted in the complete abandonment of an effective drug.

TETRACYCLINES

The tetracyclines are a large group of drugs with a common basic structure and activity. Chlortetracycline, isolated from *Streptomyces aureofaciens,* was introduced in 1948. Oxytetracycline, derived from *Streptomyces rimosus,* was introduced in 1950. Tetracycline (many trade names), obtained by catalytic dehalogenation of chlortetracycline, has been available since 1953. Demeclocycline (demethylchlortetracycline) was obtained by demethylation of chlortetracycline. The most recently developed tetracyclines have emphasized good absorption combined with prolonged blood levels.

Chemistry

All of the tetracyclines have the basic structure shown below.

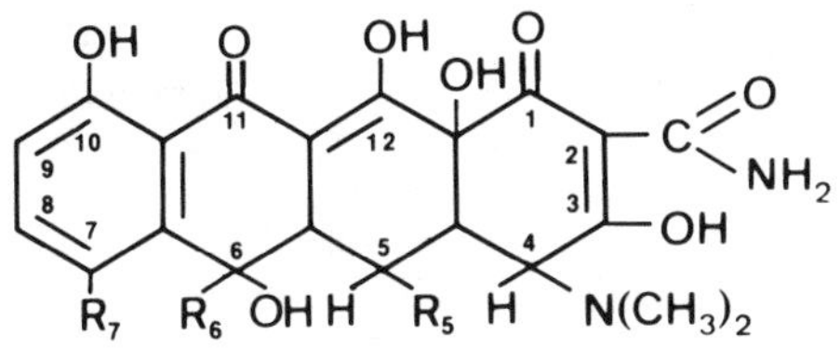

	R_7	R_6	R_5	Renal Clearance (mL/min)
Chlortetracycline	—Cl	—CH$_3$	—H	35
Oxytetracycline	—H	—CH$_3$	—OH	90
Tetracycline	—H	—CH$_3$	—H	65
Demeclocycline	—Cl	—H	—H	35
Methacycline	—H	=CH$_2$ *	—OH	31
Doxycycline	—H	—CH$_3$ *	—OH	16
Minocycline	—N(CH$_3$)$_2$	—H	—H	10

*There is no —OH at position 6 on methacycline and doxycycline.

Free tetracyclines are crystalline amphoteric substances of low solubility. They are available as hydrochlorides, which are more soluble (about 10% in water). Such solutions are acid and, with the exception of chlortetracycline, fairly stable. Chlortetracycline is very unstable in vitro, losing much of its activity in a few hours; for this reason, it is not widely used clinically at present. Tetracyclines combine firmly with divalent metal ions, and this chelation can interfere with absorption and activity of the molecule. Tetracyclines fluoresce bright yellow in ultraviolet light of 360 nm.

Antimicrobial Activity

Tetracyclines are the prototype of "broad spectrum" drugs. They are bacteriostatic for many gram-positive and gram-negative bacteria, including some anaerobes; for rickettsiae, chlamydiae, mycoplasmas, and L forms; and for some protozoa, eg, amebas.

Equal amounts of tetracyclines in body fluids or tissues have approximately equal antimicrobial activity. Minocycline may have greater lipophilic properties than other congeners. Most differences in activity claimed for individual tetracycline drugs are of small magnitude and limited importance. Differences in clinical efficacy are attributable largely to features of absorption, distribution, and excretion of individual drugs. However, great differences exist in the susceptibility of different strains of a given species of microorganism. Laboratory tests on clinical isolates may therefore be important.

Tetracyclines enter microorganisms in part by passive diffusion and in part by an energy-dependent process of active transport. As a result, susceptible cells concentrate the drug so that the intracellular drug concentration is much higher than the extracellular one. Once inside the cell, tetracyclines bind reversibly to receptors on the 30S subunit of the bacterial ribosome in a position that blocks the binding of the aminoacyl-tRNA to the acceptor site on the mRNA-ribosome complex. This effectively prevents the addition of new amino acids to the growing peptide chain, inhibiting protein synthesis. The selective inhibition of protein synthesis in microorganisms may be explained largely by the lack of concentration of tetracyclines in mammalian cells.

Resistance

Susceptible microbial populations contain small numbers of organisms resistant to tetracyclines. These lack an active transport mechanism across cell membranes and thus do not concentrate tetracycline in their cells. Alternatively, resistant bacteria may lack passive permeability to tetracyclines. The degree of resistance is variable. Among gram-negative bacterial species (especially *Pseudomonas, Proteus,* and coliforms), the selection of highly resistant types has already occurred, and tetracyclines have therefore lost some of their usefulness. Tetracycline resistance is usually transmitted by plasmids (RTF). Resistance is increasing even among what were at first highly susceptible bacterial species (eg, pneumococci, *Haemophilus,* streptococci, *Bacteroides*). This is a consequence of the intense selection pressure exerted on microbial populations by the widespread use of tetracycline drugs. The incorporation of tetracyclines in animal feeds enhances the rate of growth and weight gain in animals but also results in spread of tetracycline-resistant microorganisms among farm personnel and consumers of animal products (see p 531).

Plasmids controlling resistance may be transmitted by transduction or by conjugation. The genes for tetracycline resistance are closely associated with those for other drugs, eg, aminoglycosides, sulfonamides, and chloramphenicol. Plasmids therefore usually transmit resistance to multiple drugs rather than to tetracyclines alone.

Absorption, Metabolism, & Excretion

Tetracyclines are absorbed somewhat irregularly

from the gastrointestinal tract. A portion of an orally administered dose of tetracycline remains in the gut lumen, modifies intestinal flora, and is excreted in the feces. While only 30% of chlortetracycline and 60–80% of tetracycline, oxytetracycline, and demeclocycline are absorbed in the gut, absorption is 90–100% for doxycycline and minocycline. Absorption occurs mainly in the upper small intestine and is best in the absence of food. It is impaired by chelation with divalent cations (Ca^{2+}, Mg^{2+}, Fe^{2+}) or with Al^{3+}, especially in milk and antacids, and by alkaline pH. Specially buffered tetracycline solutions are formulated for parenteral (usually intravenous) administration in persons unable to take oral medication. The parenteral dosage is generally similar to the oral dosage.

In the blood, 40–80% of various tetracyclines is protein-bound. With oral doses of 500 mg every 6 hours, tetracycline hydrochloride and oxytetracycline reach peak levels of 4–6 μg/mL. With doxycycline and minocycline, the peak levels are somewhat lower (2–4 μg/mL). Intravenously injected tetracyclines give somewhat higher levels only temporarily. The drugs are distributed widely to tissues and body fluids, except for the cerebrospinal fluid, where concentrations are low. Minocycline is unique in reaching very high concentrations in tears and saliva—a feature that permits it to eradicate the meningococcal carrier state. Tetracyclines cross the placenta to reach the fetus and are also excreted in milk. As a result of chelation with calcium, tetracyclines are bound to growing bones and teeth.

Absorbed tetracyclines are excreted mainly in bile and urine. Concentrations in bile are 10 times higher than in serum; some of the drug excreted in bile is reabsorbed from the intestine (enterohepatic circulation) and contributes to maintenance of serum levels. Ten percent to 50% of various tetracyclines is excreted into the urine, mainly by glomerular filtration. The renal clearance of tetracyclines ranges from 10 to 90 mL/min (see p 529). From 10 to 40% of tetracyclines is excreted in feces.

Doxycycline and minocycline are almost completely absorbed from the gut and are excreted more slowly, leading to persistent serum levels. Doxycycline does not require renal excretion and does not accumulate significantly in renal failure.

Clinical Uses

Tetracyclines are the most typical "broad-spectrum" antibiotics. They are effective against a variety of microorganisms and are thus often used indiscriminately.

Tetracyclines are the drugs of choice in infections with *Mycoplasma pneumoniae*, chlamydiae, and rickettsiae. They are useful in mixed bacterial infections related to the respiratory tract, especially sinusitis and bronchitis. They may be employed in many gram-positive and gram-negative bacterial infections, including cholera and other *Vibrio* infections, provided the organism is susceptible. Tetracyclines given in full

doses for 7 days can eradicate uncomplicated infections with penicillinase-producing gonococci, and may at the same time control coexisting chlamydial infections. They have been used in pneumonias and urinary tract and skin infections, particularly acne. It is claimed that 2.5 g of tetracycline hydrochloride as a single oral dose is effective in enteritis caused by both susceptible and resistant shigellae. A single dose of doxycycline, 200 mg, may be as effective in cholera as multiple doses. However, tetracycline resistance has appeared during cholera epidemics. Tetracyclines are commonly used in plague, tularemia, brucellosis, and leptospirosis. Sometimes they are combined with an aminoglycoside.

Minocycline, 200 mg orally daily for 5 days—or rifampin—can eradicate the meningococcal carrier state.

A. Oral Dosage: The minimal effective oral dose for rapidly excreted tetracyclines, equivalent to tetracycline hydrochloride, is 0.25 g 4 times daily for adults and 20 mg/kg/d for children. For severe systemic infections, a dose 2–3 times larger for at least 3–5 days is indicated.

The minimal effective daily dose is 600 mg for demeclocycline or methacycline, 100 mg for doxycycline, and 200 mg for minocycline. Tetracyclines chelate with metals as noted above and thus should not be administered with milk, antacids, or ferrous sulfate. To avoid deposition in growing bones or teeth, tetracyclines are not usually indicated for pregnant women or children under 6 years of age.

Tetracycline hydrochloride, 250–500 mg daily, is commonly taken for many months to suppress acne, especially in adolescents and young adults. This low dose presumably suppresses lipase activity of propionibacteria and inhibits inflammatory reactions.

B. Parenteral Dosage: Several tetracyclines are available for intravenous injection in doses of 0.1–0.5 g every 6–12 hours (10–15 mg/kg/d in children). Intramuscular injection is usually unsatisfactory because of pain and inflammatory reactions. There are very few instances (eg, an unconscious patient with rickettsial disease) that warrant parenteral tetracycline administration.

Adverse Reactions

Hypersensitivity reactions (drug fever, skin rashes) to tetracyclines appear to be uncommon. Most side effects are due to direct toxicity of the drug or to alteration of microbial flora.

A. Gastrointestinal Side Effects: Nausea, vomiting, and diarrhea are the commonest reasons for discontinuing tetracycline medication. During the first few days of administration, they appear to be attributable to direct local irritation of the intestinal tract.

After a few days of oral use, tetracyclines tend to modify the normal flora. Although some coliform organisms are suppressed, *Pseudomonas*, *Proteus*, staphylococci, resistant coliforms, clostridia, and *Candida* become prominent. This can result in intestinal functional disturbances, anal pruritus, vaginal or oral candidiasis, or even enterocolitis with shock and death.

Nausea, anorexia, and diarrhea can usually be controlled by administering the drug with food or carboxymethylcellulose, reducing drug dosage, or discontinuing the drug. Pseudomembranous enterocolitis associated with *Clostridium difficile* or staphylococci must be recognized promptly and treated with oral vancomycin (see Chapter 50).

B. Bony Structures and Teeth: Tetracyclines are readily bound to calcium deposited in newly formed bone or teeth in young children. When the drug is given during pregnancy, it can be deposited in the fetal teeth, leading to fluorescence, discoloration, and enamel dysplasia; it can also be deposited in bone, where it may cause deformity or growth inhibition. If the drug is given to children under 6 years of age for long periods, similar changes can result.

C. Liver Toxicity: Tetracyclines can probably impair hepatic function, especially during pregnancy, in patients with preexisting hepatic insufficiency, and when high doses are given intravenously. Hepatic necrosis has been reported with daily doses of 4 g intravenously or more.

D. Kidney Toxicity: Renal tubular acidosis and other renal injury resulting in nitrogen retention have been attributed to the administration of outdated tetracycline preparations.

Tetracyclines given together with diuretics may produce nitrogen retention. Tetracyclines, except doxycycline, may cumulate to toxic levels in patients with impaired kidney function and may aggravate the condition.

E. Local Tissue Toxicity: Intravenous injection can lead to venous thrombosis. Intramuscular injection produces painful local irritation that can lead to infiltration and should be avoided.

F. Photosensitization: Systemic tetracycline administration, especially of demeclocycline, can induce sensitivity to sunlight or ultraviolet light, particularly in blonds.

G. Vestibular Reactions: Dizziness, vertigo, nausea, and vomiting have been particularly noted with minocycline. After doses of 200–400 mg/d of minocycline, 35–70% of patients exhibited such reactions.

Medical & Social Implications of Overuse

The widespread use of tetracyclines for minor illnesses has led to the emergence of resistance even among highly susceptible species, eg, pneumococci and group A streptococci. The large-scale use of these drugs in hospitals has resulted in the selection of tetracycline-resistant organisms as superinfecting agents. In some measure, the tetracyclines (among other antibiotics) must be blamed for the rising incidence of mycotic infection in hospitalized, severely ill patients.

Tetracyclines have been extensively used in animal feeds to increase the rate of growth. This practice has been widely blamed for the steadily increasing spread of tetracycline resistance among bacteria and of plasmids that promote it. Such use has resulted in tetracycline-resistant infections among farmers, animal handlers, slaughterhouse workers, and perhaps the general public. For this reason, some countries (eg, Britain) forbid the use of tetracyclines in animal feeds.

On the other hand, tetracyclines have been of great benefit not only for the control of existing infection but also for chemoprophylaxis in chronic bronchitis and bronchiectasis, keeping many persons well and at work.

REFERENCES

Chloramphenicol

Chloramphenicol-induced bone marrow suppression. (Editorial.) *JAMA* 1970;**213:**1183.

Dajani AS, Kauffman RE: The renaissance of chloramphenicol. *Pediatr Clin North Am* 1981;**28:**195.

Feder HM et al: Chloramphenicol: A review of its use in clinical practice. *Rev Infect Dis* 1981;**3:**479.

Gump DW: Chloramphenicol: A 1981 view. *Arch Intern Med* 1981;**141:**573.

Kucers A: Chloramphenicol, erythromycin, vancomycin, tetracyclines. *Lancet* 1982;**2:**425.

O'Brien TF et al: Molecular epidemiology of antibiotic resistance in *Salmonella* from animals and human beings in the United States. *N Engl J Med* 1982;**307:**1.

Plaut ME, Best WR: Aplastic anemia after parenteral chloramphenicol: Warning renewed. *N Engl J Med* 1982;**306:**1486.

Scott JL et al: A controlled double-blind study of the hematologic toxicity of chloramphenicol. *N Engl J Med* 1965;**272:**1137.

Snyder MJ et al: Comparative efficacy of chloramphenicol, ampicillian, and co-trimoxazole in the treatment of typhoid fever. *Lancet* 1976:**2:**1155.

Wallerstein RO et al: Statewide study of chloramphenicol therapy and fatal aplastic anemia. *JAMA* 1969:**208:**2045.

Tetracyclines

Allen JC: Drugs five years later: Minocycline. *Ann Intern Med* 1976;**85:**482.

Barza M, Schiefe RT: Antimicrobial spectrum, pharmacology and therapeutic use of antibiotics. 1. Tetracyclines. *Am J Hosp Pharm* 1977;**34:**49.

Chopra I, Howe TGB: Bacterial resistance to tetracyclines. *Microbiol Rev* 1978;**42:**707.

Drew TM et al: Minocycline for prophylaxis of infection with *Neisseria meningitidis:* High rate of side effects in recipients. *J Infect Dis* 1976;**133:**194.

Holmberg SD et al: Drug-resistant *Salmonella* from animals fed antimicrobials. *N Engl J Med* 1984:**311:**617.

Hoshiwara I et al: Doxycycline treatment of chronic trachoma. *JAMA* 1973;**224:**220.

Hurwitz S: Acne vulgaris: Current concepts of pathogenesis and treatment. *Am J Dis Child* 1979;**133:**536.

McNeil PJ et al: Evaluation of doxycycline hyclate in the treatment of nongonococcal urethritis. *Sex Transm Dis* 1981; **8:**127.

Mhalu FS et al: Rapid emergence of El Tor *Vibrio cholerae* resistant to antimicrobials during first six months of fourth cholera epidemic in Tanzania. *Lancet* 1979;**1:**345.

Neu HC: Changing mechanisms of bacterial resistance. *Am J Med* 1984;**77(Suppl 1B):**11.

Ory EM: The tetracyclines. Chap 9, pp 117–126, in: *Antimicrobial Therapy,* 3rd ed. Kagan BM (editor). Saunders, 1980.

Pickering LK et al: Single dose tetracycline therapy for shigellosis in adults. *JAMA* 1978;**239:**853.

Rockhill RC et al: Tetracycline resistance of *Corynebacterium diphtheriae* isolated from diphtheria patients in Indonesia. *Antimicrob Agents Chemother* 1982;**21:**842.

Sack DA et al: Single-dose doxycycline for cholera. *Antimicrob Agents Chemother* 1978;**14:**462.

Sauer GC: Safety of long-term tetracycline therapy for acne. *Arch Dermatol* 1976;**112:**1603.

Siegel D: Tetracyclines: New look at old antibiotic. (2 parts.) *NY State J Med* 1978;**78:**950, 1115.

Simpson MB et al: Hemolytic anemia after tetracycline therapy. *N Engl J Med* 1985;**312:**840.

Aminoglycosides & Polymyxins

45

Ernest Jawetz, MD, PhD

AMINOGLYCOSIDES

Aminoglycosides are a group of bactericidal drugs sharing chemical, antimicrobial, pharmacologic, and toxic characteristics. At present, the group includes streptomycin, neomycin, kanamycin, amikacin, gentamicin, tobramycin, sisomicin, netilmicin, and others. All of these agents inhibit protein synthesis in bacteria and suffer the disadvantage of multiple types of resistance.

All aminoglycosides are potentially ototoxic and nephrotoxic. All can accumulate in renal insufficiency; therefore, dosage adjustments must be made.

Aminoglycosides are used most widely against gram-negative enteric bacteria, especially in bacteremia, sepsis, or endocarditis. Streptomycin is the oldest and best-studied of the aminoglycosides. Neomycin and kanamycin are now largely limited to topical or oral use. Among the newer drugs, tobramycin, gentamicin, and amikacin are the most widely employed at present.

General Properties of Aminoglycosides

A. Physical and Chemical Properties: Aminoglycosides are water-soluble, stable in solution, and more active in alkaline than at acid pH. They have a hexose nucleus, either streptidine (in streptomycin) or deoxystreptamine (other aminoglycosides), to which amino sugars are attached by glycosidic linkages (Figs 45–1 and 45–2). This is why these molecules are also referred to as aminocyclitols. Each drug is characterized by the number and kind of amino sugars. Aminocyclitols may form complexes with β-lactam drugs in vitro and may lose some activity.

B. Mechanism of Action: Aminoglycosides are bactericidal for susceptible organisms by virtue of irreversible inhibition of protein synthesis. However, the precise mechanism for this bactericidal activity is not clearly evident. The initial event is penetration through the cell envelope. This is in part an active transport process, in part passive diffusion. The latter can be greatly enhanced by the presence of cell wall–active drugs, eg, penicillins. Since the active transport is an oxygen-dependent process, aminoglycosides are relatively ineffective against strict anaerobes.

Once an aminoglycoside has entered the cell, it binds to receptors on the 30S subunit of the bacterial ribosome. These receptors, some of which have been purified, are proteins under chromosomal control. Ribosomal protein synthesis is inhibited by aminoglycosides in at least 3 ways: (1) They interfere with the "initiation complex" of peptide formation; (2) they induce misreading of the code on the mRNA template, which causes incorporation of incorrect amino acids into the peptide; and (3) they cause a breakup of polysomes into nonfunctional monosomes.

C. Mechanisms of Resistance: Three principal mechanisms have been established: (1) Alteration in the cell surface, which interferes with the permeability or active transport of aminoglycoside into the

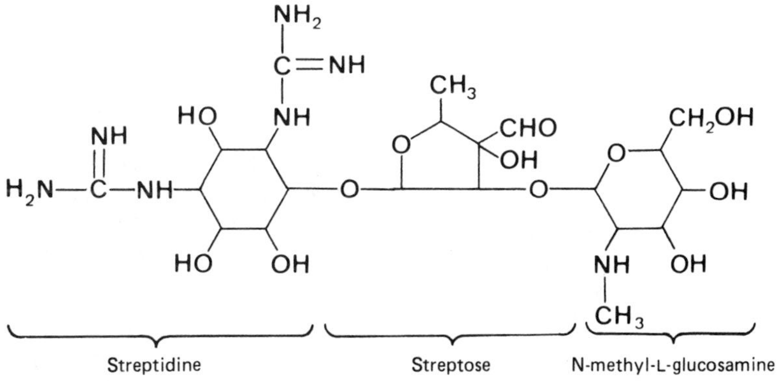

Figure 45–1. Structure of streptomycin.

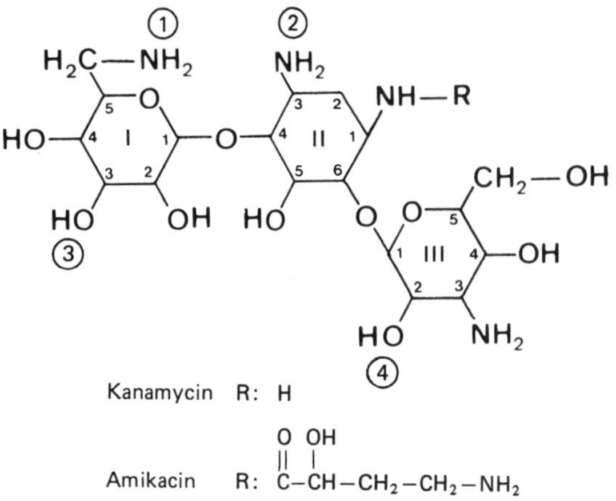

Kanamycin R: H

Amikacin R: $C-CH-CH_2-CH_2-NH_2$ (O, OH above)

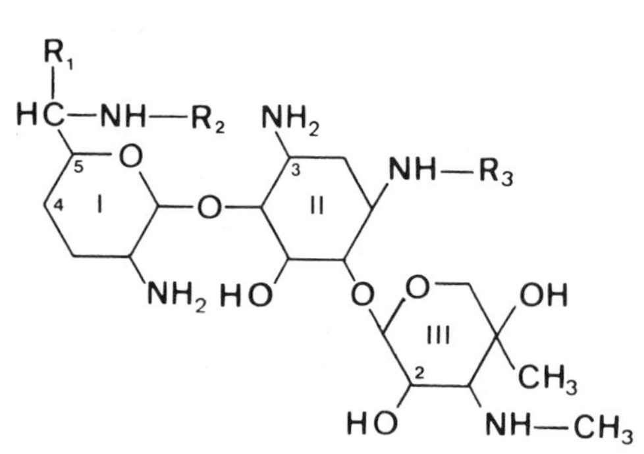

Gentamicin, netilmicin

	Ring I			Ring II
	R_1	R_2	C4–C5 bond	R_3
Gentamicin C_1	CH_3	CH_3	Single	H
Gentamicin C_2	CH_3	H	Single	H
Gentamicin C_{1a}	H	H	Single	H
Netilmicin	H	H	Double	C_2H_5

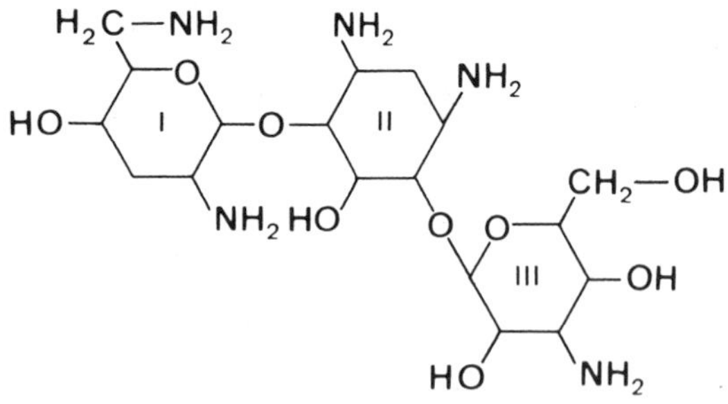

Tobramycin

Figure 45–2. Structures of several important aminoglycoside antibiotics. Ring II is 2-deoxystreptamine. The resemblance between kanamycin and amikacin and between gentamicin, netilmicin, and tobramycin can be seen. The circled numerals on the kanamycin molecule indicate points of attack of plasmid-mediated bacterial enzymes that can inactivate this drug: ① and ②, acetylase; ③, phosphorylase; ④, adenylylase. Amikacin is resistant to degradation at ②, ③, and ④.

cell. This may be chromosomal (eg, enterococci) or plasmid-controlled (eg, gram-negative bacteria). (2) The receptor (protein) on the 30S ribosomal subunit may be deleted or altered as a result of chromosomal mutation. (3) The microorganism acquires the ability to produce enzymes that destroy the aminoglycoside activity by adenylylation, acetylation, or phosphorylation. This is usually plasmid-controlled and is the principal type of resistance among gram-negative enteric bacteria. This transmissible resistance is of great clinical and epidemiologic concern. (4) In addition, facultative organisms growing under anaerobic conditions are usually resistant to aminoglycosides because of the oxygen-dependent transport process described above.

D. Absorption, Distribution, Metabolism, and Excretion: Aminoglycosides are absorbed poorly or not at all from the intact gastrointestinal tract but may be absorbed if ulcerations are present. Virtually the entire oral dose is excreted in feces. After intramuscular injection, aminoglycosides are absorbed well, giving peak concentrations in blood within 30–90 minutes. Only about 10% of the absorbed drugs are bound to plasma proteins. Occasionally, aminoglycosides are injected intravenously.

Being highly polar compounds, aminoglycosides do not enter cells readily and are largely excluded from the central nervous system and the eye. In the presence of active inflammation, cerebrospinal fluid levels reach 20% of plasma levels, and in neonatal meningitis the levels may be higher. In order to achieve greater levels of activity in these structures, the drugs must be introduced directly. Intrathecal or intraventricular injection is required for high levels in cerebrospinal fluid. After parenteral injection, concentrations of aminoglycosides are not high in most tissues except the renal cortex. Concentration in most secretions is also modest; in the bile, it may reach 30% of the blood level. Diffusion into pleural or synovial fluid may result in concentrations 50–90% of that of plasma with prolonged therapy. There is no significant metabolic breakdown. The half-life in serum is 2–3 hours. Excretion is mainly by glomerular filtration and is greatly reduced with impaired renal function. Aminoglycosides are partly and irregularly removed by hemodialysis, eg, 40–60% for gentamicin, and even less effectively by peritoneal dialysis.

In persons with impaired renal function, there is danger of drug accumulation and toxic effects. Therefore, either the dose of drug is kept constant and the interval between doses is increased, or the interval is kept constant and the dose is reduced. Nomograms and formulas have been constructed relating serum creatinine levels to adjustments in treatment regimens. The simplest formula divides the dose (calculated on the basis of normal renal function) by the serum creatinine value (mg/dL). Thus, a 60-kg patient with normal renal function might receive 300 mg/d of gentamicin given as 100 mg every 8 hours. A 60-kg patient with a serum creatinine of 3 mg/dL would receive 100 mg/d as 33.3 mg every 8 hours. However, there is considerable variation in aminoglycoside serum levels in different patients with similar serum creatinine values. Therefore, it is highly desirable, especially when using higher dosages, to monitor drug levels in blood in order to avoid severe toxicity. Peak levels should be obtained $1/2$–1 hour after infusion; trough levels should be obtained just prior to the next infusion (see Chapter 67).

E. Adverse Effects: Hypersensitivity occurs infrequently. All aminoglycosides can cause varying degrees of ototoxicity and nephrotoxicity. The ototoxicity can manifest itself either as hearing loss (cochlear damage), noted first with high-frequency tones, or as vestibular damage evident by vertigo, ataxia, and loss of balance. Nephrotoxicity results in rising serum creatinine levels or reduced creatinine clearance. In very high doses, aminoglycosides can be neurotoxic, producing a curarelike effect with neuromuscular blockade that results in respiratory paralysis. Calcium gluconate (given promptly) or neostigmine can serve as an antidote to this neurotoxic action.

F. Clinical Uses: Aminoglycosides are used most widely against gram-negative enteric bacteria or when there is suspicion of sepsis. In the treatment of bacteremia or endocarditis caused by fecal streptococci or some gram-negative bacteria, the aminoglycoside is given together with a penicillin that enhances permeability and facilitates the entry of the aminoglycoside. Aminoglycosides are selected according to recent susceptibility patterns in a given area or hospital until susceptibility tests become available on a specific isolate. All positively charged aminoglycosides and polymyxins are inhibited in blood cultures by sodium polyanethol sulfonate and other polyanionic detergents. Some aminoglycosides (especially streptomycin) are useful as antimycobacterial drugs.

STREPTOMYCINS

Streptomycin was isolated from a strain of *Streptomyces griseus* by Waksman and his associates in 1944. Dihydrostreptomycin can be produced by catalytic reduction of streptomycin trihydrochloride. Both streptomycin compounds have similar chemical and identical antimicrobial properties. However, dihydrostreptomycin is significantly more ototoxic than streptomycin and has been abandoned.

Streptomycin is a triacidic base with the empirical formula $C_{21}H_{39}N_7O_{12}$. It consists of streptidine, streptose, and N-methyl-L-glucosamine. The latter 2 components are referred to as streptobiosamine (see Fig 45–1).

Streptomycin sulfate is a white powder, quite soluble in water and insoluble in alcohol. Neutral solutions are stable for weeks at temperatures below 25 °C. Streptomycin is more active at alkaline pH. It can be inactivated by hydroxylamine or cysteine.

The antimicrobial activity of streptomycin is typical of that of other aminoglycosides, as are the mechanisms of resistance. Resistant microorganisms have emerged in most species, severely limiting the current usefulness of streptomycin, with the exceptions listed below. Streptomycin-dependent bacteria require the drug for growth. This results from a mutation in the receptor protein (P 12).

The emergence of resistance in an apparently susceptible isolate tends to be rapid, so that treatment with streptomycin as the sole drug is usually limited to 5 days.

Clinical Uses

A. Tuberculosis and Other Mycobacterial Infections: In pulmonary and other nondisseminated forms of tuberculosis, streptomycin, 1 g, is injected intramuscularly twice weekly or daily, as part of combined therapy. (When used in the treatment of tuberculosis, streptomycin is always combined with isoniazid, 5–10 mg/kg/d, or other drugs, for months.) In acute tuberculous pneumonia, miliary dissemination, or meningitis in children, up to 60 mg/kg/d intramuscularly should be administered initially in combination with isoniazid or other drugs. In meningitis, streptomycin, 25 mg dissolved in 10 mL saline, may be injected intrathecally.

B. Nontuberculous Infections: In systemic infections (eg, plague, tularemia), streptomycin, 2–4 g daily intramuscularly, is given in divided doses every 4–8 hours. A second drug may be added (see below).

C. Combined Treatment: In certain infections, penicillin plus an aminoglycoside may be required for eradication of organisms even though in vitro the bacteria appear to be resistant to serum levels of the aminoglycoside alone. For example, in enterococcal endocarditis, streptomycin, 1–2 g intramuscularly daily, may be given in addition to penicillin, 12–60 g intravenously daily (or ampicillin, 4–12 g intravenously daily), to achieve bactericidal levels in serum and clinical cure.

In *Streptococcus viridans* endocarditis, the addition of an aminoglycoside may also enhance the bactericidal action of penicillin. In tularemia and plague, streptomycin may be combined with tetracyclines.

Adverse Reactions

A. Allergy: Fever, skin rashes, and other allergic manifestations may result from hypersensitivity to streptomycin. This occurs most frequently upon prolonged contact with the drug, either in patients who receive a prolonged course of treatment (eg, for tuberculosis) or in medical personnel who handle the drug. (Nurses preparing solutions should wear gloves.) Desensitization is occasionally successful.

B. Toxicity: Pain at the injection site is common but usually not severe. The most serious toxic effect is disturbance of vestibular function—vertigo and loss of balance. The frequency and severity of this disturbance are proportionate to the age of the patient, the blood levels of the drug, and the duration of administration. Vestibular dysfunction may follow a few weeks of unusually high blood levels (eg, in individuals with impaired renal function) or months of relatively low blood levels. After the drug is discontinued, partial recovery frequently occurs.

The concurrent or sequential use of other aminoglycosides with streptomycin should be avoided to reduce the likelihood of ototoxicity. Streptomycin given during pregnancy can cause deafness in the newborn.

General Medical Problems From Overuse

Streptomycin-resistant bacteria have become prevalent as a result of widespread use of the drug, often in unnecessary combination with penicillin. Multiple drug resistance is frequent among bacteria in urinary tract infections, and the hospital transmission of such organisms aggravates treatment problems. Primary infection with streptomycin-resistant tubercle bacilli occurs in up to 15% of cases of pulmonary tuberculosis in children studied in the USA.

KANAMYCIN & NEOMYCIN

These drugs constitute a chemically and biologically closely related group. Neomycin was isolated by Waksman in 1949 from *Streptomyces fradiae;* kanamycin (Fig 45–2) was isolated by Umezawa in 1957 from *Streptomyces kanamyceticus.* Other members of the group are **framycetin** and **paromomycin.** All have similar properties.

Antimicrobial Activity

Drugs of the neomycin group are bactericidal in concentrations of 1–10 μg/mL for many gram-positive and gram-negative bacteria and mycobacteria. *Proteus* organisms are often susceptible, but *Pseudomonas* and streptococci are generally resistant. The mechanism of antibacterial action of the neomycin group is typical of the aminoglycosides. Neomycin can substitute for streptomycin in streptomycin-dependent organisms.

Resistance

Resistance mechanisms are the same as with other aminoglycosides. The widespread use of neomycin-kanamycin in bowel preparation for elective surgery of the colon has led to the selection of resistant organisms in some hospitals and outbreaks of enterocolitis. While cross-resistance between neomycin and kanamycin is complete, there is limited cross-resistance with other aminoglycosides.

Absorption, Metabolism, & Excretion

Drugs of the neomycin group are not significantly absorbed from the gastrointestinal tract. After oral administration, the intestinal flora is suppressed or modified and the drug is excreted in the feces.

After parenteral injection (0.5 g intramuscularly every 6–12 hours), serum levels reach 5–15 μg/mL. Excretion is mainly through glomerular filtration into the urine, where levels of 10–50 μg/mL may be reached. Some excretion also occurs in the bile. Because of toxicity, the parenteral administration of neomycin or kanamycin is now rarely considered.

Clinical Uses

These drugs are now limited mainly to topical and oral use.

A. Topical: Solutions containing 1–5 mg/mL are used on infected surfaces or injected into joints, the pleural cavity, tissue spaces, or abscess cavities where infection is present. The total amount of drug given in this fashion must be restricted because much of it can be absorbed, giving rise to systemic toxicity. Ointments containing 1–5 mg/g are applied to infected skin lesions or in the nares for suppression of staphylococci. Some ointments contain polymyxin and bacitracin in addition to neomycin.

B. Oral: For preoperative reduction of gut flora, 1 g every 4–6 hours is given for 1–2 days before surgery. Each dose is often combined with 1 g oral erythromycin base. In hepatic coma, the coliform flora can be suppressed for prolonged periods by giving 1 g every 6–8 hours, together with reduced protein intake, thus reducing ammonia intoxication. Paromomycin (Humatin), 1 g every 6 hours orally for 2 weeks, has been effective in intestinal amebiasis. Kanamycin or neomycin can suppress intestinal infection with enteropathogenic *Escherichia coli,* but they are not effective in the treatment of *Shigella* or *Salmonella* infections.

C. Parenteral: Kanamycin, 0.5 g every 6–12 hours intramuscularly (15 mg/kg/d), may be effective in the treatment of bacteremia caused by gram-negative enteric organisms. It is sometimes combined with clindamycin in penetrating abdominal wounds. The systemic use of kanamycin is now infrequent and largely limited to infants and children. Kanamycin is considered to be less toxic than neomycin.

Adverse Reactions

All members of the neomycin group have nephrotoxic and ototoxic side effects. Auditory function is affected more than vestibular. Deafness has occurred especially in adults with impaired renal function and prolonged elevated drug levels.

The sudden absorption of postoperatively instilled kanamycin from the peritoneal cavity (3–5 g) has resulted in curarelike neuromuscular blockade and respiratory arrest. Calcium gluconate and perhaps neostigmine can act as antidotes.

While hypersensitivity is not common, prolonged application of neomycin-containing ointments to skin and eyes has resulted in severe allergic dermatitis.

AMIKACIN

Amikacin is a semisynthetic derivative of kanamycin (Fig 45–2). It is relatively resistant to several of the enzymes that inactivate gentamicin and tobramycin, and it therefore can be employed against some microorganisms resistant to the latter drugs.

However, bacterial resistance due to impermeability to amikacin is increasing. Many gram-negative enteric bacteria, including many strains of *Proteus, Pseudomonas, Enterobacter,* and *Serratia,* are inhibited by 1–20 μg/mL amikacin in vitro. After the injection of 500 mg amikacin every 12 hours (15 mg/kg/d) intramuscularly, peak levels in serum are 10–30 μg/mL. Some infections caused by gram-negative bacteria resistant to gentamicin respond to amikacin. Central nervous system infections require intrathecal or intraventricular injection of 1–10 mg daily.

Like all aminoglycosides, amikacin is nephro- and ototoxic (particularly for the auditory portion of the eighth nerve). Its levels should be monitored in patients with renal failure. Concurrent use with diuretics (eg, furosemide, ethacrynic acid) should be avoided.

GENTAMICIN

Gentamicin is an aminoglycoside complex isolated from *Micromonospora purpurea.* It is effective against both gram-positive and gram-negative organisms, and many of its properties resemble those of other aminoglycosides. Sisomicin is very similar to the C_{1a} component of gentamicin.

Chemistry

The 3 active antibiotic components of gentamicin C have molecular weights of 450–475 and differ principally in methyl group content. The proposed structural formula is shown in Fig 45–2. The sulfate is used for intramuscular injection; it is soluble in water, and such solutions are stable for weeks.

Antimicrobial Activity

In concentrations of 0.5–5 μg/mL, gentamicin is rapidly bactericidal for many gram-positive and gram-negative bacteria. Gentamicin sulfate, 10 μg/mL, inhibits in vitro many strains of staphylococci, coliform organisms *(E coli, Klebsiella, Enterobacter),* *Pseudomonas aeruginosa, Proteus,* and *Serratia.*

The simultaneous use of carbenicillin or ticarcillin and gentamicin may result in synergistic enhancement and activity against some strains of *P aeruginosa* and may permit use of smaller doses of gentamicin. However, a penicillin and gentamicin cannot be mixed in vitro.

Resistance

Most streptococci are resistant to gentamicin but can be killed by synergistic mixtures of a cell wall–inhibitory drug (eg, penicillin) with gentamicin. This resistance is based on lack of transport of gentamicin into the cell. Among gram-negative bacteria, resistance to gentamicin is increasing somewhat in proportion to the amount of drug used in a given hospital environment. This resistance is most commonly attributable to the spread of plasmids that govern gentamicin-destroying enzymes. Organisms resistant to gentamicin are often resistant to kanamycin and sometimes to tobramycin but infrequently (as yet) to amikacin.

Clinical Uses

A. Intramuscular: Gentamicin is employed in severe infections caused by gram-negative bacteria that are likely (or proved) to be resistant to other less toxic drugs. Included are sepsis, infected burns, pneumonia, and other serious infections due to coliform organisms, *Klebsiella-Enterobacter, Proteus, Pseudomonas,* and *Serratia.* In these disorders, gentamicin is employed in full systemic doses: 5–7 mg/kg/d intramuscularly (or, rarely, intravenously) in 3 equal doses for 7–10 days. Renal, auditory, and vestibular functions should be monitored, particularly in patients with preexisting nitrogen retention. Direct enzymatic assays or radioimmunoassays of gentamicin concentration in serum are available. In renal failure, the dose must be significantly reduced (see p 534).

In urinary tract infections caused by these organisms, 0.8–1.2 mg/kg/d is injected intramuscularly in 2 or 3 equal divided doses for 10 days or more. Gentamicin may be employed together with penicillin for enhanced (synergistic) action against streptococcal endocarditis or gram-negative sepsis.

B. Topical: Creams, ointments, or solutions containing 0.1–0.3% gentamicin sulfate have been used for the treatment of infected burns, wounds, or skin lesions and the prevention of intravenous catheter infections. Topical gentamicin is partly inactivated by purulent exudates. However, such topical use must be restricted in hospitals to avoid favoring the development of resistant bacteria. Ten milligrams can be injected subconjunctivally.

C. Intrathecal: Meningitis caused by gram-negative bacteria has been treated by the intrathecal injection of gentamicin sulfate, 1–10 mg/d. In neonates, neither intrathecal nor intraventricular gentamicin was beneficial in meningitis, and intraventricular gentamicin was toxic. Epidural abscess, after aspiration, has been instilled with gentamicin, 20 mg/d for 10 days.

Adverse Reactions

These are analogous to the side effects of other aminoglycosides. Nephrotoxicity requires adjustment of regimens, especially in diminished renal function as described above. Whenever possible, gentamicin serum levels should serve as a guide in difficult clinical situations. Ototoxicity manifests itself mainly as vestibular dysfunction, perhaps due to destruction of hair cells by prolonged elevated drug levels (more than 10 μg/mL). Loss of hearing can occur and has occasionally been extensive and irreversible. The incidence of hypersensitivity reactions to gentamicin is poorly documented.

TOBRAMYCIN

This aminoglycoside (Fig 45–2) has an antibacterial spectrum similar to that of gentamicin. While there is some cross-resistance between gentamicin and tobramycin, it is unpredictable in individual strains. Separate laboratory susceptibility tests are therefore necessary.

The pharmacologic properties of tobramycin (Fig 45–2) are virtually identical to those of gentamicin. The daily dose of tobramycin is 5–7 mg/kg/d intramuscularly, divided in 3 equal amounts and given every 8 hours. About 80% of the drug is excreted by glomerular filtration into the urine within 24 hours of administration. In uremia, the drug dosage must be reduced. A formula for such dosage is 1 mg/kg every (6 × serum creatinine level) hours. However, monitoring blood levels in renal insufficiency is desirable. Tobramycin can be cleared somewhat during peritoneal dialysis and about 50% during hemodialysis.

Tobramycin has the same spectrum as gentamicin, principally against aerobic gram-negative enteric bacteria. It tends to be somewhat less active against *Serratia* and more active against *Pseudomonas*. Either tobramycin or gentamicin is the aminoglycoside most often employed in combination with ticarcillin against gram-negative bacterial sepsis or in combination with penicillin G against enterococcal endocarditis.

Like other aminoglycosides, tobramycin is ototoxic and nephrotoxic. Nephrotoxicity of tobramycin may be slightly less than that of gentamicin. It should not be used concurrently with other drugs having similar adverse effects or with diuretics, which tend to enhance aminoglycoside tissue concentrations.

NETILMICIN

This aminoglycoside became available in the USA in 1983. It shares many characteristics with gentamicin and tobramycin. However, the addition of an ethyl group to the 1-amino position of the 2-deoxystreptamine ring (ring II, Fig 45–2) sterically protects the netilmicin molecule from enzymatic degradation at the 3-amino (ring II) and 2-hydroxyl (ring III) positions. Consequently, it is expected that netilmicin will not be inactivated by many gentamicin-resistant and tobramycin-resistant bacteria.

The dosage (5–7 mg/kg/d) and the routes of administration are the same as for gentamicin. The principal indication for netilmicin may be iatrogenic infections in immunocompromised and severely ill patients at very high risk for gram-negative bacterial sepsis in the hospital setting.

It is believed that netilmicin may prove to be less ototoxic and possibly less nephrotoxic than the other aminoglycosides.

SPECTINOMYCIN

Spectinomycin is an aminocyclitol antibiotic (related to aminoglycosides) dispensed as the dihydrochloride pentahydrate for intramuscular injection. While active in vitro against many gram-positive and gram-negative organisms, spectinomycin is proposed only as an alternative treatment for gonorrhea in patients who might be hypersensitive to penicillin or whose gonococci are resistant to penicillin. Most gonococci are inhibited by 6 μg/mL of spectinomycin. About 10% of gonococci may be resistant to spectinomycin, but there is no cross-resistance with other drugs used in gonorrhea.

Spectinomycin is rapidly absorbed after intramuscular injection. A dose of 2 g injected intramuscularly once results in serum levels of 60–90 μg/mL and is said to result in cure of 90% of cases of gonorrhea. There is pain at the injection site and occasionally fever and nausea. Nephrotoxicity and anemia have been observed rarely.

THE POLYMYXIN GROUP

The polymyxins are a group of basic polypeptides selectively active against gram-negative bacilli. Polymyxins A, B, C, D, and E were derived from a spore-forming gram-positive bacillus *(Bacillus polymyxa, Bacillus aerosporus)* in 1947. All but polymyxins B and E have been discarded because of excessive nephrotoxicity. Colistin, introduced in 1950, is identical with polymyxin E.

Chemistry

All polymyxins are cationic, basic polypeptides with molecular weights of about 1400. All contain the fatty acid D-6-methyloctan-1-oic acid and the amino acids L-threonine and L-diaminobutyric acid. In addition, polymyxins B and E contain L-leucine; B contains D-phenylalanine; and E contains D-leucine. The sulfates of polymyxins are freely soluble in water and very stable. Methanesulfonate (sulfo-methyl) complexes can be prepared that slowly release the active peptide. One microgram of pure polymyxin B sulfate equals 10 units. The relationship between micrograms and units appears to be variable in the case of methanesulfonate complexes.

Antimicrobial Activity

The activity of polymyxin B sulfate is identical with that of polymyxin E (colistin) sulfate. Similarly, the methanesulfonate complexes of polymyxins B and E have the same activity. However, it is misleading to compare quantitatively the activity of the sulfate of one polymyxin with the methanesulfonate of another. Sulfates are used in disk tests and do not reflect methanesulfonate activity.

Polymyxins are active mainly against gram-negative bacilli, particularly *Pseudomonas* and coliform organisms. They are strongly bactericidal in concentrations of 1–5 μg/mL. They act by attaching to the cell membranes of bacteria and other membranes rich in phosphatidylethanolamine and disrupting the osmotic properties and transport mechanisms of the membrane. This results in leakage of macromolecules and death of the cell. This action is inhibited by cations. The action of polymyxins is markedly inhibited by purulent exudates.

Resistance

Proteus sp, gram-positive organisms, and neisseriae are highly resistant. This is probably due to the impermeability of the outer membrane to polymyxins. In susceptible bacterial populations, resistant mutants are rare. There is complete cross-resistance between polymyxin B and polymyxin E.

Absorption, Metabolism, & Excretion

Polymyxins are not absorbed from the gastrointestinal tract.

With parenterally injected polymyxins (2.5 mg/kg/d), blood levels rarely exceed 1–4 μg/mL. Tissue concentrations are even lower. Polymyxins pass the placenta but do not reach the central nervous system or cerebrospinal fluid unless injected intrathecally. They do not reach joint fluids or ocular tissues unless injected locally. Polymyxins are strongly bound by cell debris, acid phospholipids, and purulent exudates. They do not penetrate cells, and phagocytosed or intracellular bacteria are therefore unaffected.

Excretion is mainly in the urine, where concentrations of 25–300 μg/mL may be reached during prolonged administration. Excretion is impaired in renal insufficiency.

Clinical Uses

Polymyxins once were drugs of choice for the treatment of infections caused by *Pseudomonas* or coliform bacteria resistant to other antimicrobial drugs. Polymyxin treatment is now severely limited.

A. Topical: Solutions containing 1 mg/mL of polymyxin B or E sulfate can be applied to wounds, burns, sinuses, and other surfaces infected with *P aeruginosa* or other resistant microorganisms. Similar solutions (up to a total dose of 2.5 mg/kg/d) can be injected intrapleurally or intraperitoneally. Solutions of 1–10 mg/mL are inhaled as aerosols in *Pseudomonas* infections of the bronchi and lungs. Up to 20 mg of polymyxin B sulfate may be injected subconjunctivally in *Pseudomonas* infections of the eye. Ointments containing 0.5 mg/g of polymyxin B sulfate in mixture with bacitracin or neomycin (or both) are commonly applied to infected skin lesions. Solutions containing polymyxin B, 20 mg/L, and neomycin, 40 mg/L, can be employed as antiseptic for continuous irrigation of the urinary bladder through a 3-way catheter in a closed sterile system. This can delay bacterial contamination of the drainage system.

B. Intrathecal: In *Pseudomonas* meningitis, the intrathecal injection of polymyxin B or E sulfate, 2–10 mg in saline daily for 2–3 days, and then every other day for 2–3 weeks, can be curative. Polymyxin methanesulfonates are never given intrathecally.

C. Intramuscular: The intramuscular injection of polymyxin sulfates is painful and requires the simultaneous administration of a local anesthetic. For

this reason, the methanesulfonate complex, which sometimes includes a local anesthetic and slowly releases active drug after intramuscular injection, is preferred. The total systemic dose can be 2.5–5 mg/kg/d. It can be used in urinary tract infections with *Pseudomonas, Enterobacter,* or other coliforms resistant to less toxic drugs. *Salmonella* infections do not respond to polymyxins in spite of in vitro susceptibility.

D. Intravenous: In serious infections, the intravenous injection of polymyxin B sulfate is preferable. The intravenous injection by slow drip of 2.5 mg/kg/d of polymyxin B sulfate in 5% dextrose in water is indicated in *Pseudomonas* bacteremia or peritonitis (eg, after peritoneal dialysis). When renal function is impaired, the drug may be administered in full doses once every 3–5 days. Hemodialysis does not remove polymyxins rapidly.

E. Oral: Polymyxins are not absorbed from the gut but have been used to suppress aerobic gram-negative members of the intestinal flora in immunosuppressed persons for "prophylaxis."

Adverse Reactions

The general toxicity of polymyxins limits both the dose and the duration of therapy. The sulfates produce intense local pain. The principal side effects are neurotoxicity and nephrotoxicity. Hypersensitivity appears to be very rare. Very high blood levels (> 30 μg/mL) of any polymyxin can cause respiratory arrest. Respiratory paralysis caused by polymyxins can be reversed by calcium gluconate.

A. Neurotoxic Effects: Adequate systemic concentrations of any polymyxin can cause paresthesias (circumoral and stocking or glove distribution), dizziness, flushing, and incoordination. All of these disappear promptly when the drug has been discontinued and excreted.

B. Nephrotoxic Effects: Some proteinuria, hematuria, or cylindruria commonly accompanies the administration of polymyxin B or E and is evidence of tubular injury. These urinary signs usually disappear soon after the drug is discontinued. In individuals with preexisting renal disease, nitrogen retention must be monitored and the dose of polymyxin adjusted. Accidental overdosage may result in renal failure, neuromuscular paralysis, and even death.

Laboratory

The large molecules of the polymyxins diffuse poorly through agar. Consequently, disk tests reveal very narrow zones of inhibition even with fully susceptible microorganisms. Colistin disks contain sulfate, not methanesulfonate.

Use for Resistant Organisms

Polymyxins may again become important because of the increasing numbers of patients infected with *Pseudomonas* and *Enterobacter* resistant to other drugs. These are often hospitalized patients with immunosuppression and impaired renal function who require careful adjustments of a polymyxin regimen.

REFERENCES

Appel JB, Neu HC: The nephrotoxicity of antimicrobial agents. (3 parts.) *N Engl J Med* 1977;**296:**663, 722, 784.

Bennett WW et al: Drug therapy in renal failure. *Ann Intern Med* 1980;**93:**62.

Blair DC: Inactivation of amikacin and gentamicin by carbenicillin in patients with end-stage renal failure. *Antimicrob Agents Chemother* 1982;**22:**376.

Brynan LE et al: Mechanism of aminoglycoside antibiotic resistance in anaerobic bacteria. *Antimicrob Agents Chemother* 1979;**15:**7.

Calderwood SB, Moellering RC: Common adverse effects of antibacterial agents on major organ systems. *Surg Clin North Am* 1980;**60:**65.

Chan RA et al: Gentamicin therapy in renal failure: A dosage nomogram. *Ann Intern Med* 1972;**76:**773.

Davis SD: Polymyxins, colistin, vancomycin and bacitracin. Chap 6, pp 77–83, in: *Antimicrobial Therapy,* 3rd ed. Kagan BM (editor). Saunders, 1980.

Egan EA et al: Prospective controlled trial of oral kanamycin in prevention of neonatal necrotizing enterocolitis. *J Pediatr* 1976;**89:**467.

Finitzohieber T et al: Ototoxicity in neonates treated with gentamicin and kanamycin: Results of a 4-year controlled follow-up study. *Pediatrics* 1979;**63:**443.

Kaiser AB, McGee ZA: Aminoglycoside therapy of gram-negative bacillary meningitis. *N Engl J Med* 1975;**293:**1215.

Klastersky J et al: Comparative clinical study of tobramycin and gentamicin. *Antimicrob Agents Chemother* 1974;**5:**133.

Krogstad DJ et al: Plasmid-mediated resistance to antibiotic synergism in enterococci. *J Clin Invest* 1978;**61:**1645.

Love LJ et al: Randomized trial of empiric antibiotic therapy with ticarcillin in combination with gentamicin, amikacin or netilmicin in febrile patients with granulocytopenia and cancer. *Am J Med* 1979;**66:**603.

Maigaard S, Frimodt-Moller N, Madsen PO: Comparison of netilmicin and amikacin in treatment of complicated urinary tract infections. *Antimicrob Agents Chemother* 1978;**14:**554.

McCormack WM, Finland M: Spectinomycin. *Ann Intern Med* 1976;**84:**712.

McCracken GH: Clinical pharmacology of gentamicin in infants. *Am J Dis Child* 1972;**124:**884.

McCracken GH et al: Intraventricular gentamicin therapy in gram-negative bacillary meningitis of infancy. *Lancet* 1980; **1:**787.

Meyer RD: Drugs five years later: Amikacin. *Ann Intern Med* 1981;**95:**328.

Moellering RC et al: Experience with tobramycin therapy of infections due to gentamicin-resistant organisms. *J Infect Dis* 1976;**134(Suppl):**S40.

Murillo J et al: Gentamicin and ticarcillin serum levels. *JAMA* 1979;**241:**2401.

Neu HC: Tobramycin: An overview. *J Infect Dis* 1976;**134 (Suppl):**S3.

Riff LJ, Jackson GG: Conditions for gentamicin inactivation by carbenicillin. *Arch Intern Med* 1972;**130:**887.

Sarubbi FA, Hull JH: Amikacin serum concentrations: Prediction of levels and dosage guidelines. *Ann Intern Med* 1978;**89:**612.

Smith CR et al: Double-blind comparison of the nephrotoxicity and auditory toxicity of gentamicin and tobramycin. *N Engl J Med* 1980;**302:**1106.

Snavely SR, Hodges GR: The neurotoxicity of antibacterial agents. *Ann Intern Med* 1984;**101:**92.

Swartz MN: Intraventricular use of aminoglycosides in the treatment of gram-negative bacillary meningitis: Conflicting views. *J Infect Dis* 1981;**143:**293.

Tai PC et al: Streptomycin causes misreading of natural messenger by interacting with ribosomes after initiation. *Proc Natl Acad Sci USA* 1978;**75:**275.

Wolfson JS, Swartz MN: Serum bactericidal activity as a monitor of antibiotic therapy. *N Engl J Med* 1985;**312:**968.

Zaske DE et al: Wide interpatient variations in gentamicin dose requirements for geriatric patients. *JAMA* 1982;**248:**3122.

Antimycobacterial Drugs

46

Ernest Jawetz, MD, PhD

Mycobacterial infections may be symptomatic or asymptomatic but typically are very chronic. Therapy thus presents unusual problems. This chapter describes drugs used for tuberculosis (*Mycobacterium tuberculosis* infections), infections of clinical significance caused by various "atypical" mycobacteria, and leprosy (*Mycobacterium leprae* infections). Most of these mycobacterial infections are now controllable by specific chemotherapy, and earlier methods of rest, sunshine, and collapse therapy have been abandoned.

DRUGS USED IN TUBERCULOSIS

Streptomycin was the first antimicrobial drug to exhibit striking action against tubercle bacilli. It remains an important agent in the management of severe tuberculosis, but it is now rarely one of the initially selected drugs. First-line drugs now are isoniazid, rifampin, and ethambutol for initial treatment, with streptomycin as an alternative first-line drug. Several agents that are drugs of second choice in the treatment of tuberculosis are mentioned here only briefly.

Singular problems exist in the treatment of tuberculosis and related mycobacterial infections. The infections tend to be exceedingly chronic but may also give rise to hyperacute, lethal complications. The organisms are frequently intracellular, exhibit long periods of metabolic inactivity, and tend to develop resistance to any one drug. All these points contribute to the complexity of antituberculosis therapy.

To delay the rapid emergence of resistance in the large mycobacterial populations that occur in clinically active tuberculosis, combinations of first-line drugs are employed. If the organisms are susceptible to these drugs, the patient usually becomes noninfective within 2–3 weeks. While treatment in tuberculous meningitis or miliary tuberculosis is usually continued for 18–24 months, this length of treatment is no longer needed in uncomplicated pulmonary tuberculosis, the most common clinical presentation. With the most effective "bactericidal" drug combination of isoniazid and rifampin, "short-course" schedules of 6–9 months of therapy give satisfactory results. Thus, the vast majority of patients require little hospitalization.

ISONIAZID (INH)

Isoniazid, introduced in 1952, is the most active drug for the treatment of patients who can tolerate it and whose mycobacteria are susceptible.

Chemistry
Isoniazid is the hydrazide of isonicotinic acid, often called INH. It is a small (MW 137), simple molecule freely soluble in water. The structural similarity to pyridoxine is shown below.

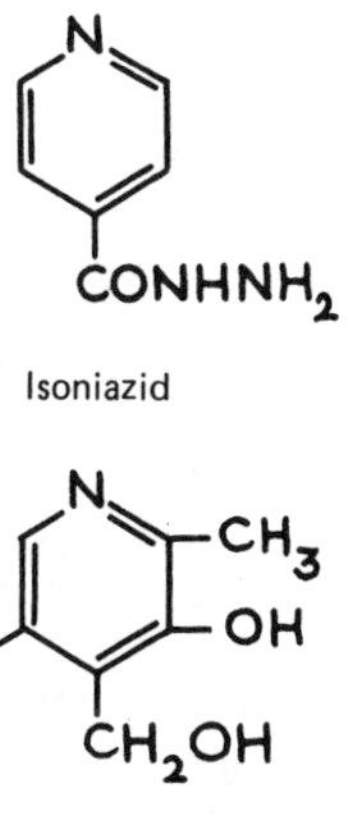

Isoniazid

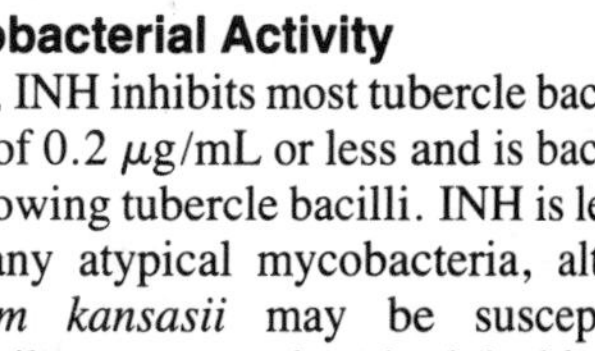

Pyridoxine

Antimycobacterial Activity
In vitro, INH inhibits most tubercle bacilli in a concentration of 0.2 μg/mL or less and is bactericidal for actively growing tubercle bacilli. INH is less effective against many atypical mycobacteria, although *Mycobacterium kansasii* may be susceptible. INH reaches similar concentrations both inside and outside animal cells and thus is able to act on intracellular mycobacteria as well as extracellular ones. Resistant mutants occur in susceptible mycobacterial populations with a frequency of about 1 in 10^6. Since tuberculous lesions often contain more than 10^7 tubercle bacilli, resistant mutants would be readily selected out if INH were to be given as the sole drug. There is no cross-resistance between INH, rifampin, and ethambutol. The simultaneous use of any 2 of these drugs markedly delays the emergence of resistance to any one of them.

The mechanism of action of INH is not fully understood. It apparently involves the inhibition of synthesis of mycolic acids, thus interfering with the formation of mycobacterial cell walls. INH and pyridoxine are structural analogs, and INH exerts competitive antagonism in pyridoxine-catalyzed reactions in *Escherichia coli*. However, this mechanism is not involved in the antituberculosis action. The administration of large doses of pyridoxine to patients receiving INH does not interfere with tuberculostatic action of INH, but it prevents neuritis.

Absorption, Metabolism, & Excretion

INH is readily absorbed from the gastrointestinal tract. The administration of usual doses (5 mg/kg/d) results in peak plasma concentrations of 3–5 μg/mL within 1–2 hours. INH diffuses readily into all body fluids and tissues. The concentration in the central nervous system and cerebrospinal fluid is about one-fifth of the plasma level. The intracellular and extracellular levels are similar.

The metabolism—particularly the acetylation—of INH is under genetic control. Two groups of people can be recognized: the "slow" and the "rapid" inactivators of the drug through acetylation. High acetyl transferase activity results in fast INH inactivation and is inherited as an autosomal dominant trait. The average concentration of active INH in the plasma of rapid inactivators is about one-third to one-half of that in slow inactivators. The average half-life of INH in rapid inactivators is less than 1½ hours, whereas in slow inactivators the half-life is 3 hours. It has been claimed that rapid acetylators are more prone to hepatic toxicity of INH, but this has not been confirmed. About half of white and of black persons in the USA are slow inactivators, whereas many Eskimos, Native Americans, and Orientals are rapid inactivators. The rate of acetylation has little influence in daily dose regimens but may impair antimycobacterial activity in intermittent (1–2 times weekly) administration of INH.

INH is excreted mainly in the urine—partly as unchanged drug, partly as the acetylated form, and partly as other conjugates. The amount of unchanged, free INH in the urine is higher in slow inactivators. In renal failure, normal doses of INH can usually be given, but in severe hepatic insufficiency the dose must be reduced.

Clinical Uses

Isoniazid is probably the most widely useful drug in tuberculosis. In active, clinically manifest disease, it is given in conjunction with ethambutol, rifampin, or streptomycin. The usual dose is 5 mg/kg/d (maximum for adults, 300 mg daily). Twice that dose is sometimes used in severe illness and meningitis, but there is little evidence that the higher dose (10 mg/kg/d) is more effective in adults. Children should receive 10 mg/kg/d, and for maintenance therapy after initial improvement, 15 mg/kg twice weekly is sometimes given. Pyridoxine, 10 mg per 100 mg of isoniazid, should be given to prevent neuritis.

Children or adults converting from negative to positive tuberculin skin tests may be given INH, 5–10 mg/kg/d (maximum 300 mg/d), for 1 year as prophylaxis against the 5–15% risk of meningitis or miliary dissemination. For prophylaxis, INH is given as the sole drug. In addition to skin test converters without active disease, prophylactic INH is also suggested for household and other very close contacts (especially children but also residents of nursing homes) of freshly recognized active cases; and for skin test–positive persons who undergo immunosuppressive or antineoplastic chemotherapy and have not received adequate antimycobacterial treatment in the past.

INH is usually given by mouth but can be injected parenterally in the same dosage.

In some parts of the world INH has been used as a single drug in the treatment of clinically active tuberculosis, with large mycobacterial populations. Predictably, INH-resistant mutants were selected out. The presence of such resistant mutants in migrants from Southeast Asia is creating major treatment problems. Tuberculosis in such migrants should be started with INH, rifampin, and ethambutol until drug susceptibility tests are completed.

Adverse Reactions

The incidence and severity of untoward reactions to INH are related to dosage and duration of administration.

A. Allergic Reactions: Fever, skin rashes, and hepatitis are occasionally seen.

B. Direct Toxicity: The most common toxic effect (10–20%) are on the peripheral and central nervous systems. These have been attributed to a relative pyridoxine deficiency, perhaps resulting from competition of INH with pyridoxal phosphate for an enzyme (apotryptophanase). These toxic reactions include peripheral neuritis, insomnia, restlessness, muscle twitching, urinary retention, and even convulsions and psychotic episodes. Most of these complications can be prevented by the administration of pyridoxine, and accidental INH overdose can be treated with pyridoxine in amounts equivalent to the INH ingested.

INH can reduce the metabolism of phenytoin, increasing its blood level and toxicity. With prolonged use on a large scale in chemoprophylaxis, INH has been associated with hepatotoxicity. Abnormal liver function tests, clinical jaundice, and multilobular necrosis have been observed. In large groups, about 1% of persons develop clinical hepatitis and up to 10% subclinical abnormalities. Some fatalities have occurred. Hepatitis with progressive liver damage is age-dependent. It occurs rarely under age 20, in 1.5% of those between 30 and 50, and in 2.5% of older persons. The risk of hepatitis with permanent damage significantly influences the decision for the prophylactic use of INH.

In glucose-6-phosphate dehydrogenase deficiency, INH may cause hemolysis.

RIFAMPIN

Rifampin is a large (MW 823), complex semisynthetic derivative of rifamycin, an antibiotic produced by *Streptomyces mediterranei*. It is active in vitro against some gram-positive and gram-negative cocci, some enteric bacteria, mycobacteria, chlamydiae, and poxviruses. While many meningococci and mycobacteria are inhibited by less than 1 μg/mL, highly resistant mutants occur in all microbial populations in a frequency of 1 in 10^7 or greater. The administration of rifampin as a single drug permits the emergence of these highly resistant organisms. There is no cross-resistance to other antimicrobial drugs. Rifampin resistance may be due to a permeability barrier or to a mutation of the DNA-dependent RNA polymerase.

Rifampin binds strongly to DNA-dependent RNA polymerase and thus inhibits RNA synthesis in bacteria and chlamydiae. Human RNA polymerase is not affected. Rifampin blocks a late stage in the assembly of poxviruses, perhaps interfering with envelope formation. When administered together with INH, rifampin is usually bactericidal for mycobacteria and tends to sterilize infected tissues, cavities, or sputum. Rifampin penetrates phagocytic cells well and can kill intracellular mycobacteria and other organisms.

Rifampin is well absorbed after oral administration, widely distributed in tissues, and excreted mainly through the liver into bile. It then undergoes enterohepatic recirculation, with the bulk excreted in feces and a small amount in the urine. Usual doses result in serum levels of 5–7 μg/mL, and cerebrospinal fluid levels are between 10 and 40% of serum levels. Rifampin is distributed widely in body fluids and tissues.

In tuberculosis, a single oral dose of rifampin, usually 600 mg daily (10–20 mg/kg), is administered together with INH, ethambutol, or another antituberculosis drug in order to delay the emergence of rifampin-resistant mycobacteria. A similar regimen may apply to atypical mycobacteria. Rifampin is effective in leprosy when used together with a sulfone.

An oral dose of 600 mg twice daily for 2 days can eliminate a majority of meningococci from carriers. Unfortunately, some highly resistant meningococcal strains are selected out by this procedure. Up to 10% of treated meningococcus carriers may exhibit rifampin-resistant organisms. Rifampin, 20 mg/kg/d for 4 days, is used as prophylaxis in contacts of children with *Haemophilus influenzae* type b disease. In urinary tract infections and in chronic bronchitis, the use of rifampin rapidly selects resistant mutants and thus has no place in clinical therapy.

Rifampin imparts a harmless orange color to urine, sweat, tears, and contact lenses. Occasional adverse effects include rashes, thrombocytopenia, nephritis, and impairment of liver function. Rifampin commonly causes light chain proteinuria and may impair antibody response. If administered less often than twice weekly, rifampin causes a "flu syndrome" of uncertain nature and anemia. Rifampin induces microsomal enzymes involved in drug metabolism. Thus, it increases the elimination of anticoagulants (eg, warfarin) and may impose a need for a higher dose of anticoagulant. Likewise, administration of rifampin with ketaconazole or with chloramphenicol results in significantly lower serum levels of these drugs. Rifampin increases the urinary excretion of methadone, lowers its plasma concentration, and may result in "methadone withdrawal" signs.

Caution: The indiscriminate use of rifampin for minor infections may favor the widespread selection of rifampin-resistant mycobacteria and thus deprive the drug of most of its usefulness.

ETHAMBUTOL

This is a synthetic, water-soluble, heat-stable compound, the D isomer of the structure shown below, dispensed as the dihydrochloride salt.

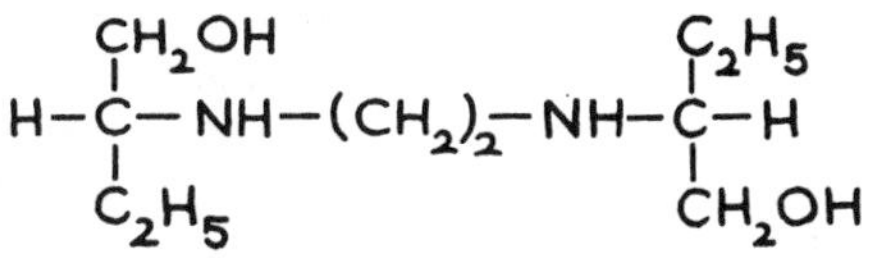

Ethambutol

Many strains of *M tuberculosis* and other mycobacteria are inhibited in vitro by ethambutol, 1–5 μg/mL. The mechanism of action is not known.

Ethambutol is well absorbed from the gut. Following ingestion of 25 mg/kg, a blood level peak of 2–5 μg/mL is reached in 2–4 hours. About 20% of the drug is excreted in feces and 50% in urine in unchanged form. Excretion is delayed in renal failure. About 15% of absorbed drug is metabolized by oxidation and conversion to a dicarboxylic acid. In meningitis, ethambutol appears in the cerebrospinal fluid to the extent of 10–40% of serum levels.

Resistance to ethambutol emerges fairly rapidly among mycobacteria when the drug is used alone. Therefore, ethambutol is given in combination with other antituberculosis drugs.

Ethambutol hydrochloride, 15 mg/kg, is usually given as a single dose in combination with INH or rifampin. At times, the dose is 25 mg/kg/d.

Hypersensitivity to ethambutol is rare. The commonest side effects are visual disturbances: reduction in visual acuity, optic neuritis, and perhaps retinal damage occur in some patients given 25 mg/kg/d for several months. Most of these changes apparently regress when ethambutol is discontinued. However, periodic visual acuity testing is desirable during treatment. With doses of 15 mg/kg/d, visual disturbances are very rare.

STREPTOMYCIN

The pharmacologic features of streptomycin have been discussed in Chapter 45. It is assumed that the mechanism of action of streptomycin against mycobacteria is the same as that against other microorganisms. Most tubercle bacilli are inhibited by streptomycin, $1-10$ μg/mL, in vitro. Most "atypical" mycobacteria are resistant to streptomycin in pharmacologic concentrations. All large populations of tubercle bacilli contain some streptomycin-resistant mutants. On the average, 1 in 10^8 to 1 in 10^{10} tubercle bacilli can be expected to be resistant to streptomycin at levels of $10-100$ μg/mL. Some of these mutants survive the in vivo exposure to therapeutic concentrations of streptomycin if given alone. This results in "treatment resistance" of clinical tuberculosis. Therefore, streptomycin is employed in combination with another drug effective against tubercle bacilli. Combined treatment can markedly delay the emergence of streptomycin-resistant mutants. It is estimated that among primary infections in children in 1970, about 15% were caused by streptomycin-resistant *M tuberculosis*.

Streptomycin exerts its action mainly on extracellular tubercle bacilli. Only about 10% of the drug penetrates cells that harbor intracellular organisms. Thus, even if the entire microbial population were streptomycin-susceptible, at any one moment a large percentage of the tubercle bacilli would be unaffected by streptomycin. Treatment for many months is therefore required.

Streptomycin sulfate remains an important drug in the treatment of tuberculosis. It is employed principally in individuals with severe, possibly life-threatening forms of tuberculosis, particularly miliary dissemination, and extensive, active pulmonary or renal involvement. The usual dosage is 1 g intramuscularly daily for adults ($20-40$ mg/kg/d for children) for several weeks, followed by 1 g intramuscularly $2-3$ times weekly for several months. Other drugs are always given simultaneously.

Intrathecal injection of streptomycin in tuberculous meningitis has been largely abandoned, because other drugs such as INH or ethambutol appear in the cerebrospinal fluid. However, the use of streptomycin must still be considered, particularly for INH-resistant mycobacteria.

The eighth nerve toxicity of streptomycin injected intramuscularly for many weeks manifests itself principally as dysfunction of the labyrinth, resulting in inability to maintain equilibrium and in deafness. The latter is often permanent, but some compensation for the former often occurs.

ALTERNATIVE SECOND-LINE DRUGS IN TUBERCULOSIS TREATMENT

Because of their antimicrobial efficacy and their relative clinical safety, first-line drugs in tuberculosis in 1985–1986 are isoniazid, rifampin, ethambutol, and streptomycin. The alternative drugs listed below are usually considered only (1) in the case of resistance to the drugs of first choice, which occurs with increasing frequency; (2) in case of failure of clinical re-

sponse to conventional therapy; and (3) when expert guidance is available to deal with the toxic side effects. For most of the second-line drugs listed below, the dosage, emergence of resistance, and long-term toxicity have not been fully established.

Capreomycin

Capreomycin is a peptide antibiotic obtained from *Streptomyces capreolus*. Daily injection of 1 g intramuscularly results in blood levels of 10 μg/mL or more. Such concentrations in vitro are inhibitory for several mycobacteria. There is some cross-resistance between capreomycin, viomycin, and kanamycin. Capreomycin (20 mg/kg/d) can perhaps take the place of the latter drugs in combined antituberculosis therapy. The most serious toxicity is for the kidney, resulting in nitrogen retention, and for the eighth nerve, resulting in deafness and vestibular disturbances. Toxicity is less marked if 1 g is given 2 or 3 times weekly, and such a schedule is sometimes used.

Cycloserine

Cycloserine is an antibiotic analog of D-alanine. Oral doses of 250 mg 3 times daily result in blood levels of $15-25$ μg/mL. This is sufficient to inhibit many strains of tubercle bacilli. The most serious toxic reactions are various central nervous system dysfunctions and psychotic reactions. Some of these can be controlled by phenytoin, 100 mg/d orally.

The dosage of cycloserine in tuberculosis is $0.5-1$ g/d. Cycloserine has been used in urinary tract infections in doses of $15-20$ mg/kg/d.

Cycloserine is discussed further in Chapter 51.

Ethionamide

This yellow crystalline substance is stable and almost insoluble in water. It is a close chemical relative of isoniazid.

In spite of this similarity, there is no cross-resistance between isoniazid and ethionamide. Most tubercle bacilli are inhibited in vitro by ethionamide, 2.5 μg/mL, or less. Many photochromogenic mycobacteria are also inhibited by ethionamide, 10 μg/mL. Such concentrations in plasma and tissues are achieved by daily oral doses of 1 g. This dosage is effective in the clinical treatment of tuberculosis, but is poorly tolerated because of the intense gastric irritation and neurologic symptoms it causes. A dose of 0.5 g orally per day is better tolerated but not very effective. Resistance to ethionamide develops rapidly in vitro and in vivo. Consequently, this drug can be used only in combination with other antituberculosis drugs.

Ethionamide

Pyrazinamide (PZA)

This relative of nicotinamide is stable, slightly soluble in water, and quite inexpensive.

At neutral pH, it is inactive in vitro, but at pH 5.0 it strongly inhibits the growth of tubercle bacilli within cells in concentrations of 15 μg/mL. Such concentrations are achieved by daily oral doses of 20–30 mg/kg, given as 0.5 g 4 times daily or 0.75 g twice daily. Pyrazinamide is well absorbed from the gastrointestinal tract and widely distributed in body tissues. Tubercle bacilli develop resistance to pyrazinamide fairly readily, but there is no cross-resistance with isoniazid. Satisfactory clinical effects can be achieved with this drug, but toxicity can be significant, particularly impairment of liver function. In general, pyrazinamide is used only in combined drug regimens against mycobacteria resistant to first-line drugs; but sometimes it is given (50mg/kg twice weekly) as a first-line drug in short-course treatment with other drugs.

Pyrazinamide (PZA)

Aminosalicylic Acid (PAS)

Among several derivatives of salicylic and benzoic acids, p-aminosalicylic acid has the most marked effect on tubercle bacilli.

The structural formula of PAS reveals its close similarity to p-aminobenzoic acid (PABA) and to the sulfonamides (see Chapter 47).

Aminosalicylic acid (PAS)

PAS is a white crystalline powder only slightly soluble in water and rapidly destroyed by heat. The sodium salt is freely soluble in water and relatively stable at room temperature.

Most bacteria are not affected by PAS. Tubercle bacilli are usually inhibited in vitro by PAS, 1–5 μg/mL, but "atypical" mycobacteria are resistant. In susceptible mycobacterial populations, resistant mutants occur and tend to emerge in vitro and in vivo during exposure to PAS. The simultaneous use of a second drug with antimycobacterial activity tends to delay this emergence of resistance.

It is likely that PAS and PABA compete for the active center of an enzyme involved in converting PABA to dihydropteroic acid. The receptors for PABA attachment must be quite specific, because PAS is ineffective against most bacteria whereas sulfonamides are ineffective against tubercle bacilli.

PAS is readily absorbed from the gastrointestinal tract. Average daily doses (8–12 g) tend to give blood levels of 10 μg/mL or more. The drug is widely distributed in tissues and body fluids except the cerebrospinal fluid. PAS is rapidly excreted in the urine, in part as active PAS and in part as the acetylated compound and other metabolic products. Very high concentrations of PAS are reached in the urine. To avoid crystalluria, the urine must be kept alkaline.

Aminosalicylic acid was employed in the past together with isoniazid or streptomycin, or both, in the long-term treatment of tuberculosis. It is used infrequently now because other oral drugs are better tolerated. The dosage is 8–12 g daily orally for adults and 300 mg/kg/d for children.

Gastrointestinal symptoms often accompany full doses of PAS. Anorexia, nausea, diarrhea, and epigastric pain and burning may all be diminished by giving PAS with meals and with antacids. Peptic ulceration and hemorrhage may occur. Kidney or liver damage, thyroid gland injury (goiter with or without myxedema), and metabolic acidosis are rare.

Drug fever, joint pains, skin rashes, granulocytopenia, and a variety of neurologic symptoms—all probably due to hypersensitivity—often occur after 3–8 weeks of PAS therapy, making it necessary to stop PAS administration temporarily or permanently.

Viomycin

This antibiotic is produced by certain *Streptomyces* organisms. It is a complex basic polypeptide dispensed as a neutral sulfate that is very soluble in water. Most strains of tubercle bacilli are inhibited in vitro by viomycin, 1–10 μg/mL. Such concentrations can be achieved by the injection of 2 g intramuscularly twice weekly. Tubercle bacilli resistant to viomycin emerge fairly rapidly. There is also some cross-resistance with streptomycin, kanamycin, and capreomycin. Therefore, viomycin—if used at all—must be used in combination with other drugs to delay the emergence of resistance. The most serious toxic side effects are damage to the kidney and to the eighth nerve, resulting in loss of equilibrium and deafness. Toxic effects are more serious than with streptomycin.

Ansamycin

This antibiotic is derived from rifamycin and is related to rifampin. It has significant activity against *M tuberculosis* and several atypical mycobacteria, especially *Mycobacterium avium-intracellulare* (see p 547). Its role in therapy and its toxicity are not well defined at present.

Other Antimycobacterial Drugs

Kanamycin and **tetracyclines** have been employed in combined therapy of tuberculosis. These drugs can inhibit tubercle bacilli in concentrations that may be achieved in vivo. However, they are much less effective than the drugs of first choice. They are at times useful in treatment of infections due to "atypical" mycobacteria (see p 547).

SHORT-COURSE TUBERCULOSIS CHEMOTHERAPY

Based on several recent trials, a marked change in chemotherapy for uncomplicated pulmonary tuberculosis has developed. Traditional treatment programs have been based on 18–24 months of drug therapy. Newer schemes of drug combinations for 6–12 months, involving daily or twice weekly therapy, have achieved good success in inducing complete remissions at least on short-term follow-up.

It must be stressed that these schemes apply *only* to uncomplicated pulmonary tuberculosis and regimens that contain *both* isoniazid (INH) and rifampin with or without other drugs. In adults, 300 mg of INH and 600 mg of rifampin are given daily. Children receive INH, 10 mg/kg/d up to 300 mg/d, and rifampin, 10–20 mg/ kg/d up to 600 mg/d. Ethambutol, 15 mg/kg/d, should be added if the patient resides in or has come from an area with a high level of initial drug resistance. This daily regimen continues for 2–8 weeks, depending on clinical and x-ray evidence of response and speed of sputum conversion. Subsequently, INH, 15 mg/kg, can be given twice weekly (eg, 900 mg of INH twice weekly for a 60-kg adult) and rifampin, 600 mg twice weekly. Intermittently, patients must be monitored for thrombocytopenia. The total treatment time is 9–12 months, at least 6 months beyond conversion of sputum culture to negative.

Other short-course treatments have been proposed.

DRUGS AGAINST ATYPICAL MYCOBACTERIA

About 10% of mycobacterial infections seen in clinical practice in the USA are not caused by *M tuberculosis* or *M leprae* but by "atypical" mycobacteria. These organisms have distinctive laboratory characteristics, occur in the environment, are generally not communicable from person to person, and are sometimes resistant to several antituberculosis drugs. Disease caused by these organisms is often not as severe as tuberculosis and occurs in individuals without contact with tuberculosis yet yielding acid-fast mycobacteria in smears. Chest x-rays may be negative. A few representative pathogens, with the clinical presentation and with the drugs to which they are often susceptible, are given in Table 46–1. Some atypical mycobacteria, especially the *M avium-intracellulare* complex, are relatively prominent in producing serious disseminated disease in acquired immunodeficiency syndrome (AIDS). Ansamycin has sometimes

been beneficial in therapy. Drug choice for most of these infections must be influenced by susceptibility testing, which requires weeks.

DRUGS USED IN LEPROSY

Mycobacterium leprae has never been grown in vitro, but animal models, such as growth in injected mouse footpads, have permitted laboratory evaluation of drugs. Only those drugs that have the widest clinical use are presented here. Because of increasing reports of dapsone resistance, treatment of leprosy with combinations of the drugs listed below is now being advocated.

DAPSONE & OTHER SULFONES

Several drugs closely related to the sulfonamides have been used effectively in the long-term treatment of leprosy. Dapsone, the most widely used, is diaminodiphenylsulfone. It probably inhibits folate synthesis. Resistance can emerge in large populations of *M leprae*, eg, in lepromatous leprosy, if very low doses are given.

Dapsone

Sulfones are well absorbed from the gut and widely distributed throughout body fluids and tissues. The serum half-life is 1–2 days, and drug tends to be retained in skin, muscle, liver, and kidney. Skin heavily infected with *M leprae* may contain several times as much of the drug as normal skin. Sulfones are excreted into bile and reabsorbed in the intestine. Excretion into urine is variable, and most excreted drug is acetylated. In renal failure, the dose may have to be adjusted.

The usual dosage in leprosy begins with one or two 25-mg tablets of dapsone per week, increasing by one tablet weekly until a full dose of 400–600 mg/wk is reached. For children the dose is proportionately less.

Untoward reactions to dapsone are common. Many patients develop some hemolysis, particularly if they have glucose-6-phosphate dehydrogenase deficiency. Methemoglobinemia is common. Gastrointestinal intolerance, fever, pruritus, and various rashes occur. During dapsone therapy of lepromatous leprosy, erythema nodosum leprosum develops often. It is sometimes difficult to distinguish reactions to dapsone from manifestations of the underlying illness. Erythema nodosum leprosum may be suppressed by corticosteroids or by thalidomide.

Acedapsone (4,4-diacetamidodiphenylsulfone) is a repository form of dapsone. A single intramuscular in-

Table 46–1. Clinical features and treatment of infections due to atypical mycobacteria.

Runyon Group	Pathogen	Frequent Clinical Features	Treatment Possibilities: Often Susceptible To—
I	*M kansasii*	Resembles tuberculous pulmonary disease.	Ethambutol + rifampin (+ INH); erythromycin, ethionamide.
	M marinum	Skin granulomas.	Minocycline, rifampin.
II	*M scrofulaceum*	Cervical adenitis in children.	Amikacin, erythromycin, rifampin, streptomycin. (Surgical excision is treatment of choice.)
III	*M avium-intracellulare*	Occasional pulmonary disease; widespread as asymptomatic infection; serious or fatal dissemination in AIDS patients.	Amikacin + rifampin, cycloserine, ethambutol, ansamycin.
IV	*M fortuitum*	Skin ulcers; rarely, lung disease.	Tetracycline, amikacin, ethionamide, capreomycin.
	M ulcerans	Skin ulcers.	Rifampin, streptomycin.

jection of 300 mg may maintain inhibitory dapsone levels in tissue for up to 3 months. Several other sulfones related to dapsone have also been used. When intolerance develops, it is to all sulfones.

RIFAMPIN

This drug (see above) in a dose of 600 mg daily can be strikingly effective in lepromatous leprosy. Because of the probable risk of emergence of rifampin-resistant *M leprae*, the drug is usually given in combination with dapsone or another antileprosy drug. A single *monthly* dose of 600 mg may be beneficial in combination therapy. The cost of rifampin is high for use in developing parts of the world where the need may be greatest.

CLOFAZIMINE

Clofazimine is a phenazine dye that can be used as an alternative drug to dapsone. Its mechanism of action is unknown, but may involve DNA binding. It is relatively expensive.

Absorption of clofazimine from the gut is variable, and a major portion of the drug is excreted in feces. Clofazimine is stored widely in reticuloendothelial tissues and skin, and its crystals can be seen inside phagocytic reticuloendothelial cells. It is slowly released, so that the serum half-life may be 2 months. Only a small proportion of each dose is excreted into urine or bile.

Clofazimine is given for sulfone-resistant leprosy or when patients are intolerant to sulfone. A common dose is 100–300 mg/d orally. In combination therapy, a dose of 50–100 mg/d has been satisfactory. The most prominent untoward effect is skin discoloration ranging from red-brown to nearly black. Gastrointestinal intolerance occurs occasionally.

Clofazimine

AMITHIOZONE

Amithiozone is a thiosemicarbazone employed as a substitute for dapsone in intolerant patients. It appears to be more effective in tuberculoid than in lepromatous leprosy. Oral administration of 150 mg daily or 450 mg twice weekly yields serum concentrations inhibitory for mycobacteria, but resistance may develop if the drug is given alone. Gastrointestinal intolerance occurs frequently and hepatic damage has been reported. The drug is currently not available in the USA.

REFERENCES

Addington WW: Treatment of pulmonary tuberculosis: Current options. *Arch Intern Med* 1979;**139**:1391.

Alvarez S, McCabe WR: Extrapulmonary tuberculosis revisited. *Medicine (Baltimore)* 1984;**63**:25.

Byrd RB et al: Toxic effects of isoniazid in tuberculosis chemoprophylaxis. *JAMA* 1979;**241**:1239.

Carpenter JL et al: Disseminated disease due to *Mycobacterium chelonei* treated with amikacin and cefoxitin. *Arch Intern Med* 1984;**144**:2063.

Cox F et al: Rifampin prophylaxis for contacts of *Haemophilus influenzae* type b disease. *JAMA* 1981;**245**:1043.

Curry FJ: Prophylactic effect of isoniazid in young tuberculin reactors. *N Engl J Med* 1967;**277**:562.

Doster B et al: Ethambutol in the initial treatment of pulmonary tuberculosis. *Am Rev Respir Dis* 1973;**107**:177.

Dutt AK, Stead WW: Present chemotherapy for tuberculosis. *J Infect Dis* 1982;**146**:698.

Eickhoff TC: Studies of resistance to rifampin in meningococci. J Infect Dis 1971;**123**:414.

Ellard GA, Mitchison DA: The hepatic toxicity of isoniazid among rapid and slow acetylators of the drug. *Am Rev Respir Dis* 1978;**118**:628.

Farr B, Mandell GL: Rifampin. *Med Clin North Am* 1982; **66**:157.

Graber CD et al: Light chain proteinuria and humoral immunoincompetence in tuberculous patients treated with rifampin. *Am Rev Respir Dis* 1973;**107**:713.

Joint Statement by American Thoracic Society and Centers for Disease Control: Guidelines for short-course tuberculosis chemotherapy. (2 parts.) *MMWR* 1980;**29**:97, 183.

Lester TW: Drug-resistant and atypical mycobacterial disease: Bacteriology and treatment. *Arch Intern Med* 1979;**139**:1399.

Maddrey WC, Boitnott JK: Isoniazid hepatitis. *Ann Intern Med* 1973;**79**:1.

McKenzie MS et al: Drug treatment of tuberculous meningitis in childhood. *Clin Pediatr* 1979;**18**:75.

Newman R et al: Rifampin in initial treatment of pulmonary tuberculosis. *Am Rev Respir Dis* 1974;**109**:216.

Pratt TH: Rifampin induced organic brain syndrome. *JAMA* 1979;**241**:2421.

Stead WW et al: Tuberculosis as an endemic and nosocomial infection among the elderly in nursing homes. *N Engl J Med* 1985;**312**:1483.

Steiner P et al: Primary isoniazid-resistant tuberculosis in children: Clinical features, strain resistance, treatment, and outcome in 26 children treated at Kings County Medical Center of Brooklyn between the years 1961 and 1972. *Am Rev Respir Dis* 1974;**110**:306.

Waters MF et al: Rifampicin for lepromatous leprosy: Nine years' experience. *Br Med J* 1978;**1**:133.

Wolinsky E: Nontuberculous mycobacteria and associated diseases. *Am Rev Respir Dis* 1979;**119**:107.

Sulfonamides & Trimethoprim

47

Ernest Jawetz, MD, PhD

SULFONAMIDES

A red dye, prontosil, synthesized in Germany by Klarer and Mietzsch in 1932, was tested but found to be ineffective against bacteria in vitro. However, Domagk reported in 1935 that it was strikingly active in vivo against hemolytic streptococcal and other infections. This was due to the conversion in the body of prontosil to sulfanilamide, the active drug. Since then the sulfonamide molecule has been chemically altered by the attachment of many different radicals, and there has been a proliferation of active compounds. Perhaps 150 different sulfonamides have been marketed at one time or another, the modifications being designed principally to achieve greater antibacterial activity, a wider antibacterial spectrum, greater solubility, or more prolonged action. In spite of the advent of the antibiotic drugs, the sulfonamides are among the most widely used antibacterial agents in the world today, chiefly because of the low cost and their relative efficacy in some common bacterial diseases. The synergistic action of sulfonamide with trimethoprim has brought about an enormous resurgence in sulfonamide use everywhere during the last decade.

Chemistry

The sulfonamides are a group of compounds whose basic formula and relationship to PABA are shown in Fig 47–1.

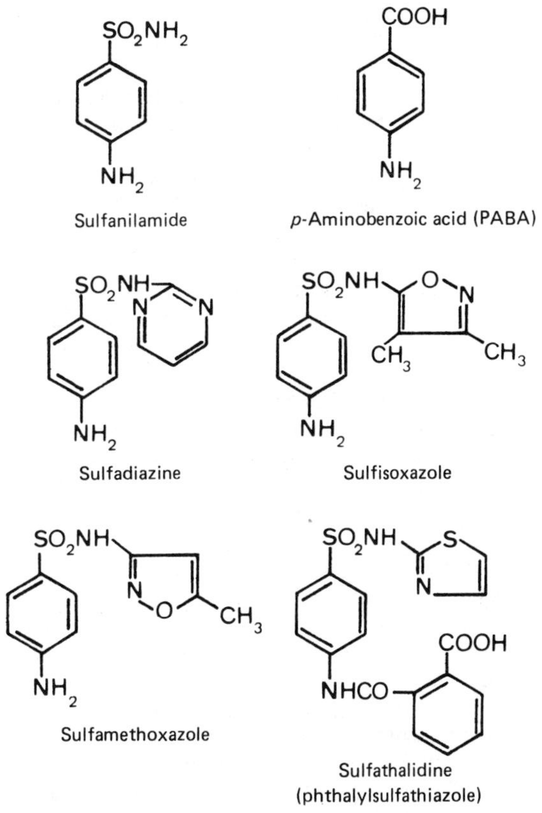

All have the same nucleus to which various R radicals in the amido group $(-SO_2NHR)$ have been attached or in which various substitutions of the amino group (NH_2) are made. These changes produce compounds with varying physical, chemical, pharmacologic, and antibacterial properties. In general, the sulfonamides are white, odorless, bitter tasting crystalline powders that are much more soluble at alkaline than at acid pH. In a mixture of sulfonamide drugs, each component drug exhibits its own solubility. Therefore, a mixture may be much more soluble, in terms of total sulfonamide present, than one drug used alone. This is the reason for the use of trisulfapyrimidines, a preparation that permits 3 times higher dosage than a single drug for comparable solubility in urine.

Most sulfonamides can be prepared as sodium salts that are moderately soluble, and these are used for intravenous administration. Such solutions are highly alkaline and not very stable, and may precipitate out of solution with polyionic electrolytes (eg, lactate-chlo-

Figure 47–1. Structures of some sulfonamides and *p*-aminobenzoic acid.

ride-carbonate). Certain sulfonamide molecules are designed for low solubility (eg, phthalylsulfathiazole) so that they will stay in the lumen of the bowel for long periods.

Antimicrobial Activity

Different sulfonamides may show quantitative but not necessarily qualitative differences in activity. Sulfonamides can inhibit both gram-positive and gram-negative bacteria, *Nocardia, Chlamydia trachomatis*, and some protozoa. Some enteric bacteria are inhibited but not *Pseudomonas, Serratia, Proteus*, and other multiresistant organisms. Sulfonamides alone are drugs of choice in previously untreated urinary tract infections, nocardiosis, and occasionally in other bacterial infections. Many strains of meningococci,

pneumococci, streptococci, staphylococci, and gonococci are now resistant. Indications for sulfonamide-
trimethoprim mixtures are given below.

Sulfonamides are structural analogs of *p*-amino-
benzoic acid (PABA). The action of sulfonamides is
bacteriostatic and is reversible by removal of the drug
or in the presence of an excess of PABA. The mode of
action of the sulfonamides is a good example of **competitive inhibition**. In brief, susceptible microorganisms require extracellular PABA in order to form folic
acid (Fig 47–2), an essential step in the production of
purines and in the ultimate synthesis of nucleic acids.
Sulfonamides can enter into the reaction in place of
PABA, compete for the enzyme dihydropteroate synthetase, and form nonfunctional analogs of folic acid.
As a result, further growth of the microorganisms is
prevented. However, growth can resume when the
sulfonamide is displaced by an excess of PABA or
when it dissociates from the enzyme.

Resistance

Animal cells (and some bacteria) are unable to synthesize folic acid but depend upon exogenous sources
and for this reason are not susceptible to sulfonamide
action. Other cells that produce a large excess of
PABA are resistant to sulfonamides, and still others
may be relatively impermeable to the drugs. Sulfonamide-resistant cells occur in most susceptible bacterial populations and tend to emerge under suitable selection pressure. Sulfonamide resistance may occur as
a result of mutation causing overproduction of PABA
or a structural change in the folic acid–synthesizing
enzyme with a lowered affinity for sulfonamides.
Most often sulfonamide resistance is under the genetic
control of a transmissible plasmid that may become
rapidly and widely disseminated. Thus, the widespread therapeutic use of sulfonamides against gonococci and meningococci has resulted in the establishment of sulfonamide-resistant strains throughout the
world. The widespread use of sulfonamides against
beta-hemolytic streptococci similarly aided the emergence of resistant strains. Other types of microorganisms—eg, many coliform organisms—are also com-

monly resistant. It should be specifically mentioned
that rickettsiae not only are not inhibited by sulfonamides but are actually stimulated in their growth.

Absorption, Metabolism, & Excretion

Most sulfonamides are given orally. They are
rapidly absorbed from the stomach and small intestine
and distributed widely to tissues and body fluids (including central nervous system and cerebrospinal
fluid), placenta, and fetus. Absorbed sulfonamides become bound to serum proteins to an extent varying
form 20% to over 90%. A varying proportion also becomes acetylated or inactivated by other metabolic
pathways. Chemical determinations performed on
serum may measure free (active) sulfonamide, the
acetylated (inactive) sulfonamide, or the total of both.
In order to be therapeutically effective after systemic
administration, a sulfonamide must generally achieve
a concentration of 8–12 mg of free drug per deciliter of
blood. Peak blood levels generally occur 2–3 hours after oral intake.

Soluble sulfonamides are excreted mainly by
glomerular filtration into the urine. Different compounds exhibit different degrees of reabsorption in the
tubules. A portion of the drug in the urine is the acetylated metabolite, but enough active drug remains for
effective treatment of infections of the urinary tract
(usually 10–20 times the concentration present in the
blood). In significant renal failure, the dose of sulfonamide must be reduced.

Sodium salts of sulfonamides are employed for intravenous administration because of their greater solubility. Their distribution and excretion are similar to
those of the orally administered drugs.

The "insoluble" sulfonamides (eg, phthalylsulfathiazole) are given orally, are absorbed only slightly
in the intestinal tract, and are excreted largely in the feces. Their action is exerted mainly on the aerobic intestinal flora.

"Long-acting" sulfonamides, eg, sulfamethoxypyridazine, are rapidly absorbed after oral intake and are
distributed widely, but urinary excretion—especially
of the free form—is very slow. This results in prolonged drug levels in serum. The slow renal excretion
is due in part to the high protein binding (more than
85%) and in part to the extensive tubular reabsorption
of the free (unacetylated) drug. These drugs are often
inadvisable because instances of severe toxicity have
resulted from their use. With the exception of sulfadoxine (in Fansidar, p 553), they have been withdrawn
in the USA but are still available elsewhere.

Sulfonamides of "intermediate action," eg, sulfamethoxazole, have no advantage except convenience of dosage, particularly when formulated in a
mixture with trimethoprim (80 mg trimethoprim plus
400 mg sulfamethoxazole per tablet).

Laboratory Studies

In order to grow bacteria from specimens obtained
from patients receiving sulfonamides, culture media
should contain an excess of PABA (5 mg/dL) to over-

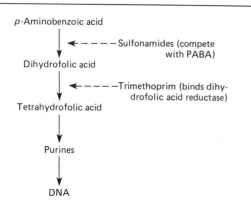

Figure 47–2. Actions of sulfonamides and trimethoprim.

come the inhibitory effect of the sulfonamide carried in the specimen.

Bacterial susceptibility testing with sulfonamide-containing disks is often unreliable because traces of PABA may be present in the medium or because uneven distribution of the bacterial inoculum gravely prejudices the results. Reliable susceptibility testing must be performed in well-defined liquid media that are completely free of PABA, contain all nutrients required for fastidious microorganisms (eg, meningococci), and permit the use of a small bacterial inoculum.

Clinical Uses

A. Topical: In general, the application of sulfonamides to the skin, in wounds, or on mucous membranes is undesirable because of their low activity and high risk of allergic sensitization. (An exception to the rule against topical application of sulfonamides may be the use of sodium sulfacetamide solution [30%] or ointment [10%] to the conjunctiva.) Oral administration of the "insoluble" sulfonamides, 8–15 g daily, results in a local effect—temporary inhibition of the intestinal aerobic microbial flora—that is of value in preparing the bowel for surgery; it must be timed so that the lowest microbial levels coincide with the time of the operation (usually on the fourth, fifth, or sixth day after administration). Mafenide acetate (*p*-amino methyl benzene sulfonamide; Sulfamylon) is a sulfonamide topically applied (as 10% cream) to burned skin surfaces. The drug is absorbed in 3 hours into tissue from the vehicle. It has been effective in reducing burn sepsis but has led to an increase of burn infections by fungi and resistant bacteria.

Mafenide causes significant pain on application. Silver sulfadiazine has been applied to burn wounds with relatively little pain. The sulfadiazine is released slowly, and only low systemic levels develop. Silver sulfadiazine appears to be effective in controlling infecting flora of most burn wounds, especially if the burns are not too deep.

Sulfasalazine (salicylazosulfapyridine) is widely used in ulcerative colitis, enteritis, and other inflammatory bowel disease. There is some evidence that this drug is more effective than soluble sulfonamides or other antimicrobials taken orally—all of which may occasionally have a beneficial effect in this type of inflammatory bowel disease. Sulfasalazine is split by intestinal microflora to yield sulfapyridine and 5-aminosalicylate. The latter may be released in the colon in a high concentration and may be responsible for an anti-inflammatory effect. Comparably high concentrations of salicylate cannot be achieved in the colon by oral intake of salicylates. The sulfapyridine is absorbed and may lead to toxic symptoms if more than 4 g of sulfasalazine is taken per day, particularly in persons who are slow acetylators.

B. Oral: The highly soluble and rapidly excreted sulfonamides are most commonly employed for the following clinical indications:

1. First (previously untreated) infections of the urinary tract–Sulfisoxazole and triple sulfonamides are highly soluble in urine and therefore preferred. Sulfisoxazole, 2–4 g initially and 0.5–1 g every 4–6 hours (150 mg/kg/d for children in divided doses), gives high levels both in tissues and in urine and is effective against a large proportion of organisms producing urinary tract infections in the community.

2. Chlamydial infections–*Chlamydia trachomatis* infections of the genital tract, eye, or respiratory tract may be effectively treated with oral sulfonamides, although tetracyclines and erythromycins may be drugs of choice. Sulfonamides are ineffective in psittacosis.

3. Bacterial infections–In nocardiosis, sulfisoxazole or sulfadiazine, 6–8 g/d, is the treatment of choice. In other bacterial infections, including those caused by beta-hemolytic streptococci, meningococci, and shigellae, sulfonamides were formerly drugs of choice. However, sulfonamide resistance is now widespread among these organisms. In underdeveloped parts of the world, sulfonamides—because of their availability and low cost—are widely used for respiratory tract infections, sinusitis, bronchitis, pneumonitis, otitis media, and bacillary dysentery. Sulfonamide-trimethoprim mixtures are widely employed for these and other bacterial infections everywhere but are much more expensive. Leprosy is treated with sulfones, eg, dapsone (see Chapter 46).

4. Dermatitis herpetiformis–This is not an infectious disorder, but it often responds to sulfapyridine, 2–4 g/d, or dapsone.

C. Intravenous: Sodium salts of many sulfonamides are available for parenteral injection, but because of their marked alkalinity are injected intravenously (not intramuscularly) in 5% dextrose in water. Intravenous sulfonamides are generally reserved for comatose patients (most commonly patients with meningitis) or patients who are otherwise unable to take medication by mouth.

Adverse Reactions

The sulfonamides can produce a wide variety of side effects that are due partly to allergy and partly to direct toxicity, and that must be considered whenever unexplained symptoms or signs occur in a patient who may have received these drugs. Up to 5% of patients may exhibit such reactions. The overall incidence of side effects is higher with the slowly excreted "long-acting" sulfonamides than with the rapidly excreted ones.

The commonest side effects are fever, skin rashes, photosensitivity, urticaria; nausea, vomiting, or diarrhea; and difficulties referable to the urinary tract (see below). Others include stomatitis, conjunctivitis, arthritis, hematopoietic disturbances (see below), hepatitis, exfoliative dermatitis, polyarteritis nodosa, Stevens-Johnson syndrome, psychosis, and many more.

A. Urinary Tract Disturbances: Sulfonamides may precipitate in urine, especially at neutral or acid pH, producing crystalluria, hematuria, or even obstruction. This is best prevented by using the most soluble sulfonamides (sulfisoxazole, trisulfapyrimidines), keeping the urine pH alkaline (5–15 g sodium bicarbonate daily), forcing fluids, and performing urinalysis every week. Sulfonamides must not be given with methenamine compounds, because a precipitate may form.

Sulfonamides have also been implicated in various types of nephrosis and in allergic nephritis. Deterioration of renal function can occur.

In renal insufficiency, the dosage of sulfonamides must be reduced and the interval between doses prolonged.

B. Hematopoietic Disturbances: Sulfonamides can produce anemia (hemolytic or aplastic), granulocytopenia, thrombocytopenia, or leukemoid reactions. These are rare except in certain high-risk patients. Sulfonamides cause hemolytic reactions, especially in patients whose erythrocytes are deficient in glucose-6-phosphate dehydrogenase. Sulfonamides taken near the end of pregnancy increase the risk of kernicterus in newborns.

Medical & Social Aspects

Sulfonamides can be made and distributed cheaply and are thus among the principal antimicrobial agents available in many developing areas of the world. They continue to be useful for the treatment of such widespread disorders as urinary tract infections and trachoma, but the emergence of drug resistance has impaired their usefulness in streptococcal, gonococcal, meningococcal, *Shigella,* and other infections. Topical use (skin) on a vast scale has contributed heavily to the sensitization of the population.

TRIMETHOPRIM & TRIMETHOPRIM-SULFAMETHOXAZOLE MIXTURES

Trimethoprim, a trimethoxybenzylpyrimidine, inhibits the dihydrofolic acid reductase of bacteria about 10,000 times more efficiently than the same enzyme of mammalian cells. **Pyrimethamine,** another benzylpyrimidine, inhibits the dihydrofolic acid reductase of protozoa more than that of mammalian cells. Dihydrofolic acid reductases are enzymes that convert dihydrofolic acid to tetrahydrofolic acid, a stage leading to the synthesis of purines and ultimately to DNA. Trimethoprim or pyrimethamine, given together with sulfonamides, produces sequential blocking in this metabolic sequence, resulting in a marked enhancement (synergism) of the activity of both drugs (Fig 47–2).

Microorganisms that lack the step inhibited by trimethoprim (dihydrofolate reductase) can emerge by mutation or by the conjugative transmission of plasmids. Such plasmids inducing trimethoprim resistance exist in coliform bacteria, *Haemophilus* sp, and others, and this resistance is increasing in frequency.

Pyrimethamine

Trimethoprim

Absorption, Distribution, & Excretion

Trimethoprim is usually given orally, alone or in combination with sulfamethoxazole. The latter combination can also be given intravenously. Trimethoprim is absorbed well from the gut and distributed widely in body fluids and tissues, including cerebrospinal fluid. When 1 part trimethoprim is given with 5 parts sulfamethoxazole, close to a 1:20 ratio in tissues is achieved, which is optimal for the combined effect in vitro. About 65–70% of each participant drug is protein-bound, and 30–50% of the sulfonamide and 50–60% of the trimethoprim (or their respective metabolites) are excreted in urine within 24 hours.

Trimethoprim concentrates by nonionic diffusion in prostatic fluid and in vaginal fluid, which are more acid than plasma. Therefore, it may have more antibacterial activity in prostatic and vaginal fluids than many other antimicrobial drugs.

Clinical Uses

A. Oral Trimethoprim: Trimethoprim is used alone (100 mg every 12 hours) in acute urinary tract infections. A majority of community-acquired organisms tend to be susceptible to the high concentrations in urine (200–600 μg/mL).

B. Oral Trimethoprim-Sulfamethoxazole (Cotrimoxazole, TMP-SMX): This combination is dispensed in a 1:5 ratio, with tablets containing either 80 mg trimethoprim plus 400 mg sulfamethoxazole or double the amount of each drug (160 mg trimethoprim plus 800 mg sulfamethoxazole). In 1986, trimethoprim-sulfamethoxazole mixtures appear to be a choice of treatment for *Pneumocystis carinii* pneumonia, symptomatic *Shigella* enteritis, systemic *Salmonella* infections (caused by ampicillin- or chloramphenicol-resistant organisms), *Serratia* sepsis, complicated urinary tract infections and prostatitis, and many others.

Two tablets of the regular size given every 12 hours can be effective in recurrent infections of the lower or upper urinary tract. The same dose may be effective in prostatitis. Two tablets daily may be sufficient for prolonged suppression of chronic urinary tract infections, and one-half or 1 regular size tablet given 3 times weekly for many months may serve as prophylaxis in recurrent urinary tract infections of some women. Two tablets of the regular size every 12 hours may be effective in some *Shigella, Salmonella,* and *H influenzae* infections, particularly if they are resistant to ampicillin and chloramphenicol. The dose for children treated for shigellosis, urinary tract infection, or otitis media is 8 mg/kg trimethoprim and 40 mg/kg sulfamethoxazole every 12 hours.

Trimethoprim-sulfamethoxazole, 9 tablets daily for 5 days, is often effective in eradicating pharyngeal gonorrhea. *Pneumocystis* pneumonia can be treated with high doses of the combination (trimethoprim, 20 mg/kg, plus sulfamethoxazole, 100 mg/kg, daily) or can be prevented in immunosuppressed patients by 2 regular tablets twice daily. The latter seems to also prevent gram-negative bacterial sepsis in some patients. In a very few cases of *Serratia* or *Pseudomonas* or other resistant sepsis, trimethoprim-sulfamethoxazole combined with polymyxin, or with rifampin, has given encouraging results.

C. Intravenous Trimethoprim-Sulfamethoxazole: A solution of the mixture containing 80 mg trimethoprim plus 400 mg sulfamethoxazole per 5 mL can be administered by intravenous infusion diluted in 125 mL of 5% dextrose in water over 60–90 minutes. It may be indicated in severe *Pneumocystis carinii* pneumonia, gram-negative bacterial sepsis, shigel-losis, or urinary tract infection when patients are unable to take the drug by mouth. The recommended dose for adults is up to 5 ampules of 5 mL each per day.

D. Oral Pyrimethamine With Sulfonamide: This combination has been used in parasitic infections. In leishmaniasis and toxoplasmosis, full doses of a sulfonamide (6–8 g/d) have been given with pyrimethamine, 50 mg/d. In falciparum malaria, a combination of pyrimethamine with a sulfonamide (Fansidar) or pyrimethamine alone has been occasionally employed (see Chapter 56).

Adverse Effects

Trimethoprim produces the adverse effects of an antifolate drug, especially megaloblastic anemia, leukopenia, and granulocytopenia (see Chapter 58). This can be prevented by the simultaneous administration of folinic acid, 6–8 mg/d. In addition, the combination trimethoprim-sulfamethoxazole may cause all of the untoward reactions associated with sulfonamides. Occasionally, there is also nausea and vomiting, drug fever, vasculitis, renal damage, or central nervous system disturbances. Patients with acquired immunodeficiency syndrome (AIDS) and *Pneumocystis* pneumonia have a particularly high frequency of untoward reactions to trimethoprim-sulfamethoxazole, especially fever, rashes, leukopenia, and diarrhea.

REFERENCES

Ballin JC: Evaluation of a new topical agent for burn therapy: Silver sulfadiazine (Silvadene). *JAMA* 1974;**230:**1884.

Bose W et al: Controlled trial of co-trimoxazole in children with urinary tract infection. *Lancet* 1974;**2:**614.

Campieri M et al: Treatment of ulcerative colitis with high-dose 5-aminosalicylic acid enemas. *Lancet* 1981;**2:**270.

Craig WA, Kunin CM: Trimethoprim-sulfamethoxazole: Effects of urinary pH and impaired renal function. *Ann Intern Med* 1973;**78:**491.

Feldman HA: Toxoplasmosis. (2 parts.) *N Engl J Med* 1968; **279:**1370, 1431.

Goldman P, Peppercorn MA: Sulfasalazine. *N Engl J Med* 1975;**293:**20.

Gurwith M et al: A prospective controlled investigation of prophylactic trimethoprim-sulfamethoxazole in hospitalized granulopenic patients. *Am J Med* 1979;**66:**248.

Hamilton HE, Sheets RF: Sulfisoxazole-induced thrombocytopenic purpura. *JAMA* 1978;**239:**2586.

Jaffe HS et al: Complications of co-trimoxazole in treatment of AIDS-associated *Pneumocystis carinii* pneumonia in homosexual men. *Lancet* 1983;**2:**1109.

Kalowski S et al: Deterioration of renal function with co-trimoxazole. *Lancet* 1973;**1:**394.

Lau WK, Young LS: Trimethoprim-sulfamethoxazole treatment of *Pneumocystis carinii* pneumonia in adults. *N Engl J Med* 1976;**295:**716.

Lawson DH, Jick H: Adverse reactions to co-trimoxazole in hospitalized medical patients. *Am J Med Sci* 1978;**274:**53.

Meares EM Jr: Long-term therapy of chronic bacterial prostatitis with trimethoprim-sulfamethoxazole. *Can Med Assoc J* 1975; **112(13):**22. [Special issue.]

Modak SM, Fox CL: Sulfadiazine silver-resistant *Pseudomonas* in burns. *Arch Surg* 1981;**116:**854.

Murray BE et al: Emergence of high-level trimethoprim resistance in fecal *Escherichia coli* during oral administration of trimethoprim or trimethoprim-sulfamethoxazole. *N Engl J Med* 1982;**306:**130.

Rubin RH, Swartz MN: Trimethoprim-sulfamethoxazole. *N Engl J Med* 1980;**303:**426.

Smego RA Jr, Moeller MB, Gallis HA: Trimethoprim-sulfamethoxazole therapy for *Nocardia* infections. *Arch Intern Med* 1983;**143:**711.

Stamey TA, Condy M: The diffusion and concentration of trimethoprim in human vaginal fluid. *J Infect Dis* 1975;**131:**261.

48

Antifungal Agents

Ernest Jawetz, MD, PhD

Most fungi are completely resistant to the action of antibacterial drugs. Only a few substances have been discovered that exert an inhibitory effect on the fungi pathogenic for humans, and most of these are relatively toxic. There is a great need for better antifungal drugs, made more pressing by the increased incidence of systemic dissemination of fungal infections in immunosuppressed patients.

Griseofulvin is effective in dermatophytosis. Nystatin, candicidin, and tolnaftate can only be applied topically. Miconazole is effective topically and has been used systemically on a very limited scale. Other imidazoles, especially ketoconazole, are useful for oral therapy of some systemic mycoses. Amphotericin is difficult to administer and has many side effects but still remains the most effective treatment for severe systemic mycoses. Because of their importance in dermatology, many of these drugs are also discussed in Chapter 65.

SYSTEMIC ANTIFUNGAL DRUGS

1. AMPHOTERICIN B

Amphotericin B is one of 2 antibiotics produced by *Streptomyces nodosus,* purified in 1956. Amphotericin A is not used in therapy.

Chemistry

Amphotericin B is an amphoteric polyene macrolide (polyene = containing many double bonds; macrolide = containing a large lactone ring of 12 or more atoms). Amphotericin B is insoluble in water. It is unstable at 37 °C, but stable for weeks at 4 °C. Microcrystalline preparations can be applied topically but are not absorbed to a significant extent. For systemic use by intravenous injection, a colloidal preparation is employed.

Antifungal Activity

Amphotericin B, 0.1–0.8 μg/mL, inhibits in vitro *Histoplasma capsulatum, Cryptococcus neoformans, Coccidioides immitis, Candida albicans, Blastomyces dermatitidis, Sporothrix schenckii,* and other organisms producing mycotic disease in humans. It has no effect on bacteria.

The mode of action of the polyene antibiotics is fairly well understood. The drug apparently is bound firmly to the fungal cell membrane in the presence of ergosterol and disturbs the permeability and transport characteristics of the membrane. This results in loss of macromolecules and ions from the cell and produces irreversible damage. Bacteria are insusceptible to polyenes because they lack the ergosterol that is essential for attachment to the cell membrane. Amphotericin resistance may result from a decrease in membrane ergosterol or a modification in its structure so that it combines less well with the drug. Some attachment of amphotericin B to cholesterol in animal cell membranes probably accounts in part for its toxicity.

Absorption, Metabolism, & Excretion

Amphotericin is poorly absorbed from the gastrointestinal tract. Orally administered amphotericin therefore is effective only on fungi within the lumen of the tract and cannot be used for the treatment of systemic disease. The intravenous injection of 0.6 mg/kg/d amphotericin B results in average blood levels of 0.3–1 μg/mL. Amphotericin is more than 90% protein-bound and is removed to a very limited extent by hemodialysis. The injected amphotericin is excreted slowly in the urine over a period of several days. The drug is widely distributed in tissues, but only 2–3% of the blood level is reached in cerebrospinal fluid. Consequently, intrathecal administration is necessary in fungal meningitis.

Clinical Uses

For the treatment of systemic fungal infections, amphotericin B is available as a colloidal dry powder to be dissolved with sodium deoxycholate in 5% dextrose in water to a concentration of 0.1 mg/mL; the solution is then given by slow intravenous infusion over a period of 4–6 hours. The initial dose is 1–5 mg/d, increasing daily by 5-mg increments until a final dosage of 0.4–0.7 mg/kg/d is reached. This is usually continued for 6–12 weeks or longer, with a daily dose rarely exceeding 60 mg. Following an initial response to treatment, doses are given only 2–3 times per week, often on an outpatient basis.

In fungal meningitis, intrathecal injection of 0.5 mg amphotericin B may be given 3 times weekly for up to 10 weeks or longer. Continuous infusion with an Ommaya reservoir is sometimes used. Fungal meningitis relapses commonly. Combined treatment with amphotericin and flucytosine is increasingly used in *Candida* and *Cryptococcus* meningitis and in systemic candidiasis. This delays emergence of resistance to flucytosine and permits use of lower doses of amphotericin. The antifungal activity of amphotericin B has also been enhanced by rifampin or tetracycline given simultaneously in certain fungal infections so that smaller doses of amphotericin may be effective.

In corneal ulcers caused by fungi, a solution (1 mg/mL) dropped onto the conjunctiva every 30 minutes can be curative. Other local administrations include injections into joints infected with coccidioidomycosis or sporotrichosis or irrigation of the bladder in *Candida* cystitis.

Adverse Reactions

The intravenous injection of amphotericin usually produces chills, fever, vomiting, and headache. The severity of adverse reactions may be diminished by reducing the dosage temporarily, administering aspirin, phenothiazines, antihistamines, or corticosteroids, or stopping injections for several days.

Therapeutically active amounts of amphotericin B commonly impair renal and hepatocellular function and produce anemia. There is a fall in glomerular filtration rate and a change in tubular function. These result in a decrease in creatinine clearance and an increase in potassium clearance. Shocklike fall in blood pressure, electrolyte disturbances (especially hypokalemia), and a variety of neurologic symptoms also occur commonly. In impaired kidney function, the dose of amphotericin must be further reduced. The methyl ester of amphotericin B is less nephrotoxic but produces such severe mental and neurologic changes (leukoencephalitis) that it has been abandoned.

2. FLUCYTOSINE

5-Fluorocytosine (flucytosine, 5-FC) is an oral antifungal compound of the formula shown below.

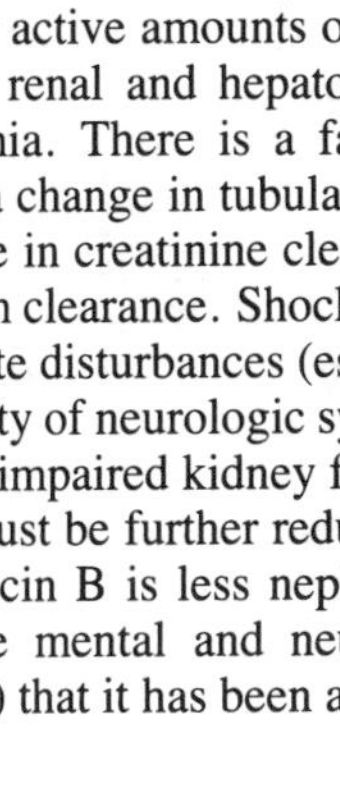

Flucytosine

Flucytosine, 5 μg/mL, inhibits in vitro many strains of *Candida, Cryptococcus,* and *Torulopsis* and some strains of *Aspergillus* and other fungi. Cells are susceptible if they convert flucytosine to fluorouracil, eventually inhibiting thymidylate synthetase and DNA synthesis. Resistant mutants emerge fairly regularly and rapidly and are selected in the presence of the drug, limiting its usefulness. For this reason, combined treatment with 5-FC and amphotericin B is being explored with some success. True synergism may occur, with enhanced antifungal effect against *Candida, Cryptococcus,* perhaps *Aspergillus,* and others.

Oral doses of 150 mg/kg/d are well absorbed and widely distributed in tissues—including the cerebrospinal fluid—where the drug concentration may be 60–80% of the serum concentration, which tends to be near 50 μg/mL. About 20% of flucytosine is protein-bound. 5–FC is largely excreted by the kidneys, and concentrations in the urine reach 10 times the concentrations in serum. In the presence of renal failure, the drug may accumulate in serum to toxic levels, but hepatic failure has no effect. Flucytosine is removed by hemodialysis.

Flucytosine appears to be relatively nontoxic for mammalian cells (perhaps because they lack a specific permease). Prolonged high serum levels often cause depression of bone marrow, loss of hair, and abnormal liver function. Uracil can inhibit the hematopoietic toxicity, manifested by bone marrow depression, but seems to have no effect on the antifungal activity of 5-FC. The untoward effects of 5-FC have been attributed to conversion to 5-fluorouracil in the body. Nausea, vomiting, and skin rashes occur occasionally. With daily amounts of 6–12 g administered in divided doses, there have been prolonged remissions of fungemia, sepsis, and meningitis caused by susceptible organisms. The combined use of flucytosine with amphotericin B has been beneficial, particularly in cryptococcal meningitis and in systemic candidiasis, and has permitted a reduction in the amphotericin dose.

3. ANTIFUNGAL IMIDAZOLES: CLOTRIMAZOLE, MICONAZOLE, & KETOCONAZOLE

These synthetic antifungal imidazoles inhibit fungi by blocking the biosynthesis of fungal lipids, especially the ergosterol in cell membranes, and perhaps by additional mechanisms. Clotrimazole as 10-mg troches 5 times daily can suppress oral candidiasis; as 1% cream it is effective topically in dermatophytosis. It is also available as vaginal tablets for candidiasis. It is too toxic for systemic use.

Miconazole has long been used as 2% cream in dermatophytosis and in vaginal candidiasis not responding to topical nystatin. Miconazole is also available for intravenous use. Up to 3.6 g/d (about 30 mg/kg/d) has been injected intravenously in disseminated candidiasis, coccidioidomycosis, cryptococcosis, paracoccidioidomycosis, blastomycosis, etc. The fungi causing these diseases tend to be inhibited by miconazole, 1–2 μg/mL, in vitro. Serum levels exceeding such concentrations have been achieved, and prolonged remissions have occurred. In meningitis due to these fungi, 10–20 mg/d of miconazole must be given intrathecally or intraventricularly, because little of the drug enters the cerebrospinal fluid from the serum. The relapse rate in fungal meningitis is high.

Miconazole produces many significant side effects, including thrombophlebitis, vomiting, anemia, thrombocytosis, hyponatremia, hyperlipidemia, and, occasionally, leukopenia and hypersensitivity reactions. Miconazole markedly increases the anticoagulant effect of coumarin drugs.

Ketoconazole is the most recent addition to this group; the formula is shown below.

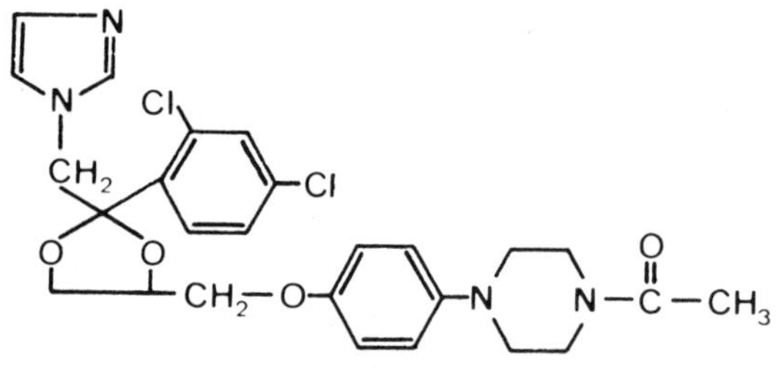

Ketoconazole

Ketoconazole is the first antifungal effective in systemic mycoses that can be given by mouth. A single daily dose of 200–400 mg is taken with food. The drug is well absorbed and widely distributed, but concentrations in the central nervous system are low unless much larger doses (up to 800 mg/d) are given. Daily dosage suppresses *Candida* infections of mouth or vagina in 1–2 weeks and dermatophytosis in 3–8 weeks. Mucocutaneous candidiasis in immunodeficient children responds in 4–10 months.

Ketoconazole, 200–600 mg/d, effectively suppresses the clinical manifestations of systemic paracoccidioidomycosis, blastomycosis, and sometimes lung, bone, or skin lesions of histoplasmosis and coccidioidomycosis, but not meningitis due to these fungi. In disease of moderate severity this oral antifungal drug has given encouraging results and administration has been without major problems.

With oral doses of 200 mg, peak levels of ketoconazole may be 2–3 μg/mL, persisting for 6 hours or more. The major toxic effects include nausea, vomiting, skin rashes, and elevation of serum transaminase levels. Very rarely, progressive hepatotoxicity has developed with high doses. Ketoconazole blocks the synthesis of adrenal steroids and can cause gynecomastia. The emergence of drug resistance has not yet been observed. The simultaneous administration of ketoconazole and rifampin tends to result in a significant reduction in the serum concentration of both drugs.

4. HYDROXYSTILBAMIDINE

Hydroxystilbamidine isethionate is an aromatic diamidine active against *B dermatitidis* in vitro and in vivo. It may be severely toxic for liver and kidneys and has been largely replaced by amphotericin B.

5. GRISEOFULVIN

Griseofulvin is a substance isolated from *Penicillium griseofulvum* in 1939. It was introduced clinically for the treatment of dermatophytoses in 1957.

Chemistry

The structure of griseofulvin is shown below. It is very insoluble in water but quite stable at high temperature, including autoclaving.

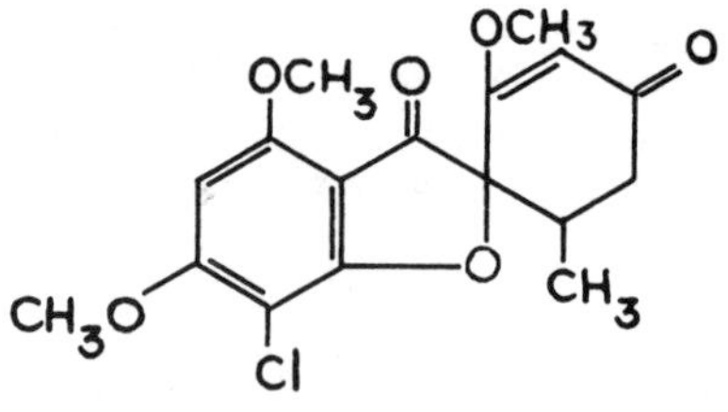

Griseofulvin

Antifungal Activity

Griseofulvin inhibits the growth of dermatophytes, including *Epidermophyton, Microsporum,* and *Trichophyton,* in concentrations of 0.5–3 μg/mL. It has no effect on bacteria, the fungi producing deep mycoses of humans, or certain fungi producing superficial lesions. Resistance can emerge among susceptible dermatophytes. (See Chapter 65.)

The mechanism of action has not been established, but it is probable that griseofulvin interferes with microtubule function or with nucleic acid synthesis and polymerization. The inhibitory effect may be partially reversed by purines.

Absorption, Metabolism, & Excretion

Absorption of griseofulvin depends greatly on the physical state of the drug and is aided by high-fat foods. Preparations containing microsize particles of the drug are absorbed twice as well as those with larger particles. Microsize griseofulvin, 1 g daily, gives, in adults, blood levels of 0.5–1.5 μg/mL. Ultramicrosize griseofulvin (Gris-PEG) is absorbed twice as well as the microsize preparation. The absorbed drug has an affinity for diseased skin and is deposited there, bound to keratin. Thus, it makes keratin resistant to fungal growth, and the new growth of hair or nails is freed of infection first. As the keratinized structures are shed, they tend to be replaced by uninfected ones. Little griseofulvin is present in body fluids or tissues. The bulk of ingested griseofulvin is excreted in feces and only a small part in urine.

Clinical Uses

Topical use of griseofulvin has little effect.

The microsize preparations of griseofulvin are given orally, 0.5–1 g daily, in divided doses (0.25–0.5 g for children weighing over 50 lb, or 15 mg/kg/d). An ultramicrosize preparation (Gris-PEG) is given in an adult dose of 0.3–0.6 g orally (7.25 mg/kg/d for children). Treatment must be continued for 3–6 weeks if only hair or skin is involved but for 3–6 months if nails are affected. Griseofulvin (Grifulvin V) is indicated for severe dermatophytosis involving skin, hair, or nails, particularly if caused by *Trichophyton ru-*

brum, which responds poorly to other measures. Other topical antifungal drugs may have to be used with griseofulvin.

Griseofulvin may increase the metabolism of coumarin, so that higher doses of the anticoagulant are required. Phenobarbital reduces absorption of griseofulvin from the gut.

Adverse Reactions

The overall frequency of side effects is low.

A. Allergic Reactions: Fever, skin rashes, leukopenia, and serum sickness–type reactions occur.

B. Direct Toxicity: Headache, nausea, vomiting, diarrhea, hepatotoxicity, photosensitivity, and mental confusion occur. Griseofulvin is teratogenic and carcinogenic in laboratory animals.

TOPICAL ANTIFUNGAL DRUGS

1. NYSTATIN

Chemistry

Nystatin is a polyene macrolide. It is slightly soluble in water but quickly decomposes in the presence of water or plasma. It is stable in dry form.

Antifungal Activity

Nystatin has no effect on bacteria or protozoa, but in vitro it inhibits many fungi, including *Candida* sp, dermatophytes, and organisms producing deep mycoses in humans. In vivo, its action is limited to surfaces where the nonabsorbed drug can be in direct contact with the yeast or mold. Resistance to nystatin does not develop in vivo, but drug-resistant strains of *Candida* sp occur.

The mode of action involves binding of nystatin to fungal membrane sterols, principally ergosterol. There it disturbs membrane permeability and transport features. This results in loss of cations and macromolecules from the cell. Resistance is due to a decrease in membrane sterols or a change in their structure and binding properties.

Absorption, Metabolism, & Excretion

Nystatin is not significantly absorbed from skin, mucous membranes, or the gastrointestinal tract. Virtually all nystatin taken orally is excreted in the feces. There are no significant blood or tissue levels after oral intake.

Clinical Uses

Nystatin can be applied topically to the skin or mucous membranes (buccal, vaginal) in the form of creams, ointments, suppositories, suspensions, or powders for the suppression of local *Candida* infections. Nystatin has been given orally for the partial suppression of *Candida* in the lumen of the bowel. This may be warranted in very small infants or persons with impaired host defenses (diabetes mellitus, leukemia, high doses of steroids), in whom the possibility of disseminated candidiasis exists. However, the addition of nystatin to oral tetracyclines is of dubious merit.

Nystatin preparations often contain antibacterial drugs.

2. TOLNAFTATE

Tolnaftate is a topical antifungal drug for use in cream, powder, or solution form in the treatment of dermatophytosis. While *Candida* is resistant, many dermatophytes are suppressed, and clinical efficacy is claimed for treatment courses of 1–10 weeks. With topical application, there appears to be no significant systemic absorption. Toxic and allergic reactions appear to be minimal.

3. CLOTRIMAZOLE & MICONAZOLE

These imidazoles are effective topical antifungals but are toxic in systemic use. They have been described above. They are used mainly in oral, vaginal, or cutaneous candidiasis, in the form of creams or troches.

4. NATAMYCIN

This is a polyene antifungal drug active against many different fungi in vitro. Topical application of 5% ophthalmic suspension can be beneficial in the treatment of keratitis caused by *Fusarium, Cephalosporium,* or other fungi. It is approved for such use but must be combined with appropriate surgical measures.

Natamycin may be effective for oral or vaginal candidiasis. The toxicity after topical application appears to be low.

5. OTHER TOPICAL ANTIFUNGAL DRUGS

Candicidin

Candicidin is a polyene antibiotic proposed solely as a topical drug (in vaginal tablets or ointment) for the treatment of candidal vaginitis. It is not absorbed systemically and produces few toxic effects. Its efficacy is currently being tested.

Fatty Acids

Fatty acids, particularly undecylenic acid and its salts, are effective topical antifungal drugs (see Chapter 54). They are widely useful in tinea pedis and corporis as powders or creams.

Haloprogin

Haloprogin is a topical drug active in vitro against many dermatophytes and in vivo against tinea corporis. It is available as a 1% cream or solution, and 10–20% of the topically applied drug may be absorbed. It occasionally causes local irritation.

REFERENCES

Bennett JE: Chemotherapy of systemic mycosis. (2 parts.) *N Engl J Med* 1974;**290:**30, 320.

Bennett JE: Flucytosine. *Ann Intern Med* 1977;**86:**319.

Bennett JE et al: A comparison of amphotericin B alone and combined with flucytosine in the treatment of cryptococcal meningitis. *N Engl J Med* 1979;**301:**126.

Block ER et al: Flucytosine and amphotericin B: Hemodialysis effects on plasma concentration in man. *Ann Intern Med* 1974;**80:**613.

Burgess JL, Birchall R: Nephrotoxicity of amphotericin B. *Am J Med* 1972;**53:**77.

Chesney PJ et al: Successful treatment of candida meningitis with amphotericin B and 5-fluorocytosine in combination. *J Pediatr* 1976;**89:**1017.

Dismukes WE et al: Treatment of systemic mycoses with ketoconazole: Emphasis on toxicity and clinical response in 52 patients. *Ann Intern Med* 1983;**98:**13.

Drutz DJ, Catanzaro A: Coccidioidomycosis. *Am Rev Respir Dis* 1978;**117:**727.

Goldman L: Griseofulvin. *Med Clin North Am* 1970;**54:**1339.

Hamilton-Miller JMT: Chemistry and biology of polyene antibiotics. *Bacteriol Rev* 1973;**37:**166.

Heiberg JK, Svejgaard E: Toxic hepatitis during ketoconazole treatment. *Br Med J* 1981;**283:**825.

Hoeprich PD et al: Development of resistance to 5-fluorocytosine in *Candida parapsilosis* during therapy. *J Infect Dis* 1974;**130:**112.

Kirkpatrick CH, Alling DW: Treatment of oral candidiasis with clotrimazole troches. *N Engl J Med* 1978;**299:**1201.

Koeffler HP, Golde DW: 5-Fluorocytosine: Inhibition of hematopoiesis in vitro and reversal of inhibition by uracil. *J Infect Dis* 1979;**139:**438.

Medoff G, Kobayashi GS: Amphotericin B. *JAMA* 1975;**232:**619.

Pont A et al: Ketoconazole blocks adrenal steroid synthesis. *Ann Intern Med* 1982;**97:**370.

Restrepo A, Stevens DA, Utz JP (editors): Symposium on ketoconazole. *Rev Infect Dis* 1980;**2:**519.

Ross JB et al: Ketoconazole for treatment of chronic pulmonary coccidioidomycosis. *Ann Intern Med* 1982;**96:**440.

Smego RA Jr: Combined therapy with amphotericin B and flucytosine for *Candida* meningitis. *Rev Infect Dis* 1984;**6:**791.

Stevens DA, Levine HB, Deresinski SC: Miconazole in coccidioidomycosis. 2. Therapeutic and pharmacologic studies in man. *Am J Med* 1976;**60:**191.

Weinstein L, Jacoby I: Successful treatment of cerebral cryptococcoma and meningitis with miconazole. *Ann Intern Med* 1980;**93:**569.

Woods RA et al: Resistance to polyene antibiotics and correlated sterol changes in isolates of *Candida tropicalis* from a patient with an amphotericin B-resistant funguria. *J Infect Dis* 1974;**129:**53.

Antiviral Chemotherapy & Prophylaxis

49

Ernest Jawetz, MD, PhD

Fundamentally, viruses are obligate intracellular parasites. Their replication depends primarily on metabolic processes of the host cell. Consequently, many chemicals that inhibit viral replication also inhibit some host cell function and possess major toxicity. Active search is under way for chemicals that inhibit virus-specific functions, as listed below.

In many viral infections, replication of the virus reaches a maximum near the time clinical symptoms first appear—or even earlier. Therefore, in order to be clinically effective, chemicals that block viral replication must be administered before the onset of disease, ie, as chemoprophylaxis. This is the case with amantadine against influenza A and methisazone against poxviruses. In some other infections, particularly those due to herpesviruses, virus replication continues for a time after symptoms and signs have manifested themselves. In those infections, inhibition of further virus replication may promote healing. This is the case with idoxuridine and other DNA inhibitors in herpetic keratitis and with vidarabine or acyclovir in disseminating herpes simplex or zoster.

Viral replication consists of the following steps: (1) adsorption to and penetration of susceptible cells; (2) synthesis of early, nonstructural proteins, eg, nucleic acid polymerases; (3) synthesis of RNA or DNA; (4) synthesis of late, structural proteins; and (5) assembly (maturation) of viral particles and their release from the cell. Antiviral drug action can be considered under these headings.

INHIBITION OF ADSORPTION & PENETRATION OF SUSCEPTIBLE CELLS

Gamma Globulin

If gamma globulin contains specific antibodies directed against superficial antigens of a given virus, it can interfere with entry of that virus particle into a cell, probably by blocking penetration rather than adsorption. The intramuscular injection of pooled gamma globulin (immune globulin USP), 0.025–0.25 mL/kg of body weight, during the early incubation period can modify infection with the viruses of measles, hepatitis, rabies, poliomyelitis, and possibly other diseases. The protective effect of a gamma globulin injection lasts 2–3 weeks. For infections that have prolonged in-

cubation periods, injections may have to be given every 2–3 weeks.

Viral replication is often only partially inhibited, so that the development of active immunity may accompany the temporary passive protection conferred by gamma globulin.

Intravenous immune globulin, containing 10% maltose or sucrose, can be given if intramuscular injection is inadvisable. Special hyperimmune globulins (concentrated from the plasma of persons with high antibody levels) are available for rabies, varicella-zoster, and hepatitis B, to be administered on specific indications (see p 592).

Amantadine (Adamantanamine)

Amantadine, a tricyclic symmetric amine, inhibits the penetration of susceptible cells or the uncoating of certain myxoviruses, eg, influenza A (but not influenza B), rubella, and some tumor viruses. It therefore inhibits the replication of these viruses in vitro and in experimental animals. Weak bases like amantadine probably act by buffering the pH of endosomes, membrane-bound vacuoles that surround virus particles as they are taken into the cell. Prevention of acidification in these vacuoles blocks the fusion of the virus envelope with the endosome membrane and thereby prevents transfer of the viral genetic material into the cytoplasm of the cell. In humans, a daily oral dose of 200 mg of amantadine hydrochloride for 2–3 days before and 6–7 days after influenza A infection reduces the incidence and severity of symptoms and the magnitude of the serologic response. There may also be a slight therapeutic effect if amantadine is started within 18 hours of the onset of symptoms of influenza. Rimantadine, an analog with a –$CHNH_2CH_3$ moiety replacing the –NH_2 in the structure below, has very similar properties.

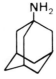

Amantadine

When given orally, amantadine is almost completely absorbed from the gut. The drug is largely

(90%) excreted by the kidneys into the urine. In persons with renal failure, amantadine may accumulate to toxic levels unless dosage is greatly reduced in proportion to the decrease in creatinine clearance. With normal serum creatinine, the half-life is about 12 hours.

Chemoprophylaxis with amantadine can be effective in household contacts, in limiting institutional spread of infection, and in protecting adults at high risk during influenza outbreaks. Rimantadine is probably equally effective and perhaps less toxic.

Amantadine has beneficial effects in some cases of Parkinson's disease (see Chapter 26).

The most marked untoward effects of amantadine are insomnia, slurred speech, dizziness, ataxia, and other central nervous system signs. The drug can cause release of stored catecholamines.

INHIBITION OF INTRACELLULAR SYNTHESIS

Inhibition of Early Protein Synthesis

Guanidine and hydroxybenzylbenzimidazole are both capable of inhibiting the replication of certain RNA enteroviruses but not of others. Both substances inhibit the formation of RNA polymerases at concentrations that appear to be harmless to host cells in vitro. Mutants resistant to the action of these compounds are frequent and are rapidly selected out in the presence of the drugs. Therefore, as expected, these compounds do not have significant therapeutic activity in vivo. Trials of biguanidines in RNA virus infections in humans were not encouraging.

Inhibition of Nucleic Acid Synthesis

A. Ribavirin: Ribavirin (ribofuranosyl-triazole-carboxamide; for structure, see p 561) can inhibit the replication of both RNA and DNA viruses in experimental models. The compound acts by interfering with guanidine monophosphate formation and subsequent nucleic acid synthesis. A therapeutic action has been noted in some experimental animal virus infections. In experimental human infections with influenza A viruses, doses of 15 mg/kg resulted in only marginal clinical benefit. However, when administered as an aerosol it appears to limit respiratory syncytial virus replication in infants and to limit the severity and duration of illness. It has also been effective as treatment for influenza A and B infection by accelerating defervescence and shortening symptoms. Ribavirin has been employed in other countries in viral respiratory infections and hepatitis but is not approved for use in the USA.

B. Pyrimidine and Purine Analogs:

1. 5-Fluorouracil (for structure, see p 676) and **5-bromouracil** effectively block the replication of DNA viruses in cell culture systems, but they are relatively ineffective in vivo. **Idoxuridine** (5-iodo-2'-deoxyuridine, IDU, IUDR) can inhibit the replication of most DNA viruses in cell culture. In vivo, it inhibits the replication of herpes simplex virus in the cornea

and thus aids in the healing of herpetic keratitis in humans. This is a special circumstance, since herpesvirus proliferates in the avascular corneal epithelium and the topically applied drug remains local and is not rapidly removed by the bloodstream. In the vascular conjunctiva the drug has little therapeutic effect; although adenoviruses are readily inhibited by idoxuridine in vitro, adenovirus conjunctivitis cannot be controlled by idoxuridine in vivo.

For treatment of herpetic keratitis, idoxuridine is applied to the cornea (every 2 hours around the clock) by instilling 1 drop of a 0.1% aqueous solution into the conjunctival sac. This tends to accelerate spontaneous healing. However, DNA synthesis of host cells is also affected, and some toxic effects on corneal cells are occasionally observed, especially if treatment is continued for more than 10 days. Ointments containing 0.5% idoxuridine provide higher drug concentrations. Idoxuridine may induce allergic contact dermatitis.

Most isolates of herpesvirus from untreated cases of herpetic keratitis are strongly inhibited in vitro by idoxuridine, 2 μg/mL. Upon prolonged exposure to idoxuridine in vitro, occasional drug-resistant mutants are selected out that are not inhibited by idoxuridine, 20 μg/mL or more. "Drug-resistant" cases of herpetic keratitis occur relatively frequently. Such patients fail to improve with prolonged idoxuridine treatment. However, many virus isolates from such cases appear to be intrinsically susceptible to idoxuridine inhibition in vitro. Such strains may escape the inhibitory effect of idoxuridine in vivo because they rapidly penetrate deep into the corneal stroma and thus become inaccessible to idoxuridine applied to the corneal surface.

In deep herpetic stromal keratitis there is little virus replication in the stroma. Corticosteroids help to reduce the inflammatory response. Idoxuridine is given simultaneously to prevent herpesvirus proliferation in the superficial epithelium.

Vaccinial keratitis responds irregularly to idoxuridine. **Trifluorothymidine** is more active than IDU but more expensive.

Topically applied idoxuridine has no effect on skin lesions of herpes simplex or zoster.

Idoxuridine is too toxic for systemic administration. **Bromvinyldeoxyuridine** is active against varicella-zoster virus in vitro and perhaps also in vivo.

2. Cytarabine (arabinofuranosylcytosine hydrochloride, cytosine arabinoside, ara-C, p 676) also inhibits DNA synthesis and interferes with the replication of DNA viruses. By weight it is about 10 times more effective than idoxuridine, but it is also 10 times more toxic for host cells. Cytarabine, 0.3–2 mg/kg intravenously as a single daily dose for 5 days, was not beneficial in disseminated herpes or varicella.

3. Vidarabine (arabinofuranosyl adenine, ara-A, adenine arabinoside) is the least toxic and most effective of the analogs. Its structure is shown below.

Vidarabine is phosphorylated in the cell to the triphosphate derivative, which inhibits viral DNA polymerase much more effectively than mammalian DNA polymerase. In vivo, vidarabine is rapidly me-

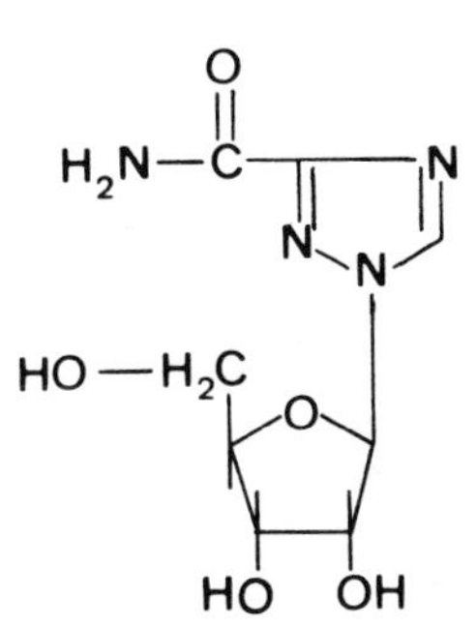

Ribavirin

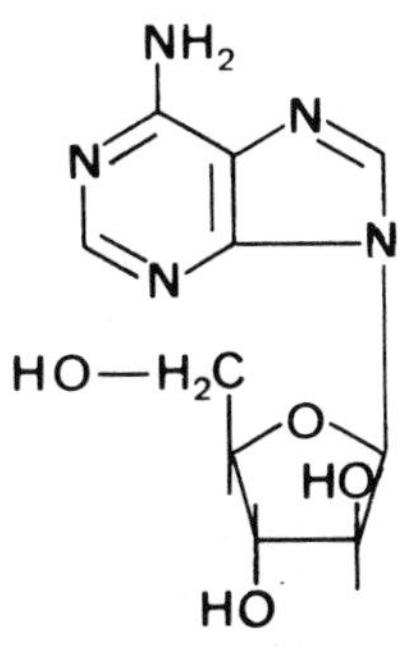

Vidarabine

Acyclovir
(acycloguanosine)

tabolized to hypoxanthine arabinoside (which is only slightly antiviral) and excreted in urine. Vidarabine monophosphate (Ara-AMP) is much more water-soluble and readily administered intravenously.

Vidarabine as 3% ointment is significantly more active against herpesvirus type 1 than against type 2. It cannot prevent recurrences but is effective treatment for herpetic and vaccinial keratitis. Topical vidarabine has no effect on skin or mucous membrane lesions (including genital lesions) of herpes simplex.

Vidarabine is also used for systemic administration because of its relatively low toxicity. There are limited effects on bone marrow and on liver and renal function, and immunosuppression appears to be minimal. Toxicity is increased in renal failure. Doses of 10–15 mg/kg/d intravenously over a 12-hour period result in substantial suppression of clinical systemic herpesvirus activity. In herpetic encephalitis proved by biopsy, use of this systemic treatment for 10 days resulted in a significant reduction in the mortality rate. However, only 40% of the treated survivors were able to resume normal life; the rest suffered from severe neurologic sequelae. The most encouraging results were observed in patients with herpetic encephalitis whose treatment was begun before onset of coma.

Systemic vidarabine (15 mg/kg/d) can limit spread of surface lesions in neonatal disseminated herpes simplex and has substantial clinical benefit. Systemic vidarabine can also inhibit the viremia in chronic active hepatitis and can inhibit the dissemination of herpes zoster in immunosuppressed cancer patients. However, prolonged systemic administration of vidarabine may produce more marked adverse gastrointestinal or neurologic side effects.

C. Other Inhibitors of Nucleic Acid Synthesis:

1. Phosphonoacetic acid–Phosphonoacetic acid inhibits herpesvirus DNA polymerase. It is effective as an inhibitor of herpesvirus proliferation in vitro and in some experimental systems. Its clinical potential is unknown.

2. Acyclovir–Acyclovir (acycloguanosine) is a guanosine derivative. Its structure is shown below.

Acyclovir is phosphorylated in herpesvirus-infected cells 30 to 100 times faster than in uninfected cells. This is due to the action of herpes-specific thymidine kinase. The product, acycloguanosine tri-

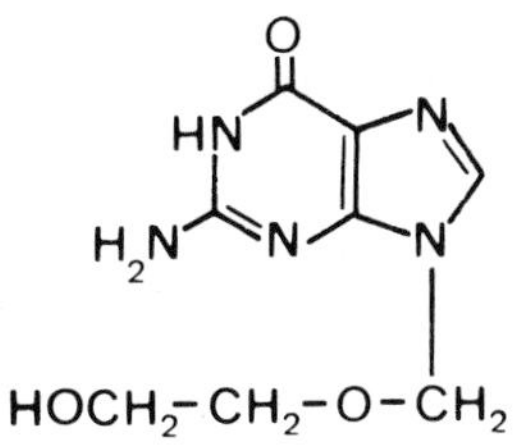

phosphate, inhibits herpesvirus DNA polymerase 10–30 times more effectively than cellular DNA polymerase. It may also have some other actions. Acyclovir inhibits many herpesviruses in cell culture and has some beneficial clinical effects. Given prophylactically before bone marrow transplants to seropositive individuals, acyclovir, 250 mg/m² every 8 hours intravenously for 18 days, significantly protected such individuals against severe herpes lesions during posttransplant immunosuppression. Given after heart transplants to prevent dissemination of herpes from existing lesions, it was effective in promoting healing of herpetic lesions but did not prevent subsequent shedding of herpesvirus. In immunocompromised patients with mucocutaneous herpetic lesions, acyclovir promoted healing of lesions and shortened viral shedding. In these trials, acyclovir, 15 mg/kg/d intravenously, produced no noticeable adverse effects in 5–18 days of administration. The same dose of acyclovir also accelerated healing of herpes zoster lesions in immunocompromised patients and perhaps reduced postherpetic pain. Intravenous acyclovir given early in the course of primary herpes simplex infections, especially of the female genital tract, reduced pain, promoted healing of lesions, and shortened viral shedding. However, such treatment did not prevent the establishment of viral latency in sensory ganglia or the frequency or intensity of recurrences. In herpetic encephalitis and in neonatal herpetic dissemination, acyclovir is more effective than vidarabine.

Oral acyclovir, 200 mg 5 times daily, has the same therapeutic effects as the intravenously administered drug, including benefit in primary genital herpes. When taken prophylactically for 4–6 months, it can reduce the frequency and severity of recurrent lesions during this period.

Topical application of 5% acyclovir ointment can limit mucocutaneous lesions of herpes simplex in immunosuppressed patients but has no effect in patients with normal immunity. Topical acyclovir can also shorten healing time and reduce pain when applied early to lesions in primary genital herpes, but it has no significant effect on recurrent genital lesions. Likewise, the frequency of recurrence is not altered.

Acyclovir-resistant herpesviruses that are thymidine kinase–deficient can emerge during treatment, but this may not alter the clinical response significantly.

3. Photodynamic inactivation–Some viruses

can be inactivated in vitro if exposed to one of several dyes and irradiated with ordinary white light. Heterotricyclic dyes, eg, neutral red or proflavine, have an affinity for the guanine base portions of DNA and are bound firmly to the DNA of some viruses. Exposure to light then leads to inactivation of the virus by producing breaks in the viral DNA.

On this theoretical basis, photodynamic inactivation has been widely applied as topical treatment to skin and mucous membrane lesions caused by herpes simplex. Controlled clinical trials have failed to show a significant benefit from this treatment. There is experimental evidence that photodynamic inactivation can result in neoplastic transformation of cells in vitro and in some animal models. While the risk incurred by treatment of humans is not defined, there is no justification for the use of this method at present.

Interferon

Interferons are a group of proteins that exert virus-nonspecific antiviral activities, at least in homologous cells, through cellular metabolic processes involving synthesis of both RNA and protein. Interferons are produced in most animal species, but they tend to be active mainly in the species in which they are produced. Among human interferons (IFN), 3 main substances are described: IFN-α represents human leukocyte interferon (type I); IFN-β represents human fibroblast interferon (type I); and IFN-γ represents human immune interferon (type II). These groupings are tentative at present. It is important to note that interferons produced by any type of cell may have more than one kind of chemical makeup and more than one type of activity.

Interferons were initially found to be produced by cells infected by viruses (type I). It was later discovered that lymphocytes also produced interferons (type II) during the immune response. Interferons express some of their activity as lymphokines and immunomodulators. Type I interferons, which act mainly as inhibitors of viral replication in cells, do so by inducing host cell ribosomes to produce cellular enzymes that subsequently block viral reproduction by inhibiting the translation of viral messenger RNA into viral proteins.

Three known enzymes are induced by interferons: (1) a protein kinase that ultimately leads to phosphorylation of elongation factor 2, resulting in inhibition of peptide chain initiation; (2) oligoisoadenylate synthetase, which ultimately leads to activation of an RNase and degradation of viral mRNA; and (3) a phosphodiesterase that can degrade the terminal nucleotides of tRNA, inhibiting peptide elongation.

In view of the broad range of viruses that are susceptible to inhibition by interferon, this agent can be considered a potentially valuable antiviral drug. Many inducers of **endogenous** interferon (eg, double-stranded RNA, synthetic polymers, small molecules such as tilorone) have been tested as topical agents applied to mucous membranes or as systemic agents given by injection. In general, the results have been

less than satisfactory: The amounts of interferon induced (or released) were small and became progressively smaller with daily inducer administration, and most inducers have exhibited some type of toxic effect. While harmless and potent inducers of endogenous interferon are still being sought, the research emphasis has been to increase production of **exogenous** human interferon on a large scale. Human interferon is now being produced in milligram quantities in pooled blood leukocytes, in fibroblasts in culture, in lymphoblastoid cells in culture, or, in gram quantities, by recombinant DNA technology, with bacteria acting as the producing cells.

Clinical studies have been performed mainly with human leukocyte interferon. If given early, interferon prevented dissemination of herpes zoster in cancer patients, reduced cytomegalovirus shedding after renal transplantation, and prevented reactivation of herpes after trigeminal root section. In chronic active hepatitis, interferon suppressed viremia with hepatitis B virus. Currently, the suggestion is being explored that interferon might have an adjunctive role in the management of certain neoplasms (Chapter 58) and might provide effective therapy in rabies and hemorrhagic fevers. The ultimate potential of interferons in human disease remains to be established. The doses used have been 10^6–10^9 units daily intravenously. Adverse effects include fatigue, weakness, anemia, and gastrointestinal disturbances. It has been postulated that these effects may be caused by interferon molecules rather than by contaminating proteins.

Inhibition of Late Protein Synthesis

A number of different amino acid analogs (eg, **fluorophenylalanine**) inhibit the synthesis of structural proteins for the coats of virus particles. The antibiotic **puromycin** has the same effect. However, these inhibitors of protein synthesis show no specificity for the synthesis of virus protein and impair protein synthesis of the host cell to such a degree that they are intensely toxic. Consequently, none of these substances are useful in chemotherapy at present.

In many poxviruses, various **thiosemicarbazones** inhibit virus replication by interfering with the synthesis of a "late" structural protein. As a result, the assembly of normal particles is blocked. **Methisazone** (N-methylisatin-β-thiosemicarbazone) can block replication of smallpox (variola) virus in humans if administered to contacts within 1–2 days after exposure. Methisazone, 2–4 g orally daily (100 mg/kg/d for children) for 3–4 days, provides striking protection against clinical smallpox. The availability of methisazone was an important consideration in abolishing smallpox vaccination. The replication of vaccinia virus can be inhibited by methisazone after symptoms have started, eg, in generalized vaccinia or in progressive vaccinia in immunologically deficient individuals. This is a valid form of antiviral chemotherapy restricted to poxviruses only.

Certain sugar analogs can inhibit the synthesis of virus-specific glycoproteins and glycolipids. Thus,

2-deoxy-D-glucose is incorporated into glycoproteins of herpes simplex virus and appears to block the cellular synthesis of major glycosylated polypeptides of herpesvirus. Clinical benefit has been claimed for topical application to initial lesions of genital herpes in women. This has not been confirmed in controlled trials.

INHIBITION OF ASSEMBLY OR RELEASE OF VIRAL PARTICLES

The assembly of intact particles can be inhibited by many agents (eg, **5-fluoro-2′-deoxyuridine** or **puro-mycin**) that induce the synthesis of defective viral constituents—whether nucleic acids or structural proteins.

Rifampin (see Chapter 46) inhibits DNA-dependent RNA polymerase in bacteria and mammalian cells. It also inhibits poxviruses, but by a different mechanism. Rifampin prevents the assembly of enveloped mature particles. The block apparently occurs during the stage of envelope formation and is reversible upon removal of the drug.

Rifampin has not been used in treatment of human poxvirus infections, but topical application can inhibit human vaccinia lesions.

REFERENCES

Balfour HH et al: Acyclovir halts progression of herpes zoster in immunocompromised patients. *N Engl J Med* 1983;**308:** 1448.

Bean B, Aeppli D: Adverse effects of high-dose intravenous acyclovir in ambulatory patients with acute herpes zoster. *J Infect Dis* 1985;**151:**362.

Bryson YJ et al: Treatment of first episodes of genital herpes simplex virus infection with oral acyclovir. *N Engl J Med* 1983;**308:**916.

Cheesman SH et al: Controlled clinical trial of prophylactic human leukocyte interferon in renal transplantation: Effects on cytomegalovirus and herpes simplex virus infections. *N Engl J Med* 1979;**300:**1345.

Coen DM et al: Biochemical and genetic analysis of acyclovir-resistant mutants of herpes simplex virus type 1. *Am J Med* 1982;**73:**351.

Dolin R et al: A controlled trial of amantadine and rimantadine in the prophylaxis of influenza A infection. *N Engl J Med* 1982;**307:**580.

Elion GB: Mechanism of action and selectivity of acyclovir. *Am J Med* 1982;**73:**7.

Fiddian AP et al: Oral acyclovir in the treatment of genital herpes. *Am J Med* 1982;**73:**335.

Hall CB et al: Aerosolized ribavirin treatment of infants with respiratory syncytial viral infection. *N Engl J Med* 1983; **308:**1443.

Hirsch MS, Swartz MN: Antiviral agents. (2 parts.) *N Engl J Med* 1980;**302:**903, 949.

Hyndiuk RA et al: Trifluridine in resistant human herpetic keratitis. *Arch Ophthalmol* 1978;**96:**1839.

Kaufman RH et al: Treatment of genital herpes simplex virus infection with photodynamic inactivation. *Am J Obstet Gynecol* 1978;**132:**861.

King DH, Galasso G: Proceedings of a symposium on acyclovir. *Am J Med* 1982;**73.** [Entire issue.]

McClung HW et al: Ribavirin aerosol treatment of influenza B virus infection. *JAMA* 1983;**249:**2671.

Merigan TC: Interferon: The first quarter century. *JAMA* 1982;**248:**2513.

Merigan TC et al: Human leukocyte interferon for the treatment of herpes zoster in patients with cancer. *N Engl J Med* 1978;**298:**981.

Mertz GJ et al: Double-blind placebo-controlled trial of oral acyclovir in first-episode genital herpes simplex virus infection. *JAMA* 1984;**252:**1147.

Nicholson KG: Antiviral agents in clinical practice. (5 parts.) *Lancet* 1984;**2:**503, 562, 617, 677, 736.

Pollard RB et al: Effect of vidarabine on chronic hepatitis B infection. *JAMA* 1978;**239:**1648.

Reichman RC et al: Topically administered acyclovir in the treatment of recurrent herpes simplex genitalis: A controlled trial. *J Infect Dis* 1983;**147:**336.

Sacks SL et al: Toxicity of vidarabine. *JAMA* 1979;**241:**28.

Saral R et al: Acyclovir prophylaxis against herpes simplex infection in patients with leukemia. *Ann Intern Med* 1983; **99:**773.

Saral R et al: Acyclovir prophylaxis of herpes simplex virus infections: A randomized, double-blind controlled trial in bone marrow transplant recipients. *N Engl J Med* 1981;**305:**63.

Spruance SL, Crumpacker CS: Topical 5 percent acyclovir in polyethylene glycol for herpes simplex labialis: Antiviral effect without clinical benefit. *Am J Med* 1982;**73:**315.

Straus SE et al: Suppression of frequently recurring genital herpes: A placebo-controlled double-blind trial of oral acyclovir. *N Engl J Med* 1984;**310:**1545.

Whitley RJ et al: Herpes simplex encephalitis: Vidarabine therapy and diagnostic problems. *N Engl J Med* 1981;**304:**313.

Whitley RJ et al: Neonatal herpes simplex infection: Follow-up evaluation of vidarabine therapy. *Pediatrics* 1983;**72:**778.

Wilson SZ et al: Treatment of influenza A (H1N1) virus infection with ribavirin aerosol. *Antimicrob Agents Chemother* 1984:**26:**200.

50 Drugs With Specialized Indications

Ernest Jawetz, MD, PhD

BACITRACIN

Bacitracin is a material first obtained from the Tracy strain of *Bacillus subtilis* in 1943. It is active against gram-positive microorganisms. Because of its marked toxicity when used systemically, it is now generally limited to topical use.

Chemistry

Bacitracin is a mixture of water-soluble polypeptides. The material is stable in the dry form or when incorporated into a petrolatum. The unit of activity is defined as the equivalent of 26 μg of a Food and Drug Administration (USA) standard.

Antibacterial Activity

Bacitracin is most active against gram-positive bacteria, including β-lactamase–producing staphylococci, in concentrations of 0.1–20 units/mL. There is no cross-resistance between bacitracin and other antimicrobial drugs.

Bacitracin inhibits cell wall formation. It interferes with the final dephosphorylation in cycling the phospholipid carrier that transfers mucopeptide to the growing cell wall (Fig 42–2).

Absorption, Metabolism, & Excretion

Bacitracin is little absorbed from gut, skin, wounds, mucous membranes, pleura, or synovia. Topical application thus results in local effects without significant systemic toxicity. After intramuscular injection, bacitracin is fairly well absorbed, widely distributed in the body, and excreted by glomerular filtration into the urine.

Clinical Uses

Because of its systemic toxicity, bacitracin is now used mainly for topical treatment. Bacitracin, 500 units/g in an ointment base (often combined with polymyxin or neomycin), is useful for the suppression of mixed bacterial flora in surface lesions of the skin, in wounds, or on mucous membranes. Solutions of bacitracin containing 100–200 units/mL in saline can be employed for instillation into joints, wounds, or the pleural cavity—often in conjunction with other drugs given systemically. In antibiotic-associated colitis, the oral administration of bacitracin, 25,000 units 4 times daily for 1–2 weeks, can be ef-

fective treatment. It is an alternative to vancomycin and is less expensive, but it has potential toxicity in this setting.

Adverse Reactions

Bacitracin is markedly nephrotoxic, producing proteinuria, hematuria, and nitrogen retention. Therefore, systemic use has been virtually abandoned. Topical application only rarely causes hypersensitivity reactions (eg, skin rashes) or produces significant systemic toxicity.

VANCOMYCIN

Vancomycin is an antibiotic produced by *Streptomyces orientalis*. It is active against gram-positive bacteria, particularly staphylococci.

Chemistry

Vancomycin is a glycopeptide with a molecular weight of 1500. The hydrochloride is a white powder, soluble in water, and very stable.

Antibacterial Activity

Vancomycin is bactericidal for gram-positive bacteria in concentrations of 0.5–3 μg/mL. Most pathogenic staphylococci including those producing β-lactamase and those resistant to nafcillin-methicillin are killed by 10 μg/mL or less. Resistant mutants are very rare in susceptible populations, and clinical resistance emerges very slowly. There is no cross-resistance with other known antibiotics.

The mechanism of action involves inhibition of cell wall mucopeptide synthesis. Vancomycin inhibits the utilization of disaccharide(-pentapeptide)-P-phospholipid (Fig 42–2). Cell membrane function is also damaged.

Vancomycin can be synergistic with aminoglycosides against certain enterococci and other gram-positive bacteria.

Absorption, Metabolism, & Excretion

Vancomycin is not absorbed from the intestinal tract and can be given orally only for the treatment of enterocolitis. Systemic doses must be administered intravenously. After intravenous injection of 0.5 g, blood levels of 7–10 μg/mL are reached in 5 minutes and maintained for 1–2 hours. The drug is widely distributed in the body. Excretion is mainly through the kidneys into the urine. In the presence of renal insufficiency, striking accumulation may occur. In functionally anephric patients, the half-life of vancomycin is between 6 and 10 days. Vancomycin may also accumulate in the presence of hepatic insufficiency. The drug is not removed by hemodialysis.

Clinical Uses

The only indication for the use of parenteral vancomycin is serious staphylococcal infection or enterococcal endocarditis not responding to other treatment. For staphylococcal bacteremia or sepsis, 0.5 g is injected intravenously in 20 minutes every 6–8 hours (20–40 mg/kg/d for children). Rarely, vancomycin is given with an aminoglycoside in enterococcal endocarditis.

Vancomycin penetrates somewhat irregularly into the central nervous system, but intravenously administered drug has been used to treat meningitis and shunt infections. Supplemental instillation into the CNS site is sometimes necessary. The role of vancomycin in prophylaxis of neurosurgical shunt infections is unsettled.

Oral vancomycin, 0.5 g every 6 hours, is used to treat antibiotic-associated enterocolitis, especially if caused by *Clostridium difficile*.

Adverse Reactions

A. Allergic Reactions: Skin rashes and anaphylaxis have been observed infrequently.

B. Direct Toxicity: Chills, fever, and phlebitis of the site of injection occur. Ototoxicity and nephrotoxicity were formerly common, but since 1970 vancomycin preparations have been relatively well tolerated.

ERYTHROMYCIN

This is a group of closely related macrolide compounds characterized by a macrocyclic lactone ring to which sugars are attached. The prototype drug, erythromycin, was obtained in 1952 from *Streptomyces erythreus*. Members of the group include carbomycin, oleandomycin, spiramycin, and many others. They act intracellularly on protein synthesis.

Chemistry

The general structure is shown below with the macrolide ring and the sugars desosamine and cladinose. The molecular weight of erythromycin is 734. It is poorly soluble in water (0.1%) but dissolves readily in organic solvents. Solutions are relatively stable at 4 °C but lose activity rapidly at 20 °C and at acid pH. Erythromycins are dispensed as various esters and salts.

Antimicrobial Activity

Erythromycins are effective against gram-positive organisms, especially pneumococci, streptococci, staphylococci, and corynebacteria, in concentrations of 0.02–2 μg/mL. Neisseriae, *Bordetella, Mycoplasma, Legionella, Chlamydia trachomatis*, and certain mycobacteria (*Mycobacterium kansasii, Mycobacterium scrofulaceum*) are also susceptible.

The antibacterial action of the erythromycins is both inhibitory and bactericidal for susceptible organisms. Activity is enhanced at alkaline pH. Inhibition of protein synthesis occurs by action on the 50S unit of ribosomes. The receptor for erythromycins, lincomycins, and perhaps other drugs is a 23S rRNA on the 50S subunit. Protein synthesis is inhibited as aminoacyl translocation reactions and the formation of initiation complexes are blocked. Resistance to erythromycins results from methylation of the rRNA receptor, which prevents attachment of the drug to the ribosome. This mechanism is under the control of a plasmid.

Resistance

In most susceptible microbial populations, organisms occur that are highly resistant to erythromycin.

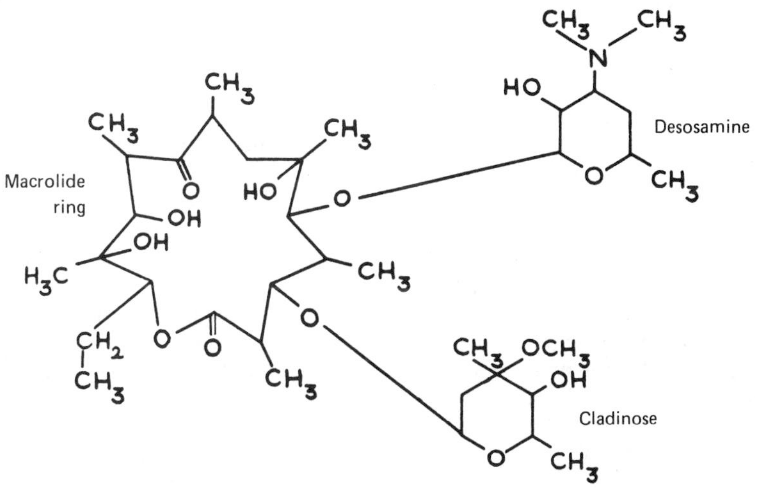

Erythromycin

Resistance is especially frequent among staphylococci, and their emergence in the course of prolonged treatment with erythromycin is highly predictable. Consequently, erythromycin should never be used as the sole drug in treating severe staphylococcal infections. Erythromycin-resistant pneumococci and streptococci are encountered occasionally.

There appears to be virtually complete cross-resistance among all members of the erythromycin group. Erythromycin resistance is based on alteration of the receptor on the 50S unit of the ribosome. Resistance does not involve destruction of drug. There is some cross-resistance to lincomycins.

Absorption, Metabolism, & Excretion

Erythromycin base is destroyed by stomach acid and must be administered with enteric coating. Stearates and esters are fairly acid-resistant and relatively well absorbed. The lauryl salt of the propionyl ester of erythromycin (erythromycin estolate) is among the best-absorbed oral preparations. Oral doses of 2 g/d result in serum levels of up to 2 μg/mL. Large amounts are lost in feces. Absorbed drug is distributed widely *except* in the brain and cerebrospinal fluid. It traverses the placenta and reaches the fetus.

Erythromycins are excreted largely in the bile, where levels may be 50 times higher than in the blood. A portion of the drug excreted into bile is reabsorbed from the intestines. Only 5% of the administered dose is excreted in the urine.

Clinical Uses

Erythromycins are the drugs of choice in corynebacterial infections (diphtheria, diphtheroid sepsis, erythrasma); in respiratory, neonatal, ocular, or genital chlamydial infections; and in pneumonias caused by *Mycoplasma* and *Legionella*. *Campylobacter jejuni* is susceptible to erythromycin, and spiramycin has some beneficial effect in diarrhea caused by *Cryptosporidium*. Otherwise, erythromycins are most useful as penicillin substitutes in individuals with streptococcal or pneumococcal infections who are hypersensitive to penicillin. In rheumatic individuals taking penicillin prophylaxis, erythromycin should be given prior to dental procedures as prophylaxis against endocarditis. Although erythromycin estolate is best absorbed, it also produces the greatest risk of adverse reactions. Therefore, the stearate or succinate may be preferred.

A. Oral Dosage: Give erythromycin base, stearate, or estolate, 0.25–0.5 g every 6 hours (for children, 40 mg/kg/d); or erythromycin ethylsuccinate, 0.4–0.6 g every 6 hours. Oral erythromycin base (1 g) is sometimes combined with oral neomycin or kanamycin for preoperative preparation of the colon.

B. Intravenous Dosage: (Eg, erythromycin gluceptate or lactobionate.) Adults, 0.5 g every 8–12 hours; children, 40 mg/kg/d.

Adverse Reactions

A. Gastrointestinal Effects: Anorexia, nausea, vomiting, and diarrhea occasionally accompany oral administration.

B. Liver Toxicity: Erythromycins, particularly the estolate, can produce acute cholestatic hepatitis (fever, jaundice, impaired liver function), probably as a hypersensitivity reaction. Most patients recover from this, but hepatitis recurs if the drug is readministered. Other allergic reactions include fever, eosinophilia, and rashes. Erythromycins can increase the effects of oral anticoagulants and of oral digoxin.

LINCOMYCIN & CLINDAMYCIN (Lincosamines)

Lincomycin is an antibiotic elaborated by *Streptomyces lincolnensis*. Clindamycin is a chlorine-substituted derivative of lincomycin.

Lincomycin resembles erythromycin in activity, but there are few if any valid indications for its use. Clindamycin is more potent and is briefly described here.

Antibacterial Activity

Many gram-positive cocci are inhibited by lincomycins, 0.5–5 μg/mL. Enterococci, *Haemophilus*, neisseriae, and *Mycoplasma* are usually resistant (in contrast to erythromycin). While lincomycins have little or no action on most gram-negative bacteria, *Bacteroides* and other anaerobes are usually susceptible. Lincomycins inhibit protein synthesis by interfering with the formation of initiation complexes and with aminoacyl translocation reactions. The receptor for lincomycins on the 50S subunit of the bacterial ribosome is a 23S rRNA, perhaps identical with the receptor for erythromycins. Thus, these 2 drug classes may block each other's attachment and may interfere with each other. Resistance to lincomycins appears slowly, perhaps as a result of chromosomal mutation. Plasmid-mediated resistance has not been established with certainty. Resistance to lincomycin is not rare among streptococci, pneumococci, and staphylococci. *C difficile* strains appear to be regularly resistant.

Absorption, Metabolism, & Excretion

Oral doses of clindamycin, 0.15–0.3 g every 6 hours (10–20 mg/kg/d for children), yield serum levels of 2–3 μg/mL. Intravenously, 600 mg clindamycin every 6–8 hours gives levels of 5–15 μg/mL. The drug is widely distributed in the body but does not appear in the central nervous system in significant concentrations. It is about 90% protein-bound. Excretion is mainly through the liver, bile, and urine.

Clinical Uses

Probably the most important indication for clindamycin is the treatment of severe anaerobic infection caused by *Bacteroides* (especially *Bacteroides frag-*

ilis) and other anaerobes that are often resistant to penicillin and that often participate in mixed infections.

Meningitis should *not* be treated with lincomycins. Clindamycin crosses the placenta and may reach the fetus in concentrations sufficient for the treatment of anaerobic intrauterine infections. Clindamycin, perhaps combined with an aminoglycoside, has also been considered for penetrating wounds of the abdomen and the gut. Clindamycin has found favor in the management of infections originating in the female genital tract, eg, septic abortion and pelvic abscesses that are populated by a variety of microbes, with heavy participation of anaerobes including *B fragilis*.

Adverse Reactions

Common side effects are diarrhea, nausea, and skin rashes. Impaired liver function (with or without jaundice) and neutropenia sometimes occur. Severe diarrhea and enterocolitis—sometimes ending fatally—have followed clindamycin administration and place a serious restraint on its use. The incidence of severe diarrhea has ranged from 2 to 20% in various studies.

The antibiotic-associated pseudomembranous colitis that has followed administration of clindamycin in some hospitals appears to be caused by toxigenic *C difficile*. This organism is infrequently part of the normal fecal flora but is selected out during administration of clindamycin (and occasionally other drugs). It grows to high numbers in the sigmoid colon and secretes a necrotizing toxin that produces pseudomembranous colitis. This potentially fatal complication must be recognized promptly and treated with oral vancomycin, 0.5 g 4–6 times daily (see above). Oral bacitracin or metronidazole may be effective as well. Variations in the local prevalence of *C difficile* may account for the great differences in incidence of antibiotic-associated colitis.

NOVOBIOCIN

Novobiocin (also called streptonivicin, cardelmycin) is an acidic antibiotic produced by *Streptomyces niveus* and purified in 1956. It is active mainly against gram-positive bacteria.

Until the advent of β-lactamase–resistant penicillins and cephalosporins, novobiocin was useful in serious staphylococcal infections. To avoid rapid emergence of resistant variants, novobiocin had to be employed in combination with another drug. At present, there appears to be no valid indication for the use of novobiocin, especially since the incidence of adverse reactions was high.

METRONIDAZOLE

This nitroimidazole drug found widespread use as an antiprotozoal agent (Chapter 56) and is effective against some anaerobic bacteria as well. Metronidazole is well absorbed after oral intake, with peak serum levels reaching 5 μg/mL 1 hour after 250 mg orally. The serum half-life is more than 8 hours. The drug diffuses well into all tissues, including the central nervous system, and enters abscesses and empyemas with little protein binding.

Metronidazole is strikingly bactericidal for many anaerobes, including *B fragilis* and clostridia. In serious anaerobic infections, the oral dose is 500–750 mg 3 or 4 times daily. An intravenous preparation is available for serious infections in a dose of 7.5 mg/kg every 6 hours. Similar doses given by rectal suppository are well absorbed and give therapeutically active levels. Thus there is little need for the intravenous form. Oral metronidazole, 0.5 g every 6–8 hours, can be effective therapy for antibiotic-associated colitis.

In trichomonal vaginitis, both sex partners can be treated with 250 mg 3 times daily by mouth for 7 days. A single dose of 2 g by mouth may be quite effective. In "nonspecific" vaginitis ("*Gardnerella*" or "*Haemophilus*" vaginitis), metronidazole is given orally, 500 mg twice daily for 7 days. In intestinal or hepatic amebiasis, 750 mg 3 times daily is given for 7–10 days.

Metronidazole is also effective in eradicating giardiasis. The drug has been used for preoperative preparation of the colon, and it seems to prevent postoperative anaerobic infections. However, metronidazole has not been approved for this purpose because of laboratory evidence of its carcinogenicity (see p 638).

Common adverse effects include stomatitis, nausea, diarrhea, and central nervous system disturbances, particularly vestibular reactions with ataxia, vertigo, and headaches. Metronidazole produces disulfiramlike reactions if taken with alcohol. Simultaneous intake of barbiturates reduces the half-life of metronidazole.

REFERENCES

Bartlett JG: Anti-anaerobic antibacterial agents. *Lancet* 1982;**2**:478.

Braun P: Hepatotoxicity of erythromycin. *J Infect Dis* 1975; **119**:300.

Chang TW et al: Bacitracin treatment of antibiotic-associated colitis and diarrhea caused by *Clostridium difficile* toxin. *Gastroenterology* 1980;**78**:1584.

Dhawan VK, Thadepalli H: Clindamycin: A review of fifteen years of experience. *Rev Infect Dis* 1982;**4**:1133.

Eichenwald HF, McCracken GH: Antimicrobial therapy in infants and children. *J Pediatr* 1978;**93**:337.

Feigen RD et al: Clindamycin treatment of osteomyelitis and septic arthritis in children. *Pediatrics* 1975;**55**:213.

Finegold SM: Metronidazole. *Ann Intern Med* 1980;**93**:585.

Freeark RJ: Penetrating wounds of the abdomen. *N Engl J Med* 1974;**291**:185.

Ginsburg CM, Eichenwald HF: Erythromycin: Review of its uses in pediatrics. *J Pediatr* 1976;**89:**872.

Goldman P: Metronidazole. *N Engl J Med* 1980;**303:**1212.

Gorbach SL, Thadepalli H: Clindamycin in pure and mixed anaerobic infections. *Arch Intern Med* 1974;**134:**87.

Hook EW, Johnson WD: Vancomycin therapy of bacterial endocarditis. *Am J Med* 1978;**65:**411.

Ioannides L et al: Rectal administration of metronidazole provides therapeutic plasma levels in postoperative patients. *N Engl J Med* 1981;**305:**1569.

Kucers A: Chloramphenicol, erythromycin, vancomycin, tetracyclines. *Lancet* 1982;**2:**425.

Ledger WJ et al: Comparison of clindamycin and chloramphenicol in treatment of serious infections of the female genital tract. *J Infect Dis* 1977;**135(Suppl):**S30.

McHenry MC, Gavan TL: Vancomycin. *Pediatr Clin North Am* 1983;**30:**31.

Meade RH: Antimicrobial spectrum, pharmacology and therapeutic use of erythromycin and its derivatives. *Am J Hosp Pharm* 1979;**36:**1185.

Moellering RC et al: Vancomycin therapy in patients with impaired renal function: A nomogram for dosage. *Ann Intern Med* 1981;**94:**343.

Pestka S et al: Induction of erythromycin resistance in *Staphylococcus aureus*. *Antimicrob Agents Chemother* 1975;**9:**128.

Portnoy D et al: Treatment of intestinal cryptosporidiosis with spiramycin. *Ann Intern Med* 1984;**101:**202.

Rosenblatt JE, Edson RS: Metronidazole. *Mayo Clin Proc* 1983;**58:**154.

Silva J et al: Treatment of *Clostridium difficile* colitis and diarrhea with vancomycin. *Am J Med* 1981;**71:**815.

Sutherland GE et al: Sterilization of Ommaya reservoir by instillation of vancomycin. *Am J Med* 1981;**71:**1068.

Teasley DG et al: Trial of metronidazole vs. vancomycin for *Clostridium difficile*: Associated diarrhea and colitis. *Lancet* 1983;**2:**1043.

Tedesco FJ: Clindamycin and colitis: A review. *J Infect Dis* 1977;**135(Suppl):**S95.

Warner JF et al: Metronidazole therapy of anaerobic bacteremia, meningitis and brain abscess. *Arch Intern Med* 1979;**139:**167.

Urinary Antiseptics[*]

Ernest Jawetz, MD, PhD

Urinary antiseptics are drugs that exert antibacterial activity in the urine but have little or no systemic antibacterial effect. Their usefulness is limited to urinary tract infections. Prolonged suppression of bacteriuria by means of urinary antiseptics may be desirable in chronic urinary tract infection where eradication of infection by short-term systemic therapy has not been possible.

NITROFURANTOIN

Chemistry

Many derivatives of furan possess antibacterial properties. Most of these substances are topical disinfectants (see Chapter 54). Nitrofurantoin is the main urinary antiseptic among nitrofurans.

Nitrofurantoin

Antibacterial Activity

Nitrofurans are bacteriostatic and bactericidal for many gram-positive and gram-negative bacteria. Susceptible bacteria are inhibited by 32 μg/mL or less—a concentration readily exceeded in urine. Although certain strains of microorganisms are resistant (eg, many strains of *Proteus vulgaris* and all strains of *Pseudomonas aeruginosa*), resistant mutants are rare in nitrofurantoin-susceptible populations. Clinical drug resistance emerges slowly. There is no cross-resistance between nitrofurans and other antimicrobial agents.

The mechanism of action of the nitrofurans is not known. The activity of nitrofurans depends to some extent upon the size of the microbial population. With very high concentrations of bacteria in the urine or in culture medium, the activity of nitrofurantoin is diminished. The activity of nitrofurantoin is greatly enhanced at pH 5.5 or below.

Absorption, Metabolism, & Excretion

Nitrofurantoin is rapidly and completely absorbed

from the gastrointestinal tract, but the absorbed drug is metabolized and excreted so rapidly that no significant levels can be detected in blood and most tissues. Thus, nitrofurantoin has no systemic antibacterial activity. In the kidneys, the drug is excreted in the urine by both glomerular filtration and tubular secretion. Tubular reabsorption occurs, and concentration in hilar lymph and renal interstitial fluid is high. With average daily doses, concentrations of 200 μg/mL are reached in urine. In renal failure, urine levels are insufficient for antibacterial action, but high blood levels may cause toxicity.

Clinical Uses

The average daily dose for urinary tract infection in adults is 50–100 mg 4 times daily by mouth (5–8 mg/kg/d for children), taken with meals or after eating. Some persons can tolerate up to 600 mg/d, but this higher dose often results in nausea or vomiting. Gastrointestinal disturbance due to nitrofurantoin can be reduced if the drug is taken with food or milk. Nitrofurantoin must never be given to patients with severe renal insufficiency. Oral nitrofurantoin can be given for weeks, months, or even years for the suppression of chronic urinary tract infection. It is desirable to keep urinary pH below 5.5 (see Acidifying Agents, below). Some women are subject to recurrent urinary tract infection as a result of sexual activity. In many of these cases, daily administration of nitrofurantoin, 100 mg, for months may result in freedom from symptoms and infection.

It is possible to administer the soluble sodium salt of nitrofurantoin intravenously, but even such injected drug has no systemic antimicrobial activity.

Another nitrofuran, furazolidone, 400 mg (5–8 mg/kg in children) daily orally, may reduce diarrhea in cholera and perhaps shorten vibrio excretion. It usually fails in shigellosis.

Adverse Reactions

A. Direct Toxicity: Anorexia, nausea, and vomiting are the principal (and frequent) side effects of orally administered nitrofurantoin. Neuropathies and hemolytic anemias (in glucose-6-phosphate dehydrogenase deficiency) are rare. Nitrofurantoin antagonizes the action of nalidixic and oxolinic acid.

B. Allergic Reactions: Various skin rashes, pulmonary infiltration, and other hypersensitivity reactions have been reported.

---

[*] The sulfonamides are discussed in Chapter 47.

NALIDIXIC ACID & OXOLINIC ACID

These are urinary antiseptics for use in the management of urinary tract infections with gram-negative bacteria. They are effective when taken orally and have no significant systemic activity. Nalidixic acid is the older and better-studied drug.

Chemistry

Nalidixic and oxolinic acids are synthetic chemicals with the formulas shown below. They are stable in dry form and poorly soluble in water.

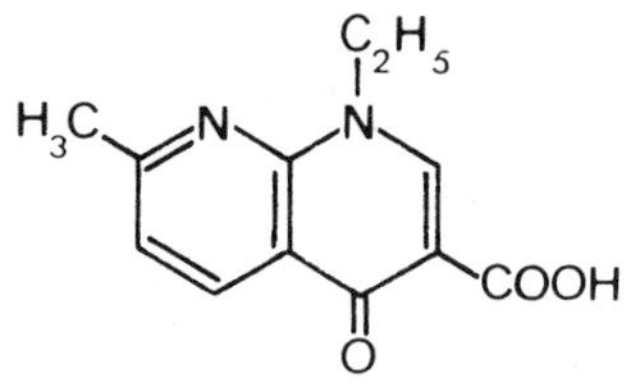

Nalidixic acid

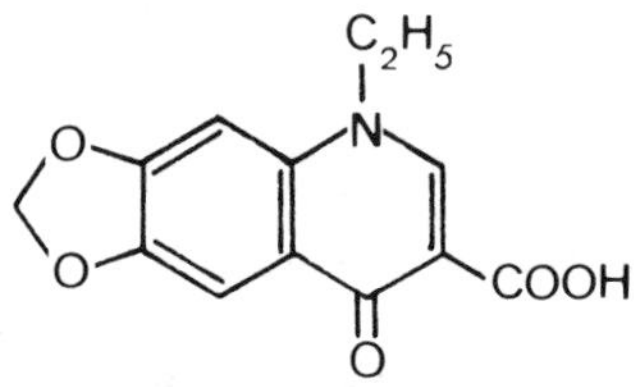

Oxolinic acid

Antibacterial Activity

Nalidixic acid inhibits many gram-negative bacteria in vitro in concentrations of 1–20 μg/mL. Much higher concentrations are necessary to inhibit gram-positive organisms. Most strains of *Escherichia coli* are inhibited, as are some strains of *Enterobacter, Klebsiella,* and *Proteus. Pseudomonas* sp are usually resistant.

The mechanism of the chemotherapeutic effect is not clear. These drugs may lower the pH of the urine sufficiently to result in inhibition of bacteria. These acids are powerful inhibitors of DNA synthesis in *E coli* (they inhibit DNA gyrase), but it is not certain that this effect is the sole basis of their therapeutic action.

Resistant microorganisms emerge rapidly during therapy, both by selection of drug-resistant mutants in the population and by superinfection with drug-resistant microorganisms of another strain or species. Plasmid-mediated resistance to nalidixic acid has not been demonstrated. There is no cross-resistance with other antimicrobial drugs.

Oxolinic acid is 2–4 times more active in vitro than nalidixic acid.

Absorption, Metabolism, & Excretion

After oral administration, the drugs are readily absorbed from the gut, rapidly metabolized, and excreted. Thus, there is no significant systemic antibacterial action. About 20% of the absorbed drug is excreted in the urine in the active form and 80% in an inactive form as a glucuronide conjugate. Levels of active drug in the urine reach 50–200 μg/mL.

Clinical Uses

The only indication for these agents is urinary tract infection with coliform organisms. The dose of nalidixic acid for adults is 1 g orally 4 times a day for 1–2 weeks (children, 30–60 mg/kg/d). The dose of oxolinic acid is 0.75 g twice a day. Cinoxacin (1 g/d), a drug related to nalidixic acid, can also be used in urinary tract infections.

Adverse Reactions

Nalidixic acid excreted in the urine may give rise to false-positive tests for glucose, but true hyperglycemia and glycosuria may also be produced. There are occasional gastrointestinal disturbances, skin rashes, sensitization to sunlight, visual disturbances, and central nervous system stimulation. Convulsions have been reported following overdosage. The central nervous system toxicity of oxolinic acid is probably higher; consequently, nalidixic acid may be preferred.

METHENAMINE MANDELATE & METHENAMINE HIPPURATE

Methenamine mandelate is the salt of mandelic acid and methenamine and possesses to some extent the properties of both of these urinary antiseptics. Methenamine hippurate is the salt of hippuric acid and methenamine. Mandelic acid ($C_6H_5CHOHCOOH$) or hippuric acid taken orally is excreted unchanged in the urine, where these drugs are bactericidal for some gram-negative bacteria if the pH can be kept below 5.5. Methenamine is absorbed readily after oral intake and excreted in the urine. If the urine is strongly acid (pH below 5.5), methenamine releases formaldehyde, which is antibacterial.

Methenamine mandelate, 1 g 4 times daily, or methenamine hippurate, 1 g twice daily by mouth (children, 50 mg/kg/d or 30 mg/kg/d), is used only as a urinary antiseptic. If necessary, acidifying agents (eg, ascorbic acid, 4–12 g daily) may be given to lower urinary pH below 5.5. Sulfonamides cannot be given at the same time because they may form an insoluble compound with the formaldehyde released by methenamine. Persons taking methenamine may exhibit falsely elevated tests for catecholamines.

The action of methenamine mandelate or hippurate is nonspecific against many different microorganisms and consists of the simultaneous effects of formaldehyde and acidity. Microorganisms such as *Proteus* that make a strongly alkaline urine through release of ammonia from urea usually are insusceptible.

ACIDIFYING AGENTS

In chronic urinary tract infections, eradication of the organisms often fails. It is then important to suppress bacteria for as long as possible.

Any substance that will produce a urine pH below 5.5 usually inhibits bacterial growth in urine. Keto-genic diets, ammonium chloride, ascorbic acid, man-delic acid, methionine, and hippuric acid (eg, from in-gestion of cranberry juice) all can be employed to that end. It is important to check urinary pH frequently and to ascertain by direct microscopic examination that the bacteriuria is actually suppressed. Prolonged suppres-sion (6–18 months) occasionally permits healing of the infection, probably because it blocks the frequent ascending reinfection of the kidneys from the lower tract.

SYSTEMICALLY ACTIVE DRUGS IN URINARY TRACT INFECTION

Many antimicrobial drugs are excreted in the urine in active form. The concentration in urine is often many times higher than the concentration in body fluids or tissues because of active secretion by the proximal tubule. Effective antibacterial concentra-tions can therefore be attained in urine with doses too low to be effective in systemic infections. This permits the use of drugs that are relatively toxic. Drugs such as gentamicin, kanamycin, amikacin, or the polymyxins can be administered in doses sufficient to achieve high urine levels without risking significant adverse effects. Even more toxic drugs such as cycloserine (see below) can be administered in a dose that produces urine lev-els sufficient to suppress highly resistant organisms, eg, *Proteus*, with only a moderate risk of serious toxi-city. Penicillins in systemic doses are excreted in the urine to yield concentrations of 60–3000 μg/mL. This may be sufficient to suppress not only gram-positive but also many gram-negative bacteria. Ampicillin and carbenicillin are particularly effective against many gram-negative bacteria in the urinary tract unless they are inactivated by high concentrations of β-lactamase in bladder urine. A single 3-g dose of amoxicillin oral-ly may be effective in uncomplicated first urinary tract infections.

Soluble sulfonamides (eg, sulfisoxazole, trisul-fapyrimidines USP) constitute a common choice for initial treatment of urinary tract infection. The dosage (0.5 g 4–6 times daily orally) is substantially smaller than the systemically active amount, yet concentra-tions in the urine are high. Even better may be the simultaneous use of sulfamethoxazole, 400 mg, with trimethoprim, 80 mg. Four such tablets daily for 1–3 days is an adequate urinary dose. One tablet daily may be useful as a prophylactic drug for sexually active women who are subject to recurrent urinary tract in-fections or the urethral syndrome.

Cycloserine

Cycloserine is an antibiotic produced by *Strepto-myces orchidaceus* in 1955 and later synthesized.

Cycloserine

The substance is water-soluble and very unstable at acid pH. Cycloserine inhibits many microorganisms, including coliforms, *Proteus*, and mycobacteria. The mode of action involves the inhibition of incorporation of D-alanine into mucopeptide of the bacterial cell wall by inhibiting the enzyme alanine racemase (Fig 42–2). After ingestion of cycloserine, 0.25 g every 6 hours, blood levels reach 20–30 μg/mL—sufficient to inhibit many strains of mycobacteria and gram-negative bac-teria. The drug is widely distributed in tissues. Most of the drug is excreted in active form into the urine, where concentrations are sufficiently high to inhibit many organisms causing urinary tract infections. The urinary tract dose is 10–15 mg/kg/d.

Cycloserine may produce serious central nervous system toxicity manifested by headaches, tremor, ver-tigo, acute psychosis, and convulsions. With careful management of oral dosage (below 0.75 g/d), these symptoms can usually be avoided. Cycloserine is occasionally employed for the treatment of tuberculo-sis or urinary tract infections. The dosage is usually 0.25 g 2–3 times daily by mouth (for children, 20 mg/kg/d). In nocardiosis, cycloserine, 0.25 g 4 times daily with full systemic doses of a sulfonamide, has been occasionally curative.

TOPICAL USE OF ANTIMICROBIAL DRUGS IN THE URINARY TRACT

Indwelling catheterization of the urinary bladder has a high risk of producing urinary tract infection. This risk can be markedly reduced if a closed, sterile collection system is employed with strictest asepsis. This is often combined with the use of an irrigating so-lution that contains 0.25% acetic acid or bactericidal concentrations of polymyxins and neomycins, admin-istered by 3-way catheter. Such systems may delay in-fection with indwelling catheterization for several weeks. They have no place in the treatment of urinary tract infections. Occasionally, amphotericin B, 20 μg/mL, is instilled into the urinary bladder for control of *Candida* infection.

REFERENCES

Bose W et al: Controlled trial of co-trimoxazole in children with urinary tract infection. *Lancet* 1974;**2**:614.

Counts GM et al: Treatment of cystitis in women with a single

dose of trimethoprim-sulfamethoxazole. *Rev Infect Dis* 1982;**4**:484.

Crumplin GC, Smith JT: Nalidixic acid: An antibacterial paradox. *Antimicrob Agents Chemother* 1974;**8:**251.

Fang LST et al: Efficacy of single dose and conventional amoxicillin therapy in urinary tract infections localized by the antibody-coated bacteria technic. *N Engl J Med* 1978;**298:**413.

Freeman RB et al: Long-term therapy for chronic bacteriuria in men. *Ann Intern Med* 1974;**83:**133.

Hamilton-Miller JM, Brumfitt W: Methenamine and its salts as urinary antiseptics. *Invest Urol* 1977;**14:**287.

Kunin CM: *Detection, Prevention, and Management of Urinary Tract Infections*, 3rd ed. Lea & Febiger, 1979.

Lohr JA et al: Prevention of recurrent urinary tract infections in girls. *Pediatrics* 1977;**59:**562.

Matthew AD et al: Prevention of bacteriuria after transurethral prostatectomy with nitrofurantoin. *J Urol* 1978;**120:**442.

Ronald AR, Harding KM: Urinary infection prophylaxis in women. *Ann Intern Med* 1981;**94:**268.

Savard-Fenton M et al: Single dose amoxicillin therapy with follow-up urine culture: Effective initial management for acute uncomplicated urinary tract infections. *Am J Med* 1982; **73:**808.

Shapera RM, Matsen JM: Oxolinic acid therapy for urinary tract infections in children. *Am J Dis Child* 1977;**131:**34.

Stamm WE: Prevention of urinary tract infections. *Am J Med* 1984;**76:**148.

Strauss WG, Griffin LM: Nitrofurantoin pneumonia. *JAMA* 1967;**199:**765.

Turck M, Anderson KN, Petersdorf RG: Relapse and reinfection in chronic bacteriuria. *N Engl J Med* 1966;**275:**70.

Vosti KL: Recurrent urinary tract infections: Prevention by prophylactic antibiotics after sexual intercourse. *JAMA* 1975; **231:**934.

Clinical Use of Antimicrobials

52

John Mills, MD, Steven L. Barriere, PharmD, & Ernest Jawetz, MD, PhD

The development of antimicrobial drugs represents one of the most important advances in therapeutics, as effective treatment of serious infections has improved the quality of life and has permitted advances in many other areas of medicine. For example, cancer chemotherapy, organ transplantation, and major surgery (especially involving insertion of prosthetic devices) are almost entirely dependent on the availability of antimicrobials. It is fortunate that most antimicrobials are relatively nontoxic; however, all have side effects (eg, allergic reactions or effects on the normal bacterial flora) that may be troublesome or even life-threatening. Thus, as with all forms of drug therapy, good clinical judgment and overall management are important to optimal patient care.

EMPIRIC ANTIMICROBIAL THERAPY

In many clinical situations in which antimicrobials are used, the pathogen causing the disease is not known at the time therapy is initiated—or, if the pathogen is known, its susceptibility to specific antimicrobials is unknown. This use of antimicrobials constitutes **empiric therapy** (also called **presumptive therapy**)—ie, therapy initiated on the presumption of infection based on broad experience with similar clinical situations rather than on specific information about a given patient's disease. The principal justification for empiric therapy is that infections are best treated early. To withhold antimicrobials until the results of cultures and susceptibility testing are available (generally 1–3 days) may expose the patient to serious morbidity or death. There are many clinical circumstances in which this is true—eg, a severely neutropenic patient who develops evidence of infection may die within a few hours if effective therapy is not begun. On the other hand, clinicians must also be cognizant of the many circumstances in which empiric therapy is unnecessary, so that antimicrobials can be withheld pending culture and susceptibility testing. For example, antimicrobial therapy of streptococcal pharyngitis only minimally shortens the duration of symptoms and will prevent rheumatic fever even if delayed for as long as 7–9 days—more than enough time to obtain microbiologic confirmation of the clinical diagnosis.

Empiric therapy has 2 main disadvantages: (1) If the patient proves not to have an infection, the expense and possible toxicity of antimicrobial drug administration have not been justified; and (2) if proper specimens for diagnosis are not obtained initially, the patient may improve but the diagnosis may be obscured, thus complicating later decisions about definitive therapy.

Initiation of empiric therapy (and, to a certain extent, all antimicrobial therapy) should conform to a well-defined protocol:

(1) Formulate a clinical diagnosis of microbial infection. Using all available data, the clinician should conclude that there is evidence of infection and should then attempt to determine the anatomic site of infection as closely as possible—eg, pneumonia, cellulitis, septicemia.

(2) Obtain specimens for laboratory examination. Examination of specimens by microscopy (Gram's stain or other methods) may provide reliable information within an hour or so about the microbial pathogen. Culture or other specialized examinations (eg, antigen detection by immunofluorescence or other methods) will provide an etiologic diagnosis within 1 or 2 days in most cases. Blood and material from the site of infection (eg, urine from patients with suspected urinary tract infection; sputum from patients with pneumonia) are commonly obtained.

Specimens for microbiologic diagnosis are best collected *before* administration of antimicrobials, because properly selected antimicrobials should eliminate or suppress the causative organisms and make specific diagnosis impossible. Identification of the causative agent permits refining antimicrobial therapy with reduction of toxicity and cost.

(3) Formulate the microbiologic diagnosis. Based on the history, physical examination, and immediately available laboratory results (eg, Gram-stained smear of sputum), the clinician should formulate as specific a microbiologic diagnosis as possible. In some instances, this may be quite specific and accurate (eg, a patient with lobar pneumonia with organisms resembling pneumococci in a Gram-stained smear of sputum); in other cases, there may be no clues to a specific bacteriologic diagnosis.

(4) Determine the necessity for empiric therapy. This is a clinical decision based partly on experience. Empiric therapy is indicated when there is a significant risk of serious morbidity if the infection is allowed to continue untreated for the time required for the laboratory to identify the causative agent and to determine its antimicrobial susceptibility pattern (usually 1–3 days).

(5) Institute treatment. Selection of empiric therapy may be based on **microbiologic diagnosis,** where antimicrobial susceptibility data are lacking (eg, based on a Gram-stained smear or preliminary culture result); on a **clinical diagnosis** without further microbiologic information (eg, cellulitis, meningitis, pneumonia); or on a combination of the two. If no microbiologic information is available, the antimicrobial spectrum of the drugs chosen must necessarily be broader than if some information about the pathogen is known.

The selection of an antimicrobial agent based on a presumed etiology is not an exact science. Selection from among several potentially active agents is dependent upon both host factors and pharmacologic factors, in addition to prescriber preference. Host factors include prior adverse drug effects, elimination or detoxification capacity (usually dependent upon renal or hepatic function), metabolic or genetic disorders predisposing to drug toxicity (eg, glucose-6-phosphate dehydrogenase deficiency), potential drug interactions resulting from other drug therapy, age of the patient, and pregnancy. Pharmacologic factors include the kinetics of absorption, distribution, and elimination, the route of elimination, ability of the drug to penetrate to the site of infection, and the potential toxicities of the drug. Finally, increasing consideration is being given to the cost of antimicrobial therapy.

Brief guides to empiric therapy based on presumptive microbial diagnosis and site of infection are given in Tables 52–1 and 52–2.

A number of clinical situations may warrant further modification of empiric therapeutic regimens. For example, in the severely leukopenic patient, 2 or 3 drugs (usually an extended-spectrum penicillin such as ticarcillin with an aminoglycoside, with or without a cephalosporin) are always used in combination. Serious gram-negative infections in these patients often respond poorly, even when 2 drugs are used; in addition, the variety of pathogens observed is great enough to warrant broad-spectrum coverage.

ANTIMICROBIAL THERAPY OF ESTABLISHED INFECTIONS

INTERPRETATION OF CULTURE RESULTS

Properly obtained and processed specimens for culture frequently yield important information about the cause of infection. Reports may be **false-negative** for a number of reasons, including sampling of the wrong sites or materials, sampling after initiation of antimicrobial therapy, overgrowth of pathogens by normal flora, and infections due to fastidious or noncultivable pathogens for which the proper tests were not performed (eg, *Rickettsia, Mycoplasma,* many viruses, *Bordetella pertussis*). **False-positive** reports may occur as a result of contamination of bacteriologic media or because the pathogen is merely colonizing the host but not causing the infection (eg, recovery of *Staphylococcus aureus* or coliforms from sputum specimens contaminated by oropharyngeal secretions). Performing semiquantitative cultures may be helpful in this latter instance, because finding large numbers of a pathogen (especially with little of the normal flora) is evidence against the organism being a commensal. Likewise, microscopic examination of stained specimens will be helpful because the presence of leukocytes and a single type of organism favors its role as a pathogen.

GUIDING ANTIMICROBIAL THERAPY OF ESTABLISHED INFECTION

Susceptibility Testing

Testing pathogens for their susceptibility to antimicrobials is now a commonplace clinical procedure. Tests measure the concentration of drug required to inhibit growth of the organism (**minimum inhibitory concentration, MIC**) or to kill the organism (**minimum lethal concentration, MLC**; with bacteria, often also called **minimum bactericidal concentration, MBC**). The results of these tests may then be compared with known drug concentrations in various body compartments and with studies correlating clinical outcome with MIC or MLC to determine whether the organism should be considered sensitive or resistant. Only MICs are routinely measured in most laboratories, as this value is adequate basis for treatment of most infections.

Two methods of susceptibility testing in common use are the disk (agar) diffusion or Kirby-Bauer method and broth dilution method. In the **disk diffusion method,** a disk containing a standardized amount of the test antimicrobial is placed on an agar plate lightly seeded with the test bacteria. The bacteria are then allowed to grow under carefully controlled conditions while the antibiotic diffuses out into the agar. The diameter of the zone of inhibition correlates with MIC, although zone sizes are not comparable from one drug to another. In the **broth dilution method,** the bacteria are inoculated into liquid medium containing graduated concentrations of the test antimicrobial for direct determination of the MIC. In general, if the MIC is one-half or less of the peak serum levels obtained routinely, the organism is considered susceptible.

Disk diffusion methods are satisfactory for determining susceptibility of many antimicrobial-organism combinations, and they are really all that is required when the susceptibility pattern of the organism is bimodal (ie, very susceptible or very resistant, with few

Table 52–1. Empiric antimicrobial therapy based on microbiologic etiology.

Suspected or Proved Disease or Pathogen	Drug(s) of First Choice	Alternative Drug(s)
Gram-negative cocci (aerobic)		
Gonococcus	Penicillin (parenteral only),[1] ampicillin,[2] tetracycline[3]	Spectinomycin,[4] cefoxitin,[4] ceftriaxone
Meningococcus	Penicillin[1]	Chloramphenicol, cefuroxime[4]
Gram-positive cocci (aerobic)		
Pneumococcus	Penicillin[1]	Erythromycin, cephalosporin[5]
Streptococcus, hemolytic groups A, B, C, G	Penicillin[1]	Erythromycin, cephalosporin[5]
Viridans streptococci	Penicillin[1] (? plus aminoglycoside)	Cephalosporin,[5] vancomycin
Staphylococcus, nonpenicillinase-producing	Penicillin[1]	Cephalosporin,[5] vancomycin
Staphylococcus, penicillinase-producing	Penicillinase-resistant penicillin[6]	Vancomycin, cephalosporin[5]
Staphylococcus, methicillin-resistant	Vancomycin	TMP-SMX[9] (? plus rifampin)
Streptococcus faecalis (enterococcus)	Ampicillin or penicillin plus aminoglycoside[7]	Vancomycin (? plus aminoglycoside[7])
Gram-negative rods (aerobic)		
Coliforms *(Escherichia coli, Klebsiella, Enterobacter, Serratia, Proteus, Providencia, Arizona,* etc)	Aminoglycoside,[7] third-generation cephalosporin[8]	TMP-SMX,[9] extended-spectrum penicillin[11]
Shigella	TMP-SMX[9]	Chloramphenicol, ampicillin
Salmonella	Chloramphenicol	TMP-SMX,[9] ampicillin
Haemophilus sp	Chloramphenicol,[4] cefuroxime,[4] third-generation cephalosporin[4,8]	TMP-SMX,[4,9] ampicillin
Brucella	Tetracycline[3]	Streptomycin plus sulfonamide[10]
Campylobacter sp	Tetracycline	Erythromycin
Yersinia pestis (plague), *Francisella tularensis* (tularemia)	Tetracycline (? plus streptomycin)	Chloramphenicol, streptomycin
Vibrio sp	Tetracycline, TMP-SMX[9]	
Pseudomonas aeruginosa	Aminoglycoside[7] plus extended-spectrum penicillin[11]	Ceftazidime or aminoglycoside[7] or both
Pseudomonas pseudomallei (melioidosis), *Pseudomonas mallei* (glanders)	Tetracycline (? plus streptomycin)	Chloramphenicol
Legionella sp	Erythromycin (? plus rifampin)	
Gram-positive rods (aerobic)		
Bacillus sp (eg, anthrax)	Penicillin[1]	Erythromycin
Listeria monocytogenes	Ampicillin (? plus aminoglycoside)	Chloramphenicol, TMP-SMX[9]
Nocardia	Sulfonamide[10]	Minocycline, TMP-SMX[9]
Anaerobes		
Gram-positive (peptococci, peptostreptococci, clostridia, etc)	Penicillin[1]	Clindamycin, tetracycline,[3] cephalosporin,[5] cefoxitin
Bacteroides fragilis (some *B bivius* and *B melaninogenicus*)	Metronidazole, clindamycin	Chloramphenicol, cefoxitin
Gram-negatives other than *B fragilis* (*Bacteroides, Fusobacterium*)	Penicillin[1]	Clindamycin, tetracycline,[3] cephalosporin,[5] cefoxitin
Mycobacteria		
Mycobacterium tuberculosis	Isoniazid (INH) plus rifampin or ethambutol or both	Streptomycin, pyrazinamide, others
Mycobacterium leprae	Dapsone plus rifampin	Clofazimine
Spirochetes		
Borrelia (relapsing fever)	Tetracycline[3]	Penicillin
Leptospira	Penicillin[1]	Tetracycline
Treponema (syphilis, yaws)	Penicillin[1]	Erythromycin, tetracycline

[1–12] See footnotes at end of table on following page.

Table 52–1 (cont'd). Empiric antimicrobial therapy based on microbiologic etiology.

Suspected or Proved Disease or Pathogen	Drug(s) of First Choice	Alternative Drug(s)
Mycoplasma pneumoniae	Tetracycline[3]	Erythromycin
Chlamydia trachomatis, Chlamydia psittaci	Tetracycline[3]	Erythromycin
Rickettsiae	Tetracycline[3]	Chloramphenicol
Fungi		
Candida sp, *Torulopsis*	Amphotericin B	Ketoconazole,[12] flucytosine
Cryptococcus neoformans	Amphotericin B plus flucytosine	Ketoconazole[12]
Coccidioidomycosis	Amphotericin B	Ketoconazole[12]
Histoplasmosis	Amphotericin B	Ketoconazole[12]
Blastomycosis	Ketoconazole[12]	Amphotericin B
Paracoccidioidomycosis	Ketoconazole[12]	Amphotericin B
Sporotrichosis	Ketoconazole[12]	Amphotericin B
Aspergillosis, mucormycosis	Amphotericin B	None

[1] Penicillin G is preferred for parenteral injection; penicillin V for oral administration. Only very susceptible microorganisms should be treated with oral penicillin.

[2] Amoxicillin or ampicillin; ampicillin esters (eg, hetacillin, bacampicillin) and cyclacillin offer no advantages. Amoxicillin is also available with potassium clavulinate as Augmentin.

[3] All tetracyclines have similar activity against microorganisms (with rare exceptions) and comparable therapeutic activity and toxicity. Dosage is determined by the rates of absorption and excretion of different preparations. Doxycycline is generally easier to administer parenterally and is more convenient to give orally (although more expensive).

[4] Effective against beta-lactamase–producing strains.

[5] First-generation cephalosporin: cephalothin, cephapirin, or cefazolin for parenteral administration; cephalexin or cephradine for oral administration.

[6] Parenteral nafcillin, oxacillin, or methicillin. Oral dicloxacillin, cloxacillin, or oxacillin.

[7] Gentamicin, tobramycin, netilmicin, or amikacin. Kanamycin can be used for some organisms other than *Pseudomonas* sp; streptomycin should be used only for drug-susceptible strains of *M tuberculosis* and streptococci (with penicillin or ampicillin).

[8] Moxalactam, cefotaxime, cefoperazone, ceftizoxime, ceftriaxone, or ceftazidime. Cefoperazone is not effective for meningitis.

[9] Trimethoprim-sulfamethoxazole (TMP-SMX) is a mixture of 1 part trimethoprim plus 5 parts sulfamethoxazole.

[10] Trisulfapyrimidines have the advantage over sulfadiazine of greater solubility in urine for oral administration; sodium sulfadiazine is suitable for intravenous injection in severely ill persons.

[11] Extended-spectrum penicillins: ticarcillin, mezlocillin, piperacillin, or azlocillin.

[12] Ketoconazole does not penetrate the central nervous system and is unsatisfactory for meningitis.

intermediate cases), as is seen with the susceptibility of *S aureus* to penicillin G. However, when there is no sharp dividing line between susceptible and resistant, determination of the MIC may be very helpful for guiding therapy.

The results of laboratory susceptibility testing generally correlate well with clinical response. However, infected patients given antimicrobials shown to be ineffective by in vitro tests may still recover satisfactorily. Host defense mechanisms may be sufficient to permit recovery in many cases, and there is ample evidence that subinhibitory concentrations of antimicrobials may have beneficial effects—eg, enhancing ingestion and killing of bacteria by phagocytes.

Drug Concentrations in Body Fluids

For most antimicrobials, the relationship of dose to resulting body fluid concentrations is well established, and the therapeutic index of most antimicrobials is high enough so that measurement of antimicrobial concentrations in body fluids is rarely necessary. Exceptions are antimicrobials with a low therapeutic index (eg, vancomycin, aminoglycosides), administration of the antimicrobial by an unreliable route for a

serious infection (oral therapy), investigation of clinical failure of apparently adequate antimicrobial therapy, and determination of drug concentrations in unusual sites (eg, central nervous system; see Table 52–3).

There are several ways in which antimicrobial concentrations can be determined. The most generally applicable method is bioassay, because it can be modified for use with any antimicrobial drug. In this method, the degree of growth inhibition of a standard organism by the clinical specimen is compared with that produced by several known concentrations of drug, and the concentration in the clinical specimen is determined by interpolation. For antimicrobials such as the aminoglycosides and vancomycin, where drug concentrations are determined frequently, a variety of automated assay methods have been developed that are not different in principle from those used to measure other drugs.

Serum Bactericidal Titers

In many infectious disorders (eg, soft tissue infections, pneumonias, enteritis), host defenses contribute materially to cure. In these conditions, drugs that

Table 52–2. Empiric antimicrobial therapy based on site of infection.

Presumed Site of Infection	Common Pathogens	Drug(s) of First Choice	Alternative Drug(s)
Bacterial endocarditis			
Acute	Staphylococci, streptococci, aerobic gram-negative rods	Penicillin plus nafcillin[1] plus gentamicin	Vancomycin plus gentamicin
Subacute	Viridans streptococci, enterococci	Penicillin plus gentamicin	Vancomycin plus gentamicin
Hematogenous osteomyelitis	*Staphylococcus aureus*	Nafcillin[1]	Clindamycin, vancomycin
Septic arthritis			
Child	*Haemophilus influenzae, S aureus, streptococci*	Cefuroxime, third-generation cephalosporin[2]	Clindamycin plus chloramphenicol
Adult	*Neisseria gonorrhoeae, S aureus, streptococci*	Cephalosporin[3]	Clindamycin plus trimethoprim-sulfamethoxazole; ampicillin
Cystitis	*Escherichia coli, Proteus mirabilis, Staphylococcus saprophyticus*	Sulfonamide, ampicillin, tetracycline	Nitrofurantoin, trimethoprim-sulfamethoxazole
Pyelonephritis	Coliforms	Trimethoprim-sulfamethoxazole	Third-generation cephalosporin,[2] aminoglycoside[4]
Otitis media and sinusitis	*H influenzae,* streptococci	Amoxicillin, ampicillin	Erythromycin plus sulfa; trimethoprim-sulfamethoxazole; cefaclor
Bronchitis (bacterial)	*H influenzae,* pneumococci	Tetracycline	Ampicillin, trimethoprim-sulfamethoxazole, cefaclor
Pneumonia (bacterial)[5]			
Neonate	Group B streptococci, *E coli, Listeria*	Ampicillin plus aminoglycoside[4]	Chloramphenicol; penicillin plus third-generation cephalosporin[2]
Child	Pneumococci, *S Aureus, H influenzae*	Cefuroxime	Clindamycin plus either chloramphenicol or trimethoprim-sulfamethoxazole
Adult	Pneumococci, *Klebsiella, S aureus*	Cephalosporin,[3] cefuroxime	Clindamycin plus aminoglycoside[4]
Cellulitis	Group A streptococci	Penicillin	Erythromycin
Abscess with cellulitis	Staphylococci	Nafcillin[1]	Clindamycin
Meningitis			
Neonate	Group B streptococci, *E coli, Listeria*	Ampicillin plus aminoglycoside[4]	Chloramphenicol; penicillin plus third-generation cephalosporin[2]
Child	*H influenzae,* pneumococci, meningococci	Chloramphenicol plus ampicillin	Cefuroxime
Adult	Pneumococci, meningococci	Penicillin	Chloramphenicol
Peritonitis due to ruptured viscus	Coliforms, *Bacteroides fragilis,* streptococci	Penicillin[6] plus clindamycin plus aminoglycoside[4]	Cefoxitin; metronidazole plus third-generation cephalosporin[2]
Septicimia	Any	Third-generation cephalosporin[2] (? plus aminoglycoside[4])	Clindamycin plus aminoglycoside[4]; ticarcillin/clavulinate
Septicemia with granulocytopenia	Any (anaerobes are uncommon)	Extended-spectrum penicillin[7] plus aminoglycoside[4]	Third-generation cephalosporin[2] plus either aminoglycoside[4] or extended-spectrum penicillin[7]

[1] Nafcillin, oxacillin, or methicillin.
[2] Moxalactam, cefotaxime, cefoperazone, ceftizoxime, ceftriaxone, or ceftazidime. Cefoperazone cannot be used for meningitis.
[3] First-generation cephalosporins: cephalothin, cephapirin, or cefazolin (for parenteral therapy).
[4] Gentamicin, tobramycin, netilmicin, or amikacin.
[5] Pneumonia may be caused by many different agents, and selection of empiric therapy is complex. Consult more specialized texts for specifics (see References).
[6] Penicillin may be omitted if patient is allergic.
[7] Extended-spectrum penicillins: ticarcillin, piperacillin, mezlocillin, or azlocillin.

Table 52–3. Penetration of selected antimicrobials into cerebrospinal fluid (CSF).

Antimicrobial	Dosage	Reported Concentration in CSF (Inflamed Meninges) (μg/mL)	Plasma Concentration (μg/mL)
Amikacin	15 mg/kg/d	0.8–9.2	5–20
Ampicillin	150–300 mg/kg/d	2–60	16–250
Carbenicillin	200–500 mg/kg/d	10–60	30–200
Cefoperazone	50–100 mg/kg/d	0–11.5	44–250
Cefotaxime	30–150 mg/kg/d	0.3–27	40–100
Cefoxitin	100–150 mg/kg/d	12.5–83	22–250
Ceftriaxone	100 mg/kg/d	0.3–42	30–260
Cefuroxime	200 mg/kg/d	1–17	60–100
Chloramphenicol	25–100 mg/kg/d	3–40	10–128
Gentamicin	2–7.5 mg/kg/d	0.5–2	0.7–7
Moxalactam	60–150 mg/kg/d	1–78	80–180
Nafcillin	150–200 mg/kg/d	2.7–88	36–176
Penicillin G	$2-3 \times 10^5$ units/kg/day	1.7–46	12–740
Sulfamethoxazole	25–50 mg/kg/d	5–40	40–85
Tobramycin	3–4.5 mg/kg/d	0.5–0.9	0.9–6.5
Trimethoprim	5–10 mg/kg/d	0.2–2.4	1.7–3.5
Vancomycin	20–30 mg/kg/d	0.1–8.5	1.4–30

merely inhibit the growth of the pathogen are often sufficient for successful treatment. In other disorders (infective endocarditis, bacteremia in the immunosuppressed host, bacterial meningitis), host defenses may contribute minimally to cure. Consequently, bactericidal drug concentrations must be achieved in the infected tissue. An assay of the titer of inhibitory as well as bactericidal activity in body fluids may be performed and will establish both susceptibility of the pathogen and adequacy of drug dosage and absorption in one simple test procedure. Serum is obtained from the patient at the appropriate time after the last dose of drug, and serial dilutions of serum are incubated with a standardized amount of the pathogen recovered from the patient. Growth inhibition and killing at a serum dilution (titer) of 1:8 or more is generally considered to be satisfactory, although the data supporting this figure are conflicting. Although this assay is not fully standardized, it is simple to perform and is useful for confirming choice of antimicrobial and dosage. It is also helpful where *bactericidal* antimicrobials are needed and where antimicrobial combinations are being studied for possible synergism (see below).

Specialized Assay Methods

A. Beta-Lactamase Assay: For some bacteria (eg, gonococci, *Haemophilus influenzae*), the susceptibility patterns of all strains are virtually identical except for production of beta-lactamase, which confers resistance to various beta-lactam antimicrobials. In these cases, extensive susceptibility testing may be omitted and a direct test for beta-lactamase done utiliz-

ing a chromogenic beta-lactam substrate. This test is sensitive, specific, rapid, and reliable.

B. Synergy Studies: These in vitro tests attempt to measure synergistic, additive, indifferent, or antagonistic drug interactions in vitro. The methods are not standardized and in general have not been correlated with clinical outcome. See section on combination chemotherapy for details.

Selection of Route of Administration

Parenteral therapy is generally preferred for acutely ill patients. The choice of intravenous over intramuscular administration is primarily determined by the drug preparations available. A few agents have such reliable oral absorption that parenteral therapy is seldom required (eg, chloramphenicol, rifampin, trimethoprim-sulfamethoxazole); however, for other agents, oral therapy is best reserved for mild to moderate infections or for definitive treatment of serious infections in situations where absorption is documented (eg, by drug levels or serum bactericidal titers).

Monitoring Therapeutic Response; Duration of Therapy

The therapeutic response should be monitored both microbiologically and clinically. Cultures of specimens taken from infected sites should show progressively smaller numbers of the pathogen during therapy and should eventually become sterile. Monitoring of cultures is also useful for detecting superinfections or the development of resistance (see below). Clinically, the patient's general manifestations of infection (malaise, fever, leukocytosis, etc) should improve and the specific findings also should abate (eg, clearing of x-ray infiltrates in pneumonia). The speed of clinical response to antimicrobial therapy is generally inversely proportionate to the duration of the illness prior to therapy.

The duration of therapy required for cure depends on the pathogen, the site of infection, and host factors; precise data on duration of therapy are available for a few infections, eg, streptococcal pharyngitis, cystitis, syphilis, gonorrhea, and tuberculosis. In many other situations, duration of therapy is determined empirically. For serious infections, continuing therapy for 7–10 days after the patient has become afebrile or cultures have become negative is a useful general rule.

Management of Antimicrobial Drug Toxicity

Because of the large number of antimicrobials available, when drug toxicity occurs it can often be managed by substitution of another drug with equivalent efficacy (Table 52–1). In the rare cases where this is not possible, continuing the drug while simultaneously treating the adverse reaction may be possible, although it is associated with some risk. For example, *Clostridium difficile* colitis induced by antimicrobials may be managed by oral administration of vancomycin without discontinuing the inducing drug. In addition, some types of drug toxicity (eg, drug fever) may be confused with manifestations of the infection.

Allergic reactions to antimicrobials are common, and management is complex. In the presence of preexisting drug allergy, avoid the suspect drug and select a substitute (see Tables 52–1 and 52–2); in virtually every instance, the alternative drugs are of equivalent efficacy. If the patient has a history of a life-threatening reaction to an antimicrobial (eg, anaphylaxis, toxic epidermal necrolysis), all related drugs should probably be avoided. Thus, in the patient with a clear history of anaphylaxis to penicillin, all beta-lactam antimicrobials are best avoided. If there is a commanding need for penicillin treatment of the patient with a history of anaphylactic penicillin reaction, desensitization may be attempted. (See Wendel reference for details.)

Clinical Failure of Antimicrobial Drug Therapy

When the patient has an inadequate clinical or microbiologic response to antimicrobial therapy selected by in vitro susceptibility testing, a systematic investigation should be undertaken to determine the cause of the problem (Table 52–4). Errors in susceptibility testing are rare, but the original results should be confirmed by repeated testing. Drug dosing and absorption should be scrutinized and tested directly with serum drug concentrations or a serum bactericidal titer. However, drug pharmacology problems rarely account for clinical failures.

The clinical data should be reviewed to make certain the patient's host defenses are adequate (adequate

Table 52–4. Common causes of failure of antimicrobial therapy.

Drug
    Inappropriate drug.
    Inadequate dose.
    Improper route of administration.
    Malabsorption.
    Accelerated drug excretion or inactivation.
    Poor penetration of drug into a privileged site of infection (eg, brain, eye, prostate).

Host
    Poor host defenses (granulocytopenia, leukopenia, AIDS, etc).
    Undrained pus (eg, abscess).
    Retained infected foreign body.
    Dead tissue (eg, sequestrum).

Pathogen
    Development of drug resistance.
    Superinfection by other pathogens.
    Dual infection initially—only one of the pathogens detected and treated.

Laboratory
    Erroneous report of susceptible pathogen.

numbers of granulocytes, etc) and that there are no abscesses requiring drainage or infected foreign bodies that need to be removed. If the patient has responded well to therapy except for persistence of fever, drug fever should be considered. Lastly, repeat cultures and susceptibility testing should be performed to determine if superinfection has occurred with another organism or if the original pathogen has developed drug resistance.

Adjunctive Measures in the Treatment of Infection

A. Surgery: It is often necessary to drain abscesses, remove foreign bodies, and close persistent sources of contamination (eg, perforated bowel). Although one is often tempted to delay surgery until the patient's systemic symptoms ("toxicity") have abated, in many cases the patient will remain ill until essential surgery is performed. On the other hand, if the patient is improving and particularly if diagnostic tests (eg, ultrasonography, CT scanning) show shrinkage of an abscess, then surgery may be postponed. Likewise, some abscesses can be drained by percutaneous needle or catheter under sonographic or CT guidance, thus avoiding an extensive surgical procedure.

B. Management of Fever: Antipyretic drugs should be used to keep the temperature below dangerous levels (40.5 °C [105 °F] in most adults; 39.5 °C [103.2 °F] in children, especially those with a history of febrile seizures) and to make the patient comfortable. If fever is not troublesome and is below dangerous levels, antipyretics are not indicated. Do not be concerned about "masking" the infection with antipyretics. In most cases of infection, antipyretic agents will lower the temperature, but some degree of fever will persist as long as the infection is active.

Antipyretics should be administered on a regular basis (usually every 4 hours), *not* given only for an elevated temperature. Intermittent administration produces wide swings in body temperature, making the patient more uncomfortable than if antipyretic drugs were not given.

C. General Supportive Measures: Rest and proper diet will improve the patient's sense of well-being. Aside from correction of obvious malnutrition, however, there is little evidence that such measures are important to recovery from a short illness if adequate antimicrobial therapy has been given.

Correction of host abnormalities associated with infection is an essential component of therapy of infectious diseases. Respiration (oxygen uptake and carbon dioxide excretion) and circulation must be supported, if inadequate. Electrolyte and acid-base disturbances should be corrected. Antitoxins to the core glycolipid (endotoxin) of gram-negative bacteria reduce shock and mortality rates in gram-negative bacterial infections. Antibodies to other bacterial components (eg, *Pseudomonas* toxins) may be beneficial as well. These approaches will doubtless be of increasing importance in the future.

CONDITIONS ALTERING ANTIMICROBIAL PHARMACOLOGY

Diseases of the major excretory organs as well as physiologic states such as infancy or pregnancy alter the disposition of antimicrobials along with other drugs. Some of these changes are shown in Tables 52–5 and 52–6. See also Chapter 63. A variety of other clinical states (puerperium, burns, cystic fibrosis) are known to alter antimicrobial pharmacokinetics; thus, measures of adequate dosing (drug concentrations or serum bactericidal titers) are advisable in patients with serious infections and significant underlying disease.

ANTIMICROBIAL DRUG INTERACTIONS

Like other classes of drugs, antimicrobials may interact with other medication being given to the patient, with possible adverse results. Some antimicrobial drug interactions of clinical importance are shown in Table 52–7. (See also Appendix I.) In addition to the interactions listed in Chapter 32, virtually all broad-spectrum antimicrobials (other than rifampin) enhance the effect of coumarin anticoagulants. Likewise, inhibition of bacterial sterol biotransformation by antimicrobial agents may decrease blood levels of contraceptive medication following oral administration (eg, pregnancy occurring in women taking birth control pills).

ANTIMICROBIAL DRUG COMBINATIONS

Possible Indications for Therapy With Multiple Antimicrobials

(1) In certain desperately ill patients with suspected infections of unknown origin, it may be desirable to administer more than one antimicrobial drug empirically in an effort to suppress all of the most likely pathogens. Thus, in suspected septicemia, an antistaphylococcal drug (eg, nafcillin) might be combined with a drug having activity against aerobic gram-negative bacilli (gentamicin, tobramycin, or amikacin) until blood cultures yield a specific microorganism (Table 52–2).

(2) In mixed infections, it is possible that 2 or 3 drugs may be required to "cover" all of the potential or known pathogens. For example, in peritonitis following perforation of the colon, a drug active against anaerobes and gram-positive bacteria (clindamycin) may be combined with one active against coliforms (an aminoglycoside).

(3) In some clinical situations, the rapid emergence of bacteria resistant to one drug may impair the chances for cure. The addition of a second drug may delay or prevent the emergence of resistant strains. This effect has been demonstrated unequivocally in tuberculosis and is the basis for the frequent use of combinations of isoniazid, ethambutol, rifampin, or other drugs in this disease.

(4) The simultaneous use of 2 drugs may in some situations achieve an effect not obtainable by either drug alone. One drug enhances the antibacterial activity of the second drug against a specific microorganism, eg, the combination of a sulfonamide with trimethoprim. Such an effect can be considered a manifestation of drug synergism. Unfortunately, such synergism is not always predictable: A given combination of drugs must be specifically tailored by laboratory tests to fit a certain strain of a given microorganism. A synopsis of the dynamics of combined antibiotic action is given below. One of the best-established examples of synergism is the cure of bacterial endocarditis caused by enterococci *(Streptococcus faecalis)* by a combination of a penicillin with an aminoglycoside, as compared to the frequent failure of treatment with a penicillin alone.

(5) Drug combinations may occasionally reduce the dosage required, and therefore the incidence or intensity of adverse reactions to single agents. A given microorganism may be susceptible to each of 2 drugs but only in doses likely to cause severe adverse reactions. If the drugs are used simultaneously, each can be used in half the dosage—perhaps below the threshold of adverse reaction. The availability of newer, more efficacious antimicrobials has made combination therapy based on this justification much less common.

Table 52–5. Antimicrobial pharmacokinetics in renal failure and during dialysis.

Drug	Drug Elimination by Indicated Route (percent)		Approximate Elimination Half-Life (hours)		Dosage Regimen[1]		
					Anuria[2]		
	Renal	Hepatic	Normal	Anuria	Initial Dose	Maintenance	Dialysis[3]
Acyclovir	30–75	. . .	2–5	Prolonged	5 mg/kg	2.5 mg/kg every 24 h	2.5 mg/kg after HD
Amantadine	90	. . .	8–18	Prolonged	100 mg	Significant reduction	No change
Amikacin	95–98	. . .	2.5	60–90	7.5 mg/kg	See footnote 4.	See footnote 5.
Amphotericin B	4–5	5–10	360	Same	No change	No change	No change
Ampicillin	75–90	5–10	0.8–1.5	8–12	3 g	1 g every 6 h	0.5 g after HD
Azlocillin	60–70	No data	1	5–6.5	3 g	2 g every 8 h	2 g after HD
Cefamandole	90–95	5–10	0.8–1	15–24	2 g	1 g every 12 h	0.5 g after HD
Cefazolin	95–98	2–5	1.4	35–56	1 g	0.5 g every 24 h	0.5 g after HD
Cefonicid	95	. . .	4.5	48–72	2 g	0.25 g twice weekly	No change
Cefoperazone	25	75	2	2	No change	No change	No change
Ceforanide	90–95	. . .	3	24–30	1 g	0.125 g every 24 h	0.5 g after HD
Cefotaxime	40–60	. . .	0.8–1	3–4	2 g	1 g every 6 h	0.5 g after HD
Cefoxitin	90	. . .	0.5–1	8–30	2 g	1 g every 12 h	0.5 after HD
Ceftriaxone	40–50	10–60	8	10–12	1 g	No change	No change
Cefuroxime	90–95	. . .	1.3	15	1.5 g	0.75 g every 12 h	0.75 g after HD
Cephalexin, cephradine	80–95	5–10	0.8–2	20–30	0.5 g	0.5 g every 24 h	0.25 g after HD
Cephalothin, cephapirin	40–60	. . .	1	3	2 g	1 g every 8 h	0.5 g after HD. Add to PD in desired serum concentration.
Chloramphenicol	5–10	. . .	2–4	4–6	No change	No change	0.25 g after HD
Clindamycin	15	. . .	2–4	4–6	No change	No change	No change
Doxycycline	20–50	. . .	15–24	Same	No change	No change	No change
Erythromycin	5–15	. . .	1.5–3	4–6	No change	No change	No change
Ethambutol	65–80	. . .	3–4	18–20	15 mg/kg	5 mg/kg every 24 h	5 mg/kg after HD or PD
Flucytosine	85–90	. . .	3–6	60–80	30 mg/kg	25 mg/kg every 24 h	15 mg/kg after HD
Gentamicin	95–98	. . .	2.5	60–80	2 mg/kg	See footnote 4.	See footnote 5.
Griseofulvin	< 1	. . .	10–20	Same	No change	No change	No data
Isoniazid	5–35	. . .	1.5 / 5(slow acetylators)	2.5 / 10 (slow acetylators)	No change	No change	No change
Kanamycin	95–98	. . .	2.5	60–90	7.5 mg/kg	See footnote 4.	See footnote 5.
Ketoconazole	< 5	50	4–8	Same	No change	No change	No data
Metronidazole	30–40	. . .	6–14	8–15	Active metabolite may accumulate: 7.5 mg/kg initially; then 7.5 mg/kg every 12–24 h.		No change
Mezlocillin	40–70	10–20	1	3.5	3 g	2 g every 6 h	2 g after HD
Miconazole	< 5	50	20–24	Same	No change	No change	No change
Minocycline	< 10	. . .	12–15	14–30	Avoid in renal failure.		No change
Moxalactam	80–90	5–10	2.5–3	20–24	2 g	1 g every 24 h	0.5 g after HD
Nafcillin	30–50	50–70	0.5	1	No change	No change	No change
Netilmicin	90–95	. . .	2.5	30–40	2.5 mg/kg	See footnote 4.	See footnote 5.
Oxacillin	50	50	0.5	1	No change	No change	No change
Penicillin G	75–90	. . .	0.5	6–20	3 million units	1 million units every 6 h	0.5 million units after HD
Piperacillin	50–90	10–40	1	3–6	3 g	2 g every 8 h	1 g after HD

[1]–[8]See footnotes at end of table on following page.

Table 52–5 (cont'd). Antimicrobial pharmacokinetics in renal failure and during dialysis.

Drug	Drug Elimination by Indicated Route (percent)		Approximate Elimination Half-Life (hours)		Dosage Regimen[1]		
					Anuria[2]		
	Renal	Hepatic	Normal	Anuria	Initial Dose	Maintenance	Dialysis[3]
Rifampin	5–15	80–90	2–3	3–5	No change	No change	No change
Sulfamethoxazole	40–50	...	9–11	18–24	See footnote 6.		See footnote 7.
Sulfisoxazole	50	...	4.5–7	6–12	15 mg/kg	7.5 mg/kg every 12 h	7.5 mg/kg after HD
Tetracycline	50	20–30	6–12	30–80	Avoid in renal failure.		No change
Ticarcillin	80–90	5–10	1	10–20	3 g	2 g every 12 h	2 g after HD
Tobramycin	95–98	...	2.5	60–80	2 mg/kg	See footnote 4.	See footnote 5.
Trimethoprim	65–80	...	10–12	24–36	See footnote 6.		See footnote 7.
Vancomycin	95	...	4–9	200–240	15 mg/kg	7.5 mg/kg once weekly.[8]	No change
Vidarabine	40–50	...	3–4	...	Daily dose should be decreased by 25%.		5 mg/kg after HD

[1] Dosages shown are for an average adult (70 kg) with a serious infection.
[2] Creatinine clearance less than 5 mL/min.
[3] HD = hemodialysis; PD = peritoneal dialysis.
[4] One-half of initial dose may be given every estimated half-life for maintenance. Serum levels should be monitored.
[5] One-half of initial dose after HD. Add to PD in desired serum concentration.
[6] Daily dose should be decreased to 25% of usual dose.
[7] One-half of daily maintenance dose should be given after HD.
[8] Serum levels should be monitored.

DYNAMICS OF COMBINED ANTIMICROBIAL DRUG ACTION IN VITRO

Problems in Measuring Antimicrobial Drug Effects

Even when technically feasible, chemical measures of antimicrobial drug concentration may not accurately reflect antibacterial activity. Direct evaluation of bacteriostasis or bactericidal activity is the only useful way of measuring the effects of these drugs. Several methods can be employed, and all may be applicable to the measurement of combined drug action.

The results of any one type of examination need not coincide with those of any other type, because the different methods may measure different events in the test system.

A. Bacteriostatic Effect: End points are expressed as the minimum amount of drug necessary to suppress visible growth for a given time.

B. Bactericidal Effect as Shown by Rate of Killing: Results are expressed as the bactericidal rate, ie, the slope of the plot of viable survivors at various time intervals after addition of drug. This is the "time-kill curve" method (Fig 52–1).

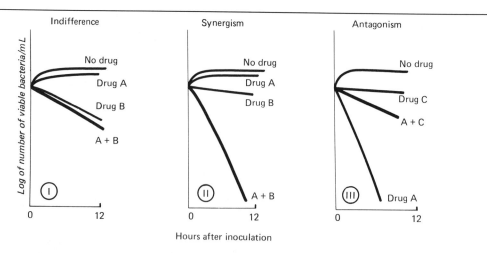

Figure 52–1. Types of combined action of antimicrobial drugs, measuring bactericidal activity by the "time-kill curve" method. *I.* Indifference (A + B = B). *II.* Synergy (A + B > > A or B). *III.* Antagonism (A + V < < A).

Table 52–6. Antimicrobial pharmacology in pregnancy and the neonatal period.

Drug Group	Pregnancy		Neonatal Period		Antibiotic Found in Breast Milk
	Pharmacology	Fetal Toxicity	Pharmacology	Toxicity	
Aminoglycosides	Accelerated excretion	Eighth nerve toxicity (especially streptomycin).	Accelerated excretion; higher dose required.	Same as adult—probably occurs less often.	Probably yes. Use if indicated, as gastrointestinal absorption is low.
Cephalosporins	Accelerated excretion	None.	No change	Same as adult.	Small amounts. Safe.
Chloramphenicol	No change	Possible cleft lip or palate.	Diminished hepatic conjugation—lower dose required.	Gray baby syndrome.	Yes. Do not use.
Erythromycins	No change	None.	No change	Same as adult. Very safe.	Some. Safe.
Ethambutol	No change	None.	No change	Same as adult.	Unknown.
Isoniazid	No change	None.	No change	Same as adult.	Yes. Use with caution.
Lincomycins	No change	None known.	Probably no change	Little experience—probably safe.	Small amounts. Safe.
Metronidazole	No change	May be mutagenic.	No change	Same as adult.	Yes. Use with caution.
Penicillins	Accelerated excretion	None.	No change	Same as adult.	Small amounts. Safe.
Rifampin	No change	None.	Probably no change	Same as adult.	Yes. Use with caution.
Sulfonamides	No change	Slight possibility of teratogenesis.	No change	Kernicterus—displaces bilirubin from serum albumin. Hemolysis (G6PD deficiency).	Yes. Use with caution.
Tetracyclines	Do not use	1. Tooth discoloration and dysplasia. 2. Inhibition of bone growth.	Do not use	Same as fetal.	Yes. Do not use. (Risk probably low owing to malabsorption by infant.)
Trimethoprim	No change	Teratogenic.	Not recommended	Same as adult.	Probably yes. Use with caution.
Vancomycin	No change	None known.	Probably no change	Same as adult.	Unknown.

C. Bactericidal Effect as Shown by Completeness of Killing: The results are expressed as the smallest concentration of drug resulting in a given number of viable survivors (eg, < 0.1%) in a given time, ie, a bactericidal end point.

D. Curative Effect as Shown in Therapeutic Trials in Vivo. The results are expressed as the smallest drug concentrations measured in patients or experimental animals whose infections are eradicated.

OUTCOMES OF COMBINED ANTIMICROBIAL ACTION

The nature of the interaction of 2 antimicrobial drugs can be judged from the plot of drug activity in an isobologram (Fig 52–2). From the results of measurements (according to any of the methods described in paragraphs A–D, above) with different doses of each drug alone and in combination acting on a given microbial population, it can be determined whether the drugs are additive, synergistic, or antagonistic. These terms can be applied to any specified intensity (the criterion) of bacteriostatic or curative effects as well as to bactericidal effects. Bactericidal action in vitro and

in vivo is important, and the 3 main results that are observed are (1) indifference or additive effect, (2) synergism, and (3) antagonism (Fig 52–1).

Indifference or Additive Effect

The most common result is indifference. The combined effect of drugs A and B is equal to that of the single more active component of the mixture A + B or is equal to the arithmetic sum of the effects of the individual drugs in their chosen doses. The same total effect could be obtained by the use of a single drug in a dose equivalent to that of the mixture.

Synergism

At times, the simultaneous action of 2 drugs results in an effect (A + B) far greater than that of either A alone or B alone in much larger dosages and also greater than could be expected from simple addition of individual drug effects.

In at least 3 types of antimicrobial synergism, the mechanism is fairly well understood (see also Chapter 42):

A. Blocking Successive Steps in a Metabolic Sequence: The best example is the combination of a sulfonamide and trimethoprim. Sulfonamides com-

Table 52–7. Interactions between antimicrobials and other drugs of clinical significance.

Antimicrobial	Other Agent(s)	Results of Interaction
Aminoglycosides	Neuromuscular blocking drugs.	Increased neuromuscular blockade.
	Other nephrotoxins or ototoxins (eg, cisplatin, amphotericin B, ethacrynic acid, vancomycin).	Increased nephrotoxicity or ototoxicity.
	Penicillins.	Inactivation of both drugs (a particular problem in renal failure and when obtaining drug levels).
Chloramphenicol	Phenytoin, tolbutamide, ethanol.	Increased blood concentration of these agents.
Erythromycin	Theophylline.	Increased blood theophylline concentration.
Isoniazid	Phenytoin.	Increased blood concentrations of both.
Ketoconazole	Antacids, cimetidine, ranitidine.	Prevent absorption.
Metronidazole (also cefamandole, moxalactam, cefoperazone)	Ethanol (including ethanol-containing medications).	Disulfiramlike reaction.
Nafcillin	Coumarin anticoagulants.	Decreased anticoagulant effect.
Penicillins and cephalosporins	Uricosuric agents (probenecid, high-dose aspirin, etc).	Block excretion of beta-lactams, causing higher serum levels.
	Copper reduction test for glycosuria (Clinitest tablets).	False-positive test for glycosuria (not seen with glucose oxidase method).
Rifampin	Coumarin anticoagulants, quinidine, digoxin, propranolol, theophylline.	Decreased effect of these drugs due to accelerated metabolism.
	Methadone.	Narcotic withdrawal.
	Oral contraceptives.	Decreased effect (pregnancy).
Sulfonamides	Sulfonylureas.	Hypoglycemia.
	Methenamine.	Precipitates in urine.
	Phenytoin.	Increased blood concentration of phenytoin.
	Oral anticoagulants (warfarin derivatives).	Enhanced hypoprothrombinemia.
Tetracyclines	Antacids, iron, calcium.	Inhibit intestinal absorption of tetracycline.

pete with *p*-aminobenzoic acid, which is required by some bacteria for the synthesis of dihydrofolate. Folate antagonists such as trimethoprim inhibit the enzyme (dihydrofolic acid reductase) that reduces dihydrofolate to tetrahydrofolate. The simultaneous presence of a sulfonamide and trimethoprim results in the simultaneous block of sequential steps leading to the synthesis of purines and nucleic acid and can result in a much more complete inhibition of growth than either component of the mixture alone.

B. One Drug Inhibits an Enzyme That Can Destroy the Second Drug: The best example of this mechanism is the noncompetitive inhibition of beta-lactamase by clavulanic acid or other substances. Organisms that produce beta-lactamase are resistant to the action of penicillin G because the drug is hydrolyzed by the enzyme. However, if the beta-lactamase is inhibited, the penicillin G is protected and can inhibit or kill the microorganism. This mechanism is an attractive one just beginning to be used clinically. Combinations of penicillins with clavulanic acid and of a carbapenem with cilastatin have recently been introduced in the USA (see Chapter 43).

C. One Drug Promotes Entry of a Second Drug Through the Microbial Cell Wall or Cell Membrane: This appears to be a widely applicable mechanism of synergism, with considerable clinical importance. For example, many streptococci exhibit a partial permeability barrier to aminoglycosides. If a cell wall–inhibitory drug is also present, it enhances the penetration of the aminoglycoside, which then acts on ribosomes and accelerates killing of the cell. This effect can occur with some viridans streptococci, group B streptococci, and group D enterococci. Combined therapy permits cure of sepsis or endocarditis caused by these organisms, whereas either drug alone often fails.

Antagonism

At times, the addition of a second drug actually diminishes the antibacterial effectiveness of the first drug, as shown by the interaction of drugs A and C in Fig 52–1. This "antagonism" can be manifested by a decrease in the inhibitory activity or in the early bactericidal rate of a drug mixture below that of one or both of its components. Antagonism can be demonstrated only when the drugs act on organisms capable of multiplication and is most marked when a barely active amount of bacteriostatic drug is added to a minimal bactericidal amount of a second drug. The bacteriostatic drug (tetracycline, chloramphenicol, erythromycin, etc) acts as an inhibitor of bacterial growth; the bactericidal drug (a penicillin, cephalosporin, or aminoglycoside) requires bacterial growth (eg, protein or cell wall synthesis) for killing. In the case of cell wall–active drugs, it has been suggested that the inhi-

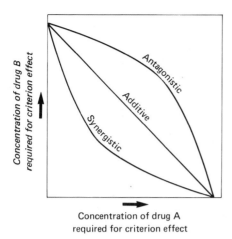

Figure 52–2. Isobologram showing possible interactions between 2 antimicrobials. The criterion effect is defined in setting up the assay and may be a specific bacteriostatic or bactericidal end point. The lines cross the ordinate at the concentration of drug B that is required to achieve the criterion effect when drug B is used alone. Similarly, the lines cross the abscissa at the concentration required for drug A alone to achieve the same effect.

bition of protein synthesis by chloramphenicol or tetracycline interferes with the production of some autolytic enzyme system postulated to be an important final step in cell lysis. A recently recognized mechanism of drug antagonism is the combined use of beta-lactamase–stable cephalosporins and extended-spectrum penicillins. The enzyme-stable cephalosporin induces the production of beta-lactamase (derepression) in certain bacteria. This enzyme may then inactivate the unstable penicillin.

CLINICAL EVIDENCE FOR ANTIMICROBIAL DRUG SYNERGISM OR ANTAGONISM

Although there are multiple in vitro instances of antimicrobial synergism and antagonism, only a few well-substantiated clinical examples are recognized.

Clinical Evidence for Synergism

The best clinical evidence for antibiotic synergism comes from the treatment of bacterial endocarditis, a disease that can be cured only if the infecting organisms are eradicated by bactericidal drugs. Endocarditis caused by enterococci *(S faecalis)* can usually not be cured by penicillin alone, since penicillin is inhibitory but not bactericidal for enterococci. The addition of an aminoglycoside is strikingly bactericidal for many strains of enterococci, and the cure of many such patients with a combination of penicillin or ampicillin with an aminoglycoside is an accepted example of clinical synergism. Beta-lactam antibiotics combined with aminoglycosides also appear to be synergistic in the treatment of endocarditis due to other streptococci

and staphylococci, although the evidence is weaker. Likewise, there is some evidence that drug combinations (usually a beta-lactam plus an aminoglycoside) selected for synergy on the basis of in vitro studies have synergistic activity in the treatment of aerobic gram-negative rod infections, especially in patients with severe granulocytopenia.

There is good clinical evidence from controlled trials that in cryptococcal meningitis, amphotericin B plus flucytosine is superior to either drug alone. This combination was selected because of in vitro evidence of synergism.

Clinical Evidence for Antagonism

Antagonism is sharply limited by time-dose relationships both in vitro and in vivo. It is readily demonstrated with single-dose treatment of animal infections but only with difficulty in multiple-dose treatment. In clinical practice, it is usual to give a large excess of antimicrobial drug in multiple doses. Consequently, antagonism cannot be expected to be a frequent outcome of clinical antimicrobial therapy, and there are few documented examples. The combination of penicillin and chlortetracycline cured fewer patients with pneumococcal meningitis than did the same dose of penicillin alone. Similarly, the addition of chloramphenicol to ampicillin resulted in more treatment failures in bacterial meningitis than did ampicillin alone.

SELECTION OF ANTIMICROBIAL COMBINATIONS IN CLINICAL PRACTICE

Antimicrobial combinations are used commonly in clinical practice, often with good justification (Tables 52–1, 52–2, and 52–8). Although the evidence for synergism is not clear in many cases, there is good evidence for clinical benefit for some combinations. On the other hand, the frequent use of antimicrobial combinations that have not been validated by clinical trials—or at least by in vitro or animal testing—should be avoided. The cost and toxicity of antimicrobials increase in direct proportion to the number of drugs used. Whenever drug combinations are employed and a clinical microbial isolate is available, it is desirable to establish the rationale for the choice by in vitro studies and to estimate the clinical effect with serum bactericidal titers.

ANTIMICROBIAL CHEMOPROPHYLAXIS

Anti-infective chemoprophylaxis is the administration of drugs to prevent the acquisition and establishment of pathogenic microorganisms. In a broader sense, it also includes the use of drugs soon after colonization by or inoculation of pathogenic microorganisms but before the development of disease.

Table 52–8. Some examples of clinically used antimicrobial combinations and their justification.

Indication	Drug Combination	Justification
Empiric therapy of various conditions (see Table 52–2)	Various	Expanded spectrum compared with single agent.
Pseudomonas aeruginosa infections	Beta-lactam plus aminoglycoside	Increased activity (additive or synergistic). Decreased toxicity. Inhibits emergence of resistant strains.
Enterococcal endocarditis	Penicillin or vancomycin plus aminoglycoside	Synergy: converts bacteriostatic drug to bactericidal.
Tuberculosis	Various—especially isoniazid (INH) plus rifampin	Inhibits emergence of resistant strains. Accelerated bacterial killing permitting shorter treatment course.
Cryptococcal meningitis	Amphotericin B plus flucytosine	Probably synergy as well as decreased toxicity.
Severely leukopenic patients	Beta-lactam plus aminoglycoside	Increased activity (additive or synergistic). Possibly decreased toxicity.

Some general principles have emerged from human and animal studies of antimicrobial prophylaxis:

(1) Prophylaxis should be directed against a specific pathogen or condition. Administration of antimicrobials cannot remove all microorganisms colonizing the host and cannot prevent all types of infections.

(2) The shorter the duration of prophylaxis, the broader the range of pathogens that may be prevented. Thus, prevention of "all" infections in severely leukopenic patients by broad-spectrum antimicrobial prophylaxis is successful only over the short term (resistance developing with long-term usage), whereas lifetime prophylaxis against group A streptococcal infections is possible.

(3) Prophylaxis is more effective and may be more widely used against pathogens that are poorly able to develop resistance to the drug used. The continued efficacy of penicillin prophylaxis against group A streptococcal infection contrasts with its rapidly dwindling efficacy against gonococcal infection.

(4) Prophylactic administration of antimicrobials generally requires doses equal to those used for therapy. In fact, since the host response to colonization or early infection may be different from that to disease, drugs effective for therapy may be relatively ineffective for prophylaxis and vice versa. For example, penicillin is highly effective treatment for meningococcal disease but is clinically ineffective for prophylaxis, because it does not eliminate colonization of the nasopharynx. Rifampin, highly effective for prophylaxis of meningococcal disease, is not recommended for therapy.

(5) As antimicrobial chemoprophylaxis entails risks (cost, drug toxicity, superinfection, and development of resistant organisms), it should be used only in situations where its efficacy has been documented.

Commonly used prophylactic regimens for nonsurgical infections are shown in Table 52–9. With the exception of the prevention of endocarditis following certain surgical procedures, the efficacy of these measures has been documented by adequate clinical trials. Prevention of endocarditis is now so widely practiced that adequately controlled studies are not possible. Data supporting this practice come from retrospective clinical trials and experiments on animal models of endocarditis. Not dealt with in this table are a multiplicity of clinical situations in which antimicrobial chemoprophylaxis was shown to be *ineffective:* heart failure, viral upper respiratory infections, comatose patients, etc.

In surgery, antimicrobials are given in the perioperative period to prevent postsurgical infectious complications. The general principles outlined above also apply to surgical prophylaxis, although there are some additional important principles that apply to the prevention of postsurgical infections:

(1) The antimicrobial agent must be active against the majority of organisms causing infections after the operation under consideration.

(2) Prophylaxis should be started immediately (not more than 6 hours) before surgery and should be continued for not more than 12–48 hours after surgery. Antimicrobial drug activity must be present in the surgical wound at the time of closure.

(3) The antimicrobial should be nontoxic and inexpensive and should not be essential for therapy of serious infections.

(4) Prophylaxis is indicated for surgical procedures in which the wound infection rate (under optimal conditions) is 5% or more except in procedures involving implantation of a foreign body, in which general usage is warranted.

Common indications for surgical prophylaxis are shown in Table 52–10.

Many second- and third-generation cephalosporins are promoted for single-dose surgical prophylaxis. There are no data proving that these agents are more effective than a single dose of cefazolin. In particular, third-generation cephalosporins should not be employed for prophylaxis because their use violates several of the principles outlined above, especially number (3).

Table 52–9. Nonsurgical antimicrobial prophylaxis of documented benefit or in common use.*

Disease or Infection to Be Prevented	Appropriate Subjects for Prophylaxis	Drugs and Adult Doses	Duration of Prophylaxis	Evidence for Efficacy	Comments
Group A strep-tococcal in-fection (post-streptococcal complications of rheumatic fever or glo-merulone-phritis)	1. Previous rheumatic fever or known rheu-matic heart disease. 2. Epidemic of strepto-coccal impetigo.	1. Benzathine penicillin, 1.2 million units IM monthly. 2. Penicillin G, 125 mg twice a day. 3. Sulfadiazine, 1 g daily.	1. For rheumatic fever, prophy-laxis should continue well into adult life. 2. For impetigo, until epidemic has abated.	Excellent (about 95%).	Does not prevent endocarditis.
Meningococcal infection	Close contacts (house-hold, sex partners, day-care center, etc) of index case.	1. Rifampin, 20 mg/kg once a day. 2. Minocycline, 100 mg twice a day. 3. Sulfisoxazole, 1 g twice a day (if organ-ism is susceptible).	Rifampin and sul-fonamide: 2 days. Minocycline: 5 days.	Excellent (about 80–90%)	Problems: 1. Rifampin resistance with widespread usage. 2. Vertiginous reactions with minocycline.
Haemophilus influenzae infection	Same as meningococci, but of susceptible age (<5–7 years old).	Rifampin, 20 mg/kg (maximum dose, 600 mg) once a day.	Four days.	Good.	Agreement on clinical use is not uniform. Emergence of resistance has occurred.
Tuberculosis	1. Close contacts of in-dex case (pending tuberculin testing). 2. Tuberculin converters. 3. Positive tuberculin test in high-risk groups (children, etc).	Isoniazid (INH), 300 mg/d.	One year.	Excellent (about 80%).	Definition of high-risk groups is variable. See Amer-ican Thoracic Society guide-lines for details.
Plague	Close contacts.	Tetracycline, 500 mg twice daily.	One week after exposure has ended.	Good.	
Gonorrhea	1. Contacts of index case. 2. All newborns.	1. As for treatment of gonorrhea. 2. Topical eye drops—silver nitrate or antimicrobial.	One dose. One dose.	Excellent. Excellent.	Required by law in USA.
Syphilis	Contacts of index case.	Benzathine penicillin, 2.4 million units IM.	Once.	Excellent (virtually 100%).	
Toxigenic *Esch-erichia coli* infection (traveler's diarrhea)	Persons traveling from nonendemic areas to endemic areas.	Many drugs effective. Doxycycline, 100 mg daily, most popular.	Duration of ex-posure.	Good.	Agreement on clinical use is not uniform. Not effective for antimicrobial-resistant strains.
Rickettsiosis	Exposure in endemic area (eg, scrub typhus).	Tetracycline (or chlor-amphenicol), 1 g/d.	Duration of ex-posure.	Good.	Recrudescence may occur when prophylaxis is discon-tinued.
Malaria	Exposure in endemic area.	Chloroquine phosphate, 500 mg weekly.	Duration of ex-posure.	Excellent.	1. Not effective for chloro-quine-resistant *Plasmo-dium falciparum*. 2. Recrudescence may occur when prophylaxis is stopped.
Influenza A	Exposure in epidemic or to index case with doc-umented infection.	Amantadine, 100 mg twice a day.	Duration of ex-posure.	Good (about 80%).	Agreement on clinical use is not uniform. Dose of 100 mg daily may be satisfactory.
Mycoplasmal pneumonia	Exposure to index case.	Tetracycline, 500 mg 4 times a day.	One week.	Poor.	Agreement on clinical use is not uniform.

*Modified, with permission, from Conte JE Jr, Sweet RW: *Infectious Diseases in Clinical Practice.* University of California, San Francisco, 1982. [Course syllabus.]

Table 52–9 (cont'd). Nonsurgical antimicrobial prophylaxis of documented benefit or in common use.*

Disease or Infection to Be Prevented	Appropriate Subjects for Prophylaxis	Drugs and Adult Doses	Duration of Prophylaxis	Evidence for Efficacy	Comments
Pneumocystis carinii infection	High-risk individual (high-dose corticosteroids, etc).	Trimethoprim, 5 mg/kg/d (with fixed ratio of sulfamethoxazole).	Uncertain. Probably duration of risk period.	Excellent.	Agreement on indications for use is not uniform.
African trypanosomiasis	Living in endemic area.	Pentamidine, 3 mg/kg IM every 3–6 months.	Duration of exposure.	Good.	
Endocarditis (endovasculitis)	Individuals with abnormal heart valves (increased susceptibility to endocarditis) or intravascular devices, undergoing a procedure known to cause bacteremia and increased risk of endocarditis (eg, dental extractions).	Penicillin or vancomycin; streptomycin or gentamicin added for gastrointestinal or genitourinary procedures.	Once for each exposure.	None.	See American Heart Association guidelines for details.
Otitis media	Individuals with recurrent otitis media.	Ampicillin or sulfonamides or trimethoprim-sulfamethoxazole.	Approximately 1 year.	Good.	
Bite wounds	Individuals bitten by humans, cats, occasionally other animals (eg, camels, gorillas).	Ampicillin or tetracycline, 0.5 g 4 times daily.	Three to 5 days.	Fair.	Close observation required even with prophylaxis.
Urinary tract infections	Individuals with a history of recurrent UTI.	Trimethoprim-sulfamethoxazole, 1 tablet twice weekly. Nitrofurantoin, 50 mg daily.	1. Continuously for uncertain duration. 2. After coitus (if a clear history of postcoital UTI).	Excellent.	Can substitute prompt, empiric treatment of each recurrence for continuous prophylaxis.
Exacerbations of chronic bronchitis	Individuals with established chronic bronchitis and frequent wintertime exacerbations.	Tetracycline, 0.5 g twice daily.	During the winter.	Good.	Not generally recommended —empiric treatment of each recurrence less toxic, equally efficacious.
Infection in the compromised host	Severely leukopenic patients (circulating granulocytes < 500/μL).	1. Oral, nonabsorbable antimicrobials (various regimens). 2. Trimethoprim-sulfamethoxazole by mouth.	Duration of leukopenia.	Variable.	Not generally recommended. Adjunctive measures required: laminar air flow, sterile hospital environment, sterilization of food, etc.

*Modified with permission, from Conte JE Jr, Sweet RW: *Infectious Diseases in Clinical Practice.* University of California, San Francisco, 1982. [Course syllabus.]

Table 52–10. Surgical prophylaxis of documented benefit or in common use.*

Disease or Operation	Usual Antimicrobial Employed	Evidence for Efficacy	Comments
Esophagus and stomach	Penicillin G parenterally, cephalosporin[1]	Good.	Needed primarily if bacterial flora (normally scanty) is increased by cancer, obstruction, or other disease.
Colon and rectum Elective	Oral, poorly absorbed antimicrobials (eg, erythromycin plus kanamycin) with mechanical bowel preparation	Good.	Example of short-term "sterilization" of normal flora to prevent infection. Addition of systemic antimicrobials probably not helpful.
Perforation	Cefoxitin alone; clindamycin plus gentamicin (see Table 52–2)	Good.	Perhaps should not be considered true prophylaxis, as gross fecal soilage of peritoneum has occurred.
Biliary tract	Ampicillin or cephalosporin	Good.	Need only for high-risk patients.
Hysterectomy Vaginal	Cephalosporin,[1] ampicillin, tetracycline	Good.	Indicated.
Routine abdominal	Cephalosporin[1]	Fair.	Use is controversial.
Radical	Various	Fair.	Probably indicated.
Cesarean section	Cephalosporin[1]	Good.	Give after cord has been clamped.
Joint replacement	Cephalosporin[1]	Good.	Benefit greater in group not using laminar flow operating room.
Open fractures	Cephalosporin[1]	Good.	Perhaps should not be considered true prophylaxis as wound is often grossly contaminated.
Cardiac valve replacement	Cephalosporin,[1] oxacillin, or nafcillin	Fair to poor.	Has become standard practice—controlled study no longer possible.

*Modified, with permission, from Conte JE Jr, Sweet RW: *Infectious Diseases in Clinical Practice.* University of California, San Francisco, 1982. [Course syllabus.]
[1]First-generation cephalosporins such as cephapirin, cephalothin, or cefazolin. Cefazolin is generally preferred. Its long serum half-life and the feasibility of intramuscular administration make this drug generally the least expensive of the group.

REFERENCES

Antimicrobials and haemostasis. (Editorial.) *Lancet* 1983;**1:** 510.

Conte JE, Barriere SL: *Manual of Antibiotics and Infectious Diseases,* 5th ed. Lea & Febiger, 1984.

Linton AL et al: Acute interstitial nephritis due to drugs. *Ann Intern Med* 1980;**93:**735.

Mandell GL, Douglas RG Jr, Bennett JE: *Principles and Practice of Infectious Diseases,* 2nd ed. Wiley, 1985.

Rahal JJ: Antibiotic combinations: The clinical relevance of synergy and antagonism. *Medicine* 1978;**57:**179.

Root RK, Sandi MA (editors): *New Dimensions in Antimicrobial Therapy.* Churchill Livingstone, 1984.

Snavely SR, Hodges GR: The neurotoxicity of antibacterial agents. *Ann Intern Med* 1984;**101:**92.

Wendel GD Jr et al: Penicillin allergy and desensitization in serious infections during pregnancy. *N Engl J Med* 1985; **312:**1229.

Wilson JT et al: Drug excretion in human breast milk: Principles, pharmacokinetics and projected consequences. *Clin Pharmacokinet* 1980;**5:**1.

53 Vaccines, Immune Globulins, & Other Complex Biologic Products

John Mills, MD, & Steven L. Barriere, PharmD

Active immunization against infectious agents, begun in the distant past with variolation for smallpox, is one of the earliest proved methods for prevention of disease. Development of antitoxins at the turn of the century permitted treatment and prevention of disease through passive immunization. Recent developments in science presage improvements in both active and passive immunization. Antigens from many infectious agents are already being produced in bacteria or yeasts using recombinant DNA technology, and within a few years it may be possible to produce large amounts of specific human immunoglobulins using the hybridoma technique. Additionally, other complex biologic products such as interferon, transfer factor, and lymphokines are being used experimentally for treatment and prevention of certain diseases; some of them (eg, interferon) show considerable promise of efficacy with minimal toxicity. Recombinant DNA technology is already permitting simplified, large-scale production of some of these materials.

PASSIVE IMMUNIZATION

Passive immunization means transfer of immunity to a host using preformed immunologic effectors. From a practical standpoint, only immunoglobulins have been utilized for passive immunization, since passive administration of immune effector cells is technically difficult and has been associated with graft-versus-host reactions. Note, however, that non-immune effector cells (eg, granulocytes) are being administered to humans with success, and cellular immunity has been transferred or augmented by other means (interferon, transfer factor).

Passive immunization with antibodies may be accomplished with either animal or human immunoglobulins in varying degrees of purity. These may contain relatively high titers of antibodies directed against a specific antigen or, as is true for pooled immune globulin, may simply contain antibodies found in most of the population.

Passive immunization is useful (1) for individuals unable to form antibodies (eg, congenital agammaglobulinemia); (2) for prevention of disease when time does not permit active immunization (eg, postexposure); (3) for treatment of certain diseases normally prevented by immunization (eg, tetanus); and (4) for treatment of conditions for which active immunization is unavailable or impractical (eg, snake bite).

Complications from administration of *human* immunoglobulins are rare. The injections may be moderately painful, and, rarely, sterile abscesses occur. Individuals with certain immunoglobulin deficiency states (IgA deficiency, etc) may occasionally develop hypersensitivity reactions to immune globulin that may limit therapy. Conventional immune globulin contains aggregates of IgG; it will cause severe reactions if given intravenously.

However, if the passively administered antibodies are derived from *animal* sera, hypsersensitivity reactions ranging from anaphylaxis to serum sickness are common. To avoid anaphylactic reactions, tests for hypersensitivity to the animal serum must be performed. If the tests give evidence of hypersensitivity, it is best to avoid that specific type of foreign protein (eg, horse serum) and obtain antibodies made in another animal (eg, human, goat, rabbit). If an alternative preparation is not available and administration of the specific antibody is deemed essential, desensitization can be carried out. A summary of tests for hypersensitivity and a desensitization protocol for antibody-containing proteins are presented below.

Antibodies derived from human serum not only avoid the risk of hypersensitivity reactions but also have a much longer half-life in humans (about 23 days for IgG antibodies) than those from animal sources (5–7 days or less). Consequently, much smaller doses of human antibody can be administered to provide therapeutic concentrations for several weeks. These advantages point to the desirability of using human antibodies for passive protection whenever possible. Materials available for passive immunization are summarized in Tables 53–1 and 53–3.

HUMAN GAMMA GLOBULIN
(Immune Globulin USP)

Immune globulin USP is a commercial preparation of gamma globulin derived from large pools of human plasma (> 1000 donors) by low-temperature ethanol fractionation. This procedure was developed by Cohn during World War II—hence the alternative name for this product, Cohn fraction II. The fractionation procedure removes most other serum proteins and infectious hepatitis viruses, thus providing a safe product for intramuscular injection. This material should not be given intravenously because it contains aggregates of IgG that may cause hypotension or other reactions. The preparation contains about 165 mg of gamma globulin per milliliter of solution (representing a 25-fold concentration of antibody-containing immunoglobulins of plasma). About 95% of the gamma globulin is IgG, with only trace amounts of IgM and IgA. Glycine is present as a stabilizing agent and thimerosal as a preservative. Immune globulin costs less than $1 per mL from commercial sources.

In addition to its use in the prevention of hepatitis, measles, and poliomyelitis, as shown in Table 53–1, immune globulin is also given in a dose of 0.6 mL/kg every 2–4 weeks to individuals with antibody immunodeficiencies. Although immune globulin has been used to prevent some other conditions (allergies, viral upper respiratory infections, and others), it is not effective and should not be so used.

Recently, immune globulin has been altered so that it is suitable for intravenous administration. Immune globulin intravenous contains 5% immune globulin in 10% maltose. This product may be useful for patients who need high levels of antibodies immediately and for those who cannot be given intramuscular injections (eg, patients with bleeding disorders). Its toxicity appears equivalent to immune globulin intramuscular, but without the local side effects. On the other hand, rare cases of non-A, non-B hepatitis have been linked to administration of some preparations of intravenous immune globulin.

ACTIVE IMMUNIZATION

Active immunization means the administration of antigens to the host to induce formation of antibodies and cell-mediated immunity. Immunization is practiced to induce protection against many infectious agents and may utilize either inactivated (killed) material or live attenuated agents (Tables 53–2 and 53–5). Desirable features of the ideal immunogen include complete prevention of disease, prevention of the carrier state, production of prolonged immunity with a minimum of immunizations, absence of toxicity, and suitability for mass immunization (ie, cheap and easy to administer). Active immunization is generally preferable to passive immunization, because host resistance is better (higher levels of antibody present at the time of exposure; coexisting cellular immunity in some cases) and the procedure need not be repeated as frequently. However, active immunization is associated with complications that do not occur with passive immunization, largely related to administering foreign proteins (eg, allergy, nonspecific toxic reactions). The advantages and disadvantages of active immunization with live attenuated and inactivated immunogens are compared in Table 53–3.

Current recommendations for routine active immunization of children are given in Table 53–4.

Legal Liability for Untoward Reactions

It is the physician's responsibility to inform the patient of the risk of immunization and to employ vaccines and antisera in an appropriate manner. Some of the risks described above are, however, currently unavoidable; on balance, the patient and society are clearly better off for accepting the risks for routinely administered immunogens (eg, poliomyelitis and tetanus vaccines).

Manufacturers should be held legally accountable for failure to adhere to existing standards for production of biologicals. However, in the present litigious atmosphere in the US, the filing of large liability claims by the statistically inevitable victims of good public health practice has caused manufacturers to abandon efforts to develop and produce low-profit but medically valuable therapeutic agents such as vaccines. Since the use and sale of these products are subject to careful review and approval by government bodies such as the Surgeon General's Advisory Committee on Immunization Practices and the Food and Drug Administration, "strict product liability" (liability without fault) may be an inappropriate legal standard to apply when rare reactions to biologicals produced and administered according to government guidelines are involved.

RECOMMENDED IMMUNIZATION OF ADULTS FOR TRAVEL

Every adult, whether traveling or not, must be immunized with tetanus toxoid and should also be fully immunized against poliomyelitis and diphtheria. In addition, every traveler must fulfill the immunization requirements of the health authorities of the countries visited. These are listed in *Health Information for International Travel*, available from the Superintendent of Documents, US Government Printing Office, Washington, DC 20402. *The Medical Letter on Drugs and Therapeutics* also offers periodically updated recommendations for international travelers (eg, see issue of April 12, 1985). Immunizations received in preparation for travel should be recorded on the International Certificate of Immunization. *Note:* Smallpox immunization is not recommended or required for travel anywhere.

[Text cont'd on p 599.]

Table 53–1. Materials available for passive immunization.

Indication	Product	Dosage	Comments
Black widow spider bite	Black widow spider anti-venin, equine.	One vial (6000 units) IM or IV.	Use should be limited to children <15 kg, the only group with significant morbidity or mortality. Available from Merck Sharp & Dohme.
Botulism	ABE polyvalent anti-toxin, equine. (Hexavalent ABCDEF, bivalent AB, and monovalent E antitoxins are also available.)	One vial IV and 1 vial IM; repeat after 2–4 hours if symptoms worsen, and after 12–24 hours.	For treatment of botulism. Available from CDC.* Twenty percent incidence of serum reactions. Only type E antitoxin has been shown to affect outcome of illness. Prophylaxis is not routinely recommended but may be given to asymptomatic persons with unequivocal exposure.
Diphtheria	Diphtheria antitoxin, equine.	20,000 (1 vial)–120,000 units IM depending on severity and duration of illness. Same dose for children and adults.	For treatment of diphtheria. Active immunization and (perhaps) erythromycin prophylaxis rather than anti-toxin prophylaxis should be given to nonimmune contacts of active cases. Contacts should be observed for signs of illness so that antitoxin may be administered if needed. Available from CDC.*
Hepatitis A ("infectious")	Immune globulin (ISG).	For postexposure prophylaxis, 0.02 mL/kg IM as soon as possible after exposure up to 2 weeks.	Modifies but does not prevent infection. Recommended for household contacts and other contacts of similar intensity. Also recommended prior to travel to endemic areas. Not recommended for office or school contacts unless an epidemic appears to be in progress.
		For chronic exposure, a dose of 0.06 mL/kg is recommended every 6 months. (0.02 mL/kg is effective for 2–3 months.)	Personnel of mental institutions, facilities for retarded children, and prisons appear to be at chronic risk of acquiring hepatitis A, as are those who work with non-human primates.
Hepatitis B ("serum")	Hepatitis B immune globulin (HBIG). Regular immune globulin may be effective as well.	0.06 mL/kg IM as soon as possible after exposure, preferably within 7 days. A second injection should be given 25–30 days after exposure, unless hepatitis B vaccine was given with first dose of HBIG.	Administer to nonimmune individuals as postexposure prophylaxis following either parenteral exposure to or direct mucous membrane contact with HBsAg-positive materials. Should not be given to persons already demonstrating anti-HBsAg antibody. Give a single dose of 0.13 mL/kg to newborns of mothers who develop hepatitis B in the third trimester and who have HBs antigenemia at time of delivery.
Hepatitis non-A, non-B	Immune globulin (ISG).	0.06 mL/kg IM as soon as possible after exposure.	Give to individuals with parenteral exposure to sera from patients with hepatitis, or other close contacts. Efficacy uncertain.
Hypogamma-globulinemia	Immune globulin (ISG).	0.6 mL/kg IM every 3–4 weeks; or 2–4 mL/kg IV every 4 weeks (only is G modified for IV use).	Give double dose at onset of therapy. Immune globulin is of no value in prevention of frequent infections in the absence of demonstrable hypogammaglobulinemia.
Measles	Immune globulin (ISG). (Measles immune globulin no longer available.)	0.25 mL/kg IM as soon as possible after exposure. This dose may be ineffective in immuno-incompetent patients, who should receive 20–30 mL.	Live measles vaccine will usually prevent natural infection if given within 48 hours following exposure. If immunoglobulin is administered, delay immunization with live virus for 3 months.
Organ transplant	Antilymphocyte or anti-thymocyte immune serum or globulin, equine.	Variable. See manufacturer's guidelines.	Used as adjunctive immunosuppressive agent in patients undergoing organ transplantation.
Pertussis	Pertussis immune globulin.	1.25 mL IM (child).	Efficacy doubtful, both for treatment as well as prophylaxis. Available from Cutter Laboratories.
Poliomyelitis	Immune globulin (ISG).	0.15 mL/kg IM.	Indicated only for exposed, unimmunized subject. Immunize with live or inactivated vaccine after 2–3 months, with subsequent boosters.

Table 53–1 (cont'd). Materials available for passive immunization.

Indication	Product	Dosage	Comments
Rabies	Rabies immune globulin. (Equine antirabies serum is available but is much less desirable and requires a higher dose of about 500 units/20 kg of body weight.)	20 IU/kg, up to half of which is infiltrated locally at the wound site, and the remainder given IM.	Give as soon as possible after exposure. Recommended for all bite or scratch exposure to carnivores, especially bat, skunk, fox, coyote, or raccoon, despite animal's apparent health, if the brain cannot be immediately examined and found rabies-free. Not recommended for individuals with demonstrated antibody response from preexposure prophylaxis. Must be combined with rabies immunization. Also available through CDC.*
Rh isoimmunization (from fetal-maternal transfusion)	Rh_o (D) immune globulin.	In an Rh_o (D)-negative woman, one dose IM within 72 hours of abortion, amniocentesis, obstetric delivery of an Rh-positive infant, or transfusion of Rh-positive blood.	For nonimmune females only. May be effective at much greater postexposure interval; therefore, give even if more than 72 hours have elapsed. One vial contains 300 μg antibody and can reliably inhibit the immune response to a fetal-maternal bleed of up to 30 mL as estimated by the Betke-Kleihauer smear technique.
Rubella	Immune globulin (ISG).	20–40 mL IM at time of exposure.	Prevents disease in recipient but *not* in fetus of exposed mother—hence *not recommended*.
Snakebite	Coral snake antivenin, equine. Crotalid (pit viper) antivenin, polyvalent, equine.	At least 3–5 vials IV (preferred) or IM.	Dose should be sufficient to reverse symptoms of envenomation. Consider antitetanus measures as well. Available from Wyeth Laboratories ([215] 688–4400) or CDC.*
Tetanus	Tetanus immune globulin. (Bovine and equine antitoxins are available but are not recommended. They are used at 10 times the dose of tetanus immune globulin.)	Prophylaxis: 250–500 units IM. Therapy: 3000–6000 units IM.	Give in separate syringe at separate site from simultaneously administered toxoid. Recommended only for major or contaminated wounds who have had fewer than 2 doses of toxoid at any time in the past (fewer than 3 doses if wound is more than 24 hours old or otherwise highly tetanus-prone).
Vaccinia	Vaccinia immune globulin.	Prophylaxis: 0.3 mL/kg IM. Therapy: 0.6 mL/kg IM. May be repeated as necessary for treatment and at intervals of 1 week for prophylaxis.	May be useful in treatment of vaccinia of the eye, eczema vaccinatum, generalized vaccinia, and vaccinia necrosum and in the prevention of such complications in exposed patients with skin disorders. Available from CDC.*
Varicella	Varicella-zoster immune globulin or zoster immune globulin. (Regular immune globulin may be effective if this is unavailable.)	Give 125 units/10 kg (patients ≤ 50 kg), up to maximum of 625 units (patients > 50 kg). Give IM within 96 hours of exposure.	For immunosuppressed or immunoincompetent children under 15 years of age, known to be nonimmune (by laboratory test if possible), and with household, hospital (same 2- or 4-bed room or adjacent beds in large ward), or playmate (>1 hour play indoors) contact with a known case of varicella-zoster; and for neonates whose mothers have developed varicella within 4 days before or 48 hours after delivery. The products modify natural disease but may not prevent the development of immunity. Expensive (about $400 to treat one adult).

*Centers for Disease Control, central number (404) 329–3311 during the day; (404) 329–2888 nights, weekends, and holidays (emergencies only).

Note: Passive immunotherapy or immunoprophylaxis should always be administered as soon as possible after exposure to the offending agent. Immune antisera and globulin are always given intramuscularly unless otherwise noted. Always question carefully and test for hypersensitivity before administering animal sera (see text).

In general, administration of live virus vaccines should be delayed at least 2 months after passive immunization with pooled human gamma globulin preparations.

Table 53–2. Materials commonly used for active immunization. (DTP = diphtheria and tetanus toxoids and pertussis vaccine; DT = diphtheria and tetanus toxoids; Td = tetanus and diphtheria toxoids, adult type; and T = tetanus toxoid.)*

Pathogen or Disease	Product (Source)	Type of Agent	Route of Administration	Primary Immunization	Duration of Effect	Comments
Cholera	Cholera vaccine.	Killed bacteria	Subcut, IM	Two doses 1 week to 1 month apart.	6 months†	Fifty percent protective. Booster doses should be given every 6 months.
Diphtheria	DTP, DT (adsorbed) for child under 6; Td (adsorbed) for all others. Also available as diphtheria toxoid alone.	Toxoid	IM	Three doses 4 weeks or more apart, with an additional dose 1 year later for a child under 6. (Can be given at the same time as polio vaccine if doses at least 8 weeks apart.)	10 years‡	Use DT if convulsions follow use of DTP. Give school children and adults third dose 6–12 months after second.
Haemophilus influenzae infection	Purified type b polysaccharide (polyribosylribitol phosphate)	Polysaccharide	IM	One dose to children age 18–24 months.	Uncertain	Efficacy best when given above age two years, but recommended for high-risk infants at age 18 months.
Hepatitis B	Hepatitis B virus and surface antigen, inactivated (human plasma from carriers).	Purified and inactivated virus coat protein	IM	Three doses: one initially, one at 1 month, and one at 6 months. Double dosage recommended for immunocompromised patients.	Years	Greater than 90% protective. Give preexposure to individuals who are not immune (ie, lack HBs antibody) and who are at high risk of acquiring disease (medical personnel, spouses of carriers, etc).
Influenza	Influenza virus vaccine, monovalent, bivalent, or trivalent (chick embryo). Composition of the vaccine is changed depending upon types of viruses causing disease.	Killed whole or split virus; types A and B	IM	One dose. (Two doses 4 weeks or more apart are preferable when a major new antigenic component is first incorporated into the vaccine. Two doses of the split virus products should be used in persons under 13 years because of a lower incidence of side effects.)	1–3 years	Give immunization by November. Recommended annually for patients with cardiorespiratory disease, diabetes, other chronic diseases, and the elderly. Patients receiving chemotherapy for malignant disease are likely to respond better if immunized between or before courses of treatment.
Measles	Measles virus vaccine, live attenuated (chick embryo).	Live virus	Subcut	One dose at age 15 months. Give earlier if risk of measles is high (eg, an epidemic).	Permanent	Reimmunize if given before 15 months of age; may prevent natural disease if given less than 48 hours after exposure.
Meningococcal meningitis	Meningococcal polysaccharide vaccine, group A, group C, or both. A tetravalent preparation is also available containing serotypes A, C, W-135, and Y.	Polysaccharide	Subcut	One dose. Since primary antibody response requires at least 5 days, antibiotic prophylaxis with rifampin (600 mg or 10 mg/kg every 12 hours for 4 doses) should be given to household contacts.	?Permanent	Recommended in epidemic situations, for use by the military to prevent outbreaks in recruits, and possibly as an adjunct to antibiotic prophylaxis in preventing secondary cases in family contacts. Not reliably effective in children less than 2 years old.
Mumps	Mumps virus vaccine, live, Jeryl Lynn strain (chick embryo).	Live virus	Subcut	One dose.	Permanent	Reimmunize if given before 1 year of age.
Pertussis	DTP; also pertussis vaccine alone.	Killed bacteria	IM	As for DTP.	See ‡	Not generally recommended after age 6.
Pneumococci	Pneumococcal polysaccharide vaccine, polyvalent (23 of the most common serotypes).	Polysaccharide	Subcut, IM	0.5 mL.	Uncertain; probably at least 5 years	Recommended for individuals at high risk of serious pneumococcal disease: asplenia, sickling hemoglobinopathies, chronic cardiorespiratory ailments, etc. Variable efficacy in children; not recommended for those less than 2 years old.

Poliomyelitis	Poliovirus vaccine, live, oral, trivalent (monkey kidney, human diploid). (Monovalent vaccines also available.)	Live virus types I, II, and III	Oral	Two doses 6–8 weeks or more apart, followed by a third dose 12 months later. (Can be given at the same time as primary DTP immunization.) A fourth dose before entering school is recommended for children immunized in the first 1–2 years of life.	Permanent	Recommended for adults only if at increased risk by travel to epidemic or highly endemic areas or occupational contact. (Inactivated vaccine may be preferable in this circumstance.) Individuals who have completed a primary series may take a single booster dose if the risk of exposure is high.
	Poliomyelitis vaccine.	Killed virus types I, II, and III	IM	Three doses 1–2 months apart, followed by a fourth dose 6–12 months later and a fifth dose before entering school.‡	2–5 years, perhaps longer	Killed virus vaccines are licensed but not readily available and are no longer recommended except for immunologically deficient patients or possibly for unimmunized adults who are at risk of exposure to poliomyelitis by reason of travel or immunization of their children.
Rabies	Rabies vaccine (human diploid cell–derived). Duck embryo or mouse brain–derived vaccine may still be available outside the USA, but are inferior to the human diploid cell–derived vaccine.	Killed virus	IM	**Preexposure:** Two doses 1 week apart, followed by third dose 2–3 weeks later. **Postexposure:** Five doses on days 0, 3, 7, 14, and 28. Always give rabies immune globulin as well (see Table 53–1).	Unknown; probably > 2 years	Preexposure immunization only for occupational or avocational risk or residence in hyperendemic area. Antibody response should be measured 3–4 weeks after last injection to ensure successful immunization, and repeat injection should be given if no response. Wounds should be copiously swabbed and flushed with soap and water. (See Table 53–1 regarding use of hyperimmune serum or immune globulin.) For animal bite, consider antitetanus measures as well.
Rubella	Rubella virus vaccine, live (human diploid).	Live virus	Subcut	One dose.	Permanent	Give after 15 months of age. Do not give during pregnancy. Women must prevent pregnancy for 3 months after immunization. Prevents disease but not infection.
Smallpox	Smallpox vaccine (calf lymph, chick embryo).	Live vaccinia virus	Intradermal	One dose.	3 years†	*The only groups for whom smallpox vaccine is indicated at the present time are* (1) military personnel and (2) laboratory personnel working with poxviruses. No longer required for international travel, as smallpox has been eradicated. Production for civilian use discontinued in May, 1983.

* Dosages for the specific product, including variations for age, are best obtained from the manufacturer's package insert. Immunizations should be given by the route suggested for the product.
† Revaccination interval required by international regulations.
‡ A single dose is a sufficent booster at any time after the effective duration of primary immunization has passed.
§ For contaminated or severe wounds, give booster if more than 5 years has elapsed since full immunization or last booster.
** Test for PPD conversion 2 months later and reimmunize if there is no conversion.

Table 53–2 (cont'd). Materials commonly used for active immunization. (DTP = diphtheria and tetanus toxoids and pertussis vaccine; DT = diphtheria and tetanus toxoids; Td = tetanus and diphtheria toxoids, adult type; and T = tetanus toxoid.)

Pathogen or Disease	Product (Source)	Type of Agent	Route of Administration	Primary Immunization	Duration of Effect	Comments
Tetanus	DTP, DT (adsorbed) for children under age 6; Td or T (adsorbed) for all others.	Toxoid	IM	Two doses 4 weeks or more apart; third dose 6–12 months after second dose.	10 years‡§	Give school children and adults a fourth dose 6–12 months after initial series of injections.
Tuberculosis	BCG vaccine (bacille Calmette-Guérin). Only the Danish substrain is available in the USA.	Live attenuated *Mycobacterium bovis*	Intradermal or subcut (per manufacturer's recommendation)	One dose (0.1 mL intradermally).	?Permanent**	Not recommended for use in USA. Has shown highly variable efficacy.
Typhoid	Typhoid vaccine.	Killed bacteria	Subcut or intradermal	Two doses 4 weeks or more apart or 3 doses 1 week apart (less desirable).	3 years‡	Seventy percent protective. Recommended only for exposure from travel, epidemic, or household carrier and not, eg, because of floods.
Yellow fever	Yellow fever vaccine (chick embryo)(17-D strain).	Live virus	Subcut	One dose.	10 years†	Recommended for residence in or travel to endemic areas of Africa and South America.

* Dosages for the specific product, including variations for age, are best obtained from the manufacturer's package insert. Immunizations should be given by the route suggested for the product.
† Revaccination interval required by international regulations.
‡ A single dose is a sufficent booster at any time after the effective duration of primary immunization has passed.
§ For contaminated or severe wounds, give booster if more than 5 years has elapsed since full immunization or last booster.
** Test for PPD conversion 2 months later and reimmunize if there is no conversion.

Table 53–3. Advantages and disadvantages of live versus dead immunogens.

Type of Immunization	Advantages	Disadvantages
Inactivated (killed) product	1. No risk of disease from infection. 2. May be highly purified (eg, toxoids). 3. Often easy to ship and store (ie, stable).	1. Immunity may be short-lived—reimmunization often required. 2. May not stimulate protective factors (eg, inactivated measles vaccine). 3. May not eliminate reinfections (without disease) or carrier state. 4. Inherent toxicity of immunogen (eg, pertussis, influenza). 5. Parenteral administration usually required.
Live attenuated product	1. Long-lasting immunity. 2. Simulate resistance induced by natural infection. 3. May not need to be given parenterally.	1. Risk of disease due to reversion to virulence (eg, polio) or failure of host restriction (eg, immunosuppressed host). 2. Mild disease often required to induce immunity. 3. Risk of carrying contaminants higher than with inactivated vaccines. 4. Attenuated agent may cause new kind of disease. 5. Generally more labile and difficult to store.

Table 53–4. Recommended schedule for active immunization and skin testing of children.

Age	Product Administered	Test Recommended
2 months	DTP[1] Oral poliovaccine,[2] trivalent	
4 months	DTP Oral poliovaccine, trivalent	
6 months	DTP Oral poliovaccine, trivalent (optional)	
15–19 months	DTP Measles vaccine[3] Mumps vaccine[4] Rubella vaccine[6] Oral poliovaccine, trivalent	
4–6 years	DTP Oral poliovaccine, trivalent	Tuberculin test[5]
12–14 years	Rubella vaccine[6] Td[7]	Tuberculin test[5]

[1] **DTP:** Toxoids of diphtheria and tetanus, alum-precipitated or aluminum hydroxide adsorbed, combined with pertussis bacterial antigen. Suitable for young children. Three doses of 0.5 mL intramuscularly at intervals of 4–8 weeks. Fourth injection of 0.5 mL intramuscularly given about 1 year later.

[2] **Oral live poliomyelitis virus vaccine:** Trivalent (types 1, 2, and 3 combined) given 3 times at intervals of 6–8 weeks and then as a booster 1 year later. Monovalent vaccine is rarely used now; it can be given at 6-week intervals, followed by a booster of trivalent vaccine 1 year later. Inactive (Salk type) trivalent vaccine is available but not recommended. *Note:* One sequence of monovalent vaccines (type 2, then 1, then 3) is in accord with the recommendations of the US Public Health Service Advisory Committee on Immunization Practices. The American Academy of Pediatrics recommends the sequence 1, 3, 2.

[3] **Live measles virus vaccine,** 0.5 mL intramuscularly. When using attenuated (Edmonston) strain, give human gamma globulin, 0.01 mL/lb, injected into the opposite arm at the same time, to lessen the reaction to the vaccine. This is not advised with "further attenuated" (Schwarz) strain vaccine. Inactivated measles vaccine should not be used.

[4] **Live mumps virus vaccine (attenuated),** 0.5 mL intramuscularly.

[5] The frequency with which **tuberculin tests** are administered depends on the risk of exposure, ie, the prevalence of tuberculosis in the population group. The intervals indicated are the recommended minimum.

[6] **Rubella live virus vaccine (attenuated)** can be given between age 1 year and puberty. Some physicians recommend rubella vaccine only for prepubertal girls. The entire contents of a single dose vaccine vial, reconstituted from the lyophilized state, are injected subcutaneously. The vaccine must *not* be given to women who are pregnant or are liable to become pregnant within 3 months of vaccination. Women must be warned that there is a possibility of developing arthralgias or arthritis after vaccination. The cell culture–grown RA 27/3 rubella virus vaccine was licensed in USA in 1979. No live vaccine should be given to immunodeficient patients.

[7] **Tetanus toxoid and diphtheria toxoid,** purified, suitable for adults, given every 7–10 years.

Table 53–5. Vaccines and other biological products of restricted availability or usage.

Material	Product	Use	Tested and Widely Used in Humans	Extensive Human Trials	Limited Human Trials
Adenovirus vaccine	Live enteric-coated vaccine against types 4, 7, and 21.	Prevents pneumonitis. Used primarily in military.	X		
Anthrax vaccine*	Protein antigen from culture filtrates, absorbed.	Occupational exposure.	X		
Arbovirus antibodies (human)*	Immune (convalescent) plasma for Ebola, Lassa, Marburg, Junin, and Machupo viruses; EEE, WEE, VEE, SLE, and California encephalitis viruses; and Russian spring-summer encephalitis virus.	Treatment of suspected or documented cases; prophylaxis of exposure to active case.			X
Arbovirus vaccines*	Inactivated vaccines—equine encephalitides.	Occupational exposure (virologists).	X		
Botulism vaccine*	Pentavalent (ABCDE) botulinum toxoid.	Occupational exposure (laboratory personnel).	X		
Cholera vaccine	Experimental antitoxins.	Prevents cholera.			X
Coccidioides immitis vaccine	Purified spherules.	Prevention of *C immitis* disease.			X
Cytomegalovirus vaccine	Live attenuated virus.	Immunocompromised, susceptible hosts.		X	
Eastern equine encephalitis (EEE) vaccine*	Inactivated virus.	Occupational exposure. Epidemics.	X		
Escherichia coli enterotoxin	Purified *E coli* enterotoxoid.	Prevents secretory diarrhea due to toxin.			X
Gonococcal vaccine	Purified gonococcal pili.	Prevents gonorrhea.			X
Haemophilus influenzae B vaccine	Outer membrane protein or protein-polysacchride conjugates.	Prevents *H influenzae* disease in children.			X
Hepatitis A vaccine	Live attenuated virus.	Prevention of hepatitis A.			X
Hepatitis B vaccine	Hepatitis B surface antigen produced in yeast by recombinant DNA technology.	Prevention of hepatitis B.			X
Herpes B (monkey B encephalitis) virus antibody (human)*	Immune (convalescent) plasma from patients.	Treatment of herpes B infection; prophylaxis of documented exposure to virus.			X
Herpes simplex vaccine	Purified herpes simplex type 2 glycoproteins.	Prevention of herpes simplex infection.			X
Influenza vaccine	Subunit vaccines. Live virus vaccines.	Prevents influenza.			X
Interferon	Leukocyte- and fibroblast-derived; also produced by recombinant DNA technology.	Antiviral—effective for zoster, hepatitis B, perhaps other viruses.		X	
		Cancer chemotherapy—enhanced cytotoxic responses; inhibition of tumor growth.		X	
Leprosy vaccine	Killed bacteria; purified subunits.	Efficacy uncertain.			X
Endotoxin antibody (human)	Human hyperimmune serum against endotoxin.	Highly effective in improving outcome of serious gram-negative infection.		X	
Malaria vaccine	Killed merozoites; sporozoite antigen.	Prevents malaria.			X
Meningococcus group B vaccine	Various experimental vaccines.	Prevents infection.		X	
Mycoplasma pneumoniae vaccine	Killed vaccines. Live attenuated vaccines.	Prevents infection.			X

Table 53–5 (cont'd). Vaccines and other biological products of restricted availability or usage.

Material	Product	Use	Tested and Widely Used in Humans	Extensive Human Trials	Limited Human Trials
Pertussis component vaccine	Purified bacterial proteins.	Prevention of pertussis.		X	
Plague vaccine	Inactivated (USA). Live attenuated (not available in the USA).	Occupational exposure; travel to epidemic area.	X		
Pseudomonas aeruginosa vaccine	Polyvalent vaccines.	For high-risk populations, eg, burn patients.		X	
Q fever vaccine	Inactivated *Rickettsia.*	Epidemics; occupational exposure.		X	
Respiratory syncytial virus vaccine	Live attenuated virus.	Prevents bronchiolitis and pneumonia in infants.			X
Shigella	Live attenuated vaccines.	High-risk groups.			X
Group A streptococcus vaccine	Purified M proteins.	High-risk groups.			X
Group B streptococcus vaccine	Polysaccharide capsule.	Infants do not respond; may need to give to mother before delivery.			X
Tularemia vaccine*	Live attenuated. (Inactivated vaccines available in some countries.)	Occupational exposure.	X		
Typhoid vaccine	Live attenuated bacterium.	Prevents infection.		X	
Varicella vaccine	Live attenuated virus.	For immunocompromised patients		X	
Venezuelan equine encephalitis (VEE) vaccine*	Live attenuated virus.	Occupational exposure.	X		
Transfer factor	Derived from leukocytes of immune donors.	Restores delayed hypersensitivity.			X
Thymic hormones (eg, thymosin)	Derived from thymic tissue.	Enhanced maturation of T lymphocytes.			X

*Available through CDC. Telephone central number (404) 329–3311 during the day, (404) 329–2888 nights, weekends, and holidays (emergencies only).

HYPERSENSITIVITY TO ANIMAL PROTEINS & DESENSITIZATION

Many persons are hypersensitive to animal proteins or drugs. If they are given such material by injection, there is a chance that anaphylaxis may develop. Therefore, tests for hypersensitivity are indicated prior to any such injection. Serum sickness can develop in anyone, independently of prior sensitization. The following steps are desirable as a safeguard against anaphylactic reactions and must be observed with biologic products administered for prophylaxis or therapy, particularly with animal sera.

Evaluation & Testing
A. Past History: Has the patient received a similar material before? Does the patient have known allergy, eg, to egg protein, which would increase the likelihood of allergy to other animal proteins?
B. Materials Available for Desensitization: Have ready the following: epinephrine, 1:1000 solution, in sterile syringe; airway; soluble corticosteroids; tourniquet; antihistamine drug (eg, diphenhydramine) for injection; oxygen; and suction. A cardiopulmonary resuscitation cart will have all the necessary materials. An intravenous catheter should be inserted before beginning desensitization.
C. Intradermal Test: About 0.02 mL of dilute (at least 1:100) test material is injected intradermally, and the site is observed for 15 minutes. The appearance of erythema and edema with wheal formation suggests specific hypersensitivity. Normal saline solution should be injected into a comparable (eg, contralateral) skin site as a control.
D. Conjunctival Test: This is a less sensitive alternative to the intradermal test. Instillation of 1 drop of 1:10 dilution of test material into a normal conjunctiva results in itching, lacrimation, and redness within 5 minutes if the person is hypersensitive. One drop of physiologic saline solution instilled into the other eye serves as a control.

A negative conjunctival or intradermal test is a reliable (but not conclusive) indication that the patient is not allergic to the test material. When the skin test or conjunctival test indicates hypersensitivity, it is preferable to avoid injection of the material in question and substitute another product. Thus, in place of diphtheria horse serum antitoxin, diphtheria antitoxin raised in goats might be administered. If an alternative product is not available and the material is essential to the patient's welfare, desensitization may be attempted as described in the following paragraphs.

Desensitization Procedure

Collect materials listed above and insert an intravenous catheter (keep open with normal saline). Inject gradually increasing doses of the product subcutaneously in an extremity every 30–60 minutes, observing for possible significant reactions. Begin with 0.1 mL of product diluted 1:100 or more. If there is no reaction, give 0.1 mL undiluted. If a significant local reaction occurs, inject the same dose, or a smaller dose together with 0.5 mL of aqueous epinephrine, 1:1000. Increase the doses of the product gradually but steadily until 2 or 3 mL of undiluted product has been administered without significant reaction. Repeat this dose every 30–60 minutes until the full prophylactic or therapeutic dose has been given.

Desensitization often permits the administration of an animal protein to which the person exhibits moderate hypersensitivity. However, if major reactions occur during the procedure, desensitization attempts generally should be abandoned.

SKIN TEST REAGENTS

Skin tests are widely employed to determine the presence of allergy (immediate hypersensitivity), to diagnose infection, or to determine if cell-mediated immunity is intact. Skin tests commonly used for determining cell-mediated immunity or the presence of past or present infection with certain pathogens are presented in Table 53–6. Recently, a device for testing cellular immunity has been marketed that simultaneously tests 6 different antigens (CMI, Multitest; Meriux).

Skin test materials for determining the presence of allergy (immediate hypersensitivity) are less standardized and are not discussed here.

Table 53–6. Some commonly used materials for assessing humoral and cell-mediated immunity.

Material	Description and Major Manufacturer	Usual intradermal Dose	(+) Response at 24–72 Hours	Interpretation and Comments
PPD-S	Purified protein derivative of *Mycobacterium tuberculosis,* stabilized with Tween-80. Potency tested by comparison with US standard tuberculin (many manufacturers).	0.1 mL, intermediate strength (5 TU).	≥ 10 mm induration (≥ 5 mm in some circumstances)	Positive reaction indicates previous infection with *M tuberculosis* or other mycobacteria. Does not indicate whether disease is present. Response to lower or higher doses (1 and 250 TU) difficult to interpret.
Candida	Partially purified and inactivated suspension of *Candida ablicans.* (Iatric Corp.)	0.1 mL of 1:500 dilution. Use 1:100 or 1:30 if negative at 1:500.	≥ 5 mm induration	Indicates presence of intact cellular immunity. Not useful for diagnosing *Candida* infection.
Diphtheria toxin (Schick test)	Diphtheria toxin. (Massachusetts Public Health Labs.)	Follow manufacturer's instructions.	Erythema and edema	*Positive* reaction indicates *lack* of circulating diphtheria antitoxin. A positive reaction after full immunization with diphtheria toxoid suggests an antibody immunodeficiency.
Trichophyton	Culture filtrate of trichophyton. (Iatric Corp.)	0.1 mL of 1:500. Use 1:100 or 1:30 if negative at 1:500.	≥ 5 mm induration	Indicates presence of intact cellular immunity; not useful for diagnosis of infection.
Mumps	Suspension of mumps virus. (Eli Lilly.)	0.1 mL (20 CF units).	≥ 1.5 cm of erythema, with induration	Not a reliable indicator of past mumps infection (many false-negatives). Induration indicates presence of intact cellular immunity.
Coccidioidin and spherulin	Purified culture filtrate of *Coccidioides immitis* mycelia or spherules, respectively. (Berkeley Biological and Iatric Corp.)	0.1 mL of 1:10 or 1:100 dilution. Use 1:100 first; use 1:10 if negative at 1:100.	≥ 5 mm induration	Indicates past infection with *C immitis*. Not useful for determining if infection is active or whether disease is present. Does not alter antibody titers. Most authorities recommend using both antigens for optimal sensitivity.
Histoplasmin	Culture filtrate of *Histoplasma capsulatum.* Standardized by comparison with histoplasmin reference standard. (Parke-Davis.)	0.1 mL of solution.	≥ 5 mm induration	Indicates past infection with *H capsulatum;* does not indicate if disease is present. Raises antibody titers that may confuse diagnosis; improved skin test reagents under development.

OTHER BIOLOGIC PRODUCTS

A number of biologic products are being used on a limited basis for treatment or prevention of infectious diseases (Table 53–5). These include **interferon** (an antiviral of proved efficacy but not yet commercially available; may also be useful as a cancer chemotherapeutic agent), **transfer factor** (transfers cell-mediated immunity without a graft-versus-host reaction; is undergoing clinical trials), and **antiendotoxic antiserum.** As our understanding of lymphokines increases and the ability to produce human proteins by tissue culture and recombinant DNA technology improves, immunotherapy with other human products will doubtless become more common.

REFERENCES

*Centers for Disease Control: *Collected Recommendations of the Advisory Committee on Immunization Practices* ("ACIP Recommendations"). [Updated at regular intervals, most recently in *MMWR* 1984;**33:**1.]

*Centers for Disease Control: Diphtheria, tetanus, and pertussis: Guidelines for vaccine prophylaxis and other preventive measures. *MMWR* 1985;**34:**405.

*Centers for Disease Control: *Health Information for International Travelers.* [Updated annually with supplemental information in *Morbidity and Mortality Weekly Report* as needed.]

*Centers for Disease Control: *Immunobiologic Agents and Drugs Available from the Centers for Disease Control: Descriptions, Recommendations and Adverse Reactions,* 3rd ed. 1982.

*Centers for Disease Control: Polysaccharide vaccine for prevention of *Haemophilus influenzae* type b disease. *MMWR* 1985;**34:**201.

*Centers for Disease Control: Recommendations for protection against viral hepatitis. *MMWR* 1985;**34:**313.

*Centers for Disease Control: Rubella prevention. *MMWR* 1984;**33:**301.

Cohen SN: Immunization. Chapter 39 in: *Basic & Clinical Immunology,* 5th ed. Stites DP et al (editors). Lange, 1984.

Committee on Immunization, American College of Physicians: *Guide for Adult Immunization.* American College of Physicians, 1985.

Conte JE, Barriere S: *Manual of Antibiotics and Infectious Diseases.* Lea & Febiger, 1985.

Cremer KJ et al: Vaccinia virus recombinant expressing herpes simplex virus type 1 glycoprotein D prevents latent herpes in mice. *Science* 1985;**228:**737.

Dreesman GR, Bronson JG, Kennedy RC (editors): *High Technology Route to Virus Vaccines.* American Society for Microbiology, 1985.

Fulginiti VA: Immunization. Chapter 5 in: *Current Pediatric Diagnosis & Treatment,* 8th ed. Kempe CH, Silver HK, O'Brien D (editors). Lange, 1984.

Fulginiti VA (editor): *Immunization in Clinical Practice.* Lippincott, 1981.

Germanier R (editor): *Bacterial Vaccines.* Beecham, 1984.

Health and Public Policy Committee, American College of Physicians: Compensation for vaccine-related injuries. *Ann Intern Med* 1984;**101:**559.

Rimland D, McGowan JE Jr, Shulman JA: Immunization for the internist. *Ann Intern Med* 1976;**85:**622.

Robbins JB, Hill JC, Sadoff JC: *Bacterial Vaccines.* Thieme-Stratton, 1982.

Sato Y, Kimura M, Fukumi H: Development of a pertussis component vaccine in Japan. *Lancet* 1984;**1:**122.

Schoenbaum SC: A perspective on the benefits, costs and risks of immunization. Chapter 9 in: *Seminars in Infectious Diseases.* Vol 3. Wernstein L, Fields BN (editors). Thieme-Stratton, 1980.

Scolnick EM et al: Clinical evaluation in healthy adults of a hepatitis B vaccine made by recombinant DNA. *JAMA* 1984;**251:**2812.

Simonsen O, Kjeldsen K, Heron I: Immunity against tetanus and effect of revaccination 25–30 years after primary vaccination. *Lancet* 1984;**2:**1240.

Stiehm ER: Standard and special human immune serum globulins as therapeutic agents. *Pediatrics* 1979;**63:**301.

*May be obtained from the CDC, Building 1, Room SB 253, Atlanta 30333.

54

Disinfectants & Antiseptics

Ernest Jawetz, MD, PhD

The antiseptics and disinfectants differ fundamentally from systemically active chemotherapeutic agents in that they possess little or no selective toxicity. Most of these substances are toxic not only for microbial parasites but for host cells as well. Therefore, they may be used to reduce the microbial population in the inanimate environment, but they can usually be applied only topically, not systemically, to humans.

The terms disinfectants, antiseptics, or germicides have been used interchangeably by some, and the definitions overlap greatly in the literature. The term **disinfectant** often denotes a substance that kills microorganisms in the inanimate environment. The term **antiseptic** often is applied to substances that inhibit bacterial growth both in vitro and in vivo when applied to the surface of living tissue under suitable conditions of contact.

The antibacterial action of antiseptics and disinfectants is largely dependent on concentration, temperature, and time. Very low concentrations may stimulate bacterial growth, higher concentrations may be inhibitory, and still higher concentrations may be bactericidal for certain organisms.

Evaluation of the antiseptics and disinfectants is difficult. Methods of testing are controversial and results are subject to different interpretations. There is a need for effective, nontoxic compounds to neutralize disinfectants in vitro. Ideally, disinfectants should be lethal for microorganisms in high dilution, noninjurious to tissues or inanimate substances, inexpensive, stable, nonstaining, odorless, and rapid-acting even in the presence of foreign proteins, exudates, or fibers. No preparation now available combines these characteristics to a high degree.

Many antiseptics and disinfectants were at one time used in medical and surgical practice. Most have now been displaced by chemotherapeutic substances. The 2 remaining areas of use are urinary antiseptics (see Chapter 51) and topical antiseptics. Most topical antiseptics do not aid wound healing but, on the contrary, often impair healing. In general, cleansing of abrasions and superficial wounds by washing with soap and water is far more effective and less damaging than the application of topical antiseptics. Substances applied topically to skin or mucous membranes are absorbed irregularly and often unpredictably. Occlusive dressings with plastic films often greatly enhance absorption. Penetration of drugs through skin epithelium is also greatly influenced by relative humidity, temperature, and occlusion.

A few chemical classes of disinfectants and antiseptics are briefly characterized in the following paragraphs.

Alcohols

Aliphatic alcohols are antimicrobial in varying degree by precipitating protein. Ethanol (ethyl alcohol) in 70% concentration is bactericidal in 1–2 minutes at 30 °C but less effective at lower and higher concentrations. Ethyl alcohol, 70%, and isopropyl alcohol (isopropanol), 90%, are at present the most satisfactory general disinfectants for skin surfaces. They may be useful for sterilizing instruments but have no effect on spores, and better agents are available for this purpose. Aerosols of 70% alcohol with 1-μm size droplets may be effective disinfectants for mechanical respirators.

Propylene glycol and other glycols have been used as vapors to disinfect air. Precise control of humidity is necessary for good antimicrobial action. Glycol vapors are rarely employed at present.

Aldehydes

Formaldehyde in a concentration of 1–10% effectively kills microorganisms and their spores in 1–6 hours. It acts by combining with and precipitating protein. It is too irritating for use on tissues, but it is widely employed as a disinfectant for instruments. Formaldehyde solution USP contains 37% formaldehyde by weight, with methyl alcohol added to prevent polymerization.

Glutaraldehyde as a 2% alkaline solution in 70% isopropanol (pH 7.5–8.5) serves as a liquid disinfectant for some optical and other instruments and for some prosthetic materials. It kills viable microorganisms in 10 minutes and spores in 3–10 hours, but the solution is unstable, and tissue contact must be avoided.

Methenamine taken orally can release formaldehyde into acid urine. It is employed as a urinary antiseptic (see Chapter 51).

Acids

Several inorganic acids have been used for cauterization of tissue. Although they are effective antimicrobial agents, the tissue destruction they cause precludes their use. Boric acid, 5% in water, or as powder, can be applied to a variety of skin lesions as an antimicrobial agent. However, the toxicity of absorbed boric acid is high, particularly for small children, and its use is not advised. Among the organic acids, benzoic acid, 0.1%, is employed as a food preservative. Esters of benzoic acid (parabens) are used as antimicrobial preservatives of certain other drugs. Acetic acid, 1%, can be used in surgical dressings as a topical antimicrobial agent; 0.25% acetic acid is a useful antibacterial agent in the external ear and for irrigation of the lower urinary tract. This can also be used with an indwelling catheter and a closed system for urinary drainage. It is particularly active against aerobic gram-negative bacteria, eg, *Pseudomonas* sp. Salicylic and undecylenic and other fatty acids can serve as fungicides on skin. They are employed particularly in dermatophytosis involving intertriginous areas, eg, "athlete's foot."

Mandelic acid is excreted unchanged in the urine after oral intake; 12 g daily taken orally can lower the pH of urine to 5.0, sufficient to be antibacterial. (See Urinary Antiseptics, Chapter 51.)

Halogens & Halogen-Containing Compounds

A. Iodine: Elemental iodine is an effective germicide. Its mode of action is not definitely known. A 1:20,000 solution of iodine kills bacteria in 1 minute and spores in 15 minutes, and its tissue toxicity is relatively low. Iodine tincture USP contains 2% iodine and 2.4% sodium iodide in alcohol. It is the most effective disinfectant available for intact skin and should be used to disinfect skin when obtaining blood cultures by venipuncture. Its principal disadvantage is the occasional dermatitis that can occur in hypersensitive individuals. This can be avoided by promptly removing the tincture of iodine with alcohol.

Iodine can be complexed with polyvinylpyrolidone to yield povidone-iodine USP. This is a water-soluble complex that liberates free iodine in solution (eg, 1% free iodine in 10% solution). It is widely employed as a skin disinfectant, particularly for preoperative skin preparation. It is an effective local antibacterial substance, killing not only vegetative forms but also clostridial spores. Hypersensitivity reactions are infrequent. Povidone-iodine (Betadine, Isodine) is available in many forms: solution, ointment, aerosol, surgical scrub, shampoo, skin cleanser, vaginal gel, vaginal douche, and individual cotton swabs. Povidone-iodine solutions can become contaminated with *Pseudomonas* sp and other aerobic gram-negative bacteria. Rarely, drops of tincture of iodine can be added for the emergency disinfection of small quantities of contaminated water.

B. Chlorine: Chlorine exerts its antimicrobial action in the form of undissociated hypochlorous acid (HOCl), which is formed when chlorine is dissolved in water at neutral or acid pH. Chlorine concentrations of 0.25 ppm are effectively bactericidal for many microorganisms except mycobacteria, which are 500 times more resistant. Organic matter greatly reduces the antimicrobial activity of chlorine. The amount of chlorine bound by organic matter (eg, water) and thus not available for antimicrobial activity is called the

"chlorine demand." The chlorine demand of relatively pure water is low, and the addition of 0.5 ppm chlorine is sufficient for disinfection. The chlorine demand of grossly polluted water may be very high, so that 20 ppm or more of chlorine may have to be added for effective bactericidal action.

Chlorine is used mainly for the disinfection of inanimate objects and particularly for the purification of water. Chlorinated lime forms hypochlorite solution when dissolved. It is a cheap (but unstable) form of chlorine used mainly for disinfection of excreta in the field. Halazone USP is a chloramine employed in tablet form for the sterilization of small quantities of drinking water. The addition of 4–8 mg halazone per liter will sterilize water in 15–60 minutes unless a large quantity of organic material is present. It may not inactivate cysts of *Entamoeba histolytica*.

Sodium hypochlorite solution USP, 0.5% NaOCl (diluted sodium hypochlorite [modified Dakin's] solution), contains about 0.1 g of available chlorine per 100 mL and can be used as an irrigating fluid for the cleansing and disinfecting of contaminated wounds. Household bleaches containing chlorine can serve as disinfectants for inanimate objects.

Oxidizing Agents

Some antiseptics exert an antimicrobial action because they are oxidizing agents. Most are of no practical importance, and only hydrogen peroxide, sodium perborate, and potassium permanganate are occasionally used.

Hydrogen peroxide solution USP contains 3% H_2O_2 in water. Contact with tissues releases molecular oxygen, and there is a brief period of antimicrobial action. There is no penetration of tissues, and the main applications of hydrogen peroxide are as a mouthwash and for the cleansing of wounds. Hydrogen peroxide can probably be used to disinfect smooth contact lenses that are subsequently applied to the eye. Hydrous benzoyl peroxide USP can be bactericidal to microorganisms. When applied to the skin as a lotion, it is also keratolytic, antiseborrheic, and irritant. It has been used in treating acne and seborrhea, but it bleaches clothing and may produce contact dermatitis.

Potassium permanganate USP consists of purple crystals that dissolve in water to give deep purple solutions that stain tissues and clothing brown. A 1:10,000 dilution of potassium permanganate kills many microorganisms in one hour. Higher concentrations are irritating to tissues. The principal use of potassium permanganate solution is in the treatment of weeping skin lesions.

Heavy Metals

A. Mercury: Mercuric ion precipitates protein and inhibits sulfhydryl enzymes. Microorganisms inactivated by mercury can be reactivated by thiols (sulfhydryl compounds). Mercurial antiseptics inhibit the sulfhydryl enzymes of tissue cells as well as those of bacteria. Therefore, most mercury preparations are highly toxic if ingested. Mercury bichloride NF

(1:100) can be used as a disinfectant for instruments or unabraded skin.

Ammoniated mercury ointment USP contains 5% of the active insoluble compound ($HgNH_2Cl$). It is a skin disinfectant in impetigo.

Some organic mercury compounds are less toxic than the inorganic salts and somewhat more antibacterial. Nitromersol USP, thimerosal USP (merthiolate), and phenylmercuric acetate or nitrate are marketed in many different liquid and solid forms as bacteriostatic antiseptics. They are also used as "preservatives" in various biologic products to reduce the chance of accidental contamination. Merbromin (Mercurochrome) is used as a 2% solution that is a feeble antiseptic but stains tissue a brilliant red color. The psychologic effect of this stain has lent support to the (otherwise negligible) antiseptic properties of this material.

B. Silver: Silver ion precipitates protein and also interferes with essential metabolic activities of microbial cells. Inorganic silver salts in solution are strongly bactericidal. Silver nitrate, 1:1000, destroys most microorganisms rapidly upon contact. Silver nitrate ophthalmic solution USP contains 1% of the salt, to be instilled into the eyes of newborns to prevent gonococcal ophthalmia. It is effective for this purpose but may cause chemical conjunctivitis by being quite acid; therefore, antibiotic ointment has been used instead at times. Other inorganic silver salts are rarely used for their antimicrobial properties because they are strongly irritating to tissues. In burns, compresses of 0.5% silver nitrate can reduce infection of the burn wound, aid rapid eschar formation, and reduce mortality. If silver nitrate is reduced to nitrite by bacteria in the burn, methemoglobinemia may result. Silver sulfadiazine 1% cream slowly releases sulfadiazine and also silver (see Chapter 47) and effectively suppresses microbial flora in burns. It may have some advantages and causes less pain than mafenide acetate (Sulfamylon) in the treatment of burns, but it has occasionally produced leukopenia.

Colloidal preparations of silver are less injurious to superficial tissues and have significant bacteriostatic properties. Mild silver protein contains about 20% silver and can be applied as an antiseptic to mucous membranes. Prolonged use of any silver preparation may result in argyria.

Other Metals

Other metal salts (eg, zinc sulfate, copper sulfate) have significant antimicrobial properties but are rarely employed in medicine for this purpose.

Soaps

Soaps are anionic surface-active agents, usually sodium or potassium salts of various fatty acids. They vary in composition depending on the specific fats or oils and on the particular alkali from which they are made. Since NaOH and KOH are strong bases, whereas most fatty acids are weak acids, most soaps when dissolved in water are strongly alkaline (pH 8.0–10.0). Thus, they may irritate skin, which has a

pH of 5.5–6.5. Special soaps (eg, Neutrogena) use triethanolamine as a base and, when dissolved, are near pH 7.0. While most common soaps are well tolerated, excessive use will dry normal skin. Admixed synthetic fragrances may cause irritation or sensitization of skin.

Most common soaps remove dirt as well as surface secretions, desquamated epithelium, and bacteria contained in them. The physical action of thorough hand washing with plain soaps is quite effective in removing transient bacteria and other contaminating microorganisms from skin surfaces. For additional antibacterial action, certain disinfectant chemicals (hexachlorophene, phenols, carbanilides, etc) have been added to certain soaps. These chemicals may be both beneficial and potentially harmful and are discussed below.

Phenols & Related Compounds

Phenol denatures protein. It was the first antiseptic employed, as a spray, during surgical procedures by Lister in 1867. Concentrations of at least 1–2% are required for antimicrobial activity, whereas a 5% concentration is strongly irritating to tissues. Therefore, phenol is used mainly for the disinfection of inanimate objects and excreta. Substituted phenols are more effective (and more expensive) as environmental disinfectants. Among them are many proprietary preparations containing cresol and other alkyl-substituted phenols. Exaggerated claims for the antibacterial and antiviral properties for some such preparations (eg, Lysol) and their possible health benefits have been made.

Other phenol derivatives such as resorcinol, thymol, and hexylresorcinol have enjoyed some popularity in the past as antiseptics. Several chlorinated phenols are much more active antimicrobial agents.

Hexachlorophene USP is a white crystalline powder that is insoluble in water but soluble in organic solvents, dilute alkalies, and soaps and is an effective bacteriostatic agent. Hexachlorophene liquid soap USP and many proprietary preparations are used widely in surgical scrub routines and as deodorant soaps. Single applications of such preparations are no more effective than plain soaps, but daily use results in a deposit of hexachlorophene on the skin that exerts a prolonged bacteriostatic action. Thus, the number of resident skin bacteria is lower on the surgeon's hands if hexachlorophene soap is used daily and if other soaps, which promptly remove the residual hexachlorophene film, are not employed.

Soaps or detergents containing 3% hexachlorophene are effective in delaying or preventing colonization of the newborn's skin with pathogenic staphylococci in hospital nurseries. However, repeated bathing of newborns (and particularly premature infants) with such preparations may permit sufficient absorption of hexachlorophene to result in toxic effects to the nervous system, especially a spongiform degeneration of the white matter in the brain. For this reason, the "routine prophylactic use" of 3% hexachlorophene preparations was discouraged. Stopping the use of hexachlorophene-containing preparations for bathing of newborns has been accompanied by a resurgence of staphylococcal infections in nursery populations.

Hexachlorophene

Other antiseptics have been added to soaps and detergents, eg, carbanilides or salicylanilides. Trichlorocarbanilide now takes the place of hexachlorophenes in several "antiseptic soaps." Regular use of such antiseptic soaps may reduce body odor by preventing bacterial decomposition of organic material in apocrine sweat. All antiseptic soaps may induce allergic reactions or photosensitization.

Chlorhexidine is a bisdiguanide antiseptic that disrupts the cytoplasmic membrane, especially of grampositive organisms. It is employed as a skin cleanser and as a constituent of disinfectant soaps. A 4% solution of chlorhexidine gluconate can be used to cleanse wounds. When incorporated into soaps it is used as an antiseptic hand-washing preparation, especially in hospitals, and for surgical scrub and preparation of skin sites for operative procedures. Repeated application of chlorhexidine-containing soap results in persistence of the chemical on the skin to give a cumulative antibacterial effect. Chlorhexidine is somewhat less effective against *Pseudomonas* and *Serratia* strains than against coliform and gram-positive organisms.

Lindane (Kwell, Scabene), previously called gamma benzene hexachloride, is employed as a 1% lotion, shampoo, or cream to treat scabies, mites, or lice. Usually it is used just twice: It is applied after the skin or hairy areas have been washed with soap and water, and the treatment is repeated one week later. Up to 10% of the chemical may be absorbed from application to the skin, and it may produce toxic effects (skin rashes, blood dyscrasias, or convulsions), especially if ingested accidentally by infants. To prevent reinfestation with mites and lice it is necessary to treat all contacts and wash all clothes of the afflicted individual (see also Chapter 65).

The use of lindane as an insecticide in agriculture has been associated with poisoning after inhalation of substantial amounts of spray or mist. Lindane is also suspected of causing nerve damage, birth defects, and aplastic anemia on rare occasion and of being a possible carcinogen.

Cationic Surface-Active Agents

Surface-active compounds are widely used as wetting agents and detergents in industry and in the home.

They act by altering the energy relationship at interfaces. Cationic surface-active agents are bactericidal, probably by altering the permeability characteristics of the cell membrane. Cationic agents are antagonized by anionic surface-active agents and thus are incompatible with soaps. Cationic agents are also strongly adsorbed onto porous or fibrous materials, eg, rubber or cotton, and are effectively removed by them from solutions.

A variety of cationic surface-active agents are employed as antiseptics for the disinfection of instruments, mucous membranes, and skin, eg, benzalkonium chloride USP (Zephiran) and cetylpyridinium chloride USP. Aqueous solutions of 1:1000–1:10,000 exhibit good antimicrobial activity but have some disadvantages. These quaternary ammonium disinfectants are antagonized by soaps, and soaps should not be used on surfaces where the antibacterial activity of quaternary ammonium disinfectants is desired. They are adsorbed onto cotton and thereby removed from solution. When applied to skin, they form a film under which microorganisms can survive. Because of these properties, these substances have given rise to outbreaks of serious infections due to *Pseudomonas* and other gram-negative bacteria. They cannot be employed safely as skin disinfectants and can only rarely be used as disinfectants of instruments.

Nitrofurans

Nitrofurazone USP (Furacin) is used as a topical antimicrobial agent on superficial wounds or skin lesions and as a surgical dressing. The preparations contain about 0.2% of the active drug and do not interfere with wound healing. However, about 2% of patients may become sensitized and may develop reactions, eg, allergic pneumonitis. Nitrofurantoin USP (Furadantin) is a urinary antiseptic (see Chapter 51).

Miscellaneous Antiseptics

Lysostaphin, a peptide enzyme, prepared for topical application, can eliminate staphylococci from the nostrils of carriers, but it is not marketed.

Many synthetic organic dyes have antimicrobial properties. Gentian violet USP is bacteriostatic and inhibits yeast growth, but it is aesthetically unappealing. Acridine dyes have been used as topical antiseptics in 1:2000 concentration. Methylene blue was formerly used as a urinary antiseptic. Pyridium, an azo dye, was used as a urinary antiseptic although it acts primarily as an analgesic in the bladder. Local anesthetics (eg, procaine, lidocaine) have some inhibitory effect on the growth of bacteria and fungi. Thus, they may interfere with culture of an etiologic agent in specimens from tissues or surfaces exposed to these agents.

Sulfur, in various preparations, is employed as a fungicide and parasiticide for topical use. Many fatty acids, especially propionic and undecylenic acids, are important topical antifungal drugs. Undecylenic acid NF, 5%, and zinc undecylenate NF, 20%, are among the least irritating and most fungistatic drugs available for treatment of dermatophytosis.

STERILIZATION PROCEDURES

It is the purpose of sterilization to make materials free from viable microorganisms, spores, and viruses. This is accomplished commonly by the application of heat under controlled conditions.

Incineration, using controlled burning, is used to dispose of infectious materials. Dry heat (160–170 °C for more than 1 hour) is employed to sterilize dry glassware, ceramics, and other materials. Moist heat or autoclaving (121 °C for 15 minutes or more at 15 lb/in^2) is used for many instruments, dressings, linens, and bacteriologic media. All of these procedures must be carefully controlled with respect to time, temperature, size of materials, air circulation, displacement of cold air by steam, permeability of packaging materials, and other features that determine the efficacy of the application of heat.

Many materials that must be sterilized do not tolerate high heat, eg, plastics, optical devices, pump oxygenators, and extracorporeal circulation devices. These materials are "gas sterilized" by exposure to **ethylene oxide,** because irradiation is not readily controllable. Ethylene oxide can destroy the viability of microorganisms, probably by the alkylation of sulfhydryl groups of proteins.

Since ethylene oxide is a highly flammable gas, it is usually employed in combinations with either 90% CO_2 or fluorinated hydrocarbons. With such a mixture at a temperature of about 40 °C and a relative humidity of 40%, about 4 hours are required for sterilization. Ethylene oxide rapidly penetrates many types of materials exposed to it in a vacuum, and sterilization is accomplished in 4 hours; it then must be removed because it leaves toxic residues, eg, ethylene glycol and ethylene chlorohydrin. For proper ethylene oxide sterilization, materials must be wrapped in cloth, paper, or polyethylene; exposed to the gas for a proper period under controlled temperature; and then evacuated to remove gas and toxic residues and aerated for a prescribed time (often 12–120 hours) before being used.

In most sterilization procedures, indicators of adequate time and temperature exposure and of sterility ("spore strips") must be employed. Careful records are essential and must be kept for years. Chemical indicators for ethylene oxide exposure must be employed.

The heating procedures employed to safeguard foods in the canning industry or in the pasteurization of dairy products and eggs are not discussed here. They are subject to specialized rules and safety precautions.

REFERENCES

Aly R, Maibach HI: Comparative study on the antimicrobial effect of 0.5% chlorhexidine gluconate and 70% isopropyl alcohol on the normal flora of hands. *Appl Environ Microbiol* 1979;**37:**610.

Ballin JC: Evaluation of a new topical agent for burn therapy. *JAMA* 1974;**230:**1184.

Beck WC: Handwashing substitute for degerming. *Am J Surg* 1978;**135:**728.

Block SS: *Disinfection, Sterilization and Preservation,* 2nd ed. Lea & Febiger, 1977.

Cason JS, Lowbury EJL: Mortality and infection in extensively burned patients treated with silver-nitrate compresses. *Lancet* 1968;**1:**651.

Dixon RE et al: Aqueous quaternary ammonium antiseptics and disinfectants: Use and misuse. *JAMA* 1976;**236:**2415.

Drewett SE et al: Skin distribution of *Clostridium welchii:* Use of iodophor as sporicidal agent. *Lancet* 1972;**1:**1172.

Fraser GL, Beaulieu JT: Leukopenia secondary to sulfadiazine silver. *JAMA* 1979;**241:**1928.

Gezon HM et al: Control of staphylococcal infections in the newborn through the use of hexachlorophene bathing. *Pediatrics* 1973;**51:**331.

Kaslow RA et al: Nosocomial pseudobacteremia: Positive blood cultures due to contaminated benzalkonium antiseptic. *JAMA* 1976;**236:**2407.

Kaul F, Jewett JR: Agents and techniques for disinfection of the skin. *Surg Gynecol Obstet* 1981;**152:**677.

Kimbrough RD: Review of evidence of toxic effects of hexachlorophene. *Pediatrics* 1973;**51:**391.

Kundsin RB, Walter CW: The surgical scrub: Practical considerations. *Arch Surg* 1973;**107:**75.

Levine AS, Labuza TP, Morley JE: Food technology. *N Engl J Med* 1985;**312:**628.

Martin-Bouyer G et al: Outbreak of accidental hexachlorophene poisoning in France. *Lancet* 1982;**1:**91.

Orkin M et al: Treatment of today's scabies and pediculosis. *JAMA* 1976;**236:**1136.

Prince AM et al: Beta-propiolactone/ultraviolet irradiation: A review of its effectiveness for inactivation of viruses in blood derivatives. *Rev Infect Dis* 1983;**5:**92.

Russell AD, Hugo WB, Ayliffe GAJ (editors): *Principles and Practice of Disinfection, Preservation and Sterilization.* Blackwell Scientific, 1982.

Basic Principles of Antiparasitic Chemotherapy

55

Ching Chung Wang, PhD

The word "parasite"* in ancient Greek denoted one who dined at the tables of the rich and tried to earn his welcome by flattery. In its general scientific sense, the term includes all of the known infectious agents such as viruses, bacteria, fungi, protozoa, and helminths, even though the infected host may not be flattered and the infectious agents may not be welcome. In this and the 2 following chapters, the term is used in a restricted sense to denote the protozoa and helminths. It has been estimated that 3 billion (3×10^9) humans suffer from parasitic infections, plus a much greater number of domestic and wild animals. Although these diseases constitute the most urgent human health problem in the world today, they have for various reasons also been the most neglected.

In theory, the parasitic infections should be relatively easy to treat because the etiologic agents are known in almost all cases. Furthermore, recent advances in cell culture techniques have made possible in vitro cultivation of many of the important parasites. These advances have not only laid to rest the traditional view that parasites somehow depend on a living host for their existence but have also enabled us to study parasites by methods similar to those employed in investigations of bacteria, including biochemistry, molecular biology, and immunologic pharmacology. However, many problems remain to be solved before effective chemotherapeutic agents will be available for all of the parasitic diseases.

A rational approach to antiparasitic chemotherapy requires comparative biochemical and physiologic investigations of host and parasite to discover differences in essential processes that will permit selective inhibition in the parasite and not in the host. One might expect that the parasite would have many deficiencies in its metabolism as a result of its parasitic nature. This is true of many parasites; the oversimplified metabolic pathways are usually indispensable for survival of the parasite and thus represent points of vulnerability. However, this is not the only opportunity for attack. Although the parasite lives in a metabolically luxurious environment and may become "lazy," the environment is not entirely friendly, so that the parasite must have defense mechanisms in order to survive—ie, to defend itself against immunologic attack, proteolytic

digestion, etc, by the host. In some instances, necessary nutrients are not supplied to the parasite from the host, though the latter can obtain the same nutrients from the diet. In this situation, the parasite will have acquired the synthetic activity needed for its survival. Finally, the great evolutionary distance between host and parasite has in some cases resulted in sufficient differences among individual enzymes or functional pathways to allow specific inhibition of the parasite. Thus, there can be 3 major types of potential targets for chemotherapy of parasitic diseases: (1) unique enzymes found only in the parasites; (2) enzymes found in both host and parasite but indispensable only for the parasite; and (3) common biochemical functions found in both parasite and host but with different pharmacologic properties. Examples of specific targets and drugs that act on them are summarized in Table 55–1. This chapter discusses antiparasitic mechanisms based upon these examples and provides background information for the drugs described in Chapters 56 and 57.

ENZYMES FOUND ONLY IN PARASITES

These enzymes would appear to be the cleanest targets for chemotherapy. Like inhibition of the enzymes involved in the synthesis of bacterial cell wall (Chapter 42), inhibition of these enzymes should have no effect on the host. Unfortunately, only a few of these enzymes have been discovered among the parasitic protozoa. Furthermore, their usefulness as chemotherapeutic targets is sometimes limited because of the development of drug resistance. Important examples of target enzymes are discussed in the following pages.

Enzymes for Dihydropteroate Synthesis

The intracellular sporozoan parasites such as *Plasmodia, Toxoplasma,* and *Eimeria* spp have long been known to respond to sulfonamides and sulfones. This has led to the assumption that sporozoans must synthesize their own folate in order to survive. The reaction of 2-amino-4-hydroxy-6-hydroxymethyl-dihydropteridine diphosphate with *p*-aminobenzoate to form 7,8-dihydropteroate has been demonstrated in cell-free extracts of the rodent malaria parasite *Plasmodium chabaudi.* 2-Amino-4-hydroxy-6-hydroxy-methyl-dihydropteridine pyrophosphokinase and 7,8-dihydrop-

---

*The word "parasite" is derived from Greek *para* "beside" + *sitos* "grain, bread."

Table 55–1. Identified targets for chemotherapy in parasites.

Targets	Parasites	Inhibitors
1. Unique enzymes		
Enzymes for dihydropteroate synthesis	Sporozoa.	Sulfones and sulfonamides.
Pyruvate:ferredoxin oxidoreductase	Anaerobic protozoa.	Nitroimidazoles.
Nucleoside phosphotransferase	Flagellated protozoa.	Allopurinol riboside and formycin B.
2. Indispensable enzymes		
Purine phosphoribosyl transferase	Protozoa.	Allopurinol.
Ornithine decarboxylase	Protozoa.	α-Difluoromethylornithine.
Glycolytic enzymes	Kinetoplastida.	Glycerol plus salicylhydroxamic acid and suramin.
3. Common biochemical functions with different pharmacologic properties		
Thiamine transporter	Coccidia.	Amprolium.
Mitochondrial electron transporter	Coccidia.	4-Hydroxyquinolines.
Microtubules	Helminth.	Benzimidazoles.
Nervous synaptic transmission	Helminth and ectoparasite.	Levamisole, piperazine, the milbemycins, and the avermectins.

teroate synthetase have also been identified, isolated, and purified. Sulfathiazole, sulfaguanidine, and sulfanilamide act as competitive inhibitors of p-aminobenzoate in this reaction. It has not been possible to demonstrate dihydrofolate synthetase activity in the parasites, which raises the possibility that 7,8-dihydropteroate may have substituted for dihydrofolate in malaria parasites. Similar lack of recognition of folate as substrate was also observed in the dihydrofolate reductase of *Eimeria tenella*, a parasite of chickens.

However, lack of utilization of exogenous folate may not fully explain the apparent indispensable nature of the synthesis of 7,8-dihydropteroate in *Plasmodium, Toxoplasma,* and *Eimeria.* It is known that most of the folate molecules in mammalian cells are linked with polyglutamates in the cytoplasm and are transported across cell membranes with difficulty. This additional factor may compound the problem of obtaining 7,8-dihydropteroate or dihydrofolate for the parasite and makes all of the enzymes involved in their synthesis attractive targets for antisporozoan chemotherapy.

The sulfones and sulfonamides synergize with the inhibitors of dihydrofolate reductase, and combinations have been effective in controlling malaria, toxoplasmosis, and coccidiosis. Although some incidents of drug resistance, especially among coccidia, have been reported, the combinations remain largely effective against malaria and toxoplasmosis. Fansidar, a combination of sulfadoxine and pyrimethamine, has been successful in controlling chloroquine-resistant *Plasmodium falciparum* malaria (see Chapter 56).

The pharmacologic properties of parasite 7,8-dihydropteroate synthetases may differ from those of the bacterial enzymes. For instance, metachloridine and 2-ethoxy-p-aminobenzoate are both ineffective against sulfonamide-sensitive bacteria, but the former has antimalarial activity and the latter is effective against infection of the chicken parasite *Eimeria acervulina;* both activities can be reversed by p-aminobenzoate.

Pyruvate:Ferredoxin Oxidoreductase

Certain anaerobic protozoan parasites lack mitochondria and mitochondrial activities for generating ATP. They possess, instead, ferredoxinlike or flavodoxinlike low-redox-potential electron transport proteins to convert pyruvate to acetyl-CoA. In trichomonad flagellates and rumen ciliates, the process takes place in a membrane-limited organelle called the hydrogenosome. By the actions of pyruvate:ferredoxin oxidoreductase and hydrogenase in the hydrogenosome, H_2 is produced by these organisms under anaerobic conditions as the major means of electron disposition. Although *Entamoeba* spp and *Giardia lamblia* have no hydrogenosome, a ferredoxin has been isolated from *Entamoeba histolytica,* and iron-sulfur and flavin centers have been detected by electron paramagnetic resonance studies on *G lamblia.*

This enzyme has no counterpart in the mammalian system. In contrast to the mammalian pyruvate dehydrogenase complex, the pyruvate:ferredoxin oxidoreductase is incapable of reducing pyridine nucleotides because of its low redox potential (approximately -400 mV). However, this low potential can also transfer electrons from pyruvate to the nitro groups of metronidazole and other 5-nitroimidazole derivatives to form cytotoxic reduced products that bind to DNA and proteins. This is apparently why these anaerobic protozoan species are highly susceptible to the compounds. Despite the recent development of drug resistance in *Trichomonas vaginalis* and the possibility of carcinogenic properties (see Chapter 56), metronidazole remains the drug of choice for anaerobic protozoan parasite infections.

Nucleoside Phosphotransferases

All of the protozoan parasites studied thus far are deficient in de novo synthesis of purine nucleotides. The various purine salvage pathways in these parasites are thus essential for their survival and growth. Among the *Leishmania* spp, a unique salvage enzyme has been identified—purine nucleoside phosphotransferase—that can transfer the phosphate group from a variety of monophosphate esters, including p-nitrophenylphosphate, to the 5′ position of purine nucleosides. This enzyme also phosphorylates purine nucleoside analogs such as allopurinol riboside, formycin B, 9-deazainosine, and thiopurinol riboside, converting them to the corresponding nucleotides. These nucleotides are either further converted to triphosphates and eventually incorporated into nucleic acid of *Leishmania* or become inhibitors of other es-

sential enzymes in purine metabolism. Consequently, allopurinol riboside, formycin B, 9-deazainosine, and thiopurinol riboside all act as potent antileishmanial agents both in vitro and in vivo. Allopurinol riboside is particularly interesting because it is remarkably nontoxic to the mammalian host; it is currently in clinical trials for use in leishmaniasis. The relevant pathways are illustrated in Fig 55–1.

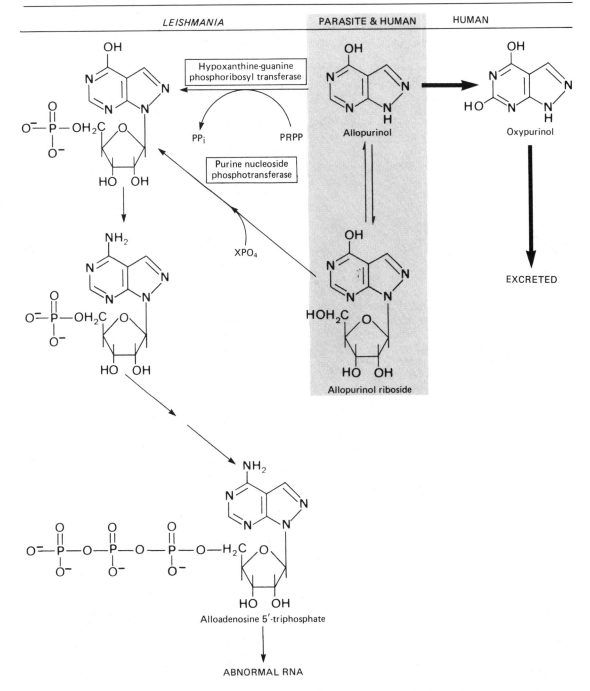

Figure 55–1. Metabolism of allopurinol and allopurinol riboside in *Leishmania* and humans. PRPP, phosphoribosylpyrophosphate; PP$_i$, inorganic pyrophosphate; XPO$_4$, a phosphate donor.

Trichomonad flagellates appear to be deficient in de novo synthesis of both purines and pyrimidines. Pyrimidine as well as purine salvage thus becomes indispensable for these parasites. Among them, *Trichomonas foetus* (the cow parasite), *T vaginalis*, and *G lamblia* also lack dihydrofolate reductase and thymidylate synthetase, a deficiency that enables them to grow normally in the presence of methotrexate, the most potent antifolate, in a concentration of 0.5 mmol/L. This metabolic deficiency leads to apparent isolation of the supply route for thymidine 5'-phosphate (TMP) from the rest of the pyrimidine ribonucleotides; TMP is provided by a single salvage pathway that converts exogenous thymidine to TMP by the action of a thymidine phosphotransferase (Fig 55–2).

The enzyme activity is not affected by thymidine kinase inhibitors such as acyclovir but is inhibitable by guanosine or 5-fluorodeoxyuridine; both compounds also inhibit the in vitro growth of the parasites. This enzyme is an attractive target for chemotherapeutic treatment of the anaerobic protozoan parasites. One could design either a false substrate or an inhibitor of the thymidine phosphotransferase; DNA synthesis in the parasites may be arrested in either case.

ENZYMES INDISPENSABLE ONLY IN THE PARASITES

Because of the many metabolic deficiencies among parasites, there are enzymes whose functions may be essential for the survival of parasites, but the same enzymes are not indispensable to the host; ie, the host may be able to achieve the same result through alternative pathways. This discrepancy opens up opportunities for antiparasitic chemotherapy.

Purine Phosphoribosyl Transferases

The absence of de novo purine nucleotide synthesis in protozoan parasites as well as in the trematode *Schistosoma mansoni* is reflected in the relative importance of hypoxanthine-guanine phosphoribosyl transferase in many species. Hypoxanthine is the obligatory base for purine nucleotide synthesis in 4 species of *Leishmania, Plasmodium berghei, E tenella, T foetus, S mansoni, Crithidia fasciculata,* and possibly other organisms as well. Unusual substrate specificity of the parasite hypoxanthine-guanine phosphoribosyl transferase (Fig 55–1) has been reported. The enzymes in *Leishmania donovani* and *Trypanosoma cruzi* can recognize allopurinol (see Chapter 34) as the substrate and convert it to allopurinol ribotide, which then accumulates in the parasites and becomes aminated, turned into triphosphate, and finally incorporated into the RNA fraction. This abnormal RNA apparently does not support normal growth (see Fig 55–1). Since allopurinol is an extremely poor substrate for the mammalian hypoxathine-guanine phosphoribosyl transferase, it has selective antileishmanial and antitrypanosomal effects in vivo. Another enzyme in *L donovani*, xanthine phosphoribosyl transferase,

has no counterpart in mammalian systems and thus could be another interesting target for antileishmanial chemotherapy.

G lamblia has an exceedingly simple scheme of purine salvage. It possesses only 2 pivotal enzymes: the adenine and guanine phosphoribosyl transferases, which convert exogenous adenine and guanine to the corresponding nucleotides. There is no salvage of hypoxanthine, xanthine, or any purine nucleosides, and no interconversion between adenine and guanine nucleotides in the parasite. Functions of the 2 phosphoribosyl transferases are thus both essential for the survival and development of *G lamblia* (Fig 55–3). The guanine phosphoribosyl transferase is an interesting enzyme because it does not recognize hypoxanthine, xanthine, or adenine as substrate. This substrate specificity distinguishes the *Giardia* enzyme from the mammalian enzyme, which uses hypoxanthine, and the bacterial one, which has xanthine as substrate. Design of a highly specific inhibitor of this enzyme is thus possible.

Ornithine Decarboxylase

Polyamines, found in almost all living organisms, are required for cellular proliferation and differentiation. Ornithine decarboxylase, the enzyme that controls the formation of the polyamine putrescine in numerous eukaryotic cells, is an enzyme characterized by its striking inducibility and very short half-life. In many species of trypanosomatids, putrescine and spermidine form the major pool of polyamines, which are synthesized rapidly from ornithine but are taken up much more slowly from extracellular sources. Intracellular levels of the polyamines fluctuate during the rapid growth cycle of the protozoa.

Alpha-difluoromethylornithine, a probable suicide inhibitor of ornithine decarboxylase with known antitumor activities, has been found to possess good activity against African trypanosomes in infected animals. DNA synthesis may be totally stopped and RNA synthesis decreased significantly in the parasites. It is thus likely that the antitrypanosomal activity of α-difluoromethylornithine is attributable to the inhibition of ornithine decarboxylase. This compound has also been found effective in controlling *E tenella* infection in chickens, in vitro schizogony of *P falciparum*, and in vitro growth of *G lamblia*. All of these activities are reversible by administration of polyamines. Alphadifluoromethylornithine is now undergoing clinical trials in Africa and has shown good therapeutic activity against *Trypanosoma brucei gambiense* infections.

It is thus apparent that because of the rapid rate of proliferation of protozoan parasites, an effective inhibition of the parasite ornithine decarboxylase may control their growth without damaging host metabolism. Further studies may uncover more enzymes involved in polyamine metabolism of protozoan parasites as suitable targets of chemotherapy.

Glycolytic Enzymes

In the bloodstream form of African trypanosomes

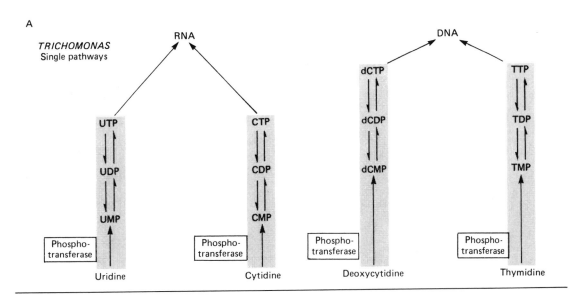

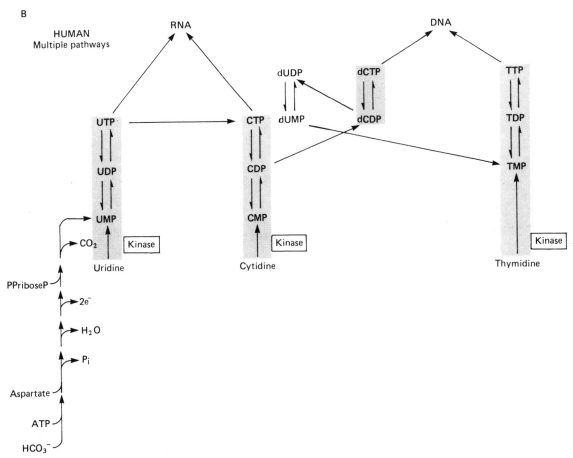

Figure 55–2. Pyrimidine metabolism in *Trichomonas vaginalis* *(A)* and in humans *(B).* Note that humans have multiple sources for thymidine monophosphate (TMP), an essential precursor for DNA synthesis. The parasite has only one source. UTP, UDP, UMP, CTP, etc = uridine triphosphate, diphosphate, monophosphate, cytidine triphosphate, etc; PPri-boseP = 1-pyrophosphorylribosyl-5-phosphate; P_i = inorganic phosphate.

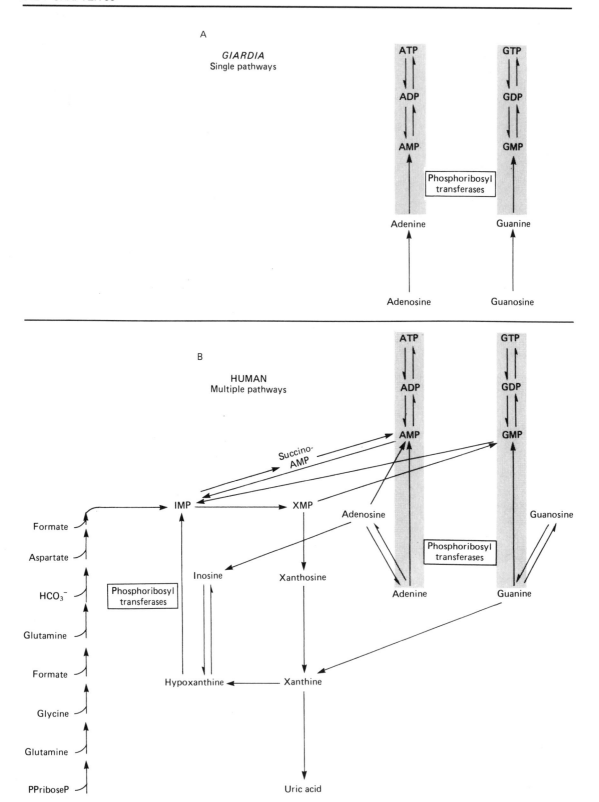

Figure 55–3. Purine metabolism in *Giardia lamblia* **(A)** and in humans **(B)**. *G lamblia* lacks enzymes both for de novo synthesis of essential purine nucleotides and for interconversion of these purine nucleotides. AMP, GMP, IMP, XMP, etc = adenosine monophosphate, guanosine monophosphate, inosine monophosphate, xanthosine monophosphate, etc.

such as *Trypanosoma brucei brucei*, the single mitochondrion has been reduced to a "peripheral canal" lacking both cytochrome and functional Krebs cycle enzymes. The organism is entirely dependent on glycolysis for its production of ATP. Under aerobic conditions, one glucose molecule can generate only 2 molecules of ATP, with 2 pyruvate molecules excreted into the host bloodstream as the end product. This low energy yield makes it necessary to have glycolysis in *T b brucei* proceed at an extremely high rate to enable the trypanosome to divide once every 7 hours. The high glycolytic rate, 50 times that in the mammalian host, is made possible not only by the abundant glucose supply in the host's blood but also by the clustering of most of the glycolytic enzymes of the parasite in membrane-bound microbody organelles, glycosomes (Fig 55–4). Since lactate dehydrogenase is absent from the parasite, the regeneration of NAD from NADH in the glycosome during glycolysis depends on a dihydroxyacetone phosphate:glycerol-3-phosphate shuttle plus a glycerol-3-phosphate oxidase. Thus, under anaerobic conditions, glycerol 3-phosphate cannot be oxidized back to dihydroxyacetone phosphate and becomes accumulated inside the glycosome. This accumulation, together with the accumulation of ADP due to depletion of NAD, eventually drives the reversed glycerol kinase-catalyzed reaction in the glycosome to generate glycerol and ATP. Thus, under anaerobic conditions, *T b brucei* generates only one ATP from each glucose molecule and excretes equimolar pyruvate and glycerol as end products.

This delicate and indispensable glycolytic system appears to be an attractive target for antitrypanosomal chemotherapy. Recent studies have demonstrated that glycerol-3-phosphate oxidase can be inhibited in the parasite with salicylhydroxamic acid (SHAM) to bring *T b brucei* into an anerobic condition. Glycolysis can then be stopped by inhibiting the reversed glycerol kinase-catalyzed reaction with added glycerol. This SHAM plus glycerol combination can lyse the African trypanosome bloodstream forms in vitro within minutes and is very effective in suppressing parasitemia in infected animals. Some of the well-known antitrypanosomal agents, discovered by random screens in the past, have been found recently to act by inhibiting glycolysis in the parasite. For example, the mechanism of action of suramin most likely consists of inhibition of glycerol-3-phosphate dehydrogenase (Fig 55–4).

Another interesting aspect of glycolysis in these parasites is the aggregation of hexokinase, phosphoglucose isomerase, phosphofructokinase, aldolase, triosephosphate isomerase, glycerol kinase, glycerol-3-phosphate dehydrogenase, glyceraldehyde phosphate dehydrogenase, and phosphoglycerate kinase in the glycosome. This close physical arrangement of the glycolytic enzymes within the confinement of the glycosomal membrane may enable substrate accumulation through the chain of reactions that makes the high glycolytic rate possible. The cumulative effect may turn a weak enzyme inhibitor into a very potent one if the inhibitor happens to be the product of the preceding enzyme in the reaction chain.

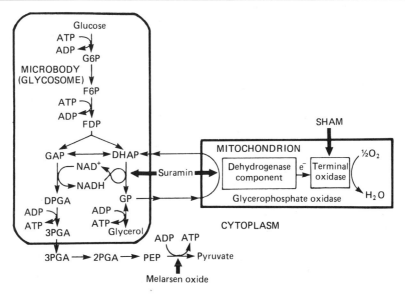

Figure 55–4. Glycolytic pathway in long, slender bloodstream forms of *Trypanosoma brucei brucei*. The principal sites of inhibition by trypanocidal drugs in vivo are indicated by bold arrows. SHAM, salicylhydroxamic acid; G6P, glucose 6-phosphate; F6P, fructose 6-phosphate; FDP, fructose 1,6-diphosphate; GAP, glyceraldehyde 3-phosphate; DHAP, dihydroxyacetone phosphate; GP, *sn*-glycerol 3-phosphate; DPGA, 1,3-diphosphoglycerate; 3PGA and 2PGA, 3- and 2-phosphoglycerate; PEP, phosphoenolpyruvate. (Modified and reproduced, with permission, from Fairlamb A: Biochemistry of trypanosomiasis and rational approaches to chemotherapy. *Trends Biochem Sci* 1982;7:249.)

BIOCHEMICAL FUNCTIONS FOUND IN BOTH PARASITE & HOST BUT WITH DIFFERENT PHARMACOLOGIC PROPERTIES

In the parasite, these functions have differentiated sufficiently to become probable targets for antiparasitic chemotherapy, not because of the parasitic nature of the organism but, more likely, because of the long evolutionary distances separating the parasite and the host. It is thus difficult to discover these targets through studying metabolic deficiency or special nutritional requirements of the parasite. They have usually been found by investigating the modes of action of some well-established antiparasitic agents discovered by screening methods in the past. The target of such drugs may not be a single well-defined enzyme but may include transporters, receptors, cellular structural components, or other specific functions essential for the survival of the parasite.

Thiamine Transporter

Carbohydrate metabolism provides the main energy source in coccidia. Diets deficient in thiamine, riboflavin, or nicotinic acid—all cofactors in carbohydrate metabolism—result in suppression of parasitic infestation of chickens by *E tenella* and *E acervulina*. A thiamine analog, amprolium (1-[(4-amino-2-propyl-5-pyrimidinyl)methyl]-2-picolinium chloride), has long been used as an effective anticoccidial agent in chickens and cattle with relatively low host toxicity. The antiparasitic activity of amprolium is reversible by thiamine and is now recognized to involve inhibition of thiamine transport in the parasite. Unfortunately, amprolium has a rather narrow spectrum of antiparasitic activity; it has poor activity against toxoplasmosis, a closely related parasitic infection.

Mitochondrial Electron Transporter

Mitochondria of *E tenella* appear to lack cytochrome c and to contain cytochrome o—a cytochrome oxidase commonly found in the bacterial respiratory chain—as the terminal oxidase. Certain 4-hydroxyquinoline derivatives such as buquinolate, decoquinate, and methyl benzoquate that have long been known to be relatively nontoxic and effective anticoccidial agents have been found to act on the parasites by inhibiting mitochondrial respiration. Direct investigation on isolated intact *E tenella* mitochondria indicated that the 4-hydroxyquinolines have no effect on NADH oxidase or succinoxidase activity but that they are extremely potent inhibitors of NADH- or succinate-induced mitochondrial respiration. On the other hand, the ascorbate-induced *E tenella* mitochondrial respiration was totally insusceptible to these 4-hydroxyquinolines. The block by the anticoccidial agents thus may be located between the oxidases and cytochrome b in the electron transport chain. A certain component at this location must be essential for mediating the electron transport and would appear to be highly sensitive to the 4-hydroxyquinolines. This

component must be a very specific chemotherapeutic target in *Eimeria* spp, since the 4-hydroxyquinolines have no effect on chicken liver and mammalian mitochondrial respiration and no activity against any parasites other than the *Eimeria* spp.

Microtubules

Microtubules are an important part of the cytoskeleton and the mitotic spindle and consist of α- and β-tubulin subunit proteins. Recent comparisons of α- and β-tubulins from several species of wide taxonomic separation (bovine kidney, sea urchin eggs, squid brain, *Pteridium* sperm flagella, *Chlamydomonas* flagella, and *Ascaridia galli*, a nematode parasite of chickens) indicated that while the β-tubulins of these organisms appeared to have the same electrophoretic migration, the α-tubulins varied widely. This variation is interesting not only in pointing out the evolutionary relations among eukaryotic cells; it is useful also in classifying the tubulins in parasites as potential targets for antiparasitic chemotherapy. A group of benzimidazole derivatives have long been established as highly effective anthelmintics. Mebendazole (methyl 5-benzoyl-2-benzimidazolecarbamate) was among the first of such anthelmintics found to act primarily by blocking transport of secretory granules and movement of other subcellular organelles in the parasitic nematode *Ascaris lumbricoides*. This inhibition coincides with the disappearance of cytoplasmic microtubules from the intestinal cells of the worm. The microtubular systems of the host cells are unaffected by the treatment. Mebendazole and fenbendazole, another anthelmintic benzimidazole, have also been shown to compete with colchicine binding to *A lumbricoides* embryonic tubulins with 250–400 times higher potencies than the binding competition to bovine brain tubulins. These differential binding affinities may explain the selective toxicity of the benzimidazoles toward the parasitic nematodes. Another anthelmintic benzimidazole derivative, thiabendazole (2-[4-thiazolyl]-1*H*-benzimidazole), also possesses antifungal activity, by binding to fungal tubulins.

Synaptic Transmission

Invertebrate nervous systems in the helminths and the arthropods differ from those of vertebrates in important ways. The motoneurons in invertebrates, for example, are unmyelinated and are thus more susceptible to disturbances of nerve membranes than are the myelinated somatic motor fibers of vertebrates. Muscle fibers in arthropods are innervated by excitatory synapses, in which L-glutamic acid is the neurotransmitter, and by inhibitory nerves, which have γ-aminobutyric acid (GABA) as transmitter. Cholinergic nerves are concentrated in the central nervous system of arthropods. In nematodes, free-living species, eg, *Caenorhabditis elegans,* and gastrointestinal parasitic species, eg, *A lumbricoides,* appear to have identical neuronal systems and synaptic transmitters. Cholinergic excitatory and GABA-ergic inhibitory synapses

Table 55–2. Some major antiparasitic agents with undefined mechanisms of action.

Antiparasitic Agents	Possibly Relevant Biochemical Activities
Antiamebiasis agents	
Diloxanide furoate	Unknown.
Emetine	Inhibitor of eukaryote protein synthesis.
Halogenated hydroxyquinolines	Unknown.
Paromomycin	Inhibitor of prokaryote protein synthesis.
Antifascioliasis agents	
Bithionol	Oxidative phosphorylation uncoupler.
Rafoxanide	Oxidative phosphorylation uncoupler.
Antifilariasis agents	
Diethylcarbamazine	Inhibitor of lipoxygenase.
Antileishmaniasis agents	
Amphotericin B	Voltage-dependent channel maker in cell membrane.
Pentavalent antimonials	Unknown.
Antimalarials	
Chloroquine	DNA binding, lysosomal neutralization, and hematoporphyrin binding.
Primaquine	Its quinoline quinone metabolite is an oxidant.
Quinacrine	DNA binding and flavoenzyme inhibition.
Quinine	DNA binding and membrane binding.
Antischistosomal agents	
Hycanthone	DNA binding.
Metrifonate	Acetylcholinesterase inhibitor.
Niridazole	Metabolites binding to DNA.
Oxamniquine	DNA binding.
Trivalent antimonials	Inhibition of phosphofructokinase.
Antitapeworm agent	
Niclosamide	Oxidative phosphorylation uncoupler.
Antitrypanosomiasis agents	
Melarsen oxide	Inhibitor of trypanothione reductase.
Aromatic diamidines	Transport can be blocked by polyamines; DNA binding.
Nifurtimox	Inducing H_2O_2 production in *Trypanosoma cruzi*.

are found at the neuromuscular junctions as well as in the central ventral cords of the worms. The mammalian hosts, on the other hand, have mainly nicotinic receptors at the neuromuscular junctions (see Chapter 5), and the GABA nerves are all confined within the central nervous system protected by the blood-brain barrier (Chapter 19).

Neurotoxicant anthelmintics must be administered systemically to mammalian hosts to reach the parasitic nematodes. Therefore, if absorbed, they must be nontoxic to the nervous system of the host. Furthermore, they must penetrate the thick cuticle of the nematodes in order to be effective. It is therefore difficult to find a useful anthelmintic that acts on the nervous system of these parasites. Nevertheless, the majority of presently available anthelmintics do act on the nerves of the nematodes. They can be classified into 2 groups: (1) those acting as ganglionic nicotinic acetylcholine agonists and (2) those acting directly or indirectly as GABA agonists. The first category includes levamisole, pyrantel pamoate, oxantel pamoate, and bephenium. The acetylcholine receptors at the neuromuscular junctions of nematodes are of the ganglionic nicotinic type; these agonists are quite effective in causing muscular contraction of the worms. Experimentally, the ganglionic nicotinic antagonist mecamylamine can reverse the action of these anthelmintics.

The second category consists of only one drug, piperazine, an older agent that apparently acts as a GABA agonist at the neuromuscular junction and causes flaccid paralysis of the nematode.

A promising new family of natural compounds, the milbemycins and avermectins, appears to act indirectly to intensify the GABA action on the ventral cord interneuron and on the motoneuron junction to immobilize nematodes, and at the neuromuscular junction of arthropods to cause paralysis. Therefore, both the milbemycins and the avermectins are potent anthelmintics, insecticides, and antiectoparasitic agents with no cross-resistance problems with agents acting on the cholinergic systems. Picrotoxin, a specific blocker of the chloride ion channel controlled by postsynaptic GABA binding, can reverse all of the physiologic effects of these drugs (see Chapter 19).

Ivermectin, a simple derivative of the mixture of avermectin B_{1a} and avermectin B_{1b}, is highly effective as an anthelmintic in domestic animals. It is also effective in controlling onchocerciasis by eliminating the microfilariae. It is currently undergoing clinical trials in West Africa and Guatemala.

Avermectins have little effect on the mammalian central nervous system because they do not cross the mammalian brain synaptosomes and synaptic membranes are used as models for investigation, specific high-affinity binding sites for the avermectins can be identified in GABA-ergic nerves. This drug binding stimulates GABA release from the presynaptic end of the GABA nerve and enhances the postsynaptic GABA binding. Avermectins also stimulate benzodiazepine binding to its receptor and enhance diazepam muscle relaxant activity in vivo. There is little doubt that milbemycins and avermectins act on the GABA nervous system and amplify GABA functions. The GABA-ergic nerves in invertebrates are thus attractive targets for chemotherapy.

Little is known about the nervous systems of cestodes and trematodes except that they probably differ from those of nematodes, since milbemycins and avermectins have no effect on them. However, a highly effective antischistosomal and antitapeworm agent, praziquantel (see Chapter 57), is known to enhance Ca^{2+} influx and induce muscular contraction in those parasites, although it exerts no action on nematodes or insects. Some benzodiazepine derivatives have activities similar to those of praziquantel; these activities are unrelated to the anxiolytic activities in the mammalian central nervous system. The nerves and muscles in schistosomes and tapeworms are thus interesting subjects for future chemotherapeutic studies.

Drugs for Which the Mechanism Has Not Been Identified

In spite of considerable progress in defining the mechanisms of action of the drugs described above, there are still wide gaps in our understanding of a number of other important antiparasitic agents. These include the compounds presented in Table 55–2. From the biochemical activities that have been identified for them, it appears that many are capable of binding DNA, and some can uncouple oxidative phosphorylation in mammals. These types of activity, which are toxic to the host but could also be involved in the antiparasitic action, may have been preferentially detectable in random screens used for antiparasitic agents in the past.

REFERENCES

Bacchi CJ et al: In vivo effects of α-DL-difluoromethylornithine on the metabolism and morphology of *Trypanosoma brucei*. *Mol Biochem Parasitol* 1983;**7**:209.

Bacchi CJ et al: Polyamine metabolism: A potential therapeutic target in trypanosomes. *Science* 1980;**210**:332.

Borgers M et al: Influence of the anthelmintic mebendazole on microtubules and intracellular organelle movement in nematode intestinal cells. *Am J Vet Res* 1975;**36**:1153.

Bowman IBR, Flynn IW: Oxidative metabolism of trypanosomes. Page 435 in: *Biology of the Kinetoplastida.* Lumsden WHR, Evans DA (editors). Academic Press, 1976.

Casida JE et al: Mechanisms of selective action of pyrethroid insecticides. *Ann Rev Pharmacol Toxicol* 1983;**23**:413.

Clarkson AB, Brohn FH: Trypanosomiasis: An approach to chemotherapy by the inhibition of carbohydrate metabolism. *Science* 1976;**194**:204.

Davidse LC, Flach W: Interaction of thiabendazole with fungal tubulin. *Biochim Biophys Acta* 1978;**543**:82.

Dawson PJ, Gutteridge WE, Gull K: Purification and characterization of tubulin from the parasitic nematode, *Ascaridia galli*. *Mol Biochem Parasitol* 1983;**7**:267.

Del Castillo J, de Mello WC, Morales T: Inhibitory action of γ-aminobutyric acid (GABA) on *Ascaris* muscle. *Experientia* 1964;**20**:141.

Fairlamb AH, Bowman IBR: Uptake of the trypanocidal drug suramin by bloodstream forms of *Trypanosoma brucei* and its effect on respiration and growth rate in vivo. *Mol Biochem Parasitol* 1980;**1**:315.

Fairlamb AJ, Opperdoes FR, Borst P: New approach to screening drugs for activity against African trypanosomes. *Nature* 1977;**256**:270.

Friedman PA, Platzer EG: Interaction of anthelmintic benzimidazoles with *Ascaris suum* embryonic tubulin. *Biochim Biophys Acta* 1980;**630**:271.

Fritz LC, Wang CC, Gorio A: Avermectin B_{1a} irreversibly blocks post-synaptic potentials at the lobster neuromuscular junction by reducing muscle membrane resistance. *Proc Natl Acad Sci USA* 1979;**76**:2062.

Kass IS et al: Avermectin B_{1a}, a paralyzing anthelmintic that affects interneurons and inhibitory motor neurons in *Ascaris*. *Proc Natl Acad Sci USA* 1980;**77**:6211.

Lewis JA et al: Levamisole-resistant mutants of the nematode *Caenorhabditis elegans* appear to lack pharmacological acetylcholine receptors. *Neuroscience* 1980;**5**:967.

Marr JJ, Berens RL: Pyrazolopyrimidine metabolism in the pathogenic Trypanosomatidae. *Mol Biochem Parasitol* 1983; **7**:339.

McCann PP et al: Effect on parasitic protozoa of α-difluoromethylornithine: An inhibitor of ornithine decarboxylase. *Adv Polyamine Res* 1981;**3**:97.

Müller M: Hydrogenosomes. *Symp Soc Gen Microbiol* 1980; **30**:127.

Opperdoes FR, Borst P: Localization of nine glycolytic enzymes in a microbody-like organelle in *Trypanosoma brucei:* The glycosome. *FEBS Lett* 1977;**80**:360.

Pax R, Bennett JL, Fetterer R: A benzodiazepine derivative and praziquantel: Effects on musculature of *Schistosoma mansoni* and *Schistosoma japonicum*. *Naunyn Schmiedebergs Arch Pharmacol* 1978;**304**:309.

Senft AW et al: Pathways of nucleotide metabolism in *Schistosoma mansoni*. 3. Identification of enzymes in cell-free extracts. *Biochem Pharmacol* 1973;**22**:449.

Smith JW, Wolfe MS: Giardiasis. *Annu Rev Med* 1980;**35**:373.

Stretton AOW et al: Structure and physiological activity of the motoneurons of the nematode *Ascaris*. *Proc Natl Acad Sci USA* 1978;**75**:3493.

Sweeney TR, Strube RE: Antimalarials. Page 333 in: *Burger's Medicinal Chemistry,* 4th ed. Wolff ME (editor). Wiley, 1979.

Visser N, Opperdoes FR, Borst P: Subcellular compartmentation of glycolytic intermediates in *Trypanosoma brucei*. *Eur J Biochem* 1981;**118**:521.

Walter RD, Königk E: Purification and properties of the 7,8-di-hydropteroate-synthesizing enzyme from *Plasmodium chabaudi*. *Hoppe Seylers Z Physiol Chem* 1974;**355:**431.

Wang CC: Biochemistry and physiology of coccidia. Page 167 in: *The Biology of the Coccidia*. Long PL (editor). University Park Press, 1982.

Wang CC, Aldritt S: Purine salvage networks in *Giardia lamblia*. *J Exp Med* 1983;**158:**1703.

Wang CC, Pong SS: Actions of avermectin B_{1a} on GABA nerves. Page 373 in: *Membranes and Genetic Disease: Progress in Clinical and Biological Research*. Vol 97. Sheppard JR, Anderson VE, Eaton JW (editors). AR Liss, 1982.

Wang CC, Simashkevich PM: Purine metabolism in a protozoan parasite *Eimeria tenella*. *Proc Natl Acad Sci USA* 1981; **78:**6618.

Wang CC et al: Pyrimidine metabolism in *Tritrichomonas foetus*. *Proc Natl Acad Sci USA* 1983;**80:**2564.

56

Antiprotozoal Drugs

Bertram G. Katzung, MD, PhD, & Robert S. Goldsmith, MD, DTM&H

MALARIA

Malaria affects hundreds of millions of people and has been called "the most important of all infectious diseases" (Sir Macfarlane Burnet). In humans, the disease can be caused by 4 species of protozoa: *Plasmodium vivax*, *Plasmodium malariae*, *Plasmodium ovale*, and *Plasmodium falciparum*. The first 2 have a secondary "exoerythrocytic" stage in the liver of the host in addition to the primary hepatic, erythrocytic, and vector (mosquito) phases that are common to all. The life cycle of the parasite and the sites of action of some of the drugs used in malaria treatment and control are shown in Fig 56–1.

Types of Antimalarial Drugs

Different antimalarials exert their effects at different stages of the parasite's life cycle (Fig 56–1). Chemoprophylaxis or therapy of acute attacks by chemosuppression of the clinical manifestations of the disease—or the elimination of all parasites at all stages (a radical cure)—may be achieved by drugs attacking at (1) the pre-erythrocytic stages (sometimes called "primary exoerythrocytic" or "tissue" stages), which take place in the liver; (2) the erythrocytic stages, in which the parasites multiply rapidly in erythrocytes; or (3) the exoerythrocytic or secondary tissue stages of the relapsing malarias (*P vivax* and *P ovale*), which also take place in the liver. In addition, some drugs may have a selectively toxic effect on the gametocytes that form in the erythrocytes and are responsible for transferring the infection to the mosquito. Other drugs, when ingested in the blood by the mosquito,

may prevent the transmission of malaria to another victim by preventing multiplication (sporogony) in the mosquito gut and salivary glands.

Antimalarial drugs are sometimes classified as follows:

(1) Primary tissue schizonticides: Drugs that destroy the primary (pre-erythrocytic) tissue schizonts in the liver soon after infection (eg, primaquine).

(2) Blood schizonticides: ("Chemosuppressive" or "clinically curative" drugs.) Drugs that suppress the symptoms of malaria by destroying the schizonts and merozoites in the erythrocytes (eg, quinine, mefloquine, chloroquine, and amodiaquine).

(3) Gametocides: Drugs that prevent infection of mosquitoes and therefore the spread of infection by mosquitoes by destroying gametocytes in the blood (eg, primaquine).

(4) Sporonticides: Drugs that help to eradicate the disease by preventing sporogony and multiplication of the parasites in the mosquito when ingested with the blood of the human host (eg, chloroguanide [proguanil] and pyrimethamine).

(5) Secondary tissue schizonticides: ("Radically curative" drugs.) Drugs used to cure the chronic relapsing fevers due to infection by *P vivax* and *P ovale* by destroying the secondary (exoerythrocytic) tissue schizonts developing in the liver (eg, primaquine).

The structures of these agents are shown in Fig 56–2.

QUININE

Of the more than 36 alkaloids found in the bark of the South American cinchona tree, 4 stereoisomers—

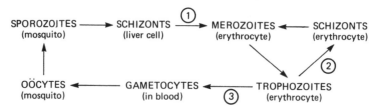

Figure 56–1. Simplified life cycle of a malaria parasite and the sites of action of some antimalarial drugs. ① Site of action of chloroguanine, primaquine, and pyramethamine. ② Site of action of chloroguanine, chloroquine, mefloquine, and quinine. ③ Site of action of chloroquine, primaquine, and quinine. Note that several drugs act at more than one site.

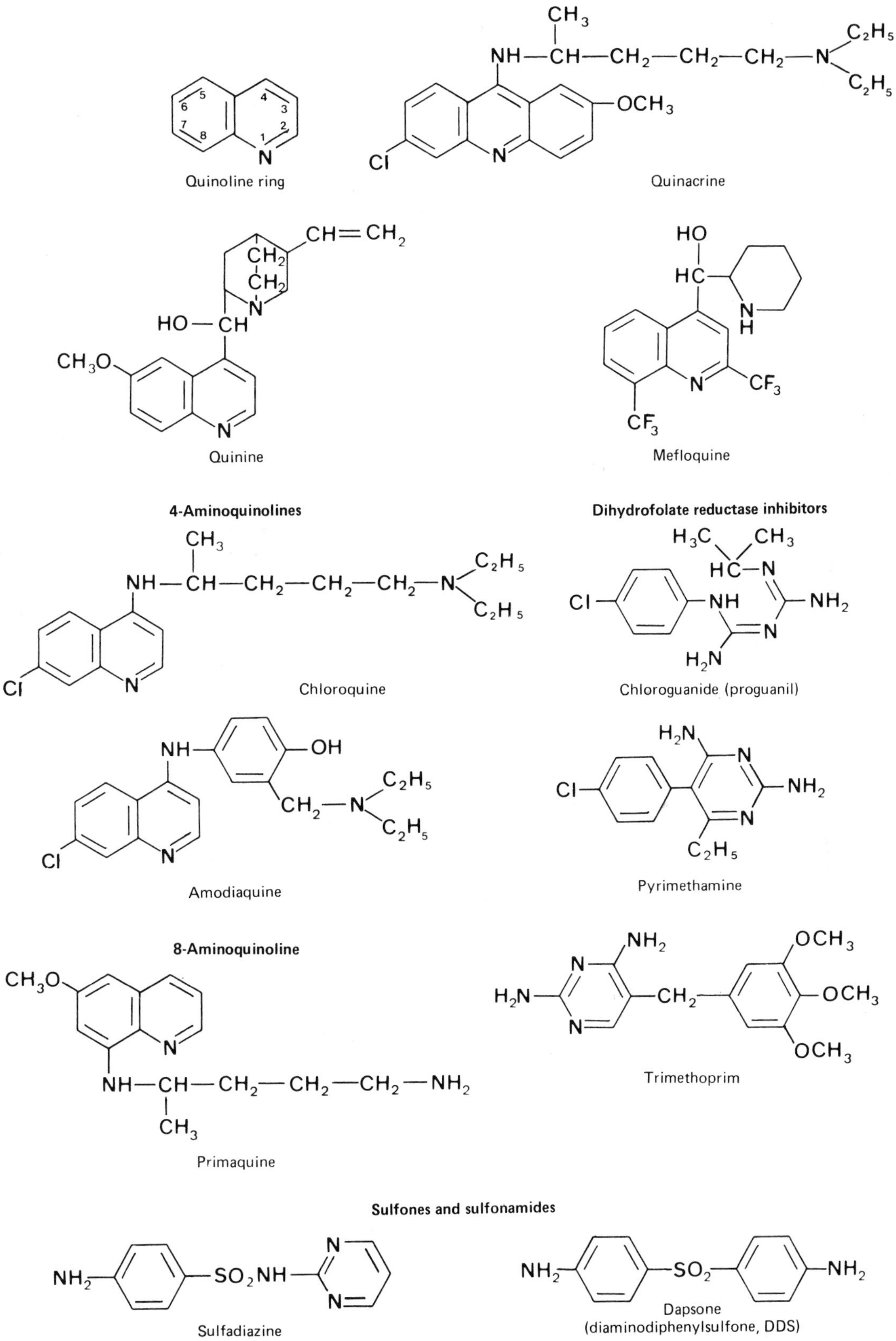

Figure 56–2. Structural formulas of antimalarial drugs.

quinine, quinidine, cinchonine, and cinchonidine—have significant antimalarial activity. Quinine (Fig 56–2) is present in highest concentration, exceeding the other active antimalarial compounds by about 10-fold. Although quinine has been synthesized, extraction from the natural source is far cheaper. Quinine and quinidine (Chapter 13) constitute the levo- and dextrorotatory members of one pair of stereoisomers, while cinchonidine and cinchonine constitute a similar pair. Although quinine and quinidine are approximately equal in potency, the larger amount of quinine in extracts of cinchona bark has made it the traditional antimalarial compound. The synthetic agent mefloquine is closely related to these drugs (Fig 56–2).

Absorption, Metabolism, & Excretion

Quinine is rapidly absorbed from the small intestine, and peak plasma concentrations are obtained 1–3 hours after ingestion. Excretion reaches a maximum after 4 hours, tapers off after another 4 hours, and is almost complete in 24 hours. Only 10% of the oral dose is excreted unchanged in the urine; the rest is metabolized. Subcutaneous or intramuscular quinine is poorly absorbed, and inflammation and sloughing may occur at the site of injection. When parenteral administration is necessary, quinine or quinidine is given intravenously.

Pharmacologic Effects

A. Mechanism of Action: The exact mechanism of quinine's antimalarial action is uncertain. Quinine can form a hydrogen-bonded complex with double-stranded DNA that inhibits protein synthesis by preventing strand separation and therefore DNA replication and transcription to RNA. However, mefloquine, which resembles quinine in many respects, does not intercalate with DNA. Both compounds bind with the characteristic "malaria pigment" produced in erythrocytes and interfere with the clumping of this pigment induced by chloroquine. The binding site for this reaction appears to be located in the digestive vacuole of the parasite. Mefloquine has also been shown to cause a generalized interruption of membrane-dependent activities in *Escherichia coli*. Since all of the quinine-related agents have a high affinity for membranes, their primary actions may occur at this organelle. Quinine has been observed to depress so many enzyme systems that it has in the past been described as a "general protoplasmic poison."

B. Effects on Malaria: Quinine, along with mefloquine, chloroquine, and amodiaquine, is classed as a "blood schizonticide." It has no effect on the primary or secondary exoerythrocytic forms of the parasites and therefore cannot bring about a radical cure of malaria caused by *P vivax* or *P ovale;* neither is it effectively gametocidal or sporonticidal to *P falciparum.* Although quinine cannot prevent infection, it can suppress the symptoms of malaria and also bring about rapid control of an acute attack. Quinine (or quinidine gluconate) by intravenous drip is now once

again the treatment of choice for acute attacks of chloroquine-resistant falciparum malaria.

C. Other Effects: The actions of quinine on the cardiovascular system are similar to those of quinidine (see Adverse Reactions, below). Quinine has little effect on smooth muscle other than a slight oxytocic action on the gravid uterus, especially during the third trimester of pregnancy. Clinically, it has no effect until labor has started, although dangerously toxic amounts may cause abortion.

In skeletal muscle, quinine has a curarelike effect on the motor end-plate and causes a lengthening of the refractory period. Tetanic contractions associated with various conditions may be diminished by quinine, and the drug has been used to lessen the contractions of myotonia congenita and to provide a diagnostic test for myasthenia gravis by aggravating the symptoms. Quinine was used for centuries to abate fevers due to any cause; its antipyretic action was due mostly to peripheral vasodilation.

Clinical Uses

A. Use in Acute Malaria: For 300 years, quinine was the drug of choice for the treatment and chemo-suppression of malaria. By 1959, quinine as an antimalarial had been totally superseded by synthetic antimalarials. However, the appearance of chloroquine-resistant strains of *P falciparum* has led to a resurgence in the use of quinine and in the search for new drugs.

B. Other Uses: Quinine is used to relieve leg cramps occurring during recumbency at night. In many parts of the world, quinine is still used as an all-purpose antipyretic. Many tonic waters and cocktail mixes contain quinine in trace amounts.

Adverse Reactions

A. Side Effects:

1. Cinchonism–This term denotes the mild toxic state that usually develops when the plasma level of quinine exceeds 10–12 mg/L. Symptoms include flushed and sweaty skin, tinnitus, blurred vision, impaired hearing, dizziness, nausea and vomiting, and diarrhea. With severe cinchonism, there may be papular or urticarial skin rashes, deafness, somnolence, diminished visual acuity or blindness (toxic amblyopia) due to ischemia of the retinal vessels, abdominal pain, and disturbances in cardiac rhythm or conduction. Marked hypotension is common, especially with intravenous therapy, and on the ECG, lengthening of the PR and QT intervals and the QRS complex is frequently observed.

2. Local irritant effect–Quinine is an irritant to the gastric mucosa, causing nausea and pain. Painful sterile abscesses frequently result from intramuscular injections. Intravenous injections may cause thrombophlebitis.

3. Hematologic effects–Hemolysis directly attributable to quinine occurs in 0.05% of people treated for acute malaria. Quinine inhibits phagocytosis and may rarely cause leukopenia, agranulocytosis, thrombocytopenic purpura, and Schönlein-Henoch purpura.

4. Blackwater fever–Blackwater fever is the syndrome of massive intravascular hemolysis, hemoglobinuria, azotemia, intravascular sludging and coagulation, renal failure, uremia, and death in 25–50% of cases. It is seldom seen in immune populations unless they have been treated with quinine. Hemoglobinuria occurs most often in patients who are also glucose-6-phosphate dehydrogenase-deficient.

B. Overdosage Toxicity: The lethal dose of quinine for adults is about 8 g, but survival has been reported after much larger doses. After overdosage, prompt gastric lavage is imperative because the drug is rapidly absorbed and death may ensue within a few hours. There is usually a profound fall of blood pressure owing to peripheral vasodilatation and myocardial depression. Respiration becomes slow and shallow, and cyanosis develops. The quinidinelike action produces the expected electrocardiographic changes and arrhythmias. Doses greater than 4 g in 24 hours usually lead to amblyopia, which is usually reversed by discontinuing the drug.

Preparations & Dosages for Chloroquine-Resistant Malaria

A. Quinine Dihydrochloride for the Parenteral Treatment of Severe *P falciparum* Infections: When parenteral administration of quinine is required for patients severely ill from a *P falciparum* infection (sensitive or resistant to chloroquine), quinine dihydrochloride or, in an emergency, when parenteral quinine or chloroquine is unavailable, quinidine gluconate (10 mg/kg in physiologic saline) is administered intravenously slowly over 2–4 hours and repeated every 8–12 hours until the patient is able to take oral medication. Blood pressure and the ECG should be monitored frequently. If it is known with certainty that the patient has not already taken the medication, a higher initial loading dose of quinine may be given (20 mg/kg). In the USA, quinine dihydrochloride is available from the Parasitic Disease Drug Service, Centers for Disease Control, Atlanta 30333. Telephone requests may be made by calling (404) 329–3670 days; (404) 329–2888 nights, weekends, and holidays.

B. Quinine Sulfate for the Oral Treatment of *P falciparum* Malaria Resistant to Chloroquine: Chloroquine-resistant strains of *P falciparum* have been reported from rural areas of Central and South America, Africa, Asia, the Indian subcontinent, and Oceania and from some urban areas as well. (For details, see CDC, *Health Information for International Travel, 1985*). All falciparum infections originating in Southeast Asia should be assumed to be resistant. Treatment of resistant strains of *P falciparum* requires oral quinine sulfate (a rapidly acting schizonticide) and a second synergistic drug (all of which are more slowly acting). One of the following regimens should be used:

(1) Quinine sulfate, 650 mg, 3 times a day for 3–7 days; on the first day, give pyrimethamine, 75 mg, and sulfadoxine, 1500 mg (Fansidar).

(2) Quinine sulfate, 650 mg, 3 times a day for 3–7 days plus pyrimethamine, 25 mg, 2 times a day for 3 days plus sulfadiazine, 500 mg, 4 times a day for 5 days; these 3 drugs must be administered concurrently.

(3) Quinine sulfate, 650 mg, 3 times a day for 3–7 days plus Bactrim Double Strength (160 mg trimethoprim and 800 mg sulfamethoxazole), 2 tablets, 2 times a day for 5 days, administered concurrently.

(4) Quinine sulfate, 650 mg, 3 times a day for 3–7 days, plus either tetracycline, 250 mg, 4 times a day for 10 days, or doxycycline, 100 mg twice daily for 7 days.

MEFLOQUINE

Mefloquine is considered to be a "third-generation" quinine derivative. Though not yet available commercially in the USA, it has been extensively studied in both resistant and nonresistant forms of malaria in humans and experimental models. It is 5–30 times more potent than quinine and may be more efficacious as well. However, it appears to be slower-acting, and it must be used orally. Like the older drug, mefloquine is inactive against the tissue stages of infection and cannot produce radical cure of the relapsing malarias. It can be used as a suppressive prophylactic against both falciparum and vivax malaria.

Mefloquine is curative in most cases of chloroquine-resistant malaria when used orally in a single dose of 1–1.5 g following a short course of quinine. It can protect against falciparum infection when given in a dose of 250–500 mg once a week. The drug has a half-life of about 2 weeks. It is much better tolerated than quinine, with no evidence of toxicity at doses up to 1.5 g and only transient nausea and dizziness at doses between 1.75 and 2 g.

Mefloquine, which is active against many but not all chloroquine-resistant strains of *P falciparum,* is a major advance in the development of drugs less toxic than quinine for this purpose. A major concern at present is that excessive use of the agent will result in the development of new strains of *P falciparum* resistant to it. Combination therapy with sulfadoxine-pyrimethamine has been recommended by some to delay the development of such resistant strains, but this involves a hazard because of the potentially serious adverse reactions of sulfadoxine. The drug is currently being used in southeast Asia as a fixed combination containing 250 mg mefloquine, 500 mg sulfadoxine, and 25 mg pyrimethamine per tablet under the name Fansimef.

AMINOQUINOLINE & ACRIDINE DERIVATIVES

These are synthetic drugs that were developed as quinine substitutes. The major agents are chloroquine and its congeners, which are 4-aminoquinolines; primaquine, an 8-aminoquinoline; and quinacrine, an acridine derivative.

1. CHLOROQUINE

From 1946 to 1966, chloroquine was the drug of choice for the treatment of malaria the world over. In 1966, chloroquine-resistant falciparum malaria began to appear in southeast Asia.

Chemistry & Nomenclature

Chloroquine (Fig 56–2) has a quinoline ring like that of quinine with a side chain identical to that of quinacrine. The chlorine atom in the seventh position appears to be crucial to the antimalarial activity of the 4-aminoquinolines and quinacrine. The D and L isomers are equally potent, but the D isomer is slightly less toxic.

Trade names include, for **chloroquine phosphate, Aralen, Avloclor,** and **Resochin;** for **chloroquine sulfate, Nivaquine;** and for **hydroxychloroquine sulfate, Plaquenil.** (See Table 56–1.)

Absorption, Metabolism, & Excretion

Absorption from the gastrointestinal tract is rapid and complete; maximum plasma concentrations are reached in 1–2 hours. The half-life of chloroquine in the body is about 5 days. Chloroquine is rapidly removed from the plasma and concentrated in those tissues where active protein synthesis and cell multiplication are greatest. The liver, spleen, kidneys, lungs, and leukocytes often contain 200–700 times the plasma concentration (whereas the brain and spinal cord contain only 10–30 times the plasma concentration). As a result, the apparent volume of distribution is very large (5–10 L/kg). For this reason, whenever an effectively schizonticidal plasma level is urgently needed, a loading dose should be given. The concentration of chloroquine in the erythrocytes is about 10–20 times greater than in the plasma and in parasitized erythrocytes about 25 times greater than in normal erythrocytes. Only 10–25% of the oral dose is excreted unchanged in the urine. The rate of excretion may be increased by acidification or decreased by alkalinization of the urine. Concomitant administration of other 4-aminoquinolines or 8-aminoquinolines prolongs and potentiates plasma levels of chloroquine.

Pharmacologic Effects

A. Mechanism of Action: Chloroquine and its congeners block the enzymatic synthesis of DNA and RNA in both mammalian and protozoal cells. The se-

Table 56–1. Drugs and oral doses for malaria chemoprophylaxis (modified from: *MMWR* [April 16]1982;**31[Suppl]:**205. (In no case should the pediatric dose exceed the adult dose.)

Generic Name	Trade Names	Adult Dose	Pediatric Dose
Amodiaquine*	Basoquin Camoquin Flavoquine	400 mg base (520 mg salt) once a week during and for 6 weeks after exposure in a malarious area.	7 mg base (9 mg salt)/kg once a week for same duration as adult dose.
Chloroguanide* (proguanil)	Paludrine, etc	100 mg once a day during and for 6 weeks after exposure in a malarious area.	1.5 mg/kg once a day for same duration as adult dose.
Chloroquine phosphate	Aralen Avloclor Resochin	300 mg base (500 mg salt) once a week 1–2 weeks before, during, and for 6 weeks after exposure in a malarious area.	5 mg base (8.3 mg salt)/kg once a week for same duration as adult dose.
Chloroquine sulfate*	Nivaquine	300 mg base (410 mg salt) once a week during and for 6 weeks after exposure in a malarious area.	5 mg base (6.8 mg salt)/kg once a week for same duration as adult dose.
Hydroxychloroquine	Plaquenil	310 mg base (400 mg salt) once a week 1–2 weeks before, during, and for 6 weeks after exposure in a malarious area.	5 mg base (6.5 mg salt)/kg once a week for same duration as adult dose.
Primaquine	None	15 mg base (26.3 mg salt) daily for 14 days, or 45 mg base (79 mg salt) weekly for 8 weeks, during the last weeks of, or just following a course of suppression with chloroquine or comparable drug.	0.3 mg base (0.5 mg salt)/kg once a day for 14 days, or 0.9 mg base (1.5 mg salt)/kg once a week for 8 weeks, during the last weeks of, or just following a course of suppression with chloroquine or comparable drug.
Pyrimethamine	Daraprim	25 mg once a week during and for 6 weeks after exposure in a malarious area.	0.5 mg/kg once a week during and for 6 weeks after exposure in a malarious area.
Pyrimethamine-sulfadoxine†	Antemal Falcidar Fansidar Methipox	25 mg pyrimethamine plus 500 mg sulfadoxine (1 tablet) once a week during and for 6 weeks after exposure in a malarious area.	0.5 mg/kg pyrimethamine plus 10 mg/kg sulfadoxine once a week for same duration as adult dose.

*Not available in the USA.

†Because of possible severe reactions to sulfonamides, this combination should be used only if there is no history of sulfonamide intolerance, and it should be discontinued immediately if any mucocutaneous symptoms occur. (*MMWR* [January 17] 1986;**35:**21.)

lective toxicity for the malarial parasites must therefore depend on a chloroquine-concentrating mechanism in parasitized cells. These drugs form a complex with DNA that prevents DNA from acting as a template for its own replication or transcription to RNA. It has been postulated that the quinoline ring of chloroquine is inserted between the base pairs of the DNA double helix so that the chlorine atom in position 7 of the quinoline ring lies in close proximity to the 2-amino group of guanine in a guanine-cytosine base pair. The diaminoaliphatic side chain of chloroquine lying across the minor groove of the DNA helix ties the 2 strands together by interacting ionically with the phosphoric acid groups of both strands.

Chloroquine is a weak base and, because it is taken up into cells in such high concentration, it has the ability to buffer the pH of intracellular endosomes and lysosomes. Since acidification of these organelles is required for the invasion of mammalian cells by some microorganisms, the high buffering capacity of chloroquine may inhibit penetration by intracellular parasites.

B. Effects:

1. In malaria—Chloroquine is an excellent blood schizonticidal drug for all 4 types of malaria. The fever and parasitemia produced by non-drug-resistant strains of plasmodia are usually controlled within 24–48 hours, and in *P falciparum* and *P malariae* infections a complete cure can be obtained. However, the drug has no effect on secondary tissue schizonts of relapsing malarias and thus cannot effect a "radical" cure of malaria caused by *P vivax* or *P ovale*.

Chloroquine, like quinine, is not lethal to the gametocytes or sporozoites of *P falciparum,* so that the blood of falciparum-infected chloroquine-treated humans can remain infective to mosquitoes for months. This may favor the emergence of drug-resistant strains of *P falciparum* in endemic areas.

Mechanism of chloroquine resistance. Parasites grown for many months in the presence of steadily increasing but sublethal doses of chloroquine will eventually become partially or totally resistant to the drug, and no concentration of chloroquine in the parasitized red cells can be demonstrated.

Plasmodial resistance to chloroquine is probably due to an impaired mechanism of drug transport across the parasite cell wall, so that the concentration of chloroquine in resistant schizonts never reaches a level sufficient to arrest nucleic acid synthesis.

2. On cardiovascular system—Chloroquine has a slight quinidinelike effect on the cardiovascular system, and changes in the T wave of the ECG may be noticeable during therapy. Chloroquine depresses myocardial excitability to approximately the same extent as quinidine, but it has hardly any effect on the conduction velocity. It has on occasion been used in place of quinidine. Toxic doses depress vasomotor function and induce circulatory collapse, shock, respiratory paralysis, and death.

3. Anti-inflammatory effects—Chloroquine has anti-inflammatory effects that have been useful in the treatment of rheumatoid arthritis and discoid lupus erythematosus. The mechanism is not understood.

Clinical Uses

A. Malaria, Acute Attacks: Chloroquine usually terminates the fever and parasitemia of acute attacks of nonresistant strains of falciparum malaria within 24–48 hours, and complete cures are usually obtained because *P falciparum* has no secondary tissue stage. Severe malaria with more than 100,000 parasites per microliter of blood or with cerebral, renal, or pulmonary complications requires immediate treatment with slow intravenous infusions of quinine. If an acute attack does not respond to chloroquine within 24 hours, a resistant strain may be involved and other antimalarial drugs must be tried (see below). For acute attacks of *P vivax* malaria, chloroquine is the drug of choice; however, because it has no effect on the exo-erythrocytic stages, radical cure requires combination therapy with primaquine.

The recommended treatment for *P vivax* infections is a total dose of 1.5 g of chloroquine (base) over a 2-day period (600 mg initial dose, followed by 300 mg at 6, 24, and 48 hours).

Most authorities believe that *P malariae* is not a relapsing species of malaria. There are no reports of *P malariae* resistance to chloroquine. Therefore, this species may be treated with chloroquine as outlined above for *P vivax;* no primaquine is indicated.

B. Suppression of Malaria: Chloroquine effectively suppresses all types of malaria except the resistant strains of *P falciparum*. If the drug is discontinued too soon after *P vivax* infections, parasitemia may recur after several days. Chloroquine is more potent, less toxic, better tolerated, and more easily administered than quinine or quinacrine. Complete suppression may be obtained with a plasma level of 5–8 μg/L. The prophylactic use of chloroquine or other 4-aminoquinolines involves the risk of the development of resistant strains.

Note: Treatment failures with chloroquine and *P falciparum* infections are occurring in many areas of the world (see above under Quinine Sulfate). CDC now recommends Fansidar (see Antifols) plus chloroquine in chemoprophylaxis.

C. Amebiasis: See p 630.

Adverse Reactions

A. Side Effects: When used in the very low doses required for the chemosuppression of malaria, chloroquine has essentially no toxic effects. During chloroquine therapy of active malaria, vertigo, malaise, anorexia, diarrhea, headache, blurring of vision, pruritus, and urticaria may occur.

After high dosage there may be macropapular eruptions, desquamation, or exfoliative lesions of the skin, and alopecia or graying of the hair. Lupus erythematosus, lichenoid skin eruptions, and leukopenia induced by chloroquine have been reported.

Toxic psychoses with hallucinations and agitation and peripheral neuropathies with loss of reflexes and muscle power in the lower limbs can occur. Electrocardiographic changes, particularly flattening or inversion of the T waves, are frequent with high doses.

Congenital deafness and mental retardation have been reported in children born to mothers who were taking large doses of chloroquine during pregnancy. Permanent nerve deafness in adults has followed high-dose chloroquine therapy.

B. Ocular Toxicity: Severe and often permanent retinal eye damage may be caused by the prolonged administration of chloroquine in high dosage. Between 10 and 33% of patients taking large doses of chloroquine develop symptomless corneal deposits, which always regress when the drug is discontinued.

C. Overdosage Toxicity: After a toxic dose, there are visual disturbances, hyperexcitability, convulsions, atrioventricular block, and death may occur within 2 hours.

There is no antidote. Because chloroquine is rapidly absorbed, gastric lavage must be done before symptoms occur if it is to be of any value. Peritoneal dialysis or hemodialysis is usually unsuccessful.

Contraindications & Cautions

Chloroquine crosses the placenta and may damage the fetus when large doses have been taken during pregnancy. Patients with porphyria and psoriasis should not use chloroquine because it may precipitate an acute attack, and chloroquine should not be combined with other drugs known to cause dermatitis. Gold or phenylbutazone therapy should be discontinued during chloroquine therapy.

Chloroquine should be used with caution in patients with a history of liver damage, or neurologic or hematologic disorders.

Resistance to chloroquine extends to the other available 4-aminoquinolines and quinacrine, and often to chloroguanide and pyrimethamine as well. However, resistance may not extend to certain experimental bis-4-aminoquinolines (hydroxypiperaquine; see Sweeney and Pick reference).

Therapy of acute attacks should never be attempted with combined chloroquine-primaquine tablets, because an adequate therapeutic dose of chloroquine cannot be achieved without also giving toxic amounts of primaquine.

2. THE CHLOROQUINE CONGENERS

None of the 200 known derivatives of 4-aminoquinoline with proved schizonticidal activity have been conclusively shown to be superior to chloroquine; therefore, chloroquine, whose potency and side effects have been abundantly documented, is the preferred preparation.

The 1972 WHO scientific group on the chemotherapy of malaria lists only 3 other 4-aminoquinolines "in common use": (1) **amodiaquine dihydrochloride (Basoquin, Camoquin, Flavoquine)** (for the prophylactic dose of amodiaquine, see Table 56–1); (2) **cy-**

cloquine (Ciklochin, Halochin); and (3) **amopyroquin (Propoquin).**

3. PRIMAQUINE

Absorption, Metabolism, & Excretion

Absorption of this 8-aminoquinoline drug (Fig 56–2) from intestine is essentially complete, and peak plasma levels are reached in 6 hours. Only trace amounts are in the plasma 24 hours later, and only about 1% is excreted in the urine unchanged.

Effective clearance of tissue schizonts does not begin until primaquine has undergone biodegradation by demethylation and oxidation to quinoline-quinone derivatives, the active antimalarial and hemolytic agents. Tissue concentrations of primaquine are higher in liver and lungs, but primaquine is also concentrated in brain, heart, and skeletal muscle.

Pharmacologic Action

A. Mechanism of Action: Unlike the 4-aminoquinolines, the 8-aminoquinolines do not inhibit DNA replication and transcription.

The quinoline-quinone intermediates derived from primaquine are electron-carrying redox compounds capable of acting as oxidants. The intermediate metabolites probably account for the hemolysis and methemoglobinemia as well as the schizonticidal action of the drug.

B. Effects: Although the 8-aminoquinolines and 4-aminoquinolines are structurally similar, their actions on malaria parasites are quite different. The 8-aminoquinolines act on the exoerythrocytic stages and have practically no effect on the erythrocytic stages (Fig 56–1).

The mode of action is probably related to the mechanism by which they produce an acute self-limiting intravascular hemolysis in individuals with an inherited glucose-6-phosphate dehydrogenase deficiency. It is postulated that, in contrast to the erythrocytic schizonts, both the tissue schizonts and the glucose-6-phosphate dehydrogenase-deficient erythrocytes have a deficiency of an enzyme or cofactor involved in the pentose phosphate pathway, making them especially susceptible to oxidative damage.

Primaquine also has an effect on the gametocytes; some are destroyed in the blood, and others cannot later mature in the mosquito gut. Primaquine is therefore a "tissue schizonticide" and the only antimalarial able to bring about "radical cures" of the relapsing malarias. Its gametocidal activity also makes it the best available drug to interrupt the transmission of malaria.

Primaquine given orally in therapeutic doses has no pharmacologic effects other than its antimalarial action and its toxic effect on erythrocyte metabolism. It is never given parenterally because it can produce electrocardiographic changes and a profound fall of blood pressure.

Clinical Uses

Primaquine is highly active against the primary exoerythrocytic stages of falciparum and vivax malaria and the secondary exoerythrocytic forms of the relapsing malarias (*P vivax* and *P ovale*). It is also highly active against the gametocytes of all 4 species causing human malaria and is therefore used to limit the transmission of malaria. It has only a slight effect on the blood schizonts and cannot be used to relieve the fever and parasitemia of acute attacks. Primaquine is at the moment the only drug able to attack the late tissue stages of *P vivax* or *P ovale* and therefore able to effect a radical cure. Unfortunately, strains of *P vivax* have now appeared in Southeast Asia that are partially resistant to primaquine.

Several programs of mass chemoprophylaxis with primaquine have been carried out in areas of heavy malaria endemicity by WHO and other public health authorities.

Adverse Reactions

A. Primaquine Sensitivity: Glucose-6-phosphate dehydrogenase deficiency, sometimes called primaquine sensitivity, is an inherited error of metabolism transmitted by a gene of partial dominance located on the X chromosome. It is estimated that over 100 million people are affected. Red cells deficient in glucose-6-phosphate dehydrogenase are sensitive in various degrees to the 8-aminoquinolines and many other drugs, eg, sulfonamides, aminosalicylic acid, aspirin, certain vitamin K derivatives, nitrofurans, and fava beans.

The enzyme glucose-6-phosphate dehydrogenase is necessary for the regeneration of NADPH, which in turn is required for the reduction of oxidized glutathione. One of the functions of reduced glutathione is to protect sulfhydryl-dependent enzymes and other cellular proteins against oxidation. The level of reduced glutathione in the red cells of glucose-6-phosphate dehydrogenase-deficient individuals fluctuates and is usually lower than normal. When primaquine brings about a further reduction of the level of reduced glutathione in cells that already have an impaired mechanism for the regeneration of NADPH, glucose metabolism may be so deranged that the red cells undergo hemolysis.

The amount of hemolysis occurring with primaquine therapy is therefore dependent on (1) the degree of glucose-6-phosphate dehydrogenase deficiency, (2) the age of the erythrocyte population, and (3) dose.

Other less common types of inherited enzyme deficiencies involving erythrocyte metabolism (eg, glutathione reductase deficiency) may also be expressed as primaquine sensitivity.

B. Side Effects: Toxic reactions, often seen when large doses (60–240 mg) are given, include nausea, headache, disturbances of visual accommodation, pruritus, and abdominal cramps (which may be relieved with antacids). Severe reactions associated with high-dose therapy include leukopenia and methemoglobinemia usually presenting as cyanosis. All patients receiving primaquine should be told to report any signs of hemolysis, such as reddening or darkening of the urine.

Contraindications & Cautions

Blacks, Greeks, Sephardic Jews, Sardinians, and Iranians, who are known to have a high incidence of glucose-6-phosphate dehydrogenase deficiency, should be watched for signs of hemolysis during primaquine therapy. Before initiating treatment with primaquine, it is recommended that all patients be screened for erythrocyte glucose-6-phosphate dehydrogenase deficiency. Periodic determinations of the hematocrit or hemoglobin are essential during therapy. Patients with active rheumatoid arthritis, lupus erythematosus, or any grave systemic disease should not receive primaquine therapy. Primaquine should not be given at the same time as quinacrine or other drugs known to have depressant effects on the bone marrow.

When primaquine was used for mass chemosuppression, drug resistance of *P falciparum* was induced. In the laboratory, strains of *Plasmodium berghei* made resistant to primaquine show significant cross-resistance to cycloguanil, pyrimethamine, and dapsone.

Dosages

For primaquine malaria chemoprophylaxis for adults and for children, see Table 56–1.

There are no indications or preparations for intravenous or intramuscular primaquine therapy.

4. QUINACRINE
(Mepacrine)

Quinacrine (Atabrine), also known as mepacrine, was the first effective synthetic antimalarial of low toxicity. Quinacrine, like quinine and the 4-aminoquinolines, is a blood schizonticide. Continuous therapy can effectively suppress all 4 types of human malaria and can effect a radical cure of *P malariae* and nonresistant strains of *P falciparum*. Until the introduction of chloroquine, it was the principal synthetic drug used for antimalarial prophylaxis.

The standard malaria suppressive dose of quinacrine is 100 mg orally. It is readily absorbed from the intestinal tract, and peak plasma levels are reached 8 hours later.

Clinical Uses

A. Treatment and Chemosuppression of Malaria: Quinacrine as an antimalarial agent was superseded in 1945 by the far more potent and less toxic 4-aminoquinolines.

B. Other Uses: See Chapters 57 and 58.

THE ANTIFOLS (DIHYDROFOLATE REDUCTASE INHIBITORS): CHLOROGUANIDE (PROGUANIL), PYRIMETHAMINE, & TRIMETHOPRIM

The discovery of the synergistic potentiation of the antimalarial activity of the antifols when combined with sulfonamides such as sulfamethoxypyridazine and sulfamethoxazole and with sulfones such as dapsone (DDS) opened a whole new field of antimalarial therapy. However, because of the rapid development of resistance, with cross-resistance to other combinations of antifols and sulfonamides, it is now recommended that these combinations be used only for the treatment of chloroquine-resistant strains.

Chemistry & Nomenclature

A. Chloroguanide (Proguanil) Hydrochloride: The structure of chloroguanide is shown in Fig 56–2. It is also known as Balusil, bigumal, biguanide, chlorguanide, Chloroguanil, Diguanyl, Drinupal, Guanatol, Lepadina, Paludrine, Palusil, Plasin, Proguanide, and Tirian. For prophylaxis, see Table 56–1.

B. Pyrimethamine: The structure of pyrimethamine is shown in Fig 56–2. It is also known by the proprietary names Chloridin, Darapram, Daraprim, Erbaprelina, and Malocide.

C. Trimethoprim: The structure of trimethoprim is shown in Fig 56–2 (see also Chapter 47). It is available as a combination of one part trimethoprim and 5 parts sulfamethoxazole, known as Bactrim or Septra.

D. Pyrimethamine-Sulfadoxine: This combination (Falcidar, Fansidar), now available in the USA, consists of a long-acting sulfonamide (sulfadoxine, 500 mg) combined with pyrimethamine, 25 mg. The preparation is recommended by WHO and CDC for chemoprophylaxis of *P falciparum* in all areas of the world where the strains are resistant to chloroquine but sensitive to antifolate-sulfonamide combinations. The dosage is 1 tablet weekly while in the endemic area and for 6 weeks after leaving. Chloroquine is given concurrently to provide chemoprophylaxis against *P vivax*, since in many areas of the world *P vivax* is resistant to the pyrimethamine in Fansidar.

The CDC, in their revised recommendations for preventing malaria in travelers (*MMWR* 1985; **34:**185), reported that since Fansidar became available in the USA in 1982, 20 cases of severe reactions had occurred, including 6 deaths. All of the reactions occurred after a series of weekly doses of Fansidar— none after a single dose. As a result, CDC now recommends that the drug only be used in chemoprophylaxis for *P falciparum* when there is a high risk of exposure. Individuals traveling through an endemic area should keep in their possession a single treatment dose of Fansidar (3 tablets = 75 mg of pyrimethamine and 1500 mg of sulfadoxine) to be taken "promptly in the event of a febrile illness [that occurs] during or after their travel *when professional medical care is not readily available.*"

Absorption, Metabolism, & Excretion

Chloroguanide, pyrimethamine, and trimethoprim are slowly but adequately absorbed from the gastrointestinal tract. Peak plasma levels are reached in 3–7 hours after an oral dose, and loading doses are not necessary. Chloroguanide is so rapidly eliminated from the body that it must be administered daily; pyrimethamine is excreted more slowly. Trimethoprim is excreted more slowly than sulfamethoxazole, with which it is combined. Sufficient pyrimethamine is excreted in maternal milk so that chemosuppressive levels of the drug may be reached in wholly breast-fed infants.

Pharmacologic Effects

When the antifols are given in therapeutic doses, no effects are seen other than the intended antiprotozoal or antibacterial effects. In excessive doses, abdominal pain, diarrhea, hematuria, and a macrocytic anemia like that of folic acid deficiency may occur.

Antimalarial Effects

All 3 of these drugs are effective schizonticides. Pyrimethamine, the most potent of the 3, has been calculated to be 2000 times as toxic to the malarial parasite as to the host. These drugs can also prevent sporogony in the mosquito gut, and a single dose of pyrimethamine given to a nonimmune person can interrupt transmission for several weeks. All 3 can provide effective antimalarial chemoprophylaxis provided they are continued for at least 6 weeks after the last infected mosquito bite and that there are no resistant strains in the area. They should not be used for the treatment of acute attacks because their blood schizonticide action is too slow. *P falciparum* malaria resistant to pyrimethamine is increasing and has been found not only in Southeast Asia and East Africa but also in West Africa. Pyrimethamine-resistant strains are usually also resistant to chloroguanide.

Mode of Action of the Antifols

Chloroguanide itself is a pro-drug; only its triazine metabolite, cycloguanil, is active. The selective toxicity of all 3 antifols depends on the fact that plasmodia, unlike humans and many other animals, have not lost the enzymes needed for the synthesis of folic acid from *p*-aminobenzoic acid (PABA), glutamic acid, and pteridine but yet cannot make use of preformed folic acid (Chapter 55). The plasmodicidal effects of these 3 antimalarials are due to a deficiency of tetrahydrofolate that results in the inhibition of cell division and schizogony. This interference with folic acid metabolism therefore explains the marked synergistic enhancement of potency that occurs when any of these drugs are combined with sulfonamides or sulfones, causing a sequential blockade of folic acid synthesis at 2 different stages along the metabolic pathway (see also Fig 47–1).

Clinical Uses

A. Malaria Chemosuppression: Chloroguanide must be taken in daily 100-mg doses because of its rapid excretion. Pyrimethamine is the most potent chemoprophylactic available (requiring only 25 mg weekly), but, like chloroguanide, it must be taken for 6 weeks after leaving the endemic area. Cures of acute attacks of malaria in nonimmune patients should not be attempted with these drugs because their action in reducing fever and parasitemia is much too slow.

B. Combination Therapy of Chloroquine-Resistant Falciparum Malaria: Various combinations such as pyrimethamine plus quinine and pyrimethamine plus sulfadoxine are advocated and have been found to be effective, but malaria resistance to these new combinations soon develops. For this reason, combinations of antifols and sulfonamides should only be used for chloroquine-resistant malaria.

C. Toxoplasmosis: Pyrimethamine, 25 mg, combined with trisulfapyrimidines, 1 g, given orally 4 times a day for 6 weeks, can be used for the treatment of toxoplasmosis. However, if toxoplasmic chorioretinitis is present or if there is a danger of congenital toxoplasmosis, corticosteroids should also be given.

Adverse Reactions

Chloroguanide occasionally induces anorexia but is the least toxic of all the antimalarials.

Pyrimethamine is also well tolerated. Large doses of pyrimethamine given for long periods sometimes lead to folic acid deficiency. Supplementary folic acid (10 mg/d in divided doses) can correct the hematologic defect without impairing the drug's therapeutic effect.

Contraindications & Cautions

Cross-resistance to chloroguanide and pyrimethamine may develop when these drugs are given singly in low doses and for long periods of chemosuppression.

Preparations & Dosages

Chloroguanide hydrochloride (proguanil, Paludrine) is available as tablets of 25, 50, 100, and 300 mg containing 87% of the base. For the chemosuppression of malaria, 100–200 mg daily is usually sufficient.

Pyrimethamine is available as 25-mg tablets. For the chemosuppression of malaria, the dosage is 1 or 2 tablets per week. For children under 14, give pyrimethamine elixir (6.25 mg/mL), 2 mL weekly. The first dose should be taken before entering endemic areas, and suppressive therapy must be continued for 6 weeks after leaving the area.

Treatment of *P Falciparum* Strains Resistant to Chloroquine

Oral treatment for strains sensitive to antifolate-sulfonamide combinations is quinine sulfate (650 mg 3 times daily for 3–7 days) plus either (1) pyrimethamine (75 mg) and sulfadoxine (1500 mg) (Fan-sidar) once only, or (2) pyrimethamine (25 mg twice daily for 3 days) and sulfadiazine (500 mg 4 times daily for 5 days). For *P falciparum* strains resistant to both chloroquine and antifolate-sulfonamide combinations, give quinine sulfate (650 mg 3 times daily for 3–7 days) plus either tetracycline (250–500 mg 4 times daily for 7 days) or doxycycline (100 mg twice daily for 7 days).

To treat severe attacks, give quinine hydrochloride intravenously. Give 600 mg in 300 mL of normal saline intravenously slowly over 2–4 hours; repeat every 6–8 hours until oral therapy is possible, but not more often than 3 times in 24 hours. Oral therapy with quinine plus a second drug should be started as soon as possible. If it is known with certainty that the patient has not already taken the medication, a higher initial loading dose of quinine is given (20 mg/kg).

QINGHAOSU (Artemisinin, Arteannuin)

This unusual heterocyclic compound is the active principle of a Chinese herbal medicine.

Qinghaosu

The compound is extremely insoluble and is usually given in suspension form, either by intramuscular injection or by mouth. More soluble derivatives are under study.

Qinghaosu has rapid blood schizonticidal activity against all types of human and most animal malarias. It has no effect on the hepatic stages and therefore cannot cure the relapsing malarias. It is effective against chloroquine-resistant *P falciparum* and has been especially useful in patients with cerebral malaria. The mechanism of action is unknown but may be related to that of the quinine derivatives. The major disadvantage reported thus far is the high rate of recurrence of malaria. It is therefore recommended that qinghaosu always be used in combination with an antifolate.

OTHER DRUGS WITH ANTIMALARIAL ACTIVITY

For chloroquine-sensitive falciparum malaria, chloroquine therapy remains the treatment of choice. Therapy should always be followed by a 6-week course of primaquine to prevent relapses due to possible concomitant *P vivax* infections.

For chloroquine-resistant malaria, quinine by intravenous infusion followed by a single dose of sulfadoxine and pyrimethamine is highly effective.

Maloprim is a fixed-combination tablet containing 100 mg dapsone with 12.5 mg pyrimethamine. The recommended prophylactic dose is 2 tablets for the week preceding exposure, followed by 1 tablet per week.

Tetracycline, 250 mg orally every 6 hours for 7 days, can clear asexual forms of the parasites of chloroquine-resistant *P falciparum* infections, but tetracycline has no effect against the gametocytes. Tetracycline may have value as an adjunctive agent to achieve radical cures of drug-resistant infections.

Clindamycin, minocycline, and **lincomycin** have shown some degree of effectiveness against resistant *P falciparum*.

THE TREATMENT OF AMEBIASIS

Robert S. Goldsmith, MD, DTM&H

Amebiasis may present as a severe intestinal infection (dysentery), a mild to moderate symptomatic intestinal infection, an asymptomatic intestinal infection, or as an ameboma, a liver abscess, or other type of extraintestinal infection.

The choice of drug depends on the clinical presentation and on the desired site of drug action. Treatment may require the concurrent or sequential use of several drugs. Table 56–2 outlines a preferred and an alternative method of treatment for each clinical type of amebiasis. Drug dosages are provided in the footnotes to the table. No drugs are recommended as safe or effective for chemoprophylaxis.

Drugs Used in Treatment

All of the antiamebic drugs act against *Entamoeba histolytica* trophozoites, but most are not effective against the cyst stage.

A. Tissue Amebicides: These are drugs that act primarily in the bowel wall, liver, and other extraintestinal tissues but are not effective against organisms in the bowel lumen.

1. Nitroimidazoles–Metronidazole (Flagyl), tinidazole* (Fasigyn), and ornidazole* are highly effective in the bowel wall and other tissues. They are, however, only partially effective and not sufficient as luminal amebicides; metronidazole, for example, when used alone fails to cure up to 50% of intestinal infections.

2. Emetines–Emetine and dehydroemetine[†] are generally given intramuscularly; in this form they act on organisms in the bowel wall and other tissues but not on amebas in the bowel lumen.

3. Chloroquine–This drug is active principally against amebas in the liver.

B. Luminal Amebicides: These are drugs that act primarily in the bowel lumen but are not effective against organisms in the bowel wall or other tissues.

1. Dichloroacetamides–Diloxanide furoate[†] (Furamide), clefamide* (Mebinol), teclozan,* etofamide.*

2. Halogenated hydroxyquinolines–Iodoquinol (diiodohydroxyquin); clioquinol (iodochlorhydroxyquin).

3. Antibiotics–The oral tetracyclines inhibit the bacterial associates of *E histolytica* in the bowel lumen and thus affect luminal amebas only indirectly, whereas paromomycin (Humatin) and erythromycin are directly amebicidal. With the exception of paromomycin, none of the antibiotics are highly effective against intestinal organisms and therefore should not be used by themselves in treatment. Given parenterally, antibiotics have little antiamebic activity in any site.

C. Other Compounds: The pentavalent arsenicals glycobiarsol,* carbarsone, difetarsone,* and acetarsone* should no longer be used because of the potential toxicity of arsenic. Emetine-bismuth-iodide* (EBI), an oral luminal amebicide, is little used at present because of its side effects, which include nausea, vomiting, and rare instances of emetine toxicity. Niridazole,* which has both luminal and tissue amebicidal actions, is not recommended because of its neurotoxicity.

Treatment of Specific Forms of Amebiasis

A. Asymptomatic Intestinal Infection: Persons with asymptomatic infection should be treated, since they may become symptomatic or transmit the infection to others. The drugs of choice, diloxanide furoate[†] and iodoquinol, give cure rates of 80–90% in a single course of treatment. Diloxanide is preferred because it causes fewer side effects. In asymptomatic infection, the additional use of a tissue amebicidal drug is not necessary.

Other alternatives for treatment or re-treatment are paromomycin or paromomycin plus iodoquinol.

B. Mild to Moderate Intestinal Infections: In this stage of intestinal disease, it is necessary to use both a luminal and a tissue amebicidal drug, since the parasites must be reached in the lumen, in the intestinal wall, and in the liver. The drug combination of choice, metronidazole plus a luminal amebicide (diloxanide furoate or iodoquinol), gives cure rates over 90%.

An alternative treatment is to combine a luminal amebicide (iodoquinol or diloxanide furoate) with a tetracycline and then follow with a short course of chloroquine. When iodoquinol is used, concomitant use of a tetracycline probably increases intestinal cure rates. It is less well established that adding a tetracycline to diloxanide therapy increases effectiveness. Chloroquine is used to destroy trophozoites carried to the liver or to eradicate an undetected early-stage ame-

---

*Not available in the USA.

[†]In the USA, available from the Centers for Disease Control, Atlanta 30333.

Table 56–2. Treatment of amebiasis.

	Drug(s) of Choice	Alternative Drug(s)
Asymptomatic intestinal infection	Diloxanide furoate[1, 2]	Iodoquinol (diiodohydroxyquin)[3]
Mild to moderate intestinal infection (nondysenteric colitis)	(1) Metronidazole[4] **plus** (2) Diloxanide furoate[2] or iodoquinol[3]	(1) Diloxanide furoate[2] or iodoquinol[3] **plus** (2) A tetracycline[5] **followed by** (3) Chloroquine[6] **or** (1) Paromomycin[7] **followed by** (2) Chloroquine[6]
Severe intestinal infection (dysentery)	(1) Metronidazole[8] **plus** (2) Diloxanide furoate[2] or iodoquinol[3] **If parenteral therapy is needed initially** (1) Intravenous metronidazole[9] until oral therapy can be started (2) Then give oral metronidazole[8] plus diloxanide furoate[2] or iodoquinol[3]	(1) A tetracycline[5] **plus** (2) Diloxanide furoate[2] or iodoquinol[3] **followed by** (3) Chloroquine[10] **or** (1) Dehydroemetine[1, 11] or emetine (see text for dosage) **followed by** (2) A tetracycline[5] plus diloxanide furoate[2] or iodoquinol[3] **followed by** (3) Chloroquine[10]
Hepatic abscess	(1) Metronidazole[8, 9] **plus** (2) Diloxanide furoate[2] or iodoquinol[3] **followed by** (3) Chloroquine[10]	(1) Dehydroemetine[1, 12] or emetine (see text for dosage) **plus** (2) Chloroquine[13] **plus** (3) Diloxanide furoate[2] or iodoquinol[3]
Ameboma or extraintestinal infection	As for hepatic abscess, but not including chloroquine	As for hepatic abscess, but not including chloroquine

[1]Available in the USA only from the Parasitic Disease Drug Service, Centers for Disease Control, Atlanta 30333. Telephone requests may be made by calling the central number (404) 329–3311 days; ((404)329–2888 nights, weekends, and holidays (emergencies only).

[2]Diloxanide furoate, 500 mg 3 times daily with meals for 10 days (for children, 20 mg/kg in 3 divided doses daily for 10 days).

[3]Iodoquinol (diiodohydroxyquin), 650 mg 3 times daily for 21 days (for children, 30–40 mg/kg [maximum 2 g] in 3 divided doses daily for 21 days).

[4]Metronidazole, 750 mg 3 times daily for 10 days (for children, 35 mg/kg in 3 divided doses daily for 10 days).

[5]A tetracycline, 250 mg 4 times daily for 10 days; in severe dysentery, give 500 mg 4 times daily for the first 5 days, then 250 mg 4 times daily for 5 days. Tetracycline should not be used during pregnancy or in children under 8 years of age; in older children, give 20 mg/kg in 4 divided doses daily for 10 days).

[6]Chloroquine, 500 mg (salt) daily for 7 days (for children, 16 mg/kg [salt] daily for 7 days).

[7]Paromomycin, 25–30 mg/kg (base) (maximum 3 g) in 3 divided doses after meals daily for 5–10 days (for children, the same dosage). Use only for mild disease.

[8]Metronidazole, 750 mg 3 times daily for 5–10 days (for children, 35–50 mg/kg in 3 divided doses daily for 10 days).

[9]An intravenous metronidazole is available; change to oral medication as soon as possible. See manufacturer's recommendation for dosage.

[10]Chloroquine, 500 mg (salt) daily for 14 days (for children, 16 mg/kg [salt] daily for 14 days).

[11]Dehydroemetine, 1 mg/kg subcut (preferred) or IM daily for the least number of days necessary to control severe symptoms (usually 3–5 days) (maximum daily dose 90 mg).

[12]Dehydroemetine, 1 mg/kg subcut (preferred) or IM daily for 8–10 days (maximum daily dose 90 mg).

[13]Chloroquine, 500 mg (salt) twice daily for 2 days and then 500 mg daily for 21 days (for children, 16 mg/kg [salt] daily for 21 days).

bic liver abscess; the minimum dose needed to accomplish this is not established.

C. Severe Intestinal Infection (Dysentery): The treatment of choice is metronidazole plus a concurrent course of diloxanide furoate or iodoquinol. For patients requiring initial parenteral therapy, an intravenous preparation of metronidazole is available.

An alternative form of treatment is a tetracycline plus diloxanide fuorate or iodoquinol. An additional alternative method, particularly for patients requiring initial parenteral therapy, is to give dehydroemetine

(or emetine) intramuscularly or subcutaneously for the minimum number of days (usually 3–5; significant toxicity usually does not occur in this period) needed to control severe symptoms. Then start an oral course of a tetracycline plus either diloxanide furoate or iodoquinol; follow these with a course of chloroquine.

Fluid and electrolyte therapy and opiates to control bowel motility are necessary adjuncts in severe amebic dysentery.

D. Hepatic Abscess: Hospitalization and bed rest are usually necessary. The treatment of choice is metronidazole, which if given for 10 days results in cures in over 95% of uncomplicated cases; however, treatment failures sometimes do occur, either during the course of treatment or after its completion. A parenteral preparation of metronidazole is available. A luminal amebicide, diloxanide furoate or iodoquinol, should also be given to eradicate intestinal infection, whether or not organisms are found in the stools. If a satisfactory clinical response has not occurred within about 3 days, and especially if the abscess has been adequately drained, therapy should be changed to the alternative mode of treatment: dehydroemetine (or emetine) plus chloroquine. When the clinical response to metronidazole is adequate, it is suggested that a 2-week course of chloroquine follow to prevent late failures. The need for adding this course of chloroquine remains to be documented. Antibiotics are added only when there is associated bacterial infection, which is rare. Metronidazole has an advantage in that it is highly effective against anaerobic bacteria, a major cause of bacterial liver abscess.

E. Ameboma or Extraintestinal Forms of the Disease: Metronidazole is the drug of choice. Dehydroemetine (or emetine) is an alternative drug; chloroquine cannot be used because it does not reach high enough tissue concentrations to be effective (except in the liver). A simultaneous course of a luminal amebicide should also be given.

CHLOROQUINE

In the treatment of amebiasis, chloroquine is used both to eradicate and to prevent amebic liver abscess. Because chloroquine reaches high liver concentrations, it is highly effective in conjunction with dehydroemetine (or emetine) in the treatment of amebic liver abscess. In the prevention of liver abscess, chloroquine is used during the treatment of moderate to severe intestinal amebiasis (and in selected mild cases) to eradicate trophozoites carried to the liver or to treat undetected early abscesses there. The minimal dose needed to prevent an abscess is not well established, nor is the minimal indication for using chloroquine in abscess prevention, although invasive amebiasis as evidenced by mucosal ulceration is a specific indication. Chloroquine is not used, however, in the treatment of intestinal amebiasis, because the drug is not active against luminal organisms and shows only moderate activity in amebic dysentery. The pharmacology, cautions, contraindications, and side effects of chloroquine are described in the section on malaria. At the dosage levels used in treatment of amebiasis, the retinopathy sometimes associated with long-term use of chloroquine does not occur.

EMETINE & DEHYDROEMETINE

Emetine hydrochloride, used for more than 70 years in the treatment of amebiasis, continues to be used for the treatment of severe intestinal infection, liver abscess, and other forms of extraintestinal disease. Emetine should not be used to treat asymptomatic or mild intestinal infections.

When available, dehydroemetine rather than emetine should be used, since the former is equally effective and may be less toxic.

Chemistry

Emetine can be derived from ipecac or synthesized. Since emetine has 4 asymmetric centers, several stereoisomers are possible, but the structure below is generally accepted as the configuration of the natural (−) alkaloid. The H atoms shaded in the structure below are absent in dehydroemetine. Emetine is usually prepared as the hydrochloride. To prevent deterioration, it should be protected from light. Racemic 2-dehydroemetine dihydrochloride, available since 1964, is a synthetic substance.

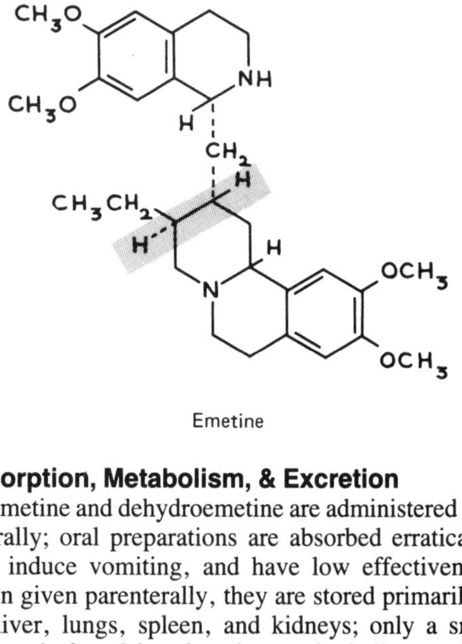

Emetine

Absorption, Metabolism, & Excretion

Emetine and dehydroemetine are administered parenterally; oral preparations are absorbed erratically, may induce vomiting, and have low effectiveness. When given parenterally, they are stored primarily in the liver, lungs, spleen, and kidneys; only a small amount is found in other tissues, including cardiac, striated, and intestinal muscle. Because they are eliminated slowly via the kidney, the drugs are cumulative; trace amounts are detectable in the urine 1–2 months after stopping therapy.

In laboratory animals, dehydroemetine disappears more rapidly from the heart (but not from the liver) than emetine and is excreted more rapidly. If this also occurs in humans, it could account for the fewer electrocardiographic changes that dehydroemetine causes when identical doses of the 2 drugs are given as reported in some studies. However, Sharad and Vakil reported comparable cardiovascular toxicity for the 2 drugs (see references). Thus, greater comparative clinical experience is needed to determine whether dehydroemetine is indeed less toxic.

Pharmacologic Effects

Emetine and dehydroemetine affect almost all tissues. They irreversibly block the synthesis of protein in eukaryotes by inhibiting the movement of the ribosome along messenger RNA; DNA synthesis is blocked secondarily. In experimental animals, emetine given parenterally in toxic doses causes cellular damage in the liver, kidneys, and skeletal and cardiac muscle. In the myocardium, cloudy swelling and necrosis of myocardial fibers occur, with focal areas of cellular infiltration and interstitial proliferation resembling Aschoff bodies. Cardiac conduction and contraction are depressed, which may result in a variety of atrial and ventricular arrhythmias, cardiac dilatation, and death.

In vitro, emetine has adrenoceptor- and cholinoceptor-blocking actions. The antiadrenoceptor action of the drug in vivo may be responsible for the hypotension that frequently accompanies its use. The nausea and vomiting common during therapy are considered central in origin. Emetine may reduce serum potassium levels in some patients. Elevated transaminase levels sometimes occur, but they do not correlate well with clinical or electrocardiographic findings.

Antiamebic Effects

In therapeutic dosages, these drugs act only against trophozoites, on which they have a direct lethal action. At high doses (beyond those tolerated by humans), the drugs may be active against cysts.

Clinical Uses

A. Severe Intestinal Disease (Amebic Dysentery): Parenterally administered emetine and dehydroemetine rapidly alleviate severe intestinal symptoms but are rarely curative even if a full course is given. For this reason and because of their toxicity, they should be given for the minimum period needed to relieve severe symptoms (usually 3–5 days). Marked toxicity is unlikely when the drugs are used for less than 7 days.

In addition to a short course of emetine or dehydroemetine, the regimen for severe intestinal amebiasis includes a tetracycline and diloxanide furoate or iodoquinol. These are followed by a course of chloroquine.

B. Amebic Liver Abscess: Emetine or dehydroemetine plus chloroquine is an alternative treatment for amebic liver abscess. A course of diloxanide furoate or iodoquinol should follow.

C. Amebomas and Extraintestinal Amebiasis: Emetine and dehydroemetine are effective in treating other forms of extraintestinal amebiasis and amebomas.

D. Other Parasites: Emetine and dehydroemetine have occasionally been useful in the treatment of infections with *Balantidium coli, Fasciola hepatica,* and *Paragonimus westermani,* but safer drugs should be used first.

Adverse Reactions

Emetine and dehydroemetine are cumulative in their toxic action. Few and (usually) mild side effects appear if the drugs are given for 3–5 days; additional mild to severe side effects appear if they are given for up to 10 days; serious toxicity is common if they are given for more than 10 days. Therefore, use of these drugs for more than 10 days is contraindicated. No fatalities have been reported after a single dose. Of the small number of deaths that have resulted from repeated doses of emetine, most were in patients given total doses of over 1200 mg; however, a few deaths occurred when the total dose did not exceed the recommended limit of 650 mg over 10 days.

A. Local Reactions: Pain, tenderness, and muscle weakness in the area of the injection are frequent, often starting 24–48 hours after the injection, and may persist for 1–2 weeks. Occasionally, eczematous or purpuric lesions or sterile abscesses develop.

B. Gastrointestinal Effects: Transient nausea occurs in about 30% of patients; vomiting is infrequent. Diarrhea is induced or exacerbated in many patients, generally beginning several days after the onset of therapy. A course of treatment can usually be completed in spite of gastrointestinal symptoms, but if these are too severe, therapy must be discontinued.

C. Cardiovascular Effects: Minor electrocardiographic changes occur frequently, but severe cardiac toxicity with significant conduction defects is rare. The most serious symptoms and findings are tachycardia and other arrhythmias, precordial pain, and congestive heart failure with dyspnea and hypotension. Electrocardiographic changes induced in more than 50% of patients include flattening and inversion of P and T waves, lengthening of the PR and QT intervals, ST elevation, premature beats, and transient atrial fibrillation. These changes usually appear about 7 days after the onset of treatment but occasionally not until 2–3 weeks after the last injection. They are generally reversible, requiring about 6 weeks to return to normal. In rare instances, emetine-induced abnormalities have persisted for several years.

D. Neuromuscular Effects: Generalized muscular weakness—sometimes associated with tenderness, stiffness, aching, or tremors—is reported by many patients. At therapeutic doses, the weakness is usually mild and reversible, but it may persist for several weeks after treatment is stopped. These symptoms are attributed to a direct action of these drugs on the muscles and not to neuritis. Although mild paresthesias are reported by patients, a true polyneuritis with objective signs of nerve damage occurs rarely.

E. Other Side Effects: Many other mild and often transient side effects may occur, including fatigue, headache, dizziness, and urticarial, eczematous, or purpuric skin lesions. Proteinuria may also be present.

Contraindications & Cautions

Hospitalization with careful supervision is essential. Considerable caution should be observed to avoid dangerous inadvertent intravenous administration. Patients should be kept at bed rest with bathroom privileges during treatment and for several days afterward. They should be examined daily for cardiovascular, neuromuscular, and gastrointestinal signs or symptoms. Pulse and blood pressure should be recorded 3 times a day and ECGs taken prior to the first injection, on the fifth and tenth days of therapy, and weekly for 2 weeks after the last injection.

Emetine and dehydroemetine should not be used in patients with cardiac or renal disease, in those with a recent history of polyneuritis, or in young children, unless alternative drugs have not been effective in controlling severe dysentery or liver abscess. They should also not be used during pregnancy.

Preparations & Dosages

Aqueous solutions of emetine hydrochloride are supplied in ampules containing 32 or 65 mg. Dehydroemetine is available in ampules of 30 or 60 mg.

The daily dose of both drugs for adults and children is 1 mg/kg subcutaneously (preferred) or intramuscularly. For children and some adults, the daily dose is divided into 2 parts. For emetine, the maximum daily dose for adults is 65 mg; for children under 8 years, 10 mg. For dehydroemetine, the maximum daily dose is 90 mg.

For the treatment of severe intestinal disease, injections are generally given for the minimum number of days needed to control severe symptoms, generally 3–5 days. See Table 56–2 for additional drugs needed to complete the course of therapy.

For the treatment of hepatic abscess, other extraintestinal disease, and ameboma, the same doses are used but for a total of 8–10 days.

If a second course of therapy is needed, an intervening period of 6–8 weeks is required.

DILOXANIDE FUROATE

Diloxanide furoate (Furamide) was introduced in 1957 and has since been extensively used outside the USA for the treatment of intestinal amebiasis. Although sufficient comparative studies are not available, the effectiveness of diloxanide is apparently not appreciably different from that of the other luminal amebicides—iodoquinol and paromomycin—but it causes the fewest side effects of the 3. Diloxanide furoate is not effective in the treatment of extraintestinal amebiasis.

Chemistry

Diloxanide is a dichloroacetamide derivative. It is tasteless and nearly insoluble in water. For stability, it should be protected from light.

Diloxanide

Pharmacology & Anthelmintic Action

Diloxanide is directly amebicidal, but its mode of action is not known. The drug has few effects in vertebrates but at very high doses has caused abortion in experimental animals. No teratogenic effects were observed.

Absorption, Metabolism, & Excretion

In the gut, diloxanide furoate is split into diloxanide and furoic acid; about 90% of the diloxanide is rapidly absorbed and then conjugated to form the glucuronide. The glucuronide reaches a peak blood level within about 1 hour, drops to low levels within 6 hours, and is rapidly excreted in the urine. The unabsorbed diloxanide is the active antiamebic substance and is not attacked by gut bacteria.

Clinical Uses

A. Asymptomatic and Mild Intestinal Amebiasis: Diloxanide furoate used alone is the drug of choice in asymptomatic infections. For the treatment of mild intestinal disease, it is used with other drugs as shown in Table 56–2. It is not clear if diloxanide used in conjunction with a tetracycline is more effective than when used alone. When diloxanide was combined with metronidazole, cure rates as high as 98% were reported.

B. Other Forms of Amebiasis: Diloxanide furoate is less effective in moderate to severe intestinal amebiasis. In the treatment of liver abscess, the drug is used to eradicate intestinal infection.

Adverse Reactions, Contraindications, & Cautions

Diloxanide furoate is free of serious side effects. Flatulence is common. Nausea and abdominal cramps are infrequent. Esophagitis, dryness of the mouth, vomiting, persistent diarrhea, pruritus, urticaria, proteinuria, and a vague tingling sensation are rarely reported.

The drug should not be used in pregnancy or administered to children under 2 years of age.

Preparations & Dosages

Diloxanide furoate (Furamide) is supplied as 500-mg tablets. See Table 56–2 for dosage. A course of treatment may be repeated in several weeks if necessary.

OTHER DICHLOROACETAMIDE DERIVATIVES

Teclozan (Falmonox; provided as 500-mg tablets) or **etofamide (Kitnos;** provided as 500-mg tablets) is given to adults at a dosage of 500 mg 3 times daily for 10 days; children are given 20 mg/kg in 3 divided doses daily for 10 days. The drugs are given after meals. These drugs are not available in the USA.

THE HALOGENATED HYDROXYQUINOLINES

Iodoquinol (diiodohydroxyquin) and clioquinol (iodochlorhydroxyquin), introduced in 1936 and 1931, respectively, are effective against organisms in the bowel lumen but not against trophozoites in the intestinal wall or extraintestinal tissues.

Chemistry

These 2 drugs are synthetic halogen-substituted 8-hydroxyquinolines—clioquinol (iodochlorhydroxyquin) (5-chloro-8-hydroxy-7-iodoquinoline) and iodoquinol (diiodohydroxyquin) (8-hydroxy-5,7-diiodoquinoline)—have had extensive clinical use. Clioquinol contains approximately 40% iodine and 12% chlorine, and iodoquinol contains approximately 64% iodine.

Clioquinol
Iodoquinol

Absorption, Metabolism, & Excretion

Knowledge is incomplete on the pharmacokinetics of the hydroxyquinolines. Clioquinol is more readily absorbed than iodoquinol. Metabolic studies in humans indicated an apparent half-life of between 11 and 14 hours.

The drugs may interfere with certain thyroid function tests by increasing protein-bound serum iodine levels, leading to a decrease in ^{131}I uptake.

Antiamebic Effects

The mechanism of action of iodoquinol and clioquinol against trophozoites is not known.

Clinical Uses

A. Intestinal Amebiasis: Iodoquinol and clioquinol are alternative drugs for the treatment of asymptomatic or mild to moderate intestinal amebiasis. However, until the question of the association of clioquinol with the SMON syndrome (see below) is resolved, only iodoquinol should be used in therapy. The drugs are not effective in the initial treatment of severe intestinal disease but are used in the subsequent eradication of the infection. They are not effective against amebomas or extraintestinal forms of the disease, including hepatic amebiasis, but are used in the eradication of concurrent intestinal infection.

B. _Trichomonas vaginalis_ Vaginitis: Clioquinol, given in vaginal inserts or insufflation powders, has been used for the topical treatment of this infection.

C. Other Intestinal Parasites: Iodoquinol (650 mg 3 times daily for 10 days) when used alone or in conjunction with a tetracycline (250 mg 4 times daily for 7 days) provides adequate treatment for _Dientamoeba fragilis_ infections. Iodoquinol has been reported also to be effective in the treatment of some cases of _Giardia lamblia_ and _B coli_ infection.

D. Travelers' Diarrhea and Nonspecific Diarrhea: Neither drug should be used in the prophylaxis or treatment of travelers' diarrhea or for the treatment of chronic nonspecific diarrhea in children and adults.

Adverse Reactions

The halogenated hydroxyquinolines can produce severe neurotoxicity, particularly if the drugs are given at greater than recommended doses and for long periods of time. The principal findings associated with this level of use are optic atrophy, visual loss, and peripheral neuropathy. Although these adverse reactions usually improve when the drug is discontinued, some patients have experienced irreversible neurologic damage.

Iodoquinol has not been implicated in producing neurotoxic side effects when used at the standard dosage of 650 mg 3 times daily for 21 days. Mild and infrequent side effects at the standard dosage include diarrhea, which usually stops after several days, and nausea and vomiting, gastritis, abdominal discomfort, constipation, pruritus ani, headache, malaise, and slight enlargement of the thyroid gland. Rarely reported side effects have been agranulocytosis, discoloration of hair or nails, hair loss, and iodine sensitivity characterized by furunculosis, chills, fever, and a variety of mild to severe skin reactions. Iodoquinol may be more toxic for infants and young children.

Clioquinol was considered nearly free of significant side effects at the standard dosage (250 mg 3 times daily for 10 days) until the question arose—as yet unresolved—about the drug's etiologic relationship to the SMON syndrome (described below). Infrequent side effects from clioquinol are the same as described for iodoquinol. The risk of neurotoxicity, however, appears to be greater and to increase with increasing dosage. At dosages of 750–1500 mg/d for less than 2 weeks, about 1% of patients had neurotoxic symptoms; at the same dosages given for over 2 weeks, symptoms appeared in approximately 35% of patients.

Controversy continues about whether a serious neurologic disease reported from Japan was due to the widespread use there of clioquinol, to a newly isolated virus, or to other factors. The syndrome is subacute myelo-optic neuropathy (SMON), characterized by chronic abdominal symptoms, peripheral polyneuritis with dysesthesia and weakness in the lower extremities, optic atrophy, and disturbances of vision. Evidence for the association of the drug with the disease included retrospective studies, animal experimental studies, the improvement of symptoms in individual patients when use of the drug was stopped, and the abrupt cessation of the epidemic with withdrawal of hydroxyquinoline drugs from the market. It is not yet possible to reach a conclusion about the cause of SMON syndrome or the risk to be attributed to the use of clioquinol. In the USA and many other countries, the drug has been withdrawn from the market because of its potential toxicity.

Contraindications & Cautions

The halogenated hydroxyquinolines should not be used for the prophylaxis or treatment of travelers' diarrhea or nonspecific diarrhea. Worldwide the drugs should be made available only on a prescription basis. When used for the treatment of amebiasis, they should be taken for the prescribed period of time and dosage.

The drugs should be discontinued when they produce a persistent diarrhea or signs of iodine reactions. They are contraindicated in patients with known intolerance to iodine, in renal and thyroid disease, and probably in severe liver disease not due to amebiasis.

When the drugs are used for young children, careful ophthalmologic assessment should be made before and during the course of therapy.

Preparations & Dosages

Iodoquinol (diiodohydroxyquin; Embequin, Lanodoxin, Savorquin, Sebaquin, Yodoxin) is available as uncoated 210-mg or 650-mg tablets. The drug is taken orally after meals. A course of treatment should not be repeated without an intervening period of 2–3 weeks.

THE ARSENICALS

The pentavalent arsenical drugs carbarsone and glycobiarsol have been used for many years for the treatment of amebiasis, but their potential toxicity no longer warrants their inclusion as alternative drugs for the treatment of intestinal infections.

The side effects of glycobiarsol and carbarsone are due to arsenical reactions. Although infrequent, the most common signs and symptoms are nausea and vomiting, diarrhea, epigastric distress, and skin rashes, which start after several days of therapy. More severe toxicity includes weight loss and polyuria. Exfoliative dermatitis, agranulocytosis, encephalitis, and hepatitis are very rare; a few fatalities have been reported.

METRONIDAZOLE

Metronidazole (Flagyl), introduced in 1959 for the treatment of trichomoniasis, was approved in the USA in 1971 for the treatment of amebiasis. Metronidazole is an excellent drug for the eradication of amebic tissue infections (liver abscess, intestinal wall and extraintestinal infections), but it requires the concomitant use of a luminal amebicide to achieve satisfactory

cure rates for luminal infections. Metronidazole kills trophozoites but does not kill cysts of *E histolytica*.

Metronidazole has been reported to increase the incidence of certain naturally occurring tumors in mice and rats given high doses over long periods of time and to induce mutagenic changes in bacterial test systems (see p 638). Metronidazole has not been shown to be teratogenic in animals or humans, but the data are not sufficient to rule this out. Overall, it appears prudent to judge metronidazole as a potentially hazardous drug.

The chemistry, pharmacokinetics, adverse reactions, and contraindications and cautions of this drug are described on pp 637–639.

Clinical Uses

Metronidazole is considered the drug of choice (in combination with other amebicides) in all symptomatic forms of amebiasis.

OTHER NITROIMIDAZOLES

Other nitroimidazole derivatives include tinidazole, nimorazole, secondizole, and ornidazole. They have similar side effects and the same mutagenic action in the *Salmonella* test systems as metronidazole. Because of its short half-life, metronidazole must be administered every 8 hours; the other drugs can be administered at longer intervals. However, with the exception of tinidazole, the other nitroimidazoles have given poorer results in the treatment of amebiasis than metronidazole.

PAROMOMYCIN SULFATE

Paromomycin sulfate (Humatin), a broad-spectrum antibiotic, is an alternative drug in the treatment of symptomatic and mild intestinal amebiasis and tapeworm infections. It is an aminoglycoside derived from *Streptomyces rimosus* and is closely related to neomycin, kanamycin, and streptomycin in properties and structure. Paromomycin is directly amebicidal in addition to its indirect effect through the inhibition of normal bacteria.

Because paromomycin is not significantly absorbed from the gastrointestinal tract, it can only be used as a luminal amebicide and has no effect in extraintestinal amebic infections. The small amount absorbed is excreted slowly and unchanged, mainly by glomerular filtration; some excretion also occurs in the bile. In the presence of ulcerative lesions of the bowel, however, and perhaps with impaired gastrointestinal motility, increased absorption may occur. In renal insufficiency, the drug may accumulate and reach a toxic level.

Mild gastrointestinal side effects are not uncommon. The number of stools increases; diarrhea, sometimes intense, has been reported in up to 16% of patients. Less frequent are anorexia, nausea and vomiting, epigastric pain, abdominal cramps, and pruritus ani. Other occasional side effects are headache, dizziness, rashes, and arthralgia. Paromomycin can cause malabsorption as well as overgrowth of nonsusceptible organisms, particularly fungi. The aminoglycosides as a group can be ototoxic (auditory and vestibular) and nephrotoxic as a result of unexpected absorption; theoretically, paromomycin has similar potential, but such reactions have apparently not been reported.

Paromomycin is supplied in 250-mg capsules and as syrup containing 125 mg/ 5 mL.

OTHER ANTIBIOTICS

Although the tetracyclines have very weak direct amebicidal action, through their effects on the gut flora they (especially oxytetracycline) are useful in conjunction with a luminal amebicide in the eradication of mild to severe intestinal disease. However, because of their potential toxicity, the tetracyclines should not be used during pregnancy or in the treatment of children under 8 years of age; when an antibiotic is needed in the treatment of amebiasis for these patients, erythromycin stearate, although somewhat less effective, can be used instead.

THE TREATMENT OF LEISHMANIASIS

Leishmaniasis includes a variety of diseases produced by protozoal parasites of the genus *Leishmania* of the family Trypanosomidae. They are transmitted to humans by the bite of several different species of phlebotomine (flesh-eating) flies, which carry the parasites directly from human to human or from infected rodents or canines to humans. Different varieties of *Leishmania* produce different lesions and require different treatments. The diseases produced by *Leishmania tropica* and *Leishmania mexicana* are characterized by cutaneous lesions only, which usually undergo spontaneous recovery. Infection with *Leishmania braziliensis* (mucocutaneous leishmaniasis) causes large destructive ulcers of the mucous membranes that rarely undergo spontaneous recovery. *Leishmania donovani* (visceral leishmaniasis, dumdum fever, tropical splenomegaly, black sickness, ponos) produces a small primary sore, often ignored, followed by hematogenous spread, causing massive enlargement of the spleen and often of the liver and recurring bouts of fever resembling brucellosis. Disease caused by *L donovani* requires hospitalization, correction of the accompanying malnutrition, and specific drug therapy (the choice of drug depending on the geographic location where the disease was encountered) with one or a combination of pentavalent antimonials and one of the aromatic diamidines.

SODIUM STIBOGLUCONATE

The standard therapy for visceral leishmaniasis is a **pentavalent antimony** compound, sodium stibogluconate, in which 2 atoms of antimony are complexed with 2 molecules of gluconate. The drug may kill the parasite by inhibiting aerobic glycosides or by binding to DNA and RNA.

The usual course of treatment with sodium stibogluconate (Pentostam) is 4 mg/kg intramuscularly daily for 10–15 days. The drug is also used in other types of leishmaniasis, but its effectiveness is not as well established in these conditions as in the visceral form. In the USA, sodium stibogluconate is available only from the Parasitic Disease Drug Service, Centers for Disease Control, Atlanta 30333.

OTHER DRUGS USED FOR THE TREATMENT OF LEISHMANIASIS

Amphotericin B (Fungizone), 25–50 mg in 500 mL of 5% glucose-saline solution, given by slow intravenous drip on alternate days for periods of weeks and even months, has led to complete healing of lesions of mucocutaneous leishmaniasis that were resistant to antimony therapy.

The suggested daily dose of amphotericin B is 0.25–1 mg/kg. (For toxicity, see Chapter 48.) Amphotericin B may be more potent as a leishmanicide than the antimonials.

Cures of *L braziliensis* and *L tropica* infections have also been obtained with intramuscular injections of the antimalarial repository drug **cycloguanil embonate** (cycloguanil pamoate), an insoluble salt of the dihydrotriazine metabolite of chloroguanide (proguanil). One or 2 intramuscular injections of 350 mg (2.5 mL) of the base have given cure rates of up to 85%.

Oral **dehydroemetine resinate (Mebadin)** in doses of 1.5 mg/kg orally after meals (to a total dose of 0.85–7 g) gave a 70% cure rate of *L tropica* infections in a study carried out in Iraq.

Metronidazole (Flagyl), 250 mg twice daily orally for 15 days, has produced an excellent cure rate of Mexican cutaneous leishmaniasis.

Allopurinol (Zyloprim) has recently been reported to be effective, alone or in combination with sodium stibogluconate, in cases of *L donovani* infections resistant to traditional therapy. This drug and other purine analogs are converted to toxic metabolites in the parasite but not in mammals (Chapter 55). Because allopurinol is essentially nontoxic in humans, this approach appears quite promising.

Nifurtimox (Lampit), a nitrofurazone derivative now used to destroy the extracellular trypanosomes in trypanosomiasis, has also been successfully used to treat mucocutaneous leishmaniasis in doses of 8–10 mg/kg daily for 3–5 weeks.

THE TREATMENT OF TRYPANOSOMIASIS

THE AROMATIC DIAMIDINES: PENTAMIDINE, STILBAMIDINE, & PROPAMIDINE

Pentamidine, stilbamidine, and propamidine are the only aromatic diamidine derivatives that are sufficiently potent as trypanosomicides and have toxicities low enough to be used for the treatment of trypanosomiasis (sleeping sickness).

Chemistry

Pentamidine is available as the isethionate (Pentam 300, M&B 800) and the methanesulfonate (Lomidine) salts. They are white, hygroscopic, crystalline powders soluble 1:10 in water.

The in vitro trypanosomicidal activity of the guanidine derivatives is associated with the terminal amidine and guanidine groups, and the activity is maximal when the amidine groups are connected by an undecane methylene chain.

Absorption, Metabolism, & Excretion

Diamidine compounds are not well absorbed from the gastrointestinal tract, but absorption after parenteral administration is satisfactory. Following intravenous injection, the drug rapidly leaves the circulation and only small amounts appear in the urine. The liver, spleen, kidneys, and adrenals maintain high levels of the diamidines for months after treatment. Single injections of pentamidine can prevent infection by *Trypanosoma brucei gambiense* for up to 6 months. A portion of the drug is metabolized in the body, and part is excreted in the urine. Intermediary metabolic products are not known.

Diamidine compounds cross the placenta but are not excreted in milk. Only trace amounts appear in the central nervous system, so that other trypanosomicides such as tryparsamide or one of the melanyl arsenicals must be used for the treatment of late stages of African trypanosomiasis with central nervous system involvement.

Pharmacologic Effects

The aromatic diamidines are highly toxic to certain species of protozoa and only slightly toxic to others. *Trypanosoma brucei rhodesiense* and *T b gambiense* infections in humans can be cured with pentamidine, but the drug has no effect on *Trypanosoma cruzi* infection in mice. The diamidines have some plasmodicidal, bactericidal, and fungicidal activity and have been used for the treatment of systemic blastomycosis.

Intravenous injections of the diamidines produce a sharp fall of blood pressure that can be only partially blocked by atropine. The peripheral vasodilatation is probably due to a release of tissue-bound histamine and peripheral adrenergic blockade.

After injection of a diamidine drug, the trypanosomes quickly take up the drug to a concentration about 1400 times that of the surrounding tissues. Trypanosomicidal effects appear only after a long latent period. The trypanosomicidal action of the diamidines is antagonized by glucose, and the addition of insulin to cultures slows trypanosome multiplication. Diamidines may interfere with glycolysis in susceptible protozoa (Chapter 55). There is also evidence that the diamidines may bind to DNA.

Clinical Uses

Pentamidine is the drug of choice for the prevention and treatment of *T b gambiense* infections. In the early stages, pentamidine can clear the organisms from the blood and lymph nodes. Diamidines cannot be given intrathecally and do not reach the central nervous system in sufficient quantities to have any therapeutic effect. Thus, other drugs such as melarsoprol or suramin must be used. In early trypanosomiasis, propamidine and stilbamidine can also be employed.

The diamidines are also used for visceral leishmaniasis (kala-azar) in patients who do not respond to or cannot tolerate antimonials.

Pentamidine is also used in the treatment of *Pneumocystis carinii* pneumonia, a protozoal infection usually associated with immunologic impairment such as the acquired immunodeficiency syndrome (AIDS).

Adverse Reactions

The diamidines may result in initial respiratory stimulation followed by respiratory depression. Intravenous injections usually produce a fall in blood pressure, dizziness, and headache together with breathlessness, tachycardia, and vomiting. Respiratory failure and death occur rarely.

The diamidines are nephrotoxic and occasionally neurotoxic, causing nystagmus, ataxia, convulsions, and death.

Delayed toxicity of stilbamidine (but not pentamidine) consists of paralysis of the trigeminal nerve and other peripheral neuropathies.

Preparations & Dosages

Pentamidine is available in the USA as the isethionate salt.

Pentamidine

For the early stages of *T b rhodesiense* and *T b gambiense* infections, pentamidine, 4 mg/kg intramuscularly, is given every 1–2 days for 10 doses. For chemoprophylaxis, give 3 mg/kg intramuscularly every 3–6 months.

For *L donovani* infections (kala-azar, visceral leishmaniasis), give pentamidine, 2–4 mg/kg intravenously or intramuscularly daily for up to 15 days.

For the late central nervous system stages of *T b rhodesiense* and *T b gambiense* infections, melarsoprol must be given.

For *P carinii* infections in patients who have failed to respond to trimethoprim and sulfamethoxazole or are unable to tolerate sulfonamides, pentamidine isethionate may be given intramuscularly in a dose of 4 mg (salt)/kg for 12–14 days.

MELARSOPROL

Melarsoprol (Mel B) is an organic arsenical, formed by condensing a toxic trivalent arsenical trypanosomicide (melarsen oxide) with an arsenic antagonist (BAL [dimercaprol]). In the product, the trypanosomicidal activity is retained while the toxicity of arsenic is mitigated. Its mode of action is probably related to an interaction with the sulfhydryl groups of enzymes essential to trypanosome metabolism.

Absorption, Metabolism, & Excretion

Melarsoprol is well absorbed from the gastrointestinal tract, but it is given only intravenously. The drug is quickly excreted.

Clinical Uses

Melarsoprol has now replaced tryparsamide (a pentavalent arsenical) as the drug of choice for the treatment of *T b gambiense* infection with CNS involvement. Tryparsamide, used for 50 years to control epidemics of trypanosomiasis, had an unfortunate tendency to cause optic atrophy.

Unlike pentamidine, melarsoprol appears in the cerebrospinal fluid in sufficient amounts to exert a trypanosomicidal effect on the late meningoencephalitic stages of human trypanosomiasis. It is also effective in the earlier stages of the disease, but it is used only for the rare pentamidine-refractory cases.

Adverse Effects

The most serious side effect of melarsoprol therapy, usually occurring at the end of the first week of therapy, is a reactive encephalopathy that may be fatal. Patients in the most advanced stages of the disease are most severely affected.

If the intravenous injections are given too fast, vomiting and colicky abdominal pains occur.

Hypersensitivity reactions can be relieved with corticosteroids.

Preparations & Dosages

Melarsoprol (Mel B) is available for intravenous injection as a solution containing 3.6% (w/v) in propylene glycol. For the therapy of the late stages of *T b rhodesiense* and *T b gambiense* infections, three 3-day courses are given with an interval of 7 days between courses. Daily injections of 90 mg are given very slowly for the first 3 days; 90–180 mg for the second 3-day course; and 180 mg for the last 3-day course.

Leakage at injection sites causes intense pain and sometimes sloughing.

In the USA, melarsoprol is available only from the Centers for Disease Control, Atlanta 30333.

OTHER TRYPANOSOMICIDAL DRUGS

Alpha-difluoromethylornithine has shown excellent trypanosomicidal activity against animal trypanosomiasis (see also Chapter 55). A recent clinical trial appears to confirm this finding (see Sjoerdsma reference). Furthermore, the compound appears to have activity against *P carinii* infections in patients with acquired immunodeficiency syndrome (AIDS).

Nifurtimox (Bayer 2502, Lampit), a nitrofurazone derivative, is the drug of choice for acute Chagas' disease *(T cruzi)*. However, serious allergic skin reactions, gastrointestinal disturbances, and neurologic toxicities are frequently noted. In chronic forms of Chagas' disease, the toxicity may outweigh the drug's usefulness. Nifurtimox may be obtained from the Centers for Disease Control, Atlanta 30333.

Suramin sodium (Bayer 205, Belganyl, Germanin, Naphuride), an organic urea compound available in the USA only from the Centers for Disease Control, is the drug of choice for the early stages of African trypanosomiasis before there is any central nervous system involvement. It is also the drug of choice for the adult forms of the filarial parasite *Onchocerca volvulus* (see Chapter 57). It is of no value in the treatment of Chagas' disease.

TREATMENT OF TRICHOMONIASIS & GIARDIASIS

METRONIDAZOLE

Metronidazole (Flagyl) is the result of a search for an effective trichomonicidal agent by French workers in the 1950s. It has become the drug of choice for *T vaginalis* infection in females and for the asymptomatic carrier state in males. It is also the drug of choice for treatment of intestinal infections with *G lamblia*, another motile protozoon.

Chemistry & Pharmacokinetics

Metronidazole is a low-molecular-weight compound that is un-ionized at physiologic pH. Eighty percent of the oral dose is absorbed within 1 hour.

Food intake does not influence its bioavailablity, and the half-life of the unchanged drug is 7 1/2 hours. Impaired renal function does not prolong the half-life, but impaired hepatic function may do so. Peak plasma concentrations are not achieved until 5–12 hours after administration by rectal suppository. Protein binding is minimal.

Metronidazole

Because of its small molecular size, metronidazole permeates all the tissues and fluids of the body, including cerebrospinal fluid and alveolar bone, and the intracellular concentration rapidly approaches extracellular concentrations. Entry into the cell is by simple diffusion and does not require active transport.

Mechanism of Action

Within anaerobic bacteria and sensitive protozoal cells, the nitro group of metronidazole is chemically reduced by ferredoxin (or ferredoxin-linked metabolic processes), and the reduction products appear to be responsible for killing the cell by reacting with various intracellular macromolecules. Thus, reduction is the driving force for the selective toxicity in anaerobic cells. Metronidazole is actively bactericidal (not bacteriostatic) in susceptible organisms. Metronidazole's narrow spectrum of activity, largely limited to anaerobic bacteria and certain protozoa, does not encourage the overgrowth of antibiotic-resistant aerobes or facultative anaerobes and should not facilitate the transmission of drug-resistance factors. However, there is some evidence for an additional aerobic antibacterial effect in mixed anaerobic/aerobic infections. Severe vaginitis caused by *Gardnerella (Haemophilus) vaginalis* (an aerobic bacterium) is clinically improved by treatment with metronidazole when other antibiotics have failed.

Metronidazole also has a radiosensitizing effect on tumor cells. This effect has been demonstrated in vitro and in rodents in vivo. As with its antibacterial action, the mechanism of action appears to be dependent on relative hypoxia in the target cells and may involve interaction with free radicals.

Clinical Uses

A. Urogenital Trichomoniasis: The treatment of choice is metronidazole, 250 mg orally 3 times a day for 7 days. A single dose of 2 g (8 tablets) is also effective. The sexual partner should be treated simultaneously. In pregnancy, treatment with metronidazole should be delayed until after the first trimester. Metronidazole-resistant strains of *T vaginalis* have been described.

B. Giardiasis: The adult dosage of metronidazole is 250 mg orally 3 times a day for 7 days. Children should receive 5 mg/kg 3 times a day for 5 days.

C. Amebiasis: See p 634.

D. Balantidiasis: If tetracycline is ineffective, give metronidazole, 750 mg 3 times a day for 7 days.

E. *Gardnerella vaginalis:* (Previously called *Corynebacterium vaginale* or *Haemophilus vaginalis*.) In refractory infections only, give metronidazole, 500 mg orally twice a day for 5 days.

F. Anaerobic Infections: Metronidazole has been reported to reduce postoperative anaerobic infections following procedures such as appendectomy, colorectal surgery, and abdominal hysterectomy. Furthermore, serious anaerobic infections involving *Bacillus fragilis* and clostridia that are refractory to other agents may respond to metronidazole, in part because of its ability to penetrate abscesses and necrotic tissue.

G. Phagedenic Leg Ulcers, Acute Ulcerative Gingivitis, Cancrum Oris, Decubitus Ulcers, and Other Indolent Lesions: Metronidazole, 250 mg orally 4 times a day, together with a penicillin or sulfonamide and appropriate topical treatment, promotes healing and provides rapid relief of pain, inflammatory edema, and purulent discharge. Anaerobic cultures of pus from these lesions often reveal fusobacteria and gram-positive cocci in addition to *B fragilis*.

Toxicity

Minor side effects of metronidazole include a metallic taste, glossitis, oral candidiasis, nausea and vomiting, and headache. The urine may be dark or reddish-brown in color.

Serious toxic effects are very uncommon. However, neurotoxic effects—including dizziness and ataxia—and leukopenia have been reported. Both effects are fully reversible when the drug is withdrawn. Metronidazole also has a disulfiramlike effect, so that nausea and vomiting occur if alcohol is consumed while the drug is still in the body.

Mutagenicity & Carcinogenicity

Metronidazole and its metabolites recovered from the urine of patients taking the drug have been proved by in vitro assays to be mutagenic in certain strains of *Salmonella typhimurium* (Ames test). Chronic oral administration of very large doses to mice has produced a statistically significant increase in the number of lung and liver tumors. This effect has not been found in any nonrodent species. Although the drug has been used in humans for 20 years, no increase of congenital abnormalities, stillbirths, or low birth weight has been reported. Culture of human lymphocytes with metronidazole, up to 10,000 μg/mL, has revealed no toxic activity. No increase in frequency of chromosomal aberration was found in patients receiving large doses for the treatment of amebic hepatitis. Nevertheless, caution should be used in prescribing the drug over long periods.

Contraindications & Cautions

Prudence dictates that metronidazole should be used in pregnant or nursing women only on clear indications.

Drug Interactions

Metronidazole has been reported to potentiate the anticoagulant effect of coumarin-type anticoagulants. Its disulfiramlike effect requires that all patients receiving it should be specifically warned not to use alcohol. The SGOT test of liver function may be depressed, and patients with severe liver disease may accumulate the drug and its metabolites in the plasma.

Preparations & Dosages

Metronidazole (Flagyl) is available in 250-mg and 500-mg tablets for oral administration. Rectal suppositories are available outside the USA. The daily dose and the duration of treatment vary with the disease being treated (see above). Should re-treatment be needed, 4–6 weeks should be allowed between courses. Metronidazole hydrochloride for intravenous injection (Flagyl IV) is available in single-dose lyophilized vials containing 500 mg. The powder is reconstituted to produce an acidic solution with a pH of 0.5–2.0. The reconstituted solution should not be given by direct injection but must be further diluted and neutralized according to the manufacturer's instructions.

REFERENCES

MALARIA

General

CDC. Health information for international travel 1985. Atlanta, Georgia: Public Health Service, U.S. Department of Health and Human Services; publication no. (CDC) 85-8280.

CDC. Revised recommendations for preventing malaria in travelers to areas with chloroquine-resistant *P. falciparum. MMWR* 1985;**34:**185.

Chemoprophylaxis of malaria. *MMWR* (April 16) 1982; **31(Suppl):**35.

Cohen S (editor): Malaria. (Symposium.) *Br Med Bull* 1982; **38:**115.

Peters W: Chemotherapy of malaria. Pages 145–283 in: *Malaria.* Vol 1: *Epidemiology, Chemotherapy, Morphology and Metabolism.* Kreier JP (editor). Academic Press, 1980.

Peters W: New answers through chemotherapy? *Experientia* 1984;**40:**1351.

Revised recommendations for malaria chemoprophylaxis for travelers to East Africa. *MMWR* (June 25) 1982;**31:**328.

World Health Organization: *Advances in malarial chemotherapy.* Report of a WHO Scientific Group. Technical Report Series No. 711, 1984.

Wyler DJ: Malaria: Resurgence, resistance, and research. (2 parts.) *N Engl J Med* 1983;**308:**875, 934.

Quinine & Congeners

Hofheinz W, Merkli B: Quinine and quinine analogs. Chap 2, pp 61–81, in: *Handbook of Experimental Pharmacology,* Vol 68/II, 1984.

Phillips RE et al: Intravenous quinidine for the treatment of severe falciparum malaria: Clinical and pharmacokinetic studies. *N Engl J Med* 1985;**312:**1273.

Sheehy TW, Reba RC: Complications of falciparum malaria and their treatment. *Ann Intern Med* 1976;**66:**807.

Sweeney TR: Drugs with quinine-like action. Chap 9, pp 267–324, in: *Handbook of Experimental Pharmacology.* Vol 68/II, 1984.

Chloroquine & Congeners

Sweeney TR, Pick RO: 4-Aminoquinolines and Mannich bases. Chap 12, pp 363–385, in: *Handbook of Experimental Pharmacology.* Vol 68/II, 1984.

8-Aminoquinolines

Cahn MM, Levy EJ: The tolerance to large weekly doses of primaquine and amodiaquine in primaquine-sensitive and non-sensitive subjects. *Am J Trop Med Hyg* 1962;**11:**605.

Peters W: The possible role of primaquine in inducing multiple drug resistance in *Plasmodium falciparum. Trans R Soc Trop Med Hyg* 1966;**60:**140.

Proguanil, Pyrimethamine, & Trimethoprim

Bushby SRM, Hitchings GH: Trimethoprim, a sulphonamide potentiator. *Br J Pharmacol* 1968;**33:**72.

Laing ABG: Treatment of acute falciparum malaria with sulphorthodimethoxine (Fanasil). *Br Med J* 1965;**1:**905.

Pearlman EJ, Hall AP: Prevention of chloroquine-resistant falciparum malaria. (Correspondence.) *Ann Intern Med* 1975;**82:**590.

Qinghaosu

Klayman DL: Qinghaosu (artemisinin): An antimalarial drug from China. *Science* 1985;**228:**1049.

AMEBIASIS

General

Adams EB, MacLeod IN: Invasive amebiasis. 1. Amebic dysentery and its complications. *Medicine* 1977;**56:**315.

Adams EB, MacLeod IN: Invasive amebiasis. 2. Amebic liver abscess and its complications. *Medicine* 1977;**56:**325.

Harries J: Amoebiasis: A review. *J R Soc Med* 1982;**75:**190.

Juniper K: Amoebiasis. *Clin Gastroenterol* 1978;**7:**3.

Knight R: The chemotherapy of amoebiasis. *J Antimicrob Chemother* 1980;**6:**577.

Masters DK, Hopkins AD: Therapeutic trial of four amoebicide regimens in rural Zaire. *J Trop Med Hyg* 1979,**82:**99.

Wolfe MS: The treatment of intestinal protozoan infections. *Med Clin North Am* 1982;**66:**707.

Emetine & Dehydroemetine

Lister GD: Delayed myocardial intoxication following the administration of dehydroemetine hydrochloride. *J Trop Med Hyg* 1968;**71:**219.

Sharad CS, Vakil BJ: Cardiovascular toxicity of emetine and dehydroemetine. *Indian Pract* 1971;**24:**237.

Wilmot AJ, Powell SJ, Adams EB: Chloroquine compared

with chloroquine and emetine combined in amebic liver abscess. *Am J Trop Med Hyg* 1959;**8**:623.

Yang WCT, Dubick M: Mechanism of emetine cardiotoxicity. *Pharmacol Ther* 1980;**10**:15.

Diloxanide Furoate

Bell S: An investigation of carriers of *Entamoeba histolytica*. *Trans R Soc Trop Med Hyg* 1967;**61**:506.

Botero RD: Treatment of intestinal amoebiasis with diloxanide furoate, tetracycline and chloroquine. *Trans R Soc Trop Med Hyg* 1967;**61**:769.

Pehrson P, Bengtsson E: Treatment of noninvasive amoebiasis: A comparison between tinidazole alone and in combination with diloxanide furoate. *Trans R Soc Trop Med Hyg* 1983;**77**:845.

Wolfe MS: Nondysenteric intestinal amebiasis: Treatment with diloxanide furoate. *JAMA* 1973;**224**:1601.

Halogenated Hydroxyquinolines & Arsenicals

Committee on Drugs: Blindness and neuropathy from diiodohydroxyquin-like drugs. *Pediatrics* 1974;**54**:378.

Inoue YK: An avian-related new herpesvirus infection in man—subacute myelo-optico-neuropathy (SMON). *Prog Med Virol* 1976;**21**:35.

Jack DB, Riess W: Pharmacokinetics of iodochlorhydroxyquin in man. *J Pharm Sci* 1973;**62**:1929.

Oakley GP Jr: The neurotoxicity of the halogenated hydroxyquinolines. *JAMA* 1973;**225**:395.

Worden AN, Heywood R: Clioquinol toxicity. (Correspondence.) *Lancet* 1978;**1**:212.

Metronidazole & Tinidazole

Beard CM et al: Lack of evidence for cancer due to use of metronidazole. *N Engl J Med* 1979;**301**:519.

Edwards DI: Mechanisms of cytotoxicity of nitroimidazole drugs. *Prog Med Chem* 1981;**18**:88.

Finegold SM: Metronidazole. *Ann Intern Med* 1980;**93**:585.

Friedman GD: Cancer after metronidazole. (Letter.) *N Engl J Med* 1980;**302**:519.

Goldman P: Metronidazole. *N Engl J Med* 1980;**303**:1212.

Kanani SR, Knight R: Experiences with the use of metronidazole in the treatment of nondysenteric intestinal amoebiasis. *Trans R Soc Trop Med Hyg* 1972;**66**:244.

Metronidazole: Proceedings of the Second International Symposium on Anaerobic Infections. Geneva, 25–27 April, 1979. Royal Society of Medicine, Series 18, 1979.

Muller M: *Metronidazole: Its Action on Anaerobes*. Rockefeller Univ Press, 1980.

Nobel JI, Tally FP: Metronidazole. Pages 255–263 in: *Antimicrobial Therapy*. Ristuccia AM, Cunha BA (editors). Raven Press, 1984.

Powell SJ, Stewart-Wynne EJ, Elsdon-Dew R: Metronidazole combined with diloxanide furoate in amoebic liver abscess. *Ann Trop Med Parasitol* 1973;**67**:367.

Roe FJC: Toxicologic evaluation of metronidazole with particular reference to carcinogenic, mutagenic, and teratogenic potential. *Surgery* 1983;**93**:158.

Scragg JN, Proctor EM: Tinidazole treatment of acute amebic dysentery in children. *Am J Trop Med Hyg* 1977;**26**:824.

Paromomycin Sulfate

Courtney KO et al: Paromomycin as a therapeutic substance for intestinal amoebiasis and bacterial enteritis. *Ann Biochem Exper Med* 1960;**20(S)**:449.

Simon M et al: Paromomycin in the treatment of intestinal amebiasis: A short course of therapy. *Am J Gastroenterol* 1967;**48**:504.

Woolfe G: The chemotherapy of amoebiasis. *Prog Drug Res* 1965;**8**:13.

LEISHMANIASIS

Beltran HF, Gutierrez FM, Biagi FF: [Treatment of Mexican cutaneous leishmaniasis with metronidazole.] *Bull Soc Pathol Exot* 1967;**60**:61.

Berman JD, Webster HK: In vitro effect of mycophenolic acid and allopurinol against *Leishmania tropica* in human macrophages. *Antimicrob Agents Chemother* 1982;**21**:887.

Hassan Abd-Rabbo: Dehydroemetine in leishmaniasis (Oriental sore). *J Trop Med Hyg* 1966;**69**:171.

Kager PA et al: Allopurinol in the treatment of visceral leishmaniasis. *Trans R Soc Trop Med Hyg* 1981;**75**:556.

Marr JJ, Berens RL: Antileishmanial effect of allopurinol. 2. Relationship of adenine metabolism in *Leishmania* species to the action of allopurinol. *J Infect Dis* 1977;**136**:724.

Prata A: Treatment of kala-azar with amphotericin B. *Trans R Soc Trop Med Hyg* 1963;**57**:266.

Reinhard M, Wacker H: [Treatment of cutaneous leishmaniasis with cycloguanil pamoate.] *Dtsch Med Wochenschr* 1970;**95**:2380.

Salem HH et al: The treatment of cutaneous leishmaniasis with oral dehydroemetine. *Trans R Soc Trop Med Hyg* 1967;**61**:776.

TRYPANOSOMIASIS

Gutteridge WE: Existing chemotherapy and its limitations. *BR Med Bull* 1985;**41**:162.

Sjoerdsma A et al: Successful treatment of lethal protozoal infections with the ornithine decarboxylase inhibitor α-difluoromethylornithine. *Clin Res* 1984;**32**:559a.

Williamson J: Chemotherapy of African trypanosomiasis. *Trop Dis Bull* 1976;**73**:531.

TRICHOMONIASIS

Metronidazole

Baker RM, Kennan AL: Therapy of trichomoniasis. *Wis Med J* 1967;**66**:370.

Diddle AW: *Trichomonas vaginalis:* Resistance to metronidazole. *Am J Obstet Gynecol* 1967;**98**:583.

Is Flagyl dangerous? *Med Lett Drugs Ther* 1975;**17**:53.

McLoughlin DK: Drug tolerance by *Trichomonas foetus*. *J Parasitol* 1967;**53**:646.

Minnesota Department of Health: *Communicable Disease Newsletter* 2(9), (Nov) 1975.

Clinical Pharmacology of the Anthelmintic Drugs

57

Robert S. Goldsmith, MD, DTM&H

CHEMOTHERAPY OF HELMINTHIC INFECTIONS

Anthelmintic drugs are used to eradicate or reduce in numbers helminthic parasites in the intestinal tract or tissues of humans and other animals. As noted in Chapter 55, these parasites have many biochemical and physiologic processes in common with their mammalian hosts, yet there are subtle differences that are beginning to yield to pharmacologic investigation. Most of the drugs described below were discovered by traditional screening methods; their mechanisms have been clarified only recently. These mechanisms (where known) are described in Chapter 55.

Table 57–1 lists the major helminthic infections and provides a guide to the drug of choice and alternative drugs for each infection. In the text that follows, these drugs are arranged alphabetically.

Most anthelmintics in use today are active against specific parasites, and some are toxic. Therefore, parasites must be identified before treatment is started, usually by finding the parasite, eggs, or larvae in the feces, urine, blood, sputum, or tissues of the host.

Administration of Anthelmintic Drugs

Unless otherwise indicated, oral drugs should be taken with water during or after meals. If pre- or posttreatment purges are necessary in conjunction with a specific drug, magnesium or sodium sulfate, 0.2–0.4 g/kg, may be used. Magnesium sulfate must not be given to persons with impaired renal function, and sodium sulfate is contraindicated in patients with congestive heart failure. Other contraindications to severe purgation are signs of intestinal obstruction, debilitation, and pregnancy. In posttreatment follow-up for intestinal nematode infections, stools should be reexamined about 2 weeks after the end of treatment.

Dosages for Children

Dosages for infants and children are on a less secure basis than for adults; when not given in milligrams per kilogram of body weight (or otherwise specified), the dosage may be based on surface area or calculated as a fraction of the adult dose based on Clark's rule or Young's rule (see Chapter 63).

Contraindications

Pregnancy and ulcers of the gastrointestinal tract are contraindications for most of the drugs listed. Specific contraindications are given in the discussions that follow.

ALBENDAZOLE (Zental)

Albendazole, introduced in 1979 as a broad-spectrum oral anthelmintic, is undergoing clinical trials. The drug is used for pinworm infection, ascariasis, trichuriases, strongyloidiasis, and infections with both hookworm species.

Chemistry, Absorption, Metabolism, & Excretion

Albendazole is shown below. The compound is nearly insoluble in water.

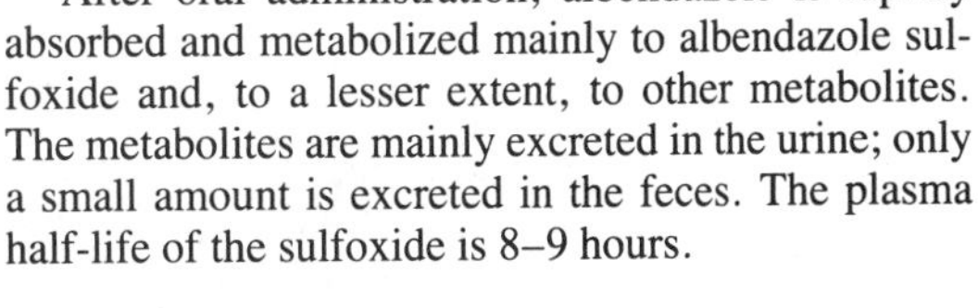

Albendazole

After oral administration, albendazole is rapidly absorbed and metabolized mainly to albendazole sulfoxide and, to a lesser extent, to other metabolites. The metabolites are mainly excreted in the urine; only a small amount is excreted in the feces. The plasma half-life of the sulfoxide is 8–9 hours.

Anthelmintic Actions & Pharmacologic Effects

A. Anthelmintic Actions: Albendazole blocks glucose uptake by larval and adult stages of susceptible parasites, depleting their glycogen stores and decreasing formation of ATP. As a result, the parasite is immobilized and dies. The drug has larvicidal effects in *Necator americanus* and ovicidal effects in ascariasis, ancylostomiasis, and trichuriasis.

B. Pharmacologic Effects: Based on most experimental animal studies, albendazole is not expected to have pharmacologic effects in humans at therapeu-

Table 57–1. Drugs for the treatment of helminthic infections.

Infecting Organism	Drug of Choice	Alternative Drugs
Roundworms (nematodes) *Ascaris lumbricoides* (roundworm)	Pyrantel pamoate	Piperazine, mebendazole, levamisole,[1] bephenium,[1] or albendazole[1,2]
Trichuris trichiura (whipworm)	Mebendazole	Oxantel/pyrantel pamoate[1,2] or albendazole[1,2,4]
Necator americanus (hookworm) *Ancylostoma duodenale* (hookworm)	Pyrantel pamoate[3] or mebendazole	Bephenium,[1] tetrachloroethylene,[1] levamisole,[1] or albendazole[1,2,4]
Combined infection with *Ascaris, Trichuris*, and hookworm	Mebendazole or oxantel/pyrantel pamoate[1,2]	Albendazole[1,2,4]
Combined infection with *Ascaris* and hookworm	Mebendazole or pyrantel pamoate	Bephenium[1] or albendazole[1,2,4]
Strongyloides stercoralis (threadworm)	Thiabendazole	Albendazole,[1,2,4] mebendazole,[3,4] or cambendazole[1,2,4]
Enterobius vermicularis (pinworm)	Mebendazole or pyrantel pamoate	Pyrvinium pamoate or albendazole[1,2]
Trichinella spiralis (trichinosis)	ACTH, corticosteroids, and thiabendazole[4] or mebendazole[3,4]	None
Trichostrongylus species	Pyrantel pamoate[3] or mebendazole[3]	Bephenium[1] or levamisole[1]
Cutaneous larva migrans (creeping eruption)	Thiabendazole	Diethylcarbamazine[4,5] or albendazole[1,2,4]
Visceral larva migrans	Thiabendazole[3,4] or mebendazole[3,4]	Diethylcarbamazine[4,5]
Angiostrongylus cantonensis	Levamisole[1,4]	None
Wuchereria bancrofti (filariasis) *Brugia malayi* (filariasis) Tropical eosinophilia *Loa loa* (loiasis)	Diethylcarbamazine[5]	None
Onchocerca volvulus (onchocerciasis)	Diethylcarbamazine[5] plus suramin[6]	Ivermectin[1,2,4]
Dracunculus medinensis (guinea worm)	Niridazole[1] or metronidazole[3]	Thiabendazole[3] or mebendazole[3,4]
Intestinal capillariasis	Mebendazole[3]	Thiabendazole[3]

[1] Not available in the USA; available in some other countries.
[2] Undergoing clinical investigation.
[3] Available in the USA but not labeled for this indication (see Unlabeled Use, p 805).
[4] Effectiveness not established.
[5] Available in the USA from Lederle Laboratories. Telephone (914) 753–5000.
[6] Available in the USA only from the Parasitic Disease Drug Service, Parasitic Diseases Branch, Centers for Disease Control, Atlanta 30333. Telephone (404) 329–3670 during the day, (404) 329–2888 nights, weekends, and holidays (emergencies only).

tic oral doses (5 mg/kg). However, high intravenous doses cause cardiovascular depression in experimental animals. In long-term (30 days) toxicity studies in rats and dogs, diarrhea, anemia, leukopenia, and elevation of alkaline phosphatase were observed in some animals given 48 mg/kg/d. Some sheep treated for 6 weeks with 10–20 mg/kg showed bone marrow depression. In pregnant rabbits and rats treated with 30 mg/kg/d, the drug was teratogenic and embryotoxic.

Clinical Uses

A. Treatment of Intestinal Nematode Infections: In multiple studies, albendazole in dosages of 400 mg once or 200 mg twice for 1 day was effective for infections with *Enterobius vermicularis, Ascaris lumbricoides, Ancylostoma duodenale, Necator americanus,* and *Trichuris trichiura.* To achieve high cure rates in ascariasis and satisfactory reduction in worm burden in moderate to heavy necatoriasis and trichuriasis will probably require repeated treatment for 2–3 days or a higher initial single dose. Optimal dosages remain to be determined.

In strongyloidiasis, 400 mg daily for 3 days resulted in cure rates of 48–81%.

B. Hydatid Disease: Following a course of albendazole, high sulfoxide levels were found in cyst fluid. Some but not all patients with liver cysts treated with 7–10 mg/kg for 1–2 months and followed for up to 30 months showed improvement with shrinkage or disappearance of cysts. Bone cysts may prove to be even more refractory to treatment.

C. Other Infections: A 400-mg dose daily for 3 days was useful in *Opisthorchis viverrini* and *Taenia saginata* infections; 400 mg for 5 days has been tried in cutaneous larva migrans infection.

Table 57–1 (cont'd). Drugs for the treatment of helminthic infections.

Infecting Organism	Drug of Choice	Alternative Drugs
Flukes (trematodes) *Schistosoma haematobium* (bilharziasis)	Praziquantel	Metrifonate[1]
Schistosoma mansoni	Praziquantel	Oxamniquine
Schistosoma japonicum	Praziquantel	Niridazole[1]
Clonorchis sinensis (liver fluke) *Opisthorchis* species	Praziquantel[3]	Mebendazole[3,4] or albendazole[1,2,4]
Paragonimus westermani (lung fluke)	Praziquantel[3]	Bithionol[6]
Fasciola hepatica (sheep liver fluke)	Bithionol[6]	Emetine, dehydroemetine,[6] or praziquantel[3,4]
Fasciolopsis buski (large intestinal fluke)	Praziquantel[3,4] or niclosamide[3]	Dichlorophen,[1,4] tetrachloroethylene,[1] or bephenium[1]
Heterophyes heterophyes and *Metagonimus yokogawai* (small intestinal flukes)	Praziquantel[3] or niclosamide[3]	Bephenium[1] or tetrachloroethylene[1]
Tapeworms (cestodes) *Taenia saginata* (beef tapeworm)	Niclosamide	Praziquantel,[3] dichlorophen,[1] paromomycin,[3] or mebendazole[3,4]
Diphyllobothrium latum (fish tapeworm)	Niclosamide	Praziquantel,[3] dichlorophen,[1] or paromomycin[3]
Taenia solium (pork tapeworm)	Niclosamide[3]	Praziquantel[3] or mebendazole[3,4]
Cysticercosis (pork tapeworm larval stage)	Praziquantel[2,3]	None
Hymenolepsis nana (dwarf tapeworm)	Praziquantel[3]	Niclosamide or paromomycin[3]
Hymenolepis diminuta (rat tapeworm) *Dipylidium cranium*	Niclosamide[3]	Praziquantel[3,4]
Echinococcus granulosus (hydatid disease) *Echinococcus multilocularis*	Mebendazole[2,3,4]	Albendazole[1,2,4]

[1] Not available in the USA; available in some other countries.
[2] Undergoing clinical investigation.
[3] Available in the USA but not labeled for this indication (see Unlabeled Use, p 805).
[4] Effectiveness not established.
[5] Available in the USA from Lederle Laboratories. Telephone (914) 753–5000.
[6] Available in the USA only from the Parasitic Disease Drug Service, Parasitic Diseases Branch, Centers for Disease Control, Atlanta 30333. Telephone (404) 329–3670 during the day, (404) 329–2888 nights, weekends, and holidays (emergencies only).

Adverse Reactions

When used for 1–3 days, albendazole appears to be nearly devoid of significant side effects. Mild transient epigastric distress, diarrhea, headache, nausea, dizziness, lassitude, and insomnia have been attributed to the drug in about 6% of patients, but placebo-controlled studies suggest that the incidence of side effects was similar in treatment and control groups. A small number of patients have shown transient low-grade transaminase elevations, fever, or mild transient neutropenia.

In patients with hydatid disease treated with albendazole for 30 days or longer, reversible leukopenia, reversible transaminase elevations, and cyst leakage with an anaphylactic reaction have been reported.

Contraindications & Cautions

The safety of albendazole has not been established in children under 2 years of age. Because the drug is teratogenic and embryotoxic in some animal species, it should not be used in pregnancy. It may be contraindicated in the presence of cirrhosis.

Preparations & Dosages

For pinworm infections, ancylostomiasis, or light necatoriasis or trichuriasis, the treatment for adults and children over 2 years is a single dose of 400 mg orally with meals. This dosage for light necatoriasis or trichuriasis infections usually reduces the worm burden to satisfactory levels. The dosage to achieve high cure rates in ascariasis or satisfactory reduction in worm burden in moderate to heavy necatoriasis or trichuriasis has not yet been determined, but 400 mg daily for 2 days may be adequate. In the treatment of strongyloidiasis, 400 mg is given daily for 3 days. When necessary, a course of treatment for any of the infections can be repeated in 3 weeks.

ANTIMONY COMPOUNDS

The trivalent antimony compounds were for many years the principal drugs for the treatment of schistosomiasis (bilharziasis) but, because of their toxicity and difficulty of administration, they should no longer be used.

BITHIONOL

Bithionol is the drug of choice for the treatment of fascioliasis (sheep liver fluke) and an alternative drug for the treatment of pulmonary paragonimiasis (lung fluke) and acute cerebral paragonimiasis. The drug has also been used successfully in some countries in the treatment of large tapeworm infections.

Bithionol (Bitin, Lorothidol) is not marketed in the USA but can be obtained from the Parasitic Disease Drug Service, Centers for Disease Control, Atlanta 30333.

Absorption, Metabolism, & Anthelmintic Actions

Bithionol is nearly insoluble in water. After ingestion, it reaches peak blood levels in 4–8 hours. At a daily dosage of 50 mg/kg orally in 3 divided doses for 5 days, a serum level of 50–200 μg/mL is maintained. Excretion appears to be mainly via the kidney. The mode of action of bithionol against *Paragonimus westermani* has not been established, but the drug does inhibit oxidative phosphorylation.

Clinical Uses

A. Pulmonary Paragonimiasis: Cure rates that range from 91–97% have been reported following alternate-day treatment with 10–50 mg/kg for 5–15 doses.

B. Cerebral Paragonimiasis: Bithionol may be useful in acute cerebral paragonimiasis, but more than one course of treatment is sometimes required. The drug has little effectiveness in chronic cerebral infections.

C. *Fasciola hepatica*: Although little information is available on the effectiveness of bithionol in fascioliasis, it should be tried first, since emetine, the alternative drug, is more toxic and praziquantel is not effective.

Adverse Reactions

Side effects occur in up to 40% of patients. They are generally mild and transient, but occasionally their severity requires interruption of therapy. Diarrhea and abdominal cramps are most common; these may diminish or stop after several days of treatment. Anorexia, nausea, vomiting, dizziness, and headache may also occur. Pruritic, urticarial, or papular skin rashes are less frequent and usually begin after a latent period of a week or more of therapy; they are probably allergic in nature, resulting from release of antigens from dying worms. Other infrequent reactions are lassitude, pyrexia, tinnitus, insomnia, proteinuria, and leukopenia.

Contraindications & Cautions

The drug should be used with caution in children under 8 years of age because of limited experience in that age group.

Serial liver function and hematologic tests should be done to observe for possible development of toxic hepatitis and leukopenia. Treatment apparently does not worsen the neurologic condition of patients with cerebral paragonimiasis, but this possibility should be kept in mind.

Preparations & Dosages

For treatment of paragonimiasis and fascioliasis, the dosage of bithionol is 30–50 mg/kg, given orally after meals on alternate days for 10–15 doses. The total daily dosage should be given in 2–3 divided doses. For pulmonary paragonimiasis, 3 negative sputum and stool specimens obtained 3 months after completion of treatment indicate eradication of the parasite. Within 4–6 months, chest film abnormalities will clear in up to 75% of cases.

DICHLOROPHEN

Dichlorophen is safe and moderately effective for the treatment of *Taenia saginata, Taenia solium*, and *Diphyllobothrium latum* infections. The drug has low efficacy in the treatment of *Hymenolepis nana* infections.

Dichlorophen has a consistent laxative effect; colic, nausea, and vomiting may also occur. Lassitude and rash are rare; jaundice has been reported.

Because of the risk of drug-induced vomiting, dichlorophen should preferably not be used for the treatment of *T solium* infections. If it is the only drug available, the same precautions should be observed as described for niclosamide—especially use of a posttreatment purge—because of the theoretical risk of cysticercosis after release of ova from disintegrating tapeworm segments. Dichlorophen is contraindicated in pregnancy and in the presence of liver disease. Alcoholic beverages should be avoided during treatment.

Dichlorophen (Anthiphen) is prepared as 0.5-g tablets. The dosage is 75 mg/kg (maximum 6 g) taken on an empty stomach in the morning for 2 days. Food may follow in 2 hours. Except for *T solium* infection, no posttreatment purge is necessary even if a search for the scolex is intended, because the drug itself has a laxative action.

Dichlorophen is not marketed in the USA.

DIETHYLCARBAMAZINE CITRATE

Diethylcarbamazine is the drug of choice for the treatment of filariasis.

Chemistry

Diethylcarbamazine is a piperazine derivative. It is marketed as the citrate salt, which contains 51% of the active base and is very soluble in water.

Diethylcarbamazine base

Absorption, Metabolism, & Excretion

Diethylcarbamazine is rapidly absorbed from the gastrointestinal tract. A single oral dose of 400 mg (salt) produces a peak blood level of 1.6 μg/mL in 1–2 hours. The minimum effective blood concentration appears to be 0.8–1 μg/mL. The plasma half-life is 2–3 hours in the presence of acidic urine, but about 10 hours if the urine is alkaline. The drug rapidly equilibrates with all tissues (including blood cells) except fat. It is excreted within 30 hours, principally in the urine, either as unchanged drug or as a variety of degradation products. The drug does not accumulate with repeated doses, except in patients with persistent urinary alkalosis or renal impairment.

Pharmacologic Effects

The biochemical mechanism of the filaricidal action of diethylcarbamazine is unknown. It appears that the effect on microfilariae is first to immobilize them and then to alter their surface structure, making them more susceptible to destruction by host defense mechanisms. The mode of action of diethylcarbamazine against adult worms is unknown. Not all species are susceptible (see below).

Headache, sleepiness, and vomiting observed in humans are probably due to effects on the central nervous system. Diethylcarbamazine has shown in vivo and in vitro immunologic suppressive actions; the mechanism is imperfectly understood. This may explain reports of relief of respiratory symptoms when the drug was used in asthmatics. The drug has shown no teratogenic effects in experimental animals. In the treatment of onchocerciasis, the presence of circulating immune complexes may be important in the pathogenesis of ocular and systemic complications.

Clinical Uses

A. W bancrofti, B malayi, B timori, L loa: Diethylcarbamazine is the drug of choice for treatment of these parasites, given its high order of therapeutic efficacy and relative lack of serious toxicity. Microfilariae are rapidly killed by diethylcarbamazine. Adult parasites are killed more slowly, often requiring several courses of treatment. The drug is highly effec-tive against adult *L loa*, but the extent to which *W bancrofti* and *B malayi* adults are killed is not known. However, if therapy is adequate, microfilariae do not reappear in the majority of patients, which suggests that the adult worms are killed or at least permanently sterilized.

B. O volvulus: Diethylcarbamazine is not effective against the adult worms but does kill the microfilariae. Since the adults survive, the reduction in microfilariae is only temporary.

C. Tropical Eosinophilia: Diethylcarbamazine is effective when given orally in a variety of dosage schedules.

D. Other Parasites: Diethylcarbamazine is effective in *Mansonella streptocerca* infections for it kills both adults and microfilariae. Limited information suggests that the drug is not effective, however, against adult *M ozzardi* and *M perstans* and that it has only a low order of effectiveness or is inactive against microfilariae of these parasites. Diethylcarbamazine is not active against *Dirofilaria immitis*.

In toxocariasis, diethylcarbamazine may be tried, but efficacy is not established. The drug has been used in the treatment of *Ascaris* infections and cutaneous larva migrans, but other drugs are superior.

E. Mass Therapy: An important application of diethylcarbamazine therapy has been its use for mass treatment of *W bancrofti* infections to reduce transmission. A common regimen is one dose each week or month for 12 doses. Often, because of side effects, patients will not return for repeated doses. However, when the drug is administered in low doses in medicated salt, it is stable in cooking and appears to be free of side effects and is active as a microfilaricide and possibly also as a macrofilaricide.

F. Prophylaxis: For the prevention of *L loa* infections, a regimen of 2–2.5 mg/kg twice daily for 3 consecutive days once a month may be tried. In the prophylaxis of bancroftian and malayan filariasis, 50 mg monthly has been recommended.

Adverse Reactions

A. Drug-Induced Reactions: Diethylcarbamazine is a safe drug at therapeutic levels. Only a few mild, transient side effects that start in 2–4 hours can be attributed directly to the drug: headache, malaise, anorexia, and weakness. Nausea, vomiting, and sleepiness occur less often.

B. Reactions Induced by Dying Parasites: Side effects also occur as a result of the release of foreign proteins from dying microfilariae, larvae, or adult worms in sensitized patients. Eosinophilia and leukocytosis are usually intensified.

1. Reactions in onchocerciasis—In onchocerciasis, a cluster of symptoms known as the "Mazzotti reaction" occurs in most patients and is often severe, especially in heavy infections. The reaction usually affects the skin (localized or generalized pruritus, rash) but may also be systemic (fever, headache, malaise to prostration, nausea and vomiting, joint and muscle pains, vertigo, tachycardia, cough and respiratory distress, and hypotension). The lymph glands draining affected skin areas may become swollen, tender, and painful. Symptoms may start within 30 minutes to 24 hours after the initial dose of diethylcarbamazine, persist for 3–7 days, and then subside, after which high doses can be tolerated without further symptoms. Reversible proteinuria may occur. A few deaths have been reported.

Patients with many microfilariae in the cornea, conjunctiva, and uveal tissues and the posterior ocular tissues may experience rapid exacerbation of lacrimation, photophobia, punctate keratitis, iridocyclitis, chorioretinitis, and optic neuritis.

2. Reactions in *W bancrofti*, *B malayi*, and *L loa* infections–Reactions to dying microfilariae are usually mild for *W bancrofti* (in up to 25% of patients), more intensive for *B malayi*, and occasionally severe for *L loa* infections. Reactions include fever, malaise, papular rash, headache, gastrointestinal symptoms, cough, chest pains, and muscle or joint pains. In *W bancrofti* and *B malayi* infections, symptoms are most likely to occur in patients with heavy loads of microfilariae but may also occur even if the patient is apparently amicrofilaremic. In loiasis, retinal hemorrhages have been described and, rarely, central nervous system involvement that can be life-threatening.

Local reactions may occur in the vicinity of dying adult or immature worms between the third and 12th days of treatment. Lymphangitis—with localized swellings or nodules—and lymph abscesses may occur in *W bancrofti* and *B malayi*; small wheals appear in the skin at the site of dying worms in *L loa*; and flat papules appear in *M streptocerca* infections. There appear to be no long-term sequelae from these inflammatory reactions.

Contraindications & Cautions

There are no absolute contraindications to the use of diethylcarbamazine, but caution is advised in patients with hypertension and renal disease.

Patients suspected of having malaria should be treated with chloroquine before they are given diethylcarbamazine, since the latter drug may provoke a relapse in nonsymptomatic malaria infections.

A. *W bancrofti*, *B malayi*, *L loa*: Patients with attacks of lymphangitis due to *W bancrofti* or *B malayi* infection should be treated in a quiescent period between attacks.

In loiasis, reactions are more likely in patients with pretreatment microfilariae counts greater than $50/\mu L$ of blood; exchange transfusion has been suggested to reduce such counts.

B. *O volvulus*: Severe reactions may occur when diethylcarbamazine is used in the treatment of onchocerciasis, particularly in heavy infections, if microfilariae are producing symptoms in the skin, or if they are found in or near the eyes. Such patients should be hospitalized and treated by experienced physicians.

Preparations & Dosages

Diethylcarbamazine citrate (Banocide, Caricide, Hetrazan, Notézine) is available as 50-mg tablets or as a syrup containing 24 mg/mL to be taken after meals. The drug has also been given by intramuscular injection. It is available in the USA only directly from Lederle Laboratories (telephone [914] 753–5000).

A. *W bancrofti*, *B malayi*, *L loa*: These infections are treated with 2 mg of the citrate salt per kilogram given orally 3 times a day for 2–4 weeks. For *W bancrofti* infections, to reduce the incidence of allergic reactions to dying microfilariae, a single dose (2 mg/kg) is administered on the first day, 2 doses on the second day, and 3 doses on the third day and thereafter. For *B malayi* or *L loa* infection (with the risk of encephalopathy), the same schedule should be used, but individual doses should start at 1 mg/kg once on the first day and gradually increase over 4–5 days.

Antihistamines may be given for the first 4–5 days of diethylcarbamazine therapy to reduce the incidence of allergic reactions. Corticosteroids should be started and doses of diethylcarbamazine temporarily lowered or interrupted if severe reactions occur.

Blood should be checked for microfilariae several weeks after treatment is completed; a course may be repeated after 3–4 weeks. Cure may require several courses of treatment over 1–2 years.

B. *O volvulus*: If possible, treatment with diethylcarbamazine should be started in the hospital. Because local inflammatory reactions induced by diethylcarbamazine around microfilariae in the eye can produce permanent retinal damage, there is controversy about whether a course of diethylcarbamazine should precede suramin treatment. If a preliminary course of diethylcarbamazine is used, it should be given in the presence of steroid immunosuppression (see below).

A schedule for the use of diethylcarbamazine is as follows: Give 25 mg once and wait several days for the reaction to subside. Then give 25 mg twice on 1 day, followed by 50 mg twice on the next day and 100 mg twice on the third day; thereafter, continue 200 mg once daily until the microfilarial load in the skin has been reduced to near zero, a process that takes about 7–14 days. Suramin treatment is then started to kill the adult worms. During the course of suramin, repeat diethylcarbamazine, 200 mg twice daily, for 3–5 days every 2–4 weeks. At the end of the suramin treatment, repeat diethylcarbamazine, 200 mg twice daily for 3–5 days at 3- to 4-week intervals until pruritic skin reactions no longer occur.

If suramin is *not* used, diethylcarbamazine may be used as a microfilarial suppressive by initially giving the standard course of therapy and then continuing the drug indefinitely at weekly intervals in a dosage of 50–200 mg; in these weekly treatments, allergic reactions will usually be insignificant.

In mild infections, symptomatic relief of pain, fever, and headache is sometimes possible with aspirin and codeine, but use of corticosteroids may become necessary. Antihistamines have not been useful.

However, all patients with heavy infections should receive a corticosteroid, eg, betamethasone, 1–2 mg 3 times daily starting 1–2 days before the first dose of diethylcarbamazine, continued through the major part of the reaction, and then tapered off over 4 days. If keratoconjunctivitis occurs, administer betamethasone eye drops; if iridocyclitis occurs, administer both eye drops and atropine, with appropriate caution to avoid precipitating acute glaucoma.

EMETINE HYDROCHLORIDE

Emetine and dehydroemetine are alternative drugs for the treatment of *Fasciola hepatica* infection. Both drugs may be effective in removing the parasite, but they are more toxic than bithionol (the drug of choice) or praziquantel (currently under investigation). Dehydroemetine is probably less toxic than emetine; general pharmacologic information, dosage, and precautions in their usage are presented in Chapter 56.

LEVAMISOLE

Levamisole hydrochloride is a synthetic imidazothiazole derivative and the L isomer of DL-tetramisole. It is highly effective in eradicating *Ascaris* and *Trichostrongylus* and moderately effective against both species of hookworm. The drug is not marketed in the USA.

Absorption, Metabolism, & Excretion

Levamisole is highly soluble in water. Following an oral dose, the drug is rapidly and extensively absorbed. In humans, a single oral dose of 150 mg produces a peak plasma level of 0.5 μg/mL in 2–4 hours. The drug is widely distributed to the tissues and reaches a high concentration in the liver, where it is extensively metabolized. Blood levels fall rapidly: the plasma half-life is 4 hours, and elimination is nearly complete in 48 hours. Less than 5% of an administered dose is excreted unchanged in the urine. Levamisole apparently crosses the blood-brain barrier, for it is effective against *Angiostrongylus cantonensis* in rats.

Pharmacologic Effects & Anthelmintic Actions

At relatively high concentrations, levamisole has a reversible ganglion-stimulating effect on mammalian tissue at both parasympathetic and sympathetic sites. In general, this results in stimulation of the central and autonomic nervous systems and skeletal muscle; as a result, the drug has some mood-elevating effects.

Levamisole is an immunomodulating agent (see Chapter 59) under investigation to determine its effectiveness in various cancers, autoimmune diseases, chronic bacterial infections, and herpetic keratitis. It affects host defenses by modulating cell-mediated immune responses, including polymorphonuclear leukocyte, macrophage, and T cell functions. In theory, the drug is useful only when cell-mediated immunity is depressed; it has little effect on normal immune mechanisms except at dosages that greatly exceed therapeutic concentrations. The immune reactivity increases promptly after only a single dose and is thought to persist from days to months. However, the responses to levamisole are not always predictable.

Toxicologic studies in pregnant animals do not indicate any teratogenic or embryotoxic effects, but in mice, high doses of the drug (25 mg/kg) increase the rate and intensity of spontaneous lymphomas. In vitro and in vivo studies of the effect of levamisole on human chromosomes show a slight increase in gaps and chromatid and chromosome breaks.

In nematodes, levamisole stimulates ganglionlike structures, causing contraction of muscle and then neuromuscular paralysis of the depolarizing type. The worms are then eliminated by peristalsis. There is some indication that the anthelmintic action of levamisole may also stem from its inhibiting action on fumarate reductase. Levamisole has little ovicidal action on *Trichuris* and none on *Ascaris*.

Adverse Reactions

When levamisole is used in a single dose for the treatment of *Ascaris* and hookworm infections, side effects are mild and transient. They include nausea, vomiting, mild abdominal cramping pain, headache, dizziness, weakness, and skin rash.

Clinical Uses, Preparations, & Dosages

Levamisole (Decaris, Ethnor, Ketrax, Solaskil) is available in 50- and 150-mg tablets and as a syrup. Adults receive a single dose of 150 mg and children a single dose of 3 mg/kg.

MEBENDAZOLE

Mebendazole, a synthetic benzimidazole like albendazole, has a wide spectrum of anthelmintic activity and a low incidence of side effects. It is a drug of choice in trichuriasis, pinworm infection, trichostrongyliasis, and infection with either of the hookworm species. It is particularly useful in mixed infections with trichurids, ascarids, and hookworms. It does not produce satisfactory cure rates in strongyloidiasis. Mebendazole is also highly effective in capillariasis and has shown promise in the treatment of trichinosis and some cases of echinococcosis.

Flubendazole, the parafluoro analog of mebendazole, continues in clinical trials. It is similar to mebendazole in its anthelmintic spectrum and paucity of side effects, but in addition it appears to be active in the treatment of strongyloidiasis and has shown no teratogenic effect in rats or rabbits.

Chemistry, Absorption, Metabolism, & Excretion

Mebendazole is nearly insoluble in water and not unpleasant in taste.

Mebendazole

Less than 10% of orally administered mebendazole is absorbed. Absorbed drug is rapidly metabolized and mostly excreted in the urine either unchanged or as decarboxylated derivatives within 24–48 hours. In addition, a portion of conjugated unchanged drug and its derivatives are excreted in the bile. Higher absorption occurs if the drug is ingested with a fatty meal.

With administration of 100 mg twice daily for 3 days, peak plasma levels of both the drug and its principal metabolites are reached in 2–4 hours and never exceed 30 ng/mL and 90 ng/mL, respectively.

Pharmacologic Effects & Anthelmintic Actions

Mebendazole and related benzimidazoles inhibit microtubule synthesis in nematodes and impair their uptake of glucose (Chapter 55). As a result, intestinal parasites are immobilized or die slowly, and their clearance from the gastrointestinal tract may not be complete until several days after treatment. Efficacy of the drug varies with gastrointestinal transit time, intensity of infection, whether or not the drug is chewed, and perhaps with the strain of parasite. The drug also kills hookworm, *Ascaris*, and *Trichuris* eggs.

In humans, mebendazole is almost inert. Acute and chronic toxicologic studies in animals indicate a wide range between therapeutic and toxic doses. However, in pregnant rats the drug has embryotoxic and teratogenic activity at single oral doses as low as 10 mg/kg.

Clinical Uses

A. A lumbricoides, T trichiura, Hookworm, and Trichostrongylus: A 3-day course of 100 mg twice daily produces cure rates of 90–100% for *Ascaris* and *Trichostrongylus* infections, 70–95% for hookworm infections by both species, and 60–90% for asymptomatic to moderate *Trichuris* infections, with a marked reduction in the worm burden in those not cured.

B. Enterobius vermicularis (Pinworm): Reports from various studies indicate cure rates of 90–100%. Thus, mebendazole compares favorably with the single-dose regimen of pyrvinium pamoate and pyrantel pamoate but has the advantages of fewer side effects and the absence of staining properties.

C. Hydatid Disease: Results of mebendazole therapy of hydatid disease have been highly variable. Subjective improvement is reported for most patients and evidence of regression of cysts in some; in other patients, particularly after long-term follow-up, cysts have continued to grow or have proved viable. Unpredictable plasma levels of the drug may contribute to

variability in response. For patients with hydatid disease who are unable to undergo surgery (the procedure of choice) or whose cysts have ruptured, mebendazole treatment can be considered at a dosage of 50 mg/kg in 3 divided doses daily for 3 months. When possible, mebendazole blood levels should be monitored; serum levels in excess of 100 mg/kg 1–3 hours after an oral dose may be necessary for parasite killing.

Occasional side effects associated with high-dose treatment of hydatid disease are pruritus, rash, eosinophilia, reversible neutropenia, musculoskeletal pain, fever, and acute pain in the cyst area. Although some of these findings may be due to cyst leakage or rupture with release of antigen, no deaths or instances of anaphylaxis or dissemination have been described in humans. Spontaneous cyst rupture does occur when mebendazole is used to treat experimental animals, and some workers have expressed concern that this might also occur in humans. Gastric irritation, cough, transient liver function abnormalities, and alopecia have also been reported. In addition, 6 cases of glomerulonephritis and 3 cases of drug-induced agranulocytosis (with one death) have been reported. Side effects are most apt to occur in the first month of treatment.

D. Other infections: For treatment of **intestinal capillariasis**, mebendazole is the drug of choice at a dosage of 400 mg/d in divided doses for 21 or more days.

In **trichinosis**, limited reports suggest therapeutic efficacy against adult worms in the intestinal tract, migrating larvae, and larvae in muscle. The following treatment schedule has been recommended for adults: 600 mg initially, increasing stepwise to 1200–1500 mg, continuing with the maximum dose for 10 days. Daily doses should be given in 3 divided portions.

Very high dosage (30 mg/kg daily for 3–4 weeks) has been reported to result in an approximately 90% cure rate of **opisthorchiasis**.

Mebendazole at a dosage of 300 mg twice daily for 3 days has been used in the treatment of **taeniasis** with variable effectiveness. In the treatment of *T solium* infection, mebendazole has one theoretical advantage over niclosamide—proglottids are expelled intact after therapy.

Cure rates for **strongyloidiasis** using the standard 3-day course of therapy are usually less than 50%; higher doses or longer courses of therapy are being investigated.

In **dracontiasis**, efficacy has been variable and needs further study. The use of mebendazole and mebendazole plus levamisole in **filariasis** and **onchocerciasis** is still under study. Mebendazole may be the first drug available for the treatment of *D perstans*.

Adverse Reactions

Low-dose, short-term mebendazole usage (1–3 days) for intestinal nematode therapy has been remarkably free of side effects, even in debilitated patients. Mild nausea, vomiting, diarrhea, and abdominal pain have been reported infrequently but more often in children heavily parasitized by *Ascaris*. Slight headache and dizziness occur rarely. Oral passage of ascarids in children under 5 years of age has been reported.

Contraindications & Cautions

In severe hepatic parenchymal disease, mebendazole is poorly detoxified and should be used with caution. The drug is contraindicated in pregnant women. It should be used with caution in children under 2 years of age because of limited experience.

Preparations & Dosage

Mebendazole (Vermox) is available as tablets of 100 mg, and in some countries as a suspension containing 100 mg/5 mL. The drug can be taken before or after meals, and it may be therapeutically advantageous that the tablets be chewed before they are swallowed. To increase absorption in the treatment of hydatid disease, trichinosis, and dracontiasis, the drug should be taken with food containing fat, which enhances absorption.

The same dosage is used for adults and for children over age 2 years. For the treatment of ascariasis, trichuriasis, and hookworm infections, give 100 mg twice daily for 3 days. Treatment can be repeated in 2–3 weeks. For the treatment of pinworm infection, give 100 mg once only. Repeat the dose at 2 and 4 weeks. No pretreatment or posttreatment purging is necessary.

In the USA, mebendazole has been approved for use in ascariasis, trichuriasis, and hookworm and pinworm infection. It is investigational for other uses.

METRIFONATE

Metrifonate, an organophosphorus compound, was introduced as the insecticide trichlorfon (Dipterex) and then as an oral drug for the treatment of *S haematobium* infections, for which it remains an effective, safe, low-cost alternative drug. It is not active against *S mansoni* or *S japonicum*.

Chemistry, Absorption, Metabolism, & Excretion

Metrifonate is rapidly absorbed after oral administration. Following a standard oral dose, peak blood levels are reached in 1–2 hours; the half-life is about $1\frac{1}{2}$ hours; and the drug is detectable for about 8 hours. Clearance appears to be through nonenzymatic transformation to dichlorvos. The amount of dichlorvos in the plasma is about 1% of the metrifonate level. The drug and its derivatives are well distributed to the tissues and are completely eliminated in 24–48 hours.

Pharmacologic Effects & Anthelmintic Actions

Metrifonate acts against both the mature and immature stages of *S haematobium* as a result of its transformation into its active metabolite dichlorvos. Dichlorvos's mode of action is not established but is thought to be due in part to its function as a cholinesterase inhibitor. The cholinesterase inhibition temporarily paralyzes the adult worms, resulting in their shift from the bladder venous plexus to small arterioles of the lungs, where they are trapped and encased and then die. The drug is not effective against *S haematobium* eggs, and live eggs will therefore continue to pass in the urine for several months after all adult worms have been killed.

Therapeutic dosages of metrifonate in humans produce no untoward physiologic or chemical abnormalities except for cholinesterase inhibition (see below). Following oral ingestion of 7.5–12.5 mg/kg of metrifonate by infected persons, there is an almost complete inhibition of plasma butyrylcholinesterase and a marked reduction (about 50%) of erythrocytic acetylcholinesterase. Plasma recovery is usually 70% or more by 2 weeks and is completed by 4 weeks, but erythrocyte recovery may take up to 15 weeks.

Some organophosphorus compounds are known to have mutagenic properties. Metrifonate or perhaps impurities associated with its manufacture show weak mutagenicity in the *Salmonella typhimurium* direct test system. It induces gene mutations in *Escherichia coli* but causes no chromosomal abnormalities in animals or humans. Reproduction toxicity studies showed negative results except for suggestions of impaired spermatogenesis.

Clinical Uses

In the treatment of *S haematobium* infections, cure rates ranged from 44 to 93% when 3 doses of 7.5–10 mg/kg were given orally at 14- to 28-day intervals. Those not cured showed a marked reduction in ovum counts. Metrifonate was also effective as a prophylactic when given monthly to children in a highly endemic area, or as mass treatment every 6 months.

In mixed infections with *S haematobium* and *S mansoni*, metrifonate has been successfully combined with oxamniquine.

Adverse Reactions

Some studies report no side effects; others note mild and transient cholinergic symptoms, including nausea and vomiting, diarrhea, abdominal pain, bronchospasm, headache, sweating, fatigue, weakness, and vertigo. These symptoms may begin within 30 minutes and persist up to 12 hours. The drug is well tolerated by patients in advanced stages of the disease.

One case of typical organophosphate poisoning following a standard dose has been reported; the patient responded well to the use of atropine.

Contraindications & Cautions

Metrifonate should not be used after recent exposure to insecticides or drugs that might potentiate cholinesterase inhibition. The use of muscle relaxants, particularly as part of general anesthesia, should be avoided for 48 hours after administration of the drug. The drug is contraindicated in pregnancy.

Preparations & Dosages

Metrifonate (Bilarcil) is supplied in 100-mg tablets and is taken orally at a dosage of 7.5 mg/kg once (maximum 600 mg), and then repeated twice at 2-week intervals. The drug is not marketed in the USA.

NICLOSAMIDE

Niclosamide, a salicylamide derivative, has been for many years the drug of choice for the treatment of most tapeworm infections.

Chemistry, Absorption, & Metabolism

Niclosamide is minimally absorbed from the gastrointestinal tract. The unaltered drug has not been recovered from the blood or urine.

Niclosamide

Pharmacologic Effects & Anthelmintic Actions

Following oral administration in animals and humans, no hematologic, renal, or hepatic abnormalities have been noted.

The scoleces and segments of cestodes, but not the ova, are rapidly killed on contact with niclosamide. This may be due to the drug's inhibition of oxidative phosphorylation or to its ATPase-stimulating property. Associated with the death of the parasite is release of the scolex from the intestinal wall. Even if a purge is used to expel the tapeworm, the scolex and proglottids may be partially digested and difficult to identify.

Clinical Uses

A. T saginata (Beef Tapeworm), T solium (Pork Tapeworm), and D latum (Fish Tapeworm): A single dose of niclosamide results in cure rates of over 85% for *D latum* and about 95% for *T saginata*; it is probably equally effective for *T solium*.

B. H nana (Dwarf Tapeworm): Niclosamide is effective against the adult parasites in the lumen of the intestine but not against cysticercoids embedded in the villi. For the drug to be successful, it must be given until all of the cysticercoids have emerged (about 4 days). Thus, the minimum course of treatment must be 5–7 days; some workers repeat the course 5 days later. The overall cure rate with niclosamide is about 75%.

C. Other Tapeworms: Results have been promising in patients treated for *Hymenolepis diminuta* and *Dipylidium caninum* infections. Most patients are cured with a 5- to 7-day course; a few require a second course of treatment. Niclosamide is not effective against cysticercosis or hydatid disease.

D. Intestinal Fluke Infections: Niclosamide can be used as an alternative drug for the treatment of *F buski, H heterophyes*, and *M yokogawai* infections.

Adverse Reactions

Side effects are infrequent, mild, and transitory. Nausea, vomiting, diarrhea, and abdominal discomfort occur in less than 4% of patients. Rarely described are headache, skin rash, urticaria, pruritus ani, and vertigo, some of which may be related to absorption of antigen from disintegrating parasites.

Contraindications & Cautions

The consumption of alcohol should be avoided on the day of treatment and for 1 day afterward.

There are no contraindications to the use of niclosamide. In children under 2 years of age, the safety of the drug has not been established. Reproductive studies in animals were negative, but there are no adequate studies in pregnant women.

Preparations & Dosages

Niclosamide (Niclocide, Yomesan) is prepared as chewable tablets, each containing 0.5 g of the drug. The adult dosage is 2 g. Children weighing more than 34 kg are given 3 tablets; children 11–34 kg, 2 tablets.

Pre- and posttreatment purges are not necessary except for an occasional patient with chronic constipation. Niclosamide should be given in the morning on an empty stomach. The tablets *must be chewed thoroughly* and then swallowed with water. For small children, pulverize the tablets and then mix with water. The patient may eat 2 hours later. In the treatment of infections with the large tapeworms, segments may continue to pass for several days with normal peristalsis. For taeniasis, if the scolex is not found or is not searched for after treatment, cure can be presumed only if regenerated segments have not reappeared after 3–5 months.

A. T saginata, D latum, and D caninum: Treatment requires only a single dose. Although not usually necessary, a purge may be given 2 hours after treatment in an attempt to recover and identify the scolex before it disintegrates and to confirm that the entire worm has passed and will not regenerate.

B. T solium: Treatment requires only a single dose. However, 2 hours after treatment, an effective purge (such as 15–30 g of magnesium sulfate) must be given to eliminate all mature segments before ova can be released. The patient should be monitored to ensure that prompt evacuation occurs. Cysticercosis is theoretically possible after treatment of *T solium* infections if tapeworm segments disintegrate and release eggs, because niclosamide is not lethal to the eggs. It is unknown whether larvae are released from ova in the large bowel. If so, they could penetrate the intestinal wall and reach the tissues. However, no cases of cysticercosis have been reported after use of niclosamide.

C. H nana and H diminuta: A variety of dosage schedules have been proposed. A typical recommendation for adults is 2 g daily for 7 days. The dosage for children weighing over 34 kg is 1.5 g as a single dose on the first day and then 1 g daily for the next 4–6 days; for children 11–34 kg, the dosage is 1 g on the first day and then 0.5 g daily for 4–6 days. Some workers repeat the course of treatment after 5 days.

D. F buski, H heterophyes, and M yokogawai: The standard dosage is given every other day for 3 doses.

NIRIDAZOLE

Niridazole, a nitrothiazole derivative, has been used for over 20 years in the oral treatment of schistosomiasis. Most persons experience side effects, sometimes severe. Mutagenic and carcinogenic properties have been reported. For these reasons, niridazole is at most an alternative drug, to be used when the preferred drugs are not available. Niridazole is also used in the treatment of dracontiasis. The drug is not marketed in the USA.

Absorption, Metabolism, & Excretion

Following oral administration, niridazole is absorbed slowly; the maximum blood concentration is reached in 6 hours. Higher blood levels are reached if the drug is given in 2 divided doses 12 hours apart rather than in one single larger dose. Niridazole has a half-life of only a few hours, whereas the drug metabolites, which are largely bound to serum proteins, have half-lives of about 40 hours. The drug is eliminated mostly as metabolites, principally in the urine and through bile into feces.

The concentration of the unmetabolized drug (the active agent against the parasite) is 5 times higher in the portal blood than in the peripheral circulation because most of the drug is metabolized in the first cycle through the liver. High blood concentrations of the unmetabolized drug are found in patients with hepatic dysfunction and in portal-systemic shunts. This factor contributes to the high incidence of side effects of niridazole.

Pharmacologic Effects

A. Actions in Experimental Animals and Humans: Niridazole produces temporary inhibition of spermatogenesis. It has been shown to have a glycogen-lowering effect in monkey muscle; such glycogen depletion may be responsible for some of the drug's side effects in humans. Niridazole also has uricosuric effects.

In addition to its antiparasitic actions, niridazole has antibacterial and anti-inflammatory properties and suppresses various manifestations of cell-mediated immunity.

In animals, damage to the hematopoietic system has been noted following several weeks of niridazole therapy, but in humans there have been no reports of adverse effects on peripheral blood counts or bone marrow, nor have there been reports of increased susceptibility to infection.

B. Anthelmintic Actions: The mechanism of action of niridazole is not known. In experimental animals infected with *Schistosoma mansoni*, niridazole causes a "liver shift" of adult worms that is followed by their death. Niridazole is rapidly concentrated in adult worms, resulting in the inhibition of phosphorylase inactivation followed by glycogen depletion of the parasite. Niridazole also inhibits or interrupts egg production.

In dracontiasis, animal studies suggest that the drug's action is anti-inflammatory rather than parasiticidal.

Clinical Uses

A. Schistosomiasis: Niridazole is an alternative drug for the treatment of *S japonicum* infections. In the treatment of *S mansoni* and *S haematobium* infections, niridazole should be considered a tertiary drug, to be used only if the preferred drugs are not available.

Efforts to reduce side effects but retain effectiveness by giving niridazole over longer periods than the standard course and at reduced daily doses have had variable success.

B. Dracunculus medinensis: Niridazole may provide effective treatment for dracontiasis (guinea worm infection). Reduction of swelling and rapid relief of pain follow treatment, often facilitating spontaneous expulsion or retraction of the worm as well as increasing the rate of healing.

Adverse Reactions

Side effects are transient and occur in more than 70% of patients. The most common adverse reactions are anorexia, nausea and vomiting, diarrhea, abdominal pain, fatigue, headache, dizziness, myalgia, arthralgia, sweating, palpitation, and skin rashes. Paresthesias and insomnia may also occur. With the death of parasites, there may be cough, pulmonary infiltrates, and marked eosinophilia. The urine may become dark brown or dark red, with an unpleasant musty odor. Liver function tests may become abnormal. Niridazole can provoke hemolysis in persons with glucose-6-phosphate dehydrogenase deficiency. Epistaxis, gastrointestinal hemorrhage, and Stevens-Johnson syndrome have rarely been reported. Tachycardia and minor electrocardiographic changes (flattening or inversion of T waves and ST depression) occur frequently but have not been associated with impairment of cardiac function.

Neuropsychiatric symptoms are uncommon (< 6%) in patients who have normal hepatic function; however, in advanced schistosomal liver disease, up to 60% may have symptoms. Initial symptoms may include mild headache, paresthesias, insomnia, and anxiety. Marked mood changes (agitation, anxiety, depression), slurred speech, confusion, psychosis (auditory or visual hallucinations, violent behavior), and convulsions have been reported.

Liver function tests and blood counts should be followed during the course of therapy.

Niridazole and its metabolic derivatives in urine have been shown to have both mutagenic and carcinogenic properties, but no teratogenic effects have been observed in limited follow-up of patients.

Contraindications & Cautions

Niridazole should always be used under close daily medical supervision. Patients with the following conditions generally should not receive the drug: glucose-6-phosphate dehydrogenase deficiency; a history of liver disease; impaired liver function; the hepatosplenic form of schistosomiasis; cardiac or renal disease; hypertension; age over 50; or a history of psychiatric disorders, epilepsy, or gastrointestinal hemorrhage or ulcer. Patients with severe malnutrition, anemia, infections, and other debilitating conditions should have these problems corrected before therapy is begun. Niridazole should not be administered concurrently with isoniazid.

Preparations & Dosages

Niridazole (Ambilhar) is prepared as 100- and 500-mg tablets. The dosage for schistosomiasis and dracontiasis is 25 mg/kg (maximum 1.5 g) daily for 7 days, divided into 2–3 fractions and given with meals. Adult patients should receive phenobarbital, 100–150 mg daily in divided doses, to reduce the incidence of central nervous system side effects. For the treatment of *S japonicum* infections, it is currently recommended that the course of treatment be stopped in 5 days.

Children infected with *S mansoni* receive the above dosage. However, children infected with *S haematobium* can be treated for 5 days if daily doses of 30–35 mg/kg are administered in divided doses.

OXAMNIQUINE

Oxamniquine, a semisynthetic tetrahydroquinoline, has been in clinical use since 1975. It is an alternative drug for the treatment of *S mansoni* infections, including patients with advanced disease. Except for its high cost, the drug is excellent for mass treatment because of its high level of effectiveness, oral administration, and freedom from significant side effects. It is not effective against *S haematobium* or *S japonicum*.

Absorption, Metabolism, & Excretion

Oxamniquine is sparingly soluble in water and readily absorbed orally. It is no longer given intramuscularly, because it causes intense and prolonged local pain. After oral administration of therapeutic doses, peak plasma concentrations—in the range of 850 ng/mL—are reached in 1–1.5 hours, with a plasma half-life of about 2.5 hours. The drug is extensively metabolized and excreted in the urine within 12 hours.

Intersubject variations in serum concentration have been noted, which could explain some treatment failures. Although the drug is taken with food to decrease side effects, food does delay its absorption.

Pharmacologic Effects & Anthelmintic Actions

Oxamniquine is active against both mature and immature stages of *S mansoni* but does not appear to be cercaricidal. Although the exact mechanism is not known, the drug may act by DNA binding. It induces a shift of the worms from the mesentery to the liver, where many die; surviving females that return to the liver cease to lay eggs.

Clinical Uses

Oxamniquine is effective only against *S mansoni*. The drug is safe and effective in all stages of the disease. In the acute (Katayama) syndrome, treatment results in disappearance of acute symptoms and subsequent failure to develop patent infection. In chronic infections, following a single dose of 15–20 mg/kg in adults, cure rates of 70–95% were reported in Brazil, and in those not cured there was marked reduction in egg excretion. In Egypt and other parts of Africa, however, a larger dose—about 60 mg/kg given over 2–3 days—was needed to achieve similar cure rates. The drug is generally less effective in children than in adults.

In mixed infections with *S mansoni* and *S haematobium*, oxamniquine has been successfully used in combination with metrifonate. Oxamniquine's potential for suppressive prophylaxis as shown in animals needs further study in humans.

Adverse Reactions

The drug has been administered to millions of patients and found nearly free of significant toxicity, but mild symptoms lasting for several hours do occur in more than one-third of patients. Dizziness is most common; drowsiness, nausea and vomiting, diarrhea, abdominal colic, headache, and pruritus are less so. A low-grade fever starting on the second day of treatment or several days later is frequently reported in Egypt but occurs less often in Brazil. An orange to red discoloration of the urine, proteinuria, erythrocytes, and a transient decrease of leukocytes and lymphocytes may appear. Central nervous system stimulation may occur very rarely, resulting in behavioral changes, seizures, or hallucinations. Usually the seizures appear in patients with a history of convulsive disorders.

Instances of mild to moderate liver enzyme abnormalities, eosinophilia, transient pulmonary infiltrates (sometimes associated with cough and rhonchi), and urticaria occurring from several days to a month after treatment, have been ascribed to the death of parasites rather than to a direct toxic effect of the drug.

Oxamniquine has shown low mutagenicity in the *S typhimurium* test system and in the host-mediated assay system in mice, but chromosomal abnormalities were not found in animals or humans. Oxamniquine has also been shown to have an embryocidal effect in rabbits and mice when given in doses 10 times the equivalent human dose.

Contraindications & Cautions

It appears prudent to observe patients for about 3 hours after ingestion of the drug for signs of central nervous system disturbances. Patients with a history of epilepsy should be hospitalized for treatment, or an alternative drug should be used. Since the drug makes many patients dizzy or drowsy, it should be used with caution in patients whose work or activity requires mental alertness.

Oxamniquine is contraindicated in pregnancy.

Preparations & Dosages

Oxamniquine (Mansil, Vansil) is prepared for oral use as 250-mg capsules and as a syrup containing 50 mg/mL. The drug is better tolerated if given with food.

Optimal dosage schedules vary for different regions of the world. In the Western Hemisphere, 12–15 mg/kg is given once; for children under 30 kg, 20 mg/kg is given in divided doses. For African strains, the total dosage for adults and children varies by region from 40 to 60 mg/kg given in divided doses over 2–3 days.

OXANTEL PAMOATE & OXANTEL/PYRANTEL PAMOATE

Oxantel pamoate (Telopar), a tetrahydroxypyrimidine and meta-oxyphenol analog of pyrantel pamoate (combantrin), is effective only in the treatment of trichuriasis infections. Since trichuriasis commonly occurs as a multiple infection with the other soil-transmitted helminths, oxantel is now being marketed in combination with pyrantel pamoate because the latter is active against *Ascaris* and hookworm infections. Neither oxantel nor oxantel/pyrantel is effective in strongyloidiasis. The drugs are not available in the USA.

In trichuriasis infections, oxantel or oxantel/pyrantel given once at a dosage of 10–20 mg/kg (base) resulted in cure rates of 53–100%. Dosages of 10 mg/kg continued daily for 3 days gave better cure rates. In all studies, there was a marked reduction in egg counts in patients not cured. Cure rates for ascariasis and hookworm using the combined drug were the same as for pyrantel pamoate alone.

Absorption, Metabolism, & Excretion

Oxantel pamoate is poorly absorbed from the gastrointestinal tract. Following an oral dose of 750 mg, 6–8% is absorbed and a peak serum concentration is reached in 2–4 hours. Excretion is for the most part in the urine within 12 hours.

Adverse Reactions, Contraindications, & Cautions

Oxantel is free of major side effects. Side effects, contraindications, and cautions are the same as described for pyrantel pamoate (below). The drug has not been studied in pregnant patients.

Preparations & Dosages

Oxantel/pyrantel pamoate (Quantrel) is available in tablets that contain 100 mg (base) of each drug and as oral suspensions that contain 20 mg or 50 mg (base) of each drug per milliliter.

A. Asymptomatic Trichuriasis, Pinworm Infection, Ascariasis, Ancylostomiasis, Trichostrongyliasis, Necatoriasis (Light to Moderate Infection): These conditions are treated with a single oral dose of 10–20 mg/kg (base) of each drug given with or without food. The maximum for children weighing less than 6.2 kg is 10 mg/kg (base) of each drug.

B. Symptomatic Trichuriasis: Give the above dose consecutively for 2 days.

C. Necatoriasis (Heavy Infection): Give the above dose consecutively for 3 days.

PAROMOMYCIN SULFATE

Paromomycin, an aminoglycoside antibiotic (see Chapter 45), is effective in the treatment of infection with the large tapeworms and may be tried in *H nana* infections. It is also used in the treatment of amebiasis and to reduce the number of intestinal bacteria.

Although paromomycin is poorly absorbed from the gastrointestinal tract, side effects, especially nausea, abdominal cramps, and diarrhea, are not uncommon; they may be reduced by giving the drug after meals. Although nephrotoxicity, ototoxicity, central nervous system toxicity, and superinfection are possible with paromomycin as with other members of the neomycin group, such complications (except for superinfections) have not been reported.

One-day courses of paromomycin used in the treatment of a small number of *T saginata*, *T solium*, and *D latum* infections resulted in cure rates of about 95%. A recommended dosage for adults is 1 g every 15 minutes for 4 doses; for children, 11 mg/kg every 15 minutes for 4 doses. Paromomycin, however, should not be used for *T solium* infections, because drug-induced vomiting may result in regurgitation of proglottids into the stomach, which could be followed by cysticercosis.

In the treatment of *H nana* infections, there is limited evidence for efficacy of paromomycin at a dosage of 45 mg/kg/d (maximum 4 g) in 2 divided doses for 5–7 days.

In the USA, the drug is marketed for other conditions, and its use for tapeworm infections is considered investigational.

PIPERAZINE

Piperazine salts continue to be alternative drugs in the treatment of ascariasis. Piperazine is not useful for treatment of hookworm infection, trichuriasis, or strongyloidiasis and is no longer recommended in this text in the treatment of pinworm infection.

Chemistry

Piperazine is available as the hexahydrate (which contains about 44% of the base) and as a variety of salts: citrate, phosphate, adipate, tartrate, and others.

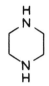

Piperazine base

Absorption, Metabolism, & Excretion

Piperazine is readily absorbed from the gastrointestinal tract, and maximum plasma levels are reached in 2–4 hours. Most of the drug is excreted unchanged in the urine in 2–6 hours, and excretion is complete within 24 hours.

Pharmacologic Effects & Anthelmintic Actions

Orally administered piperazine is almost free of pharmacologic action in the host. The formation of a potentially carcinogenic nitrosamine derivative, N-mononitrosopiperazine, has recently been demonstrated in gastric contents and urine of volunteers given therapeutic doses of piperazine; the significance of this finding remains to be determined.

Piperazine causes a paralysis of *Ascaris* by blocking acetylcholine at the myoneural junction. Piperazine has a similar (but of low order) myoneural blocking action on mammalian skeletal muscle. When the drug is used in humans, the paralyzed roundworms are unable to maintain their position in the host and are expelled live by normal peristalsis.

Clinical Uses

A. *Ascaris lumbricoides*: Piperazine is an alternative drug for roundworm infections. When patients are treated once daily for 2 days, cure rates are over 90%. Longer courses are needed for equivalent cure rates in patients with heavy infections. Piperazine syrup, administered via an intestinal drainage tube, is used in the nonsurgical management of intestinal obstruction due to heavy *Ascaris* infection.

Pyrantel pamoate is the preferred drug for treatment of ascariasis, because it is as effective as piperazine and has a similar low level of side effects but is given only once.

B. *E (Oxyuris) vermicularis*: Although effective, piperazine is no longer recommended here for pinworm infections because it requires a 7-day course of treatment.

Adverse Reactions

There is a wide range between the therapeutic and toxic doses of piperazine. Mild side effects occur occasionally, including nausea, vomiting, diarrhea, abdominal pain, and headache. Neurotoxic side effects are rare and include vertigo, incoordination, blurring of vision, muscular weakness, tremors, paresthesias, hyporeflexia, lethargy, and confusional states. Patients with epilepsy may have an exacerbation of seizures. Although piperazine is potentially allergenic, it rarely results in urticaria, erythema multiforme, purpura, fever, hepatitis, hemolysis, and arthralgia. Serum sickness–like syndromes have been reported 2–14 days after an initial dose of piperazine.

Contraindications & Cautions

Piperazine compounds should not be given to patients with impaired renal or hepatic function or with a history of epilepsy or chronic neurologic disease. Piperazine and phenothiazines should not be given together. Caution should be exercised in patients with severe malnutrition or anemia. Piperazine has not been fully evaluated for teratogenic potential. Therefore, the drug should be given to pregnant women only if clearly indicated.

Preparations & Dosages

The therapeutic effectiveness of the various piperazine salts is about the same; in solution, all form piperazine hexahydrate. Among the many preparations are tablets, wafers, and syrups.

Piperazine citrate (Antepar) is prepared as a syrup containing 110 mg/mL (the equivalent of 100 mg of piperazine hexahydrate) or as tablets containing 550 mg (the equivalent of 500 mg of piperazine hexahydrate).

For ascariasis, the dosage of piperazine (as the hexahydrate) is 75 mg/kg (maximum dose, 3.5 g) for 2 days in succession, giving the drug orally before or after breakfast. For heavy infestations, treatment should be repeated after 1 week. No pre- or posttreatment cathartics are used.

PRAZIQUANTEL

Praziquantel has the unique characteristic of being effective in the treatment of schistosome infections of all species and many trematode and cestode infections. The drug's safety and effectiveness as a single oral dose has also made it promising in mass treatment of several of the infections. Praziquantel is the first drug to be useful in the treatment of neurocysticercosis. It is not effective against *Fasciola hepatica* or in hydatid disease.

Chemistry, Absorption, Metabolism, & Excretion

Praziquantel is a synthetic isoquinoline-pyrazine derivative and is slightly soluble in water. It is rapidly absorbed (about 80%) after oral administration. Peak serum concentrations of 1 μg/mL are reached 1–2 hours after an oral dose of 50 mg/kg. Praziquantel passes the blood-brain barrier, which results in cerebrospinal fluid concentrations of 14–20% of the drug's plasma concentration; the concentration in bile (in dogs) is nearly 3 times that in venous blood. Most of the drug is rapidly metabolized to mono- and polyhydroxylated products after a first pass in the liver; the half-life of the drug is 1–1.5 hours, while that of its metabolites is 4–6 hours. Excretion is mostly via the kidneys.

Praziquantel

Pharmacologic Effects

In humans, no major alterations in biochemical or hematologic tests have been described, and the drug has not caused reactions in patients with glucose-6-phosphate dehydrogenase deficiencies or hemoglobinopathies. Transient elevations in liver function tests may occur and, rarely, minor electrocardiographic changes, but no significant damage to vital organs has been reported.

In experimental animals, no effects are seen until doses approximately 100 times the therapeutic range are reached; signs of cerebral toxicity are then noted.

In a wide variety of mutagenicity studies, no abnormalities have been found. Tests for carcinogenicity, embryotoxicity, and teratogenicity have also been negative. Several reports suggest that praziquantel acts as a comutagen in *S typhimurium* and mammalian cell test systems; the significance of these findings has not been determined.

Anthelmintic Actions

In spite of its short half-life, praziquantel is the active agent; its metabolites are inactive.

The threshold serum concentration of praziquantel for therapeutic effect is about 0.3 μg/mL. Praziquantel's in vitro action on all platyhelminths appears to be the same—the drug increases cell membrane permeability to calcium, resulting in marked contraction, followed by paralysis of worm musculature. Vacuolization and disintegration of the tegmen occur, and parasite death follows. In cestodes, the sites of vacuolization are restricted to the neck of the strobila, but in trematodes, vacuoles occur in numerous areas over the entire surface. Only a slight reaction occurs with *P westermani*. Although *F hepatica* does absorb the drug, no reaction occurs. In vitro studies with *H diminuta* and with schistosomes have shown that praziquantel also inhibits glucose uptake under anaerobic and aerobic conditions; however, this effect is thought to be secondary.

In schistosome infections of animals, praziquantel is effective against adult worms of both sexes and against the immature stages; adult worms are rapidly immobilized and then passively shift to the liver. In addition, when a single high dose of praziquantel is given concurrent with an infecting dose of cercariae, all immature forms are killed; thus, praziquantel has a prophylactic effect.

Clinical Uses

A. Schistosomiasis: Praziquantel is one of the drugs of choice for the treatment of all forms of schistosomiasis, because of its high efficacy, low toxicity, and ease of oral administration. The drug is effective in adults and children and is well tolerated by patients in the hepatosplenic stage of advanced schistosomiasis. At various dosage schedules, high cure rates (80–95%) are achieved at 3–6 months, with marked reduction in ovum counts in those not cured.

Two studies that compared praziquantel and oxamniquine in the treatment of *S mansoni* infections showed no significant differences in efficacy or side effects. Another study that compared praziquantel with metrifonate in the treatment of *S haematobium* infections showed no important differences in side effects, but praziquantel was more effective.

B. Clonorchiasis and Opisthorchiasis: For *Clonorchis* infections, "apparent" cure rates (disappearance of ova) at 2 months posttreatment have ranged from 87% to 100% of patients after a 1-day course of treatment; however, some patients failed to be cured when reexamined at 1 year. No failures have been reported at 1-year follow-up among an equivalent group treated for 2 days.

Praziquantel may be more effective against *Opisthorchis* infections; at 2 months the 1-day course results in 98–100% cure rates.

C. Paragonimiasis: When treated with 25 mg/kg 3 times daily for 1 day, 71–75% of patients with pulmonary paragonimiasis were cured; 89–100% were cured when treated for 2–3 days.

D. Taeniasis and Diphyllobothriasis: Single-dose therapy (10 mg/kg) is curative in 97–100% of cases.

E. Neurocysticercosis and Subcutaneous Cysticercosis: Praziquantel continues under clinical investigation for use in neurocysticercosis, infection with the larval stage of *T solium*. Live cysts are killed in subcutaneous tissue, muscle, and brain, but the drug does not appear to affect calcified cysts. In subcutaneous cysticercosis, initial changes start at about 2 weeks after conclusion of a course of treatment; thereafter, the cysts tend to diminish in size, and the majority disappear after about 3 months. In many (not all) cases of neurocysticercosis, therapy has resulted in reduction in cerebral hypertension, amelioration of seizures, and either disappearance or reduction in size of lesions on cerebral tomograms. Not yet established, however, are criteria for the type of cases that will benefit from praziquantel treatment or the optimal dosage.

F. H nana: Praziquantel is the drug of choice and the first drug to be highly effective. Higher doses and re-treatment may be required.

G. Other Parasites: Limited trials indicate a high order of effectiveness of praziquantel against several other infections: fasciolopsiasis, metagonimiasis, and other forms of heterophyiasis. At standard dosages, praziquantel has not been effective against hepatica.

Adverse Reactions

Mild and transient side effects directly attributable to the drug are not uncommon. They begin within several hours after ingestion and may persist for hours to 1 day. Most common are malaise, headache, dizziness, and anorexia. Other side effects are drowsiness, nausea, vomiting, abdominal pain, loose to mushy stools, pruritus, urticaria, arthralgia, myalgia, and low-grade fever. Low-grade fever, pruritus, and skin rashes (macular and urticarial), sometimes associated with augmented eosinophilia, may also appear several days after starting the medication and are more likely to be due to the release of foreign proteins from dying worms than to a direct action of the drug.

Praziquantel appears to be better tolerated in children than in adults. Side effects may be more frequent in heavily infected patients. The intensity and frequency of side effects also increase with dosage: They are mild and infrequent at dosages of 10 mg/kg given once but occur in up to 50% of patients who receive 25 mg/kg 3 times in 1 day.

Contraindications & Cautions

The only specific contraindication is ocular cysticercosis; parasite destruction in the eye may cause irreparable damage. The drug can be used in the presence of liver impairment due to parasitic infection. Safety of the drug in children under 4 years is not established.

Because the drug induces dizziness and drowsiness, patients should not drive and should be so warned if their work requires physical coordination or alertness.

The drug should preferably not be taken during pregnancy; an increase in abortion rate was found in rats treated with 3 times the human dose. In lactating women, although praziquantel appears in milk at about one-fourth plasma levels, the drug may be given to the mother provided the infant is not nursed on the day of treatment and for 3 subsequent days.

Preparations & Dosages

Praziquantel (Biltricide, Ceneride, Cesol, Cysticide) is prepared in various strengths by different manufacturers—150-mg, 500-mg, and 600-mg tablets. The tablets are taken with liquid after a meal, should not be chewed because of their bitterness, and should be swallowed immediately because the bitterness of unchewed tablets can induce retching and vomiting. If the drug is taken more than once on the same day, the interval between doses should be no less than 4 and no more than 6 hours.

Optimal dosage schedules are still being determined for some parasites.

A. Schistosomiasis: The dosage for all forms of schistosomiasis is 20 mg/kg 3 times daily for 1 day. Lower dosages have been reported as highly effective in some parts of the world and for some species.

B. *Clonorchis sinensis*, *Opisthorchis* Species, and *Paragonimus* Species: A 2-day course of treatment of 25 mg/kg 3 times daily is recommended.

C. *T saginata* and *D latum*: A single dose of 10 mg/kg has been used successfully for *T saginata* infections and 25 mg/kg for *D latum* infections. Within 24–48 hours after treatment, a disintegrating worm is usually passed by normal peristalsis. Pre- and post-treatment purges are not necessary. If the scolex is searched for but not found—or is not searched for—cure can be presumed only if regenerated segments have not reappeared 3–5 months after treatment.

D. *T solium*: Give a single dose of 10 mg/kg. At present, it is recommended that an effective purge (such as magnesium sulfate, 15–30 g) be given 2 hours after treatment to eliminate all mature segments before ova can be released from disintegrating segments. Since praziquantel does not kill the ova, it is theoretically possible that larvae released from ova in the large bowel could penetrate the intestinal wall and give rise to cysticercosis. As with use of niclosamide, this hazard is probably minimal, but the precaution of a post-treatment purge is advised.

E. Neurocysticercosis: This disorder should be treated in the hospital by a specialist. Current suggested treatment is 50 mg/kg/d in 2–3 divided doses for 15 days. To decrease or block cerebral and meningeal tissue inflammatory reactions and edema that result from dying parasites, steroids (4–16 mg/d in divided doses of dexamethasone, or equivalent) should be administered concurrently and for about 3 days afterward and then gradually reduced. Adverse reactions to praziquantel are similar to those described above but occur with greater frequency. A few deaths from intracranial hypertension or venticular blockage have occurred during or shortly after treatment.

F. H nana: *H nana* infections are treated with a single dose of praziquantel, 25 mg/kg.

PYRANTEL PAMOATE

Pyrantel pamoate is highly effective for the treatment of pinworm, *Ascaris*, and *T orientalis* infections. It is moderately effective against both species of hookworm but less so against *N americanus*. It is not effective in trichuriasis or strongyloidiasis. Oxantel pamoate, an analog of pyrantel, has been used successfully in the treatment of trichuriasis.

Chemistry

Pyrantel pamoate is a tetrahydropyrimidine derivative.

Pyrantel base

Absorption, Metabolism, & Excretion

Pyrantel is poorly absorbed from the gastrointestinal tract. Peak plasma levels are reached in 1–3 hours. Over half of the administered dose is recovered unchanged in the feces.

Pharmacologic Effects & Anthelmintic Actions

Pyrantel is effective against the mature and immature forms of susceptible helminths within the intestinal tract but not against the migratory stages of the worms. The anthelmintic action is probably due to inhibition of neuromuscular transmission. In the helminth, a spastic neuromuscular paralysis occurs, and the worm is subsequently expelled from the host's intestinal tract. In both vertebrate neuromuscular preparations and strip preparations of *Ascaris*, pyrantel shows the activity typical of depolarizing neuromuscular blocking agents. Pyrantel also inhibits cholinesterases.

Clinical Uses

A. *E vermicularis:* Pyrantel given as a single dose and repeated in 2 weeks is effective in curing pinworms in over 95% of patients. Pyrantel and pyrvinium pamoate are equally effective, but pyrantel may have fewer side effects and (unlike pyrvinium) does not stain stool or clothing red. Mebendazole is equally effective and is without significant side effects. Piperazine, which is effective and safe, requires a 7-day course of treatment.

B. *A lumbricoides:* Pyrantel given as a single dose has been reported to be curative in 85–100% of patients.

C. Hookworm and *T orientalis:* A single dose produces cures in over 90% of *A duodenale* and *T orientalis* infections and a marked reduction in the worm burden in the remainder. However, for *N americanus* infections, the cure rate depends on the intensity of infection. A single dose may give a satisfactory cure rate in light infections, but for moderate or heavy infections (over 2000 ova per gram of feces), a 3-day course is necessary to give cure rates near 90%. Hookworm burdens should be markedly reduced, but it is not always possible or essential to eradicate the infection. If iron deficiency disease accompanies the infection, it should be treated with iron medication and a high-protein diet.

Adverse Reactions, Contraindications, & Cautions

Side effects, which occur in 4–20% of children and adults, are infrequent, mild, and transient. They include nausea, vomiting, diarrhea, abdominal cramps, dizziness, drowsiness, headache, insomnia, rash, fever, and weakness. No important effects on hematologic, renal, or hepatic function have been recorded.

There are no contraindications to pyrantel, but it should be used with caution in patients with liver dysfunction, since low, transient SGOT elevations have been noted in a small number of patients. Experience with the drug in children under age 2 years is limited. Safety in pregnancy is undetermined.

Preparations & Dosages

Pyrantel pamoate (pyrantel embonate, Antiminth, Combantrin) is prepared as a suspension containing 50 mg of pyrantel base per milliliter and as tablets containing 125 mg of the base.

For the treatment of pinworm infections and ascariasis, a single oral dose of 10 mg of pyrantel base per kilogram (maximum 1 g) is given with or without food. For pinworm infections, repeat the dose at 2 and 4 weeks; for ascariasis, repeat only if ova are still found 2 weeks after treatment.

For hookworm infections due to *A duodenale*, a single oral dose of 10 mg of pyrantel base per kilogram (maximum 1 g) is used. For infections due to *N americanus* or when the species is unknown, a single dose may be sufficient for light infections, but for moderate or heavy infections the dose should be repeated daily for 3 days. A course of treatment can be repeated in 2 weeks. In the USA, pyrantel is considered an investigational drug when used for hookworm or *T orientalis* infections.

PYRVINIUM PAMOATE

Pyrvinium pamoate, a cyanine dye, is an effective alternative drug for the treatment of pinworm infections. It has only a low order of anthelmintic action against *T trichiura* and hookworm infections and is not effective against *A lumbricoides* infection.

Chemistry, Absorption, Metabolism, & Excretion

Pyrvinium pamoate (viprynium embonate, pyrvinium embonate) is a quaternary amine. The drug is not appreciably absorbed from the gastrointestinal tract.

Anthelmintic Actions

The cyanine dyes contain the amidinium ion system, which may be responsible for their anthelmintic activity. Pyrvinium appears to exert its effect by preventing the parasite from using exogenous carbohydrates. The parasite dies when its endogenous reserves are depleted. The drug does not kill *Enterobius* ova.

Clinical Uses

A. *E vermicularis* (Pinworm): Pyrvinium is an alternative drug for pinworm infections. Reported cure rates after a single dose range from 90% to 100%. Pyrvinium is as effective as the drugs of first choice, pyrantel and mebendazole; each of the drugs requires only one dose in treatment (followed by repeat doses at 2 and 4 weeks), but pyrvinium produces more side effects.

B. *S stercoralis* (Threadworm): There are few reports of the use of pyrvinium for the treatment of strongyloidiasis. The safety and effectiveness of this treatment have yet to be confirmed.

Adverse Reactions

Pyrvinium is well tolerated, but it may cause nausea, vomiting, diarrhea, and dizziness, particularly in older children and adults. Photosensitization and other allergic reactions have been reported rarely. Parents and patients should be told that posttreatment stools are often stained red for several days and that the suspension, if spilled, will stain most materials red.

Pyrvinium contains a promutagen capable of yielding a mutagenic metabolite. Further testing of the compound is needed. In similar testing of pyrantel pamoate, test results were negative.

Cautions

Tablets should be swallowed intact to avoid transient staining of the teeth. The drug should be used cautiously in children weighing less than 10 kg (22 lb); experience with the drug is limited in young children. It is preferable not to use the drug in the presence of inflammatory gastrointestinal tract disorders that theoretically might facilitate absorption.

Preparations & Dosage

Pyrvinium pamoate (Povan) is available in tablets containing 50 mg of pyrvinium base and as a suspension (Povan Suspension) containing 10 mg of base per milliliter. For the treatment of pinworm infections, a single dose is administered orally before or after meals. The dosage is 5 mg/kg (maximum, 350 mg) of pyrvinium base. No pre- or posttreatment purges are used. Treatment should be repeated at 2 and 4 weeks.

QUINACRINE HYDROCHLORIDE

Quinacrine (Atabrine) was formerly an alternative drug for the treatment of tapeworm infections. Because of its toxicity, it should no longer be used unless niclosamide or alternative drugs (praziquantel, mebendazole, paromomycin, or dichlorophen) are not available.

SURAMIN

Suramin is the drug of choice to eradicate adult parasites of *Onchocerca volvulus* infections and the drug of choice in the treatment of the hemolymphatic stage of African trypanosomiasis due to *Trypanosoma brucei gambiense* and *Trypanosoma brucei rhodesiense*. The drug is not marketed in the USA but can be obtained from the Parasitic Disease Drug Service, Centers for Disease Control, Atlanta 30333.

Chemistry, Absorption, Metabolism, & Excretion

Suramin, a complex derivative of urea, is freely soluble in water. Because it is poorly absorbed from the gastrointestinal tract and causes intense local irritation when given subcutaneously or intramuscularly, it should be given intravenously. Suramin persists in the plasma firmly bound to plasma proteins and accumulates in the reticuloendothelial cells throughout the body, especially in the Kupffer cells of the liver and in the epithelium of the renal proximal convoluted tubules. The plasma concentration falls during the first few hours to become constant for several days; this is followed by a low concentration for up to 6 months. The drug appears to be relatively resistant to catabolism, and active metabolites are not known. After a single dose, a small amount is excreted in the urine in the first few days, but thereafter most of the dose cannot be recovered. Sequential doses have a variable cumulative effect. Because suramin does not cross the blood-brain barrier in appreciable amounts, it is not effective if the central nervous system is involved in African trypanosomiasis.

Pharmacologic Effects & Anthelmintic Actions

Suramin's tendency to bind to proteins results in nonspecific inhibition of many enzymes. As a result, it is a potent ATPase inhibitor, and it has multiple actions on clotting through its effects on complement, on fibrinolysis, and on kinin formation.

The drug's action on enzymes concerned with DNA and RNA metabolism may be the basis for its antiparasitic action. In onchocerciasis, the drug acts principally on adult female worms, initially sterilizing them and then causing their death after about the fifth week of treatment; male worms live much longer. Some microfilariae (but not all) are also killed. However, unlike the rapidly acting diethylcarbamazine, suramin kills microfilariae slowly over several weeks, and the reaction is more prolonged and less severe. Although suramin will initially worsen ocular anterior chamber disease and may cause some changes in the posterior chamber, it is not thought to cause as significant changes as diethylcarbamazine.

Suramin inhibits reverse transcriptase in retroviruses, including HTLV-III/LAV/ARV virus, the agent etiologically linked to acquired immunodeficiency syndrome. Suramin is currently being tested for use in this disease.

Suramin has an abortifacient action and is teratogenic in pregnant rats.

Clinical Uses

A. *O volvulus:* Suramin and Mel W (melarsonyl potassium) are the only drugs effective against adult *Onchocerca* worms. Unpredictable deaths have occurred with both compounds, but suramin is the safer of the two. An effective therapeutic program for individual patients consists of nodulectomy for accessible *Onchocerca* nodules (particularly those on the head) plus drug therapy in the form of suramin against adult worms and diethylcarbamazine to kill the microfilariae. However, treatment must be individualized to determine whether the patient can tolerate the side effects of suramin and whether clinical findings warrant its use. If the eyes are not endangered, many authorities limit treatment to nodulectomy and an initial intensive course of diethylcarbamazine, followed by weekly doses indefinitely.

B. *T b gambiense* and *T b rhodesiense:* See Chapter 56.

Adverse Reactions

Side effects of suramin during treatment of onchocerciasis are attributable to pharmacologic reactions to the drug itself and to allergic reactions resulting from release of antigen following death of adult worms or microfilariae.

A. Drug-Induced Reactions: The drug-induced reactions are both immediate and delayed. The immediate reactions ($< 0.5\%$ of patients) are characterized by nausea, vomiting, colic, urticaria, and, rarely, circulatory collapse and loss of consciousness. Delayed drug-induced reactions are fever; renal irritation manifested by albumin, red blood cells, and casts in the urine; polyuria and increased thirst; anorexia and tiredness; photophobia and lacrimation; and hyperesthesia of the palms and soles, sometimes accompanied by desquamation. Rarely, one or more of the following severe reactions may occur: nephrotoxicity leading to renal shutdown, agranulocytosis, hemolytic anemia, jaundice, prolonged high fever, prostration, peripheral neuritis, arthritis, persistent diarrhea, exfoliative dermatitis (which must be differentiated from the inconsequential desquamation due to microfilariae dying in the skin), and severe ulcerations of the mouth and pharynx, sometimes extending to the bronchus. The mortality rate following use of suramin has varied in different parts of the world, but no deaths were reported among 27,000 persons treated in Venezuela.

B. Reactions Due to Dying Parasites: Allergic reactions due to dying parasites tend to occur after the fourth or fifth week but may start with the first dose and increase as the course of treatment proceeds.

Within an hour of the first injection, urticaria and swelling can occur over parts of the body where adult parasites are located. Later, superficial and deep abscesses can develop around the worms; if near a large joint, pain and immobilization may result.

Reactions due to dying microfilariae include fever, skin reactions (pruritus, inflammation, papular and vesicular eruptions), and eye findings (photophobia, itching, lacrimation, keratitis, iridocyclitis, and postneuritic optic atrophy with loss of peripheral vision).

Most reactions are not severe, but they can be so annoying that the patient may refuse to complete the course of treatment. Minor symptoms may be partially relieved by aspirin; severe systemic reactions require a corticosteroid for several days. The development of iridocyclitis requires prompt treatment with topical steroid drops.

Contraindications & Cautions

Patients receiving suramin must be closely watched, preferably in the hospital. Those with heavy loads of microfilariae in the ocular tissues should be treated under the supervision of a physician with adequate ophthalmologic experience. The drug is contraindicated for those intolerant to a test dose, for pregnant patients, and for patients with hypertension or preexisting hepatic and renal insufficiency; it should be used with caution in children under age 10 years, in those with a history of allergy, and in the aged or debilitated.

The patient's condition must be checked before each dose, including examination of skin, liver function, and urine for protein, red cells, and casts. Slight to moderate proteinuria is not an indication to stop therapy, as it usually clears within 2 months and there is no residual damage to the kidneys. However, the presence of protein equivalent to 20 mg or more per deciliter or formed elements in the urine calls for skipping a dose, reducing subsequent doses, or ceasing therapy. Other indications for discontinuation of treatment are prolonged high fever, severe prostration, marked arthritis, exfoliative dermatitis, ulceration of the buccal mucosa, and persistent diarrhea (over 3 days).

Preparations & Dosages

Suramin (Antrypol, Bayer 205, Belganyl, Germanin, Naphuride) is marketed in ampules containing 0.5 and 1 g dry powder that must be stored dry, cool, and sealed in dark bottles. A 10% solution in water or physiologic saline should be prepared for injection and used within 30 minutes.

A. Onchocerciasis: To reduce reactions resulting from the slow death of microfilariae during suramin therapy, it is advisable before starting suramin to treat all cases, whether lightly or heavily infected, with a course of diethylcarbamazine (see p 644) to eliminate most of the microfilariae.

An initial dose of suramin, 0.1 g, is given intravenously very slowly over 3 minutes to test for intolerance to the drug—recognized by the immediate reactions noted above. If the drug is tolerated, a course that results in an 80% or higher reduction in adult worms and microfilariae is 6 successive weekly intravenous doses (injected slowly) of 0.2 g, 0.4 g, 0.6 g, 0.8 g, 0.8–1 g, 0.8–1 g. These dosages are for adults weighing over 60 kg; proportionate reductions should be made for persons weighing less. A second course of treatment should not be given for 3 months after the first course.

About 3–4 weeks after the course of suramin is completed, remaining microfilariae in the skin are killed by giving a course of diethylcarbamazine and then repeating the course at 3- to 4-week intervals until pruritic skin reactions no longer occur.

B. African Trypanosomiasis: See Chapter 56.

TETRACHLOROETHYLENE

Tetrachloroethylene was introduced in 1925 for the treatment of hookworm infections due to *N americanus* or *A duodenale*. Other drugs with fewer side effects are now preferred, but tetrachloroethylene remains an effective and inexpensive alternative drug.

The chemical is also widely used as a cleaning agent in the dry cleaning industry, where toxic exposure has led to damage of the liver, kidneys, and other organs.

Chemistry

Tetrachloroethylene ($Cl_2C=CCl_2$; perchloroethylene), an unsaturated halogenated hydrocarbon, is a colorless, volatile liquid that is slowly decomposed by light and by various metals. To preserve its potency, it must be stored in a cool dark place.

Although the drug is nearly insoluble in water, its solubility is increased by the presence of alcohol or lipids in the gastrointestinal tract.

Absorption, Metabolism, & Excretion

Absorption of tetrachloroethylene is minimal in the normal gastrointestinal tract if the drug is taken in the absence of lipids or alcohol. The small amount absorbed is excreted in the expired air.

Pharmacologic Effects & Anthelmintic Actions

The mode of anthelmintic action of tetrachloroethylene has not been clearly established; it may depress muscle cells or neighboring nerve structures. Paralysis results, causing the hookworms to release their attachment to the intestinal mucosa. Tetrachloroethylene is not effective against *A lumbricoides*.

Teratogenic and carcinogenic effects have been reported in mice.

Clinical Uses

A. Hookworm Infection: Up to 80% of patients infected with *N americanus* and 25–65% with *A duodenale* are cured by one treatment with tetrachloroethylene; in the remaining patients, the worm load is reduced.

B. Intestinal Flukes: Tetrachloroethylene is often effective in the eradication of *H heterophyes, M yokogawai, F buski, Echinostoma* spp, and *Gastrodiscoides hominis.* The drug is used in the same dosages and in the same manner as for hookworm infections, except that for *F buski* infections, a saline purge is given 2 hours after treatment.

Adverse Reactions

Tetrachloroethylene has had extensive use as an anthelmintic without causing serious side effects. However, mild gastrointestinal symptoms (nausea, vomiting, epigastric burning, abdominal cramps) and central nervous system symptoms (dizziness, vertigo, headache, drowsiness) occur frequently. Transient loss of consciousness has been reported, and hypotensive episodes have occurred in severely anemic patients.

Contraindications & Cautions

Although it is frequently claimed that tetrachloroethylene stimulates ascarids and causes their migration, this has not been substantiated. Nevertheless, in mixed infections with both roundworms and hookworms, the roundworms should be eliminated first or, preferably, a drug should be used that is effective against both parasites. Patients with severe anemia should have this condition partially corrected before administration of the drug.

The drug is contraindicated in the treatment of small, severely ill children. It should be avoided in pregnancy, hepatic disease, gastroenteritis, alcoholism, and severe constipation.

Preparations & Dosages

Tetrachloroethylene is marketed in a liquid form or in soft gelatin capsules that contain 0.2, 1, and 5 mL. The gelatin capsules are preferred because they prevent irritation of the oral mucous membranes. Tetrachloroethylene is not marketed in the USA for human use.

The patient should be told to avoid alcohol and fatty foods for 24 hours before and 3 days after medication. Food, but not water, is withheld for a minimum of 6 hours before the drug is administered. The dosage is 0.12 mL/kg up to a maximum of 5 mL and is taken orally in capsule form in the morning or, preferably, at bedtime. The patient should be kept at bed rest for 4 hours following treatment, and food may then be started. Purgation following treatment is not advised, for it may increase side effects and decrease effectiveness of the drug. One treatment may be sufficient for necatoriasis, but for ancylostomiasis 2 or more treatments at intervals of 4–7 days may be required to clear the infection or reduce the worm burden to levels at which the remaining parasites cause no significant blood loss.

THIABENDAZOLE

Thiabendazole is the drug of choice for the treatment of strongyloidiasis and cutaneous larva migrans infections. It may also be tried in trichinosis and visceral larva migrans infections, given the absence of other effective drugs. It is no longer recommended for the treatment of pinworm, ascarid, trichurid, or hookworm infection unless the safer alternative drugs are not available.

Chemistry

Thiabendazole is a benzimidazole compound related to mebendazole. It is tasteless and nearly insoluble in water. Although it is a chelating agent that forms stable complexes with a number of metals, including iron, it does not bind calcium.

Absorption, Metabolism, & Excretion

Thiabendazole is rapidly absorbed after an oral dose. Drug concentrations in plasma peak within 1–2 hours and are barely detectable after 8 hours. Excretion is mainly via the urine. The drug is almost completely metabolized to the 5-hydroxy form, which appears in the urine largely as the glucuronide or sulfate conjugate. Thiabendazole can also be absorbed from the skin.

In some clinical situations, it may be useful to monitor serum drug concentrations.

Pharmacologic Effects & Anthelmintic Actions

Thiabendazole does not appear to produce significant effects on the cardiovascular or respiratory system. It has anti-inflammatory properties, which may be an important factor in its ability to relieve symptoms in some parasitic diseases, particularly dracontiasis. It also has immunomodulating effects on T cell function: It appears to be an immunorestorative agent, demonstrating maximum immunopotentiation in the immunosuppressed host. Thiabendazole also has antipyretic and mild antifungal and scabicidal actions. Carcinogenicity and mutagenicity have not been found, but the drug has not been shown to be safe in pregnancy. Thiabendazole may act on parasites by interfering with microtubule aggregation (see Chapter 55) and through inhibition of the enzyme fumarate reductase.

Clinical Uses

A. S stercoralis: With a dosage of 25 mg/kg twice daily for 2–3 days, cure rates are about 93%.

B. Cutaneous Larva Migrans (Creeping Eruption): Thiabendazole is highly effective in the treatment of cutaneous larva migrans, an infection caused by either *Ancylostoma braziliense* or *Ancyclostoma caninum*.

C. Trichinosis: Information is limited on the effect of thiabendazole on the intestinal phase of trichinosis in humans. During the invasive stage, biopsy evidence suggests that the drug destroys some (though not all) larvae in muscle during the first 2 months of the disease. Amelioration or remission of signs and symptoms is usual without equivalent improvement in abnormal laboratory findings.

Corticosteroids or ACTH are also effective in controlling the clinical manifestations of trichinosis and may be lifesaving in severe infections.

D. Ascariasis, Trichuriasis, and Hookworm and Pinworm Infections: Because of its potential toxicity, thiabendazole is no longer recommended for treatment of these conditions unless the preferred drugs are not available.

E. Other Infections: Intestinal capillariasis has been successfully treated with thiabendazole at a dosage of 12 mg/kg given twice daily for 30 days.

For the treatment of **dracontiasis**, high effectiveness is reported when the drug is used at a dosage of 50–75 mg/kg/d in 2 divided doses for 1 day. Local inflammation subsides rapidly, followed by death of the worms in 4–6 days. Most worms are then spontaneously extruded or can be extracted manually. Retreatment is occasionally needed.

The effectiveness of thiabendazole in **visceral larva migrans** has not been established. Several reports have indicated the usefulness of topical thiabendazole for the treatment of **scabies** and **tinea nigra palmaris**.

Adverse Reactions

At the standard dosage of 25 mg/kg twice daily for 2 days, side effects occur in 7–50% of patients, generally 3–4 hours after ingestion of the drug, and last 2–8 hours. Higher doses or extension of treatment beyond 2 days increases symptoms. Side effects are generally mild and transient but can be severe; the most common are dizziness, anorexia, nausea, and vomiting. Less frequent are epigastric pain, abdominal cramps, pruritus, headache, drowsiness, giddiness, and other neuropsychiatric symptoms. Perianal rashes, tinnitus, paresthesias, bradycardia, hypotension, and visual disturbances are rare, as are liver function abnormalities. Seven cases of erythema multiforme have been associated with thiabendazole therapy in children; in 2 severe cases (Stevens-Johnson syndrome), fatalities occurred.

Other side effects have been reported, but some may represent manifestations of the disease or reactions to dying parasites rather than drug reaction. They include fever, chills, conjunctival injection, angioneurotic edema, lymphadenopathy, skin rashes, toxic epidermal necrolysis, and anaphylaxis.

Occasionally reported during thiabendazole treatment have been leukopenia, crystalluria, hematuria, and elevations of serum aspartate aminotransferase and cephalin flocculation values, all of which subsided when therapy was discontinued.

Some patients may excrete a metabolite that imparts an asparaginelike odor to the urine during therapy and for 24 hours thereafter.

Contraindications & Cautions

Experience with thiabendazole is limited in children weighing less than 15 kg. It may be best to use alternative drugs in patients with hepatic or renal dysfunction. The drug should be used with caution where drug-induced vomiting may be dangerous. There are a few reports of ascarids becoming hypermotile after treatment and appearing at the nose or mouth.

Since the drug makes some patients dizzy or drowsy, it should not be used during the day for patients whose work or activity requires mental alertness.

Discontinue the drug immediately if hypersensitivity symptoms appear.

Preparations & Dosages

Thiabendazole (Mintezol) is available as a suspension containing 100 mg of the drug per milliliter and as tablets containing 500 mg of the drug. The standard dose is 25 mg/kg (maximum, 1.5 g). The drug should be given after meals, and the tablet formulation *should be chewed well*. Pre- and posttreatment purges and dietary restrictions are not necessary.

In the treatment of strongyloidiasis, the standard dose is given twice daily for 2 successive days. A second course may be given 1 week later if indicated. In the hyperinfection syndrome, the standard dose is continued twice daily for 5–7 days.

In the treatment of cutaneous larva migrans, the standard dose is given twice daily for 2–5 days. If active lesions are still present 2 days after completion of therapy, a second course should be given. Excellent results have also followed daily application for about 5 days of a cream containing 15% thiabendazole in a hygroscopic base.

For the treatment of trichinosis, the standard dose is given twice daily for 2–5 days; for visceral larval migrans, twice daily for up to 7 days.

REFERENCES

General References

Drugs for parasitic infections. *Med Lett Drugs Ther* 1984; **26**:27.

Mansfield JM (editor): *Parasitic Diseases*. Vol 2: *The Chemotherapy*. Marcel Dekker, 1984.

Stürchler D: Chemotherapy of human intestinal helminthiases: A review, with particular reference to community treatment. *Adv Pharmacol Chemother* 1982;**19**:124.

Vanden Bossche H, Thienpont D, Janssens PG (editors): *Chemotherapy of Gastrointestinal Helminths*. Springer-Verlag, 1985.

Albendazole

Albendazole: Worms and hydatid disease. (Editorial.) *Lancet* 1984;**2**:675.

Firth M (editor): Symposium on albendazole in helminthiasis. *Royal Society of Medicine International Congress and Symposium Series*, No. 57. The Royal Society of Medicine, Academic Press, and Grune & Stratton, 1983.

Morris DL et al: Albendazole: Objective evidence of response in human hydatid disease. *JAMA* 1985;**253**:2053.

Ramalingam S, Sinniah B, Krishnan U: Albendazole, an effective single dose, broad spectrum anthelmintic drug. *Am J Trop Med Hyg* 1983;**32**:984.

Rossignol JF, Maisonneuve H: Albendazole: Placebo-controlled study in 870 patients with intestinal helminthiasis. *Trans R Soc Trop Med Hyg* 1983;**77**:707.

Schantz PM: Effective medical treatment for hydatid disease? *JAMA* 1985;**253**:2095.

Bithionol

Coleman DL, Barry M: Relapse of *Paragonimus westermani* lung infection after bithionol therapy. *Am J Trop Med Hyg* 1982;**31**:71.

Grados O, Berrocal LA: Chemotherapy of fascioliasis with bithionol. *Rev Inst Med Trop Sao Paulo* 1977;**19**:425. [English summary.]

Kim JS: Treatment of *Paragonimus westermani* infections with bithionol. *Am J Trop Med Hyg* 1970;**19**:940.

Miyazaki I, Nishimura K: Cerebral paragonomiasis. Pages 109–132 in: *Topics on Tropical Neurology*. Hornabrook R (editor). Davis, 1975.

Yokogawa M: *Paragonimus* and paragonimiasis. Pages 375–387 in: *Advances in Parasitology*. Vol 7. Dawes B (editor). Academic Press, 1969.

Dichlorophen

Gemmell MA, Johnstone PD: Cestodes. Pages 54–114 in: *Antibiotics and Chemotherapy*. Vol 30. Schonfeld H (editor). Karger, 1981.

Seaton DR: On the use of dichlorophen as a taenifuge for *Taenia saginata*. *Ann Trop Med Parasitol* 1960;**54**:338.

Turner PP: The treatment of tapeworm infestation with "Anthiphen." *J Trop Med Hyg* 1963;**66**:259.

Diethylcarbamazine

Adjepon-Yamoah KK et al: The effect of renal disease on the pharmacokinetics of diethylcarbamazine in man. *Br J Clin Pharmacol* 1982;**13**:829.

Bryceson ADM, Warrell DA, Pope HM: Dangerous reactions to treatment of onchocerciasis with diethylcarbamazine. *Br Med J* 1977;**1**:742.

Greene BM et al: Ocular and systemic complications of diethylcarbamazine therapy for onchocerciasis: Association with circulating immune complexes. *J Infect Dis* 1983; **147**:890.

Hawking F: Diethylcarbamazine and new compounds for the treatment of filariasis. *Adv Pharmacol Chemother* 1979; **16**:129.

Ottesen EA: Efficacy of diethylcarbamazine in eradicating infection with lymphatic-dwelling filariae in humans. *Rev Infect Dis* 1985;**7**:341.

Stanley SL Jr, Kell O: Ascending paralysis associated with diethylcarbamazine treatment of *M loa loa* infection. *Trop Doct* 1982;**12**:16.

Levamisole

Kilpatrick ME et al: Levamisole compared to mebendazole in the treatment of *Ancylostoma duodenale* in Egypt. *Trans R Soc Trop Med Hyg* 1981;**75**:578.

Levamisole: A cautionary note. (Editorial.) *Lancet* 1979;**2**: 291.

Miller JM: Use of levamisole in parasitic infections. *Drugs* 1980;**19**:122.

Moens J et al: Levamisole in ascariasis: A multicenter controlled evaluation. *Am J Trop Med Hyg* 1978;**27**:897.

Symoens J et al: Levamisole. Pages 407–464 in: *Pharmacological and Biochemical Properties of Drug Substances*. Vol 2. Goldberg ME (editor). American Pharmaceutical Association, 1979.

Mebendazole

Jaroonvesama N et al: Treatment of *Opisthorchis viverrini* with mebendazole. *Southeast Asian J Trop Med Pub Health* 1981;**12**:595.

Kammerer WS, Schantz PM: Long term follow-up of human hydatid disease (echinococcus granulosus) treated with a high-dose mebendazole regimen. *Am J Trop Med Hyg* 1984;**33**:132.

Keystone JS, Murdoch JK: Diagnosis and treatment. Drugs five years later: Mebendazole. *Ann Intern Med* 1979; **91**:582.

Mravak S, Schopp W, Bienzle U: Treatment of strongyloidiasis with mebendazole. *Acta Tropica* 1983;**40**:93.

Schantz PM, Van den Bosche H, Eckert J: Chemotherapy for larval echinococcosis in animals and humans: Report of a workshop. *Z Parasitenkd* 1982;**67**:5.

Van den Bossche H, Rochette F, Hörig C: Mebendazole and related anthelmintics. *Adv Pharmacol Chemother* 1982; **19**:67.

Wilson KH, Kauffman CA: Persistent *Strongyloides stercoralis* in a blind loop of bowel: Successful treatment with mebendazole. *Arch Intern Med* 1983;**143**:357.

Metrifonate

Farid Z et al: Urinary schistosomiasis in Egyptian farmers treated with metrifonate (Bilarcil). *Ann Trop Med Parasitol* 1981;**75**:459.

Feldmeier H et al: Efficacy of metrifonate in urinary schistosomiasis: Comparison of reduction of *Schistosoma haematobium* and *S mansoni* eggs. *Am J Trop Med Hyg* 1982; **31**:1188.

Jewsbury JM: Metrifonate in schistosomiasis. *Acta Pharmacol Toxicol* 1981;**49(Suppl 5)**:123.

Symposium: Metrifonate and dichlorvos: Theoretical and practical aspects. Aldridge WN, Holmstedt B (editors). *Acta Pharmacol Toxicol* 1981;**49(Suppl 5)**:3.

Tswana SA, Mason PR: Eighteen-month follow-up on the treatment of urinary schistosomiasis with a single dose of metrifonate. *Am J Trop Med Hyg* 1985;**34**:746.

Metronidazole

Nik-Akhtar B, Tabibi V: Metronidazole in fascioliasis: Report of four cases. *J Trop Med Hyg* 1977;**80**:179.

Niclosamide

Jones WE: Niclosamide as a treatment for *Hymenolepis diminuta* and *Dipylidium caninum* infection in man. *Am J Trop Med Hyg* 1979;**28**:300.

Most H et al: Yomesan (niclosamide) therapy of *Hymenolepis nana* infections. *Am J Trop Med Hyg* 1971;**20**:206.

Pearson RD, Hewlett EL: Niclosamide therapy for tapeworm infections. *Ann Intern Med* 1985;**102**:550.

Perera DR et al: Niclosamide treatment of cestodiasis: Clinical trials in the United States. *Am J Trop Med Hyg* 1970;**19**:610.

Niridazole

Kale OO: A controlled field trial of the treatment of dracontiasis with metronidazole and niridazole. *Ann Trop Med Parasitol* 1974;**68**:91.

The pharmacological and chemotherapeutic properties of niridazole and other antischistosomal compounds. (Conference.) *Ann NY Acad Sci* 1969;**160**:426.

Roxe DM et al: Mutagenic activity or urinary pigments from patients on antischistosomal therapy with niridazole. *Mutat Res* 1980;**77**:367.

Saif M et al: On the treatment of urinary bilharziasis with ni-

ridazole. *J Egypt Med Assoc* 1974;**57**:83.

Sy FS: Niridazole in the treatment of schistosomiasis japonicum. *J Philippine Med Assoc* 1977;**53**:151.

Oxamniquine

Kilpatrick ME et al: Treatment of schistosomiasis mansoni with oxamniquine: Five years experience. *Am J Trop Med Hyg* 1981;**306**:1219.

Krajden S, Keystone JS, Glenn C: Safety and toxicity of oxamniquine in the treatment of *Schistosoma mansoni* infections, with particular reference to electroencephalographic abnormalities. *Am J Trop Med Hyg* 1983;**32**:1344.

Lambertucci JR et al: A double blind trial with oxamniquine in chronic schistosomiasis mansoni. *Trans R Soc Trop Med Hyg* 1982;**76**:751.

Oxamniquine symposium. *Rev Inst Med Trop Sao Paulo* 1980;**22(Suppl 4)**:1. [Entire issue.]

Oxantel Pamoate

Dissanaike AS: A comparative trial of oxantel-pyrantel and mebendazole in multiple helminth infection in school children. *Drugs* 1978;**15(Suppl 1)**:11.

Sinniah B, Sinniah D: The anthelmintic effects of pyrantel pamoate, oxantel-pyrantel pamoate, levamisole and mebendazole in the treatment of intestinal nematodes. *Ann Trop Med Parasitol* 1981;**75**:315.

Paromomycin

Botero D: Paromomycin as effective treatment of *Taenia* infections. *Am J Trop Med Hyg* 1970;**19**:234.

Pawlowski Z, Schultz AG: Taeniasis and cysticercosis *(Taenia saginata)*. *Adv Parasitol* 1972;**10**:292.

Tanowitz HB, Wittner M: Paromomycin in the treatment of *Diphyllobothrium latum* infection. *Am J Trop Med Hyg* 1973;**76**:151.

Wittner M, Tanowitz H: Paromomycin therapy of human cestodiasis with special reference to hymenolepiasis. *Am J Trop Med Hyg* 1971;**20**:433.

Piperazine

Bellander BTD, Hagmar LE, Osterdahl BG: Nitrosation of piperazine in the stomach. *Lancet* 1981;**2**:372.

Brown HW, Chan KF, Hussey KL: Treatment of enterobiasis and ascariasis with piperazine. *JAMA* 1956;**161**:515.

Bumbalo TS, Plummer LJ: Piperazine (Antepar) in the treatment of pinworm and roundworm infections. *Med Clin North Am* 1957;**41**:575.

Fernando MA, Balasuriya S: Control of ascariasis by mass treatment with piperazine citrate. *Ceylon Med J* 1977; **22**:120.

Ukadgaonkar NG, Bjagwat RB, Kulkarni MU: Transient cerebellar syndrome due to piperazine citrate. *Clinician* 1982;**46**:461.

Praziquantel

Bell DR: Cysticercosis: A new hope. *Br Med J* 1984;**289**:857.

Campos R, Bressnan MCRV, Evangelista MGBF: Activity of praziquantel against *Hymenolepis nana*, at different development states, in experimentally infected mice. *Rev Inst Med Trop Sao Paulo* 1984;**26**:334.

Chen C-Y, Hsieh W-C: Clinical investigation of praziquantel in the treatment of clonorchiasis sinensis. *J Formosan Med Assoc* 1982;**81**:1434.

Classen HG, Schramm V (editors): Praziquantel (Embay 8440, Biltricide). Given at the Biltricide Symposium on African Schistosomiasis, Nairobi, 24–26 February 1980. *Drug Res* 1981;**31**:535.

Classen HG, Schramm V (editors): Symposium Proceedings: International Symposium on Human Trematode Infections in Southeast and East Asia. Given in Kyongju, Republic of Korea, 19–21 October 1983. *Drug Res* 1984;**34**:1115.

Davis A, Wegner DHG: Multicentre trials of praziquantel in human schistosomiasis: Design and techniques. *Bull WHO* 1979;**57**:767.

Farid Z, Ayad El-Masry N, Wallace CK: Treatment of *Hymenolepis nana* with a single oral dose of praziquantel. *Trans R Soc Trop Med Hyg* 1984;**78**:280.

Groll EW: Chemotherapy of human cysticercosis with praziquantel. In: *Cysticercosis: Present State of Knowledge and Perspective.* Academic Press, 1982.

Johnson RJ et al: Paragonimiasis: Diagnosis and the use of praziquantel in treatment. *Rev Infect Dis* 1985;**7**:200.

Katz N, Rocha RS: Double-blind clinical trial comparing praziquantel with oxamniquine in schistosomiasis mansoni. *Rev Inst Med Trop Sao Paulo* 1982;**24**:310.

McMahon JE: A comparative trial of praziquantel, metrifonate and niridazole against *Schistosoma haematobium. Ann Trop Med Parasitol* 1983;**77**:139.

Nash TE, Neva FA: Recent advances in the diagnosis and treatment of cerebral cysticercosis. *N Engl J Med* 1984; **311**:1492.

Robles C (editor): International Symposium on the Medical Treatment of Neurocysticercosis, Mexico, 10–11 September 1982. Symposium Internacional sobre Tratamiento Medico de la Neurocisticercosis. *Salud Publica de Mexico* 1982;**24**:605.

Sotelo J et al: Therapy of parenchymal brain cysticercosis with praziquantel. *N Engl J Med* 1984;**310**:1001.

World Health Organization: Multicentre trials of praziquantel in human schistosomiasis. *Bull WHO* 1979;**57**:767.

Zhejiang Clinical Cooperative Research Group for Praziquantel: Clinical evaluation of praziquantel in treatment of schistosomiasis japonicum. *Chin Med J* 1980;**93**:375.

Pyrantel Pamoate

Botero D, Castaño A: Comparative study of pyrantel pamoate, bephenium hydroxynaphthoate, and tetrachlorethylene in the treatment of *Necator americanus* infections. *Am J Trop Med Hyg* 1973;**22**:45.

Davis A: *Drug Treatment in Intestinal Helminthiases.* World Health Organization, 1973.

Kale OO: Controlled comparative study of the efficacy of pyrantel pamoate and a combined regimen of piperazine citrate and bephenium hydroxynaphthoate in the treatment of intestinal nemathelminthiasis. *Afr J Med Sci* 1981; **10**:63.

Sinniah B, Sinniah D: The anthelmintic effects of pyrantel pamoate, oxantel-pyrantel pamoate, levamisole and mebendazole in the treatment of intestinal nematodes. *Ann Trop Med Parasitol* 1981;**75**:315.

Pyrvinium Pamoate

Buchanan RA et al: Pyrvinium pamoate. *Clin Pharmacol Ther* 1974;**16**:716.

Macphee DG, Podger DM: Mutagenicity tests on anthelmintics: Microsomal activation of viprynium embonate to a mutagen. *Mutat Res* 1977;**48**:307.

Turner JA, Johnson PE Jr: Pyrinium pamoate in the treatment of pinworm infection (enterobiasis) in the home. *J Pediatr* 1962;**60**:243.

Wang CC, Galli GA: Strongyloidiasis treated with pyrvinium pamoate. *JAMA* 1965;**193**:847.

Suramin

Anderson J, Fuglsang H: Further studies on the treatment of ocular onchocerciasis with diethylcarbamazine and suramin. *Br J Ophthalmol* 1978;**62**:450.

Hawking F: Suramin: With special reference to onchocerciasis. *Adv Pharmacol Chemother* 1978;**15**:289.

Mitsuya H et al: Suramin protection of T cells in vitro against infectivity and cytopathic effect of HTLV-III. *Science* 1984;**226**:172.

Research and Control of Onchocerciasis in the Western Hemisphere: Proceedings of an International Symposium, Washington, D.C., 18–21 November 1974. Pan American Health Organization Scientific Publication No. 298, 1974.

Scharlau G: Onchocerciasis-chemotherapy: A risk-approach. *Trop Doct* 1981;**11**:8.

Thylefors B, Rolland A: The risk of optic atrophy following suramin treatment of ocular onchocerciasis. *Bull WHO* 1979;**57**:479.

Tetrachloroethylene

Ikeda M: Metabolism of trichloroethylene and tetrachloroethylene in human subjects. *Environ Health Perspect* 1977; **21**:239.

Senewiratne B et al: A comparative study of the relative efficacy of pyrantel pamoate, bephenium hydroxynaphthoate and tetrachloroethylene in the treatment of *Necator americanus* infection in Ceylon. *Ann Trop Med Parasitol* 1975;**69**:233.

Thiabendazole

Grove DI: Treatment of strongyloidiasis with thiabendazole: An analysis of toxicity and effectiveness. *Trans R Soc Trop Med Hyg* 1982;**76**:114.

Kale OO, Elemile T, Enahoro F: Controlled comparative trial of thiabendazole and metronidazole in the treatment of dracontiasis. *Ann Trop Med Parasitol* 1983;**77**:151.

Perrin J et al: Thiabendazole treatment of presumptive visceral larva migrans. *Clin Pediatr* 1975;**14**:147.

Rex D et al: Intrahepatic cholestasis and sicca complex after thiabendazole. *Gastroenterology* 1983;**85**:718.

Sastry SC, Kumar KJ, Lakshminarayana V: The treatment of dracontiasis with thiabendazole. *J Trop Med Hyg* 1978; **81**:32.

Winter PAD, Fripp PJ: Treatment of cutaneous larva migrans (sandworm disease). *S Afr Med J* 1978;**54**:556.

Cancer Chemotherapy

58

Sydney E. Salmon, MD, & Alan C. Sartorelli, PhD

Cancer is a group of neoplastic diseases that occur in humans of all age groups and races as well as in all animal species. The incidence, geographic distribution, and behavior of specific types of cancer are related to multiple factors including sex, age, race, genetic predisposition, and exposure to environmental carcinogens. Of these factors, the last is probably most important. Chemical carcinogens (particularly those in tobacco smoke) as well as agents such as azo dyes, aflatoxins, and benzene have been clearly implicated in cancer induction in humans as well as in animals. Identification of potential carcinogens in the environment has been greatly simplified by the widespread use of the "Ames test" for mutagenic agents. Ninety percent of carcinogens can be shown to be mutagenic on the basis of this assay. Ultimate identification of potential human carcinogens requires, however, testing in 2 animal species. Certain herpes and papilloma group DNA viruses and type C RNA viruses have also been implicated as causative agents in animal cancers and might be responsible for some human cancers as well. Oncogenic RNA viruses all appear to contain a "reverse transcriptase" enzyme that permits translation of the RNA message of the tumor virus into the DNA code of the infected cell. Thus, the information governing transformation can become a stable part of the genome of the host cell. Expression of virus-induced neoplasia probably also depends on additional host and environmental factors that modulate the transformation process. A specific human T cell leukemia virus (HTLV-I) has been identified as causative of this specific type of leukemia. A closely related virus (HTLV-III/LAV/ARV) causes acquired immunodeficiency syndrome (AIDS). Cellular genes homologous to the transforming genes of the retroviruses, a family of RNA viruses, are known that induce oncogenic transformation. These mammalian cellular genes, known as "oncogenes," have been shown to code for specific growth factors and may be amplified (increased number of gene copies) or modified by a single nucleotide in malignant cells. While some RNA tumor viruses have apparently "picked up" cellular oncogenes at some point in phylogeny and have capitalized on these genes for oncogenic transformation, other RNA tumor viruses (eg, HTLV-I) are oncogenic despite the absence of known oncogenes.

Whatever the cause, cancer is basically a disease of cells characterized by a shift in the control mechanisms that govern cell proliferation and differentiation. Cells that have undergone neoplastic transforma-

tion usually express cell surface antigens that appear to be of normal fetal type and have other signs of apparent "immaturity" and may exhibit qualitative or quantitative chromosomal abnormalities, including various translocations and the appearance of amplified gene sequences. Such cells proliferate excessively and form local tumors that can compress or invade adjacent normal structures. A small subpopulation of cells within the tumor can be described as **tumor stem cells.** They retain the ability to undergo repeated cycles of proliferation as well as to migrate to distant sites in the body to colonize various organs in the process called **metastasis.** Such tumor stem cells thus can express **clonogenic** or colony-forming capability. Maintenance of the clonogenic potential of tumor stem cells can be demonstrated in animals or in vitro by recovering tumor colonies and reseeding the cells that comprise them, thus showing that the cells can renew themselves and give rise to secondary colonies. Fig 58–1 depicts a typical human tumor colony cloned from a tumor stem cell in vitro. Tumor stem cells often have chromosome abnormalities reflecting their genetic instability, which leads to progressive selection of subclones that can survive more readily in the multicellu-

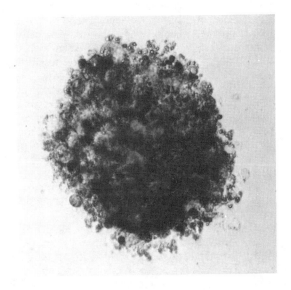

Figure 58–1. Human colon tumor "stem cell" colony in soft agar grown from clonogenic cells from a biopsy of a previously untreated patient. Such tumor colony–forming cells can be tested with standard and new anticancer drugs with respect to inhibition of clonogenicity.

lar environment of the host. Quantitative abnormalities in various metabolic pathways and cellular components accompany this neoplastic progression. The invasive and metastatic processes as well as a series of metabolic abnormalities resulting from the cancer cause illness and eventual death of the patient unless the neoplasm can be eradicated with treatment.

Next to heart disease, cancer is the major cause of death in the USA, causing over 500,000 fatalities annually. With present methods of treatment, one-third of patients are cured with local measures (surgery or radiation therapy), which are quite effective when the tumor has not metastasized by the time of treatment. Earlier diagnosis might lead to cure of 50% of patients with such local treatment; however, in the remaining cases, early micrometastasis is a characteristic feature of the neoplasm, indicating that a systemic approach such as can be attained with chemotherapy will be required (often along with surgery or radiation) for effective cancer management. At present, about 50% of patients with cancer can be cured, with chemotherapy contributing to cure in about 17% of patients.

Cancer chemotherapy as currently employed can be curative in certain disseminated neoplasms that have undergone either gross or microscopic spread by the time of diagnosis. These include testicular cancer, diffuse histiocytic lymphoma, Hodgkin's disease, and choriocarcinoma as well as childhood tumors such as acute lymphoblastic leukemia, Burkitt's lymphoma, Wilms' tumor, and embryonal rhabdomyosarcoma. Of major importance are recent demonstrations that use of chemotherapy along with initial surgery can increase the cure rate in relatively early-stage breast cancer, soft tissue, and osteogenic sarcoma. Common carcinomas of the lung and colon are generally refractory to currently available treatment and have usually disseminated by the time of diagnosis.

At present, chemotherapy provides palliative rather than curative therapy for many other forms of disseminated cancer. Effective palliation results in temporary clearing of the symptoms and signs of cancer and prolongation of useful life. In the past decade, advances in cancer chemotherapy have also begun to provide evidence that chemical control of neoplasia may become a reality for many forms of cancer during the 1980s. This will probably be achieved first through combined therapy in which optimal combinations of surgery, radiotherapy, and chemotherapy are used to eradicate both the primary and its occult micrometastases before gross spread can be detected on physical or x-ray examinations.

Drug research may provide the ultimate cure for cancer, although many of the currently available agents fall short of this goal. A major effort to develop anticancer drugs through both empiric screening and rational design of new compounds has now been under way for 3 decades. Recent advances in this field have included the synthesis of peptides and proteins with the recombinant DNA technique and monoclonal antibodies. The drug development program has employed testing in a few well-characterized transplantable animal tumor systems. The development of a simple in vitro colony assay for measuring drug sensitivity of human tumor stem cells may augment and shorten the testing program in the near future. An example of such an in vitro assay for standard anticancer drugs is presented in Fig 58–2. Once new drugs with potential anticancer activity are identified, they are subjected to preclinical toxicologic and limited pharmacologic studies in animals as described in Chapter 4. Promising agents that do not have excessive toxicity are then advanced to phase I clinical trials wherein their pharmacologic and toxic effects are tested in patients with advanced cancer. Phase II clinical trials are then used to establish the tumor types for which the drug is useful, followed by phase III trials to compare the new agent with the best standard therapy. Subsequently, the drug may be licensed by the FDA for use in practice.

Ideal anticancer drugs would eradicate cancer cells without harming normal tissues. Unfortunately, no currently available agents meet this criterion, and clinical use of these drugs involves a weighing of benefits against toxicity in a search for a favorable therapeutic index.

Information on cell and population kinetics of cancer cells in part explains the limited effectiveness of

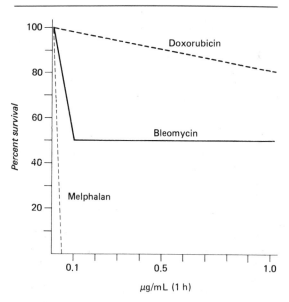

Figure 58–2. Example of an in vitro sensitivity assay with pharmacologically achievable doses of cytotoxic anticancer drugs tested against tumor colony–forming stem cells from a patient's tumor biopsy sample. The cells were incubated in various concentrations of the drugs for 1 hour prior to plating in soft agar and then cultured for 1 week prior to counting the survival of tumor colony–forming units. The results demonstrate sensitivity to melphalan, resistance to doxorubicin, and heterogeneity in response to bleomycin. Fifty percent of the colony-forming cells showed sensitivity to bleomycin at the lowest dose tested, while the remaining 50% were resistant to the highest dose.

most available anticancer drugs. A schematic summary of cell cycle kinetics is presented in Fig 58–3. This information is relevant to the mode of action, indications, and scheduling of cell cycle–specific (CCS) and cell cycle–nonspecific (CCNS) drugs. Agents falling in these 2 major classes are summarized in Table 58–1. Other classes of drugs have recently also entered development, including the following: inducers of differentiation, intended to force neoplastic cells past a maturation block to form end-stage cells with little or no neoplastic potential; antimetastatic drugs, designed to perturb surface properties of malignant cells and thus alter their invasive and metastatic potential; hypoxic tumor stem cell–specific agents, designed to exploit the greater capacity for reductive reactions in these therapeutically resistant cells created by oxygen deficiency of solid tumors; tumor radiosensitizing and normal tissue radioprotecting drugs, aimed at increasing therapeutic effectiveness of radiation therapy; and "biologic response modifiers," which alter tumor-host metabolic and immunologic relationships. Patients with widespread cancer (eg, acute leukemia) may have 10^{12} (1 trillion) tumor cells

throughout the body at the time of diagnosis. If tolerable dosing of an effective drug is capable of killing 99.9% of clonogenic tumor cells, this would induce a clinical remission of the neoplasm associated with symptomatic improvement. However, there would still be many logs (10^9) of tumor cells remaining in the body, including some that may be inherently resistant to the drug because of heterogeneity, while others might reside in pharmacologic sanctuaries (eg, the central nervous system) where effective drug concentrations may be difficult to achieve. When CCS drugs are used, the tumor stem cells must also be in the sensitive phase of the cell cycle (and not in G_0), so scheduling of these agents is of particular importance. In common bacterial infections, a 3-log reduction in microorganisms might be curative, because host resistance factors can eliminate residual bacteria through immunologic and microbicidal mechanisms; however, host mechanisms for eliminating moderate numbers of cancer cells appear to be generally ineffective. To overcome the limited "log kill" of individual anticancer drugs, combinations of agents with differing toxicities and mechanisms of action have been em-

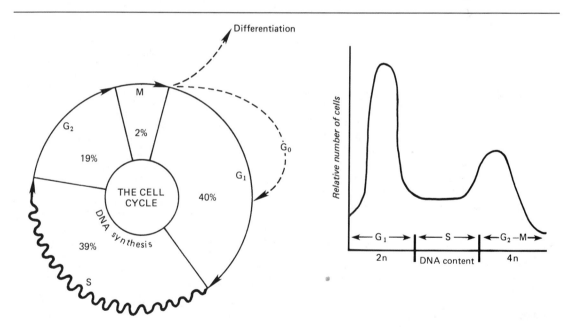

Figure 58–3. The cell cycle and cancer. The illustration at left is a conceptual depiction of the cell cycle phases that all cells—normal and neoplastic—must traverse prior to cell division. The relative durations of the various phases of the cycle are given in approximate percentages spent in each phase by a typical malignant cell; the duration of G_1, however, can vary markedly. At right is a histogram of DNA content of an unperturbed population of tumor cells as determined by flow microfluorimetry (FMF), a technique that permits quantitation of the proportion of cells in the major phases of the cell cycle. Many of the effective anticancer drugs exert their action on cells traversing the cell cycle and are called cell cycle–specific (CCS) drugs (Table 58–1). A second group of agents called cell cycle–nonspecific (CCNS) drugs can sterilize tumor cells irrespective of whether they are cycling or resting in the G_0 compartment. G_1 is the initial phase of the cell cycle of a cell committed to proliferation and is associated with synthesis of enzymes required for function and for DNA synthesis. The S (synthesis) phase is the time during which the DNA genome is duplicated. The G_2 phase is associated with synthesis of cellular components required for mitosis followed by the brief M (mitotic) phase of cell division. CCNS drugs are capable of killing both G_0 and cycling cells (although cycling cells are more sensitive). The damage induced by CCNS drugs is often manifested as a lengthening of the S phase and an irreversible G_2 block. An FMF curve of cells treated with a CCNS drug would be reduced in size in comparison to that seen above, and with a shift in DNA content of intact cells to a 4n accumulation.

Table 58–1. Cell cycle relationships of major classes of drugs.

Cell Cycle–Specific (CCS) Agents	Cell Cycle–Nonspecific (CCNS) Agents
Antimetabolites (azacitidine, cytarabine, fluorouracil, mercaptopurine, methotrexate, thioguanine)	Alkylating agents (busulfan, cyclophosphamide, mechlorethamine, melphalan, thiotepa)
Bleomycin peptide antibiotics	Antibiotics (dactinomycin, daunorubicin, doxorubicin, mithramycin, mitomycin)
Podophyllin alkaloids (etoposide, VP-16; teniposide, VM-26)	Cisplatin
Vinca alkaloids (vincristine, vinblastine, vindesine)	Nitrosoureas (BCNU, CCNU, methyl-CCNU)

ployed. If the drugs do not have too much overlap in toxicity, they can be used at almost full dosage, and at least additive cytotoxic effects can be achieved with combination chemotherapy; furthermore, subclones resistant to only one of the agents can potentially be eradicated. Some combinations of anticancer drugs also appear to exert true synergism wherein the effect of the 2 drugs is greater than additive. The efficacy of combination chemotherapy has now been validated in many forms of human cancer, and the scientific rationale appears to be sound. As a result, combination chemotherapy is now the standard approach to curative treatment of testicular cancer and lymphomas and improved palliative treatment of many other tumor types. This important therapeutic approach was first formulated by Skipper and Schabel and described as the "log-kill hypothesis." It is depicted in Fig 58–4.

In general, CCS drugs have proved most effective in hematologic malignancies and other tumors in which a relatively large proportion of the cells are proliferating or are in the **growth fraction.** CCNS drugs (many of which bind to DNA and damage these macromolecules) are useful in low-growth-fraction "solid tumors" as well as in high-growth-fraction tumors. In all instances, effective agents sterilize or inactivate tumor stem cells, which are often only a small fraction of the cells within a tumor. Non–stem cells (eg, those that have irreversibly differentiated) are considered sterile by definition and are not a significant component of the cancer problem.

Resistance to Cytotoxic Drugs

A major problem in cancer chemotherapy is **drug resistance.** Some tumor types, eg, non–small cell lung cancer and colon cancer, exhibit *primary* resistance, ie, absence of response on the first exposure, to currently available standard agents. *Acquired* resistance develops in a number of drug-sensitive tumor types. Experimentally, drug resistance can be observed that is highly specific to a single drug and usually is based on a change in the tumor cell's genetic apparatus with *amplification* of one or more specific genes. In other instances, a multidrug-resistant phenotype occurs—resistance to a variety of natural product anticancer drugs developing after exposure to a single agent. This form of multidrug resistance is associated

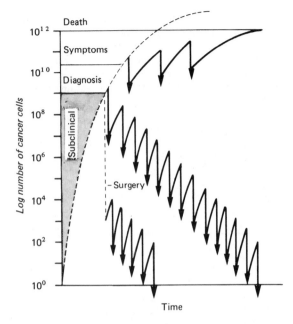

Figure 58–4. The "log-kill hypothesis." Relationship of tumor cell number to time of diagnosis, symptoms, treatment, and survival. Three alternative approaches to drug treatment are shown for comparison with the course of tumor growth when no treatment is given (dotted line). In the protocol diagrammed at top, treatment (indicated by the arrows) is given infrequently, and the result is manifested as prolongation of survival but with recurrence of symptoms between courses of treatment and eventual death of the patient. The combination chemotherapy treatment diagrammed in the middle section is begun earlier and is more intensive. Tumor cell kill exceeds regrowth, drug resistance does not develop, and "cure" results. In this example, treatment has been continued long after all clinical evidence of cancer has disappeared (1–3 years). This approach has been established as effective in the treatment of childhood acute leukemia, testicular cancers, and Hodgkin's disease. In the treatment diagrammed near the bottom of the graph, early surgery has been employed to remove the primary tumor, and intensive adjuvant chemotherapy has been administered long enough (up to 1 year) to eradicate the remaining tumor cells that comprise the occult micrometastases.

with changes in cell surface glycoproteins and intracellular drug accumulation.

POLYFUNCTIONAL ALKYLATING AGENTS

History

This group of agents evolved from the sulfur mustard vesicant gas dichloroethyl sulfide used in World War I. During World War II, the nitrogen mustards were developed (but never used) as chemical warfare agents. In addition to their vesicant effect upon the skin, these compounds produced atrophy of lymphoid tissue and bone marrow. Because of these latter effects, they were introduced for the treatment of malignant lymphomas and leukemias and were later found to be effective against bronchogenic carcinoma and carcinoma of the ovary as well. Since the introduction of the parent nitrogen mustard "HN2"—methylbis(β-chloroethyl)amine, mechlorethamine, Mustargen—new and more stable polyfunctional alkylating drugs have been developed in the search for more effective and less toxic agents. It is now recognized that different alkylating agents have some specificity for selected neoplasms, largely because of differences in reactivity that alter patterns of absorption, distribution, and excretion.

Chemistry

The major clinically useful alkylating agents (Fig 58–5) have a structure containing a bis(chloroethyl)-amine, ethyleneimine, or nitrosourea moiety. Among the bis(chloroethyl)amines, cyclophosphamide, mechlorethamine, melphalan, and chlorambucil have the greatest utility. Ifosfamide is an investigational agent closely related to cyclophosphamide. The aziridine thiotepa and the alkylsulfonate busulfan are used for specialized purposes for ovarian cancer and chronic myeloid leukemia, respectively. The major nitrosoureas are BCNU (carmustine), CCNU (lomustine), and methyl-CCNU (semustine). A variety of investigational alkylating agents have been synthesized that link various carrier molecules such as amino acids, nucleic acid bases, hormones, or sugar moieties to a group capable of alkylation; however, successful "site-directed" alkylation has not to date been achieved.

As a class, the alkylating agents act by exerting cytotoxic effects via transfer of their alkyl groups to various cellular constituents. Alkylations of DNA within the nucleus probably represent the major interactions that lead to cellular lethality. However, these drugs react chemically with sulfhydryl, amino, hydroxyl, carboxyl, and phosphate groups of all cellular nucleophiles as well. The general mechanism of action of these drugs involves intramolecular cyclization to form an **ethyleneimonium ion** that may directly or through formation of a **carbonium ion** transfer an alkyl group to a cellular constituent. In addition to

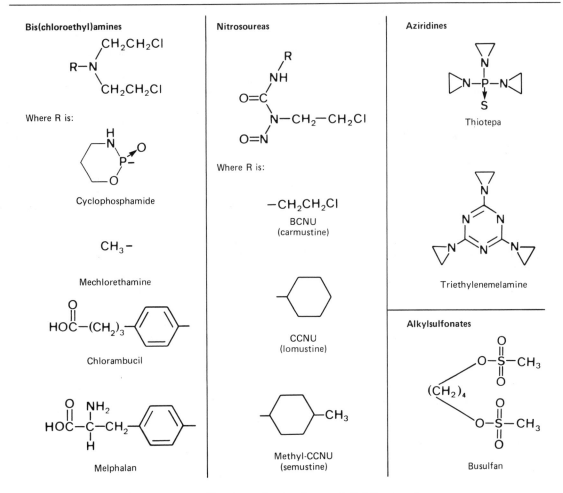

Figure 58–5. Structures of major classes of alkylating agents.

alkylation, a secondary mechanism that occurs with nitrosoureas involves carbamoylation of lysine residues of proteins through formation of isocyanates. The major site of alkylation within DNA is the N7 position of guanine (Fig 58–6); however, other bases are also alkylated to lesser degrees, including N1 and N3 of adenine, N3 of cytosine, and O6 of guanine, as well as phosphate atoms and proteins associated with DNA. These interactions can occur on a single strand or both strands of DNA through cross-linking, as most major alkylating agents are bifunctional, with 2 reactive groups. Alkylation of guanine can result in miscoding through abnormal base pairing with thymine, or in depurination by excision of guanine residues. The latter effect leads to DNA strand breakage through scission of the sugar-phosphate backbone of DNA. Cross-linking of DNA appears to be of major importance to the cytotoxic action of alkylating agents, and replicating cells are most susceptible to these drugs. Thus, although alkylating agents are not cell cycle–specific, cells are most susceptible to alkylation in late G_1 and S phases of the cell cycle and express blockage in G_2.

Drug Resistance

The mechanism of acquired resistance to alkylating agents may involve increased capacity to repair DNA lesions, decreased permeability of the alkylating drug, and increased production of low-molecular-weight thiols that serve as a trap for the alkylating agents.

Pharmacologic Effects

Active alkylating agents have direct vesicant effects and can damage tissues at the site of injection as well as produce systemic toxicity. Toxicities are generally dose-related and occur particularly in rapidly growing tissues such as bone marrow, gastrointestinal tract, and gonads. After intravenous injection, nausea and vomiting usually occur within 30–60 minutes with mechlorethamine, cyclophosphamide, or BCNU. The emetic effects are of central nervous system origin and can be reduced by pretreatment with phenothiazines or cannabinoids (tetrahydrocannibinol, nabilone). Subcutaneous injection of mechlorethamine or BCNU leads to tissue necrosis and sloughing. Cyclophosphamide does not have direct vesicant effects and must be activated to cytotoxic forms by microsomal enzymes in the liver (Fig 58–7).

The liver microsomal cytochrome P-450 mixed function oxidase system converts cyclophosphamide to 4-hydroxycyclophosphamide, which is in equilibrium with aldophosphamide. These active metabolites are believed to be carried by the bloodstream to tumor and normal tissue, where nonenzymatic cleavage of aldophosphamide to the cytotoxic forms—phosphoramide mustard and acrolein—occurs. The liver appears to be protected through the enzymatic formation of the inactive metabolites 4-ketocyclophosphamide and carboxyphosphamide. The major toxicity of alkylating agents is on the bone marrow and results in dose-related suppression of myelopoiesis. The white blood count and absolute granulocyte count reach their low point 10–12 days after injection of mechlorethamine or cyclophosphamide, with subsequent recovery within 21 days (cyclophosphamide) to 42 days (mechlorethamine). The white count nadir with nitrosoureas is delayed to 28 days, with recovery by 42 days. Effects on megakaryocytes and platelets parallel those on granulocytes. Because of the long life span of the erythrocyte, effects on erythropoiesis are minor, and the red cell count is usually only mildly reduced. Side effects on the bone marrow may be more severe when an alkylating agent is given along with other myelosuppressive drugs or radiation therapy, and dose reductions are often required in such circumstances to avoid excessive toxicity.

Following hematopoietic recovery, these agents may be given again on an intermittent dosage schedule at sufficient intervals to permit blood count recovery. Ovarian or testicular failure is a common late sequela

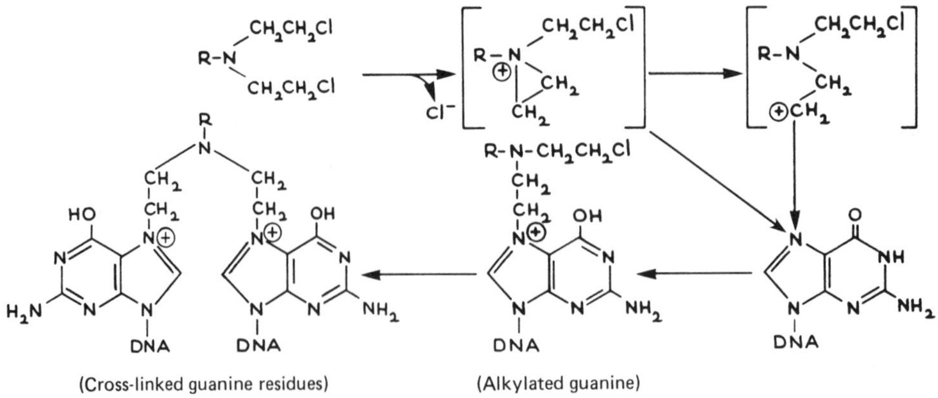

Figure 58–6. Mechanism of alkylation of DNA guanine. A bis(chloroethyl)amine forms an ethyleneimonium ion and a carbonium ion that react with a base such as N7 of guanine in DNA, producing an alkylated purine. Alkylation of a second guanine residue, through the illustrated mechanism, results in cross-linking of DNA strands.

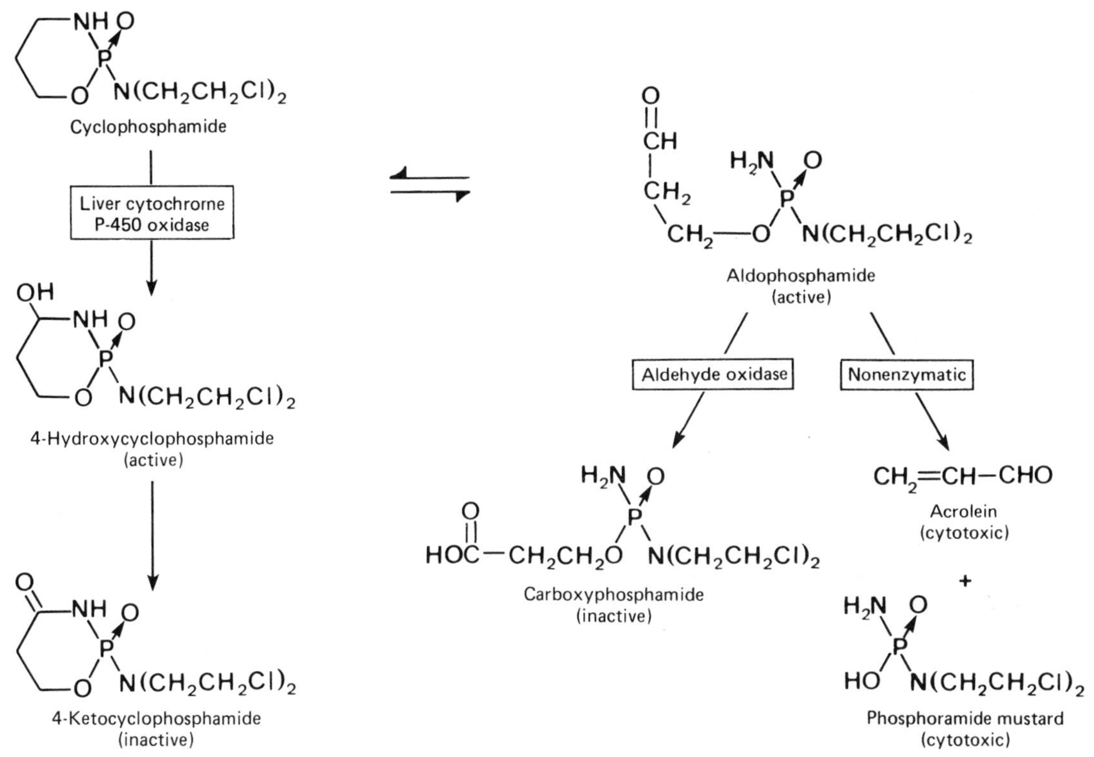

Figure 58–7. Cyclophosphamide metabolism.

of alkylating agent therapy, while acute leukemia is a relatively rare complication of use of these mutagenic agents (see Boice reference).

Oral dosage forms of alkylating agents have been of great value and have been developed using relatively less reactive alkylating drugs. Oral administration of cyclophosphamide, melphalan, chlorambucil, busulfan, and CCNU represents the most common route of administration of these agents and produces effects similar to those observed with parenteral administration. In general, if a tumor is resistant to one alkylating agent, it will be relatively resistant to other agents of this class (although not necessarily to nitrosoureas); however, there are distinct exceptions to this rule for specific tumor types. Overall, cyclophosphamide is the most useful alkylating agent currently available. The oral drug busulfan has a major degree of specificity for the granulocyte series and therefore is of particular value in therapy of chronic myelogenous leukemia. Busulfan does not cause nausea or vomiting despite uniform absorption. Increased skin pigmentation is common with this drug, and rarer syndromes of pulmonary fibrosis or adrenal insufficiency or wasting have been reported often enough so that they can be attributed to busulfan. With all oral alkylating agents, some degree of leukopenia is necessary to provide evidence that the drug has been absorbed adequately. Repeated blood counts are essential during administration of these agents, as the development of severe leukopenia or thrombocytopenia necessitates interruption of therapy.

NITROSOUREAS

Carmustine (BCNU), lomustine (CCNU), and semustine (methyl-CCNU) appear to be non–cross-reactive (as regards tumor resistance) with other alkylating agents; all appear to require biotransformation for antitumor activity, which occurs by nonenzymatic decomposition to liberate derivatives with both alkylating and carbamoylating activities. The nitrosoureas are highly lipid-soluble and cross the blood-brain barrier, making them useful in the treatment of brain tumors. The nitrosoureas appear to function by cross-linking through alkylation of DNA. The drugs may be more effective against plateau phase cells than exponentially growing cells, although within a cycling cell population the drugs appear to slow cell progression through the DNA synthetic phase. After oral administration of lomustine or semustine, plasma metabolites account for virtually all the administered drug, with peak plasma levels of metabolites appearing within 1–4 hours, and prompt central nervous system appearance of 30–40% of the activity present in the plasma. While the initial plasma $t\,\frac{1}{2}$ is in the range of 6 hours, a second $t\,\frac{1}{2}$ is in the range of 1–2 days, and 15–20% of the metabolites are still in the body at 5 days. Urinary excretion appears to be the major route of elimination from the body. One naturally occurring sugar-containing nitrosourea, streptozocin (Zanosar), is interesting because it has minimal bone marrow toxicity but is frequently effective in the treatment of insulin-secreting islet cell carcinoma of the pancreas and occasionally in non-Hodgkin lymphomas.

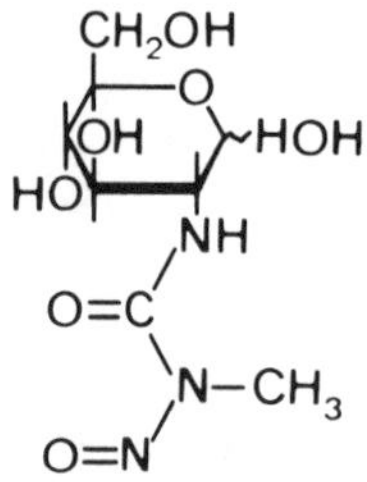

Streptozocin

RELATED DRUGS POSSIBLY ACTING AS ALKYLATING AGENTS

A variety of other compounds have mechanisms of action that involve alkylation. These include procarbazine, dacarbazine, hexamethylmelamine, and cisplatin.

1. PROCARBAZINE

The oral agent procarbazine (Matulane) is a methylhydrazine derivative with chemotherapeutic activity (particularly in Hodgkin's disease). The drug is also leukemogenic and has teratogenic and mutagenic properties.

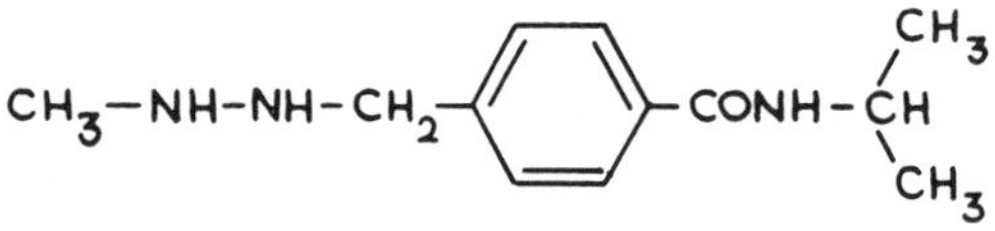

CH$_3$—NH—NH—CH$_2$—⟨ ⟩—CONH—CH⟨CH$_3$, CH$_3$⟩

N-Isopropyl-a-(2-methylhydrazino)-
p-toluamide (procarbazine)

The mechanism of action of procarbazine is uncertain; however, the drug inhibits the syntheses of DNA, RNA, and protein, prolongs interphase, and produces chromosome breaks. Oxidative metabolism of this drug by microsomal enzymes generates azoprocarbazine and H$_2$O$_2$, which may be responsible for DNA strand scission. A variety of other metabolites of the drug are formed that may be cytotoxic. One metabolite is a monoamine oxidase (MAO) inhibitor, and adverse side effects can occur when procarbazine is given with other MAO inhibitors. In addition to predictable nausea, vomiting, and myelosuppression, hemolytic anemia, pulmonary reactions, and adverse responses with alcohol (disulfiramlike) have also been reported, as have skin rashes when procarbazine is given with phenytoin.

Procarbazine has had major use in combination chemotherapy of Hodgkin's disease, as it is not cross-resistant with *Vinca* alkaloids or conventional alkylating agents. However, its leukemogenic properties may eventually lead to its replacement with drugs that have lesser carcinogenic potential.

2. DACARBAZINE

Dacarbazine is a synthetic compound that functions as an alkylating agent following metabolic activation

by liver microsomal enzymes by oxidative N-demethylation to the monomethyl derivative that spontaneously decomposes to 5-aminoimidazole-4-carboxamide, which is excreted in the urine, and diazomethane. The diazomethane generates a methyl carbonium ion that is believed to be the likely cytotoxic species. Dacarbazine is administered parenterally and is not schedule-dependent. It produces marked nausea, vomiting, and myelosuppression. Its major applications are in melanoma, Hodgkin's disease, and some soft tissue sarcomas. In the latter 2 tumors, its activity is potentiated by doxorubicin.

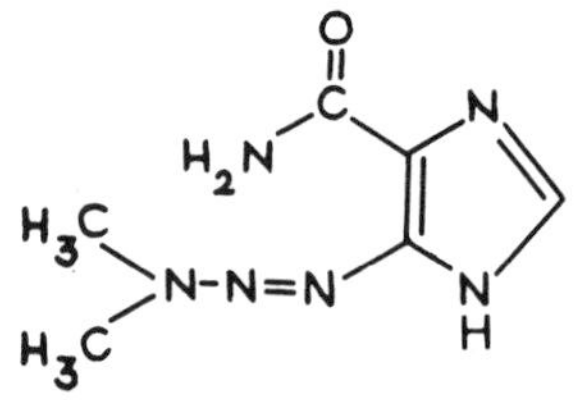

Dacarbazine
(dimethyl imidazole carboxamide)

3. HEXAMETHYLMELAMINE

Hexamethylmelamine is an investigational drug structurally similar to triethylenemelamine. It is relatively insoluble and available only in oral form. A related compound, pentamethylmelamine, which is a major metabolite of hexamethylmelamine, is more soluble and is now in clinical trial in an intravenous form. Both agents are rapidly biotransformed by demethylation, presumably to active intermediates. These agents cause nausea, vomiting, and central and peripheral nervous system neuropathies but relatively mild myelosuppression. They are currently classed as investigational. Hexamethylmelamine is useful in alkylating agent–resistant ovarian carcinoma and will probably be approved by the FDA for use in that disorder in the near future.

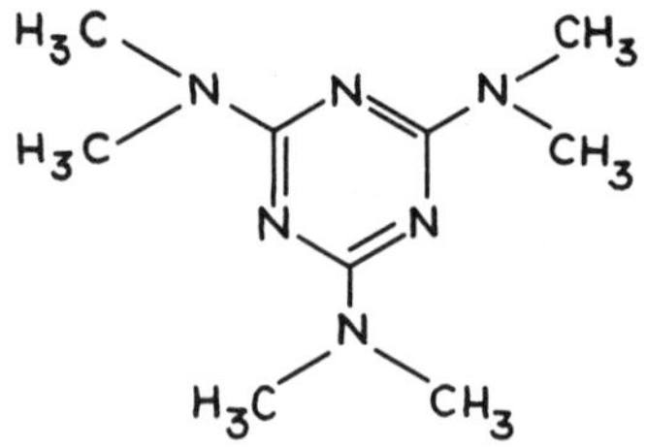

Hexamethylmelamine

4. CISPLATIN

Cisplatin (cis-diamminedichloroplatinum [II], Platinol) is an inorganic metal complex discovered by Rosenberg and his colleagues, who made the serendipitous observation that neutral platinum complexes inhibit division and induce filamentous growth of *Escherichia coli*. A whole series of platinum analogs have been synthesized, but cisplatin is the only one currently in clinical use. While the precise mechanism of action of cisplatin is still to be defined, it is thought to act analogously to alkylating agents. It kills cells in all stages of the cell cycle, inhibits DNA biosynthesis, and binds DNA through the formation of interstrand cross-links. The primary binding site is the N7 of guanine, but covalent interaction with adenine and cytosine also occurs. The platinum complexes appear to synergize with certain other anticancer drugs. After intravenous administration, the major acute toxicity is nausea and vomiting. Cisplatin has relatively little effect on the bone marrow, but it can induce significant renal dysfunction and occasional acoustic nerve dysfunction. Hydration with saline infusion—alone or with mannitol or other diuretics—appears to minimize nephrotoxicity.

$$H_3N \diagdown \quad \diagup Cl^-$$
$$Pt^{2+}$$
$$H_3N \diagup \quad \diagdown Cl^-$$

Cisplatin

Cisplatin has major antitumor activity in genitourinary cancers, particularly testicular, ovarian, and bladder cancer. Its use along with vinblastine and bleomycin has been a major advance in the development of curative therapy for nonseminomatous testicular cancers. Several platinum analogs with less gastrointestinal and renal toxicity are currently in clinical trial.

DOSAGE & TOXICITY OF POLYFUNCTIONAL ALKYLATING AGENTS

The alkylating agents are used in the treatment of a wide variety of hematologic and solid cancers, generally as components of combination chemotherapy (Table 58–7). These are discussed under various specific tumors. Dosages and major toxicities are listed in Table 58–2.

Nausea and vomiting are almost universally reported with intravenously administered mechlorethamine, cyclophosphamide, and carmustine and occur with moderate frequency with oral cyclophosphamide.

The important toxic effect of therapeutic doses of virtually all the alkylating drugs is depression of bone marrow and subsequent leukopenia and thrombocytopenia. Severe infections and septicemia may result, with granulocytopenia below 600 PMNs/μL. Platelet depression below 40,000/μL may be accompanied by induced hemorrhagic phenomena. Cyclophosphamide may produce slight to severe alopecia in up to 30% of patients. It may also cause hemorrhagic cystitis. The cystitis can often be averted with adequate hydration.

The hematopoietic effects of toxic doses of alkylating drugs are treated by discontinuing the agent. Red cell and platelet transfusions and antibiotics to control infections are employed as needed until the marrow has regenerated.

ANTIMETABOLITES (Structural Analogs)

The development of drugs with actions on intermediary metabolism of proliferating cells has been important both clinically and conceptually. While biochemical properties unique to all cancer cells have yet to be discovered, neoplastic cells do have a number of quantitative differences in metabolism from normal cells that render them more susceptible to a number of antimetabolites or structural analogs. Many of these agents have been rationally designed and synthesized, based on knowledge of cellular processes, although a few have been discovered as antibiotics. The prototype for inhibiting malignant growth is the folic acid antagonist methotrexate, which acts directly as a substitute for a normal metabolite.

Biochemical Mechanisms

Antimetabolites or their active products (after biotransformation) can work by any of a number of different mechanisms to inhibit cell proliferation. For example, the antimetabolite may be metabolized instead of the normal substrate for a biosynthetic pathway, so that the antimetabolite is incorporated into a critical macromolecule that then cannot function properly. A second mechanism involves competition with a normal metabolite that acts at either the catalytic site of an enzyme or at an allosteric (regulatory) site. Binding to either of these sites on the enzyme may be reversible or irreversible depending on the specific structure and function of the antimetabolite. One form of antimetabolite that binds to the catalytic site of an enzyme will strongly inhibit it when the enzyme is in a transition state with respect to the substrate. In some instances, inhibition of an enzyme will cause cell death by causing toxic products to accumulate; however, this mechanism appears to be relatively uncommon.

The biochemical pathways that have thus far proved to be most exploitable with antimetabolites have been those relating to nucleotide and nucleic acid synthesis. In a number of instances, when an enzyme is known to have a major effect on pathways leading to cell replication, inhibitors of the reaction it catalyzes have proved to be useful anticancer drugs. A summary of sites of action of some of the antimetabolites affecting DNA synthesis is depicted in Fig 58–8.

These drugs and their doses and toxicities are shown in Table 58–3. The principal drugs are discussed below.

Table 58–2. Polyfunctional alkylating agents and probable alkylating agents: Dosages and toxicity.

Alkylating Agent	Single-Agent Dose	Acute Toxicity	Delayed Toxicity
Nitrogen mustard (HN2, mechlorethamine, Mustargen)	0.4 mg/kg IV in single or divided doses	Nausea and vomiting	Moderate depression of peripheral blood count. Excessive doses produce severe bone marrow depression with leukopenia, thrombocytopenia, and bleeding. Alopecia and hemorrhagic cystitis occasionally occur with cyclophosphamide. Cystitis can be prevented with adequate hydration.
Chlorambucil (Leukeran)	0.1–0.2 mg/kg/d orally; 6–12 mg/d	None	
Cyclophosphamide (Cytoxan)	3.5–5 mg/kg/d orally for 10 days; 1 g/m² IV as single dose	Nausea and vomiting	
Melphalan (Alkeran)	0.25 mg/kg/d orally for 4 days every 4–6 weeks	None	
Thiotepa (triethylenethiophosphoramide)	0.2 mg/kg IV for 5 days	None	
Busulfan (Myleran)	2–8 mg/d orally; 150–250 mg/course	None	
Carmustine (BCNU)	200 mg/m² IV every 6 weeks	Nausea and vomiting	Leukopenia and thrombocytopenia. Rarely hepatitis.
Lomustine (CCNU)	150 mg/m² orally every 6 weeks	Nausea and vomiting	
Semustine (methyl-CCNU)	150 mg/m² orally every 6 weeks	Nausea and vomiting	
Hexamethylmelamine	10 mg/kg/d for 21 days	Nausea and vomiting	Leukopenia, thrombocytopenia, and peripheral neuropathy.
Procarbazine (Matulane)	50–200 mg/d orally	Nausea and vomiting	Bone marrow depression, central nervous system depression.
Dacarbazine	300 mg/m² daily IV for 5 days	Nausea and vomiting	Bone marrow depression.
Cisplatin (Platinol)	20 mg/m²/d IV for 5 days or 50–70 mg/m² as single dose every 3 weeks	Nausea and vomiting	Renal dysfunction. Acoustic nerve dysfunction.

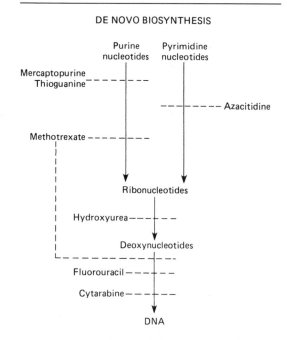

Figure 58–8. Sites of action of antimetabolites on DNA synthetic pathways.

METHOTREXATE

Methotrexate (MTX) is a folic acid antagonist that binds to the active catalytic site of dihydrofolate reductase (DHFR), interfering with the synthesis of the reduced form that accepts one-carbon units. Lack of this cofactor interrupts the synthesis of thymidylate, purine nucleotides, and the amino acids serine and methionine, thereby interfering with the formation of DNA, RNA, and protein. The enzyme binds methotrexate extremely tightly, and at pH 6 virtually no dissociation of the enzyme-inhibitor complex occurs (inhibition constant about 1 nmol/L). At physiologic pH, reversible competitive kinetics occur (inhibition constant about 1 μmol/L). Intracellular formation of polyglutamate derivatives appears to be important in the therapeutic action of methotrexate (see Jolivet reference, p 699). The polyglutamates are equivalent to methotrexate as inhibitors of DHFR and are retained by cells longer than methotrexate, making them important determinants in the duration of action of methotrexate.

Drug Resistance

Tumor cell resistance to methotrexate has been attributed to (1) decreased drug transport, (2) altered

Table 58–3. Structural analogs: Dosages and toxicity.

Chemotherapeutic Agent	Single-Agent Dose	Delayed Toxicity*
Methotrexate (amethopterin, MTX)	2.5–5 mg/d orally; 10 mg intrathecally 1–2 times weekly	Oral and gastrointestinal tract ulceration, bone marrow depression, leukopenia, thrombocytopenia.
Mercaptopurine (Purinethol, 6-MP)	2.5 mg/kg/d orally	Usually well tolerated. Larger dosages may cause bone marrow depression.
Thioguanine (6-TG)	2 mg/kg/d orally	Usually well tolerated. Larger dosages may cause bone marrow depression.
Fluorouracil (5-FU)	15 mg/kg/d IV for 5 days by 24-hour infusion; 15 mg/kg weekly IV	Nausea, oral and gastrointestinal ulceration, bone marrow depression.
Cytarabine (ara-C, Cytosar-U)	100 mg/m²/d for 5–10 days, either by continuous IV infusion or subcutaneously every 8 hours	Nausea and vomiting, bone marrow depression, megaloblastosis, leukopenia, thrombocytopenia.
Azacitidine	200 mg/m²/d IV for 5 days	Nausea and vomiting, diarrhea, fever, hypotension, prolonged marrow hypoplasia.
Supportive Agent With All Drugs	**Dose**	**Delayed Toxicity**
Allopurinol (Zyloprim)	300–800 mg/d orally for prevention or relief of hyperuricemia	Usually none. Enhances effects and toxicity of 6-MP when used in combination.

*These drugs do not cause acute toxicity.

DHFR with lower affinity for methotrexate, and (3) synthesis of increased levels of DHFR. This occurs through gene amplification and results in a marked increase in DHFR messenger RNA. It remains to be established whether this genetic resistance mechanism is relevant for other drugs or for resistant tumors in patients receiving methotrexate.

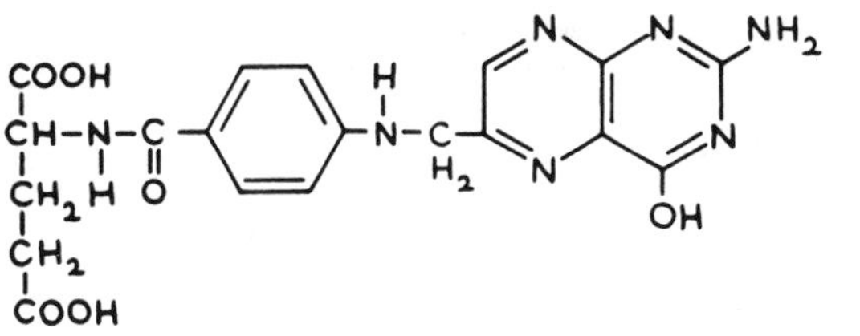

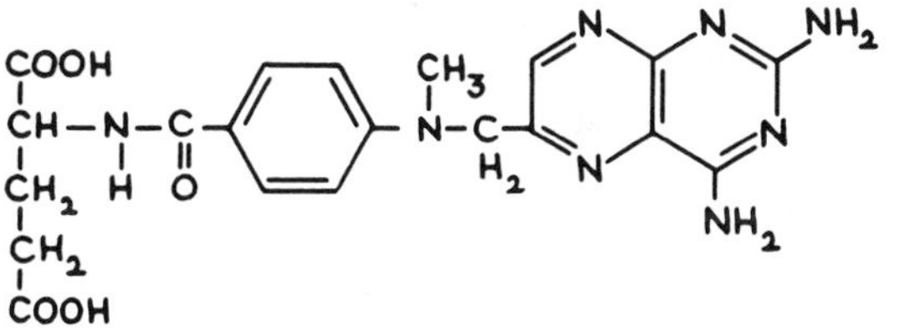

Dosage & Toxicity

Methotrexate is administered clinically by the intravenous or oral route (Table 58–3). Up to 90% of an oral dose is excreted in the urine within 12 hours. The drug is not subject to metabolism, and serum levels are therefore proportionate to dose as long as renal function and hydration status are adequate. Toxic side effects to proliferating tissues are usually observed on the bone marrow and to a lesser extent on the skin and gastrointestinal mucosa. The effects of methotrexate can be reversed by administration of leucovorin (citrovorum factor). Leucovorin "rescue" has been used with accidental overdose or experimentally along with high-dose methotrexate therapy in a protocol intended to rescue normal cells while still leaving the tumor cells subject to its cytotoxic action.

PURINE ANTAGONISTS

Mercaptopurine (Purinethol, 6-MP) was the first of the thiopurine series found useful as an anticancer drug. Like other thiopurines, it must be anabolized by hypoxanthine-guanine phosphoribosyl transferase (HGPRT) to the nucleotide form (6-thioinosinic acid), which in turn inhibits a number of the enzymes of purine interconversion. Significant amounts of thioguanylic acid and 6-methylmercaptopurine ribotide

Folic acid

Methotrexate

(MMPR) also are formed from 6-MP. These metabolites may also contribute to the action of the mercaptopurine. 6-MP is used primarily in the treatment of childhood acute leukemia, and a closely related analog, azathioprine, is used as an immunosuppressive agent (Chapter 59).

Thioguanine (6-TG) inhibits several enzymes in the purine nucleotide pathway. A variety of metabolic lesions are associated with the cytotoxic action of the purinethiols. These include inhibition of purine nucleotide interconversion; decrease in intracellular levels of guanine nucleotides, which leads to inhibition of glycoprotein synthesis; interference with the formation of DNA and RNA; and incorporation of purinethiols into both DNA and RNA. 6-TG has a synergistic action when used together with cytarabine in the treatment of adult acute leukemia.

Drug Resistance

Resistance to both 6-MP and 6-TG occurs most commonly by decrease in HGPRT activity; an alternative mechanism in acute leukemia involves elevation of levels of alkaline phosphatase, which results in dephosphorylation of thiopurine nucleotide and cellular loss of the resulting ribonucleoside.

Dosage & Toxicity

Mercaptopurine and thioguanine are both given orally (Table 58–3), absorbed rapidly from the gut, and excreted mainly in the urine. However, 6-MP is converted to an inactive metabolite (6-thiouric acid) by an oxidation catalyzed by xanthine oxidase, whereas 6-TG requires deamination before metabolism by this enzyme. This factor is important because the purine analog allopurinol (Zyloprim), a potent xanthine oxidase inhibitor, is frequently used along with chemotherapy in hematologic cancers. Simultaneous therapy with allopurinol and 6-MP results in excessive mercaptopurine toxicity unless the dose of mercaptopurine is reduced to 25–30% of the usual level. This effect does not occur with 6-TG, which can be used in full doses despite administration of allopurinol. Allopurinol plays an important supportive role in chemotherapy of the leukemias and lymphomas. Even though it is noncytotoxic, it prevents toxicity from purine bases released through tumor lysis by inhibition of xanthine oxidase activity. This allows excretion of cellular purines relatively more soluble than uric acid. Nephrotoxicity and acute gout produced by excessive uric acid is thereby prevented.

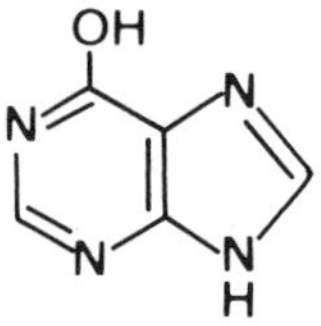

Hypoxanthine 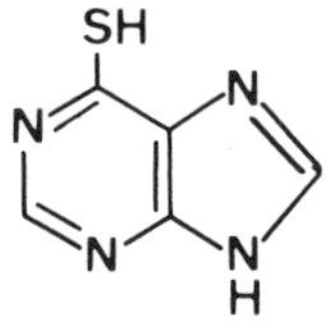   6-Mercaptopurine 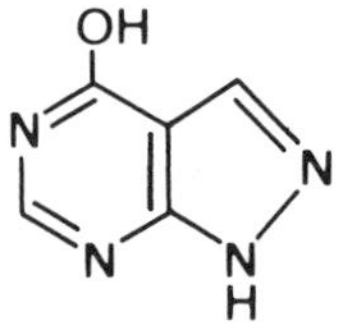   Allopurinol

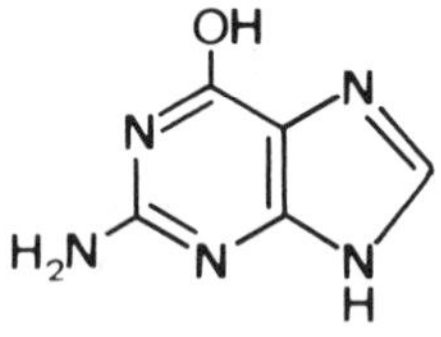

Guanine 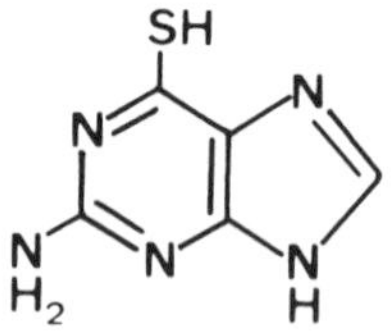   6-Thioguanine

PYRIMIDINE ANTAGONISTS

1. FLUOROURACIL

Fluorouracil (5-FU) undergoes anabolic biotransformation to ribosyl and deoxyribosyl nucleotide metabolites. One of these metabolites, 5-fluoro-2′-deoxyuridine 5′-phosphate (FdUMP), forms a covalently bound ternary complex with the enzyme thymidylate synthetase and its cofactor $N^{5,10}$-methylenetetrahydrofolate, a reaction critical for the synthesis of thymine nucleotides. This results in inhibition of DNA synthesis through "thymineless death." 5-FU after conversion to 5-fluorouridine triphosphate is incorporated into RNA and interferes with RNA processing and function. Cytotoxicity of 5-FU is thus due to its effects on both DNA and RNA.

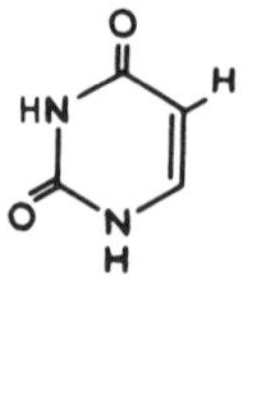

Uracil 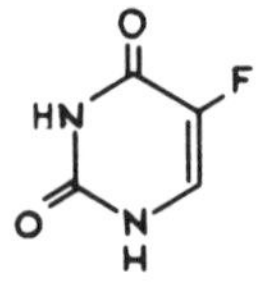   5-FU 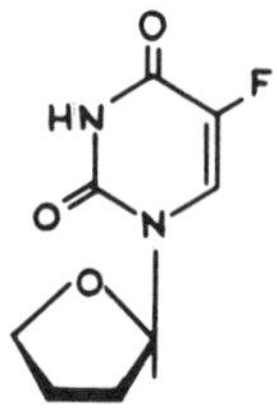   Ftorafur

5-FU is normally given intravenously (Table 58–3) and has a short metabolic half-life. Although it is active when given orally, its bioavailability is erratic by that route of administration. Floxuridine (5-fluorodeoxyuridine, FUDR) has an action similar to that of 5-FU and is used for hepatic artery infusions. A cream incorporating 5-FU (Efudex) is used topically for treating skin cancers. A related investigational drug, tegafur (ftorafur), appears to release 5-FU slowly after it is injected. However, this new agent has neurotoxicity that may limit its utility. Fluorouracil is used systemically in the treatment of a variety of adenocarcinomas. Its major toxicities are myelosuppression and mucositis.

2. CYTARABINE

Cytarabine (cytosine arabinoside, ara-C, Cytosar-U) is an S phase–specific antimetabolite that is converted by deoxycytidine kinase to the 5′-mononucleotide (AraCMP). AraCMP is further anabolized to the triphosphate (AraCTP), which competitively inhibits DNA polymerase. This results in blockage of DNA synthesis while RNA and protein formation continues and leads to unbalanced growth. Cytarabine is also incorporated into RNA and DNA. Incorporation into DNA leads to interference with chain elongation and defective ligation of fragments of newly synthesized DNA. The cellular retention time for AraCTP appears to correlate with its lethality to malignant cells.

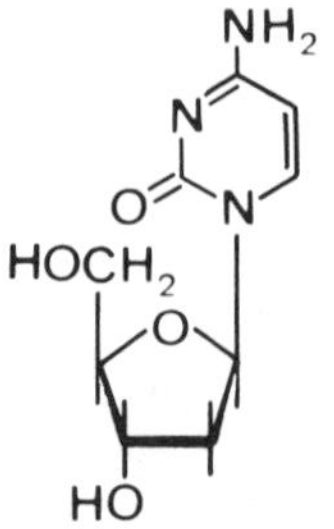

Cytosine deoxyriboside 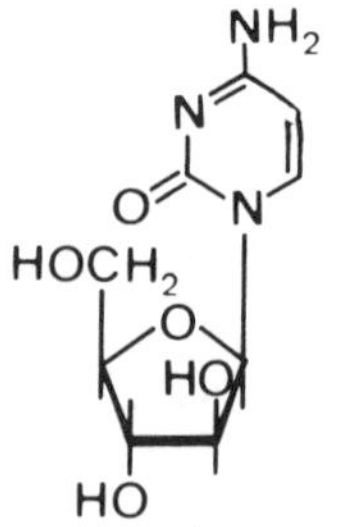   Cytosine arabinoside

After intravenous administration (Table 58–3), the drug is cleared rapidly, with most of it being deaminated to an inactive form. The ratio of the anabolic enzyme deoxycytidine kinase to the inactivating catalyst cytidine deaminase is important to the cytotoxicity of cytarabine.

In view of cytarabine's S phase specificity, the drug is highly schedule-dependent and must be given either by continuous infusion or every 8–12 hours for 5–7 days. Its activity is limited almost entirely to treatment of acute myelogenous leukemia, for which it is a major drug. Side effects include nausea, severe myelosuppression, and varying degrees of stomatitis or alopecia.

3. AZACITIDINE

Azacitidine (5-azacytidine) produces multiple effects associated with its cytotoxicity. It is phosphorylated to the mononucleotide form by uridine-cytidine kinase. Azacitidine 5'-phosphate then inhibits orotidylate decarboxylase, which reduces production of pyrimidine nucleotides. Further metabolism results in incorporation of azacitidine into DNA and RNA as well as inhibition of DNA, RNA, and protein synthesis.

Azacitidine is administered intravenously (Table 58–3) and must be shielded from light and kept at slightly acid pH, as it is unstable and can undergo ring opening. Nausea and fever are observed during drug administration. The half-life is 3–6 hours, with most of the drug excreted either unchanged or in deaminated form.

Cytidine   5-Azacytidine

Azacitidine is currently an investigational agent in the USA, but it is a recognized "second-line agent" in the treatment of acute leukemia. Optimal dosage schedules have yet to be developed. The drug can produce profound myelosuppressive toxicity of long duration.

PLANT ALKALOIDS

VINBLASTINE

Vinblastine (Velban) is an alkaloid derived from *Vinca rosea*, the periwinkle plant (see below). Its mechanism of action involves depolymerization of mi-

crotubules, which are an important part of the cytoskeleton and the mitotic spindle. It binds specifically to the microtubular protein tubulin in dimeric form; the drug-tubulin complex adds to the forming end of the microtubules to terminate assembly, and depolymerization of the microtubules then occurs. This results in mitotic arrest at metaphase, dissolution of the mitotic spindle, and interference with chromosome segregation. It produces nausea and vomiting and marrow depression as well as alopecia. It has value in the treatment of systemic Hodgkin's disease and other lymphomas. See clinical section below and Table 58–4. Several related agents, including desacetylvinblastine (vindesine) and vinzolidine, are currently in clinical trial as investigational drugs.

R is: O=C–H   R is: CH₃

Vincristine   Vinblastine

VINCRISTINE

Vincristine (Oncovin), also an alkaloid derivative of *Vinca rosea*, is closely related in structure to vinblastine. Its mechanism of action is considered to be identical to that of vinblastine, and it also appears to be a "spindle poison" and to cause arrest of the mitotic cycle. Despite these marked similarities to vinblastine, vincristine has a strikingly different spectrum of clinical activity and qualitatively different toxicities.

Vincristine has been used with considerable success in combination with prednisone for remission induction in acute leukemia in children. It is also useful in certain other rapidly proliferating neoplasms. It causes a significant incidence of neurotoxicity (Table 58–4), which limits its use to short courses. It occasionally produces bone marrow depression.

PODOPHYLLOTOXINS

Two compounds, VP-16 (etoposide) and a related drug, VM-26 (teniposide), are semisynthetic derivatives of podophyllotoxin, which is extracted from the root of the mayapple or mandrake (*Podophyllum peltatum*). Etoposide (VePesid) is now approved for clinical use in the USA; an oral formulation is still investigational.

Etoposide and teniposide are quite similar in chemical structure, in their block of cells in the late S–G2 phase of the cell cycle, and clinically. The mode of

Table 58–4. Natural product cancer chemotherapy drugs: Dosages and toxicity.

Drug	Single-Agent Dose	Acute Toxicity	Delayed Toxicity
Bleomycin (Blenoxane)	Up to 15 mg/m^2 twice weekly to a total dose of 200 mg/m^2	Allergic reactions, fever, hypotension	Edema of hands, pulmonary fibrosis, stomatitis, alopecia.
Dactinomycin (actinomycin D, Cosmegen)	0.04 mg/kg IV weekly	Nausea and vomiting	Stomatitis, gastrointestinal tract upset, alopecia, bone marrow depression.
Daunorubicin (daunomycin, Cerubidine)	30–60 mg/m^2 daily IV for 3 days, or 30–60 mg/m^2 IV weekly	Nausea, fever, red urine (not hematuria)	Cardiotoxicity, bone marrow depression, alopecia.
Doxorubicin (Adriamycin)	60 mg/m^2 IV every 3 weeks to a maximum total dose of 550 mg/m^2	Nausea, red urine (not hematuria)	Cardiotoxicity, alopecia, bone marrow depression, stomatitis.
Etoposide (VePesid)	50–100 mg/m^2 daily for 5 days	Nausea, vomiting, hypotension	Alopecia, bone marrow depression.
Mithramycin (Mithracin)	25–50 μg/kg IV every other day for up to 8 doses	Nausea and vomiting	Thrombocytopenia, hepatotoxicity.
Mitomycin (Mutamycin)	20 mg/m^2 every 6 weeks	Nausea	Thrombocytopenia, leukopenia.
Vinblastine (Velban)	0.1–0.2 mg/kg IV weekly	Nausea and vomiting	Alopecia, loss of reflexes, bone marrow depression.
Vincristine (Oncovin)	1.5 mg/m^2 IV (maximum: 2 mg weekly)	None	Areflexia, muscle weakness, peripheral neuritis, paralytic ileus, mild bone marrow depression, alopecia.

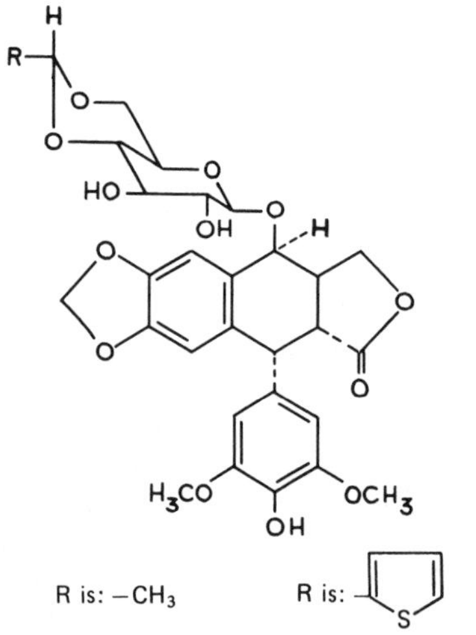

VP-16-213, etoposide
(4'-demethyl-epipodophyllotoxin-
β-D-ethylidene glucoside)

VM-26
(teniposide)

R is: —CH$_3$

R is: (thiophene)

action is thought to involve degradation of DNA (possibly via topoisomerase), inhibition of nucleoside transport, and inhibition of mitochondrial electron transport. The drugs are water-insoluble and require a solubilizing vehicle for clinical formulation. After intravenous administration (Table 58–4), they are protein-bound and evenly distributed throughout the body, except for the brain. Excretion is predominantly in the urine, with a lesser amount excreted in bile. In addition to nausea, vomiting, and alopecia, significant toxicity occurs to the hematopoietic and lymphoid systems. Thus far, etoposide has shown activity in monocytic leukemia, testicular cancer, and oat cell carcinoma of the lung, and teniposide has activity in various lymphomas.

ANTIBIOTICS

Screening of microbial products has led to the discovery of a number of growth inhibitors that have proved to be clinically useful in cancer chemotherapy. Many of these antibiotics bind to DNA through intercalation between specific bases and block the synthesis of new RNA or DNA (or both), cause DNA strand scission, and interfere with cell replication. All of the clinically useful antibiotics now available are products of various strains of the soil fungus *Streptomyces*. These include the anthracyclines, actinomycin, bleomycin, mitomycin, and mithramycin.

ANTHRACYCLINES

The anthracycline antibiotics, isolated from *Streptomyces peucetius* var *caesius,* are among the most useful cytotoxic anticancer drugs. Two congeners— doxorubicin (Adriamycin) and daunorubicin (Cerubidine)—are FDA-approved and in general use. Their structures are shown below.

Other anthracyclines are currently being developed, including semisynthetic agents. Daunorubicin (the first agent in this class to be isolated) is used in the treatment of acute leukemia. Doxorubicin has a broad spectrum of potent activity against many different types of cancers.

R is: $-\overset{O}{\overset{\|}{C}}-CH_3$ R is: $-\overset{O}{\overset{\|}{C}}-CH_2OH$

Daunorubicin   Doxorubicin

Mechanism of Action

Three major actions have been documented for the organ and tumor toxicities of the anthracyclines. These include (1) high-affinity binding to DNA through intercalation with consequent blockade of the synthesis of DNA and RNA, and DNA strand scission; (2) binding to membranes, to alter fluidity and ion transport; and (3) generation of the semiquinone free radical and oxygen radicals through a cytochrome P-450–mediated reductive process. This latter action may be responsible for cardiac toxicity through oxygen radical–mediated damage to membranes, since the free radical scavenger α-tocopherol (vitamin E) lessens cardiac damage of doxorubicin in experimental systems without decreasing anticancer activity.

Absorption, Metabolism, & Excretion

Clinically useful anthracyclines are administered only by the intravenous route (Table 58–4). Peak blood concentration decreases by 50% within the first 30 minutes after injection, but significant levels persist for up to 20 hours. The anthracyclines are metabolized by the liver, with reduction and hydrolysis of the ring substituents. An alcohol form is an active metabolite, whereas the aglycone is inactive. Most of the drug and its metabolites are excreted in bile, and about one-sixth is excreted in urine. Some metabolites retain antitumor activity. The biliary route of excretion includes enterohepatic recirculation of cytotoxic moieties. In patients with significant elevations of serum bilirubin (greater than 2.5 mg/dL), the initial dose of anthracyclines must be reduced by 75%.

Clinical Uses

Doxorubicin is one of the most important anticancer drugs, with major clinical application in carcinomas of the breast, endometrium, ovary, testicle, thyroid, and lung and in treatment of many sarcomas, including neuroblastoma, Ewing's sarcoma, osteosarcoma, and rhabdomyosarcoma. It is useful also in hematologic cancers, including acute leukemia, multiple myeloma, Hodgkin's disease, and the diffuse non-Hodgkin lymphomas. It is used in adjuvant therapy in osteogenic sarcoma and breast cancer. It is generally used in combination with other agents (eg, cyclophosphamide, cisplatin, and nitrosoureas), with which it often synergizes, yielding longer remissions than are observed when it is used as a single agent. This approach can also minimize some of the toxicities that would otherwise be associated with use of higher dosages of doxorubicin. The major use of daunorubicin is in acute leukemia, and for this purpose the drug may have slightly greater activity than doxorubicin. However, daunorubicin appears to have a far narrower spectrum of utility, as its efficacy in solid tumors appears to be limited.

A series of new anthracycline analogs has recently entered clinical trial as investigational agents. These include aclacinomycin A, 4-epiadriamycin, 4'-deoxy-doxorubicin, and 4-demethoxydaunorubicin. These new agents may have differing spectrums of action and somewhat less toxicity. For example, initial reports indicate that aclacinomycin A, 4'-deoxydoxorubicin, and 4-demethoxydaunorubicin cause far less alopecia and cardiac toxicity than other anthracyclines. Antitumor activity is only now being defined for these new agents.

Adverse Reactions

In common with many other cytotoxic drugs, the anthracyclines cause bone marrow depression, which is of short duration with rapid recovery. Toxicities more pronounced with anthracyclines (doxorubicin and daunorubicin) than with other agents include a potentially irreversible, cumulative dose–related cardiac toxicity. The mechanism of cardiac toxicity is still under study but appears to involve excessive intracellular production of free radicals within the myocardium by doxorubicin. This is rarely seen at doxorubicin dosages below 500 mg/m². Use of lower weekly doses or continuous infusions of doxorubicin that avoid high peak plasma concentrations appear to reduce the frequency of cardiac toxicity as compared to intermittent (every 3–4 weeks) higher dosage schedules.

A second toxicity of doxorubicin and daunorubicin is the almost universal occurrence of severe or total alopecia at standard dosages.

DACTINOMYCIN

Dactinomycin (actinomycin D, Cosmegen) is an antitumor antibiotic isolated from a *Streptomyces*. The drug is composed of 2 identical cyclic polypeptides linked to an aromatic planar phenoxazone ring system. A number of analogs have been devised naturally and semisynthetically, but most have not been tested carefully for antitumor activity.

Mechanism of Action

Dactinomycin binds tightly to double-stranded DNA through intercalation between adjacent guanine-cytosine base pairs. Dactinomycin inhibits all forms of DNA-dependent RNA synthesis, with ribosomal RNA formation being most sensitive to drug action. DNA replication is much less reduced, but protein synthesis is blocked in affected cells. The degree of responsiveness to dactinomycin appears to be dependent on the cellular capacity for accumulation and retention of the antibiotic.

Absorption, Metabolism, & Excretion

Approximately half of the intravenous dose of dactinomycin (Table 58–4) remains unmetabolized and is excreted in the bile; a small amount is lost by urinary excretion. The plasma half-life is short. Because the drug is irritating to tissues, it is usually administered with caution to avoid extravasation and with "flushing" with normal saline to wash out the vein.

Clinical Uses

Dactinomycin is used in combination with surgery and vincristine (with or without radiotherapy) in the adjuvant treatment of Wilms' tumor. It is also used along with methotrexate to provide potentially curative treatment for patients with localized or disseminated gestational choriocarcinoma.

Adverse Reactions

Bone marrow depression, the major dose-limiting toxicity of this agent, is usually evident within 7–10 days. All blood elements are affected, but platelets and leukocytes are affected most profoundly, and severe thrombocytopenia sometimes occurs. Nausea and vomiting, diarrhea, oral ulcers, and skin eruptions may also be noted. The agent is also immunosuppressive, and patients receiving this drug should not receive live virus vaccines during that time. Alopecia and various skin abnormalities occur occasionally. As with anthracyclines, dactinomycin can interact with radiation, producing a "radiation recall" skin abnormality associated with inflammation at sites of prior radiation therapy.

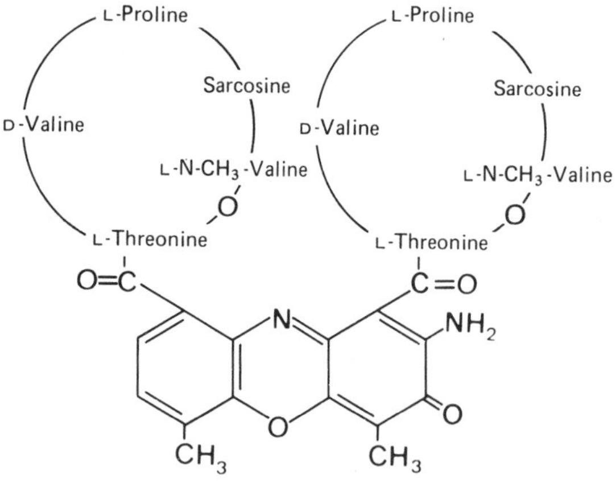

Dactinomycin

MITHRAMYCIN

Mithramycin (Mithracin) is one of the chromomycin antibiotics isolated from *Streptomyces plicatus*. The mechanism of action of mithramycin is thought to involve binding of the drug to DNA, possibly through an antibiotic-Mg^{2+} complex; this interaction interrupts DNA-directed RNA synthesis. Additionally, the drug causes a calcium-lowering effect, apparently

through an action on osteoclasts that is independent of its action on tumor cells (Chapter 41). The drug has some usefulness in testicular cancers refractory to standard treatment, but it is of greater utility in reversing severe hypercalcemia associated with malignant disease.

Toxic side effects of mithramycin include nausea and vomiting, thrombocytopenia, leukopenia, hypocalcemia, bleeding disorders, and liver toxicity. Aside from its use in management of hypercalcemia, mithramycin currently has few other indications.

Other chromomycin antibiotics (eg, toyomycin) have been studied in Japan but appear to be of limited utility.

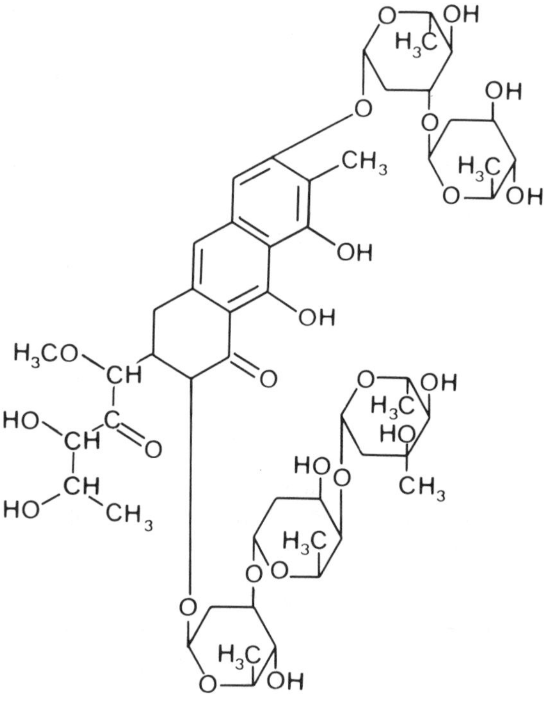

Mithramycin

MITOMYCIN

Mitomycin (mitomycin C, Mitocin-C, Mutamycin) is an antibiotic isolated from *Streptomyces caespitosus*. It contains quinone, carbamate, and aziridine groups, all of which may contribute to its activity. The drug is a "bioreductive" alkylating agent that undergoes metabolic activation through a cytochrome P-450 reductase–mediated reduction to generate an alkylating agent that cross-links DNA. Hypoxic tumor stem cells of solid tumors exist in an environment conducive to reductive reactions and are more sensitive to the cytotoxic actions of mitomycin than normal and oxygenated tumor cells. Mitomycin is thought to be a CCNS alkylating agent. While this agent is one of the more toxic drugs available for clinical use, it is the best available drug for use against hypoxic tumor cells and appears to have increasing usefulness in combination chemotherapy (with bleomycin and vincristine) for squamous cell carcinoma of the cervix and for adenocarcinomas of the stomach, pancreas, and lung (along with doxorubicin and fluorouracil). The drug also has some usefulness as a second-line agent for metastatic colon cancer. A special application of mitomycin has been in topical intravesical treatment of small bladder papillomas. Instillations of the agent in distilled water are usually held in the bladder for 3 hours, and the procedure is repeated over a course of weeks. Very little of the agent is absorbed systemically, and it can be quite effective at reducing the frequency of such bladder tumors.

Mitomycin

When mitomycin is administered intravenously, it is cleared rapidly from the vascular compartment; it appears to be eliminated primarily by liver metabolism. Mitomycin causes severe myelosuppression with relatively late toxicity against all 3 formed elements from the bone marrow, with increasingly profound toxicity after repeated doses. This late form of toxicity suggests an action on hematopoietic stem cells as opposed to later progenitors. Nausea, vomiting, and anorexia commonly occur shortly after injection, and occasional instances of renal toxicity and interstitial pneumonitis have also been reported.

BLEOMYCIN

The bleomycins are a series of antineoplastic antibiotics produced by *Streptomyces verticillus*. The clinically used material (Blenoxane) is a mixture of 11 different glycopeptides with the major components being bleomycin A_2 and bleomycin B_2. Bleomycin appears to act through binding to DNA, which results in single- and double-strand breaks following free radical formation, and inhibition of DNA biosynthesis. The fragmentation of DNA seems to be due to oxidation of a DNA-bleomycin-Fe(II) complex and leads to chromosomal aberrations. Bleomycin is a CCS drug that causes accumulation of cells in G_2. It appears to be schedule-dependent, and chronic low-dose administration by repeated injection or continuous infusion seems to be the most effective schedule. The drug synergizes with other drugs such as vinblastine and cisplatin, thus comprising one-third of the curative regimen used for testicular cancers. It is also used in squamous cell carcinomas of the head and neck, cervix, skin, penis, and rectum, and has utility in combination chemotherapy for the lymphomas. A special use has been for intracavitary therapy of malignant effusions in ovarian and breast cancer. Its efficacy in this latter setting may be associated with intrinsic sensitivity of the tumor stem cells in these effusions, as opposed to a nonspecific vesicant effect. The drug can be given subcutaneously, intramuscularly, or intravenously as well as by the intracavitary route (Table 58–4). Peak blood levels of bleomycin after intramuscular injection appear within 30–60 minutes. Intravenous injection of similar dosages yields higher peak concentrations and a terminal half-life of about 2½ hours. Although there is some metabolic inactivation of this agent through an aminopeptidase B–like activity in tumor and normal tissues, approximately 50% can be recovered as the active drug in the urine within 24 hours.

A number of toxic side effects have been described, including lethal anaphylactoid reactions and a high incidence of fever, with or without chills, particularly in patients with lymphoma. Fever may result in dehydration and hypotension in susceptible patients, and small test doses of the drug are commonly used to anticipate this potentially serious toxicity. More common toxic side effects include anorexia and blistering and hyperkeratosis of the palms. A form of pulmonary fibrosis is an uncommon but sometimes fatal adverse

Bleomycins

Bleomycin components (R is):

A_1: $-NH-CH_2-CH_2-CH_2-SO-CH_3$

$DM \cdot A_2$: $-NH-CH_2-CH_2-CH_2-S-CH_3$

A_2: $-NH-CH_2-CH_2-CH_2-S^+(CH_3)_2$

$A_2' \cdot a$: $-NH-CH_2-CH_2-CH_2-CH_2-NH_2$

$A_2' \cdot b$: $-NH-CH_2-CH_2-CH_2-NH_2$

B_2: $-NH-CH_2-CH_2-CH_2-CH_2-NH-\underset{\underset{NH}{\parallel}}{C}-NH_2$

B_4: $-NH-(CH_2)_4-NH-\underset{\underset{NH}{\parallel}}{C}-NH-(CH_2)_4-NH-\underset{\underset{NH}{\parallel}}{C}-NH_2$

A_5: $-NH-(CH_2)_3-NH-(CH_2)_4-NH_2$

A_6: $-NH-(CH_2)_3-NH-(CH_2)_4-NH-(CH_2)_3-NH_2$

effect seen particularly in older patients who have received a total dose over 200 mg/m^2; they may develop a reduced diffusion capacity for oxygen. Patients receiving large doses should undergo serial pulmonary function studies, so that the drug can be discontinued before severe pulmonary toxicity develops. Cough and pulmonary infiltrates are additional indications for discontinuing bleomycin and initiating therapy with antibiotics and corticosteroids. The drug does not have significant myelosuppressive effects, which means that it may be incorporated into a number of different combination chemotherapy programs with no significant addition to bone marrow toxicity.

HORMONAL AGENTS

STEROID HORMONES & ANTISTEROID DRUGS

Sex hormones and adrenocortical hormones are employed in the management of several types of neoplastic disease. The sex hormones are concerned with the stimulation and control of proliferation and function of certain tissues, including the mammary and prostate glands. Cancer arising from and retaining properties of these tissues may be inhibited or stimulated by appropriate changes in hormone balance. Cancer of the breast and cancer of the prostate have been effectually palliated with sex hormone therapy or ablation of certain endocrine organs. The relationship between hormones and hormone-dependent tumors was initially demonstrated by Beatson in 1896 when it was shown that oophorectomy produced improvement in women with advanced breast cancer.

The adrenal corticosteroids (particularly the glucocorticoid analogs) have been useful in the treatment of acute leukemia, lymphomas, myeloma, and other hematologic cancers as well as in advanced breast cancer, and as supportive therapy in the management of hypercalcemia resulting from many types of cancer (Table 58–7). These steroids cause dissolution of lymphocytes, regression of lymph nodes, and inhibition of growth of certain mesenchymal tissues.

The most useful steroid hormones in cancer chemotherapy are listed in Table 58–5.

Pharmacologic Effects

The mechanisms of action of steroid hormones on lymphoid, mammary, or prostatic cancer have been partially clarified. Recent observations indicate that

Table 58–5. Hormonally active agents: Dosages and toxicity.

	Usual Adult Dose	Acute Toxicity	Delayed Toxicity
Androgens			
Testosterone propionate	100 mg IM 3 times weekly	None	Fluid retention, masculinization.
Fluoxymesterone (Halotestin)	10–20 mg/d orally	None	Cholestatic jaundice in some patients receiving fluoxymesterone.
Estrogens			
Diethylstilbestrol	1–5 mg 3 times a day orally	Occasional nausea and vomiting	Fluid retention, feminization, uterine bleeding.
Ethinyl estradiol (Estinyl)	3 mg/d orally		
Antiestrogen			
Tamoxifen (Nolvadex)	20 mg daily orally	None	None.
Progestins			
Hydroxyprogesterone caproate (Delalutin)	1 g IM twice weekly	None	None.
Medroxyprogesterone (Provera)	100–200 mg/d orally; 200–600 mg orally twice weekly	None	None.
Megestrol acetate (Megace)	40 mg 4 times daily orally	None	Fluid retention.
Adrenocorticosteroids			
Hydrocortisone	40–200 mg/d orally	None	Fluid retention, hypertension, diabetes, increased susceptibility to infection, "moon facies."
Prednisone	20–100 mg/d orally or, when effective, 50–100 mg every other day orally as single dose	None	
Gonadotropin-releasing hormone agonists			
Leuprolide (Lupron)	1 mg/d subcutaneously	Hot flashes	None.
Aromatase inhibitors			
Aminoglutethimide (Cytadren)	250 mg twice daily orally, with hydrocortisone, 20 mg twice daily	Dizziness, rash	None.

steroid hormones bind to receptor proteins in cancer cells and that high levels of receptor proteins are predictive for responsiveness to endocrine therapy. Highly specific receptor proteins have been identified for estrogens, progesterone, corticosteroids, and androgens in certain neoplastic cells. As in normal cells (Chapter 35), steroid hormones form a mobile steroid-receptor complex that ultimately binds directly to nuclear nonhistone protein of DNA to activate transcription of associated clusters of genes.

Most steroid-sensitive cancers have specific receptors. Prednisone-sensitive lymphomas and estrogen-sensitive breast and prostatic cancers contain, respectively, specific receptors for corticosteroids, estrogens, and androgens. It is now possible to assay biopsy specimens for steroid receptor content and to predict which individual patients are likely to benefit from steroid therapy. Measurement of the estrogen receptor (ER) protein in breast cancer tissue is now a standard clinical test (Fig 58–9). ER positivity does predict responsiveness to endocrine ablation or additive therapy, whereas patients whose tumors are ER-negative generally fail to respond to such treatment. Similar observations have been reported in prostatic carcinoma. On the basis of animal studies, it appears likely that conversion of a tumor from steroid sensitivity to steroid resistance is associated with loss of specific receptor protein production, presumably as a result of selection.

Clinical Uses

The sex hormones are employed in cancer of the female and male breast, cancer of the prostate, and cancer of the endometrium of the uterus (Table 58–7). Extensive studies with the androgenic, estrogenic, and progestational sex hormones have demonstrated their value in advanced inoperable mammary cancer, cancer of the prostate, and cancer of the endometrium (see pp 687 and 693–696).

Adverse Reactions

Androgens, estrogens, and adrenocortical hormones all can produce fluid retention through their sodium-retaining effect. Prolonged use of androgens and estrogens will cause masculinization and feminization, respectively. Extended use of the adrenocortical steroids may result in hypertension, diabetes, increased susceptibility to infection, and the development of cushingoid appearance ("moon facies") (see Chapter 38 and Table 58–5).

ANTIESTROGEN

The antiestrogenic compound tamoxifen has proved to be extremely useful for the treatment of breast cancer. As an antiestrogen, it inhibits estrogen-stimulated increases in uterine weight and vaginal cornification. Tamoxifen functions as a competitive inhibitor of estrogen and binds to the cytoplasmic estrogen receptor (ER) protein of estrogen-sensitive tissues and tumors. Translocation of the receptor complex to the nucleus appears to occur normally, suggesting that the antiestrogen acts at the nuclear level Studies in tissue culture have shown that in the absence of estrogen, tamoxifen is cytotoxic to ER-positive and progesterone receptor (PR)–positive breast cancer cells. This provides evidence that the antiestrogen has a potent direct effect. However, tamoxifen has a 100- to 1000-fold lower affinity constant for ER than does estradiol, indicating the importance of ablation of endogenous estrogen for optimal antiestrogen effect.

Excellent plasma levels of tamoxifen are obtained after oral administration, and the agent has a much longer biologic half-life than estradiol. The usual dosages in breast cancer treatment are in the range of 10 mg twice daily (Table 58–5), although doses up to 100 mg/m^2 have been administered without major toxicity. Because it may take several weeks to achieve a steady-state level of the active metabolite (monohydroxytamoxifen) with the dosage of 20 mg daily, it is advisable to give an 80-mg "loading course" on the first day to achieve good blood levels rapidly.

Side effects in the usual dose range are quite mild. Hot flashes are the most frequent side effect. Nausea is observed occasionally, as is fluid retention and mild

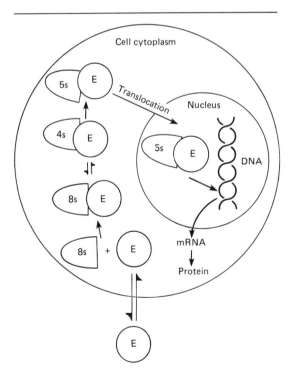

Figure 58–9. Prototype cancer cell that is estrogen receptor–positive. Estrogen (E) binds to an 8s receptor, which then undergoes metabolic transformations, with reduction in molecular weight, after which it is translocated to the cell nucleus. The complex is then bound to chromatin, and RNA synthesis and protein synthesis are initiated. A similar process appears to apply for progesterone and androgen receptors. Cells bearing such steroid hormone receptors often respond to endocrine therapy.

hematologic toxicity. Occasional "flares" of breast cancer are observed, but it is uncertain if this is a side effect or a manifestation of preexisting rapid tumor growth.

Tamoxifen has recently proved to have significant antitumor activity in estrogen-resistant prostatic cancer and progesterone-resistant endometrial cancer. A lesser degree of activity has also been observed in metastatic melanoma, and a variety of tumor types are now being studied for their content of estrogen receptor to determine whether they might also be amenable to growth inhibition with tamoxifen.

Tamoxifen

In advanced breast cancer, clinical improvement is observed in 40–50% of patients who receive tamoxifen. Patients who show objective benefit with treatment are largely those who (1) lack endogenous estrogens (oophorectomy or postmenopausal state) and (2) have breast cancers in which the cytoplasmic ER or PR protein is demonstrable on radioreceptor assay. Thus, it is not rational therapy to use tamoxifen in patients who are known to be ER-negative or have endogenous estrogen production. Tamoxifen has also been effective at prolonging survival when used as surgical adjuvant therapy for postmenopausal women with ER-positive breast cancer.

GONADOTROPIN-RELEASING HORMONE AGONISTS

Leuprolide acetate (Lupron) is a synthetic peptide composed of 9 amino acids and an analog of naturally occurring gonadotropin-releasing hormone (GnRH, LHRH). It is portrayed in Chapter 36.

This analog is more potent than the natural hormone and functions as a GnRH agonist, with paradoxic results on the pituitary—initial stimulation followed by inhibition of release of follicle-stimulating hormone and luteinizing hormone. This results in reduced testicular androgen synthesis. The latter effect underlies the efficacy of this agent in the treatment of metastatic carcinoma of the prostate.

Leuprolide (1 mg subcutaneously daily) has been directly compared to standard endocrine therapy of prostatic cancer with diethylstilbestrol (DES, 3 mg orally daily). Suppression of androgen synthesis and reductions in serum prostatic acid phosphatase (a marker of metastatic tumor burden) are comparable with both leuprolide and DES. However, painful gy-

necomastia, nausea, vomiting, edema, and thromboembolism occur significantly less frequently with leuprolide than with DES. Leuprolide is more costly than DES in terms of drug cost per se, but that is more than offset by the overall cost of complications of DES or the surgical and hospitalization costs associated with surgical orchiectomy. The endocrine effects of leuprolide may also prove useful in the management of hormone receptor–positive breast cancer, but this application remains to be established.

AROMATASE INHIBITORS

Aminoglutethimide (Cytadren) is an inhibitor of adrenal steroid synthesis at the first step (conversion of cholesterol to pregnenolone; Chapter 38). Aminoglutethimide also inhibits the extra-adrenal synthesis of estrone and estradiol. Aside from its direct effects on adrenal steroidogenesis, aminoglutethimide is a specific inhibitor of an aromatase enzyme that converts the adrenal androgen androstenedione to estrone. This aromatization of an androgenic precursor into an estrogen can occur in body fat. Since estrogens promote the growth of many breast cancers, estrogen synthesis in extragonadal (fat) tissue can be important in breast cancer growth in postmenopausal women. Therapeutically, aminoglutethimide has proved to be an effective agent for the treatment of metastatic breast cancer in women whose tumors contain significant levels of estrogen or progesterone receptors. Aminoglutethimide is normally administered along with adrenal replacement doses of hydrocortisone to avoid symptoms of adrenal insufficiency. Hydrocortisone is preferable to dexamethasone, as the latter agent accelerates the rate of catabolism of aminoglutethimide. Side effects of aminoglutethimide include dizziness, lethargy, visual blurring, and a pruritic rash.

The use of aminoglutethimide plus hydrocortisone has been compared to both surgical adrenalectomy and hypophysectomy and has been found to be as good as or better than either in its action against metastatic breast cancer. Aminoglutethimide plus hydrocortisone is normally used as second-line therapy for women who have been treated with tamoxifen, largely because aminoglutethimide causes somewhat more side effects than tamoxifen. However, it can be used as primary endocrine therapy also.

MISCELLANEOUS ANTICANCER DRUGS (See Table 58–6.)

AMSACRINE

Amsacrine is a 9-anilinoacridine derivative that causes chromosome breakage. This drug intercalates between base pairs in DNA, distorts the double helix, and produces single- and double-strand breaks in

Table 58–6. Miscellaneous anticancer drugs: Dosages and toxicity.

Drug	Usual Dose	Acute Toxicity	Delayed Toxicity
Amsacrine	90 mg/m² intravenously for 5 days (leukemia)	Nausea	Bone marrow depression.
Asparaginase	20,000 IU/m² daily IV for 5–10 days	Nausea and fever, allergic reactions	Hepatotoxicity, mental depression, pancreatitis.
Hydroxyurea	300 mg/m² orally for 5 days	Nausea and vomiting	Bone marrow depression.
Mitotane	6–15 g/d orally	Nausea and vomiting	Dermatitis, diarrhea, mental depression.
Mitoxantrone	10–12 mg/m² intravenously every 3–4 weeks	Nausea	Bone marrow depression, occasional cardiac toxicity, mild alopecia.
Quinacrine	100–300 mg/d by intracavitary injection for 5 days	Local pain and fever	None.

DNA and DNA-protein cross-links. DNA strand breaks appear to be mediated by formation of topoisomerase II–DNA complexes trapped by amsacrine in the breaking-sealing action of the enzyme.

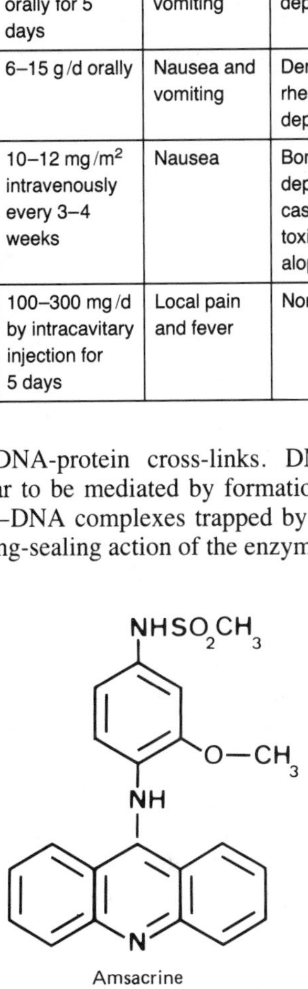

Amsacrine

The plasma clearance of amsacrine is biphasic, with an initial plasma decay half-life of 10–15 minutes and a terminal half-life of 8–9 hours; unchanged drug and metabolites are excreted in the urine and the bile. Amsacrine is predominantly metabolized by the liver; thus, liver impairment causes considerable prolongation of plasma concentrations. Amsacrine has significant activity against anthracycline- and cytarabine-refractory acute myelogenous leukemia, advanced ovarian carcinomas, and lymphomas. Hematologic toxicity is dose-limiting, and cardiac arrest has been reported during amsacrine infusions.

ASPARAGINASE

Asparaginase (L-asparagine amidohydrolase, Crasnitin, Elspar) is an enzyme that is isolated for clinical use from various bacteria (eg, *E coli, Erwinia carotovora*). The active enzyme has a molecular weight of 133,000 and a tetrameric structure containing 4 identical subunits. The drug is used to treat childhood acute leukemia. Asparaginase acts indirectly by catabolic depletion of serum asparagine to aspartic acid and ammonia. Blood glutamine levels are also reduced. This results in inhibition of protein synthesis in neoplastic cells requiring an external source of asparagine because of low or deficient levels of asparagine synthase, and cell proliferation is blocked. Most normal cells are capable of synthesizing asparagine and thus are less susceptible to the action of asparaginase.

HYDROXYUREA

Hydroxyurea ($H_2NCONHOH$, Hydrea) is an analog of urea whose mechanism of action is through inhibition of DNA synthesis, exerting its lethal effect on cells in S phase. This action is through inhibition of the enzyme ribonucleotide reductase, with resulting depletion of deoxynucleoside triphosphate pools. The drug is administered orally and is available in capsules (0.5 g). Its major uses are in melanoma and chronic myelogenous leukemia; however, it plays a secondary role in both of these circumstances. Its role in combination chemotherapy has yet to be defined. The major side effect of this agent is bone marrow depression. At high dosages (greater than 40 mg/kg/d), megaloblastosis unresponsive to vitamin B_{12} or folic acid may appear. Gastrointestinal symptoms, including nausea, vomiting, and diarrhea, are common in patients receiving high dosages of the drug. Less common reactions include skin reactions and mucositis and occasional renal dysfunction or central nervous system abnormality.

MITOXANTRONE

Mitoxantrone (Novantrone, dihydroxyanthracenedione, DHAD) binds to DNA to produce strand breakage and inhibits both DNA and RNA biosynthesis. The plasma half-life in patients is approximately 32 hours; the predominant route of mitoxantrone excretion is in the feces. Mitoxantrone is active in both pediatric and adult acute myelogenous leukemia, non-Hodgkin lymphomas, and breast cancer. Leukopenia is the dose-limiting toxicity, and mild nausea and vomiting, stomatitis, and alopecia also occur.

MITOTANE (LYSODREN)

This drug (see Fig 38–5) is a DDT congener that was first found to be adrenolytic in dogs. Subsequently, it was found to be of use in the treatment of adrenal carcinoma. The drug produces tumor re-

Mitoxantrone

gression and relief of the excessive adrenal steroid secretion that often occurs with this malignancy. Toxicities include skin eruptions, diarrhea, and mental depression.

About 40% of an oral dose is absorbed, and 60% is excreted in stool. Of the amount reaching the tissues, most is stored in fat for several weeks. About 25% of an absorbed dose is excreted as a urinary metabolite. It produces anorexia, nausea, somnolence, and dermatitis.

The utility of mitotane appears to be limited to adrenal carcinoma, and it is marketed for that one indication.

QUINACRINE

This antimalarial drug has been found to be of occasional use in the control of malignant pleural, pericardial, and abdominal effusions. It is instilled directly into the fluid-containing cavity. Although its exact mechanism of action is uncertain, it is a local irritant and leads to the production of local fibrous adhesions. Amsacrine (AMSA) is a structural analog of quinacrine that is investigational for use in lymphomas and myelogenous leukemia (see above).

INVESTIGATIONAL AGENTS

Several of the drugs mentioned in the text remain in an investigational status in the USA until their efficacy and safety for cancer chemotherapy can be established. In specific instances where treatment with one of these agents seems warranted, it usually can be arranged through a university hospital or cancer center or by contacting the Division of Cancer Treatment of the National Cancer Institute, which can provide further information and identify investigators who are authorized to administer these drugs.

This status applies to deoxycoformycin, 5-fluoro-AMP, 4-demethoxydaunorubicin, and amsacrine, agents useful in acute leukemias. Other products still in the investigational phase include mitoxantrone, bisantrene, hexamethylmelamine, azacitidine, tegafur (ftorafur), desacetylvinblastine, carboplatin, and teniposide. Several hexitol sugar derivatives that may act as alkylating agents are under study; these include mitobronitol, mitolactol, and dianhydrogalactilol. All

of these drugs have substantial toxicities. Until their pharmacology is more completely understood and their net effects have proved to be beneficial, their use will be restricted to clinical research. New inhibitors of nucleoside metabolism include the adenosine deaminase inhibitor deoxycoformycin. Of the biologic response modifiers, the vitamin A analogs (isotretinoin, etretinate; see p 772) and biologicals (human interferon, tumor necrosis factor, and monoclonal antibodies) appear to be particularly promising. It is likely that amsacrine, mitoxantrone, and interferon will have major uses in cancer therapy.

CLINICAL PHARMACOLOGY OF CANCER CHEMOTHERAPEUTIC DRUGS
(See Table 58–7.)

Knowledge of the kinetics of tumor cell proliferation and total body tumor cell number, as well as information on the pharmacology and mechanism of action of cancer chemotherapeutic agents, has become important in designing optimal chemotherapeutic regimens for patients with advanced cancer. The strategy for developing drug regimens requires a knowledge of the particular characteristics of specific tumors—eg, Is there a high growth fraction? Is there a high spontaneous cell death rate? Are most of the cells in G_0? Is a significant fraction of the tumor composed of hypoxic stem cells? Are their normal counterparts under hormonal control? Similarly, knowledge of the pharmacology of specific drugs is equally important—eg, Does the drug have a particular affinity for uptake by the tumor cells (streptozocin)? Are the tumor cells sensitive to the drug? Is the drug cycle-phase specific?

Drugs that affect cycling cells can often be used most effectively after treatment with a cycle-nonspecific agent (eg, alkylating agents); this principle has been tested in only a few human tumors, but with increasing success. Similarly, recognition of true drug synergism (tumor cell kill by the drug combination greater than the additive effects of the individual drugs) or antagonism is important in the design of combination chemotherapeutic programs. The combination of cytarabine with 6-thioguanine in the treatment of acute myelogenous leukemia, the use of doxorubicin and cyclophosphamide in breast cancer, and the use of vinblastine or etoposide along with cisplatin and bleomycin in testicular tumors are good examples of true drug synergism against cancer cells but not against normal tissues.

In general, it is preferable to use cytotoxic chemotherapeutic agents in intensive "pulse" courses every 3–4 weeks rather than to give continuous daily dosage schedules. This allows for maximum effects against neoplastic cell populations with complete hematologic and immunologic recovery between courses rather than leaving the patient continuously sup-

Table 58–7. Malignancies responsive to chemotherapy.

Diagnosis	Current Treatment of Choice	Other Valuable Agents
Acute lymphocytic leukemia	Induction: vincristine plus prednisone. Remission maintenance: mercaptopurine, methotrexate, and cyclophosphamide in various combinations	Asparaginase, daunorubicin, carmustine, doxorubicin, cytarabine, allopurinol,* craniospinal radiotherapy
Acute myelocytic and myelomonocytic leukemia	Combination chemotherapy: doxorubicin, vincristine, cytarabine, prednisone or thioguanine, cytarabine, and daunorubicin	Methotrexate, thioguanine, mercaptopurine, allopurinol,* azacitidine,† amsacrine†
Chronic myelogenous leukemia	Busulfan	Vincristine, mercaptopurine, hydroxyurea, vindesine,† melphalan, interferon, allopurinol*
Chronic lymphocytic leukemia	Chlorambucil and prednisone (if indicated)	Vincristine, androgens,* allopurinol,* doxorubicin
Hodgkin's disease (stages III and IV)	Combination chemotherapy: mechlorethamine, vincristine, procarbazine, prednisone ("MOPP")	Vinblastine, doxorubicin, lomustine, dacarbazine, teniposide,† bleomycin
Non-Hodgkin lymphomas	Combination chemotherapy: cyclophosphamide, doxorubicin, vincristine, prednisone	Bleomycin, lomustine, carmustine, teniposide,† BCG,† amsacrine,† interferon
Multiple myeloma	Melphalan plus prednisone or multiagent combination chemotherapy	Cyclophosphamide, vincristine, carmustine, interferon, doxorubicin, androgens*
Macroglobulinemia	Chlorambucil	Melphalan
Polycythemia vera	Busulfan, chlorambucil, or cyclophosphamide	Radioactive phosphorus 32
Carcinoma of lung	Cyclophosphamide plus doxorubicin, methotrexate, and lomustine	Cisplatin, quinacrine,* hexamethylmelamine,† vindesine,† vincristine, etoposide
Carcinomas of head and neck	Fluorouracil plus cisplatin	Methotrexate, bleomycin, hydroxyurea, doxorubicin, vinblastine
Carcinoma of endometrium	Progestins or tamoxifen	Fluorouracil
Carcinoma of ovary	Cyclophosphamide and cisplatin	Doxorubicin, melphalan, fluorouracil, vincristine, hexamethylmelamine,† bleomycin

*Supportive agent, not oncolytic.
†Investigational agent. Treatment available through qualified investigators and centers authorized by National Cancer Institute and Cooperative Oncology Groups.

pressed with cytotoxic therapy. This approach reduces side effects and does not reduce therapeutic efficacy.

The application of these principles is well illustrated in the current approach to the treatment of acute leukemia, lymphomas, Wilms' tumor, and testicular neoplasms.

ADJUVANT CHEMOTHERAPY FOR MICROMETASTASES: MULTIMODALITY THERAPY

The most important role for effective cancer chemotherapy is undoubtedly as an "adjuvant" to initial or "primary field" treatment with other methods of treatment such as surgery or radiation therapy. Failures with primary field therapy are due principally to occult micrometastases outside the primary field. With the currently available treatment modalities, this form of multimodality therapy appears to offer the greatest chance of curing patients with solid tumors.

Distant micrometastases are usually present in patients with one or more positive lymph nodes at the time of surgery (eg, in breast cancer) and in patients with tumors having a known propensity for early hematogenous spread (eg, osteogenic sarcoma, Wilms' tumor). The risk of recurrent or metastatic disease in such patients can be extremely high (80%). Only systemic therapy can adequately attack micrometastases. Chemotherapy regimens that are at least moderately effective against advanced cancer may have curative potential (at the right dosage and schedule) when combined with primary therapy such as surgery. Recent studies show prolongation of disease-free and overall survival in patients with osteogenic sarcoma, rhabdomyosarcoma, or breast cancer who receive adjuvant chemotherapy. In osteogenic sarcoma, methotrexate with leucovorin (folinic acid) rescue, doxorubicin alone, and doxorubicin in combination with other drugs have proved effective. Similar comments apply to the use of 3 cycles of combination chemotherapy (MOPP, p 691) prior to total nodal radiation in stage IIB Hodgkin's disease.

In breast cancer, premenopausal women with positive lymph nodes at the time of mastectomy have benefited from combination chemotherapy. It has been

Table 58–7 (cont'd). Malignancies responsive to chemotherapy.

Diagnosis	Current Treatment of Choice	Other Valuable Agents
Carcinoma of cervix	Mitomycin plus bleomycin, vincristine, and cisplatin	Lomustine, cyclophosphamide, doxorubicin, methotrexate
Breast carcinoma	(1) Combination chemotherapy alone or plus tamoxifen (see text) if lymph nodes are positive at mastectomy (2) Combination chemotherapy or hormonal manipulation for late recurrence (see text)	Cyclophosphamide, doxorubicin, vincristine, methotrexate, fluorouracil, mitoxantrone,[†] quinacrine,[*] prednisone,[*] megestrol, androgens,[*] aminoglutethimide
Choriocarcinoma (trophoblastic neoplasms)	Methotrexate, alone or in combination with vincristine, dactinomycin, and cyclophosphamide	Cisplatin, vinblastine, mercaptopurine, chlorambucil, doxorubicin
Carcinoma of testis	Combination therapy: cisplatin, bleomycin, and etoposide	Methotrexate, dactinomycin, mithramycin, vinblastine, doxorubicin, cyclophosphamide, etoposide
Carcinoma of prostate	Estrogens or leuprolide	Aminoglutethimide, doxorubicin, cisplatin, prednisone,[*] estramustine, fluorouracil, progestins
Wilms' tumor	Vincristine plus dactinomycin after surgery and radiotherapy	Methotrexate, cyclophosphamide, doxorubicin
Neuroblastoma	Cyclophosphamide plus doxorubicin and vincristine	Dactinomycin, daunorubicin, cisplatin
Carcinoma of thyroid	Radioiodine (^{131}I), doxorubicin	Bleomycin, fluorouracil, melphalan
Carcinoma of adrenal	Mitotane	Doxorubicin
Carcinoma of stomach or pancreas	Fluorouracil plus doxorubicin and mitomycin	Hydroxyurea, lomustine, cisplatin
Carcinoma of colon	Fluorouracil	Cyclophosphamide, mitomycin, nitrosoureas
Carcinoid	Doxorubicin plus cyclophosphamide	Interferon, dactinomycin, methysergide,[*] streptozocin
Insulinoma	Streptozocin	Doxorubicin, fluorouracil, mitomycin, streptozocin
Osteogenic sarcoma	Doxorubicin, or methotrexate with citrovorum rescue initiated after surgery	Cyclophosphamide, dacarbazine, interferon
Miscellaneous sarcomas	Doxorubicin plus dacarbazine	Methotrexate, dactinomycin, cyclophosphamide, vincristine, vinblastine
Melanoma	Dacarbazine	Lomustine, hydroxyurea, mitomycin, dactinomycin, interferon

[*]Supportive agent, not oncolytic.

[†]Investigational agent. Treatment available through qualified investigators and centers authorized by National Cancer Institute and Cooperative Oncology Groups.

established that several programs of cytotoxic chemotherapy achieve prolonged disease-free and overall survival times and as a result have increased the cure rate in high-risk primary breast cancer. Active regimens have included, in various combinations, the agents cyclophosphamide (C), methotrexate (M), fluorouracil (F), doxorubicin (D), and vincristine (V). In general, regimens with at least 3 active drugs have been useful. The end results obtained with combination chemotherapy have already proved superior to results obtained with single agents, because combination chemotherapy can cope with tumor cell heterogeneity and produces a greater tumor cell log kill. Full protocol doses of cytotoxic agents are required to maximize the likelihood of efficacy. The CMFVP regimen appears to be effective in both pre- and postmenopausal women, perhaps because of the greater potency of these combinations against breast cancer. Early results of ongoing clinical trials of tamoxifen alone or in combination with chemotherapy have yielded encouraging results in postmenopausal women with positive estrogen receptor tests on the primary tumor. Whether tamoxifen suppresses or eradicates micrometastases remains to be established. Adjuvant chemotherapy should definitely be considered as part of standard and indicated therapy in premenopausal women, and use of tamoxifen is now standard in node-positive postmenopausal women with positive ER or PR tests on tumor specimens.

Other areas of current investigation include adjuvant chemotherapy for "Dukes C" stage colorectal cancer (fluorouracil in combination with semustine or radiotherapy) and in testicular (vinblastine, bleomycin, and cisplatin), head and neck, and gynecologic neoplasms (various drugs). Thus, adjuvant chemotherapy (with curative intent) should now be given serious consideration for patients who undergo primary surgical staging and therapy and are found to have a stage and histologic type of cancer known to be associated with a high risk of micrometastasis. This policy is germane to those tumor types for which palliative chemotherapy has already been developed and been shown to induce complete remissions in advanced stages of the disease. In each instance, the benefit/risk ratio must be closely examined.

ACUTE LEUKEMIA

Acute leukemia is a general term for a group of malignant disorders of blood leukocytes. Age at onset of disease and certain morphologic characteristics have significant implications for patient survival and responsiveness to chemotherapy. With current agents, childhood acute leukemia is more treatable than that which occurs later in life. In all leukemic patients, major emphasis must be given to intensive support of the patient with necessary red cell and platelet transfusions, and prevention of hyperuricemia and infection.

Leukemia of Childhood

Acute lymphoblastic leukemia (ALL) is the predominant form of leukemia in childhood and the most common form of cancer in children. The usual cell of origin appears to be a "null" lymphocyte. These children now have a relatively good prognosis. A subset of patients with a poor prognosis have neoplastic lymphocytes expressing surface antigenic features of T lymphocytes (see Chapter 59). A cytoplasmic enzyme expressed by normal thymocytes, terminal deoxycytidyl transferase (terminal transferase), is also expressed in many cases of ALL. T cell ALLs also express high levels of the enzyme adenosine deaminase (ADA). (This led to interest in the use of the ADA inhibitor deoxycoformycin for treatment of such T cell cases.) Until 1948, the median survival in ALL was 3 months. With the advent of the folic acid antagonists, a major increase in survival was achieved. Subsequently, corticosteroids, mercaptopurine, cyclophosphamide, vincristine, daunorubicin, and asparaginase were all found to have activity in this disease. In general, current practice is to employ a combination of vincristine and prednisone for initial induction of remission. Over 85% of children enter complete remission with this therapy, with only minimal toxicity. Because circulating tumor stem cells often lodge in the brain, such cells are not killed by these drugs, as they do not cross the blood-brain barrier. The value of "prophylactic" intrathecal methotrexate therapy for prevention of central nervous system leukemia (a major mechanism of relapse) has been clearly demonstrated. Intrathecal therapy with methotrexate should therefore be considered as a standard component of the induction regimen for children with ALL. Alternative approaches for prevention of central nervous system leukemia that also appear to be efficacious are intrathecal cytarabine and craniospinal irradiation. Radiation therapy to the neuraxis can cause skeletal growth retardation as a side effect. Once a complete remission has been induced (greater than a 3-log cell kill), "maintenance" or "consolidation" therapy is always indicated. This usually consists of a combination of oral methotrexate, mercaptopurine, and cyclophosphamide, administered either in pulses, simultaneously, or in various sequences. Some centers employ periodic "reinforcements," with repeated courses of the inducing agents (vincristine and prednisone) several times each year. Such efforts at "total therapy" should be considered as the standard approach to treatment, because they have resulted in a substantial increase in the cure rate of children with acute leukemia. Although many of the clinical trials are still under way, such therapy appears to offer the best hope of cure for an increasing percentage of patients. The median survival in childhood acute leukemia is now approaching 4 years. Many centers discontinue intensive chemotherapy in patients who have shown no sign of relapse after 3 years of intensive chemotherapy. Such children are markedly immunosuppressed during therapy; however, both humoral and cell-mediated immunity usually return to normal within 6 months after cessation of chemotherapy. Cell-mediated immunity to ALL can definitely be demonstrated—more readily when the patient enters complete remission. Children who survive for 5 years in complete remission have a greater than 50% chance of having a permanent remission or cure.

If leukemia does recur in a patient in remission, an attempt is made to reinduce the remission with the same drugs used initially. If resistance is observed, reinduction is attempted with different agents (daunorubicin, vincristine, asparaginase, methotrexate, etc) in various combinations. The possibility of cure of this dread disease of young patients has imparted great impetus to current investigations of intensive combination chemotherapy with proved agents plus asparaginase, daunorubicin, and other experimental agents and has led to increased interest in combination chemotherapy of other kinds of neoplastic diseases.

Leukemia in Adults

Acute leukemia in adults is predominantly of the myelocytic variety, although some cases of lymphoblastic leukemia are also seen. Acute myelogenous leukemia (AML) has been quite difficult to treat, and until recently the median survival was in the range of 3 months. Unlike ALL, induction therapy in AML requires the use of drugs toxic to normal bone marrow cells. The single most active agent for AML is cytarabine; however, it is best used in combination. Combinations of cytarabine, thioguanine, and daunorubicin or of cytarabine and daunorubicin are capable of inducing remissions in over 50% of previously untreated cases. Doxorubicin has had similar activity to daunorubicin and may act synergistically when used in combination with prolonged cytarabine infusions. Recent trials with combinations of anthracyclines with cytarabine have induced complete remissions in about 70% of patients. Currently, cytarabine is being tested at doses 10 times those used conventionally in the treatment of leukemia ("high-dose cytarabine"). The patient often requires intensive supportive care during the toxic period of induction chemotherapy before remission is achieved. Such supportive care includes platelet transfusions to prevent bleeding due to thrombocytopenia and combinations of bactericidal antibiotics plus granulocyte transfusions to combat infections. Patients over 60 respond less well to chemotherapy, primarily because their resistance to infection is lower. Remission maintenance is usually with thioguanine and cytarabine courses. Azacitidine and amsacrine are utilized as secondary agents for patients who develop resistance to standard therapy. The median life expectancy of patients with AML who enter complete remission is now in excess of 1 year, and some patients are in remission for over 3 years. About 20% of adult patients who achieve complete remission with current standard chemotherapy appear to remain free of recurrent leukemia and are probably cured. For patients under age 30 who have an HLA-matched sibling (or identical twin), use of total body irradiation and bone marrow transplantation while in remission has become an increasingly successful treatment strategy.

CHRONIC MYELOGENOUS LEUKEMIA

Chronic myelogenous leukemia (CML) arises from a chromosomally abnormal hematopoietic stem cell. An abnormal chromosome 22 with deletion of a short arm or translocation to the long arm of chromosome 9 is present in 90% of cases. The clinical symptoms and course are related to the leukocyte level and its rate of increase. Most patients with leukocyte counts over $50,000/\mu L$ should be treated. The goal of treatment is to reduce the granulocytes to normal levels, to raise the hemoglobin concentration to normal, and to relieve metabolic symptoms. The most useful form of treatment is chemotherapy with busulfan, although other oral alkylating agents can also be used. Local splenic x-ray therapy is occasionally used. In the early stages of the disease, treatment produces a prompt decrease in spleen size and a fall in the leukocyte count associated with subjective well-being. Current therapy does not prolong survival, but it markedly relieves symptoms. Efforts to achieve better results with combination chemotherapy plus splenectomy have thus far been unsuccessful.

Initial chemotherapy consists of giving busulfan, 4 mg daily orally, until the number of leukocytes falls to $12,000/\mu L$. If the initial white count is higher than $100,000/\mu L$, allopurinol should be used prophylactically to prevent the development of hyperuricemia. Maintenance therapy is advisable if the leukocyte count doubles within 1 month after discontinuance of the initial course of treatment. A maintenance dose of 2 mg of busulfan daily is usually sufficient, but as the disease progresses it may be necessary to increase the dose to 6 or 8 mg daily.

Resistance to busulfan eventually develops. The hemoglobin falls, the spleen enlarges, and the differential count shows increasing cellular immaturity, with large numbers of blast cells. At this point, busulfan is discontinued and agents such as hydroxyurea or mercaptopurine may be of some value, but only partial and temporary success can be anticipated. This blastic transformation, or "blast crisis," generally occurs 3–4 years after diagnosis, and the disease converts to acute leukemia. Therapy at that point is still investigational, but combination chemotherapy, including cytarabine, vincristine, vindesine, or hydroxyurea with or without prednisone, and asparaginase, may have some benefit in a subset of patients. True remissions rarely occur in patients who have undergone blast crisis. Bone marrow transplantation is now showing promise for CML patients who have an HLA-matched donor.

CHRONIC LYMPHOCYTIC LEUKEMIA

Treatment of chronic lymphocytic leukemia is markedly different from that of chronic myelogenous leukemia. Whereas chronic myelogenous leukemia is a proliferative neoplasm requiring chemotherapy for symptomatic control, chronic lymphocytic leukemia appears to result from a gradual accumulation of monoclonal B lymphocytes rather than from rapid neoplastic cell proliferation. Chronic lymphocytic leukemia is often detected accidentally long before the development of symptoms. Although the average life expectancy is only 3 years, the disease occurs frequently in elderly patients, which skews the survival data. Many patients who are asymptomatic may have prolonged survival (eg, 5–15 years) without any therapy. In patients whose disease is restricted to lymphocytosis in the peripheral blood, it is reasonable to withold treatment because in chronic lymphocytic leukemia one does not "treat the lymphocyte count" unless it is well above $150,000/\mu L$. When anemia, immunodeficiency, weight loss, fever, and generalized organ and bone marrow involvement do occur, treatment is indicated.

The therapeutic resources available for the treatment of chronic lymphocytic leukemia include corticosteroids and low-dose total body irradiation or alkylating agent chemotherapy. Prednisone is often quite effective, and after an initial course of 80 mg/d for several weeks the dose can be tapered to low levels or switched to an intermittent (every other day) schedule, which virtually eliminates side effects. Hemolytic anemia may respond dramatically to prednisone, although thrombocytopenia is often more refractory. Alkylating agents will also decrease the number of lymphocytes and organ enlargement in most patients, and the choice between corticosteroids and alkylating agents is frequently based on relative contraindications of one drug or the other.

Chlorambucil (Leukeran) is probably the most easily administered oral alkylating agent and has fewest side effects. The dose is usually 0.1 mg/kg/d, with monitoring of blood counts at weekly intervals. Alternatively, cyclophosphamide can be given in "pulse courses" of 1 g/m^2 orally over 4 days every 4–6 weeks. More aggressive therapy, eg, with cyclophosphamide, vincristine, and prednisone, is indicated in instances of severe hemolytic anemia and rapidly progressive disease. The goal of therapy is to eliminate the systemic manifestations of the disease, and complete normalization of the lymphocyte count is not necessary. Therapy can be discontinued once the patient's condition has stabilized, but maintenance therapy should be considered if symptoms reappear quickly. Local x-ray therapy is useful for shrinking symptomatic enlarged lymph nodes but is only occasionally indicated. It is important not to overtreat these usually elderly patients, because of their poor host resistance.

THE LYMPHOMAS

1. HODGKIN'S DISEASE

Although remarkably little is known about the cause of Hodgkin's disease, its therapy has undergone revolutionary improvement. Hodgkin's disease is a lymphoma with certain unique characteristics in its natural history: its apparent tendency to progress from a single involved node to anatomically adjacent nodes in a somewhat "orderly" fashion, and its tendency to appear confined to the lymphoid system for a long period of time, with progression to involve retroperitoneal nodes and spleen. Extranodal involvement may also occur, and involvement of the liver, bone marrow, lungs, or other sites is taken as evidence of more "malignant" behavior of the tumor. A concerted attempt at adequate staging of the extent of disease is essential to effective treatment of this disorder, and newly diagnosed cases must be adequately studied with x-rays, lymphography, and exploratory laparotomy and splenectomy (looking for occult disease) in order to prepare a rational treatment plan. Widespread involvement is manifested by symptoms such as sweats, fever, anorexia, and weight loss and infiltration of other organs, including the lungs, liver, and bone marrow.

Intensive x-ray therapy with supervoltage equipment is curative in most cases of early Hodgkin's disease confined to one lymph node area or several adjacent areas above the diaphragm (stages I and II). Radiation therapy is also of some use in asymptomatic patients with more generalized Hodgkin's disease limited to the lymphoid system above and below the diaphragm (stage III), and occasionally in stage IV for palliation of symptoms due to enlarging lymph nodes. As can be seen in Table 58–7, a variety of chemotherapeutic agents are active in Hodgkin's disease; however, it is now clear that optimal treatment is with combination chemotherapy.

Combination chemotherapy is now indicated in patients presenting with stage III or stage IV Hodgkin's disease. The results have been sufficiently promising to lead to present trials of combination chemotherapy along with x-ray therapy in stage I and stage II disease. Results in stage IIIA Hodgkin's disease with 3 cycles of chemotherapy (see below) followed by total nodal radiotherapy are clearly superior to those achieved with radiotherapy alone. The most effective form of chemotherapy at present is with a 4-drug combination known as MOPP, consisting of mechlorethamine (HN2, Mustargen), Oncovin (vincristine), procarbazine (Matulane), and prednisone. This form of treatment, developed by DeVita and his associates at the National Cancer Institute, is given repeatedly for at least 6 months and sometimes for as long as a year. Over 80% of previously untreated patients with advanced Hodgkin's disease (stages III and IV) go into complete remission, with disappearance of all symptoms and objective evidences of tumor.

A popular schedule for use of MOPP includes repeated courses every 2 months with M (mechlorethamine), 6 mg/m^2 intravenously on days 1 and 8; O (vincristine), 1.4 mg/m^2 intravenously on days 1 and 8; P (procarbazine), 50 mg orally on day 1, 100 mg orally on day 2, and 100 mg/m^2 on days 3–10; and P (prednisone), 40 mg/m^2 orally on days 1–10. A "non–cross-resistant" alternative to the MOPP regimen developed by Bonadonna consists of doxorubicin (Adriamycin), bleomycin, vinblastine, and dacarbazine (ABVD). The ABVD program appears to be similar in efficacy to MOPP and, more importantly, has been of value in treatment of MOPP failures. Complex treatment regimens such as these should be under the direction of a medical oncologist who is familiar with the individual and synergistic toxicities and contraindications for each of the drugs involved. Frequent blood counts are obtained, and treatment is modified or suspended temporarily in the event of severe depression of the white cell or platelet count. After remission induction with at least 6 courses of MOPP or ABVD, approximately 50% of patients will remain free of all signs of Hodgkin's disease for over 2 years. The ABVD combination has thus far been free from association with late development of acute leukemia, perhaps because of the lack of alkylating agents and procarbazine from this combination.

Theoretical calculations based on the number of logs of tumor cells likely to be killed with this type of intensive therapy suggest that a cellular cure of Hodgkin's disease may be accomplished in some of these cases, but follow-ups of 5–15 years after cessation of all chemotherapy are required for confirmation. Thus far, about half of patients who have achieved complete remission with MOPP appear to remain disease-free at 10 years. This form of chemotherapy therefore represents a major improvement in the management of advanced Hodgkin's disease, and patients should be afforded every chance to achieve complete remission.

Some of the reasons for the success of MOPP and

ABVD chemotherapy were the previously demonstrated antineoplastic activity of each of the individual drugs used in Hodgkin's disease, the differing modes of action of the drugs in these combinations, and the lack of cross-resistance of tumors to these different drugs. Even better results than those obtained with MOPP or ABVD have been achieved by alternating cycles of MOPP and ABVD with more than 90% of advanced Hodgkin's disease patients achieving complete remission. This is the first clinical use of alternating non–cross-resistant combination chemotherapy.

Nitrosoureas such as lomustine are also effective in Hodgkin's disease and have been combined with other drugs for reinduction of remission in patients who relapse from the standard regimens. New agents observed to be active in Hodgkin's disease include mitoxantrone and isotopically labeled ferritin antibody.

2. NON-HODGKIN LYMPHOMAS

The clinical characteristics of non-Hodgkin lymphomas are related to major histopathologic features and the immunologic origin of the neoplastic cells. The simplest useful pathologic classification is one based on cell type plus the presence or absence of nodularity in the lymphomatous tissues. Thus, a non-Hodgkin lymphoma may be of any one of a number of cell types and may have either a diffuse or a nodular architectural pattern. This histopathologic classification has great prognostic significance in terms of clinical features, sites of involvement, response to irradiation or chemotherapy, and overall survival. In general, the nodular lymphomas have a far better prognosis (median survival up to 7 years) than do the diffuse ones (median survival about 1–2 years). Diffuse large cell ("histiocytic") lymphoma is the most rapidly progressive of the diffuse lymphomas and is the prototype "high-grade" lymphoma. Immunologic classifications have been worked out, and it has been determined that 80–90% of all non-Hodgkin lymphomas (and all nodular lymphomas) are B cell neoplasms. T cell lymphomas have been identified, with the major variants being mycosis fungoides and other cutaneous lymphomas and a T cell lymphoma arising in the mediastinum.

Careful clinical, radiographic, laboratory, and surgical evaluation of patients with non-Hodgkin lymphoma prior to treatment appears justified, since as many as one-third are still localized (stages I and II). Despite this apparent localization, dissemination is usually present but covert, since better results have been obtained with multiagent chemotherapy alone or chemotherapy plus radiotherapy than with radiotherapy alone. Abdominal CT scans and bone marrow core biopsy techniques are useful during initial staging to define the extent of spread. Liver and bone marrow, gastrointestinal, and localized extralymphatic involvement are all observed more commonly in these tumors than in Hodgkin's disease, and a higher fraction of patients (about a third) therefore have stage IV

disease at presentation—in contrast to 15% of patients with Hodgkin's disease.

Alkylating agents, doxorubicin, vincristine, and prednisone all have a place in management of the advanced stages of high-grade diffuse lymphomas. Combination chemotherapy is clearly preferred to single-agent therapy for diffuse but not for nodular lymphomas. The nodular lymphomas are "low grade" and indolent tumors and respond much better to palliative treatment with single agents than do the diffuse lymphomas. However, some of the diffuse lymphomas are curable with available drugs, whereas nodular lymphomas are not. In fact, there is no evidence that combination chemotherapy is any better than single-agent chlorambucil in the treatment of low-grade nodular lymphomas. Complete remission in diffuse lymphomas is a major objective, since it not only leads to relief of all symptoms but also significantly lengthens useful life expectancy. Once complete remission is attained, it appears desirable to continue the same form of chemotherapy.

Doxorubicin has been found to be extremely active in the treatment of non-Hodgkin lymphomas. At present, diffuse large cell lymphomas are being tested very aggressively with sequential combinations—including doxorubicin, vincristine, cyclophosphamide, prednisone, cytarabine, bleomycin, methotrexate, and etoposide—with excellent results. These intensive drug combinations induce complete remissions in over 80% of cases of non-Hodgkin lymphomas. Currently available data suggest that one-third to one-half of patients with diffuse histiocytic lymphomas will remain in permanent remission after intensive combination chemotherapy has been discontinued. For patients with nodular lymphomas, adding doxorubicin has not improved results over those obtained with alkylating agents. The new agent mitoxantrone also appears to be quite active in non-Hodgkin lymphomas, and with limited toxicity. Human interferon has been observed to cause tumor regression in some nodular lymphomas, and this will undoubtedly be an area of further investigation, particularly with the introduction of highly purified interferon prepared synthetically with recombinant DNA techniques. Monoclonal antisera directed against T cell antigens have recently been tested in a few patients with T cell leukemias or lymphomas, and some antitumor effects have been observed.

MULTIPLE MYELOMA

This plasma cell tumor is now one of the "models" of neoplastic disease in humans because the tumor arises from a single tumor stem cell, and the tumor cells all produce a marker protein (myeloma immunoglobulin) that allows for quantitation of the total body burden of tumor cells. The tumor grows principally in the bone marrow and the surrounding bone, causing anemia, bone pain, lytic lesions, bone fractures, and anemia as well as increased susceptibility to infection. It has been clear for about 10 years that patients do improve if treated with oral alkylating agents such as melphalan or cyclophosphamide and that intermittent high doses of prednisone also have an oncolytic effect. Relatively simple combination chemotherapy was therefore developed by combining melphalan and prednisone, administering both drugs for courses of 4 days every 4–6 weeks. More recently, better results have been obtained in advanced-stage cases with the use of more intensive regimens containing alkylating agents, doxorubicin, a nitrosourea, and a *Vinca* alkaloid. About 75% of myeloma patients improve with this treatment, and patients who have the greatest reduction in total body tumor cell number (generally only 1–2 logs) have significant relief of symptoms and prolongation of survival with this treatment and return to a more active life. Such therapy, although beneficial, is far from optimal, because between 10^{10} and 10^{11} myeloma cells persist in a "plateau," and resistance to chemotherapy usually occurs after 2–3 years of treatment in most responding cases.

Other drugs with definite activity in myeloma now being evaluated in combination are doxorubicin and carmustine. This latter combination has proved useful for reinduction of remission for patients who initially respond to melphalan and subsequently relapse. Approximately 50% of such cases can be brought back into remission (at least briefly) with this treatment. The best long-term survival results in patients with stage III myeloma have been obtained with aggressive administration of multiagent chemotherapy combinations and alternating combination programs. Human interferon has been observed to induce remissions in 30% of myeloma patients in relapse from cytotoxic drugs. With the advent of gene-cloning techniques, large-scale production of human interferons has become feasible, and such interferons are now in clinical trial in multiple myeloma.

Treatment of complications of myeloma is another important aspect of comprehensive therapy, and this effort is most important shortly after diagnosis, when they are most likely to be present.

Similar comments apply to Waldenström's macroglobulinemia, which is a related plasma cell neoplasm. The growth characteristics of this tumor are more analogous to those of chronic lymphocytic leukemia; treatment need not be quite so aggressive, because the macroglobulin-producing cells rarely attack the skeleton. In most instances, low-dosage chlorambucil therapy proves adequate, and the patients have a relatively long life expectancy. Plasmapheresis using a blood cell separator can also be utilized to remove the excessive amounts of macroglobulin that produce many of the symptoms and signs of the disorder.

CARCINOMA OF THE BREAST

Stage I & Stage II Neoplasms

The management of primary carcinoma of the breast is currently undergoing remarkable change as a result of major efforts at early diagnosis (through encouragement of self-examination as well as through the use of cancer detection centers) and the implementation of multimodality clinical trials incorporating systemic chemotherapy as an adjuvant to surgery. Women with stage I lateral lesions at the time of breast surgery (small primaries and negative axillary lymph node dissections) are currently treated with surgery and have an 80% chance of cure with surgery alone. A current trend is toward more conservative surgery. The mutilating radical and extended radical mastectomies have largely been abandoned. While the standard surgical procedure is now the modified radical mastectomy, recent studies suggest that segmental mastectomy (lumpectomy) plus an axillary lymph node sampling may prove to be of equivalent value.

Women with one or more positive lymph nodes have a very high risk of systemic recurrence and death from breast cancer (approaching 90% at 10 years) if treated with surgery alone, and 80% of cases with 4 or more positive lymph nodes will recur within 5 years. Thus, lymph node status can be taken as a direct indication of the risk of occult distant micrometastasis of a few (10^0–10^1) or a moderate number (10^1–10^4) of tumor stem cells. In this setting, postoperative use of cycles of combination chemotherapy sufficient to eradicate this order of magnitude of tumor stem cells is warranted. Such clinical trials have now reached the 10-year mark; the results obtained with monthly cycles of cyclophosphamide-methotrexate-fluorouracil (CMF) show a reduced relapse rate in the treated group (over 150 women) as compared to 65% relapse rate in a similar number of patients randomized to a control group. As a result of this study and other clinical tests, much fewer women are now being treated with surgery alone when they have lymph node involvement. The CMFVP (cyclophosphamide-methotrexate-fluorouracil plus vincristine and prednisone) program appears quite effective in both pre- and postmenopausal women. All of these chemotherapy regimens have been of most benefit in women with stage II breast cancer with 1–3 involved lymph nodes. Women with 4 or more involved nodes have had limited benefit thus far from adjuvant chemotherapy. Long-term analysis has clearly shown improved survival in node-positive premenopausal women who have been treated aggressively with multiagent combination chemotherapy. The antiestrogen tamoxifen may also prove very useful either alone or in combination with chemotherapy; results in the National Surgical Adjuvant Breast Project (which has utilized this approach) are quite positive, as are those from a British trial of tamoxifen alone. In elderly women with ER-positive tumors, long-term use of tamoxifen as an adjuvant also appears reasonable and lacks significant toxicity. A recent analysis of very large numbers of postmenopausal women treated with adjuvant tamoxifen has shown clear improvement in long-term survival. At present, the optimal adjuvant combination cannot be specified, since long-term effects (5 and 10 years) on overall survival and the potential delayed toxicity of chemotherapy have yet to be assessed. It is not established whether local radiotherapy (in addition to surgery and chemotherapy) will play any role as an adjuvant. The major benefit of radiotherapy appears to be as a substitute for radical surgery, thus allowing far better cosmetic results associated with limited breast surgery.

Advanced Breast Cancer (Stage III & Stage IV)

Until such multimodality programs as those discussed above are fully effective in the population at risk, the treatment of women with advanced breast cancer remains a major problem. Indeed, some women still present with inoperable "local" lesions with suspected metastases (stage III) or overt distant metastases (stage IV). Currently, most women with local or distant recurrence have had prior breast cancer surgery or surgery plus radiotherapy.

Efforts at treatment of advanced breast cancer are entirely palliative inasmuch as the available treatment modalities are not capable of eliminating the overt 10^{10}–10^{12} tumor cells in the body. In addition to local radiotherapy for stage III lesions, 2 major (and complementary) systemic approaches are available: hormonal manipulation and combination chemotherapy. When compared directly in an unselected population, combination chemotherapy was more effective than hormonal management. Consideration of hormonal procedures (ablation or addition) can now potentially be made on a rational basis through the direct measurement of estrogen (and progesterone) receptors in breast cancer tissue. While a spectrum of receptor levels has been observed, the presence of such receptor proteins appears to reflect the more biochemically differentiated tumors that appear to be present in about half of women with breast cancer. Biochemically differentiated breast cancers (as determined with this test) retain many of the intrinsic hormonal sensitivities of the normal breast—including the growth stimulatory response to ovarian, adrenal, and pituitary hormones. While oophorectomy and perhaps other hormonal ablation procedures seem most reasonable in premenopausal women with skin, lymph node, pleural, or bone metastases, only two-thirds of women with positive hormone receptor assays show subjective and objective benefit from such procedures. Patients who show improvement with ablative procedures also respond to the addition of the antiestrogen drug tamoxifen. Patients with moderate to severe lung, liver, brain, or visceral involvement generally have biochemically undifferentiated metastases and rarely benefit to any great extent from hormonal maneuvers, which means that initial systemic chemotherapy is indicated in such cases. Irrespective of sites of involvement, if the estrogen receptor is absent, the likelihood of observing a response to hormonal therapy is less than 5%. Premenopausal patients who respond objectively to oophorectomy may have remissions of 1–2 years and constitute the group that responds best also to adrenalectomy or hypophysectomy and to antiestrogens. Males with breast cancer

show similar therapeutic responses to castration at almost any age.

Androgenic Hormones

Androgens are used as palliative agents predominantly in premenopausal women who have responded to oophorectomy, but they are also useful beyond the menopause. Testosterone propionate, 100 mg intramuscularly 3 times weekly, results in subjective improvement characterized by euphoria and relief of pain from bone metastases within 1–2 weeks after therapy is started. Soft tissue metastases are less responsive to androgens, and lesions in the liver or brain rarely respond. Oral halogenated androgens such as fluoxymesterone produce similar results but carry a risk of cholestatic jaundice.

Unpleasant side effects of androgens include virilism, hirsutism, deepening of the voice, acne, flushing, sodium retention, and increased libido. The oral androgen derivative calusterone appears to be less virilizing than other preparations and of similar therapeutic efficacy. Hypercalcemia, which occurs in about 10% of patients with extensive osteolytic metastases, may increase with androgen treatment, and in such patients androgens should be discontinued.

Estrogenic Hormones

Estrogens (as well as antiestrogens) are useful in both men and women with widespread breast cancer. In women, estrogens are rarely used until several years after the menopause. It is likely that only those patients whose primary tumors arose in an estrogen-free environment and also possess the estrogen receptor will respond to estrogen therapy. In responsive patients, large doses may produce tumor regression lasting for many months. It generally takes a 3-month trial to determine if estrogens will be effective, and, as in the case of androgen, it is unreasonable to expect a response in rapidly progressive disease, particularly in patients with extensive visceral involvement. Side effects of estrogens include sodium retention and edema, anorexia, uterine bleeding, occasional depression, nausea and vomiting, breast tenderness, hypercalcemia, and tumor growth.

Antiestrogens

The antiestrogen tamoxifen has proved to be a virtually nontoxic alternative to conventional endocrine therapy of breast cancer and has already supplanted the use of other agents in many settings and can be considered the drug of choice for hormone receptor–positive breast cancer. "Flare" of disease is observed occasionally with tamoxifen and can herald the subsequent achievement of an excellent remission, but meticulous supportive care (eg, for bone pain or hypercalcemia) is required. Tamoxifen is effective in both pre- and postmenopausal women who are ER- or PR-positive. However, oophorectomy may be preferable in premenopausal ER-positive patients, and in premenopausal patients, tamoxifen may be ineffective in the presence of the ovaries.

Aromatase Inhibitors

Aminoglutethimide plus hydrocortisone is effective in hormone receptor–positive breast cancers. It is often used in women who have previously responded to tamoxifen or who have ER- or PR-positive breast cancers.

Systemic Chemotherapy

Use of cytotoxic drugs and hormones has become a highly specialized and increasingly effective means of treating cancer. Combination chemotherapy has improved considerably for patients with visceral involvement from advanced breast cancer. Doxorubicin is the most active single agent, with an average response rate of 40%. The use of combination chemotherapy has been found to induce much more durable remissions in 50–80% of patients. Non–doxorubicin-based combination regimens have generally employed cyclophosphamide plus methotrexate and fluorouracil (CMF) alone or plus vincristine and prednisone (CMFVP). Doxorubicin-based combinations have generally included cyclophosphamide and either vincristine or fluorouracil in addition. In most combination chemotherapy regimens, partial remissions have a median duration of about 10 months and complete remissions a duration of about 15 months. Unfortunately, only 10–20% of patients achieve complete remissions with any of these regimens, and complete remissions are not usually very long-lasting in metastatic breast cancer. Addition of the antiestrogen tamoxifen to such programs yields only modest additional improvement. When doxorubicin is used in such combinations, it is generally discontinued before the patient reaches cardiotoxic limits. At that point, other drugs are generally substituted.

CARCINOMA OF THE CERVIX

The incidence of invasive squamous carcinoma of the cervix has decreased markedly as a result of improved early diagnosis with cervical cytologic surveillance by Papanicolaou smear. Invasive lesions that do occur are still difficult to treat. Stage II (and stage III) lesions are generally treated with surgery and radiotherapy. Until recently, there was virtually no systemic chemotherapy of value, although occasional responses to nitrosoureas or bleomycin were observed. Now, a useful 4-drug regimen (mitomycin-vincristine-bleomycin plus cisplatin) has been developed with a high objective response rate. The combination f fluorouracil and cisplatin also shows promise. Some of the patients appear to have prolonged complete remissions, so this regimen can be recommended as initial therapy for patients with stage III and stage IV metastatic cervical carcinomas.

CARCINOMA OF THE ENDOMETRIUM OF THE UTERUS

The incidence of endometrial carcinoma appears to be increased approximately 5-fold in women who have had prolonged conjugated estrogen therapy.

Progesterone derivatives cause dramatic objective tumor regression and symptomatic improvement lasting for several years in about 30% of patients with stage IV metastatic endometrial carcinoma. Those tumors that regress on progesterone probably have cytoplasmic progesterone receptors expressed, with prognostic significance similar to that of the estrogen receptor in breast cancer. Tamoxifen has also proved useful in this patient population and is relatively nontoxic. Remissions can also be achieved with the combination of doxorubicin and cyclophosphamide. It therefore appears reasonable to combine hormones with chemotherapy in such patients and to consider this combination along with local radiotherapy in multimodality approach to patients with stage II endometrial carcinoma (endocervical extension), since such patients may have distant micrometastases at the time of primary therapy.

CHORIOCARCINOMA OF THE UTERUS

This is a rare tumor of women arising from fetal trophoblastic tissue and was the first metastatic cancer cured with chemotherapy. It has been found that massive doses of methotrexate—25 mg daily for 4–5 days—will produce a high percentage of cures associated with complete regression of metastatic lesions and disappearance of chorionic gonadotropic hormones in the urine. Therapy should be given repeatedly until some months after all evidence of the disease has disappeared. In some cases, combination or sequential chemotherapy with methotrexate, chlorambucil, vincristine, cisplatin, dactinomycin, and mercaptopurine is required to achieve cure if methotrexate alone is not adequate.

CARCINOMA OF THE OVARY

This neoplasm often remains occult until it has metastasized to the peritoneal cavity; it may present with malignant ascites. It is important to stage such patients accurately, using laparoscopy, ultrasound, lymphangiography, or [57]cobalt-bleomycin scanning. Stage I patients appear to benefit from pelvic radiotherapy and might receive additional benefit from combination chemotherapy. Radiotherapy (including whole abdomen radiotherapy) does not improve the survival of patients with higher stages of involvement and is generally not indicated. Combination chemotherapy is now the standard approach to stage III and stage IV disease. The most useful combinations include cyclophosphamide and cisplatin, wherein 70–80% of patients achieve remission, with approximately 40% complete remissions. Multimodality therapy utilizing surgery, radiotherapy, and combination chemotherapy in adjuvant fashion in stage I and stage II patients appears rational and has shown promising signs of efficacy in current clinical trials. Assays of tumor stem cells are being utilized increasingly to aid in tailoring treatment regimens for individual patients with ovarian cancer.

TESTICULAR NEOPLASMS

Single-agent chemotherapy has produced some impressive tumor regressions in advanced nonseminomatous testicular neoplasms but few complete responses lasting more than 1 year. The introduction of combination chemotherapy with cisplatin (Platinol), vinblastine, and bleomycin (PVB) has made an impressive change in these statistics. Ninety-five percent of patients respond to chemotherapy, with approximately 90% entering complete remission. It now seems likely that over half of patients achieving complete remission are cured with chemotherapy. Alternative regimens combining etoposide are also being tested in hope of reducing toxicity. Recent reports indicate that substituting etoposide for vinblastine yields similar remission and cure rates with significantly less toxicity. Because of the effectiveness of this treatment in advanced disease, its use in the adjuvant setting for patients who have positive lymph nodes is currently under investigation. Use of chemotherapy in an adjuvant setting is quite controversial, inasmuch as not all patients relapse after primary treatment and the apparent salvage rate in advanced disease has been quite good.

CARCINOMA OF THE PROSTATE

Carcinoma of the prostate was one of the first forms of cancer shown to be responsive to hormonal manipulation. Orchiectomy or low-dose estrogen therapy (or both) has resulted in prolonged improvement in patients with bone lesions. Similar results have also been obtained with the gonadotropin-releasing hormone agonist leuprolide. This agent appears to be less toxic but significantly more expensive than estrogens. Hormonal treatment produces symptomatic benefit in 70–80% of patients and a significant degree of regression of established metastases. Subjective relief of bone pain, objective evidence of normalization of involved bones, and reduction of the prostatic fraction of alkaline phosphatase are common criteria of response to therapy for this disorder. Responsive patients are treated indefinitely until relapse occurs. At that point, use of progestins, doxorubicin, fluorouracil, or other agents is often warranted.

CARCINOMA OF THE THYROID

Until recently, only radioactive iodine (^{131}I) had therapeutic activity in metabolic thyroid cancer, and its effects were limited to well-differentiated tumors that could concentrate iodine. It is now clear that doxorubicin has significant activity in thyroid cancer of a variety of histologic types (particularly anaplastic lesions), induces excellent regressions of tumor, and prolongs survival. Bleomycin also has some activity, although of lesser magnitude. The use of combination chemotherapy in thyroid cancer appears promising in conjunction with ^{131}I therapy for high-risk patients who have anaplastic cell characteristics on histologic examination or vascular invasion of the thyroid gland.

GASTROINTESTINAL CARCINOMAS

This group of neoplasms has only limited sensitivity to available chemotherapeutic agents. It is of interest that all of these lesions release carcinoembryonic antigen (CEA), and radioimmunoassay can be used to detect recurrence after surgery as well as response (or relapse) with systemic chemotherapy. Colorectal adenocarcinoma is the most common type, and only 43% of cases are curable with surgery. Fluorouracil is the most active single agent for patients with metastatic disease, but it induces only a 21% patient remission rate and virtually no complete remissions. Lomustine, mitomycin, and cyclophosphamide all have definite but lesser degrees of activity. Mitomycin or carmustine also has activity in combination with fluorouracil. All of these regimens induce substantial hematologic toxicity. Because these combinations (1) do not induce complete remission, (2) do not prolong survival, and (3) are rather toxic, their use should be limited to patients with symptomatic metastatic disease. Their use in the adjuvant setting with postoperative patients with Dukes stage C colon cancer is currently a matter for investigation, and routine application should be discouraged because of the substantial risk of major or life-threatening toxicity. Fluorouracil alone has been extensively tried as a surgical adjuvant and has produced only a minor reduction in the relapse rate observed with surgery alone.

Gastric carcinoma and pancreatic carcinoma are less common but far more aggressive lesions that usually cannot be completely resected surgically and are generally grossly metastatic at the time of surgery. The combination of fluorouracil, doxorubicin, and mitomycin has a 40% response rate in advanced stomach cancer. Responses are less frequent in pancreatic cancer.

Islet cell carcinoma of the pancreas arising from B cells and secreting insulin has been found to be exquisitely sensitive to the antibiotic streptozocin. The results have been good in this rare tumor, and this therapy may be curative in some patients. Streptozocin is often used in combination with several other agents, eg, fluorouracil, doxorubicin, and mitomycin.

BRONCHOGENIC CARCINOMA

The management of epidermoid cancers, large cell cancers, and adenocarcinomas of the lung is very unsatisfactory, and prevention (primarily through avoidance of cigarette smoking) remains the most important means of control. The average life expectancy after diagnosis has been 8 months. The tumor can rarely be cured by surgery, and x-ray therapy is used primarily for palliation of pain, obstruction, or bleeding. However, in most cases of lung cancer, distant metastases (including spread to the bone marrow) have often occurred by the time of diagnosis, and chemotherapy therefore appears to be the most feasible approach.

Although lung cancer had been notoriously resistant to all conventional forms of cancer chemotherapy, several novel approaches now show promise. Histologic examination of tumor tissue has been found to be important in identifying subgroups of patients who will respond to chemotherapy. For non–small cell lung cancer, combinations of a *Vinca* alkaloid and cisplatin have recently been advocated, but they are of limited benefit. Patients with small cell (oat cell) lung cancer (the most rapidly growing type) show the best responses to combination chemotherapy with agents such as doxorubicin, cyclophosphamide, etoposide, methotrexate, and nitrosoureas.

Small cell carcinoma patients with limited extent of disease respond best to such regimens. They also require whole brain irradiation to sterilize occult central nervous system metastases, which are usually present in such patients.

Several local complications also deserve mention. Patients with superior vena caval compression often benefit from local radiotherapy alone or in combination with chemotherapy. Pleural effusion due to carcinomatous metastasis may be controlled by intrapleural injection of mechlorethamine, quinacrine, or tetracycline (see below).

MALIGNANT MELANOMA & MISCELLANEOUS SARCOMAS

Metastatic melanoma is one of the most difficult neoplasms to treat. Most chemotherapeutic agents are reported to induce regression in at least 10% of melanoma patients; however, spontaneous regressions also occur, especially in skin metastases, and regressions of cutaneous lesions thus may not necessarily imply sensitivity to chemotherapy. Immunologic reactivity to the tumor by host lymphocytes may partially explain the evanescent changes in skin lesions, but "spontaneous regression" of visceral disease is rare, and metastases occur in virtually every organ in the body. Alkylating agents such as melphalan, semustine, and hydroxyurea occasionally cause visceral regressions. Dacarbazine is the most active single drug, although human leukocyte interferon (natural or recombinant) may have a similar order of activity. Combinations of carmustine and vincristine have been tried with limited success. The addition of nonspecific immunotherapy with BCG (to chemotherapy or surgery or both) has not improved therapy significantly.

Osteogenic sarcoma and Ewing's sarcoma respond to doxorubicin, and a combination of doxorubicin and dacarbazine may induce substantial regressions in about 40% of cases of rhabdomyosarcoma, fibrosarcoma, osteogenic sarcoma, and related tumors. The use of doxorubicin as part of adjuvant therapy after primary surgery for osteosarcoma has already increased the median survival time and now appears likely to increase the long-term salvage rate for this otherwise almost uniformly fatal neoplasm. Similar results have recently been reported for patients with soft tissue sarcomas of the extremities, for whom adjuvant chemotherapy has clearly improved disease-free survival. Significantly, this approach has been applied in concert with limb-salvage surgery and has reduced the need for amputation as part of initial surgery.

BRAIN TUMORS

Stage III and stage IV astrocytomas (predominantly glioblastoma multiforme) are the most common primary brain tumors, and they have been extraordinarily refractory to surgical therapy. Although advances in diagnostic methods such as CT scan have better delineated the site of primary involvement for surgical therapy, the median survival time with surgery alone is still in the range of 20 weeks. As shown by the National Brain Tumor Study Group, the addition of whole brain radiotherapy (approximately 5500 R) or carmustine alone (220 mg/m^2 every 6–8 weeks) increases the median survival time to 36 weeks, whereas the use of multimodality therapy (surgery plus radiotherapy plus carmustine) increases it to 50 weeks, with approximately 25% of patients still alive at 18 months. This multimodality approach, although still limited in efficacy, can be recommended as palliation for patients with such tumors until more effective regimens are developed by investigative teams particularly interested in research on the treatment of brain tumors.

CONTROL OF MALIGNANT EFFUSIONS & ASCITES

The direct injection of mechlorethamine or other anticancer drugs into the involved cavity will eliminate or suppress an effusion in about two-thirds of patients with ascites and effusions due to carcinoma. The method is useful irrespective of the type of primary tumor.

The procedure is as follows: Most of the pleural or ascitic fluid is withdrawn, and the drug is injected into the cavity. The dose of mechlorethamine employed intrapleurally is 0.4 mg/kg, or a total dose of 20–30 mg in the usual patient. The solution is prepared immediately before administration so as to avoid loss of potency through hydrolysis. A free flow of fluid from the cavity must be established before the drug is injected to avoid injection into the tissues. Pleural or peritoneal effusions due to ovarian or breast carcinoma are frequently responsive to an intracavitary dose of 60 mg/

m² of bleomycin. After the drug is injected, the patient is placed in a variety of positions in order to distribute the drug throughout the pleural cavity. On the following day, the remaining fluid is withdrawn.

Pain, nausea, and vomiting sometimes occur following injection of mechlorethamine into the pleural cavity. Nausea and vomiting can often be controlled with an intramuscular dose of a phenothiazine given immediately before the procedure and at intervals following the injection. Bone marrow depression is mild with this method of administration, except in patients who have received extensive radiation therapy. Agents such as bleomycin or thiotepa are preferable to mechlorethamine for intraperitoneal use, since they cause significantly less peritoneal irritation and pain.

Quinacrine and tetracycline have been employed intrapleurally with similar therapeutic benefit. Local pain and fever are commonly noted. There is no systemic hematopoietic depression.

EVALUATION OF TUMOR RESPONSE

Inasmuch as cancer chemotherapy can induce clinical improvement, significant toxicity, or both, it is extremely important to assess critically the beneficial effects of treatment to determine that the net effect is favorable. Preliminary evidence regarding predictive selection of chemotherapy with the tumor stem cell assay is quite encouraging, particularly with respect to rejecting drugs that would probably cause toxicity without compensating clinical benefit. The assay also appears to be relatively accurate (70%) in identifying drugs that will prove useful in the patient. The most valuable signs to follow after initiation of therapy include the following:

A. Tumor Size: Demonstration of significant shrinkage in tumor size on physical examination, chest film or other x-ray, or special scanning procedure such as bone scanning (breast, prostate cancer), CT scan, magnetic resonance imaging (MRI), or ultrasonography.

B. Marker Substances: Significant decrease in the quantity of a tumor product or marker substance that reflects the amount of tumor in the body. Examples of such markers include paraproteins in the serum or urine in multiple myeloma and macroglobulinemia, chorionic gonadotropin in choriocarcinoma and testicular tumors, urinary steroids in adrenal carcinoma and paraneoplastic Cushing's syndrome, 5-hydroxyindoleacetic acid in carcinoid syndrome, and prostatic acid phosphatase in prostatic carcinoma. Secreted tumor antigens such as alpha-fetoprotein can be found in hepatoma, in teratoembryonal carcinoma, and in occasional cases of gastric carcinoma and the carcinoembryonic antigen in carcinomas of the colon, lung, and breast. Techniques for measurement of these fetal proteins are now generally available.

C. Organ Function: Normalization of function of organs that were previously impaired as a result of the presence of a tumor is a useful indicator of drug effectiveness. Examples of such improvement include the normalization of liver function (eg, increased serum albumin) in patients known to have liver metastases and improvement in neurologic findings in patients with cerebral metastases. Disappearance of the signs and symptoms of the paraneoplastic syndromes often falls in this general category and can be taken as an indication of tumor response.

D. General Well-Being and Performance Status: A valuable sign of clinical improvement is the general well-being of the patient. Although this finding is a combination of subjective and objective factors and may be subject to placebo effects, it nonetheless serves as an obvious and useful sign of clinical improvement and can be used in reassessment of some of the objective observations listed above. Factors included in the assessment of general well-being include improved appetite and weight gain and improved "performance status" (eg, ambulatory versus bedridden). Evaluation of factors such as activity status has the advantage of summarizing beneficial and toxic effects of chemotherapy and enables the physician to judge whether the net effect of chemotherapy is worthwhile palliation.

SECOND MALIGNANCIES & CANCER CHEMOTHERAPY

Second malignancy is a late complication of some types of cancer chemotherapy. The most frequent second malignancy is acute myelogenous leukemia (AML). Aside from AML, other second malignancies are sporadic. AML has been observed in up to 15% of patients with Hodgkin's disease who have received radiotherapy plus MOPP, or patients with multiple myeloma, ovarian, or breast carcinoma treated with melphalan. Several alkylating agents (as well as ionizing radiation) are considered to be leukemogenic. Additionally, procarbazine (a component of the MOPP combination) is known to be mutagenic to bacteria and carcinogenic in animals. The mechanisms of carcinogenesis with these other agents remain poorly understood. While the risk of AML is relatively small, the benefit of complete remission or cure of Hodgkin's disease or remission in other neoplasms is considerable. However, the benefit/risk ratio of adjuvant therapy of stage I breast cancer with melphalan could be relatively small if over 5% of women developed AML, because only 15–20% of women treated would be likely to have recurrent cancer. As further advances are made in chemical control and cure of cancer, the problem of the second malignant tumor assumes greater importance. There are already hints that certain alkylating agents (eg, cyclophosphamide) may be less carcinogenic than others. Systematic testing of carcinogenicity of anticancer drugs in several animal species allows selection of agents to be substituted for other more carcinogenic ones in chemotherapy regimens. In this fashion, the risk of second tumors should be reduced without sacrifice of therapeutic benefit.

REFERENCES

General

Bonadonna G, Valagussa P: Adjuvant systemic therapy for resectable breast cancer. *J Clin Oncol* 1985;**3**:259.

Capizzi RL (editor): The pharmacological basis of cancer chemotherapy. *Semin Oncol* 1977;**4**:131.

Cooper GM: Cellular transforming genes. *Science* 1982; **218**:801.

DeVita VT Jr: The relationship between tumor mass and resistance to chemotherapy. *Cancer* 1983;**51**:1209.

DeVita VT Jr, Hellman S, Rosenberg SA (editors): *Principles and Practice of Oncology,* 2nd ed. Lippincott, 1985.

DeVita VT et al: The drug development and clinical trials program of the Division of Cancer Treatment, National Cancer Institute. *Cancer Clin Trials* 1979;**2**:195.

Doolittle RF et al: Simian sarcoma virus onc gene, v-sis, is derived from the gene (or genes) encoding a platelet-derived growth factor. *Science* 1983;**221**:275.

Dorr RT, Fritz WL: *Cancer Chemotherapy Handbook.* Elsevier/North Holland, 1980.

Goldie JH, Coldman AJ: A mathematical model for relating drug sensitivity of tumors to their spontaneous mutation rate. *Cancer Treat Rep* 1979;**63**:1727.

Hamlyn P, Sikora K: Oncogenes. *Lancet* 1983;**2**:326.

Haskell CM: *Cancer Treatment.* Saunders, 1980.

Holland JF: Breaking the cure barrier. *J Clin Oncol* 1983; **1**:75.

Kennedy KA et al: The hypoxic tumor cell: A target for selective cancer chemotherapy. *Biochem Pharmacol* 1980;**29**:1.

Krontiris J: The emerging genetics of human cancer. *N Engl J Med* 1983;**309**:404.

MacKillop WJ et al: A stem cell model of human tumor growth: Implications for tumor cell clonogenic assays. *J Natl Cancer Inst* 1983;**70**:9.

Rosenberg SA: The low grade non-Hodgkin's lymphomas: Challenges and opportunities. *J Clin Oncol* 1985;**3**:299.

Salmon SE: Malignant disorders. Chap 32, pp 1065–1080, in: *Current Medical Diagnosis & Treatment 1985.* Krupp MA, Chatton MJ, Tierney LM Jr (editors). Lange, 1985.

Salmon SE, Trent J (editors): *Human Tumor Cloning.* Grune & Stratton, 1984.

Salmon SE et al: Quantitation of differential sensitivity of human-tumor stem cells to anticancer drugs. *N Engl J Med* 1978;**298**:1321.

Sartorelli AC, Johns DG (editors): *Antineoplastic and Immunosuppressive Agents.* 2 vols. Springer, 1975.

Sartorelli AC et al (editors): *Molecular Actions and Targets for Cancer Chemotherapeutic Agents.* Academic Press, 1981.

Von Hoff DD et al: Prospective clinical trial of a human tumor cloning system. *Cancer Res* 1983;**43**:1926.

Alkylating Agents

Boice JD Jr et al: Leukemia and preleukemia after adjuvant treatment of gastrointestinal cancer with semustine (methyl-CCNU). *N Engl J Med* 1983;**309**:1079.

Connors TA et al: Regression of human lung tumor xenografts induced by water-soluble analogs of hexamethylmelamine. *Cancer Treat Rep* 1977;**61**:927.

Hayes DM et al: High dose cis-platinum diammine dichloride: Amelioration of renal toxicity by mannitol diuresis. *Cancer* 1977;**39**:1372.

Von Hoff DD et al: Estramustine phosphate: A specific chemotherapeutic agent? *J Urol* 1977;**117**:464.

Antimetabolites

Bloch A (editor): Chemistry, biology and clinical uses of nucleoside analogs. *Ann NY Acad Sci* 1975;**255**:1.

Frei E et al: New approaches to cancer chemotherapy with methotrexate. *N Engl J Med* 1975;**292**:845.

Haghbin M: Antimetabolites in the prophylaxis and treatment of central nervous system leukemia. *Cancer Treat Rep* 1977;**61**:661.

Jolivet J et al: The pharmacology and clinical use of methotrexate. *N Engl J Med* 1983;**309**:1094.

Stoller RG et al: Use of plasma pharmacokinetics to predict and prevent methotrexate toxicity. *N Engl J Med* 1977; **297**:630.

Antibiotics & Other Agents

Alberts DS et al: Bleomycin pharmacokinetics in man: 2. Intracavitary administration. *Cancer Chemother Pharmacol* 1979;**2**:127.

Carter SK et al (editors): *Bleomycin: Current Status and New Developments.* Academic Press, 1978.

Creagan ET, Moertel CG, O'Fallon JR: Failure of high dose vitamin C to benefit patients with advanced cancer. *N Engl J Med* 1979;**301**:687.

Garnik MB, Ensminger WD, Israel M: A clinical-pharmacological evaluation of hepatic arterial infusion. *Cancer Res* 1979;**39**:4105.

Gralla RJ et al: Phase II evaluation of vindesine in patients with non-small cell carcinoma of the lung. *Cancer Treat Rep* 1979;**63**:1343.

Louie AC, Issell BF: Amsacrine (AMSA): A clinical review. *J Clin Oncol* 1985;**3**:562.

Marmor JB, Kozak D, Hahn G: Effects of systemically administered bleomycin or adriamycin with local hyperthermia on primary tumor and lung metastases. *Cancer Treat Rep* 1979;**63**:1279.

Radice PA, Bunn PA Jr, Idhe DC: Therapeutic trials with VP-16-213 and VM-26. *Cancer Treat Rep* 1979;**63**:1231.

Rozencweig M et al: VM26 and VP16-213: A comparative analysis. *Cancer* 1977;**40**:334.

Vindesine International Workshop (multiple authors). *Cancer Chemother Pharmacol* 1979;**2**:229.

Young RC et al: The anthracycline antineoplastic drugs. *N Engl J Med* 1981;**305**:139.

Hormonally Active Agents

Allegra JC et al: Association between steroid hormone receptor status and disease-free interval in breast cancer. *Cancer Treat Rep* 1979;**63**:1271.

Clark GM et al: Progesterone receptor as a prognostic factor in stage II breast cancer. *N Engl J Med* 1983;**309**:1343.

Eckman P et al: Steroid receptor content in human prostatic carcinoma and response to endocrine therapy. *Cancer* 1979;**44**:1173.

Jensen EV et al: The role of estrophilin in estrogen action. *Vitam Horm* 1974;**32**:89.

Kaiser N et al: Glucocorticoid receptors and the mechanisms of resistance in the cortisol-sensitive and resistant lines of lymphosarcoma. *Cancer Res* 1974;**34**:621.

Leuprolide Study Group: Leuprolide versus diethylstilbestrol for metastatic prostate cancer. *N Engl J Med* 1984; **311**:1281.

Lippman M et al: In vitro models for the study of hormone-dependent human breast cancer. *N Engl J Med* 1977;**296**:154.

McGuire W, Carbone P, Vollmer E (editors): *Estrogen Receptors in Human Breast Cancer*. Raven, 1975.

Tamoxifen Workshop. *Cancer Treat Rep* 1976;**60**:1409.

Yamomoto K, Stampfer M, Tomkins GM: Receptors from glucocorticoid-sensitive lymphoma cells: Physical and DNA-binding properties. *Proc Natl Acad Sci USA* 1974; **71**:3901.

Biologic Response Modifiers & Immunologic Agents

Krown SE et al: Preliminary observations on the effect of recombinant leukocyte A interferon in homosexual men with Kaposi's sarcoma. *N Engl J Med* 1983;**308**:1071.

Lenhard RE et al: Isotopic immunoglobulin: A new systemic therapy for advanced Hodgkin's disease. *J Clin Oncol* 1985;**3**:1296.

Merrigan TC, Sikora K, Breeder JH: Preliminary observations on the effects of human leukocyte interferon in non-Hodgkin's lymphoma. *N Engl J Med* 1979;**299**:149.

Miller RA, Levy R: Response of cutaneous T cell lymphoma to therapy with hybridoma monoclonal antibody. *Lancet* 1981;**2**:226.

Clinical Oncology: Combined Modality or Drug Combinations

Alberts DS, Durie BGM, Salmon SE: Doxorubicin/BCNU chemotherapy for multiple myeloma in relapse. *Lancet* 1976;**1**:926.

Bagley CW et al: Advanced lymphosarcoma: Intensive cyclical combination chemotherapy with cyclophosphamide, vincristine, and prednisone. *Ann Intern Med* 1972;**76**:227.

Baum M: Controlled trial of tamoxifen as adjuvant agent in management of early breast cancer (for Nolvadex Adjuvant Trial Organisation). *Lancet* 1983;**1**:257.

Bonadonna G, Mathé G, Salmon SE (editors): Adjuvant therapies and post surgical markers of minimal residual disease. In: *Recent Results in Cancer Research*. Vols 67 and 68. Springer-Verlag, 1979.

Bonadonna G, Veronesi V (editors): Breast cancer. *Semin Oncol* 1978;**5**:341. [Entire issue.]

Bonadonna G et al: Combination chemotherapy as an adjuvant treatment in operable breast cancer. *N Engl J Med* 1976;**294**:405.

Bonadonna G et al: Combination chemotherapy (MOPP or ABVD)—radiotherapy approach in advanced Hodgkin's disease. *Cancer Treat Rep* 1977;**61**:7169.

Cortes EP et al: Amputation and adriamycin in primary osteosarcoma. *N Engl J Med* 1974;**291**:998.

De Vita VT Jr et al: Combination chemotherapy in the treatment of advanced Hodgkin's disease. *Ann Intern Med* 1970;**73**:881.

Einhorn LH, Donohue J: Cis-diammine-dichloroplatinum, vinblastine and bleomycin combination chemotherapy in disseminated testicular cancer. *Ann Intern Med* 1977; **87**:293.

Einhorn LH, Williams SD: Current concepts in cancer: The role of cisplatinum in solid tumor chemotherapy. *N Engl J Med* 1979;**300**:289.

Fisher B et al: Treatment of primary breast cancer with chemotherapy and tamoxifen. *N Engl J Med* 1981;**305**:1.

Greenspan EM: Combination cytotoxic chemotherapy in advanced disseminated breast carcinoma. *J Mt Sinai Hosp* 1966;**33**:1.

Jaffe N: The potential of combined modalities approaches for the treatment of malignant bone tumors in children. *Cancer Treat Rev* (March) 1975;**2**:33.

Jones SE, Durie BGM, Salmon SE: Combination chemother-

apy with adriamycin and cyclophosphamide for advanced breast cancer. *Cancer* 1975;**36**:90.

Jones SE, Salmon SE (editors): *Adjuvant Therapy of Cancer IV*. Grune & Stratton, 1984.

Kaplan HS: Hodgkin's disease: Multidisciplinary contributions to the conquest of a neoplasm. *Radiology* 1977; **123**:551.

Macdonald JS et al: 5-Fluorouracil, adriamycin, and mitomycin C (FAM) combination chemotherapy in the treatment of advanced gastric cancer. *Cancer* 1979;**44**:42.

Miller TP, Jones SE: Initial chemotherapy for clinically localized lymphomas of unfavorable histology. *Blood* 1983;**62**:413.

Rainey JM, Jones SE, Salmon SE: Combination chemotherapy for advanced breast cancer utilizing vincristine, adriamycin and cyclophosphamide (VAC). *Cancer* 1979; **43**:66.

Rosenberg SA et al: Prospective randomized evaluation of adjuvant chemotherapy in adults with soft tissue sarcomas of the extremities. *Cancer* 1983;**52**:424.

Rubens RD et al: Controlled trial of adjuvant chemotherapy with melphalan for breast cancer. *Lancet* 1983;**1**:839.

Santoro A et al: Alternating drug combinations in the treatment of advanced Hodgkin's disease. *N Engl J Med* 1982; **306**:770.

Young RC et al: Advanced ovarian carcinoma: A prospective clinical trial of melphalan (L-PAM) versus combination chemotherapy (Hexa-CAF). *N Engl J Med* 1978;**299**:1261.

Clinical Oncology: Miscellaneous

Bell DR et al: Detection of *p*-glycoprotein in ovarian cancer: A molecular marker associated with multidrug resistance. *J Clin Oncol* 1985;**3**:311.

Brennan M: Total parenteral nutrition in the cancer patient. *N Engl J Med* 1981;**305**:375.

Bunn PA et al: Clinical course of retrovirus-associated adult T-cell lymphoma in the United States. *N Engl J Med* 1983; **309**:257.

Dean JC, Salmon SE, Griffith KS: Prevention of doxorubicin-induced alopecia with scalp hypothermia. *N Engl J Med* 1979;**301**:1427.

DeVita VT Jr: The consequences of the chemotherapy of Hodgkin's disease: The 10th David A. Karnofsky Lecture. *Cancer* 1981;**47**:1.

Friedman EL et al: Therapeutic guidelines and results in advanced seminoma. *J Clin Oncol* 1985;**3**:1325.

Gale RP: Advances in the treatment of acute myelogenous leukemia. *N Engl J Med* 1979;**300**:1189.

Glucksberg H et al: Combination chemotherapy (CMFVP) versus L-phenylalanine mustard (L-PAM) for operable breast cancer with positive axillary nodes. *Cancer* 1982; **50**:423.

Gottlieb JA, Hill CS Jr: Chemotherapy of thyroid cancer with adriamycin. *N Engl J Med* 1974;**290**:193.

Hamburger AW, Salmon SE: Primary bioassay of human tumor stem cells. *Science* 1977;**197**:461.

Hutter AM, Kayhoe DE: Adrenal cortical carcinoma: Clinical features of 138 patients. *Am J Med* 1966;**41**:572.

Kersey J et al: Clinical usefulness of monoclonal antibody phenotyping in childhood acute lymphoblastic leukemia. *Lancet* 1982;**2**:1419.

Macdonald JS et al: 5-Fluorouracil, adriamycin, and mitomycin C (FAM) combination chemotherapy in the treatment of advanced gastric cancer. *Cancer* 1979;**44**:42.

McIntyre OR: Current concepts in cancer: Multiple myeloma. *N Engl J Med* 1979;**301**:193.

Phillips TL et al: The hypoxic cell sensitizer programme in the

United States. *Br J Cancer* 1978;**37(Suppl 3):**276.

Reifenstein E: Hydroxyprogesterone caproate therapy in advanced endometrial cancer. *Cancer* 1971;**27:**485.

Salmon SE et al: Alternating combination chemotherapy improves survival in multiple myeloma: A southwest oncology study. *J Clin Oncol* 1983;**1:**453.

Seyberth HS et al: Prostaglandins as mediators of hypercalcemia associated with cancer. *N Engl J Med* 1975;**293:**1283.

Stahel RA et al: Detection of bone marrow metastasis in small cell lung cancer by monoclonal antibody. *J Clin Oncol* 1985;**3:**445.

Storring RA et al: Oral non-absorbed antibiotics prevent infection in acute non-lymphoblastic leukaemia. *Lancet* 1977;**2:**837.

Veronesi U et al: Inefficacy of immediate node dissection in stage I melanoma of the limbs. *N Engl J Med* 1977;**297:**627.

Warren RD, Bender RA: Drug interactions with antineoplastic agents. *Cancer Treat Rep* 1977;**61:**1231.

Wilson CB: Current concepts in cancer: Brain tumors. *N Engl J Med* 1979;**300:**1469.

Ziegler JL, Magrath IT, Olweny CLM: Cure of Burkitt's lymphoma. *Lancet* 1979;**2:**936.

Drugs & the Immune System

Sydney E. Salmon, MD

IMMUNOSUPPRESSIVE AGENTS

THE IMMUNE MECHANISM

Agents that suppress the immune response now play an important role in tissue transplantation procedures and in certain diseases associated with disorders of immunity. Although some of the details of the overall immune mechanism are still uncertain, a general scheme of the steps involved in the genesis of specific immunity can be sketched (Figs 59–1 and 59–2) as a means of placing the effects and toxicities of immunosupportive agents in perspective.

Specific immunity appears to result from the interaction of antigens (substances the host normally recognizes as foreign) with mononuclear cells that circulate in the blood and lymph. The nature of self-recognition, or "tolerance," is complex, but it appears to be defined in utero, during the development of the lymphoid tissues. Mechanisms that have been implicated in tolerance include clonal deletion, blockade of antigen receptor by antigen-antibody complex, antibody to cell surface immunoglobulin, and active T cell-mediated suppression. Although lymphoid cells derived embryologically from the thymus and bone marrow play the major role in the development of specific immunity, a critical initial "antigen-processing" step occurs in a dendritic mononuclear phagocyte (thought to be derived from the blood monocyte or the

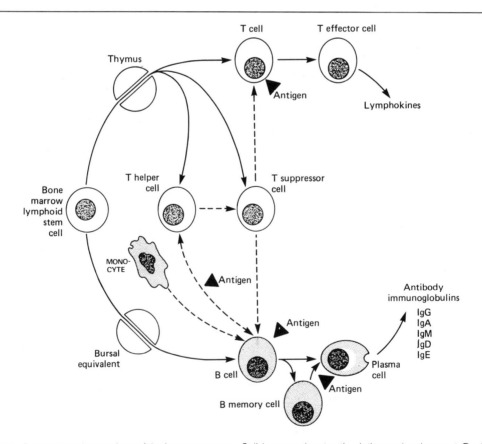

Figure 59–1. Genesis and interactions of the immune system. Solid arrows denote stimulation or development. Dashed arrows indicate inhibition.

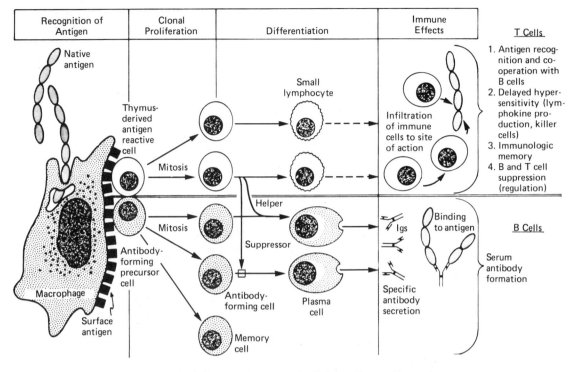

Recognition of Antigen	Clonal Proliferation	Differentiation	Immune Effects

Figure 59–2. A theoretical scheme of cellular and humoral immunity.

tissue macrophage), which then makes the antigen more readily recognizable or available to lymphoid cells. Macrophages or supernatants from macrophage cultures also can stimulate or inhibit immunoproliferative reactions. Several peptide growth factors have also been identified that promote proliferation of either B cells or T cells. Additionally, monocytes and macrophages secrete prostaglandin E_2, which has been found to inhibit immunoproliferation of B and T cell precursors. The ability of lymphoid cells to interact with specific antigens appears to be genetically determined, with different lymphoid clones having individual specificities for different antigenic determinants. The genetic regulation of immunoproliferation also appears to reside in macrophages that express Ia antigens that signal or control lymphoid proliferation.

A basic dualism seems to govern the function of the lymphoid system. Two different types of lymphoid cells—**T and B cells**—mediate cellular immunity and serologic immunity, respectively. Both types of cells are found in the blood as well as in peripheral lymphoid tissues. Long-lived clones of small lymphoid cells derived from or influenced by the thymus (T cells) appear to recognize the antigen and presumably bind to it. The T cell specificity of this line of cells appears to arise from a bone marrow progenitor under the influence of thymic hormone, which is produced by the epithelioid component of the thymus. T cell function seems to be modulated also by histamine, and T cells bear a histamine type 2 receptor that can be blocked with H_2 blockers but not with "classic" antihistamines such as diphenhydramine. The prolifera-

tion of clones of antigen recognition T cells, which occurs after contact with antigen, is responsible for the development of "cellular immunity," which can be demonstrated in delayed hypersensitivity reactions and is important in tissue graft rejection. Specific subsets of T cells also influence or modulate antibody synthesis by B cells. These include both "helper" and "suppressor" T cells. The T cell subsets can be assayed functionally, but can now be identified with monoclonal antibodies directed against specific cell surface antigens that differ on the T helper and suppressor cells. T cells also have surface receptors that allow them to recognize a foreign antigen and react to it. T cells appear to exert their effects by direct cytotoxic interaction (eg, with tumor cells or transplants) and by release of various effector substances, or **lymphokines,** including the interleukins and interferons (Table 59–1).

The genesis of specific antibody **immunoglobulins** resides in the progeny of a second type of lymphoid cell, the antibody precursor cell (B cell), derived from the bone marrow. B cells can be identified by the presence of monoclonal immunoglobulins on their surfaces that are located in "spots" on the cell membrane and, through their antibody function, appear to serve as antigen receptors. B cells also have receptors for complement components and immune complexes as well as having cell surface "Ia-like" receptors that relate to the genetics of the immune response and are linked to the major histocompatibility complex. Prior to contact with antigen, lymphocyte surface immunoglobulin is predominantly of the IgD and IgM

Table 59–1. The lymphokines produced by lymphocytes.

Substance	Effect
Transfer factor (TF)	Transfer of cutaneous hypersensitivity.
Migration inhibitory factor (M I F)	Inhibits macrophage migration.
Interleukin II	Stimulates growth of T lymphocytes.
Lymphotoxin (LT)	Cytotoxicity against target cells.
Chemotactic factor	Stimulates chemotactic migration of macrophages.
Interferon	Inhibits intracellular viral replication and modulates immunoproliferation.
Immunoglobulin (Ig)	Specific antibody molecules.

classes. By the time of birth, lymph node and splenic architecture includes parafollicular cuffs of thymus-derived lymphocytes and follicular nests of immunoglobulin-synthesizing cells that form germinal centers. Intimate cell-cell interaction between macrophages bearing the antigen in an immunogenic form on the cell surface and complementary clones of T cells and B cells are thought to be required before the clonal proliferation of T cells can develop cellular immunity and the B cells can form antibody-forming cells (Figs 59–1 and 59–2). The primary immunoproliferative response is augmented or inhibited by T cells with helper or suppressor function. Natural killer (NK) cells may play an important role in tumor rejection. NK cells are morphologically large granular lymphocytes that are surface immunoglobulin–negative and Fc receptor–positive, with low affinity for sheep red blood cells. Studies with monoclonal antisera suggest that NK cells may be of T cell or monocytic origin, but they may represent an entirely separate lineage of lymphoid cells. NK cells have reactivity against tumor and normal cells and may play an important role in host defense. However, their in vivo relevance remains uncertain.

Antibody-forming cells can increase their synthetic capacity by further differentiation into plasma cells, clones of which specifically secrete large amounts of antibody of one of the immunoglobulin classes—**IgG, IgA, IgM, IgD, or IgE**. During the course of this differentiation, individual clones may "switch" their immunoglobulin type from IgD to IgM to IgG or IgA, even though the active site of the secreted antibody retains the identical structure after this "switch." Finally, specific antibody binds to the foreign antigen, leading to its precipitation, inactivation (eg, virus), lysis (eg, red cells), or phagocytosis (eg, bacteria). In some of these circumstances, complement is bound to the antigen-antibody complex and facilitates the destruction or phagocytosis of the antigen. Once an antibody response is established, reexposure to antigen leads to an immediate chemical combination of antigen and antibody and also serves to provide a "booster" for a rapid secondary wave of cell proliferation and antibody synthesis.

The dual nature of immunity is underscored by certain "experiments of nature," or **genetic diseases**. For example, DiGeorge's syndrome, resulting from absence of the third branchial cleft, is associated with absent thymic development and impaired delayed hypersensitivity but normal antibody formation, whereas delayed hypersensitivity is usually normal in X-linked congenital agammaglobulinemia, which presents as an antibody deficiency syndrome. Infants with DiGeorge's syndrome or those with severe combined immunodeficiency (missing both cellular and humoral immunity) lack circulating thymic hormone activity. Studies of circulating T and B cells in the blood have shown that patients with DiGeorge's syndrome lack T cells, whereas those with congenital agammaglobulinemia lack B cells. Patients with later onset of agammaglobulinemia may have circulating B cells that seem to be inhibited from undergoing terminal differentiation into plasma cells. This inhibition may be due to the action of suppressor T cells.

The acquired immunodeficiency syndrome due to infection with the lymphocytotropic retrovirus (HTLV III/LAV/ARV) has also underscored the profound defect that can occur in host immunity to both infection and cancer that occurs when T helper cells are depleted.

The complexity of the immune system appears to provide a sufficient number of control points to render the emergence of a "forbidden clone," which is reactive against the host's own constituents, a relatively rare event. Normally, most components of the lymphoid system remain in a highly "repressed" state until they are selectively activated for a specific immune response. The numerous steps of the process also imply that immunosuppressive agents can be directed at various steps along this pathway (Fig 59–3), including the induction of specific tolerance. Because the immune system provides a major barricade against invading microorganisms (including oncogenic viruses), toxins, and foreign cells, generalized immunosuppression can potentially be very dangerous to the host.

With only one notable exception—Rh_o (D) immune globulin—the clinically useful immunosuppressive agents that are now available may have general immunosuppressive properties and must be used with caution. Generalized immunosuppression increases the risk of infection and may also increase the risk of development of lymphoreticular and other forms of cancer. In general, it is easier to prevent or attenuate a primary immune response with immunosuppressive drugs than to suppress an established immune response.

Even with these limitations and cautions, immunosuppression is of proved usefulness in a number of acquired immune disorders as well as in organ transplantation.

TESTS OF IMMUNOCOMPETENCE

A wide variety of techniques have been used to test immunologic competence and its drug-induced sup-

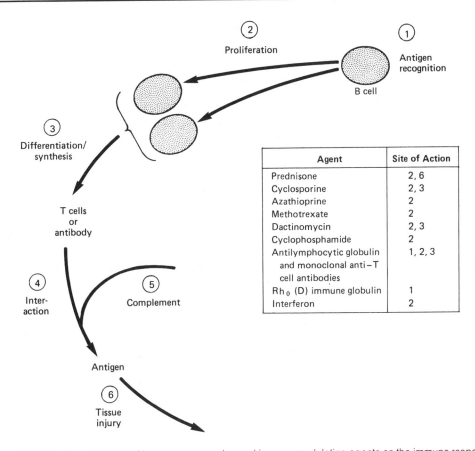

Agent	Site of Action
Prednisone	2, 6
Cyclosporine	2, 3
Azathioprine	2
Methotrexate	2
Dactinomycin	2, 3
Cyclophosphamide	2
Antilymphocytic globulin and monoclonal anti–T cell antibodies	1, 2, 3
Rh_0 (D) immune globulin	1
Interferon	2

Figure 59–3. The sites of action of immunosuppressive and immunomodulating agents on the immune response.

pression. The simplest tests that can be used to detect the effects of immunosuppressive or immunostimulating agents include the following:

(1) Delayed hypersensitivity testing with skin test antigens to detect the ability to respond to mumps, streptokinase-streptodornase, *Candida albicans,* and other antigens to which most individuals have been exposed or to respond to sensitizing chemicals such as dinitrochlorobenzene.

(2) Measurement of serum immunoglobulins, serum complement, and specific antibodies to various natural and acquired antibodies.

(3) Serial measurements of antibody response after primary immunization or a secondary booster injection (Fig 59–4).

(4) Absolute circulating lymphocyte counts.

(5) Measurement of the percentages of B cells, T cells, and "null cells" (eg, with monoclonal antibodies or "rosette tests") that comprise the circulating blood lymphocyte count.

These relatively simple tests plus the evaluation of clinical responses in organ transplantation and autoimmune disorders have provided most of the current information on the in vivo effects of the immunosuppressive agents in humans. However, evidence of immunosuppression as measured by these tests of immune response does not always correlate well with the clinical response of the disease state being treated. The

relevance to in vivo events of cell responses in various in vitro tests of lymphoid function, such as lymphocyte transformation testing, is less clear. Lymphocyte stimulation with phytohemagglutinin (PHA) measures the proliferative capacity of T cells; pokeweed mitogen measures the response of both B and T cells.

RELATIONSHIP BETWEEN IMMUNOSUPPRESSIVE THERAPY & CANCER CHEMOTHERAPY

Although there is definite overlap between the drugs used for immunosuppression (Fig 59–3) and those used in cancer chemotherapy (see Chapter 58), different principles govern their use in these 2 disease categories. The general pharmacologic properties and toxicities of several of these agents (corticosteroids, alkylating agents, and certain structural analogs) were described in Chapter 58. Since many cytotoxic drugs (eg, structural analogs) act primarily on proliferating cells, there is, in a sense, a similarity between their uses against proliferating cancer cells and against proliferating immune cells. However, the character and kinetics of cancer cell proliferation (see Chapter 58) are not identical to immune cell proliferation and allow different features to be exploited in immunosuppression. For example, whereas cancer cell prolifera-

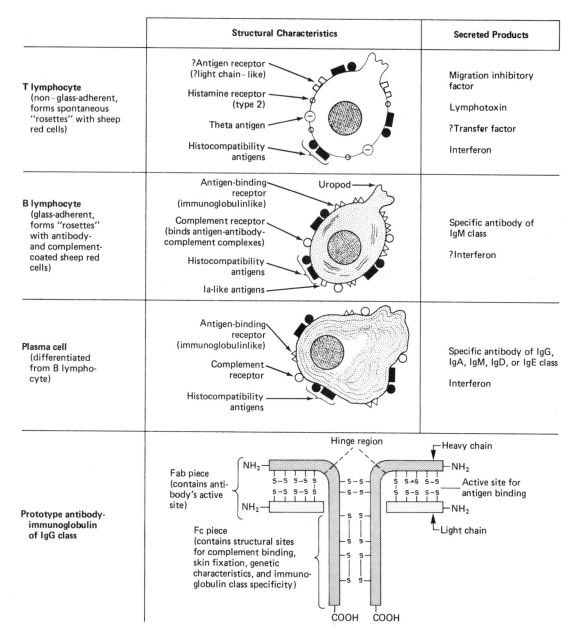

Figure 59-4. Effectors in the immune response. Specific cell types including T lymphocytes, B lymphocytes, and plasma cells—as well as secreted antibody-immunoglobulin—have binding sites for specific antigen as well as differential genetic and functional characteristics. Membrane features as well as secreted products can thus be seen to have important functions in the immune response.

tion appears to be "unstimulated," immune cell proliferation usually occurs in response to the presence of a specific antigen. While division of individual malignant cells within a large cancer cell population appears to occur randomly in an apparently unsynchronized way, immune cell proliferation appears to be "synchronized" in a burst of mitotic division that occurs after introduction of the antigen, with a large fraction of the responding cells going through the generation cycle in order to produce specific immunity. Thus, when cytotoxic drugs are used at the time of ini-

tial exposure to foreign antigen (eg, a kidney transplant), a very high percentage of an initially small number of precursor cells can be destroyed, because the antigen stimulates selected relevant clones to proliferate rather than all clones of immune cells. Therefore, a greater degree of selective toxicity can be initially obtained against the unwanted immune clone, whereas this objective is harder to achieve in cancer chemotherapy. Additionally, when cytotoxic drugs are used for immunosuppression, they are generally administered in a low-dosage daily schedule to block immunoproliferation continuously. In contrast, when these same drugs (eg, cyclophosphamide) are used for cancer chemotherapy, they are administered intermittently in high-dosage "pulse" courses every 3–6 weeks. Such "pulse" administration permits rapid immune rebound between treatments, which is desirable for augmentation of tumor immunity but undesirable in immunosuppressive therapy.

The selective nature of immunosuppression in a synchronized response can result in less damage to other normal cells, and dosages of the drugs are sometimes lower than those used in cancer chemotherapy. When dealing with an established immune response, the selective advantage in immunosuppression is not so great as in the instance of the primary immune response. Lymphoid cells can still be damaged somewhat more than other host tissues, however, because they are generally more sensitive to cytotoxic drugs and radiation than are other types of normal cells. Macrophages are relatively radioresistant cells and presumably also are less affected by immunosuppressive drugs than are lymphoid cells. However, macrophage function is inhibited by corticosteroids and perhaps also by prostaglandin inhibitors such as indomethacin.

CORTICOSTEROIDS

Corticosteroids were the first class of hormonal agents that were recognized to have lympholytic properties. Administration of a glucocorticoid (eg, prednisone, dexamethasone) reduces the size and lymphoid content of the lymph nodes and spleen, although it has essentially no toxic effect on proliferating myeloid or erythroid stem cells in the bone marrow. Glucocorticoids are thought to interfere with the cell cycle of activated lymphoid cells. The mechanism of their action is described in Chapter 58. Prednisone is quite cytotoxic to certain subsets of T cells but can suppress both cellular immunity and antibody as well as prostaglandin and leukotriene synthesis. Limited data currently available suggest that some of the diverse effects of prednisone may be attributable to lysis of either "suppressor" or "helper" T cells. Plasma cells seem to be less sensitive to the effects of corticosteroids. However, since the precursor lymphoid cells are sensitive to this agent, the primary response can be diminished, and, with continued use, previously established antibody responses are also decreased. Additionally, continuous administration of prednisone does increase the fractional catabolic rate of IgG, the major class of antibody immunoglobulins, thus lowering the effective concentration of specific antibodies. Corticosteroids also appear to interfere with the ability of reticuloendothelial macrophages to phagocytose antibody-coated cells and reduce the rate of cell destruction (eg, in hemolytic anemias).

Prednisone is used in a wide variety of clinical circumstances where it is thought that the immunosuppressive properties of the drug account for its beneficial effects. Indications include autoimmune disorders such as autoimmune hemolytic anemia, idiopathic thrombocytopenic purpura, and lupus erythematosus and some cases of Hashimoto's thyroiditis. Additionally, corticosteroids also modulate allergic reactions and are used in bronchial asthma, as will be discussed later in this chapter. Corticosteroids are also used liberally in organ transplant recipients and are of particular value during rejection crises because the dosage can be increased without fear of bone marrow toxicity. The usual dose range for prednisone as an immunosuppressive agent is 10–100 mg orally daily. The potential side effects of corticosteroids, including adrenal suppression (see Chapters 38 and 58), are also relevant when these agents are used chronically for immunosuppression.

CYCLOSPORINE
(Cyclosporin A)

Cyclosporine (Fig 59–5) is a recently approved immunosuppressive agent that has shown impressive efficacy in human organ transplantation and in the treatment of graft-versus-host (GVH) syndrome after bone marrow transplantation. Patients in whom it is used as the only immunosuppressant or combined with prednisone have similar graft survival frequency and a lower incidence of rejection and infectious complications than patients treated with combinations such as azathioprine, prednisone, and antilymphocyte antibodies. Substantial investigation in animals has also shown excellent results. The drug is a fat-soluble peptide antibiotic that appears to act at an early stage in the differentiation of T cells and has been hypothesized to cause clonal deletion of T helper cells. Recent in vitro studies have indicated that cyclosporine inhibits the *production* of factors that stimulate T lymphocyte growth, but it does not block the *effect* of such factors on primed T cells. However, its exact mechanism of action is unknown.

Cyclosporine (Sandimmune) has been given orally on a daily basis at a dosage of 10–25 mg/kg. Toxicities have included nephrotoxicity (which may be preventable with mannitol diuresis), some increase in incidence of viral infections, and transient liver dysfunction. There is very little bone marrow toxicity. While a slightly increased incidence of lymphoma has been seen in transplant recipients receiving cyclosporine, there is also an increased incidence of lymphoma in other transplant recipients who have received other immunosuppressive agents.

Recent reports suggest that cyclosporine may be of sufficient potency and efficacy to obviate the need for simultaneous use of corticosteroids, azathioprine, cyclophosphamide, or other immunosuppressive drugs. It has been used with apparent success as the sole immunosuppressant for cadaveric transplants of the kidney, pancreas, and liver, and it has proved extremely useful in cardiac transplants as well.

Little is known about the pharmacokinetics of this

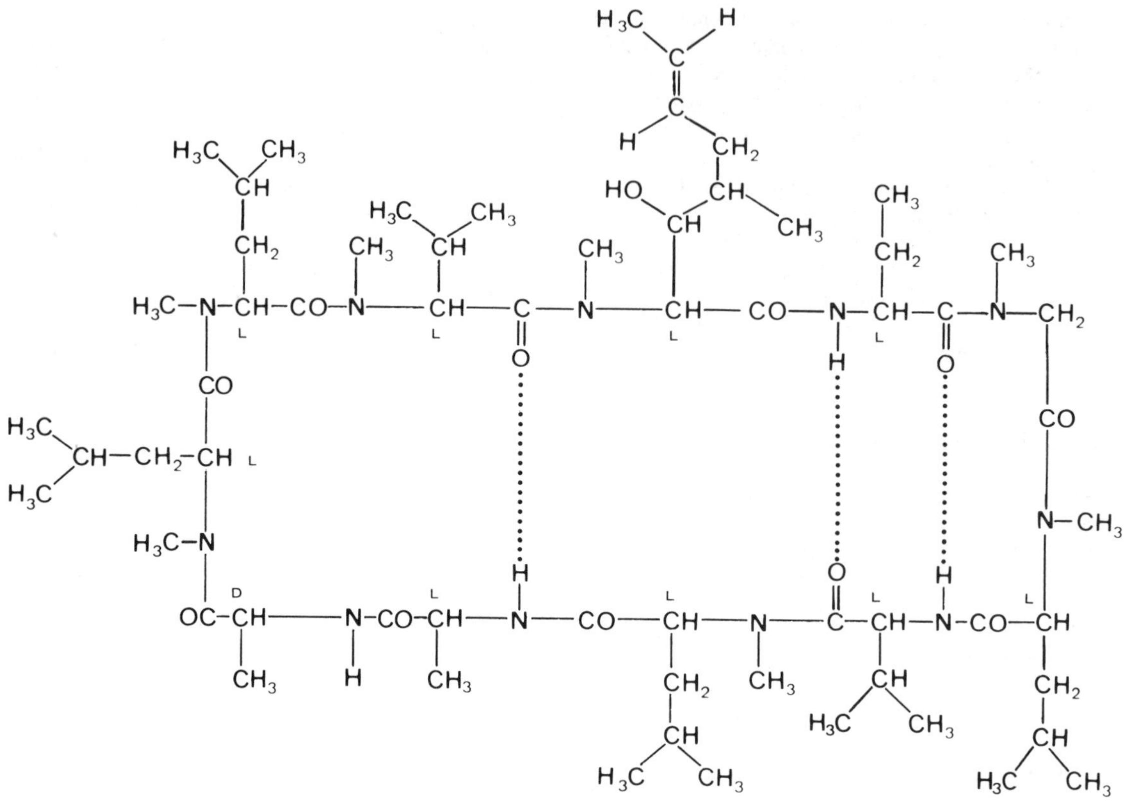

Figure 59–5. Cyclosporine (cyclosporin A). "L" and "D" refer to levo- and dextrorotatory forms of the indicated specific amino acids in the molecule.

agent at present. Preliminary studies suggest that the drug is slowly and incompletely absorbed after oral administration. It has a half-life of about 19 hours after either oral or intravenous administration. Most of the administered dose is metabolized and excreted in the bile.

Cyclosporine appears to be a major step in the direction of a more specific and selective agent effective against a subpopulation of lymphocytes, but its side effects are still considerable—although perhaps less than those of corticosteroids and other cytotoxic agents used for immunosuppression. Experimental studies suggest that the effects of cyclosporine for suppression of graft-versus-host syndrome may be greater if the agent is begun prior to grafting.

CYTOTOXIC AGENTS

1. AZATHIOPRINE

Azathioprine is an imidazolyl derivative of mercaptopurine (6-mercaptopurine, 6-MP) and functions as a structural analog or "antimetabolite" (see Chapter 58). Although its action is presumably mediated by mercaptopurine as the active form, it has received more widespread use than mercaptopurine for im-

munosuppression in humans. These agents represent prototypes of the structural analog or cytotoxic types of immunosuppressive drugs, and many other agents that kill proliferative cells seem to work at a similar level in the immune response.

Azathioprine is absorbed well from the gastrointestinal tract and is metabolized in vivo, primarily into mercaptopurine (portion below the dashed line in figure). Xanthine oxidase splits much of the active material to 6-thiouric acid prior to excretion in the urine. After administration of azathioprine, small amounts of unchanged drug and mercaptopurine are also excreted by the kidney, and as much as a 2-fold increase in toxicity may occur in anephric or anuric patients. Since much of the drug's inactivation depends on xanthine oxidase, patients who are also receiving allopurinol (see Chapter 58) for control of hyperuricemia should have the dose of azathioprine reduced to one-fourth to one-third the usual dose to prevent excessive toxicity.

Immunosuppression with azathioprine or mercaptopurine therapy seems to result from interference with nucleic acid metabolism at steps that are required for the wave of cell proliferation that follows antigenic stimulation. The purine analogs are thus cytotoxic agents that destroy stimulated lymphoid cells. Although continued messenger RNA synthesis is necessary for sustained antibody synthesis by plasma cells, these analogs appear to have less effect on this process than on nucleic acid synthesis in proliferating cells. Cellular immunity as well as primary and secondary serum antibody responses can be blocked by these cytotoxic agents. Animal studies have shown that, if a course of mercaptopurine therapy is completed prior to exposure to a new antigen, the subsequent antibody response may actually be potentiated rather than suppressed. Although this latter phenomenon has yet to be substantiated clinically, such observations emphasize the need for precise timing of therapy relative to organ transplantation.

Azathioprine and mercaptopurine appear to be of definite benefit in maintaining renal homografts and may also be of value in transplantation of other tissues. These analogs have also been used with some success in the management of acute glomerulonephritis and in the renal component of systemic lupus erythematosus.

As with mercaptopurine, the chief toxicity of azathioprine is bone marrow depression, usually manifest as leukopenia, although anemia, thrombocytopenia, and bleeding may also occur. Skin rashes, drug fever, nausea and vomiting, and sometimes diarrhea occur, with the gastrointestinal symptoms seen mainly at higher dosages. Hepatic dysfunction, manifested by very high serum alkaline phosphatase levels and mild jaundice, occurs occasionally.

Although these agents are potentially toxic to bone marrow elements, including the megakaryocytes and red cell precursors, the favorable effects sometimes outweigh the toxic effects. The drugs have been of occasional use in prednisone-resistant antibody-mediated idiopathic thrombocytopenic purpura and autoimmune hemolytic anemias.

Azathioprine

2. CYCLOPHOSPHAMIDE

The alkylating agent cyclophosphamide (Cytoxan) has recently been the focus of considerable interest as an immunosuppressive agent in animals and humans. It is perhaps the most potent immunosuppressive drug that has been synthesized. Cyclophosphamide destroys proliferating lymphoid cells but also appears to alkylate some resting cells. It has been observed that very large doses (eg, > 120 mg/kg intravenously over several days) may induce an apparent specific tolerance to a new antigen if the drug is administered simul-

taneously with—or shortly after—the antigen. In smaller doses, it has been very effective in autoimmune disorders (including systemic lupus erythematosus), in patients with acquired factor XIII antibodies and bleeding syndromes, in those with antibody-induced pure red cell aplasia, and in patients with Wegener's granulomatosis.

Although treatment with large doses of cyclophosphamide carries considerable risk of pancytopenia and hemorrhagic cystitis, the drug has aided in "takes" of bone marrow transplants and may have value in other types of organ transplantation also. Although cyclophosphamide appears to induce tolerance for marrow or immune cell grafting, its use does not prevent the subsequent graft-versus-host syndrome, which may be serious or lethal if the donor is a poor histocompatibility match. Specialized medical care and supportive facilities are mandatory for patient survival during the period of intensive therapy.

3. OTHER CYTOTOXIC AGENTS

Other cytotoxic agents, including vincristine, methotrexate, and cytarabine (see Chapter 58), also have immunosuppressive properties. Although these agents can be used for immunosuppression, they have not received as widespread use as the purine antagonists and their indications for immunosuppression are less certain. The use of methotrexate (which can be given orally) appears reasonable in patients with idiosyncratic reactions to purine antagonists. The antibiotic dactinomycin has also been used with some success at the time of impending renal transplant rejection. Vincristine appears to be quite useful in idiopathic thrombocytopenic purpura refractory to prednisone, but it is not yet certain whether this effect is immunologically mediated. The related *Vinca* alkaloid vinblastine has been shown to prevent mast cell degranulation in vitro by binding to microtubule units within the cell and to prevent release of histamine and other vasoactive compounds.

ANTIBODIES AS IMMUNOSUPPRESSIVE AGENTS

Until recently, development of specific antibodies required immunization and collection of antisera with subsequent purification of the gamma globulin or IgG fraction. The development of "hybridoma" technology by Milstein and Köhler has revolutionized this field and radically increased the purity and specificity of antibodies used for immunosuppression and other applications. Hybridomas consist of antibody-forming cells fused to plasmacytoma cells. Hybrid cells that are stable and produce the required antibody can be cloned for mass culture for antibody production. Fermentation facilities in the pharmaceutical industry are now being used for this purpose.

1. ANTILYMPHOCYTE ANTIBODIES

Although antisera directed against lymphocytes have been prepared sporadically since Metchnikoff's first observations just before the turn of the century, detailed evaluation was not made of antilymphocytic serum until the 1960s. With the era of human organ homotransplantation, heterologous antilymphocytic globulin (ALG) suddenly took on new importance. ALG and antithymocyte globulin and monoclonal anti–T cell antibodies are now in clinical use in many medical centers that have organ transplantation programs.

The antiserum is usually obtained by immunization of large animals with human lymphoid cells or with the hybridoma technique for monoclonal antibody generation. Extremely potent antisera have been obtained by immunization with human fetal thymus. The potency of each batch of ALG is estimated by lymphocyte agglutination and cytotoxicity testing in vitro. Cytotoxicity titers correspond somewhat to the clinical responses, but the activity of ALG has yet to be adequately standardized. Standardization of the monoclonal antibodies is far more readily achieved.

Antilymphocytic antibody acts primarily on the small, long-lived peripheral lymphocytes that circulate between the blood and lymph. With continued administration, the "thymus-dependent" lymphocytes from the cuffs of lymphoid follicles are also depleted, as they normally participate in the recirculating pool. Antilymphocytic antibody binds to the surface of these small "antigen recognition" T cells (Fig 59–2), and cytotoxic destruction of the cells then takes place, mediated by serum complement. As a result of the destruction of the T cells, a rather specific impairment of delayed hypersensitivity and cellular immunity occurs while humoral antibody formation remains relatively intact. The selectivity of ALG for the cellular immune system accounts for its usefulness in preventing rejection of transplanted organs. ALGs produced by immunization with fetal thymus appear to be the most effective anti–T cell immunosuppressive agents. Application of the hybridoma technology to production of anti–T cell antibodies is now well established, and various immunologic specificities have been identified. Murine hybridoma monoclonal antibodies directed against T cell antigens have entered clinical trial for T cell leukemias and lymphomas as well as for their immunosuppressive properties in prevention of graft rejection (many organs) and the graft-versus-host syndrome that follows bone marrow transplantation. One very useful strategy in bone marrow transplantation, to prevent graft-versus-host syndrome, has been to "purge" the marrow in vitro with one or more anti–T cell monoclonal antibodies prior to marrow infusion in the recipient.

Since such antibodies have not been adequately standardized, only generalizations about dosage and treatment can be given. After transplantation of an organ such as the kidney, ALG is often administered (by intramuscular injection) first on a daily basis and subsequently cut back in frequency. Because ALG is usually administered along with azathioprine and prednisone, it has not been possible to assess the effect of ALG alone in human kidney transplants. Investigators who treat their renal transplant recipients with ALG believe that it reduces the dosage requirements for the other immunosuppressive drugs and improves survival in patients who receive kidneys from unrelated or cadaver donors. However, cyclosporine is finding increasing use in renal transplants, and the role of other agents (including ALG) may decrease. There has been some limited success in the use of ALG alone for recipient preparation for bone marrow transplantation. In this procedure the recipient is treated with ALG in large doses for 7–10 days, followed by transplantation of $1-3 \times 10^{10}$ bone marrow cells from the donor. Residual ALG appears to destroy the T cells in the donor marrow graft, and the severe graft-versus-host syndrome has not been observed. These limited data do indicate that ALG given alone is a potent immunosuppressive agent in humans.

The side effects of ALG are mostly those of the injection of a foreign protein obtained from heterologous serum. Local pain and erythema often occur at the injection site. Since the humoral antibody mechanism remains active, skin-reactive and precipitating antibodies can be formed against the foreign IgG. Similar reactions occur with monoclonal antibodies of murine origin. For this reason, development of human-human hybridomas is a major current research objective, since it should eliminate most heterologous protein reactions.

Anaphylactic and serum sickness reactions have been observed and usually require cessation of ALG or monoclonal antibody therapy. In addition, complexes of host antibodies with horse ALG may precipitate and localize in the glomerulus of the transplanted kidney. Even more disturbing has been the development of histocytic lymphoma in the buttock at the site of ALG injection. The incidence of lymphoma as well as other forms of cancer is increased in kidney transplant patients, and it may be as high as 2% in long-term survivors. It appears likely that part of the increased risk of cancer is related to the suppression of a normally potent defense system against oncogenic viruses or transformed cells. Thus, it remains to be seen whether ALG is any more carcinogenic than the other immunosuppressive agents.

Standardization of antilymphocytic antibody with antithymocyte globulin (ATG) of monoclonal origin offers considerable promise, because some of these antisera are selective for T cell subsets and are potentially available in unlimited quantities with very well defined specificity. For example, monoclonal antibodies with anti–T cell activity against murine thy1.2 specificity have been conjugated with the toxic plant lectin ricin. In an in vivo murine model, pretreatment of allogeneic bone marrow with this antibody-ricin conjugate has prevented otherwise fatal graft-versus-host disease following bone marrow transplantation. Clinical studies have recently been reported that used a murine monoclonal antibody (OKT3) directed against a molecule on the surface of human thymocytes and mature T cells. In vitro, OKT3 blocks both killing by cytotoxic human T cells and the generation of other T cell functions. In a prospective randomized multicenter trial with cadaveric renal transplants, use of OKT3 (along with lower doses of steroids or other immunosuppressive drugs) proved more effective at reversing acute rejection than did conventional steroid treatment. This was associated also with a better 1-year survival (62% with OKT3) as compared to steroid therapy (45%).

2. Rh$_o$ (D) IMMUNE GLOBULIN

One of the major advances in immunopharmacology was the development of a technique for preventing Rh hemolytic disease of the newborn. The technique is based on the observation that a primary antibody response to a foreign antigen can be blocked if specific antibody is administered passively at the time of exposure to antigen.

Rh$_o$ (D) immune globulin (RhoGAM) is a concentrated (15%) solution of human IgG globulin containing a high titer of antibodies against the Rh$_o$ (D) antigen of the red cell. The IgG is prepared by cold alcohol fractionation of carefully selected plasma from Rh$_o$ (D)–negative, D^u-negative mothers sensitized by repeated Rh-incompatible pregnancies or from Rh-negative volunteers who have been deliberately immunized for plasma collection.

Sensitization of Rh-negative mothers to the D antigen occurs usually at the time of birth of an Rh$_o$ (D)–positive or D^u-positive infant, when fetal red cells may leak into the mother's bloodstream. Sensitization might also occur occasionally with miscarriages or ectopic pregnancies. With subsequent pregnancies, maternal antibody against Rh-positive cells is transferred to the fetus during the third trimester, leading to the development of erythroblastosis fetalis or hemolytic disease of the newborn.

If an injection of Rh$_o$ (D) antibody is administered to the mother within 72 hours after the birth of an Rh-negative baby, the mother's own antibody response to the foreign Rh$_o$ (D)–positive cells is suppressed. When the mother has been treated in this fashion, Rh hemolytic disease of the newborn has not been observed in the subsequent pregnancy. For this prophylactic treatment to be successful, the mother must be Rh$_o$ (D)–negative and D^u-negative and must not already be immunized to the Rh$_o$ (D) factor. Treatment is also often advised for Rh-negative mothers who have had miscarriages, ectopic pregnancies, or abortions in which the blood type of the fetus is unknown.

Note: Rh$_o$ (D) immune globulin is administered to the mother and must not be given to the infant.

The usual dose of RhoGAM is 2 mL intramuscularly. Adverse reactions are infrequent and consist of local discomfort at the injection site or, rarely, a slight temperature elevation.

The mechanism of suppression of the immune response by passive administration of specific antibody may consist of prompt elimination of the foreign antigen after combination with the antibody or may be a type of "feedback immunosuppression" in which a change in the antigen results from its combination with antibody, so that it is no longer recognized as foreign. If antibody produces "feedback" immunosuppression, it presumably acts on the macrophage, the T lymphocyte, or the B lymphocyte (Figs 59–1 to 59–3).

CLINICAL USES OF IMMUNOSUPPRESSIVE DRUGS

Immunosuppressive agents are currently used in 3 clinical circumstances: (1) organ transplantation, (2) autoimmune disorders, and (3) isoimmune disorders (Rh hemolytic disease of the newborn). The agents used differ somewhat for the specific disorders treated (see specific agents and Table 59–2), as do administration schedules. Optimal treatment schedules have yet to be established in many clinical situations in which these drugs are used.

Organ Transplantation

In organ transplantation, tissue typing, based on donor and recipient histocompatibility matching with the human leukocyte antigen (HLA) haplotype system and in vitro mixed lymphocyte culture (MLC), is of definite value. Close histocompatibility matching reduces the likelihood of graft rejection and may also reduce the requirements for intensive immunosuppressive therapy. Response to transplantation and immunosuppressive drugs in renal disease may be dependent on the nature of the primary renal lesions in patients undergoing transplant.

Primary renal disease itself is frequently immunologic in nature. Two major types of glomerular injury are mediated by immune mechanisms. The first type results from the passive deposition of antigen-antibody complexes from the circulation as blood is filtered through the glomerulus. Deposition of antigen-antibody complexes, which may fix complement, in a "lumpy-bumpy" or discontinuous pattern, is associated with the renal disease of systemic lupus erythematosus and with most cases of acute glomerulonephritis. The second form of glomerulonephritis is associated with linear deposition of specific anti–basement membrane antibody in the glomerulus.

Although immunosuppressive therapy may be of benefit in both of these circumstances, the data are incomplete. Since patients with severe glomerulonephritis are often candidates for kidney transplantation, pathologic factors that might persist and also damage the transplanted kidney are of great importance. It has been observed that patients with anti–basement membrane antibody may experience an acute graft rejection when they receive a kidney transplant. Patients with anti–basement membrane antibodies are likely to need immunosuppressive therapy for 6–8 weeks after bilat-

Table 59–2. Clinical uses of immunosuppressive agents.

Disease	Immunosuppressive Agents Used	Response
Autoimmune		
Idiopathic thrombo-cytopenic purpura	Prednisone,* vincristine, occasionally mercapto-purine or azathioprine, high-dose gamma globulin	Usually good
Autoimmune hemo-lytic anemia	Prednisone,* cyclophos-phamide, chlorambucil, mercaptopurine, azathio-prine	Usually good
Acute glomerulo-nephritis	Prednisone,* mercaptopu-rine, cyclophosphamide	Usually good
Acquired factor XIII antibodies	Cyclophosphamide plus factor XIII	Usually good
Miscellaneous "auto reactive" disorders[†]	Prednisone, cyclophos-phamide, azathioprine, cyclosporine	Often good
Isoimmune		
Hemolytic anemia of the newborn	Rh_o (D) immune globulin*	Excellent
Organ transplantation		
Renal	Cyclosporine, azathio-prine, prednisone, ALG, OKT3 monoclonal anti-body, dactinomycin, cyclo-phosphamide	Very good
Heart		Good
Liver	Cyclosporine, prednisone	Fair
Bone marrow (HLA-matched)	Cyclosporine, cyclophos-phamide, prednisone, methotrexate, ALG, total body irradiation, donor marrow purging with monoclonal anti–T cell antibodies	Increasing success

* Drug of choice.
[†] Systemic lupus erythematosus, rheumatoid arthritis, Wegener's granulomatosis, chronic active hepatitis, lipoid nephrosis, inflammatory bowel disease.

eral nephrectomy, being maintained on a dialysis program, before transplantation of a donor kidney can be considered. Similarly, patients with a disease such as systemic lupus erythematosus are poor candidates for renal transplant until the systemic cause of the renal injury is under control.

Even with all these considerations, the response to renal transplantation has become increasingly gratifying, including that with unmatched kidneys from cadaver donors. Patients who have received prior blood transfusion have a higher success rate with cadaveric renal grafts. At present, over 80% of carefully selected but nonrelated recipients may survive beyond 2 years after the transplant, and 5-year survival is not an unrealistic hope. As discussed above, use of the monoclonal anti–T cell antibody OKT3 has reduced acute graft rejection significantly.

Recently, increasing success has been achieved with bone marrow transplantation in patients with aplastic anemia, refractory acute leukemia, or severe combined immunodeficiency disease (congenital) who have an HLA- and MLC-matched donor. Patients with aplastic anemia or leukemia require intensive immunosuppression prior to transplantation. Monoclonal antibodies to leukemia-associated antigens in childhood acute lymphocytic leukemia have been used to "clean up" patients' bone marrow for autologous bone marrow storage and reinfusion after high-dose chemotherapy. Use of monoclonal antibody–immunotoxin conjugates appears particularly promising in this regard and may markedly broaden the use of autologous bone marrow transplantation. Patients who do not receive autologous bone marrow or a graft from an identical twin require postengraftment immunosuppression to minimize the graft-versus-host syndrome attributable to donor immunocytes in the marrow graft. Recent investigations indicate that anti–T cell antiserum or cyclosporine can modify or abrogate established graft-versus-host syndrome in a significant proportion of cases.

Cyclosporine has proved to be an effective immunosuppressive drug for use in renal, cardiac, hepatic, and bone marrow transplantation. It is now being evaluated as an alternative to other more complex immunosuppressive regimens.

Autoimmune Disorders

The effectiveness of immunosuppressive drugs in autoimmune disorders varies widely. Most of these disorders are of unknown cause and the rationale for immunosuppression is sometimes strained, although it is usually thought that faulty recognition mechanisms of antibody cross-reactivity account for the proliferation of unneeded lymphoid clones. Studies of the NZB/NZW mouse strain suggest that there may be a deficiency in a soluble immune response suppressor substance (SIRS) in some autoimmune disorders. In the autoimmune diseases, unlike the situation in immunosuppression for transplantation, the unwanted immune response is already established when the disease is diagnosed, and a large proliferating mass of lymphoid cells must be dealt with. Nonetheless, with immunosuppressive therapy, remissions can be obtained in most instances of autoimmune hemolytic anemia, idiopathic thrombocytopenic purpura, Hashimoto's thyroiditis, and temporal arteritis. Apparent improvement is also often seen in patients with systemic lupus erythematosus, acute glomerulonephritis, acquired factor VIII inhibitors (antibodies), and certain other autoimmune states. Some cases of idiopathic aplastic anemia also appear to have an autoimmune basis. In some instances, it appears to be the result of increased activity of OKT8-positive T suppressor cells. In such instances, gamma interferon produced by T suppressor cells may be the humoral mediator of hematopoietic expression. A recent series of aplastic anemia patients showed significant clinical improvement and prolonged survival with thymocyte globulin (ALG) alone. Some prior cases treated with bone marrow transplantation after conditioning with cyclophosphamide or ALG have also shown prolonged improvement in blood counts even though there was evidence of graft rejection and recovery of recipient marrow function, again supporting an autoimmune basis for some cases of aplastic anemia. Recently, the use of high doses of normal gamma globulin (administered intravenously) has been found useful in therapy of refractory idiopathic thrombocytopenic purpura. The presumed mechanism of action is through reticuloendothelial cell blockade, thus reducing the distribution of antibody-damaged platelets.

In most instances it is only assumed that it is the immunosuppressive properties of drugs such as prednisone, cyclophosphamide, mercaptopurine, or ALG that produce these improvements. Anti-inflammatory effects of some of these drugs may also contribute to their efficacy. Cyclosporine has also entered clinical trial in the therapy of various autoimmune disorders. For example, the drug may prove useful in suppressing pancreatic islet cell destruction in early juvenile diabetes.

Hemolytic Disease of the Newborn

Prevention of Rh hemolytic disease of the newborn is a landmark in the development of immunosuppressive therapy. It is hoped that this example of precise suppression without side effects will also apply to other disease states once the offending antigens can be identified.

IMMUNOMODULATING AGENTS

A new frontier in pharmacology—still in the stage of exploration and debate—is the development of agents that modulate the immune response rather than suppress it. The rationale underlying all research into the development of these agents is that they can be used to increase the immunoresponsiveness of patients who have either selective or generalized immunodeficiency. The major potential uses are in (1) immunodeficiency disorders, (2) chronic infectious disease, and (3) cancer. At present, all immunostimulating or immunomodulating agents are classed as investigational drugs. The recent appearance of the acquired immunodeficiency syndrome (AIDS), caused by an RNA-retrovirus (HTLV-III/LAV/ARV), has greatly increased interest in developing more effective immunomodulatory drugs. This retrovirus resides in and destroys T-4 helper cells, leading to progressive immunologic paralysis.

Thymosin

This protein hormone, which is synthesized by the epithelioid component of the thymus, has recently been isolated and purified from bovine and human thymus glands. Thymosin, which has a molecular weight of approximately 10,000, appears to convey T cell specificity to uncommitted lymphoid stem cells. Lower-molecular-weight fractions may also have thymic hormone–like activity. Thymosin levels are

high through normal childhood and early adulthood, begin to fall in the third to fourth decades, and are low in elderly people. Serum levels are also low in DiGeorge's syndrome of T cell deficiency. In vitro treatment of lymphocytes with thymosin increases the number of cells that manifest T cell surface markers and function. Mechanistically, thymosin is considered to induce the maturation of pre–T cells. The effects of fetal thymus transplantation in DiGeorge's syndrome are probably attributable to the action of thymosin. The purified hormone therefore has potential therapeutic applications in DiGeorge's syndrome and other T cell deficiency states. Over 60 children with various immunodeficiencies have been treated with thymosin, and favorable responses are reported in over half of cases.

Interferons & Interleukins*

Interferons were first described as antiviral proteins produced by host cells. Subsequently, the interferons were found to have antiproliferative activity and to modulate the function of other immune cells (eg, macrophages and natural killer cells). Significant amounts of interferon have been extracted from leukocytes harvested at the time of routine blood donation using a process developed in Finland by Cantell. Interferon might be useful in the treatment of certain infections (eg, hepatitis; see p 562) as well as in some autoimmune diseases (eg, rheumatoid arthritis) and certain forms of cancer, particularly hairy cell leukemia but also myelomas and lymphomas arising from B cells (see Chapter 58). At present, 3 types of interferon are being produced (see p 562). Several pharmaceutical firms are currently producing standardized natural interferon in adequate quantities for clinical trial. What is more, recombinant DNA cloning technology has been successfully applied to producing alpha, beta, and gamma interferons. The cloned interferons have been introduced into clinical trials and are now being studied extensively. Interleukin-1 (IL-1) has been identified as the "endogenous pyrogen" and interleukin-2 (IL-2) as a hormone that stimulates the proliferation of T lymphocytes as well as exhibiting a variety of immunomodulatory and immunoregulatory processes.

Transfer Factor (TF)

This agent is a small RNA molecule or peptide (MW about 5000) derived from normal human lymphoid cells. Transfer factors are apparently immunologically specific for given antigens, although they may serve as adjuvants or "superantigens." Transfer factors also appear to be species-specific. Cell-mediated immunity to the specific antigen required should be present in the potential transfer factor donor. TF often converts negative delayed hypersensitivity skin tests to positive. The effect of a TF dose lasts for up to 6 months. The effects of transfer factor

*Interferons and interferon inducers are discussed also in Chapter 49 as antiviral agents.

therapy may be dramatic in some cases of chronic mucocutaneous candidiasis. Claims also have been made for the possible usefulness of transfer factor in the treatment of leprosy and the Wiskott-Aldrich syndrome. These reports are preliminary and will require detailed confirmation before a clear role for transfer factor therapy can be established for any of these disease states. Transfer factor dosage is based on the number of lymphocytes from which the TF has been prepared. Therapeutic doses require that at least 10^9 lymphocytes be used for TF preparation, although the TF from as many as 40×10^9 lymphocytes has been administered as a single dose without incident. The TF is not immunogenic, and only very rare reactions have occurred on repeated injection.

Synthetic Agents

Several synthetic chemical agents have been discovered to have immunomodulating properties. The chemical agent levamisole was first synthesized for the treatment of parasitic infections. Recent studies suggest that it increases the magnitude of delayed hypersensitivity or T cell–mediated immunity in humans. In immunodeficiency associated with Hodgkin's disease, levamisole has been noted to increase the number of E rosette–forming lymphoid cells (T cells) in vitro and to enhance skin test reactivity in vivo. Levamisole has also been widely tested in rheumatoid arthritis and found to have some efficacy but not without toxicity (see Chapter 34). More recently, inosiplex (isoprinosine) has been found to have immunomodulating activities also, and in various preclinical and clinical settings this agent has increased natural killer cell cytotoxicity as well as T cell and monocyte functional activities. It has been tested in acquired immunodeficiency syndrome (AIDS), with some (slight) benefit observed.

BCG (Bacille Calmette Guérin) & Other Adjuvants

BCG is a viable strain of *Mycobacterium bovis* that has been used for immunization against tuberculosis. Recently, it has been employed as a nonspecific adjuvant or immunostimulant in cancer therapy. BCG appears to act—at least in part—via activation of macrophages to make them more effective killer cells in concert with lymphoid cells in the efferent limb of the immune response. Macrophage activation with BCG also appears to increase the rate of clearance of immune complexes (eg, antibody-soluble tumor antigen) from the blood and thereby may overcome "tolerance" to the tumor. Immune T cells are also necessary for BCG's anticancer action, since, in animals pretreated with anti–T cell sera, the immunotherapeutic effect of BCG is blocked. It is being tried in studies of melanomas, lung and ovarian cancer, and other neoplasms. Some beneficial "local" immunotherapy effects appear likely. Systemic effects are unproved. Lipid extracts of BCG (eg, methanol-extractable residue) as well as nonviable preparations of *Corynebacterium parvum* may also have similar nonspecific immunostimulant properties. Both of these agents prepare macrophages for the release of a cytotoxic molecule currently known as "tumor necrosis factor" (TNF). TNF is released into the serum of BCG-treated animals after endotoxin challenge. TNF has also been synthesized using recombinant DNA technology.

IMMUNOLOGIC REACTIONS TO DRUGS & DRUG ALLERGY

The basic immune mechanism and the ways in which it can be suppressed or stimulated by drugs are discussed in the foregoing sections of this chapter. Drugs often serve also to *activate* the immune system in undesirable ways that appear as adverse drug reactions. These reactions are generally lumped in a broad classification as "drug allergy." Indeed, many drug reactions such as those to penicillin, iodides, phenytoin, and sulfonamides are allergic in nature. These drug reactions are manifested as skin eruptions, edema, anaphylactoid reactions, fever, and eosinophilia. The underlying mechanism of the allergic sensitization to drugs was clarified by the discovery of the IgE class of immunoglobulins and by a better understanding of the process of sensitization and activation of blood basophils and tissue mast cells.

Other drug reactions mediated by immune mechanisms may have different mechanisms. Thus, any one of the 4 major types of hypersensitivity can be associated with an allergic drug reaction:

Type I: IgE-mediated allergic reactions to stings and drugs, including anaphylaxis, urticaria, and angioedema.

Type II: Allergic reactions that are complement-dependent and therefore involve IgG or IgM antibodies in which the antibody is fixed to a circulating blood cell subject to complement-dependent lysis.

Type III: Drug reactions are exemplified by serum sickness, which involves IgG and is a multisystem complement-dependent vasculitis.

Type IV: Cell-mediated allergy is the mechanism involved in allergic contact dermatitis from topically applied drugs.

In a number of drug reactions, more than one of these hypersensitivity reactions may present itself simultaneously. Some adverse reactions to drugs may be mistakenly classified as allergic or immune when they are in reality genetic deficiency states or are idiosyncratic and not mediated by immune mechanisms (eg, hemolysis due to primaquine in glucose-6-phosphate dehydrogenase deficiency, or aplastic anemia due to chloramphenicol).

MECHANISMS OF IMMEDIATE (TYPE I) DRUG ALLERGY

The mechanisms of immune activation that are operative in drug allergy are similar to the normal hu-

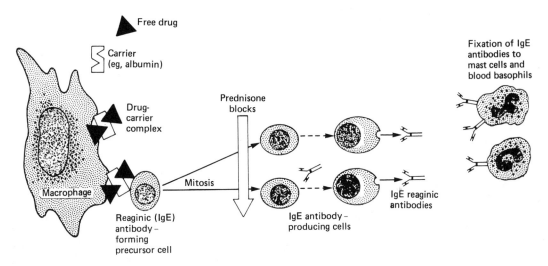

Figure 59–6. Induction of IgE-mediated allergic sensitivity to drugs and other allergens.

moral antibody responses to foreign macromolecules. These mechanisms can now be placed in a theoretical construct that includes an afferent limb of the immune response (Fig 59–6) as well as an efferent limb that includes the pharmacologic mediators of allergy (Fig 59–7). Landsteiner and his associates first demonstrated that animals could be sensitized to simple chemicals such as picric acid (a hapten) if the chemical was linked to a carrier protein. This linkage can occur in the body with a normal tissue or serum protein serving as the carrier. The subsequent immune response will be specific for the hapten even though linkage to a carrier is necessary for immune recognition. Surprisingly, carrier recognition is genetically determined even though the host does not produce antibodies against the carrier protein. When drugs serve as hap-

tens, the antibody-forming precursor cells that respond are often the precursors of cells that produce antibodies of the IgE class. IgE class–specific antibody responses are very dependent on helper T cell effects. Suppressor T cells may also function in modulating or inhibiting the IgE response. In nonallergic individuals, IgE globulin levels are the lowest of any immunoglobulin (< 1 μg/mL), whereas in allergy they may be increased 10-fold or more. IgE antibodies have the interesting property of fixing to blood basophils and tissue mast cells and are described as skin-sensitizing or reaginic antibodies.

The fixation of the IgE antibody to blood basophils or their tissue equivalent (mast cells) sets the stage for an acute allergic reaction. When the offending drug is reintroduced into the body, IgE antibody molecules on

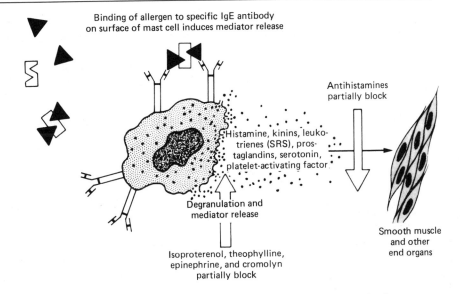

Figure 59–7. Response of IgE-sensitized cells to subsequent exposure to allergens.

the surface of sensitized basophilic leukocytes bind to the antigenic form of the drug (Fig 59–7). Sensitized tissue mast cells or blood basophils are stimulated to release mediators (eg, histamine, leukotrienes; Chapters 15, 17) from granules. Mediator release is associated with a fall in intracellular cAMP within the mast cell. Many of the drugs that block mediator release appear to act through the cAMP mechanism (eg, catecholamines, corticosteroids, theophylline), with different loci of action in the pathway of cAMP synthesis or degradation. Other vasoactive substances such as kinins may also be generated during histamine release. These mediators initiate immediate skin and smooth muscle responses and thus initiate tissue injury and the inflammatory response. Mediator-induced reactions can be devastating or lethal to the patient, especially when they produce laryngospasm, bronchospasm, or hypotension.

DRUG TREATMENT OF IMMEDIATE ALLERGY

One can test an individual for possible sensitivity to a drug by a simple scratch test, ie, by applying an extremely dilute solution of the drug to the skin. If allergy is present, an immediate wheal and flare will often occur. However, in many instances the skin test may be negative in spite of marked hypersensitivity to a hapten or to a metabolic product of the drug, or at times when the antibody may be of a class other than IgE. Skin reactivity to a specific drug can also be transferred from an allergic individual to a normal recipient (human or primate) with serum that contains the reaginic IgE antibodies (the Prausnitz-Küstner reaction).

Drugs that modify allergic responses act at several links in this chain of events. Prednisone, which is often used in severe allergic reactions, is immunosuppressive and probably blocks proliferation of the IgE-producing clones and could inhibit function of helper T cells in the IgE response. In the efferent limb of the allergic response, isoproterenol, epinephrine, and theophylline block the release of mediators from mast cells and basophils and produce bronchodilatation, whereas antihistamines competitively inhibit histamine, which would otherwise produce bronchoconstriction and increased capillary permeability in the end organ. Corticosteroids may also act to reduce tissue injury and edema in the inflamed tissue, as well as "unblocking" β-blocked cells, thereby facilitating the actions of catecholamines in cells that may have become refractory to epinephrine or isoproterenol. Several agents directed toward the inhibition of leukotriene synthesis are currently in clinical trial, with the view that they may be useful in acute allergic and inflammatory disorders. Cromolyn sodium, a drug that is useful for treatment of allergic asthma, appears to inhibit the liberation of the mediators of anaphylaxis that are released after antibody-antigen interaction

(see Chapter 18). However, its complete mechanism of action is still obscure.

DESENSITIZATION TO DRUGS

When reasonable alternatives are not available, certain drugs (eg, penicillin) must be used for life-threatening illnesses even in the presence of known allergic sensitivity. In such cases, desensitization can sometimes be accomplished by starting with minute dosages of the drug and gradually increasing the dose over a period of hours or days to the full therapeutic range. This practice is hazardous, and one must always be ready to treat the patient for an episode of acute anaphylactic shock before desensitization has been achieved. This form of desensitization differs from immunosuppression in that the immune mechanism often appears to be stimulated and reactivity is only predictably diminished while the treatment is continued. With the advent of cephalosporins and other antibodies, the need for such desensitization procedures to administer penicillin has been essentially eliminated.

The exact mechanism of desensitization to drugs is complex and incompletely understood. It may be due to controlled anaphylaxis (with gradual depletion of mast cells and basophils) while symptoms are suppressed or to antigen excess, which can under certain circumstances block mediator release. In some instances, allergic desensitization appears to be accomplished by the stimulation of competing clones of cells that produce "blocking" antibodies, often of the IgG or IgA immunoglobulin class. Additionally, desensitization with antigen could induce the generation of specific suppressor T cells.

AUTOIMMUNE (TYPE II) REACTIONS TO DRUGS

Certain autoimmune syndromes can be induced by drugs. Examples of this phenomenon include systemic lupus erythematosus following hydralazine or procainamide therapy, "lupoid hepatitis" due to cathartic sensitivity, autoimmune hemolytic anemia resulting from methyldopa administration, thrombocytopenic purpura due to quinidine, and agranulocytosis due to a variety of drugs. In these drug-induced autoimmune states, antibodies to tissue constituents or to the drug can be demonstrated. Immune mechanisms also appear to be involved in many additional cases of so-called idiopathic thrombocytopenic purpura, but it is more difficult to demonstrate the specific antibodies. The blood platelet or granulocyte is sometimes an innocent bystander to an immunologic reaction to a drug but manages to be damaged or activated by antigen-antibody complexes or destroyed by the reticuloendothelial system, leading to the development of "idiopathic" thrombocytopenic purpura or agranulocytosis.

Fortunately, autoimmune reactions to drugs usually subside within several months after the offending drug is withdrawn. Immunosuppressive therapy is warranted only when the autoimmune response is unusually severe.

SERUM SICKNESS & VASCULITIC (TYPE III) REACTIONS

Serum sickness reactions to drugs are more common than immediate anaphylactic responses. The clinical features of serum sickness include urticarial skin eruptions, arthralgia or arthritis, lymphadenopathy, and fever. The reactions generally last 6–12 days and usually subside once the offending drug is eliminated. Although IgE antibodies may play some role, complement-fixing antibodies of the IgM or IgG class are usually involved. Corticosteroids are useful in attenuating severe serum sickness reactions to drugs.

Immune vasculitis can also be induced by drugs. The sulfonamides, penicillin, thiouracil, anticonvulsants, and iodides have all been implicated in the initiation of hypersensitivity angiitis. Erythema multiforme is a relatively mild vasculitic skin disorder that may be secondary to drug hypersensitivity. Stevens-Johnson syndrome is probably a more severe form of this hypersensitivity reaction and includes erythema multiforme, arthritis, nephritis, central nervous system abnormalities, and myocarditis. It has frequently been associated with sulfonamide therapy.

CLINICAL IDENTIFICATION OF IMMUNOLOGIC REACTIONS TO DRUGS

In view of the multiplicity of drugs administered to hospitalized patients, it is not always easy to determine which drug has initiated an allergic or immune syndrome of drug sensitivity. Careful questioning about the history of prior drug sensitivities is an important part of every patient's medical record, and errors of omission can be dangerous. In almost all instances, once an offending drug is identified, its use is discontinued. If an alternative drug is to be used (eg, an antibiotic), it is important to select one from a different class of agents to avoid cross-sensitivity reactions. Since certain commonly used drugs such as the penicillins are frequent offenders, direct questions about penicillin sensitivity should always be included in the patient's history. Skin testing may be very useful in confirming drug allergy when the history is equivocal and the proper antigens are available. Skin testing is considerably less hazardous than a therapeutic trial and is usually indicated where there is an equivocal allergic history and a strong clinical indication for treatment with the drug. An alternative to skin testing that is increasingly available is the radioallergosorbent test (RAST), a form of radioimmunoassay procedure.

Warnings of known sensitivities should be prominently displayed in the patient's record or hospital chart. When drug intolerance is suspected, an assessment of the patient's anaphylactic potential should be made, since delayed rashes carry a different prognosis from that of urticaria and angioedema. Once a drug allergy is defined, this information should always be conveyed to the patient in clear language to prevent repeated challenges with the same agent in the future, when the reaction may be much more severe. In the case of known severe sensitivity to common drugs, the patient should be advised to carry a clearly written notice of the sensitivity to lessen the chance of being given the agent during incapacitation, as after an accident.

REFERENCES

Current Concepts in Immunology

Bockman RS, Rothschild M: Prostaglandin E inhibition of T-lymphocyte colony formation. *J Clin Invest* 1979;**64**:812.

Bodmer WF et al: The structure of HLA. *Transplant Proc* 1983;**15**:36.

Botazzo GF et al: In situ characterization of autoimmune phenomena and the expression of HLA molecules in the pancreas in diabetic insulinitis. *N Engl J Med* 1985;**313**:353.

Cosimi AB: The clinical usefulness of antilymphocytic antibodies. *Transplant Proc* 1983;**15**:583.

Gale RP (editor): *Recent Advances in Bone Marrow Transplantation.* AR Liss, 1983.

Hymes JL et al: Macrophages synthesize and release prostaglandins in response to inflammatory stimuli. *Nature* 1977;**269**:149.

Köhler O, Milstein C: Continuous cultures of fused cells secreting antibody of defined specificity. *Nature* 1975; **55**:495.

Ledbetter J et al: Evolutionary conservation of surface molecules that distinguish T lymphocyte helper/inducer and cytotoxic/suppressor subpopulation in mouse and man. *J Exp Med* 1981;**153**:310.

Melchers F, Potter M, Warner NL (editors): *Lymphocyte Hybridomas.* Springer, 1978.

Origins of lymphocyte diversity. (2 parts.) *Cold Spring Harbor Symp Quant Biol* 1977;**41**:1, 417.

Ortaldo JR et al: Determination of surface antigens on highly purified human NK cells by flow cytometry with monoclonal antibodies. *J Immunol* 1981;**127**:2401.

Roitt I, Brostoff J, Male D (editors): *Immunology.* Mosby, 1985.

Stites DP et al (editors): *Basic & Clinical Immunology*, 5th ed. Lange, 1984.

Unanue ER: The regulation of lymphocyte function by the macrophage. *Immunol Rev* 1978;**40**:227.

Vogelsang G et al: An in vitro predictive test for graft versus host disease in patients with genotypic HLA-identical bone marrow transplants. *N Engl J Med* 1985;**313**:645.

Waldmann TA, Broder S: Suppressor cells in the regulation of the immune response. Pages 155–199 in: *Progess in Clinical Immunology.* Schwartz RS (editor). Grune & Stratton, 1977.

Immunosuppressive Agents

Atkinson K et al: Cyclosporin A associated nephrotoxicity in the first 100 days after allogeneic bone marrow transplantation. *Br J Haematol* 1983;**54**:59.

Beveridge T: Cyclosporin A: An evaluation of clinical results. *Transplant Proc* 1983;**15**:433.

European Multicentre Trial Group: Cyclosporine in cadaveric renal transplantation. *Lancet* 1983;**2**:986.

Fehr J, Hofmann V, Kappeler CM: Transient reversal of thrombocytopenia in idiopathic thrombocytopenia purpura by high-dose intravenous gamma globulin. *N Engl J Med* 1982;**306**:1254.

Freda VJ et al: Prevention of Rh hemolytic disease: Ten years' experience with Rh immune globulin. *N Engl J Med* 1975; **292**:1014.

Goodwin JS, Messner RP: Sensitivity of lymphocytes to prostaglandin E$_2$ increases over the age of 70. *J Clin Invest* 1979;**64**:434.

Harris KR et al: Azathioprine and cyclosporine: Different tissue matching criteria needed? *Lancet* 1985;**2**:802.

Hendricks GFJ et al: Excellent outcome after transplantation of renal allografts from HLA-DR-W6-positive donors, even in HLA-DR mismatches. *Lancet* 1983;**2**:187.

Hess AD, Tutschka PJ, Santos GW: Effect of cyclosporin A on human lymphocytes in vitro. *J Immunol* 1982;**128**:355.

Imbach P et al: Intravenous immunoglobulin versus oral corticosteroids in acute immune thrombocytopoenic purpura in childhood. *Lancet* 1985;**2**:464.

Jansen FK, Blythmann H, Carriere D: Immunotoxins: Hybrid molecules combining high specificity and potent cytotoxicity. *Immunol Rev* 1982;**62**:185.

Kahan BD: Cyclosporine: The agent and its actions. *Transplant Proc* 1985;**17(Suppl 1)**:5.

Merion RM et al: Cyclosporine: Five years' experience in cadaveric renal transplantation. *N Engl J Med* 1984;**310**:148.

Ortho Multicenter Transplant Study Group: Randomized trial of OKT3 monoclonal antibody for acute rejection of cadaveric renal transplants. *N Engl J Med* 1985;**313**:337.

Powles RL et al: Cyclosporin-A in patients receiving renal allografts from cadaver donors. *Lancet* 1978;**2**:1327.

Ramsay NK et al: A randomized study of the prevention of graft-versus-host disease. *N Engl J Med* 1982;**306**:392.

Speck B et al: Treatment of aplastic anemia by anti-lymphocytic globulin with and without allogeneic bone marrow infusions. *Lancet* 1977;**2**:1145.

Stadecker MJ et al: Synthesis and release of thymidine by macrophages. *J Immunol* 1977;**199**:1738.

Starzl TE et al: Liver transplantation with the use of cyclosporin A and prednisone. *N Engl J Med* 1981;**305**:266.

Vallera DA et al: Monoclonal antibody toxin conjugates for experimental graft-versus-host disease prophylaxis. *Transplantation* 1983;**36**:73.

Wagner H: Cyclosporin A: Mechanism of action. *Transplant Proc* 1983;**15**:523.

Willebrand EV, Hagry P: Cyclosporin A deposits in renal allografts. *Lancet* 1983;**2**:189.

Immunomodulating Agents

Dinarello CA: Interleukin-1. *Rev Infect Dis* 1984;**6**:51.

Goldstein G: Isolation of bovine thymin: A polypeptide hormone of the thymus. *Nature* 1974;**247**:11.

Gresser I (editor): *Interferon.* Academic Press, 1981.

Lewis V: Circulating thymic-hormone activity in congenital immunodeficiency. *Lancet* 1977;**2**:471.

Vilcek J, Gresser I, Merrigan TC (editors): Regulatory functions of interferons. *Ann NY Acad Sci* 1980;**350**:1. [Entire issue.]

Wybran J: Immunomodulatory properties of isoprinosine in man: In vitro and in vivo data. *Int J Immunopharmacol* 1980;**2**:197.

Immunologic Reactions to Drugs & Allergy

Askenase PW: Effector and regulatory mechanisms in delayed type hypersensitivity. Chap 9, pp 147–165, in: *Allergy Principles and Practice,* 2nd ed. Middleton E Jr, Reed C, Ellis EF (editors). Mosby, 1983.

Lichtenstein LM, Norman PS: Human allergic reactions. *Am J Med* 1969;**46**:163.

Parker CW: Drug allergy. *N Engl J Med* 1975;**292**:732.

Plaut M, Lichtenstein LM, Henney C: Properties of a subpopulation of T cells bearing histamine receptors. *J Clin Invest* 1975;**55**:856.

Russell AS, Lessoff MH: Hypersensitivity to drugs. *Clin Allergy* 1971;**1**:179.

Samuelsson B et al: Leukotrienes and slow reacting substance of anaphylaxis (SRS-A). *Allergy* 1980;**35**:375.

Spiegelberg HL et al: Lymphocytes with immunoglobulin E FC receptors in patients with atopic disorders. *J Clin Invest* 1979;**64**:714.

Tijo AH, Hull WM, Gleich JG: Production of human immunoglobulin E in vitro. *J Immunol* 1979;**122**:2131.

Introduction to Toxicology: Occupational & Environmental Toxicology

60

Gabriel L. Plaa, PhD

Humans live in a chemical environment. Estimates indicate that more than 60,000 chemicals are in common use and about 500 new chemicals are said to enter the commercial market annually. One needs to know how these chemicals can be utilized by society without being hazardous to its members and the environment.

Pollution has paralleled technologic advances. Industrialization and the creation of large urban centers have led to the contamination of air, water, and soil. The principal causes of pollution are related to the production and use of energy, the production and use of industrial chemicals, and increased agricultural activity.

TOXICOLOGY & ITS SUBDIVISIONS

Toxicology is concerned with the deleterious effects of chemical and physical agents on all living systems. In the biomedical area, however, the toxicologist is primarily concerned with adverse effects in humans resulting from exposure to drugs and other chemicals as well as the demonstration of safety or hazard associated with their use.

Occupational Toxicology

Occupational toxicology deals with the chemicals found in the workplace. Industrial workers may be exposed to these agents during the synthesis, manufacturing, or packaging of these substances or through their use in an occupational setting. Agricultural workers, for example, may be exposed to harmful amounts of pesticides during their application in the field. The major emphasis of occupational toxicology is to identify the agents of concern, define the conditions leading to their safe use, and prevent absorption of harmful amounts.

Guidelines have been elaborated to establish safe ambient air concentrations for many chemicals found in the workplace. The American Conference of Governmental Industrial Hygienists periodically prepares lists of recommended **threshold limit values (TLV)** for about 600 such chemicals. Three different categories of air concentrations (expressed in "parts per million" [ppm] or "milligrams per cubic meter"

[mg/m^3]) have been elaborated to cover various exposure conditions: (1) threshold limit value–time-weighted average (TLV-TWA) is the concentration for a normal 8-hour workday or 40-hour workweek to which workers may be repeatedly exposed without adverse effect; (2) threshold limit value–short-term exposure limit (TLV-STEL) is the maximum concentration (a value greater than the TLV-TWA) that should not be exceeded at any time during a 15-minute exposure period; and (3) threshold limit value–ceiling (TLV-C) is the concentration that should not be exceeded even instantaneously. These guidelines are reevaluated as new information becomes available.

Environmental Toxicology

Environmental toxicology deals with the potentially deleterious impact of chemicals, present as pollutants of the environment, to living organisms. The term "environment" includes all the surroundings of an individual organism, but particularly the air, soil, and water. A "pollutant" is a substance that occurs in the environment, at least in part as a result of human activity, and which has a deleterious effect on living organisms. While humans are considered a target species of particular interest, other terrestrial and aquatic species are of considerable importance as potential biologic targets.

Air pollution is a product of industrialization, technologic development, and increased urbanization. Humans may also be exposed to chemicals used in the agricultural environment as pesticides—or in food processing—that may persist as residues or ingredients in food products. The Food and Agriculture Organization and the World Health Organization (FAO/WHO) Joint Expert Commission on Food Additives adopted the term **acceptable daily intake (ADI)** to denote "the daily intake of a chemical which, during an entire lifetime, appears to be without appreciable risk on the basis of all the known facts at the time." After evaluation of the pertinent scientific data, the FAO/WHO periodically lists ADI values (expressed in milligrams per kilogram of body weight per day) for many pesticides and food additives that may enter the human food chain. These guidelines are reevaluated as new information becomes available.

Ecotoxicology

Ecotoxicology has evolved recently as an extension of environmental toxicology. It is concerned with the toxic effects of chemical and physical agents on living organisms, especially on populations and communities within defined ecosystems; it includes the transfer pathways of those agents and their interactions with the environment. Traditional toxicology is concerned with toxic effects on *individual* organisms; ecotoxicology is concerned with the impact on *populations* of living organisms or on ecosystems. It is possible that an environmental event, exerting severe effects on individual organisms, has no important impact on populations or an ecosystem. Thus, the terms "environmental toxicology" and "ecotoxicology" are not interchangeable.

TOXICOLOGIC TERMS & DEFINITIONS

Toxicity, Hazard, & Risk

Toxicity is the ability of an agent to cause injury. It is a qualitative term. Whether or not these injuries occur depends on the amount of chemical absorbed (severity of the exposure, dose). Hazard, on the other hand, is the *likelihood that injury will occur* in a given situation or setting; the conditions of use and exposure are primary considerations. To assess hazard, one needs to have knowledge about both the inherent toxicity of the substance (qualitative aspect) and the amounts to which individuals are liable to be exposed (quantitative aspect). Humans can safely use potentially toxic substances when the necessary conditions minimizing absorption are established and respected. The presence of a potentially toxic substance in the workplace or in the environment does not necessarily mean that a hazardous situation exists.

Risk is defined as the *expected frequency of the occurrence of an undesirable effect* arising from exposure to a chemical or physical agent. Estimation of risk makes use of dose-response data and extrapolation from the observed relationships to the expected responses at doses occurring in actual exposure situations. The quality and suitability of the biologic data used in such estimates are major limiting factors. A number of mathematical models have been devised and are often used for calculating risk of carcinogenesis; they may also be used to assess the risk involved with other forms of toxicity.

Routes of Exposure

The route of entry for chemicals into the body differs in different exposure situations. In the industrial setting, inhalation is the major route of entry. The transdermal route is also quite important, but oral ingestion is a relatively minor route. Consequently, preventive measures are largely designed to eliminate absorption by inhalation or by topical contact. Atmospheric pollutants gain entry by inhalation, whereas for pollutants of water and soil, oral ingestion is the principal route of exposure for humans.

Duration of Exposure

Toxic reactions may differ qualitatively depending on the duration of the exposure. A single exposure—or multiple exposures occurring over 1 or 2 days—represents **acute exposure.** Multiple exposures continuing over a longer period of time represent a **chronic exposure.** In the occupational setting, both acute (eg, accidental discharge) and chronic (eg, repetitive handling of chemical) exposures may occur, whereas with chemicals found in the environment, chronic exposure (eg, pollutants in ground water) is more likely. Society is also concerned with the possible harmful effects of contact with small concentrations of chemicals over long periods of time; this type of chronic situation is called **low-level, long-term exposure.** The appearance of the toxic effect after acute exposure may appear rapidly or after a variable interval; the latter is called **delayed toxicity.** With chronic exposures, the toxic effect may not be discernible until after several months of repetitive exposure. The harmful effect resulting from either acute or chronic exposure may be reversible or irreversible. The relative reversibility of the toxic effect depends on the recuperative properties of the affected organ.

Presence of Mixtures

Humans normally come in contact with several (or many) different chemicals concurrently or sequentially. This complicates the assessment of potentially hazardous situations encountered in the workplace or in the environment. The resulting biologic effect of combined exposure to several agents can be characterized as **additive, supra-additive** (synergistic), or **infra-additive** (antagonistic). Another type of interaction, **potentiation** (a special form of synergism), may be observed. In cases of potentiation, one of 2 agents exerts no effect upon exposure; but when exposure to both together occurs, the effect of the active agent is increased. All of these types of interactions have been observed in humans. In the absence of contrary evidence, one usually assumes that the toxic effects of mixtures of chemicals are likely to be additive.

ENVIRONMENTAL CONSIDERATIONS

Certain chemical and physical characteristics are known to be of importance for estimating the potential hazard involved for environmental toxicants. In addition to information regarding effects on different organisms, knowledge about the following properties is essential to predict the environmental impact: The **degradability** of the substance; its **mobility** through air, water, and soil; whether or not **bioaccumulation** occurs; and its transport and **biomagnification** through food chains. Chemicals that are poorly degraded (by abiotic or biotic pathways) exhibit *environmental persistence* and thus can accumulate. Lipophilic substances tend to bioaccumulate in body fat, resulting in tissue residues. When the toxicant is incorporated into the food chain, biomagnification occurs as one species feeds upon others and concentrates the chemical. The pollutants that have the widest environmental impact are poorly degradable; are relatively mobile in air, water, and soil; exhibit bioaccumulation; and also exhibit biomagnification.

In ecotoxicology there are 3 interacting components: the toxicant, the environment, and the organisms (community, population, or ecosystem). The environment may modify the toxicant or may modify the response of the organism to the toxicant; the toxicant may affect the organism directly or may modify the environment; and the organism may modify the toxicant or the environment. Ecotoxicologic studies are designed to determine emission and entry of the toxicant in the abiotic environment, including distribution and fate; entry and fate of the toxicant in the biosphere; and the qualitative and quantitative toxic consequences to the ecosystem.

Table 60–1. Threshold limit values of some common air pollutants and solvents.

Compound	TLV (ppm)	
	TWA*	STEL*
Benzene	10	25
Carbon monoxide	50	400
Carbon tetrachloride	5	20
Chloroform	10	50
Nitrogen dioxide	3	5
Ozone	0.1	0.3
Sulfur dioxide	2	5
Tetrachloroethylene	50	200
Toluene	100	150
1,1,1-Trichloroethane	350	450
Trichloroethylene	50	200

*See text for definitions.

SPECIFIC CHEMICALS

AIR POLLUTANTS

The 5 major pollutants that account for about 98% of air pollution are carbon monoxide (about 52%), sulfur oxides (about 18%), hydrocarbons (about 12%), particulate matter (about 10%), and nitrogen oxides (about 6%). The sources of these chemicals include transportation, industry, generation of electric power, space heating, and refuse disposal. The "reducing type" of pollution (sulfur dioxide and smoke resulting from incomplete combustion of coal) has been associated with acute adverse effects, particularly among the elderly and individuals with preexisting cardiac or respiratory disease. The association of acute adverse effects, other than severe irritation of the eyes, is less striking with the "oxidizing or photochemical type" of pollution (hydrocarbons, nitrogen oxides, and photochemical oxidants). Ambient air pollution has been implicated as a contributing factor in bronchitis, obstructive ventilatory disease, pulmonary emphysema, bronchial asthma, and lung cancer.

1. CARBON MONOXIDE

Carbon monoxide (CO) is a colorless, tasteless, odorless, and nonirritating gas, a byproduct of incomplete combustion. The average concentration of CO in the atmosphere is about 0.1 ppm; in heavy traffic, the concentration may exceed 100 ppm. The recommended threshold limit values (TLV-TWA and TLV-STEL) are shown in Table 60–1.

Mechanism of Action

CO combines reversibly with the oxygen-binding sites of hemoglobin and has an affinity for hemoglobin which is about 220 times that of oxygen. The product formed, carboxyhemoglobin, cannot transport oxygen. Furthermore, the presence of carboxyhemoglobin interferes with the dissociation of oxygen from the remaining oxyhemoglobin, thus reducing the transfer of oxygen to tissues. The brain and the heart are the organs most affected. Normal nonsmoking adults have carboxyhemoglobin levels of less than 1% saturation (1% of total hemoglobin is in the form of carboxyhemoglobin); this level has been attributed to the endogenous formation of CO from heme catabolism. Smokers may exhibit 5–10% saturation, depending on their smoking habits. An individual breathing air containing 0.1% CO (1000 ppm) would have a carboxyhemoglobin level of about 50%.

Clinical Effects

The principal signs of CO intoxication are those of hypoxia and progress in the following sequence: (1) psychomotor impairment; (2) headache and tightness in the temporal area; (3) confusion and loss of visual acuity; (3) tachyardia, tachypnea, syncope, and coma; and (4) deep coma, convulsions, shock, and respiratory failure. Individual variability in response to a given carboxyhemoglobin concentration is quite high. Carboxyhemoglobin levels below 15% rarely produce symptoms; collapse and syncope may appear around 40%; above 60%, death may ensue. Prolonged hypoxia and posthypoxic unconsciousness can result in residual irreversible damage to the brain and the myocardium. The clinical effects may be aggravated by heavy labor, high altitudes, and high ambient temperatures.

While CO intoxication is usually thought of as a form of acute toxicity, there is evidence that chronic exposure to low levels can lead to undesirable effects, including the development of atherosclerotic coronary disease in cigarette smokers. The fetus may be quite susceptible to the effects of CO exposure.

Treatment

In cases of acute intoxication, removal of the individual from the exposure source and maintenance of respiration is essential, followed by administration of oxygen—the specific antagonist to CO—within the limits of oxygen toxicity. With room air at 1 atm, the elimination half-time of CO is about 320 minutes; with 100% oxygen, the half-time is about 80 minutes; and with hyperbaric oxygen (2–3 atm), the half-time can be reduced to about 20 minutes.

2. SULFUR DIOXIDE

Sulfur dioxide (SO_2) is a colorless, irritant gas generated primarily by the combustion of sulfur-containing fossil fuels. The TLV-TWA and TLV-STEL are given in Table 60–1.

Mechanism of Action

On contact with moist membranes, SO_2 forms sulfurous acid, which is responsible for its severe irritant effects on the eyes, mucous membranes, and skin. It is estimated that approximately 90% of inhaled SO_2 is absorbed in the upper respiratory tract, the site of its principal effect. The inhalation of SO_2 causes bronchial constriction; altered smooth muscle tone and parasympathetic reflexes appear to be involved in this reaction (Chapter 18). Exposure to 5 ppm for 10 minutes leads to increased resistance to air flow in most humans. Exposures to 5–10 ppm are reported to cause severe bronchospasm; 10–20% of the healthy young adult population is estimated to be reactive to even lower concentrations. The phenomenon of adaptation to irritating concentrations is a recognized occurrence in workers.

Clinical Effects & Treatment

The signs and symptoms of intoxication include irritation of the eyes, nose, and throat and reflex bronchoconstriction. If severe exposure has occurred, delayed onset of pulmonary edema may be observed. Cumulative effects from chronic low-level exposure to SO_2 are not striking, particularly in humans. Treatment is not specific for SO_2 but depends on therapeutic maneuvers utilized in the treatment of irritation of the respiratory tract.

3. NITROGEN OXIDES

Nitrogen dioxide (NO_2) is a brownish irritant gas sometimes associated with fires. It is formed also from fresh silage; exposure of farmers to NO_2 in the confines of a silo can lead to "silo-filler's disease." The 1984 TLV-TWA and TLV-STEL are shown in Table 60–1.

Mechanism of Action

NO_2 is a deep lung irritant capable of producing pulmonary edema. The type I cells of the alveoli appear to be the cells chiefly affected on acute exposure. Exposure to 25 ppm is irritating to some individuals; 50 ppm is moderately irritating to the eyes and nose.

Exposure for 1 hour to 50 ppm can cause pulmonary edema and perhaps subacute or chronic pulmonary lesions; 100 ppm can cause pulmonary edema and death.

Clinical Effects & Treatment

The signs and symptoms of acute exposure to NO_2 include irritation of the eyes and nose, cough, mucoid or frothy sputum production, dyspnea, and chest pain. Pulmonary edema may appear within 1–2 hours. In some individuals, the clinical signs may subside in about 2 weeks; the patient may then pass into a second stage of abruptly increasing severity, including recurring pulmonary edema. Chronic exposure of laboratory animals to 10–25 ppm NO_2 has resulted in emphysematous changes; thus, chronic effects in humans are of concern. There is no specific treatment for acute intoxication to NO_2; therapeutic measures for the management of deep lung irritation and noncardiogenic pulmonary edema are employed.

4. OZONE

Ozone (O_3) is a bluish irritant gas that occurs normally in the earth's atmosphere, where it is an important absorbent of ultraviolet light. In the workplace, it can occur around high-voltage electrical equipment and around ozone-producing devices used for air and water purification. It is also an important oxidant found in polluted urban air. See Table 60–1 for TLV-TWA and TLV-STEL values.

Clinical Effects & Treatment

O_3 is an irritant of mucous membranes and can cause deep lung irritation, with pulmonary edema, when inhaled at sufficient concentrations. Some of the effects of O_3 resemble those seen with radiation, suggesting that O_3 toxicity may result from the formation of reactive free radicals. The gas causes shallow, rapid breathing and a decrease in pulmonary compliance. Enhanced sensitivity of the lung to bronchoconstrictors is also observed. Exposures around 0.1 ppm for 10–30 minutes causes irritation and dryness of the throat; above 0.1 ppm, one finds changes in visual acuity, substernal pain, and dyspnea. Pulmonary function is impaired at concentrations exceeding 0.8 ppm. Long-term exposure in animals results in morphologic and functional pulmonary changes. Chronic bronchitis, bronchiolitis, fibrosis, and emphysematous changes have been reported in a variety of species exposed to concentrations above 1 ppm. There is no specific treatment for acute O_3 intoxication. Management depends on therapeutic measures utilized for deep lung irritation and noncardiogenic pulmonary edema.

SOLVENTS

1. HALOGENATED ALIPHATIC HYDROCARBONS

These agents find wide use as industrial solvents, degreasing agents, and cleaning agents. The substances include carbon tetrachloride, chloroform, trichloroethylene, tetrachloroethylene (perchloroethylene), and 1,1,1-trichloroethane (methyl chloroform). See Table 60–1 for recommended threshold limit values.

Mechanism of Action & Clinical Effects

In laboratory animals, the halogenated hydrocarbons cause central nervous system depression, liver injury, kidney injury, and some degree of cardiotoxicity. These substances are depressants of the central nervous system in humans, although their relative potencies vary considerably; chloroform is the most potent and was widely used as an anesthetic agent. Chronic exposure to tetrachloroethylene can cause impaired memory, numbness of the extremities, and peripheral neuropathy. Hepatotoxicity is also a common toxic effect that can occur in humans after acute or chronic exposures, the severity of the lesion being dependent on the amount absorbed. Carbon tetrachloride is the most potent of the series in this regard. Nephrotoxicity can occur in humans exposed to carbon tetrachloride, chloroform, and trichloroethylene. With chloroform, carbon tetrachloride, trichloroethylene, and tetrachloroethylene, carcinogenicity has been observed in lifetime exposure studies performed in rats or mice. The potential effects of low-level, long-term exposures to humans, however, are yet to be determined.

Treatment

There is no specific treatment for acute intoxication resulting from exposure to halogenated hydrocarbons. Management depends upon the organ system involved.

2. AROMATIC HYDROCARBONS

Benzene is widely used for its solvent properties and as an intermediate in the synthesis of other chemicals. The 1984 recommended TLV-TWA and TLV-STEL values are given in Table 60–1. The acute toxic effect of benzene is depression of the central nervous system. Exposure to concentrations larger than 3000 ppm may cause euphoria, nausea, locomotor problems, and coma; vertigo, drowsiness, headache, and nausea may occur at concentrations ranging from 250 to 500 ppm. No specific treatment exists for the acute toxic effect of benzene.

Chronic exposure to benzene can result in very serious toxic effects, the most significant being an insidious and unpredictable injury to the bone marrow; aplastic anemia, leukopenia, pancytopenia, or thrombocytopenia may occur. Bone marrow cells in early stages of development appear to be most sensitive to benzene. The early symptoms of chronic benzene intoxication may be rather vague (headache, fatigue, and loss of appetite). Epidemiologic data suggest an association between chronic benzene exposure and an increased incidence of leukemia in workers; such effects have yet to be produced in laboratory animals.

Toluene (methylbenzene) does not possess the myelotoxic properties of benzene, nor has it been associated with leukemia. It is, however, a central nervous depressant. See Table 60–1 for the TLV-TWA and TLV-STEL values.

INSECTICIDES

1. CHLORINATED HYDROCARBON INSECTICIDES

These agents are usually classified in 4 groups: DDT (chlorophenothane) and its analogs, benzene hexachlorides, cyclodienes, and toxaphenes (Table 60–2). They are aryl, carbocyclic, or heterocyclic compounds containing chlorine substituents. The individual compounds differ widely in their biotransformation and capacity for storage; toxicity and storage are not always correlated. They can be absorbed through the skin as well as by inhalation or oral ingestion. There are, however, important quantitative differences between the various derivatives; DDT in solution is poorly absorbed by the skin, whereas dieldrin absorption from the skin is very efficient.

Human Toxicology

The acute toxic properties of the chlorinated hydrocarbon insecticides in humans are qualitatively simi-

Table 60–2. Chlorinated hydrocarbon insecticides.

Chemical Class	Compounds	Toxicity Rating[*]	ADI[†]
DDT and analogs	Dichlorodiphenyl-trichloroethane (DDT)	4	0.005
	Methoxychlor	3	0.1
	Tetrachlorodiphenyl-ethane (TDE)	3	—
Benzene hexachlorides	Benzene hexachloride (BHC; hexachlorocyclohexane)	4	—
	Lindane	4	0.01
Cyclodienes	Aldrin	5	0.0001
	Chlordane	4	0.001
	Dieldrin	5	0.0001
	Heptachlor	4	0.0005
Toxaphenes	Toxaphene (camphechlor)	4	—

[*]Toxicity rating: Probable human oral lethal dosage for class 3 = 500–5000 mg/kg, class 4 = 50–500 mg/kg, and class 5 = 5–50 mg/kg. (See Gosselin reference.)

[†]ADI = acceptable daily intake (mg/kg body weight/d).

lar. These agents interfere with inactivation of the sodium channel in excitable membranes and cause rapid repetitive firing in most neurons. The major effect is central nervous stimulation. With DDT, tremor may be the first manifestation, possibly continuing on to convulsions, whereas with the other compounds convulsions often appear as the first sign of intoxication. There is no specific treatment regimen for the acute intoxicated state, treatment being symptomatic. Chronic administration of some of these agents to laboratory animals over long periods has resulted in enhanced tumorigenicity; there is no agreement regarding the potential carcinogenic properties of these substances, and extrapolation of these observations to humans is controversial. Evidence of carcinogenic effects in humans has not been established.

Environmental Toxicology

The chlorinated hydrocarbon insecticides are considered "persistent" chemicals. Degradation is quite slow when compared to other insecticides, and bioaccumulation, particularly in aquatic ecosytems, is well documented. Their mobility in soil depends on the composition of the soil; the presence of organic matter favors the adsorption of these chemicals onto the soil, whereas adsorption is poor in sandy soils. Once adsorbed, they do not readily desorb.

2. ORGANOPHOSPHORUS INSECTICIDES

These agents, some of which are listed in Table 60–3, are utilized to combat a large variety of pests. They are useful pesticides when in direct contact with insects or when used as "plant systemics," where the agent is translocated within the plant and exerts its effects on insects that feed on the plant. Some of these agents are used in human and veterinary medicine as local or systemic antiparasitics or in circumstances in which prolonged inhibition of cholinesterase is indicated (Chapter 6). The compounds are absorbed by the skin as well as by the respiratory and gastrointestinal tracts. Biotransformation is rapid, particularly when

Table 60–3. Organophosphorus insecticides.

Compound	Toxicity Rating*	ADI†
Azinphos-methyl	5	0.0025
Chlorfenvinphos	—	0.002
Diazinon	4	0.002
Dichlorvos	—	0.004
Dimethoate	4	0.02
Fenitrothion	—	0.005
Leptophos	—	—
Malathion	4	0.02
Parathion	6	0.005
Parathion-methyl	5	—
Trichlorfon	4	0.01

*Toxicity rating: Probable human oral lethal dosage for class 4 = 50–500 mg/kg, class 5 = 5–50 mg/kg, and class 6 = < 5 mg/kg. (See Gosselin reference.)
†ADI = acceptable daily intake (mg/kg body weight/d).

compared to the rates observed with the chlorinated hydrocarbon insecticides.

Human Toxicology

In mammals as well as insects, the major effect of these agents is inhibition of acetylcholinesterase, because of phosphorylation of the esteratic site. The signs and symptoms that characterize acute intoxication are due to inhibition of this enzyme, resulting in the accumulation of acetylcholine; some of the agents also possess direct cholinergic activity. These effects and their treatment are described in Chapter 6.

In addition to—and independent of—inhibition of acetylcholinesterase, some of these agents are capable of phosphorylating another enzyme present in neural tissue, the so-called "neurotoxic esterase." This results in development of a delayed neurotoxicity characterized by polyneuropathy, associated with paralysis and axonal degeneration; hens are particularly sensitive to these properties and have proved very useful for studying the pathogenesis of the lesion and for identifying potentially neurotoxic organophosphorus derivatives. In humans, neurotoxicity has been observed with triorthocresyl phosphate (TOCP), a noninsecticidal organophosphorus compound, and is thought to occur with the insecticides merphos, mipafox, trichlorfon, and leptophos. The polyneuropathy usually begins with burning and tingling sensations, particularly in the feet, with motor weakness following a few days later. Sensory and motor difficulties may extend to the legs and hands. Gait is affected, and ataxia may be present. There is no specific treatment for this form of delayed neurotoxicity.

Environmental Toxicology

Organophosphorus insecticides are not considered to be "persistent" pesticides. As a class they are considered to have a small impact on the environment.

3. CARBAMATE INSECTICIDES

These compounds (Table 60–4) inhibit acetylcholinesterase by carbamoylation of the esteratic site. Thus, they possess the toxic properties associated with inhibition of this enzyme as described for the organophosphorus insecticides. The effects and treatment are described in Chapter 6. Generally speaking, the clinical effects due to carbamates are of shorter duration than those observed with organophosphorus compounds. The range between the doses that cause minor intoxication and those which result in lethality is larger with carbamates than that observed with the organophosphorus agents. Spontaneous reactivation of cholinesterase is more rapid after inhibition by the carbamates.

The carbamate insecticides are considered to be "nonpersistent" pesticides in the environment, and they are thought to exert a small impact on the environment.

Table 60–4. Carbamate insecticides.

Compound	Toxicity Rating*	ADI†
Aldicarb	6	0.005
Aminocarb	5	—
Carbaryl	4	0.01
Carbofuran	5	0.01
Dimetan	4	—
Dimetilan	4	—
Isolan	5	—
Methomyl	5	—
Propoxur	4	0.02
Pyramat	4	—
Pyrolan	5	—
Zectran	5	—

*Toxicity rating: Probable human oral lethal dosage for class 4 = 50–500 mg/kg, class 5 = 5–50 mg/kg, and class 6 = < 5 mg/kg. (See Gosselin reference.)

†ADI = acceptable daily intake (mg/kg body weight/d).

4. BOTANICAL INSECTICIDES

Insecticides derived from natural sources include **nicotine, rotenone,** and **pyrethrum.** Nicotine is obtained from the dried leaves of *N tabacum* and *N rustica.* It is rapidly absorbed from mucosal surfaces; the free alkaloid, but not the salt, is readily absorbed from the skin. Nicotine reacts with the acetylcholine receptor of the postsynaptic membrane (sympathetic, parasympathetic ganglia, neuromuscular junction), resulting in depolarization of the membrane. Toxic dosages cause stimulation rapidly followed by blockade of transmission. These actions are described in Chapter 6. Treatment is directed toward maintenance of vital signs and suppression of convulsions.

Rotenone is obtained from *Derris elliptica, Derris mallaccensis, Lonchocarpus utilis,* and *Lonchocarpus urucu.* The oral ingestion of rotenone produces gastrointestinal irritation. Conjunctivitis, dermatitis, pharyngitis, and rhinitis can also occur. Treatment is symptomatic.

Pyrethrum consists of 6 known insecticidal esters: pyrethrin I, pyrethrin II, cinerin I, cinerin II, jasmolin I, and jasmolin II. Pyrethrum may be absorbed after inhalation or ingestion; absorption from the skin is not significant. The esters are extensively biotransformed. The major site of toxic action is the central nervous system; excitation, convulsions, and tetanic paralysis can occur by a mechanism resembling that of DDT. Treatment is with anticonvulsants. The most frequent injury reported in humans results from the allergenic properties of the substance. Contact dermatitis is the most frequently observed manifestation.

HERBICIDES

1. CHLOROPHENOXY HERBICIDES

2,4-Dichlorophenoxyacetic acid (2,4-D), 2,4,5-trichlorophenoxyacetic acid (2,4,5-T), and their salts and esters are the major compounds of interest as herbicides used for the destruction of weeds. They have been assigned toxicity ratings of 4 or 3, respectively, which place the probable human lethal dosages at 50–500 or 500–5000 mg/kg, respectively. (See Gosselin reference.)

In humans, 2,4-D in large doses can cause coma and generalized muscle hypotonia. Rarely, muscle weakness and marked myotonia may persist for several weeks. With 2,4,5-T, coma may occur, but the muscular dysfunction is less evident. In laboratory animals, signs of liver and kidney dysfunction have also been reported. The toxicologic profile for these agents, particularly with 2,4,5-T, has been confusing because of the presence of chemical contaminants (**dioxins**) produced during the manufacturing process. The presence of 2,3,7,8-tetrachlorodibenzo-*p*-dioxin (TCDD) is believed to be largely responsible for the teratogenic effects detected in some animal species as well as the contact dermatitis and chloracne observed in workers involved in the manufacture of 2,4,5-T. In spite of exhaustive studies, no long-term toxic effects of TCDD have been documented in humans. With pure 2,4-D and 2,4,5-T, documentation of long-term effects is also lacking.

2. BIPYRIDYL HERBICIDES

Paraquat is the most important agent of this class. It has been given a toxicity rating of 4, which places the probable human lethal dosage at 50–500 mg/kg. A number of lethal human intoxications (accidental or suicidal) have been reported.

In humans, the first signs and symptoms are attributable to gastrointestinal irritation (hematemesis and bloody stools). Within a few days, however, respiratory distress may appear (delayed toxicity) with the development of congestive hemorrhagic pulmonary edema accompanied by widespread cellular proliferation. Evidence of hepatic, renal, or myocardial involvement may also be present. The interval between ingestion and death may be several weeks. Because of the delayed pulmonary toxicity, prompt removal of paraquat from the digestive tract is important. Gastric lavage, the use of cathartics, and the use of adsorbents to prevent further absorption have all been advocated; after absorption, treatment is successful in fewer than 50% of cases.

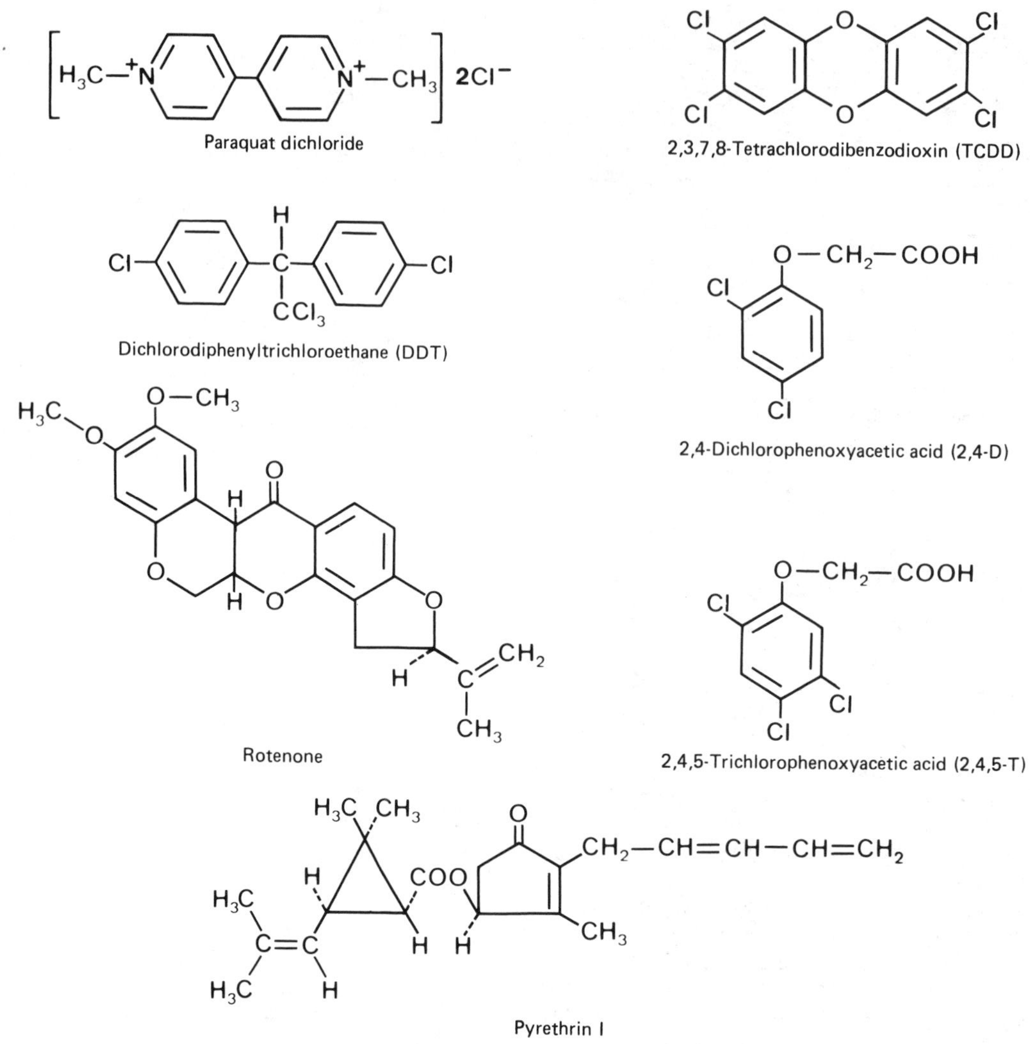

Figure 60–1. Chemical structures of selected agents.

ENVIRONMENTAL POLLUTANTS

The **polychlorinated biphenyls (PCBs)** have been used in a large variety of applications as dielectric and heat transfer fluids, plasticizers, wax extenders, and flame retardants. Their industrial use and manufacture in the USA was terminated by 1977. Unfortunately, they persist in the environment. The products used commercially were actually mixtures of PCB isomers and homologs containing 12–68% chlorine. These chemicals are highly stable and highly liphophilic, poorly metabolized, very resistant to environmental degradation, and bioaccumulate in food chains. Food is the major source of PCB residues in humans.

A serious exposure to PCBs, lasting several months, occurred in Japan as a result of cooking oil contamination with PCB-containing transfer medium (Yusho disease). It is now known that the contami-

nated cooking oil contained not only PCBs but also polychlorinated dibenzofurans (PCDFs) and polychlorinated quaterphenyls (PCQs). Consequently, the effects that were initially attributed to the presence of PCBs are now thought to have been largely caused by the other contaminants. Workers occupationally exposed to PCBs have exhibited the following clinical signs: dermatologic problems (chloracne, folliculitis, erythema, dryness, rash, hyperkeratosis, hyperpigmentation), some hepatic involvement, and elevated plasma triglycerides. Effects on reproduction and development, as well as carcinogenic effects, have yet to be established in humans, even though some subjects have been exposed to very high levels of PCBs. The bulk of the evidence from human studies indicates that PCBs pose little hazard to human health except in situations where food is contaminated with high concentrations of these congeners.

REFERENCES

General

Doull J, Klaassen CD, Amdur MO: *Casarett and Doull's Toxicology,* 2nd ed. Macmillan, 1980.

Loomis TA: *Essentials of Toxicology,* 3rd ed. Lea & Febiger, 1978.

Lu FC: *Basic Toxicology: Fundamentals, Target Organs, and Risk Assessment.* Hemisphere, 1985.

Air Pollution

Amdur MO: Air pollutants. Pages 608–611 in: *Casarett and Doull's Toxicology,* 2nd ed. Doull J, Klaassen CD, Amdur MO (editors). Macmillan, 1980.

Occupational Toxicology

Proctor NH, Hughes JP: *Chemical Hazards of the Workplace.* Lippincott, 1978.

Environmental Toxicology & Ecotoxicology

Butler GC: *Principles of Ecotoxicology.* Wiley, 1978.

Kimbrough RD: Studies in defined populations exposed to PCBs and related chemicals. *Environ Health Perspect* 1984;**59**:99.

Moriarty F: *Ecotoxicology.* Academic Press, 1983.

Plaa GL: Present status: Toxic substances in the environment. *Can J Physiol Pharmacol* 1982;**60**:1010.

Reggiani G, Bruppacher R: Symptoms, signs and findings in humans exposed to PCBs and their derivatives. *Environ Health Perspect* 1985;**60**:225.

Smeets J: New challenges to ecotoxicology. *Ecotoxicol Environ Safety* 1979;**3**:116.

Truhaut R: Ecotoxicology: Objectives, principles and perspectives. *Ecotoxicol Environ Safety* 1977;**1**:151.

Pesticides

Hayes WJ Jr: *Pesticides Studied in Man.* Williams & Wilkins, 1982.

Hayes WJ Jr: *Toxicology of Pesticides.* Williams & Wilkins, 1975.

Clinical Toxicology

Arena JM: *Poisoning,* 4th ed. Thomas, 1979.

Gosselin RE et al: *Clinical Toxicology of Commercial Products,* 4th ed. Williams & Wilkins, 1976.

61

Chelators & Heavy Metal Intoxication

Maria Almira Correia, PhD, & Charles E. Becker, MD

Heavy metals in the environment have posed a hazard to biologic organisms since life began. Some of the oldest diseases of humans can be traced to heavy metal poisoning associated with the development of metal mining, refining, and use. Even with the present recognition of the hazards of heavy metals, the incidence of intoxication remains significant and the need for effective therapy remains high.

I. PHARMACOLOGY OF CHELATORS

Chelating agents are the most versatile and effective antidotes for metal intoxication. These compounds are usually flexible molecules with 2 or more electronegative groups that form stable coordinate-covalent bonds with the cationic metal atom. The complexes thus formed are then excreted by the body. The action of these drugs provides an excellent application of the principle of chemical antagonism.

The efficiency of the chelator is partly determined by the number of ligands available for metal binding. Edetate (ethylenediamine-tetraacetate, Fig 61–1) is an important example. The greater the number of these ligands, the more stable the metal-chelator complex. Depending on the number of metal-ligand bonds, the complex may be referred to as mono-, bi-, or polydentate. The chelating ligands include functional groups such as –OH, –SH, and –NH, which can donate electrons for coordination with the metal. Such bonding effectively prevents interaction of the metal with similar functional groups of enzymes, coenzymes, cellular nucleophiles, and membranes. Unfortunately, chelators are often nonspecific and may chelate essential metals such as Ca^{2+} and Zn^{2+}, which are vital for body function. Such interactions are determined by the relative affinities of the toxic metal and the essential metal for the chelator. Thus, the toxicity associated with administration of some chelators may be associated with chelation of essential metals. This problem may be circumvented by judicious administration of the essential metal along with the chelating agent.

The relative efficacy of various chelators in facilitating excretion of metals from the body is also deter-

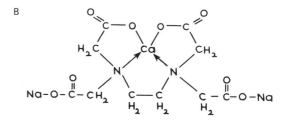

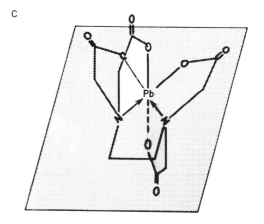

Figure 61–1. Salt and chelate formation with ethylenediamine-tetraacetate (EDTA). *A:* In a solution of the disodium salt of EDTA, the sodium and hydrogen ions are chemically and biologically available. *B:* In solutions of calcium disodium edetate, calcium is bound by coordinate-covalent bonds with nitrogens as well as by the usual ionic bonds. Calcium ions are effectively removed from solution. *C:* In the lead-edetate chelate, lead is incorporated into 5 heterocyclic rings. (Modified and reproduced, with permission, from Meyers FH, Jawetz E, Goldfien A: *Review of Medical Pharmacology,* 7th ed. Lange, 1980.)

mined in part by the pharmacokinetics of the chelator in vivo. For any significant metal sequestration to occur, the affinity of the metal for the chelator must be greater than its affinity for endogenous ligands, and the relative rate of exchange of the metal between the endogenous ligands and the chelator must be faster than the rate of elimination of the chelator. If a chelator is eliminated more rapidly than the dissociation of the metal–endogenous ligand complex, it may not be present in sufficient concentrations for effective competition with the endogenous binding sites. This would be particularly critical if sequestration occurred via a ternary complex (endogenous ligand–metal–exogenous chelator). The above considerations also dictate that efficient mobilization can be accomplished only when the physiologic distribution of the chelator is the body compartment containing the metal. Following absorption, the tissue distribution profile of the metal may change markedly with time. For example, lead is first distributed to soft tissue such as bone marrow, liver, kidneys, and testes. Distribution to bone occurs subsequently. Therefore, the choice of chelator may also be determined on the basis of its distribution to primary and secondary tissue sites. Combination therapy with 2 or more chelating agents, each capable of permeating different target tissue compartments, may prove useful.

SPECIFIC AGENTS

BIDENTATE

DIMERCAPROL
(2,3-Dimercaptopropanol)

Dimercaprol (BAL) (Fig 61–2) is a colorless oily liquid with an offensive odor of rotten eggs. It is soluble in water, but aqueous solutions are unstable and oxidize readily. Dimercaprol is therefore dispensed in 10% solution in peanut oil and must be administered intramuscularly. It interacts directly with metals in blood and tissue fluids and reactivates cellular sulfhydryl-containing enzymes. However, it is most efficient if administered immediately following exposure to the metals. This indicates that its salutary effects may be due primarily to *prevention* of metal binding to cellular constituents rather than *removal* of metal already bound.

Indications & Toxicity
Dimercaprol is a useful antidote in arsenic, mercury, and lead poisoning. Given intramuscularly, it is readily absorbed, metabolized, and excreted by the kidney within 4 hours. It produces a variety of side effects of which the cardiovascular (hypertension and tachycardia) are most significant. It also causes head-

ache, nausea, vomiting, lacrimation, salivation, paresthesias, and pain. Because of the high incidence of these untoward side effects, several congeners are currently being investigated. One of them is the 2,3-dimercaptopropane-1-sulfonate (DMPS), which, owing to its relatively greater polarity, may remain confined to the extracellular space to a greater extent and thus reduce cellular toxicity. However, for the same reason, its relative efficacy as compared to dimercaprol may also prove to be inferior. A second analog is 2,3-dimercaptosuccinic acid (DMSA), which has been found to be relatively less toxic than dimercaprol and effective by the oral route (see Aposhian reference).

PENICILLAMINE
(D-β,β-Dimethylcysteine)

Penicillamine (Cuprimine) (Fig 61–2) is a white crystalline, water-soluble product of degradation of penicillin. The D isomer is relatively nontoxic compared to the L form and consequently is the preferred form of the antidote. Penicillamine is readily absorbed from the gut and is resistant to metabolic degradation. Greater resistance to metabolic degradation has also been achieved by N-acetylation, as in N-acetylpenicillamine.

Indications & Toxicity
Penicillamine is used chiefly for poisoning with copper or to prevent copper accumulation, as in Wilson's disease. It is also used as adjunctive therapy in the treatment of lead and arsenic poisoning.

Pyridoxine deficiency is a frequent toxic effect of other forms of the drug but is rarely seen with the D form. Acute allergic reactions, especially in patients allergic to penicillin, may preclude the continued use of the drug. Nephrotoxicity with proteinuria has also been reported and with protracted use of the drug may result in renal insufficiency. Bone marrow toxicity resulting in aplastic anemia has been associated with prolonged drug intake. Autoimmune diseases, including lupus erythematosus and hemolytic anemia have been reported also.

POLYDENTATE

EDETATE CALCIUM DISODIUM

Ethylenediamine-tetraacetic acid (EDTA, Versenate) (Fig 61–1) is an efficient chelator of many divalent and trivalent metals in vitro. However, chelation of essential calcium in vivo—due to this very property—limits its clinical use. This limitation has been partially circumvented by administration of its calcium disodium salt.

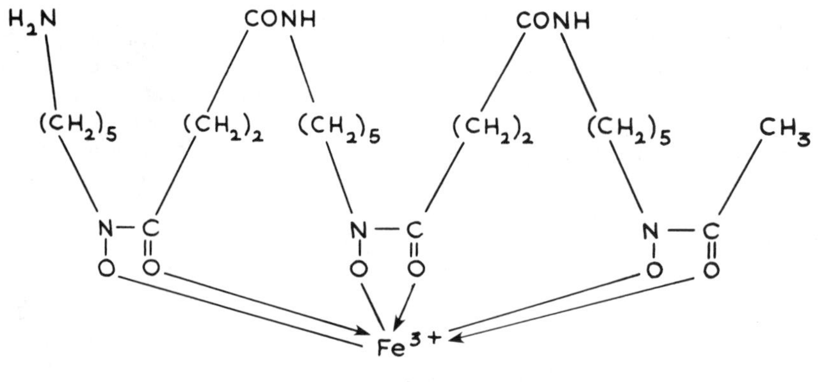

Ferroxamine

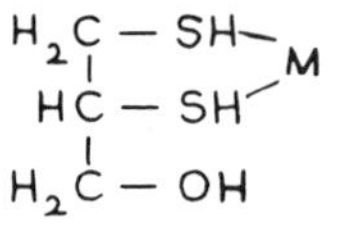

Dimercaprol
(2,3-dimercaptopropanol)

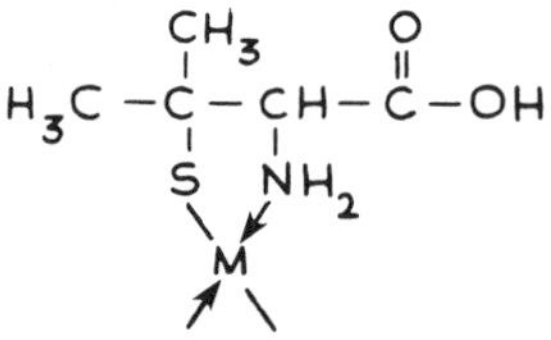

Penicillamine
(D-β,β-dimethylcysteine)

Figure 61–2. Chemical structures of several metal chelates. Ferroxamine without the chelated ions is deferoxamine. It is represented here to show the functional groups; the iron is actually held in a caged system. Dimercaprol incorporates the metal into a stable heterocyclic ring by covalent bonding. A single molecule of copper or other metal may be held by 2 molecules of penicillamine. M = metal molecules. (Modified and reproduced, with permission, from Meyers FH, Jawetz E, Goldfien A: *Review of Medical Pharmacology*, 7th ed. Lange, 1980.)

EDTA penetrates cell membranes relatively poorly, thus serving primarily as an extracellular rather than an intracellular chelator.

The highly polar ionic character of EDTA precludes significant oral absorption, and consequently the chelator (calcium disodium salt) is administered either by slow intravenous infusion or intramuscularly. It is excreted by glomerular filtration in the urine almost completely unchanged over 24 hours. Therefore its effect (including renal toxicity; see below) may be prolonged in patients in renal failure.

Indications & Toxicity

Metals such as lead and a few other heavy metals capable of binding EDTA and displacing Ca^{2+} are effectively chelated. EDTA-induced mobilization of mercury, in contrast to that of lead, is unsuccessful, perhaps owing to the relatively poor distribution of the chelator into tissue compartments where mercury is found as well as to the less successful competition of mercury with the chelated calcium.

EDTA is toxic to the kidney, and the renal tubules appear relatively sensitive to its toxic effects, which include hydropic degeneration of the proximal tubules, progressing into total destruction. Mild effects disappear with cessation of therapy. Other (rare) toxic effects include chills, fever, nausea, vomiting, myalgia, allergic reactions, and glycosuria.

TRIENTINE

Trientine (trien, Cuprid) is a polydentate chelating agent that has affinity for copper and is useful in the treatment of Wilson's disease (hepatolenticular degeneration). It has recently been approved for use in the USA. Early reports suggest that it may be less toxic than penicillamine in this application.

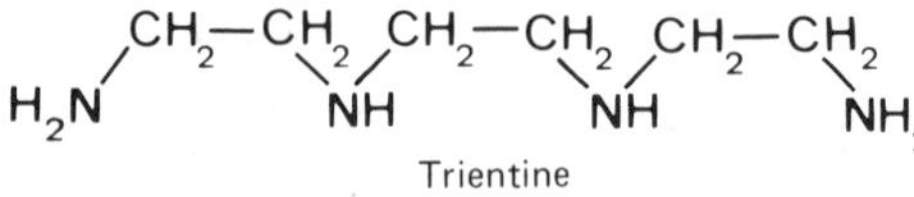

Trientine

DEFEROXAMINE

Deferoxamine mesylate (Desferal) is isolated from *Streptomyces pilosus*. It binds iron avidly but essential trace metals poorly. Furthermore, while competing for loosely bound iron in iron-carrying proteins (hemosiderin and ferritin), it fails to compete with biologically chelated iron, as in microsomal and mitochondrial cytochromes and hemoproteins. Consequently, it is the chelator of choice for iron poisoning. Recent studies suggest that it may also be useful in the treatment of aluminum toxicity induced by chronic dialysis.

Deferoxamine is poorly absorbed when administered orally. To be effective, it must be administered intramuscularly or intravenously. It is believed to be metabolized, but the pathways are unknown. The products are excreted almost completely in the urine. Intravenous administration may result in hypotensive shock owing to histamine release, especially if given rapidly.

Use of deferoxamine in iron poisoning is described in Chapter 31.

II. TOXICOLOGY OF HEAVY METALS

LEAD

The toxic effects of lead probably constitute the oldest occupational disease in the world. Lead is now widely distributed in air, food, and water, so that a completely lead-free environment would be difficult or impossible to achieve. With a greater understanding of the kinetics and toxicology of lead, acute lead poisoning is fortunately much less frequent than in the past. Hazardous working conditions have been improved, exposure of children to flaking lead-base paints has been reduced, and adult exposure to illicit whiskey and battery casings is less frequent (see Annest reference). However, important public health questions remain concerning environmental pollution and the hazard to reproductive, hematopoietic, and neurologic function imposed by chronic lead exposure.

Pharmacokinetics

Metallic lead is slowly but consistently absorbed by all routes except through the skin. *Organic* lead compounds are well absorbed through the skin. Absorption of lead dust via the respiratory tract is the most common cause of industrial poisoning. The intestinal tract is the primary route of entry in nonindustrial exposure (Table 61–1). Absorption via the gastrointestinal tract varies with the nature of the lead compound, but in general, about 10% of ingested inorganic lead is absorbed. Dietary calcium, iron, and phosphorus may alter gastrointestinal lead absorption. Studies in laboratory animals demonstrate that a diet low in calcium increases lead retention and that there are associated biochemical and morphologic manifestations of enhanced lead toxicity.

Once absorbed from the respiratory or gastrointestinal tract, lead is bound to erythrocytes and widely distributed initially to soft tissues such as bone marrow, liver, kidney, and testes. Its half-life in these tissues is about 30 days. Lead also crosses the placenta and poses a potential hazard to the fetus. Most lead entering the body is eventually bound in the skeleton; the half-life of elimination from bone is in excess of 20 years. Lead is also bound in hair and nails, which could theoretically be a useful method of estimating the body burden. However, external contamination creates special problems in interpreting these levels. Ingested lead is excreted in the stool (over 90%) and urine. Most of the absorbed lead is excreted via renal elimination. Lead is also eliminated through sweat and in mother's milk.

Pharmacodynamics

Lead is capable of forming complex ligands with many compounds. It interferes with the activity of enzymes and affects a variety of organ systems.

A. Blood: The organ system most sensitive to lead is the hematopoietic system. Hypochromic microcytic anemia is common, but not all patients with lead poisoning are anemic. Lead induces critical derangements in heme biosynthesis, leading to excretion of porphyrins and their precursors in urine. The enzymes most sensitive to lead inhibition are delta-aminolevulinic acid dehydratase and ferrochelatase. Inhibition of the first enzyme blocks conversion of delta-aminolevulinic acid to porphobilinogen. Delta-aminolevulinic acid is excreted in the urine, and the urine concentration can be used as a diagnostic test. Inhibition of ferrochelatase results in decreased production of heme and accumulation of its precursor, protoporphyrin IX. In addition, the shortened life span of erythrocytes contributes to lead-induced anemia.

B. Nervous System: Lead also affects the peripheral and central nervous systems. The lowest concentration of lead associated with neurologic damage is still uncertain. Even at very high blood levels and marked alterations of hematopoietic function, some individuals may have no neurologic manifestations. The most common sign of peripheral neuropathy is painless weakness of the extensor muscles of the hand (wristdrop). The lower limb is less often involved. Sensory function is usually not affected. Lead-induced neuropathy usually develops after months of chronic exposure but may occur subacutely in 2–3 weeks.

Lead encephalopathy is an important acute disorder usually seen in children who have eaten lead-base paints. It is rare in adults. Encephalopathy most often begins with convulsions and is associated with increased intracranial pressure and brain edema. The mortality rate is high, and urgent chelation therapy is required.

C. Kidneys: Lead may cause kidney damage. Acutely, lead may affect uric acid metabolism and cause both acute gout and gouty nephropathy. Lead nephropathy itself develops only after years of prolonged lead exposure. Recent studies suggest that renal damage, hypertension, or both in adults may result from childhood lead exposure.

D. Reproductive Organs: Lead also affects reproductive function. It has long been known that lead poisoning is associated with decreased fertility in women and an increased incidence of stillbirths. Little is known about the effects of lead on male reproductive function, though sterility and testicular atrophy have been noted in severe cases, and asymptomatic lead exposure has been associated with dose-related alteration of sperm.

Table 61–1. Toxicology of lead, mercury, and arsenic.

	Form Entering Body	Route of Absorption	Distribution	Target Organs for Toxicity	Metabolism	Elimination
Lead	Inorganic lead oxides and salts.	Gastrointestinal, respiratory, skin (minor).	Bone (90%), teeth, hair, blood (erythrocytes), liver, kidney.	Hematopoietic tissues and liver, CNS, kidney, neuromuscular junction.	Dissociation and binding of lead to critical tissue sulfhydryl groups.	Urine and feces (major); sweat (minor).
	Organic (tetraethyl lead).	Skin (major), gastrointestinal.	Liver.	CNS.	Hepatic dealkylation (fast) → trialkylmetabolites (slow) → dissociation to lead.	Urine and feces (major); sweat (minor).
Mercury	Elemental mercury.	Respiratory tract.	CNS (where it is trapped as Hg^{2+}), kidney (following conversion of elemental Hg to Hg^{2+}).	CNS (neuropsychiatric due to elemental Hg and its Hg^{2+} metabolite), kidney (substantial due to conversion of elemental Hg to Hg^{2+}).	Elemental Hg converted to Hg^{2+}.	Urine (major); feces (minor).
	Inorganic: Hg^+ (less toxic); Hg^{2+} (more toxic).	Gastrointestinal, skin (minor).	Kidney (predominant), blood, brain (minor).	Kidney, GI.	Hg^{2+} plus R–SH converted to Hg^+–S–R, $Hg(S-R)_2$.	Urine.
	Organic: alkyl, aryl, alkoxyalkyl.	Gastrointestinal, skin (substantial).	Kidney, brain, blood.	CNS.	$R-Hg^+$ converted to Hg^{2+} plus R (slow).	Urine.
Arsenic	Inorganic arsenic salts.	Gastrointestinal, skin, respiratory (all mucous surfaces).	Red cells (95–99% bound to globin) (24 hours); then to liver, lung, kidney, wall of gastrointestinal tract, spleen, muscle, nerve tissue (2 weeks); then to skin, hair, and bone (years).	Increased vascular permeability leading to vasodilatation and vascular collapse. Uncoupling of oxidative phosphorylation resulting in impaired cellular metabolism.	Binds avidly to cellular sulfhydryl groups of various critical enzymes to form stable cyclic thioarsenicals. Substitutes for inorganic phosphorus in synthesis of high-energy phosphates.	Principally renal. Sweat and feces minor.

E. Gastrointestinal Tract: Lead poisoning may cause loss of appetite, epigastric distress, abdominal colicky pains, and constipation. The mechanism of lead colic is unclear but involves contraction of smooth muscles of the intestinal wall. The gastrointestinal symptoms are reversible with chelation therapy.

Major Forms of Lead Intoxication
A. Inorganic Lead Poisoning:
1. Acute–Acute inorganic lead poisoning is very uncommon. It usually results from industrial inhalation of large quantities of lead oxide or, in small children, from ingestion of a large oral dose of lead in lead-based paints. Acute intoxication is associated with severe gastrointestinal distress that progresses to marked central nervous system abnormalities and anemia. If absorption of lead is slower, abdominal colic and encephalopathy may develop over days. The diagnosis of acute inorganic lead poisoning may be difficult. Disorders that simulate lead poisoning include appendicitis, peptic ulcer, and pancreatitis.

2. Chronic–The most common manifestations of chronic inorganic lead poisoning are weakness, anorexia, nervousness, tremor, weight loss, headache, and gastrointestinal symptoms. The association of re-

current abdominal pain and extensor muscle weakness without sensory disturbances suggests the possibility of lead poisoning. The most characteristic neurologic finding in chronic lead poisoning is wristdrop.

The diagnosis is confirmed by measuring lead in the blood and identifying abnormalities of porphyrin metabolism. The zinc erythrocyte protoporphyrin test is especially valuable if iron deficiency anemia can be ruled out. Peripheral blood smears may show basophilic stippling. Lead deposits in long bones are uncommon, as are lead lines on the gums.

Treatment is discussed below.

B. Organic Lead Poisoning: Organic lead poisoning is usually caused by tetraethyl or tetramethyl lead, which is used as an "antiknock" agent in gasoline. Organic lead is highly volatile and lipid-soluble. Thus, it can be readily absorbed through the skin and respiratory tract. Severe poisoning has resulted from deliberate "sniffing" of gasoline. Acute central nervous system disorders result. These can progress rapidly, causing hallucinations, insomnia, headache, and irritability (similar to severe alcohol withdrawal). Organic lead causes relatively few hematologic abnormalities. Tetraethyl and tetramethyl lead are metabolized by the liver to trialkyl lead and inorganic lead.

Trialkyl lead is thought to be responsible for the acute poisoning syndrome. Chronic poisoning with organic lead is fortunately uncommon. Most organic lead exposures occur in the course of cleaning gasoline storage tanks. With massive organic lead exposure, seizures may terminate in coma and death. Blood and urine lead levels are relatively unreliable in organic lead poisoning but may be elevated.

Treatment is discussed below.

Treatment

A. Inorganic Lead Poisoning: Treatment of inorganic lead poisoning involves immediate termination of exposure and use of chelation therapy. The more severe the symptoms, the more urgent the need for chelation therapy. For severe intoxication, use an intravenous infusion of calcium disodium EDTA in a dose of approximately 8 mg/kg; dimercaprol, 2.5 mg/kg/dose intramuscularly, may also be given. Blood and urine levels of lead should be monitored as a guide to therapy. For less severe acute intoxication, chronic therapy with penicillamine (Cuprimine), 1 g over 24 hours orally in divided doses, may be repeated until blood and urine lead levels are reduced. Treating asymptomatic patients with chelating agents is not recommended. Prophylactic use of chelating agents in workers exposed to lead is contraindicated. After discontinuing chelation therapy, blood lead and porphyrin function should be assessed by serial analysis in order to identify a rebound increase in lead as lead is mobilized from bone.

B. Organic Lead Poisoning: Initial treatment consists of decontaminating the skin and preventing further exposure. Treatment of seizures requires judicious use of anticonvulsants.

ARSENIC

Elemental arsenic and arsenic compounds are widely distributed in nature. Arsenic is a common contaminant of coal and of many metal ores, especially copper, lead, and zinc. The 2 largest sources of industrial arsenic are coal-burning power plants and smelters. Approximately 1.5 million employees in the USA are potentially exposed to arsenic compounds.

The chemical forms of arsenic of toxicologic importance are elemental arsenic, inorganic arsenic, organic arsenicals, and arsine gas (AsH_3).

Arsenic was used as both a therapeutic agent and poison in ancient Greek and Roman times. More recently (until the advent of penicillin), arsenic was used in the treatment of syphilis and as a tonic in Fowler's solution. Its only therapeutic use today is in the treatment of trypanosomiasis involving the central nervous system. The most common nonmedical uses of arsenic compounds are as insecticides, herbicides, fungicides, algicides, and wood preservatives. Arsenic is also used for doping semiconductors, alloying, and in glassmaking.

Pharmacokinetics

Environmental and dietary exposure to arsenic and its compounds is possible, since arsenic is present in ocean water, especially near the mouths of estuaries draining industrial areas. Alcoholic beverages when improperly prepared occasionally contain large amounts of arsenic. Many types of seafood contain high levels of pentavalent arsenic. These environmental contaminants may account for elevated urinary arsenic levels. The average daily intake of arsenic from environmental sources is less than 1 mg. The total body burden of arsenic in adults is about 20 mg, mostly in bone and to a lesser extent in hair and skin. Inorganic arsenic can be absorbed from the lungs, the gut, and rarely through intact skin (Table 61–1).

Gastrointestinal absorption of arsenic compounds is a function of their water solubility. Trivalent arsenites are poorly soluble and pentavalent arsenates more soluble. Organic arsenicals are usually poorly absorbed from the gastrointestinal tract. Arsenic can cross the placenta and may cause fetal damage. The trivalent form of arsenic is excreted slowly, chiefly by the fecal route, whereas the pentavalent form is more rapidly excreted in urine in a methylated form. Absorption of arsenic through the skin is a function of lipid solubility, with the trivalent form being more lipid-soluble than the pentavalent form. Trivalent inorganic arsenicals are partially oxidized in the body to the pentavalent form, and some is methylated.

Pharmacodynamics

All of the major toxicologic effects of inorganic arsenical compounds are attributable to the trivalent form of arsenic. Trivalent arsenic inhibits sulfhydryl enzymes and is corrosive to epithelium lining the respiratory and gastrointestinal tracts, to skin, and to other tissues. The primary target organs for trivalent arsenic are the nervous system, bone marrow, liver, skin, and respiratory tract.

Major Forms of Arsenic Intoxication

A. Acute and Subacute Inorganic Arsenic Poisoning: Acute and subacute forms of inorganic arsenic poisoning may produce acute violent nausea, vomiting, abdominal pain, skin irritation, laryngitis, and bronchitis. The gastroenteritis may be so severe as to be hemorrhagic. A sweet metallic garlicky odor is imparted to breath and feces. Vomiting may be severe, and diarrhea may be characterized as "rice water stool." The trivalent form of arsenic also damages capillaries, causing increased permeability, dehydration, shock, and death. If patients survive the acute episodes, bone marrow depression, encephalopathy, and a crippling sensory neuropathy may follow.

Treatment of acute arsenic poisoning includes induction of emesis or gastric lavage, correction of dehydration and electrolyte imbalance, and supportive care for liver and other tissue injury. In severe cases, give also immediate chelation therapy with dimercaprol, 3–5 mg/kg intramuscularly every 4 hours for 48 hours. Dimercaprol is continued every 12 hours for

10 days while monitoring urinary excretion of arsenic. Occasionally, oral penicillamine therapy may be used as an adjunctive measure if dimercaprol injections cause intolerable pain.

B. Chronic Inorganic Arsenic Poisoning: Chronic inorganic arsenic poisoning may present as perforation of the nasal septum, irritation of the skin, sensory neuropathy, hair loss, bone marrow depression, fatty infiltration of the liver, or renal damage. The skin manifestations include cutaneous vasodilatation and pallor (from anemia), resulting in a characteristic "milk and roses" complexion. Prolonged arsenic exposure may lead to hyperkeratosis of the palms and soles, increased skin pigmentation, hair loss, and white lines over the nails. Patients may become cachectic owing to chronic nausea and gastrointestinal complaints. Conjunctivitis and irritation of the mucous membranes, larynx, and respiratory passages are common.

Laboratory diagnosis of inorganic arsenic poisoning may be difficult. Urinary arsenic measurements and hair and nail analyses are indications of exposure but not intoxication. Urinary arsenic levels are influenced by intake of seafood. Most unexposed persons taking an average amount of seafood in the diet will excrete less than 100 μg of arsenic per 24 hours in the urine. Laboratory evidence of bone marrow suppression, abnormal liver function tests, proteinuria, and hematuria may also be diagnostically useful.

C. Organic Arsenic Poisoning: Organic arsenical poisoning is rare. Organic arsenicals are absorbed to a varying extent depending on their valences and are usually rapidly excreted. Benzene arsenicals are not converted to inorganic arsenic compounds under most circumstances. The mechanism of organic arsenical toxicity involves inhibition of sulfhydryl enzymes, especially in the central nervous system. Cerebral lesions are occasionally observed in both gray and white matter.

D. Arsine Gas Poisoning: Arsine gas (AsH_3) is one of the most powerful hemolytic agents known. It is absorbed primarily through inhalation. Arsine combines with hemoglobin and is oxidized to a hemolytic compound. Dramatic destruction of red blood cells leads to hemoglobinuria, causing acute renal failure. Extensive renal tubular damage occurs, along with thickening of glomerular basement membranes. Initial symptoms are dark urine, jaundice, and severe abdominal pain. Severe arsine exposure will lead to high arsenic levels in the urine. Laboratory findings consist of hemolysis and severe anemia. Chelation therapy is generally not useful to prevent red cell destruction. Supportive care, including exchange transfusion and hemodialysis for renal failure, determines the outcome with acute arsine poisoning.

E. Other Manifestations of Arsenic Poisoning: Increased incidence of skin cancer is recognized in patients undergoing prolonged treatment for psoriasis and other skin disease with inorganic arsenicals, especially Fowler's solution. A study of smelter workers in the USA suggests an increased risk of respiratory system cancer that is probably dose-related. Since smelter workers have multiple exposures and confounding variables for enhanced risk of respiratory cancer, further studies are required to define the risk. Attempts to demonstrate the carcinogenic potential of arsenic compounds in animals have generally been unrewarding. Mutagenic testing, especially with the Ames test, has failed to show any mutagenic effects of arsenic compounds.

MERCURY

Metallic mercury as "quicksilver"—the only metal that is liquid under ordinary conditions—has attracted scholarly and scientific interest from earliest times. It was quickly recognized that the mining of mercury was hazardous to health. As industrial uses of mercury became common during the past 200 years, new forms of toxicity were recognized that were found to be associated with inorganic compounds of the element or with the metal itself. In 1953, a mysterious epidemic occurred in the Japanese fishing village of Minamata. The village is located near the effluent of a large factory in which vinyl plastic is manufactured. The epidemic of poisoning was traced to the consumption of fish contaminated by the effluent discharged by the factory. The causative agent was methylmercury, formed in ocean water by bacterial action on inorganic mercury from the effluent.

The main sources of inorganic mercury as a toxic hazard include materials used in dental laboratories, wood preservatives, herbicides, insecticides, spermicidal jellies, fireworks, batteries, thermometers, barometers, gauges, and preparations of chlorine and sodium hydroxide. Organic mercury compounds are used as seed dressings, as fungicides, and in preventing mold.

Pharmacokinetics

The absorption of mercury varies considerably depending on the chemical form of the metal. Elementary mercury is poorly absorbed from the gastrointestinal tract but is quite volatile and can be absorbed from the lungs (Table 61–1). Inhaled mercury is the primary source of occupational exposure. Organic short-chain alkyl mercury compounds are volatile and potentially harmful by the same route. After absorption, mercury is distributed to the tissues in a few hours, with the highest concentration occurring in the proximal renal tubules. Mercury is readily bound to sulfhydryl groups. Excretion of mercury is primarily through the urine, although some is removed through the gastrointestinal tract and the sweat glands. Most inorganic mercury gaining entrance into the body is excreted over a 1-week period, but the kidney and the brain retain mercury for longer periods.

The acute and chronic poisoning syndromes with mercury depend on the form of the metal. Oral metallic mercury has little effect. Oral mercurous chloride has relatively low toxicity. Mercuric chloride is very toxic and causes acute kidney damage. Organic mercurials, especially methyl mercury, are more completely absorbed from the gastrointestinal tract. The short-chain organic mercury compounds are usually distributed to the central nervous system and are devoid of renal toxicity.

Major Forms of Mercury Intoxication

A. Acute: Acute mercury poisoning most frequently occurs from inhalation of high concentrations of mercury vapor. Symptoms include chest pain and shortness of breath, metallic taste, and nausea and vomiting. Acute damage to the kidney occurs next. If the patient survives, severe gingivitis and gastroenteritis occur on the third to fourth days. In the most severe cases, severe muscle tremor and psychopathology develop.

B. Chronic: Chronic mercury poisoning may be difficult to diagnose. Complaints of mouth and gastrointestinal disorders may be reported, and signs of renal insufficiency may be present. Gingivitis, discolored gums, and loosening of the teeth are common. The salivary glands may be enlarged. Tremor involving the fingers, arms, and legs if often present. Chronic mercury poisoning may also simulate drug intoxication, cerebellar dysfunction, or Wilson's disease. An alteration of handwriting is frequently observed. Ocular changes, including deposition of mercury in the lens, are reported. Personality changes with unusual fearfulness, inability to concentrate, and irritability have been described. This psychologic disorder is known as erethism.

Diagnosis of chronic mercury poisoning depends primarily on a history of exposure. Assays of mercury in the body vary widely, apparently owing to pharmacokinetic factors.

Treatment

A. Acute: Treatment of acute mercury poisoning consists of removal from exposure and chelation treatment with dimercaprol, usually in a dosage of 3–5 mg/kg intramuscularly every 4 hours for 48 hours and then every 12 hours for 10 days. If renal damage occurs, hemodialysis will be required. Oral charcoal therapy is probably not useful in binding mercury in the gastrointestinal tract.

B. Chronic: With chronic mercury poisoning, oral penicillamine or N-acetylpenicillamine (250–500 mg orally 4 times a day for 10 days) is usually required. Urinary mercury levels should be monitored to observe enhanced removal. Treatment of organic mercury poisoning has been poorly studied. Administration of chelating agents requires further study.

REFERENCES

Chelating Agents

Aposhian HV: DMSA and DMPS: Water soluble antidotes for heavy metal poisoning. *Annu Rev Pharmacol Toxicol* 1983; **23**:193.

Brown DJ et al: Treatment of dialysis osteomalacia with desferrioxamine. *Lancet* 1982;**2**:343.

Catsch A, Hartmuth-Hoehne AE: Pharmacology and therapeutic applications of agents used in heavy metal poisoning. *Pharmacol Ther [A]* 1976;**1**:1.

Gordon MH: Penicillamine for treatment of rheumatoid arthritis. *JAMA* 1974;**229**:1342.

Penicillamine: More lessons from experience. *Br Med J* 1975;**3**:120.

Walshe JM: Treatment of Wilson's disease with trientine (triethylene tetramine) dihydrochloride. *Lancet* 1982;**1**:643.

Heavy Metals

Greenhouse AH: Heavy metals and the nervous system. *Clin Neuropharmacol* 1982;**5**:45.

Landrigan PJ: Occupational and community exposures to toxic metals: Lead, cadmium, mercury and arsenic. *West J Med* 1982;**137**:531.

Lead

Annest JL et al: Chronological trend in blood lead levels between 1976 and 1980. *N Engl J Med* 1983;**308**:1373.

Brangstrup-Hanse JP: Chelatable lead burden by calcium disodium EDTA and blood lead concentration in man. *J Occup Med* 1981;**93**:39.

Bushnell PJ, Jaeger RJ: Hazards from environmental lead exposure: A review of recent literature. *Vet Hum Toxicol* 1986;**28**:255.

Chisolm JJ: The continuing hazard of lead exposure and its effects in children. *Neurotoxicology* 1985;**5**:23.

Craswell PW et al: Chronic renal failure with gout: A marker of chronic lead poisoning. *Kidney Int* 1984;**26**:319.

Hernberg SL: Lead in occupational medicine. Chap 30, pp 715–769, in: *Principles and Practical Approach of Occupational Medicine*. Zenz C (editor). Year Book, 1975.

Oheme FW: Mechanism of heavy metal toxicity. *J Clin Toxicol* 1972;**5**:151.

Pirkle JL et al: The relationship between blood lead levels and blood pressure and its cardiovascular risk implication. *Am J Epidemiol* 1985;**121**:246.

Settle DM: Lead in albacore: Guide to lead pollution in America. *Science* 1980:**207**:1167.

Arsenic

Martin DW Jr, Woeber KA: Arsenic poisoning. *Calif Med* (March) 1973;**118**:13.

National Institute of Safety and Health: *Occupational Exposure to Inorganic Arsenic: New Criteria*. US Department of Health, Education, and Welfare Publication No. 75–140, 1975.

Peterson RG, Rumack BH: D-Penicillamine therapy of acute arsenic poisoning. *J Pediatr* 1977;**91**:661.

Mercury

Done AK: The toxic emergency: The many faces of mercurialism. *Emerg Med* (Jan) 1980;**12**:137.

Jung RC, Aaronson J: Death following inhalation of mercury vapor at home. *West J Med* 1980;**132**:539.

Kahn A, Denis R, Blum D: Accidental ingestion of mercuric sulphate in a 4-year-old child. *Clin Pediatr* 1977;**16**:956.

Krohn IT et al: Subcutaneous injection of metallic mercury. *JAMA* 1980;**243:**548.

Roels H et al: Surveillance of workers exposed to mercury vapor: Validation of previously proposed biological threshold limit value for mercury concentration in the urine. *Am J Ind Med* 1985;**7:**45.

Snodgrass W et al: Mercury poisoning from home gold ore processing. *JAMA* 1981;**246:**1929.

Management of the Poisoned Patient

62

Charles E. Becker, MD, & Kent R. Olson, MD

Many thousands of cases of acute poisoning occur each year. Most of the deaths were due to intentional suicidal overdose with a drug or toxic substance. Childhood deaths due to accidental ingestion of a toxic product have been markedly reduced in the past 10 years as a result of safety packaging and effective poisoning prevention education.

In spite of the large number of deaths that occur every year, poisoning is rarely fatal if the victim receives medical attention promptly and good supportive care is given. Careful management of airway obstruction, respiratory failure, hypotension, seizures, and thermoregulatory disturbances has resulted in improved survival of overdosed patients who reach the hospital alive.

This chapter reviews some of the basic principles of poisoning, the pathophysiology of lethal poisoning, initial management of the overdose, diagnosis of toxic syndromes, and specialized treatment of poisoning including methods of increasing the elimination of drugs and toxins.

TOXICOKINETICS & TOXICODYNAMICS

Toxicologic problems are best viewed in a classic pharmacologic model. This model is based on the pharmacologic properties of chemical agents and the effects of "normal" doses on "normal" people. Toxicology extends this information to excessive doses.

The term "toxicokinetics" has been coined to denote the absorption, distribution, excretion, and metabolism of toxins, toxic doses of therapeutic agents, and their metabolites. "Toxicodynamics" can be used to denote the injurious effects of these substances on vital function. Although there are many similarities between the pharmacokinetics and toxicokinetics of most substances, there are also important differences. The same caution applies to pharmacodynamics and toxicodynamics.

SPECIAL ASPECTS OF TOXICOKINETICS

Volume of Distribution

The volume of distribution (V_d) is defined as the "apparent" volume into which a substance is distributed. It is calculated from the dose given and the resulting plasma concentration: V_d = dose/concentration, as described in Chapter 3. If a chemical is highly tissue-bound or otherwise sequestered outside of the plasma, then the plasma concentration will be low and the V_d very large. A large V_d implies that the drug is not readily accessible to measures aimed at purifying the blood, such as hemodialysis.

Clearance

Clearance is a measure of the volume of plasma that is "cleared" of drug per unit time. In order to calculate the rate at which the drug is actually eliminated from the body, one needs to know the volume of distribution. For example, if the clearance of drug A by hemodialysis is 100 mL/min and its V_d is 40 L in an average-sized person, then it will theoretically take 40/0.10 or 400 minutes of dialysis to eliminate all of drug A. In contrast, if drug B has the same clearance but its V_d is 400 L, it would take 4000 minutes (almost 3 days of dialysis) to eliminate it.

The body has intrinsic mechanisms for clearing drugs, and the total clearance is the sum of clearances by excretion by the kidneys, metabolism by the liver, and elimination by sweat, feces, and expired air (see Chapter 3). In planning detoxification strategy, it is important to know the contribution of each organ to total clearance. For example, if a drug is 95% cleared by liver metabolism and only 5% cleared by renal excretion, then even a dramatic increase in urinary output would have little effect on overall elimination.

Overdosage of a drug can alter the usual pharmacokinetic values, and this must be considered when applying kinetics to poisoned patients. For example, dissolution of tablets or gastric emptying time may be altered so that peak effects of the toxin are delayed. Drugs may injure the gastrointestinal tract and thereby alter absorption. If the capacity of the liver to metabolize a drug is exceeded, then more drug will be delivered to the circulation. With a dramatic increase in the concentration of drug in the blood, tissue-binding and protein-binding capacity may be exceeded, resulting in an increased fraction of free drug and a smaller volume of distribution. At normal dosage, most drugs are eliminated at a rate proportionate to the plasma concentration (first-order kinetics). If the plasma concentration is very high and normal metabolism is saturated, the rate of elimination may become fixed (zero-order kinetics). This may markedly prolong the serum half-life.

SPECIAL ASPECTS OF TOXICODYNAMICS

Knowledge of basic pharmacology may also help the physician anticipate important toxicodynamic problems in the diagnosis and management of the intoxicated patient. The general dose-response principles described in Chapter 2 are of crucial importance in determining the severity of the intoxication. When considering **quantal dose-response** data, both the therapeutic index and the overlap of therapeutic and toxic response curves must be considered. The standardized safety margin, if known, takes the latter factor into account. For instance, as shown in Fig 62–1, drugs A and B have the same therapeutic index. However, drug B is much more liable to cause inadvertent intoxication, because its toxic response curve overlaps the therapeutic dose range much more than in the case of drug A. For some drugs, eg, sedative-hypnotics, the major toxic effect is a direct extension of the therapeutic action, as shown by their **graded dose-response curves** (Fig 62–2). In the case of a drug with a flat dose-response curve (drug A), lethal effects may require 100 times the normal therapeutic dose. In contrast, a drug with a steeper curve (drug B) may be lethal at 10 times the normal dose.

For many drugs, at least part of the toxicity may be

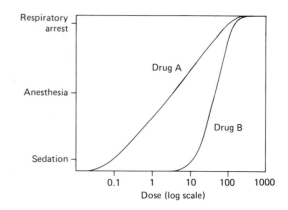

Figure 62–2. Graded dose-response comparison of 2 sedative-hypnotic drugs. A much larger multiple of the normal prescription dose of drug A is required to cause respiratory arrest, ie, it is safer than drug B.

distinct from the therapeutic action yet interact with it. For example, intoxication with drugs that have atropinelike effects (eg, tricyclic antidepressants) will block sweating, making it more difficult to dissipate heat. In tricyclic antidepressant intoxication, there may also be increased muscular activity or seizures; the body's production of heat is thus enhanced, and lethal hyperpyrexia may result. Overdoses of drugs that depress the cardiovascular system, eg, beta-adrenoceptor–blocking agents or barbiturates, can profoundly alter not only target organ function but all functions that are dependent on blood flow. These include renal and hepatic elimination of the toxin and any other drugs that may be given.

Conversely, lack of tissue perfusion with falling blood pressure may lead to a transient decrease in target organ drug levels. When the blood pressure is restored, enhanced delivery of the toxin can lead to an increase in the degree of intoxication. The result is a confusing waxing and waning of the signs and symptoms. Thus, an appreciation of the toxicodynamics of an agent will allow for better understanding of changes in the clinical course of intoxicated patients.

APPROACH TO THE POISONED PATIENT

HOW DOES THE POISONED PATIENT DIE?

In the majority of cases of poisoning, supportive measures alone are the mainstay of treatment. An understanding of common mechanisms of death due to poisoning can help prepare the physician to treat patients effectively.

Most lethal toxins depress the central nervous system, resulting in obtundation or coma. Comatose pa-

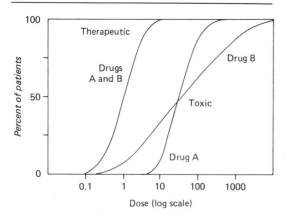

Figure 62–1. Quantal dose-response comparison of 2 drugs with differing safety margins. Both drugs have the same therapeutic index (TD50/ED50). However, at the dose required for therapeutic effects in 90% of patients, less than 1% of patients receiving drug A have toxicity, but 20% of those taking drug B have toxicity.

tients frequently lose their reflexive airway protection and their respiratory drive. Thus, they are likely to die as a result of airway obstruction by the flaccid tongue, aspiration of gastric contents into the tracheobronchial tree, or simple respiratory arrest. These are the most common causes of death due to overdoses of narcotics, barbiturates, alcohol, and other sedative-hypnotic drugs.

Cardiovascular toxicity is also frequently encountered in poisoning. Hypotension may be due to direct depression of cardiac contractility; hypovolemia, due to fluid sequestration or fluid or blood loss; peripheral vascular collapse, due to blockade of alpha-adrenoceptor–mediated vascular tone; and brady- and tachyarrhythmias, due to direct cardiac effects. Hypotension is common with overdoses of tricyclic antidepressants, phenothiazines, theophylline, phenobarbital, and other sedative-hypnotic drugs. Hypothermia due to exposure as well as the temperature-dysregulating effects of many drugs can also produce hypotension. Asystole and lethal arrhythmias such as ventricular tachycardia and fibrillation can occur with overdoses of many cardioactive drugs such as tricyclic antidepressants, digitalis, and theophylline.

Systemic hypoxemia may occur in spite of adequate ventilation and high inspired oxygen administration when poisoning is due to cyanide, hydrogen sulfide, carbon monoxide, and other poisons that interfere with transport or utilization of oxygen. In such patients, hypoxemia is evident, in the absence of cyanosis, by the development of lactic acidosis and signs of ischemia on the ECG.

Seizures, muscular hyperactivity, and rigidity may result in death. Seizures result in pulmonary aspiration and hypoxia and lactic acidosis. Hyperthermia may result from sustained muscular hyperactivity and can lead to muscle breakdown and myoglobinuria, renal failure, lactic acidosis, hyperkalemia, and brain damage, features typical of heat stroke. Drugs and toxins that often induce seizures are tricyclic antidepressants, theophylline, isoniazid (INH), phenothiazines, cocaine, lithium, phencyclidine (PCP), strychnine, and chlorinated hydrocarbons such as camphor and lindane.

Other organ system damage may occur after poisoning. Paraquat characteristically attacks lung tissue, resulting in pulmonary fibrosis. Massive hepatic necrosis due to poisoning by acetaminophen or certain mushrooms results in hepatic encephalopathy and death.

Finally, some patients may die before hospitalization because of the behavioral effects of the ingested drug. Intoxication with alcohol and other sedative-hypnotic drugs is a frequent contributing factor to vehicle accidents. Patients under the influence of hallucinogens such as phencyclidine (PCP) may die in gun battles or in leaps from high places.

INITIAL MANAGEMENT OF THE POISONED PATIENT

The initial management of a patient with coma, seizures, or otherwise altered mental status should follow a standard approach regardless of the poison involved. Attempting to make a specific toxicologic diagnosis only delays the application of supportive measures that form the basis of poisoning treatment.

First, the **airway** should be cleared of vomitus or any other obstruction and an oral airway or endotracheal tube inserted if needed. For many patients, simple positioning in the lateral decubitus position is sufficient to move the flaccid tongue out of the airway. Adequacy of **breathing** should be assessed by observation and by measuring arterial blood gases. Patients with respiratory insufficiency should be intubated and mechanically ventilated. Adequacy of the **circulation** should be assessed by measurement of pulse rate, blood pressure, urinary output, and evaluation of peripheral perfusion. An intravenous line should be placed and blood drawn for serum glucose and other routine determinations.

At this point, every patient with altered mental status should receive a challenge with concentrated **dextrose.** Adults are given 25 g or 50 mL of 50% dextrose intravenously. This should be routine, because patients comatose from hypoglycemia are rapidly and irreversibly losing brain cells. Hypoglycemic patients may appear to be intoxicated, and there is no reliable way to distinguish them from poisoned patients. It is not harmful to give glucose while awaiting the blood sugar determination. Alcoholic patients should also receive 100 mg of thiamine intramuscularly at this time to prevent Wernicke's syndrome.

The narcotic antagonist naloxone (Narcan) may be given in a dose of 0.4–2 mg (1–5 ampules) intravenously. Naloxone will reverse respiratory and central nervous system depression due to all varieties of narcotic drugs and has been reported to be effective in some cases of ethanol and sedative-hypnotic overdose. It is useful to remember that these drugs cause death primarily by respiratory depression; therefore, if airway and breathing assistance have already been instituted, naloxone may not be necessary.

History & Physical Examination

Once these essential initial interventions have been carried out, one can begin a more detailed evaluation to make a specific diagnosis. This includes gathering any available history and performing a toxicologically oriented brief physical examination. Other causes of coma or seizures such as head trauma, meningitis, or metabolic abnormalities should be looked for and treated.

A. History: Oral statements about the amount and even the type of drug ingested in toxic emergencies are often unreliable. Even so, family members, police, and fire department or paramedical personnel should be asked to describe the environment in which the toxic emergency occurred and should bring to the emergency room all syringes, empty bottles, household products, or over-the-counter medications in the immediate vicinity of the possibly poisoned patient.

B. Physical Examination: A brief examination should be performed emphasizing those areas most likely to give clues to the toxicologic diagnosis. These include vital signs, eyes and mouth, skin, abdomen, and nervous system.

1. Vital signs–Careful evaluation of vital signs (blood pressure, pulse, respirations, and temperature) is essential in all toxicologic emergencies. Hypertension and tachycardia are typical with amphetamines, cocaine, phencyclidine (PCP), nicotine, and antimuscarinic drugs. Hypotension and bradycardia are characteristic features of overdose with narcotics, clonidine, sedative-hypnotics, and beta blockers. Tachycardia and hypotension are common with tricyclic antidepressants, phenothiazines, and theophylline. Rapid respirations are typical of amphetamines and other sympathomimetics, salicylates, carbon monoxide, and other toxins that produce metabolic acidosis. Hyperthermia may be due to sympathomimetics, antimuscarinics, salicylates, and drugs producing seizures or muscular rigidity. Hypothermia can be caused by narcotics, phenothiazines, and sedative drugs, especially when accompanied by exposure to a cold environment.

2. Eyes–The eyes are a valuable source of toxicologic information. Constriction of the pupils (miosis) is typical of narcotics, clonidine, phenothiazines, organophosphate insecticides and other cholinesterase inhibitors, and deep coma due to sedative drugs. Dilation of the pupils (mydriasis) is common with amphetamines, cocaine, LSD, and atropine and other antimuscarinic drugs. Horizontal nystagmus is characteristic of intoxication with phenytoin, alcohol, barbiturates, and other sedative drugs. The presence of both vertical and horizontal nystagmus is pathognomonic of phencyclidine (PCP) poisoning. Ptosis and ophthalmoplegia are features of botulism.

3. Mouth–The mouth may show signs of burns due to caustic substances, or soot from smoke inhalation. Typical odors of alcohol, hydrocarbon solvents, paraldehyde, or ammonia may be noted. Poisoning due to cyanide can be distinguished by some examiners as an odor like bitter almonds. Arsenic and organophosphates have been reported to produce a garlicky odor.

4. Skin–The skin often appears flushed, hot, and dry in poisoning with atropine and other antimuscarinics. Excessive sweating occurs with organophosphates, nicotine, and sympathomimetic drugs. Cyanosis may be caused by hypoxemia or by methemoglobinemia. Icterus may suggest hepatic necrosis due to acetaminophen or *Amanita phalloides* poisoning.

5. Abdomen–Abdominal examination may reveal ileus, which is typical of poisoning with antimuscarinic, narcotic, and sedative drugs. Hyperactive bowel sounds, abdominal cramping, and diarrhea are common in poisoning with organophosphates, iron, arsenic, theophylline, and *A phalloides*.

6. Nervous system–A careful neurologic examination is essential. Focal seizures or motor deficits suggest a structural lesion (such as intracranial hemorrhage due to trauma) rather than toxic or metabolic encephalopathy. Nystagmus, dysarthria, and ataxia are typical of phenytoin, alcohol, barbiturate, and other sedative intoxication. Rigidity and muscular hyperactivity are common with methaqualone, haloperidol, phencyclidine (PCP), and sympathomimetic drugs. Seizures are often caused by overdose with tricyclic antidepressants, theophylline, isoniazid, and phenothiazines. Flaccid coma with absent reflexes and even an isoelectric EEG may be seen with deep coma due to narcotic and sedative-hypnotic drugs and may mimic brain death.

Toxic Syndromes

Based on the initial physical examination, a tentative diagnosis of the type or class of poisoning might be possible. Table 62–1 lists some important toxic syndromes.

Laboratory & X-Ray Procedures

Routine laboratory tests that are valuable in toxicologic diagnosis include the following:

A. Arterial Blood Gases: Hypoventilation will result in an elevated P_{CO_2}, (hypercapnia). The P_{O_2} may be low with aspiration pneumonia or drug-induced pulmonary edema. Poor tissue oxygenation due to hypoxia, hypotension, or cyanide poisoning will result in metabolic acidosis. The P_{O_2} measures only oxygen dissolved in the plasma and not total blood oxygen content and therefore may appear normal despite significant oxyhemoglobin deficiency in carbon monoxide poisoning.

B. Electrolytes: Sodium, potassium, chloride, and bicarbonate should be measured. The anion gap is then calculated by subtracting the measured anions from cations:

$$Anion\ gap = (Na^+ + K^+) - (HCO_3^- + Cl^-)$$

It is normally no greater than 12–16 meq/L. A larger-than-expected anion gap is caused by the presence of unmeasured anions accompanying metabolic acidosis. This is caused by, for example, diabetic ketoacidosis, renal failure, or shock-induced lactic acidosis. Drugs that may induce an elevated anion gap metabolic acidosis (Table 62–2) include aspirin, methanol, ethylene glycol, isoniazid, and iron.

C. Renal Function Tests: Some toxins have direct nephrotoxic effects; in other cases, renal failure is due to shock, disseminated intravascular coagulation (DIC), or myoglobinuria. Blood urea nitrogen and creatinine levels should be measured and urinalysis performed. Elevated serum creatine phosphokinase (CPK) and myoglobin in the urine suggest muscle necrosis due to seizures or muscular rigidity. Oxalate

Table 62–1. Toxic syndromes.

Acetaminophen
Mild anorexia, nausea, vomiting, delayed jaundice, renal failure.

Alcohol
Depressed sensorium, odor on breath, metabolic acidosis (anion gap), osmolar gap.

Amphetamines
Toxic psychosis, hyperthermia, flushing, increased blood pressure, dilated pupils, hallucinations, seizures, tachycardia, rhabdomyolysis.

Antifreeze (ethylene glycol)
Renal failure, crystals in urine, anion and osmolar gap, initial central nervous system excitation, but eye examination normal.

Arsenic
Early: garlic on breath, vomiting, profuse bloody diarrhea, burning tears. Delayed: hair loss, lines on nails, neuropathy, increased skin pigmentation. Arsine gas: hemolysis.

Barbiturates
Nystagmus, hypotension, hypothermia. Prognosis depends on systolic blood pressure on admission and blood pH.

Botulism
Dysphagia, dysarthria, ptosis, ophthalmoplegia, muscle weakness. Incubation period 12–36 hours.

Bromide
Increased pigmentation, acne, dementia, psychosis, hyperchloremia.

Cadmium
Metallic taste, delayed pulmonary edema; late, kidney and lung disease.

Carbon monoxide
Coma, metabolic acidosis, normal P_{aO_2}, retinal hemorrhages.

Chloral hydrate
Pearlike odor, cardiac arrhythmias, radiopaque tablets (seen on x-ray film).

Clonidine
Miosis, decreased blood pressure, decreased pulse, no response to naloxone.

Cocaine
Perforated nasal septum, dilated pupils, psychosis, tachycardia, scarred veins (cocaine burns).

Cyanide
Bitter almond odor, convulsions, coma, abnormal ECG.

Digitalis
Visual disturbances, delirium, abnormal ECG, nausea, increased serum potassium levels, normal kidney function.

Ethchlorvynol (Placidyl)
Deep coma, pungent aromatic odor, slow pulse, decreased blood pressure, pink gastric aspirate.

Gasoline
Distinctive odor, coughing, pulmonary infiltrates.

Glutethimide (Doriden)
Dilated pupils, coma, prolonged respiratory depression.

Heroin
Coma, decreased blood pressure, bradycardia, hypoventilation, miosis, needle marks, rapid response to naloxone.

Hydrocarbons
Pneumonia, tinnitus, convulsions, ventricular fibrillation, unique odor.

Hydrogen sulfide
Rotten egg smell, loss of sense of smell, sudden collapse and death.

Iron
Bloody diarrhea, coma, radiopaque material in gut (seen on x-ray film), high leukocyte count, hyperglycemia.

Isoniazid
Coma, seizures, severe acidosis.

Isopropyl alcohol
Gastritis, acetonemia with normoglycemia, osmolar gap.

Lead
Abdominal pain, increased blood pressure, convulsions, muscle weakness, metallic taste, anorexia, encephalopathy, delayed motor neuropathy, subtle changes in renal and reproductive function.

Lithium
Tremor, seizures, polyuria, delayed central nervous system and renal toxicity, prolonged coma.

LSD
Hallucinations, dilated pupils, hypertension.

Mercury
Acute renal failure, tremor, salivation, gingivitis, colitis, erethism (fits of crying, irrational behavior), nephrotic syndrome.

Methadone
Miosis, coma, slow pulse, decreased blood pressure and respiration, transient response to naloxone.

Methaqualone (Quaalude)
Hyperreflexia, tonic-clonic spasms.

Methyl alcohol (methanol)
Rapid respirations, visual symptoms, osmolar gap, severe metabolic acidosis (anion gap).

Methylene chloride
History of paint-stripping exposure; confusion, increased carbon monoxide level.

Methylphenidate (Ritalin)
Eosinophilia, wheezing, scarred veins, abscess.

Table 62–1 (cont'd). Toxic syndromes.

Mushrooms Severe nausea and vomiting 8 hours after ingestion; delayed hepatic and renal failure with *Amanita phalloides*.	**Plants, poisonous (cont'd)** **Oleander and foxglove** Digitalislike poisoning.
Nitrogen oxides History of silo or cave exposure; delayed pulmonary edema.	**Predatory bean (rosary pea, jequirity bean); castor bean** Delayed severe gastrointestinal distress, seizures, hemolytic anemia, renal failure, death.
Organophosphates or carbamates Miotic pupils, abdominal cramps and diarrhea, salivation, lacrimation, urination, increased bronchial secretions, muscle fasciculations.	**Propoxyphene (Darvon)** Seizures, miosis, limited response to naloxone.
Paraquat History of exposure to herbicide; oropharyngeal burning, vomiting, delayed pulmonary fibrosis, and death.	**Salicylates** Hyperventilation, vomiting, fever, bleeding, acidosis, tinnitus.
Phencyclidine (PCP) Coma with eyes open, hyperacusis, myoclonic jerks, vertical nystagmus, violent behavior.	**Strychnine** Stiff neck, status epilepticus, hyperacusis.
Phenothiazines Postural hypotension, hypothermia, miosis, tremor, radiopaque material on abdominal film, increased QT interval.	**Thallium (rat poison)** Alopecia, gastrointestinal distress, motor and sensory neuropathy, hematologic examination normal.
	Theophylline Gastrointestinal distress, seizures, hypotension, tachycardia, hypokalemia.
Phosgene History of exposure to burning plastics or welding; pulmonary edema.	**Tricyclic antidepressants** Coma, convulsions, conduction disturbances, prolonged QRS.
Plants, poisonous **Nightshade family, jimsonweed** Hallucinations, dilated pupils, seizures (contain atropinelike alkaloids).	**Vacor (rat poison)** Ketoacidosis, postural hypotension.
	Vanadium Green tongue, severe pulmonary irritation.

crystals in the urine are characteristic of ethylene glycol poisoning.

D. Serum Osmolality: The calculated serum osmolality is dependent mainly on the serum sodium and glucose and the blood urea nitrogen and can be estimated from the following formula:

$$(2 \times Na^+ \text{ [meq/L]}) + (\text{Glucose [mg/dL]} \div 18)$$
$$+ (\text{BUN [mg/dL]} \div 3)$$

This value is normally 280–290 mosm/kg. Ethanol and other alcohols may contribute significantly to the measured serum osmolality but, since they are not included in the calculation, cause an "osmolar gap":

$$\text{Osmolar gap} = \text{Measured osmolality} - \text{Calculated osmolality}$$

In the absence of significant levels of an osmotically active intoxicant molecule, the osmolar gap is zero. Table 62–3 lists the molecular weight, dose, and expected contribution to the serum osmolality in ethanol, methanol, ethylene glycol, and isopropanol poisonings.

E. Electrocardiogram: Widening of the QRS complex duration to greater than 0.1 s is typical of tri-

cyclic antidepressant and quinidine overdoses. The QT interval may be prolonged in quinidine, phenothiazine, and tricyclic antidepressant poisoning. Variable atrioventricular block and multiple ventricular arrhythmias are common with digitalis poisoning. The ECG may show typical abnormalities when hypothermia and electrolyte abnormalities accompany overdose. Hypoxemia due to carbon monoxide poisoning may result in ischemic changes on the ECG.

F. X-Ray Findings: A plain film of the abdomen should be obtained, since some toxins, particularly iron and enteric-coated drugs, may be radiopaque. Chest x-ray may reveal aspiration pneumonia, hydrocarbon pneumonia, or pulmonary edema. When head trauma is suspected, a CT scan is recommended.

Table 62–2. Drug-induced anion gap acidosis.

Type of Elevation of the Anion Gap	Agents
Metabolic acidosis	Methanol, ethylene glycol, salicylates.
Lactic acidosis	Any drug-induced seizures, iron, phenformin, hypoxia.
Ketoacidosis	Ethanol.

Note: The normal anion gap calculated from $(Na^+ + K^+) - (HCO_3^- + Cl^-)$ is 12–16 meq/L; calculated from $(Na^+) - (HCO_3^- + Cl^-)$, it is 8–12 meq/L.

Table 62–3. Substances that cause osmolar gap.

	Molecular Weight (g/mol)	Lethal Level (mg/dL)	Corresponding Osmolar Gap (mosm/kg)
Ethanol	46	350	75
Methanol	32	80	25
Ethylene glycol	62	200	35
Isopropanol	60	350	60

Example: For ethanol (the commonest cause of osmolar gap), a gap of 30 mosm/kg would indicate an ethanol level of 30 × 46 ÷ 10 = 138 mg/dL. See text for the basis of this calculation.
Note: Most laboratories use the freezing point method of determining osmolality. If the vaporization point method is used, the alcohols will be driven off and their contribution to osmolality will be lost.

Screening Tests

It is a common misconception that a "stat" toxicology "screen" is the best way to diagnose and manage an acute poisoning. The "screen" is time-consuming, expensive, and often unreliable; many drugs are not tested for. The clinical examination of the patient and selected routine laboratory tests are usually sufficient to generate a tentative diagnosis and an appropriate treatment plan. When a specific antidote or invasive therapy such as hemodialysis is under consideration, in-depth laboratory testing may be indicated. For example, quantitative determination of acetaminophen is useful in determining antidotal therapy with N-acetylcysteine. Serum levels of theophylline, lithium, salicylates, and other drugs may indicate the need for hemodialysis or hemoperfusion (Table 62–7).

Time of Ingestion of Poison

To estimate the severity of poisoning, it is important to estimate the time since ingestion and compare it with the plasma level. The importance of time in evaluating plasma levels has been particularly well demonstrated for aspirin poisoning. An aspirin concentration of 50 mg/dL 4–6 hours after ingestion is associated with only mild intoxication; the same level obtained 36 hours after ingestion is associated with very severe poisoning. The basis for this relationship lies in the fact that the clinical manifestation of toxic effects in some target organs such as the brain may lag significantly behind the peak levels in the blood.

Blood Levels of Toxins

Note: Treatment should not be delayed while waiting for laboratory reports.

There are 5 acute toxic emergencies in which measurement of blood levels is necessary to monitor treatment: acetaminophen, aspirin, lithium, carbon monoxide, and theophylline poisoning. Poisoning with ethanol, methanol, ethylene glycol, and digoxin can usually be diagnosed on clinical grounds but must be confirmed by the toxicology laboratory. Quantitative analysis of blood and urine for sedative-hypnotic drugs is important when simple supportive procedures do not appear adequate and especially when dialysis is being considered, eg, in phenobarbital poisoning. Table 62–4 lists common sedative-hypnotic drugs, their kinetic parameters, and treatment methods.

A special role of the toxicology laboratory involves forensic toxicology and confirmation of brain death. Some toxic emergencies can mimic brain death. Therefore, decisions about depth and length of sup-

Table 62–4. Toxicologic features of sedative-hypnotic overdose.

Drug	V_d (L/kg)	Normal Doses $t_{1/2}$ (hours)	Overdoses $t_{1/2}$ (hours)	Maximum Therapeutic Level (μg/mL)	Treatment	Comments
Phenobarbital	0.75	60–100	70–120	20	Supportive. Repeat administrations of charcoal by nasogastric tube are useful.	Avoid fluid overload.
Pentobarbital	1–2	20–30	50	50	Supportive.	Short-acting.
Chloral hydrate	0.6	4–8	10–20	15	Supportive.	Gastritis, arrhythmias. Radiopaque pills.
Glutethimide (Doriden)	20–25	8–12	24–40	0.5	Supportive.	Cyclic variation in coma; mydriasis.
Ethchlorvynol (Placidyl)	3–4	10–20	20–100	100	Supportive.	Pink or green gastric aspirate with pungent odor. Prolonged coma with overdose.
Methaqualone (Quaalude)	1–2	10–40	?	20	Supportive.	With severe overdose, muscular rigidity and myoclonus may occur.
Diazepam (Valium)	1–2	30–70	50–140	5	Supportive.	Severe overdose uncommon unless combined with other drugs.

portive care must be reviewed in light of thorough toxicology laboratory assessments.

Decontamination

Decontamination procedures should be undertaken after initial diagnostic assessment and laboratory evaluation. Decontamination involves removing toxins from the skin or gastrointestinal tract.

A. Skin: Contaminated clothing should be completely removed and saved for analysis. Percutaneous penetration by toxins has been poorly studied but should be anticipated. Vigorous washing with copious amounts of water and soap should be carried out.

B. Gastrointestinal Tract: *Caution:* It is essential to protect the airway. All necessary emergency equipment such as suction must be readily available. Seizures, absence of the gag reflex, and ulcerated oral mucous membranes are contraindications to emesis. Gastric lavage is contraindicated if the airway is at risk (eg, unconscious patient with no gag reflex). Acid and alkaline corrosives should be diluted but not neutralized.

Decontamination procedures have important clinical consequences. "Universal antidote" is not an antidote and certainly not a universal one. Therapists should not put their fingers in the patient's throat and should not use salt water or mustard as emetic agents.

1. Emesis–If the airway is protected by a gag reflex, there is no ulceration of mucous membranes, and the patient is not having seizures, induce emesis by oral administration of **ipecac syrup,** 30 mL for adults or 10–15 mL (in fruit juice) for children, repeated once after 15 minutes if necessary. (Ipecac fluid extract should be avoided because of its cardiac toxicity.) Home use of ipecac, an emetinelike alkaloid, has been documented to be safe and effective and should be part of the home treatment of children in poisoning emergencies. Ipecac is effective even when antiemetic medications have been taken in overdose. Apomorphine is much more toxic than ipecac, especially in children, because of its persistent emetic effects and the central nervous system depression it causes. Apomorphine should not be used.

2. Gastric lavage–In adults, if the airway is protected by an endotracheal tube, gastric lavage may be performed. Gastric lavage is usually not successful in children, because of the necessity of using small-bore tubes; as large a tube as possible should be used in adults. Lavage solutions (usually 0.9% saline) should be at body temperature to prevent hypothermia.

3. Catharsis–Administration of a cathartic agent should hasten removal of toxins from the gastrointestinal tract and reduce absorption, though no controlled studies have been done. Pediatricians have reported finding whole tablets—especially enteric-coated ones—in stools after administration of cathartic agents. If charcoal is also administered, this procedure marks the stool with charcoal, so that total gastrointestinal transit time can be estimated. **Sorbitol (70%)** is the preferred cathartic agent if heart failure is not present. **Magnesium sulfate** may be used if renal function is unimpaired. Cathartic agents with an oil base are of no value and are potentially harmful. Table 62–5 lists some common cathartics.

4. Activated charcoal–Administration of activated charcoal is a valuable decontamination procedure if given in sufficient quantity because it binds many toxins. It is best to give it in a ratio of at least 10:1 of charcoal to estimated dose of toxin. It is believed that charcoal does not bind cyanide, iron, or alcohols. Generally, charcoal is underutilized and given in insufficient doses. Charcoal should not be administered simultaneously with ipecac, because it binds ipecac. In most studies in humans, charcoal was administered after normal therapeutic doses of drug; controlled studies of the use of charcoal after overdose are few. Recent studies suggest that serial administration of charcoal every 4 hours may be of value in shortening coma in sedative-hypnotic poisoning, especially in cases of phenobarbital overdose.

Specific Antidotes

There is a popular misconception that there is an antidote for every poison. The opposite is true—relatively selective antidotes are available for only 8 classes of toxins. The major antidotes and their characteristics are listed in Table 62–6. These drugs are supplemented by the immunologic agents such as snake antivenin (see below) and digoxin antibodies.

Methods of Enhancing Elimination of Toxins

After appropriate diagnostic and decontamination procedures and administration of antidotes, it is important to consider measures for enhancing elimination, such as forced diuresis, dialysis, or exchange procedures. If a patient is able to eliminate a toxin rapidly, the period of coma will be shortened, metabolites removed, and organ damage reduced. It is thus

Table 62–5. Usual doses of cathartics in decontamination.*

Magnesium citrate (10%) (magnesium = 1.6 meq/mL)	Adult: 150–250 mL Child: 1–2 mL/kg
Magnesium sulfate (10%) (magnesium = 0.8 meq/mL)	Adult: 150–250 mL Child: 1–2 mL/kg
Milk of magnesia	Adult: 15–60 mL Child: 0.1–0.2 mL/kg
Sodium sulfate (10%) (sodium = 1.4 meq/mL)	Adult: 150–250 mL Child: 1–2 mL/kg
Sorbitol (70%)	Adult: 100–150 mL Child: 1–2 mL/kg

*Modified and reproduced, with permission, from Riegel JM, Becker CE: Use of cathartics in toxic ingestions. *Ann Emerg Med* 1981;**10**:254.
Note:
1. Avoid magnesium cathartics in renal disease and cases of nephrotoxin ingestion.
2. Avoid sodium cathartics in congestive heart failure and hypertension.
3. *Never* use oil-based cathartics.

Table 62–6. Specific antidotes.

Antidote	Poison(s)	Comments
Acetylcysteine (Mucomyst)	Acetaminophen.	Best results if given within 12 hours of overdose. Follow liver function tests and acetaminophen blood levels. Little recognized toxicity. Dose: 140 mg/kg orally as loading dose, then 70 mg/kg orally every 4 hours for 17 doses in severe cases. Intravenous acetylcysteine has been used successfully in Europe and is currently under trial in the USA.
Atropine	Anticholinesterases, organophosphates, physostigmine.	A test dose of 2 mg (for children, 0.05 mg/kg) is given IV until symptoms of atropinism appear (tachycardia, dilated pupils, ileus). Dose may be repeated every 10–15 minutes, with decrease of secretions as therapeutic end point.
Deferoxamine (Desferal)	Iron salts: toxic dose, 60–70 mg/kg; lethal dose, 60–180 mg/kg. Judge severity by white blood count, elevated blood sugar, severe vomiting and diarrhea, central nervous system depression, and plain film of abdomen.	If poisoning is severe, give 15 mg/kg/h IV *after* blood has been drawn for serum iron and iron-binding capacity determination. Maximum dose: 80 mg/kg/d. Urine will become wine-red. 100 mg of deferoxamine binds 8.5 mg of iron.
Ethanol	Methanol, ethylene glycol.	Ethanol therapy is begun before laboratory diagnosis is confirmed. A loading dose is calculated so as to give a blood level of at least 100 mg/dL (42 g/70 kg in adults).
Metal chelators N-Acetyl-D, L-penicillamine	Mercury.	Excreted rapidly by kidney. Side effects: loss of taste, nephrotic syndrome, trace metal deficiencies.
Calcium disodium ethylenediaminetetraacetate (CaEDTA)	Lead.	Give 50–75 mg/kg/d IM or IV in 3–6 divided doses for up to 5 days in cases of lead encephalopathy. Modify dose in renal failure. Toxicity: zinc depletion and vitamin B_6 deficiency. Avoid oral therapy.
Dimercaprol (BAL)	Arsenic, gold, mercury.	Give 3–5 mg/kg every 4 hours IM for 2 days, then 2.5–3 mg/kg every 6 hours for 7 days. When urine arsenic falls below 50 μg/24 h, antidote may be stopped. After 5 days off all chelation, repeat urine arsenic determination. Not effective for arsine gas. Side effects: increased blood pressure, burning lips. Try to keep urine pH alkaline.
Penicillamine	Lead, gold, arsenic.	Give 1 g orally daily in 4 divided doses before meals.
Naloxone (Narcan)	Narcotic drugs, propoxyphene, pentazocine, diphenoxylate.	A specific antagonist of narcotics; 0.4 mg (1 mL) may be given by IV, IM, or subcutaneous injection and repeated every 2–3 minutes for 2 or 3 doses. Larger doses may be needed to reverse the effects of overdose with propoxyphene.
Physotigmine salicylate	"Suggested" for antimuscarinic anticholinergic agents.	Adult dose is 1 mg IV slowly (usually 0.5 mg first). May cause bradycardia, miosis, fasciculations, salivation, lacrimation, increased bronchial secretions, urination, or diarrhea. Maximum initial doses: 4 mg for adults and 2 mg for children. The effects are transient (30–60 minutes), and the lowest effective dose may be repeated when symptoms return. Have atropine ready to reverse excess effects. Nonspecific central nervous system stimulation culminating in seizures may occur. Dangerous antidote.
Pralidoxime (2-PAM)	Anticholinesterases, organophosphates.	Adult dose is 1 g IV, which may be repeated every 8–12 hours as needed. Pediatric dose is approximately 250 mg. No benefit in carbamate poisoning.

important to have knowledge of the toxicokinetics of the poison.

In cases of massive overdose, elimination pathways often involve enzyme and carrier systems with limited capacities. Elimination of even normal doses of ethanol, salicylate, and phenytoin is limited by saturation of the elimination mechanism. Drugs that have been demonstrated to exhibit concentration-dependent toxicokinetics in the overdose setting are chloral hydrate, ethchlorvynol, some barbiturates, theophylline, and acetaminophen. In cases of toxic ingestion of these drugs, methods of enhancing elimination that contribute to total body clearance can significantly improve the clinical outcome.

A. Techniques Available:

1. Dialysis procedures, including peritoneal dialysis, hemodialysis, and hemoperfusion, are theoretically appealing as a means of removing toxins that are eliminated through metabolic mechanisms that cannot be enhanced.

2. Renal elimination of a few toxins is enhanced by forced diuresis or alteration of urinary pH. Forced alkaline diuresis is useful in cases of salicylate or phenobarbital overdose. Forced acid diuresis may be useful in strychnine and amphetamine intoxication. Increasing renal elimination of most sedative-hypnotic drugs may increase the urinary concentration of the drug but contributes little to total body clearance. Such forced diuresis also enhances the risk of fluid and electrolyte imbalance and of worsening pulmonary function.

B. Dialyses:

1. Peritoneal dialysis–This is a relatively simple and available technique but is inefficient in removing most drugs.

2. Hemodialysis–Hemodialysis is more efficient than peritoneal dialysis and has been well studied. It assists in correction of fluid and electrolyte imbalance and may also enhance removal of toxic metabolites, eg, formate in cases of methanol poisoning. The efficiency of both peritoneal dialysis and hemodialysis is a function of the molecular weight, water solubility, protein binding, endogenous clearance, and distribution in the body of the specific toxin. Removal of drug with these procedures can be enhanced by increasing the time on dialysis or by altering the dialysis medium to bind the toxin. However, the complications of these procedures also increase with the length of time of dialysis. Hemodialysis is especially useful in overdose cases in which fluid and electrolyte imbalances are present or when toxic by-products are removable.

a. Salicylate, methanol, and ethylene glycol are 3 toxins in which hemodialysis is the preferred method of treatment.

b. Because lithium overdose is extremely dangerous when sufficient to cause seizures and prolonged coma, prolonged hemodialysis is probably valuable but has not been adequately studied.

C. Hemoperfusion: Hemoperfusion for treatment of drug intoxication has been used increasingly in the past 5 years. Blood is pumped from the patient via a venous catheter through a column of adsorbent material and then recirculated to the patient. Systemic anticoagulation with heparin is required to prevent the blood from clotting in the cartridge. Hemoperfusion does not alter fluid and electrolyte balance and does not remove all toxic products. However, it does remove many high-molecular-weight toxins that have poor water solubility, because the perfusion cartridge has a large surface area for adsorption that is directly perfused with the blood and is not impeded by a membrane. The rate-limiting factors in removal of toxins by hemoperfusion are the affinity of the adsorbent resin for the drug, the rate of blood flow through the cartridge, and the rate of equilibration of the drug from the peripheral tissues to the blood. Many different hemoperfusion cartridges are now being studied for use in various toxic circumstances.

Although relatively few toxins have been studied, there is evidence that hemoperfusion may enhance whole body clearance of salicylate, phenytoin, ethchlorvynol, phenobarbital, and, in the early stages, theophylline and paraquat. Complications such as embolization of adsorbed particles, depletion of blood cells, and removal of proteins, solutes, and steroids have been minimized with increasing clinical experience.

D. Selection of Technique to Be Used: Drugs or toxins with extremely large volumes of distribution such as tricyclic antidepressants and digoxin are poorly removed by hemodialysis or hemoperfusion. Therefore, critical review of kinetic parameters and dialysis capability is required before undertaking dialysis procedures. Table 62–7 lists intoxications requiring immediate dialysis, those in which it is used only if supportive measures fail, and those for which dialysis is not indicated. The toxicology laboratory should monitor methanol, ethylene glycol, salicylate, theophylline, phenobarbital, paraquat, and lithium blood levels during dialysis.

The problems of enhancing elimination are well illustrated in PCP intoxication. Studies in laboratory animals suggest that there is limited renal clearance and little effect of blood pH changes on the distribution of the drug. However, urinary acidification has been demonstrated to increase the renal clearance of phencyclidine. Gastric acidification and gastric suction increase the diffusion of phencyclidine into gastric contents. Based on these preliminary data, large numbers of patients have been treated by acidification of the urine and gastric suction but with little documentation of the effectiveness of these techniques. Because intoxication with PCP has a waxing and waning clinical response, it has been difficult to evaluate improvement in the clinical status. Because phencyclidine poisoning

Table 62–7. Indications for hemodialysis (HD) and hemoperfusion (HP).

	Toxin	Procedure
Indicated immediately if significant intoxication	Ethylene glycol	HD
	Lithium	HD
	Methanol	HD
	Salicylate	HD
	Theophylline	HP
	Paraquat	HP
Indicated if supportive measures fail or if prolonged coma is expected	Digitoxin	HP
	Ethchlorvynol	HP
	Phenobarbital	HP
Not indicated	Amphetamines, PCP, cocaine	
	Benzodiazepines (chlordiazepoxide, diazepam)	
	Chlorpromazine, haloperidol, other antipsychotics	
	Digoxin	
	Glutethimide	
	Narcotics	
	Quinidine, procainamide	
	Short-acting barbiturates	
	Tricyclic antidepressants	

is associated with muscle destruction and excretion of myoglobin in the urine, inappropriate acidification of the urine may increase the likelihood of precipitation of myoglobin, thereby increasing the likelihood of renal failure.

Supportive Care

Management of poisoning requires thorough knowledge of how to treat hypoventilation, coma, shock, seizures, and psychosis. Sophisticated toxicokinetic considerations are of little value if vital functions are not maintained. Hypoventilation and coma require particular attention to airway management. Arterial blood gases must be checked frequently, and aspiration of gastric contents must be prevented.

Fluid and electrolyte management may be complex. Monitoring body weight, central venous pressure, pulmonary capillary wedge pressure, and arterial blood gases is necessary to ensure adequate but not excessive administration of fluid.

With appropriate support for coma, shock, seizures, and agitation, additional areas of supportive care may be checked. If bowel sounds are decreased or if excessive quantities of toxin are noted on the plain abdominal film, serial administration of activated charcoal may be required. Monitoring of renal and hepatic function is essential. Muscle destruction (rhabdomyolysis) may result in acute renal failure. Inadvertent acidification of the urine may increase the likelihood of renal insufficiency resulting from myoglobin destruction and excretion. Catheters in veins and arteries or in the bladder may become sources of infection. Large amounts of fluid at room temperature or dialysis procedures may lower body temperature and worsen cardiovascular function. Apparent worsening of the patient's status may follow administration of an antidote with a short half-life such as naloxone. Appropriate supportive treatment may on occasion result in physiologic survival of a neurologically impaired patient, so that lumbar puncture and CT scans are needed and EEGs may be required to confirm brain death. One must be extremely cautious in diagnosing brain death, however, especially in cases of sedative-hypnotic drug overdose.

Treatment of Snake, Spider, & Scorpion Envenomation

The venoms of several snakes and scorpions and (in very small children) that of black widow spiders are important toxicologic emergencies. In the USA, rattlesnake bite is by far the most important, because of the amount of venom that may be injected, its intrinsic toxicity, and the fact that victims may be far from medical help when the bite occurs.

Evidence of envenomation includes local bleeding, severe pain, superficial edema of rapid onset, hemorrhagic bleb formation, lymphadenitis, and obvious fang marks. Many studies have shown that emergency field remedies such as incision and suction, tourniquets, and ice packs are far more damaging than useful. Avoidance of unnecessary motion, on the other hand, does help to limit the spread of the venom. Definitive therapy relies on antivenins and should be started as soon as possible.

Three antivenins are available in the USA: (1) mixed crotalid snake antivenin, (2) coral snake antivenin (used rarely), and (3) black widow spider antivenin (of little documented therapeutic value).

Blood should be typed and cross-matched before antivenin is administered. Clotting and bleeding times should be monitored. Dose of the antivenin should be adjusted according to the presence or absence of signs of systemic intoxication, including nausea, vomiting, paresthesias, bleeding disorder, shock, arrhythmias, renal failure, and pulmonary edema. For rattlesnake bite, at least 5 vials of mixed crotalid antivenin should be administered; if envenomation is severe, 10–20 vials may be required. Skin testing is important because the antivenins are made in horses; signs of serum sickness usually develop 10–12 days after treatment. It is important to avoid ice packs, incisions, tourniquets, fasciotomies, and steroids in snakebite management. Steroids are useful only for severe serum sickness.

Common Errors in Management of Poisoning

"Universal antidote" (burnt toast, magnesium oxide, tannic acid) is of no value and may be harmful. If ipecac syrup is to be used, it should be given at once and not postponed until arrival at the hospital or during the evaluation procedure in the emergency room. Ipecac should not be administered simultaneously with charcoal. Clinical experience, especially in pediatrics, suggests that ipecac can be administered by a lay person, especially when instructed by the physician over the telephone.

In the past, ingested acid and alkaline substances were neutralized; this liberates heat and increases tissue destruction. Dilution of caustics or acid substances is preferred. Inducing emesis by placing a finger in the throat or with copper salts or hypertonic salt solution is hazardous to the mouth and esophagus. Use of oil-based cathartic agents may cause lipid pneumonia. Lavage fluids containing large quantities of sodium and phosphate may cause severe electrolyte imbalances. Excessive hydration may worsen pulmonary function. Large amounts of glucose may lower phosphate and potassium. Respiratory stimulants and analeptic agents are of no value and are harmful in toxic emergencies.

REFERENCES

Basic Texts

Casarett LJ, Doull J (editors): *Toxicology: The Basic Science of Poisons*. Macmillan, 1980.

Gosselin RE et al: *Clinical Toxicology of Commercial Products,* 5th ed. Williams & Wilkins, 1985.

Haddad LM, Winchester JF (editors): *Clinical Management of Poisoning and Drug Overdose*. Saunders, 1983.

Mills J et al (editors): *Current Emergency Diagnosis & Treatment,* 2nd ed. Lange, 1985.

Proctor NH, Hughes JP: *Chemical Hazards of the Workplace*. Lippincott, 1978.

Other Sources

Berg GL (editor): *Farm Chemicals Handbook 1983*. Meister, 1983. [Annual publication.]

Rumack BH (editor): *Poisindex*. Micromedex, Inc., 1984. [National Center for Poison Information, Denver 80204. Revised quarterly.]

Winchester JF et al: Dialysis and hemoperfusion of poisons and drugs: Update. *Trans Am Soc Artif Intern Organs* 1977;**23:**762.

Handbooks of Poisoning

Dreisbach RH: *Handbook of Poisoning: Prevention, Diagnosis, & Treatment,* 11th ed. Lange, 1983.

Goldfrank LR (editor): *Toxicologic Emergencies*. Appleton-Century-Crofts, 1986.

Hanenson IB (editor): *Quick Reference to Clinical Toxicology*. Lippincott, 1980.

Matthew H, Lawson AAH: *Treatment of Common Acute Poisonings,* 4th ed. Churchill Livingstone, 1979.

Useful Phone Numbers

Poison Control Centers:
    San Francisco: (415) 476–6600
    Denver: (303) 629–1123
    Boston: (617) 232–2120
Teratogen Registry (California): (714) 294–3584

Special Aspects of Perinatal & Pediatric Pharmacology

63

Martin S. Cohen, MD

The effects of drugs on the fetus and newborn infant are based on the general principles set forth in Chapter 1–3 of this book. However, the contexts in which these pharmacologic laws operate are different in pregnant women and in rapidly maturing infants. At present, the special pharmacokinetic factors are beginning to be understood, whereas information regarding pharmacodynamic differences (eg, receptor affinities and number) is still quite fragmentary.

This chapter presents the basic principles of pharmacology in the special context of perinatal and pediatric therapeutics.

DRUG THERAPY IN PREGNANCY

Many drugs taken by pregnant women can cross the placenta and expose the developing embryo and fetus to their pharmacologic and teratogenic effects. Critical factors affecting placental drug transfer and drug effects on the fetus include the following: (1) The physicochemical properties of the drug. (2) The rate at which the drug crosses the placenta and the amount of drug reaching the fetus. (3) The duration of exposure to the drug. (4) How the drug is distributed in different fetal tissues. (5) The stage of placental and fetal development at the time of exposure to the drug. (6) The effects of drugs used in combination.

As is true also of other biologic membranes, drug passage across the placenta is dependent on the lipid solubility and degree of drug ionization. Lipophilic drugs tend to diffuse readily across the placenta and enter the fetal circulation. For example, thiopental, a drug commonly used for cesarean sections, crosses the placenta almost immediately and can produce sedation or apnea in the newborn infant. Highly ionized drugs such as succinylcholine and d-tubocurarine, also used for cesarean sections, cross the placenta slowly and achieve very low concentrations in the fetus.

Impermeability of the placenta to polar compounds is relative rather than absolute. If high enough maternal-fetal concentration gradients are achieved, polar compounds can cross the placenta. Salicylate, which is almost completely ionized at physiologic pH, crosses the placenta rapidly. This occurs because the small amount of salicylate that is not ionized is highly lipid-soluble.

The molecular weight of the drug also influences the rate and amount of drug transferred across the placenta. Drugs with molecular weights of 250–500 can cross the placenta easily, depending upon their lipid solubility and degree of ionization; those with molecular weights of 500–1000 cross the placenta with more difficulty; and those with molecular weights greater than 1000 cross very poorly. The apparent exceptions are maternal antibody globulins and certain polypeptides that cross the placenta by some selective mechanism as yet unknown.

The degree to which a drug is bound to plasma proteins (particularly albumin) also affects the rate and amount transferred. If a compound is very lipid-soluble (eg, anesthetic gases), it is not affected greatly by protein binding. Transfer of these drugs and their overall rates of equilibration are more dependent on (and proportionate to) placental blood flow. This is because very lipid-soluble drugs diffuse across placental membranes so rapidly that their overall rates of equilibration do not depend on the free drug concentrations becoming equal on both sides.

If a drug is poorly lipid-soluble and is ionized, its transfer is slow and will probably be impeded by its binding to maternal plasma proteins. Protein binding is also important, since some drugs exhibit greater protein binding in maternal plasma than in fetal plasma because of a lowered binding affinity of fetal proteins. This has been shown for sulfonamides, barbiturates, phenytoin, and local anesthetic agents.

Two mechanisms help to protect the fetus from drugs in the maternal circulation: (1) The placenta itself plays a role both as a semipermeable barrier and as a site of metabolism of some drugs passing through it. Several different types of aromatic oxidation reactions (eg, hydroxylation, N-dealkylation, demethylation) have been shown to occur in placental tissue. Ethanol and pentobarbital are oxidized in this way. (2) Drugs that have crossed the placenta enter the fetal circulation via the umbilical vein. About 40–60% of umbilical venous blood flow enters the fetal liver; the remainder bypasses the liver and enters the general fetal circulation. A drug that enters the liver may be partly metabolized there before it enters the fetal circulation. In addition, a large proportion of drug present in the umbilical artery (returning to the placenta) may be shunted through the placenta back to the umbilical vein and into the liver again. It should be noted that metabolites of some drugs may be more active than the parent compound and may affect the fetus adversely.

A single intrauterine exposure to a drug can affect structures undergoing rapid development at the time of exposure. Thalidomide is an example of a drug that profoundly affects the development of the limbs after only brief exposure. This exposure, however, must be at a critical time in the development of the limbs. Continued exposure may produce cumulative effects or may affect several organs going through varying stages of development.

Chronic consumption of ethanol during pregnancy, particularly during the first and second trimesters, results in the fetal alcohol syndrome (Chapter 21). In this syndrome, the central nervous system, growth, and facial development are all affected. Another example of the effects of continued exposure is chronic use of opiate narcotics by the mother, which produces narcotic dependence in the fetus and newborn. This dependence is manifested after delivery as neonatal narcotic withdrawal.

Some drugs with known adverse effects in pregnancy are listed in Table 63–1.

Fetal therapeutics is an emerging area in perinatal pharmacology. This involves drug administration to the pregnant woman with the fetus as the target of the drug. At present, corticosteroids are used to stimulate fetal lung maturation when premature birth is expected. Phenobarbital, when given to pregnant women near term, can induce fetal hepatic enzymes responsible for the glucuronidation of bilirubin, and the incidence of jaundice is lower in newborns whose mothers are given phenobarbital than when phenobarbital is not used. Drugs have also been given to mothers for treatment of fetal cardiac arrhythmias.

DRUG DISPOSITION IN INFANTS & CHILDREN

Drug Absorption

Drug absorption in infants and children follows the same general principles as in adults. Unique factors that influence drug absorption include blood flow at the site of administration as determined by the physiologic status of the infant or child; and (for orally administered drugs) gastrointestinal function, which changes rapidly during the first few days after birth. The effects of age after birth on gastrointestinal function also influence the regulation of drug absorption.

A. Blood Flow at the Site of Administration: Absorption after intramuscular or subcutaneous injection depends mainly, in neonates as in adults, on the rate of blood flow to the muscle or subcutaneous area injected. Physiologic conditions that might reduce blood flow to these areas are cardiovascular shock, vasoconstriction due to sympathomimetic agents, and heart failure. However, sick premature infants may require intramuscular injections and have very little muscle mass. This is further complicated by dimin-

Table 63–1. Drugs with significant adverse effects on the fetus.

Drug	Trimester	Effect
Aminopterin	First	Multiple gross anomalies.
Barbiturates	All	Chronic use can lead to neonatal dependence.
Chloramphenicol	Third	Increased risk of gray baby syndrome.
Chlorpropamide	All	Prolonged symptomatic neonatal hypoglycemia.
Cortisone	First	Increased risk of cleft palate.
Diazepam	All	Chronic use leads to neonatal dependence.
Diethylstilbestrol	All	Vaginal adenosis, clear cell vaginal adenocarcinoma.
Ethanol	All	High risk of fetal alcohol syndrome.
Heroin	All	Chronic use leads to neonatal dependence.
Iodide	All	Congenital goiter, hypothyroidism.
Methadone	All	Chronic use leads to neonatal dependence.
Methyltestosterone	Second and third	Masculinization of female fetus.
Methylthiouracil	All	Hypothyroidism.
Norethindrone	All	Masculinization of female fetus.
Phenytoin	All	Cleft lip and palate.
Propylthiouracil	All	Congenital goiter.
Tetracycline	All	Discoloration of teeth.
Thalidomide	First	Phocomelia.
Trimethadione	All	Multiple congenital anomalies.
Warfarin	First	Hypoplastic nasal bridge, chondrodysplasia.
	Third	Risk of bleeding. Discontinue use 1 month before delivery.

ished peripheral perfusion to these areas. In this case, absorption becomes irregular and difficult to predict, because the drug may remain in the muscle and be absorbed more slowly than expected. In this way, it acts like a reservoir. However, if perfusion suddenly improves, there can be a sudden and unpredictable increase in the amount of drug entering the circulation, resulting in high and often toxic concentrations of drug. Examples of drugs especially hazardous in this situation are cardiac glycosides, aminoglycoside antibiotics, and anticonvulsants.

B. Gastrointestinal Function: Significant biochemical and physiologic changes occur in the neonatal gastrointestinal tract shortly after birth. Within the first 24 hours of life, there is a marked increase in gastric acidity. Therefore, drugs that are partially or totally inactivated by the low pH of gastric contents should not be administered orally.

Gastric emptying time is prolonged in the first day or 2 of life (up to 6 or 8 hours). Therefore, drugs that are absorbed primarily in the stomach may be absorbed more completely than anticipated. However, in the case of drugs absorbed in the small intestine, absorption—and therefore therapeutic effect—is delayed. Peristalsis in the neonate is irregular and may be slow. The amount of drug absorbed in the small intestine is therefore unpredictable in neonates; eg, more than the usual amount of drug may be absorbed if peristalsis is slowed, and this could result in toxicity from an otherwise normal dose. Table 63–2 lists the absorption of various drugs in the neonate as compared with older children and adults.

An increase in peristalsis, as in diarrheal conditions, tends to decrease overall absorption, since contact time with the large absorptive surface of the intestine is decreased.

Drug Distribution

As body composition changes with development, the relative volume into which a drug is distributed also changes. The neonate has a higher percentage (70–75%) of its body weight in the form of water than does the adult (50–60%). Differences can also be observed between the full-term neonate (70% of body weight as water) and the small premature neonate (85% of body weight as water). In addition, extracellular water is 40% of body weight in the neonate, compared with 20% in the adult. Most neonates will have a diuresis in the first 24–48 hours of life. Since most drugs become distributed throughout the extracellular water space in order to reach their receptors, the size (volume) of the extracellular water compartment is important in determining the concentration of drug at the receptor sites.

Premature infants have much less fat than full-term infants. Total body fat in premature infants is about 1% of total body weight, compared with 15% in full-term neonates. Therefore, organs that generally accumulate high concentrations of lipid-soluble drugs in adults and older children may accumulate smaller amounts of these drugs in more immature infants.

Another major factor determining drug distribution is drug binding to plasma proteins. Albumin is the plasma protein with the greatest binding capacity. In general, protein binding of drugs is reduced in the neonate. This has been seen with local anesthetic

Table 63–2. Oral drug absorption (bioavailability) of various drugs in the neonate compared with older children and adults.

Drug	Oral Absorption
Acetaminophen	Decreased
Ampicillin	Increased
Diazepam	Normal
Digoxin	Normal
Gentamicin	Decreased
Nafcillin	Increased
Penicillin G	Increased
Phenobarbital	Decreased
Phenytoin	Decreased
Sulfonamides	Normal

drugs, phenytoin, ampicillin, and phenobarbital. Therefore, the concentration of free (unbound) drug in plasma is increased. This can result in greater drug effect or toxicity despite a normal or even low plasma concentration of total drug (bound plus unbound).

As a practical example, consider 100 mg of drug X given to a patient. The concentration of total drug in the plasma is 100 μg/mL. If the drug is 50% protein-bound in an older child or adult, then 50 μg/mL is the concentration of free drug. Assume that this concentration of free drug produces the desired effect in the patient without producing toxicity. However, if this drug is given to a premature infant in a dosage adjusted for body weight and it produces a total drug concentration of 100 μg/mL, the concentration of free drug could be as high as 75 μg/mL because of reduced plasma protein binding. This concentration might be toxic.

Some drugs compete with serum bilirubin for binding to albumin. Drugs given to a neonate with jaundice can displace bilirubin from albumin. Because of the greater permeability of the neonatal blood-brain barrier, significant amounts of bilirubin may enter the brain and cause kernicterus. This was in fact observed when sulfonamide antibiotics were given to premature neonates as prophylaxis against sepsis. Conversely, as the serum bilirubin rises for physiologic reasons or because of a blood group incompatibility, bilirubin can displace a drug from albumin and significantly raise the free drug concentration. This would occur without altering the total drug concentration and would result in greater drug effects or toxicity at normal drug concentrations. This has been shown to happen with phenytoin.

Drug Metabolism

The metabolism of most drugs occurs in the liver (Chapter 3). The drug-metabolizing activities of the cytochrome P-450–dependent, mixed-function oxidases and the conjugating enzymes are substantially lower in early neonatal life than later. The point in development at which enzymatic activity is maximal depends upon the specific enzyme system in question. Because of the neonate's decreased ability to metabolize drugs, many drugs have slow clearances and prolonged half-lives in the body. If drug doses and dosing schedules are not altered accordingly, this immaturity predisposes the neonate toward adverse drug responses from drugs that are metabolized by the liver.

The data in Table 63–3 demonstrate how neonatal and adult drug half-lives can differ and how the half-lives of phenobarbital and phenytoin decrease as the neonate gets older. The process of maturation must be considered when administering drugs to this age group, especially if the drug or drugs are administered over long periods.

Another consideration for the neonate is whether or not the mother was receiving a drug such as phenobarbital, which can induce early maturation of fetal hepatic enzyme. In this case, the ability of the neonate to metabolize certain drugs will be greater than expected,

Table 63–3. Approximate half-lives of various drugs in neonates and adults.

Drug	Neonatal Age	Neonates $t_{1/2}$ (hours)	Adults $t_{1/2}$ (hours)
Acetaminophen		2.2–5	1.9–2.2
Diazepam		25–100	15–25
Digoxin		60–107	30–60
Phenobarbital	0–5 days 5–15 days 1–30 months	200 100 50	64–140
Phenytoin	0–2 days 3–14 days 14–50 days	80 18 6	12–18
Salicylate		4.5–11	2–4
Theophylline	Neonate Child	13–26 3–4	5–10

and one may see less therapeutic effect and lower plasma drug concentrations when the usual neonatal dose is given.

Drug Excretion

The glomerular filtration rate is much lower in newborns than in older infants, children, or adults, and this limitation persists during the first few days of life. Calculated on the basis of surface area, glomerular filtration in the neonate is only 30–40% and tubular secretion 20–30% of adult values. Function improves substantially during the first week of life. At that time, the glomerular filtration rate and renal plasma flow have increased 50% from the first day. By the end of the third week, glomerular filtration is 50–60% of the adult value; by 6–12 months, it reaches adult values. Therefore, drugs that depend on renal function for elimination are cleared from the body very slowly in the first weeks of life.

Penicillins, for example, are cleared from premature infants at 17% of the adult rate based on comparable surface area and 34% of the adult rate when adjusted for body weight. The dose of ampicillin for a neonate less than 7 days old is 50–100 mg/kg/d in 2 doses at 12-hour intervals. The dose for a neonate over 7 days old is 100–200 mg/kg/d in 3 doses at 8-hour intervals. A decreased rate of renal elimination in the neonate has also been observed with aminoglycoside antibiotics (kanamycin, gentamicin, neomycin, streptomycin). The dose of gentamicin for a neonate less than 7 days old is 5 mg/kg/d in 2 doses at 12-hour intervals. The dose for a neonate over 7 days old is 7.5 mg/kg/d in 3 doses at 8-hour intervals. Total body clearance of digoxin is directly dependent upon adequate renal function, and accumulation of digoxin can occur when glomerular filtration is decreased.

Since renal function in a sick infant may not improve at the predicted rate during the first weeks and months of life, appropriate adjustments in dose and dosing schedules may be very difficult. In this situation, adjustments are best made on the basis of plasma drug concentrations, determined at intervals throughout the course of therapy.

In summary, physiologic processes in the infant change significantly in the first year of life and particularly in the first few weeks. These changes must be considered when any drug is administered in the neonatal period.

PEDIATRIC DOSAGE FORMS & COMPLIANCE

The form in which a drug is manufactured and the way in which the parent dispenses the drug to the child determine the actual dose administered. Many drugs prepared for children are in the form of elixirs or suspensions. Elixirs are alcoholic solutions in which the drug molecules are dissolved and evenly distributed. No shaking is required, and the first dose from the bottle and the last dose should contain equivalent amounts of drug.

Suspensions contain undissolved particles of drug that must be distributed throughout the vehicle by shaking. If shaking is not thorough each time a dose is given, the first doses from the bottle will contain less drug than the last doses, with the result that less than the expected plasma concentration or effect of the drug may be achieved early in the course of therapy. Conversely, toxicity may occur late in the course of therapy when not expected. It is thus essential that the prescriber know the form in which the drug will be dispensed.

Compliance may be more difficult to achieve in pediatric practice than otherwise, since it involves not only the parent's conscientious effort to follow directions but such practical matters as measuring errors, spilling, and spitting out. (The measured volume of "teaspoons" ranges from 2.5 to 7.8 mL.) The parents should obtain a calibrated medicine spoon or syringe from the pharmacy. These devices improve the accuracy of dose measurements and simplify administration of drugs to children.

When evaluating compliance, it is often helpful to ask if an attempt has been made to give a further dose after the child has spilled half of what was offered. The parents may not always be able to say with confidence how much of a dose the child actually received. The parents must be told whether or not to wake the baby for its every-6-hour dose day or night. In the first 3 days of antibiotic therapy for otitis media, it may be important to maintain a relatively constant concentration of antibiotic in the blood and middle ear. If that is the goal, it is important that the parent give the medication on schedule no matter who is sleeping at the time. During the second week of treatment, since a constant concentration of antibiotic is then less important, a strict 6-hour schedule is not obligatory. These matters should be discussed with the parents and made clear to them, and no assumptions should be made about what the parents may or may not do. Noncompliance frequently occurs when antibiotics are prescribed to treat otitis media or urinary tract infections and the child feels well after 4 or 5 days of therapy. The parents may not feel there is any reason to continue giving the medicine even though it was prescribed for 10 or 14 days. This common situation should be anticipated so the parents can be told why it is important to continue the medicine for the prescribed period even if the child seems to be "cured."

Practical and convenient dosage forms and dosing schedules should be chosen to the extent possible. The easier it is to administer and take the medicine and the easier the dosing schedule is to follow, the more likely it is that compliance will be achieved.

Consistent with their abililty to comprehend and cooperate, children should also be given some responsibility for their own health care and for taking medications. This should be discussed in appropriate terms both with the child and the parents. Possible side effects and drug interactions with over-the-counter medicines or foods should also be discussed.

DRUG USE DURING LACTATION
(Table 63–4)

Drugs should be used conservatively during lactation, and the physician must know which drugs enter breast milk and are potentially dangerous to nursing infants (Table 63–4). Most drugs administered to lactating women are detectable in breast milk. Fortunately, the concentration of drug achieved in breast milk is usually low. Therefore, the total amount the infant would receive in a day is likely to be less than what would be considered a "therapeutic dose." If the nursing mother must take medication and the drug is a relatively safe one, she should take it 30–60 minutes after nursing and 3–4 hours before the next feeding. This allows time for many drugs to be cleared from the mother's blood, and the concentrations in breast milk will be relatively low. Drugs for which no data are available on safety during lactation should be avoided or breast feeding discontinued while they are given.

Most antibiotics taken by nursing mothers can be detected in breast milk. Sulfonamides should not be taken in the early neonatal period, because they compete with bilirubin for binding to plasma albumin and increase the risk of kernicterus. Tetracycline concentrations in breast milk are approximately 70% of maternal serum concentrations and present a risk of permanent tooth staining in the infant. Chloramphenicol concentrations in breast milk are not sufficient to cause gray baby syndrome, but there is a remote possibility of causing bone marrow suppression, and chloramphenicol should be avoided during lactation. Isoniazid reaches a rapid equilibrium between breast milk and maternal blood. The concentrations achieved in breast milk are high enough so that pyridoxine deficiency may occur in the infant if the mother is not given pyridoxine supplements.

Most sedatives and hypnotics achieve concentrations in breast milk sufficient to produce a pharmaco-

logic effect in the infant. Barbiturates taken in hypnotic doses by the mother can produce lethargy, sedation, and poor suck reflexes in the infant. Chloral hydrate can produce sedation if the infant is fed at peak milk concentrations. Diazepam can have a sedative effect on the nursing infant, but most importantly, its long half-life can result in significant drug accumulation.

Narcotics such as heroin, methadone, and morphine enter breast milk in quantities sufficient to induce a state of prolonged neonatal narcotic dependence if the drug was taken chronically by the mother during pregnancy. If conditions are well controlled and there is a good relationship between the mother and the physician, an infant could breast-feed while the mother is taking methadone. She should not, however, stop taking the drug abruptly; the infant can be tapered off the methadone as the mother's dose is tapered. The infant should be watched for signs of narcotic withdrawal.

Moderate use of alcohol by the mother should not be harmful to a nursing infant. Excessive amounts of alcohol, however, can produce alcohol effects in the infant. Nicotine concentrations in the breast milk of smoking mothers are low and do not produce effects in the infant. Very small amounts of caffeine are excreted in the breast milk of coffee-drinking mothers.

Lithium enters breast milk in concentrations equal to those in maternal serum. Clearance of this drug is almost completely dependent upon renal elimination, and women who are receiving lithium should not breast-feed.

Drugs that can alter endocrine function such as thiouracil and tolbutamide enter breast milk in quantities sufficient to affect endocrine function in the infant. They should be avoided if possible or breast feeding discontinued.

Radioactive substances such as iodinated ^{125}I albumin and radioiodine can cause thyroid suppression in infants and may increase the risk of subsequent thyroid cancer as much as 10-fold. Breast feeding is contraindicated after large doses and should be withheld for days to weeks after small doses.

In general, drug use by nursing mothers should be avoided if possible, and they should be cautioned against excessive use of over-the-counter medications, since the effects on nursing infants have not been studied extensively.

PEDIATRIC DRUG DOSAGE

Because of differences in pharmacokinetics in infants and children, simple linear reduction in the adult dose is rarely adequate in achieving a safe and effective pediatric dose. The most reliable pediatric dose information is usually that provided by the manufacturer in the package insert. If such information is not available for a given product, an approximation can be made by any of several methods based on age, weight, or surface area. These rules are not precise and should

Table 63–4. Commonly used drugs and their excretion into breast milk.

Drug	Effect on Infant	Comments
Ampicillin	Minimal	No significant side effects; possible occurrence of diarrhea or allergic sensitization.
Aspirin	Minimal	Occasional doses probably safe; high doses may produce significant concentration in breast milk.
Caffeine	Minimal	Caffeine intake in moderation is safe; concentration in breast milk is about 1% of total dose taken by mother.
Chloral hydrate	Significant	May cause drowsiness if fed at peak concentration in milk.
Chloramphenicol	Significant	Concentrations too low to cause gray baby syndrome; possibility of bone marrow suppression does exist; recommend not taking chloramphenicol while breast feeding.
Chlorothiazide	Minimal	No side effects reported.
Chlorpromazine	Minimal	Appears insignificant.
Codeine	Minimal	No side effects reported.
Diazepam	Significant	Will cause sedation in breast-fed infants; accumulation can occur in newborns.
Dicumarol	Minimal	No adverse side effects reported; may wish to follow infant's prothrombin time.
Digoxin	Minimal	Insignificant quantities enter breast milk.
Ethanol	Moderate	Moderate ingestion by mother unlikely to produce effects in infant; large amounts consumed by mother can produce alcohol effects in infant.
Heroin	Significant	Enters breast milk and can prolong neonatal narcotic dependence.
Iodine (radioactive)	Significant	Enters milk in quantities sufficient to cause thyroid suppression in infant.
Isoniazid (INH)	Minimal	Milk concentrations equal maternal plasma concentrations. Possibility of pyridoxine deficiency developing in the infant.
Kanamycin	Minimal	No adverse effects reported.
Lithium	Significant	Avoid breast feeding.
Methadone	Significant	(See heroin.) Under close physician supervision, breast feeding can be continued. Signs of opiate withdrawal in the infant may occur if mother stops taking methadone or stops breast feeding abruptly.
Oral contraceptives	Minimal	Will suppress lactation in high doses.
Penicillin	Minimal	Very low concentrations in breast milk.
Phenobarbital	Moderate	Hypnotic doses can cause sedation in the infant.
Phenytoin	Moderate	Amounts entering breast milk may be sufficient to cause side effects in infant.
Prednisone	Moderate	Low maternal doses probably safe. Doses 2 or more times physiologic amounts should probably be avoided.
Propranolol	Minimal	Very small amounts enter breast milk.
Propylthiouracil, thiouracil	Significant	Can suppress thyroid function in infant.
Spironolactone	Minimal	Very small amounts enter breast milk.
Tetracycline	Moderate	Possibility of permanent staining of developing teeth in the infant. Should be avoided during lactation.
Theophylline	Moderate	Can enter breast milk in moderate quantities but not likely to produce significant effects.
Thyroxine	Minimal	No adverse effects in therapeutic doses.
Tolbutamide	Minimal	Low concentrations in breast milk.
Warfarin	Minimal	Very small quantities found in breast milk.

not be used if the manufacturer provides a pediatric dose. Most drugs approved for use in children have recommended pediatric doses, generally stated as so many milligrams per kilogram or per pound. When pediatric doses are calculated (either from one of the methods set forth below or from a manufacturer's dose), the pediatric dose should never exceed the adult dose.

Surface Area

Calculations of dosage based on age or weight (see below) are conservative and tend to underestimate the

Table 63–5. Determination of drug dosage from surface area.[*][†]

Weight		Approximate Age	Surface Area (m²)	Percent of Adult Dose
(kg)	(lb)			
3	6.6	Newborn	0.2	12
6	13.2	3 months	0.3	18
10	22	1 year	0.45	28
20	44	5.5 years	0.8	48
30	66	9 years	1	60
40	88	12 years	1.3	78
50	110	14 years	1.5	90
65	143	Adult	1.7	102
70	154	Adult	1.76	103

[*]Reproduced, with permission, from Silver HK, Kempe CH, Bruyn HB: *Handbook of Pediatrics,* 14th ed. Lange, 1983.
[†]If adult dose is 1 mg/kg, dose for 3-month-old infant would be 2 mg/kg.

required dose. Doses based on surface area (Table 63–5) are more likely to be adequate. A more accurate estimate of surface area derived from data on weight and height may be obtained by reference to the nomograms on p 845.

Age

Young's rule:

$$\text{Dose} = \text{Adult Dose} \times \frac{\text{Age (years)}}{\text{Age} + 12}$$

Weight

Somewhat more precise is Clark's rule:

$$\text{Dose} = \text{Adult Dose} \times \frac{\text{Weight (kg)}}{70}$$

or

$$\text{Adult dose} \times \frac{\text{Weight (lb)}}{150}$$

REFERENCES

Drug toxicity in the newborn. (Symposium.) *Fed Proc* 1985; **44:**2301.

Hansten PD: *Drug Interactions,* 5th ed. Lea & Febiger, 1985.

McCracken HH, Nelson JD: *Antimicrobial Therapy for Newborns.* Grune & Stratton, 1977.

Mirkin BL (editor): *Clinical Pharmacology and Therapeutics: A Pediatric Perspective.* Year Book, 1978.

Mirkin BL (editor): *Perinatal Pharmacology and Therapeutics.* Academic Press, 1976.

Pagliaro LA, Levin RH (editors): *Problems in Pediatric Drug Therapy.* Drug Intelligence, 1979.

Rementeria JL (editor): *Drug Abuse in Pregnancy and Neonatal Effects.* Mosby, 1977.

Roberts RJ: *Drug Therapy in Infants: Pharmacologic Principles and Clinical Experience.* Saunders, 1984.

Wilson JT (editor): *Drugs in Breast Milk.* ADIS Press, 1981.

Yaffe SJ (editor): *Pediatric Pharmacology: Therapeutic Principles in Practice.* Grune & Stratton, 1980.

64

Special Aspects of Geriatric Pharmacology

Bertram G. Katzung, MD, PhD

Society often classifies everyone over 65 as "elderly," but most authorities consider the field of geriatrics to apply to persons over 75, even though this too is an arbitrary definition. Furthermore, chronologic age is only one determinant of most of the changes pertinent to drug therapy that occur in older adults. Important changes in drug responses occur with increasing age in most individuals. Drug usage patterns also change as a result of the increasing incidence of disease with age, the tendency to prescribe heavily for patients in nursing homes, and general changes in the lives of older people that have significant effects on the way drugs are—or should be—used. Among the latter are the increased incidence with advancing age of multiple diseases, nutritional problems, reduced financial resources, and the possibility of decreased dosing compliance for a variety of reasons.

The health practitioner thus should be aware of the changes in pharmacologic responses that may occur in older people and how to deal with these changes.

PHARMACOLOGIC CHANGES ASSOCIATED WITH AGING

Measurements of functional capacity of most of the major organ systems show a decline beginning in young adulthood and continuing throughout life. As shown in Fig 64–1, there is no "middle-age plateau" but rather a linear decrease beginning no later than age 45. Thus, the elderly do not lose specific functions at an accelerated rate compared to young and middle-aged adults but rather accumulate more deficiencies with the passage of time. Some of these changes result in altered pharmacokinetics. For the pharmacologist, the most important of these is the decrease in renal function. Other changes—and concurrent diseases—may alter the pharmacodynamic characteristics of the patient.

Pharmacokinetic Changes

A. Absorption: There is little evidence that there is any major alteration in drug absorption with age. However, conditions associated with age may alter the rate at which some drugs are absorbed. Such conditions include altered nutritional habits, greater con-

sumption of nonprescription drugs (eg, antacids, laxatives), and changes in gastric emptying.

B. Distribution: As noted in Chapters 1 and 3, the distribution of a drug is a function of the chemical characteristics of the drug molecule and the size and composition of the compartments of the body. The elderly have reduced lean body mass, reduced total and percentage body water, and an increase in fat as a percentage of body mass. Some of these changes are shown in Table 64–1. There is usually a decrease in serum albumin, which binds many drugs, especially weak acids. There may be a concurrent increase in serum orosomucoid (α-acid glycoprotein), a protein that binds many basic drugs. Thus, the ratio of bound to free drug may be significantly altered. As explained in Chapter 3, these changes may alter the appropriate loading dose of a drug. However, since both the clearance and the effects of drugs are related to the free concentration, the steady-state effects of a maintenance dosage regimen should not be altered by these factors

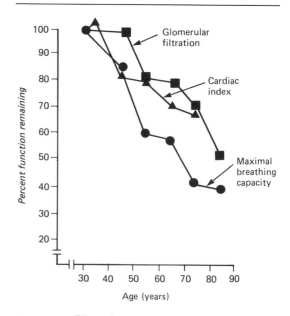

Figure 64–1. Effect of age on some physiologic functions. (Modified and reproduced, with permission, from Kohn RR: *Principles of Mammalian Aging.* Prentice-Hall, 1978.)

Table 64–1. Some changes related to aging that affect pharmacokinetics of drugs.*

Variable	Young Adults (20–30 years)	Geriatric Adults (60–80 years)
Body water (% of body weight)	61	53
Lean body mass (% of body weight)	19	12
Body fat (% of body weight)	26–33 (women) 18–20 (men)	38–45 36–38
Serum albumin (g/dL)	4.7	3.8
Kidney weight (% of young adult)	100	80
Hepatic blood flow (% of young adult)	100	55–60

*Compiled from various sources.

alone. For example, the loading dose of digoxin in an elderly patient with congestive heart failure should be reduced because of the decreased apparent volume of distribution. The maintenance dose may have to be reduced because of reduced clearance of the drug.

C. Metabolism: The capacity of the liver to metabolize drugs does not appear to decline consistently with age for all drugs. Animal studies and some clinical studies have suggested that certain drugs are metabolized more slowly; some of these drugs are listed in Table 64–2. It would appear that the greatest changes are in phase I reactions, ie, those carried out by the microsomal mixed function oxidase system; there are much smaller changes in the ability of the liver to carry out conjugation (phase II) reactions. (See Chapter 3.) Some of these changes may be caused by decreased liver blood flow (Table 64–1), an important

Table 64–2. Effects of age on hepatic clearance of some drugs. **(1)** Phase I metabolism by hepatic mixed function oxidase system; **(2)** phase II metabolism (conjugation) or phase I metabolism by nonmicrosomal systems. (For details, see Benet and Sheiner; Greenblatt, Sellars, and Shader; and Vestal references.)

Age-Related Decrease in Hepatic Clearance Found	No Age Difference Found
Alprazolam (1)	Ethanol (2)
Barbiturates (1)	Isoniazid (2)
Carbenoxolone (1)	Lidocaine (1)
Chlordiazepoxide (1)	Lorazepam (2)
Chlormethiazole (1)	Nitrazepam (2)
Clobazam (1)	Oxazepam (2)
Desmethyldiazepam (1)	Prazosin (1)
Diazepam (1)	Salicylate (2)
Flurazepam (1)	Warfarin (1)
Imipramine (1)	
Meperidine (1)	
Nortriptyline (1)	
Phenylbutazone (1)	
Propranolol (1)	
Quinidine, quinine (1)	
Theophylline (1)	
Tolbutamide (1)	

variable in the clearance of drugs that have a high hepatic extraction ratio. In addition, there is a decline with age of the liver's ability to recover from injury, eg, that caused by alcohol or viral hepatitis. Therefore, a history of recent liver disease in an older person should lead to caution in dosing with drugs that are cleared primarily by the liver, even after apparently complete recovery from the hepatic insult. Finally, diseases that affect hepatic function, eg, congestive heart failure, are more common in the elderly. Congestive heart failure may dramatically alter the ability of the liver to metabolize drugs and may also reduce hepatic blood flow. Similarly, severe nutritional deficiencies, which occur more often in old age, may impair hepatic function.

D. Elimination: Because the kidney is the major organ for clearance of drugs from the body, the "natural" decline of renal functional capacity referred to above is very important. As shown in Table 64–3, there is an age-related decline in creatinine clearance. It is important to note that this decline is not reflected in an equivalent rise in serum creatinine because the production of creatinine is also reduced as muscle mass declines with age. The decrease in clearance is rather consistent, so direct measurements of creatinine clearance need be made only if there is suspicion of actual renal disease or a disturbance of salt and water metabolism, eg, severe dehydration. The practical result of this change is marked prolongation of the half-life of many drugs (Fig 64–2) and the possibility of accumulation to toxic levels if dosage is not reduced in size or frequency. Dosing recommendations for the elderly often include an allowance for reduced renal clearance. If only the young adult dosage for a drug is known, correction can be made as described in Chapter 67. As indicated above, nutritional changes alter pharmacokinetic parameters. A patient who is severely dehydrated (not uncommon in patients with stroke or other motor impairment) may have an additional severe reduction in renal clearance of drugs that is completely reversible by rehydration.

The lungs are important for the excretion of gaseous drugs. As a result of reduced respiratory capacity (Fig 64–1) and the increased incidence of active

Table 64–3. Effects of age on creatinine clearance, serum concentration, and total body creatinine production.*

Age (years)	Creatinine Clearance (mL/min)†	Serum Creatinine Concentration (mg/dL)	Creatinine Production (mg/24 h)
17–24	140	0.81	1790
25–34	140	0.81	1862
35–44	133	0.81	1746
45–54	127	0.83	1689
55–64	120	0.84	1580
65–74	110	0.83	1409
75–84	97	0.84	1259

*Modified and reproduced, with permission, from Rowe JW et al: *J Gerontol* 1976;**31**:155.
†Normalized to 1.73 m² body surface area.

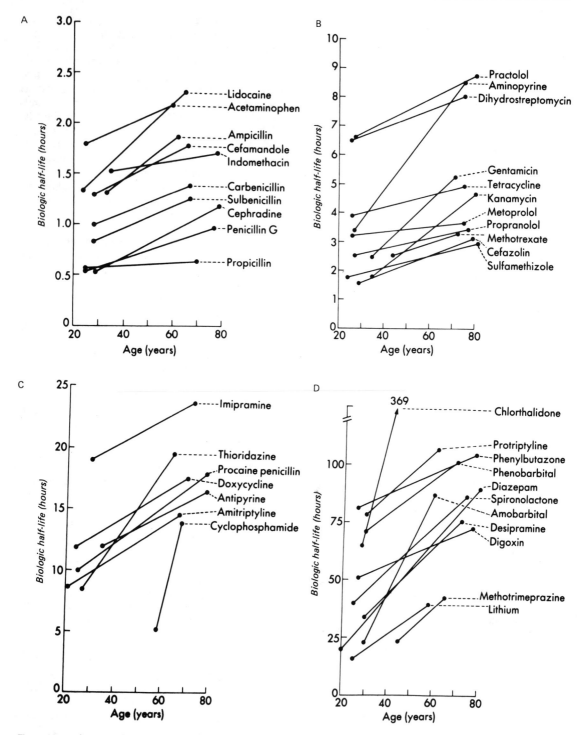

Figure 64–2. Increase in half-life of some drugs with age. The drugs have been grouped on the basis of half-life: *A:* 0.5–3 hours; *B:* 1–10 hours; *C:* 5–25 hours; *D:* 20–370 hours. Note that the lines merely connect the end points of the age range; they do not imply a linear relationship between age and half-life. (Modified and reproduced, with permission, from Ritschel WA: Pharmacokinetics in the aged. Chapter 10 in: *Pharmacologic Aspects of Aging.* Pagliaro LA, Pagliaro AM [editors]. Mosby, 1983.)

pulmonary disease in the elderly, the use of inhalation anesthesia is less common and parenteral agents more common in this age group. (See Chapter 23.)

Pharmacodynamic Changes

It was long believed that geriatric patients were much more "sensitive" to the action of many drugs, implying a change in the pharmacodynamic interaction of the drugs with their receptors. It is now recognized that many—perhaps most—of these apparent changes result from altered pharmacokinetics or diminished homeostatic responses. Clinical studies have supported the idea that the elderly are more sensitive to *some* sedative-hypnotics and analgesics. In addition, there are some data from animal studies that suggest actual changes with age in the characteristics or numbers of certain types of receptors. The most extensive studies show a decrease in responsiveness to beta-adrenoceptor stimulants and blockers. Other examples are discussed below.

Certain homeostatic control mechanisms appear to be blunted in the elderly. Since homeostatic responses are often important components of the total response to a drug, these physiologic alterations may change the pattern or intensity of drug response. In the cardiovascular system, average blood pressure goes up with age (in most Western countries), but the incidence of symptomatic orthostatic hypotension also increases markedly. Similarly, the average 2-hour postprandial blood sugar increases by about 1 mg/dL for each year of age above 50. Temperature regulation is also impaired, and hypothermia is poorly tolerated in the elderly.

MAJOR DRUG GROUPS

CENTRAL NERVOUS SYSTEM DRUGS

Sedative-Hypnotics

The half-lives of many benzodiazepines and barbiturates increase 50–150% between age 30 and age 70. Much of this change occurs during the decade from 60 to 70. For most of the benzodiazepines, both the parent molecule and its metabolites (produced in the liver) are pharmacologically active (Chapter 20). The age-related decline in renal function and liver disease both contribute to the reduction in elimination of these compounds. In addition, an increased volume of distribution has been reported for some of these drugs. Lorazepam and oxazepam may be less affected by these changes than most of the benzodiazepines. In addition to these pharmacokinetic factors, it is generally believed that the elderly are more variable in their sensitivity to the sedative-hypnotic drugs on a pharmacodynamic basis as well. Among the toxicities of these drugs, ataxia should be particularly watched for in order to avoid accidents.

Analgesics

The opioids (narcotic analgesics) show variable changes in pharmacokinetics with age. However, the elderly are often markedly more sensitive to the respiratory effects of these agents because of age-related changes in respiratory function. Therefore, this group of drugs should always be used with caution until the sensitivity of the particular patient has been evaluated. On the other hand, there is no reason to withhold opioids from the elderly if a proper indication for their use is present (see Chapter 29).

Antipsychotic & Antidepressant Drugs

The antipsychotic agents (phenothiazines and haloperidol) have been very heavily used (and probably misused) in the management of a variety of psychiatric diseases in the elderly. There is no doubt that they are useful in the management of schizophrenia in old age, and they are probably useful also in the treatment of symptoms associated with delirium or dementia, agitation and combativeness, and a paranoid syndrome that appears in some geriatric patients. However, they are not fully satisfactory in these geriatric conditions, and dosage should not be increased on the assumption that full control is possible. There is no evidence that these drugs have any beneficial effects in Alzheimer's dementia, and on theoretical grounds the antimuscarinic effects of the phenothiazines might be expected to worsen memory impairment and intellectual dysfunction (see below). Much of the apparent improvement in agitated and combative patients may simply reflect the sedative effects of the drugs. When a sedative antipsychotic is desired, a phenothiazine such as thioridazine is appropriate. If sedation is to be avoided, haloperidol is more appropriate. The latter drug has increased extrapyramidal toxicity, however, and should be avoided in patients with preexisting extrapyramidal disease. The phenothiazines, especially older drugs such as chlorpromazine, often induce orthostatic hypotension in young adults because of their alpha-adrenoceptor–blocking effects. They are even more prone to do so in the elderly. (See also Chapter 27.)

Because of increased responsiveness to all these drugs, dosage should usually be limited to a fraction of that used in young adults. The half-lives of some phenothiazines are increased in the geriatric population. The thioridazine half-life, for example, is more than doubled. Plasma protein binding of fluphenazine is reduced, which results in an increase of the free drug: total drug ratio.

Lithium is often used in the treatment of mania in the aged. Because it is cleared by the kidneys, doses should be adjusted appropriately. Concurrent use of thiazide diuretics reduces the clearance of lithium and should be accompanied by further reduction in dosage and measurement of lithium blood levels.

Psychiatric depression is thought to be underdiagnosed and undertreated in the elderly. The suicide rate in the over-65 age group (twice the national average) supports this view. Unfortunately, the apathy, flat affect, and social withdrawal of major depression may be mistaken for senile dementia. Limited evidence suggests that the elderly are as responsive to the antidepressants (both tricyclic agents and MAO inhibitors) as younger patients but are more sensitive to their toxic effects. This factor—along with the reduced clearance of some of these drugs—underlines the importance of careful dosing and strict attention to the appearance of toxic effects.

Drugs Used in Alzheimer's Disease

Alzheimer's disease is characterized by progressive impairment of memory and cognitive functions and may lead to a completely vegetative state. The biochemical defects responsible for these changes have not been identified, but there is considerable evidence that there is a marked decrease in choline acetyltransferase and other markers of cholinergic neuron activity. Decreases in brain dopamine, norepinephrine, serotonin, and somatostatin concentrations have also been reported. Eventually, cholinergic and possibly other neurons die or are destroyed (see Cutler reference). Many methods of treatment have been explored, but there is no convincing evidence that they are effective. The most promising (all of which are investigational at present) include methods for transmitter repletion and facilitation of cholinergic transmission. So-called cerebral vasodilators are quite ineffective.

CARDIOVASCULAR DRUGS

Antihypertensive Drugs

As noted above, blood pressure, especially systolic pressure, increases with age in Western countries and in most cultures in which salt intake is high. The increase is especially marked after age 50 in women. The high frequency and rather benign course of this form of late-onset systolic hypertension encourage a conservative approach to its treatment. On the other hand, diastolic hypertension and significant elevation of the systolic pressure above the age-corrected norm should be vigorously treated since they are associated with a marked increase in the incidence of stroke, congestive heart failure, and renal failure, and because effective treatment has been clearly shown to reduce the incidence of these sequelae.

The basic principles of therapy are not different in the geriatric age group from those described in Chapter 10, but the usual cautions regarding altered pharmacokinetics and sensitivity apply. Because of its safety, nondrug therapy (weight reduction in the obese and salt restriction) should be encouraged. Thiazides are a reasonable first step in drug therapy. The hypokalemia, hyperglycemia, and hyperuricemia toxicities of these agents are more relevant in the elderly because of the higher incidence of arrhythmias, non–insulin-dependent diabetes, and gout in these patients. Thus, use of low antihypertensive doses, rather than maximum diuretic doses, is important (see also Chap-

ter 14). Beta-blocking agents are effective and safe if titrated to the appropriate response. They are especially useful if the patient also has atherosclerotic angina (Chapter 11) but potentially hazardous in patients with obstructive airway disease. For more severe hypertension, methyldopa and hydralazine have proved effective and safe. The most powerful drugs, such as guanethidine and minoxidil, are rarely needed.

Positive Inotropic Agents

Congestive heart failure is a common and particularly lethal disease in the elderly. Fear of this condition may be one reason why physicians overuse cardiac glycosides in this age group. In one study, 90% of a group of elderly patients who were withdrawn from digoxin therapy had no recurrence of symptoms or signs of failure, ie, the drug was being used unnecessarily. The toxic effects of this drug group are particularly dangerous in the geriatric population, since the elderly are more susceptible to arrhythmias. The clearance of digoxin appears to be decreased in the older age group, and while the volume of distribution is often decreased, the half-life of this drug may be increased by 50% or more. Because the drug is cleared by the kidneys, renal function must be considered in designing a dosage regimen. There is no evidence that there is any increase in pharmacodynamic sensitivity to the therapeutic effects of the cardiac glycosides; in fact, animal studies suggest a possible decrease in therapeutic sensitivity. On the other hand, as noted above, there is probably an increase in sensitivity to the toxic arrhythmogenic actions. Hypokalemia, hypomagnesemia, hypoxemia (from pulmonary disease), and coronary atherosclerosis all contribute to the high incidence of digitalis-induced arrhythmias in geriatric patients. The less common toxicities of digitalis such as delirium, visual changes, and endocrine abnormalities (Chapter 12) also occur more often in the elderly.

Antiarrhythmic Agents

The treatment of arrhythmias in the elderly is particularly challenging because of the lack of good hemodynamic reserve, the frequency of electrolyte disturbances, and the high incidence of severe coronary disease. The clearances of quinidine and procainamide decrease and their half-lives increase with age. Disopyramide should probably be avoided in the geriatric population, because its major toxicities—antimuscarinic action, leading to voiding problems in men; and negative inotropic cardiac effects, leading to congestive heart failure—are particularly undesirable in these patients. The clearance of lidocaine appears to be little changed, but the half-life is increased in the elderly. Although this observation implies an increase in the volume of distribution, it has been recommended that the loading dose of this drug be reduced in geriatric patients because of their greater sensitivity to its toxic effects.

ANTIMICROBIAL DRUGS

Several age-related changes contribute to the high incidence of infections in geriatric patients. There appears to be a reduction in host defenses in the elderly; this is manifested in the increase in both serious infections and cancer. This may reflect an alteration in T lymphocyte function. In the case of the lungs, a major age- and tobacco-dependent decrease in mucociliary clearance significantly increases susceptibility to infection. In the urinary tract, the incidence of serious infection is greatly increased by urinary retention and catheterization in men. Since 1940, the antimicrobial drugs have contributed more to the prolongation of life than any other drug group, because they can compensate to some extent for this deterioration in natural defenses.

The basic principles of therapy of the elderly with these agents are no different from those applicable in younger patients and have been presented in Chapter 52. The major age-dependent changes relate to the decrease in renal function that has been described above; because most of the lactam and aminoglycoside antibiotics are excreted by this route, important changes in half-life may be expected. This is particularly important in the case of the aminoglycosides, because they cause concentration-dependent toxicity in the kidney and in other organs. For gentamicin, kanamycin, and netilmicin, the half-lives are more than doubled. According to one study, the increase may not be so marked for tobramycin.

ANTI-INFLAMMATORY DRUGS

Osteoarthritis is a very common disease of the elderly, and its treatment is often an exercise in geriatric pharmacology. Rheumatoid arthritis is less exclusively a geriatric problem, but the same drug therapy is usually applicable. The basic principles laid down in Chapter 34 and the properties of the anti-inflammatory drugs described there apply fully here.

The nonsteroidal anti-inflammatory agents must be used with special care in the geriatric patient because they cause toxicities to which the elderly are very susceptible. In the case of aspirin, the most important of these is gastrointestinal irritation and bleeding. In the case of the newer NSAIDs, they include renal damage, which may be irreversible, and a lesser degree of gastrointestinal intolerance. Because they are cleared primarily by the kidneys, they will accumulate more rapidly in the geriatric patient and especially in the patient whose renal function is already compromised beyond the normal limits for his or her age. A vicious cycle is easily set up in which cumulation of the NSAID causes more renal damage, which causes more cumulation, and so on. Benoxaprofen, a very efficacious NSAID, was withdrawn shortly after it was released because several elderly patients died in renal failure as a result of improper dosing. Elderly patients receiving high doses of any NSAID should be carefully monitored for changes in renal function.

Corticosteroids are extremely useful in elderly patients who cannot tolerate full doses of NSAIDs. However, they consistently cause a dose- and duration-related osteoporosis, an especially hazardous toxic effect in the elderly. It is not certain whether this drug-induced effect can be reduced by increased calcium and vitamin D intake, but it would seem prudent to use these agents and to encourage frequent exercise in any patient taking corticosteroids. (See also Chapter 41.)

ADVERSE DRUG REACTIONS IN THE ELDERLY

The positive relationship between number of drugs taken and the incidence of adverse reactions to them has been well documented. In long-term care facilities, which have a high population of the elderly, the average number of prescriptions per patient varies between 6.6 and 7.7. Studies have shown that the percentage of patients with adverse reactions increases from about 10% when a single drug is being taken to nearly 100% when 10 drugs are taken. Thus, it may be expected that about half of patients in long-term care facilities will have recognized or unrecognized reactions at some time. The overall incidence of drug reactions in geriatric patients is estimated to be at least twice that in the younger population. Reasons for this high incidence undoubtedly include errors in prescribing on the part of the practitioner and errors in drug usage by the patient.

Practitioner errors sometimes occur because the physician does not appreciate the importance of changes in pharmacokinetics with age and age-related diseases. Some errors occur because the practitioner is unaware of incompatible drugs prescribed by other practitioners for the same patient. For example, cimetidine, a drug heavily prescribed to the elderly, has a much higher incidence of untoward effects (eg, confusion, slurred speech) in the geriatric population when used alone. It also inhibits the hepatic metabolism of many drugs, including phenytoin, warfarin, beta blockers, and other agents. A patient who has been taking one of the latter agents without ill effect may develop markedly elevated blood levels and severe toxicity if cimetidine is added to the regimen without adjustment of dosage of the other drugs. Additional examples of drugs that inhibit liver microsomal enzymes and lead to adverse reactions are described in Appendix I.

Patient errors may result from noncompliance for reasons described below. In addition, they often result from use of nonprescription drugs that are taken without the knowledge of the physician. As noted in Chapter 68, many OTC agents contain "hidden ingredients" with potent pharmacologic effects. For example, many antihistamines have significant sedative effects and are inherently more hazardous in patients with impaired cognitive function. Similarly, their antimuscarinic action may precipitate urinary retention in the geriatric male or glaucoma in a patient with a narrow anterior chamber. If the patient is also taking a metabolism inhibitor such as cimetidine, the probability of an adverse reaction is greatly increased.

PRACTICAL ASPECTS OF GERIATRIC PHARMACOLOGY

The quality of life in elderly patients can be greatly improved—and life can be prolonged—by the intelligent use of drugs. However, there are several practical obstacles to compliance that the prescriber must recognize.

The expense of drugs can be a major disincentive in patients receiving marginal retirement incomes who are not covered by health insurance. The prescriber must be aware of the cost of the prescription and of cheaper alternative therapies. For example, leuprolide, a promising new peptide hormone for the treatment of advanced prostatic cancer (Chapter 36), costs more than $130 for a 14-day supply. Diethylstilbestrol, an older agent used for the same condition, costs about $4 for the same period. The monthly cost of arthritis therapy with newer NSAIDs exceeds $25, while that for generic aspirin is about $2 and for ibuprofen, an older NSAID, about $10–15.

Noncompliance may result from forgetfulness or confusion, especially if the patient has several prescriptions and different dosing intervals. Surveys show that the elderly receive 25% of the prescriptions written although they represent only 11% of the population. Since the prescriptions are often written by several different practitioners, there is usually no attempt to design "integrated" regimens that use drugs with similar dosing intervals for the conditions being treated. Patients may forget instructions regarding the need to complete a fixed duration of therapy when a course of treatment is being given, eg, for an infection. The disappearance of symptoms is often regarded as the best reason to halt drug-taking, especially if the prescription was expensive.

Noncompliance may also be deliberate. A decision not to take a drug may be based on prior experience with it. There may be excellent reasons for such "intelligent" noncompliance, and the practitioner should try to elicit them. Such efforts may also improve compliance with alternative drugs, because enlisting the patient as a participant in therapeutic decisions tends to increase motivation to succeed.

Some errors in drug-taking are caused by physical disabilities. Arthritis, tremor, and visual problems may all contribute. Liquid medications that are to be measured out "by the spoonful" are especially inappropriate for patients with any type of tremor or motor disability. "Childproof" containers are often "patient-proof" if the patient has arthritis. Cataracts and macular degeneration occur in a large number of patients over 70; therefore, labels on prescription bottles should be large enough for the patient with diminished vision to read—or color-coded if the patient can no longer read.

As noted above, drug therapy has considerable potential for both helpful and harmful effects in the geriatric patient. The balance may be tipped in the right direction by adherence to a few principles:

(1) Take a careful drug history. The disease to be treated may be drug-induced, or drugs being taken may lead to interactions with drugs to be prescribed.

(2) Prescribe only for a specific diagnosis. Do not prescribe cimetidine for "dyspepsia."

(3) Start with small doses and titrate to the response desired. Wait at least 3 geriatric half-lives before increasing the dose. If the expected response does not occur at the normal adult dosage, check blood levels. (See Chapter 67.)

(4) Maintain a high index of suspicion regarding drug reactions and interactions. Know what other drugs the patient is taking.

(5) Simplify the regimen as much as possible. When multiple drugs are prescribed, try to use drugs that can be taken at the same time of day. Whenever possible, reduce the number of drugs being taken.

REFERENCES

Benet LZ, Sheiner LB: Design and optimization of dosage regimens: Pharmacokinetic data. Appendix 2, pp 1663–1733, in: *Goodman and Gilman's The Pharmacological Basis of Therapeutics,* 7th ed. Gilman AG et al (editors). Macmillan, 1985.

Cutler NR et al: Alzheimer's disease and Down's syndrome: New insights. *Ann Intern Med* 1985;**103**:566.

Feldman RD et al: Alterations in leukocyte β-receptor affinity with aging: A potential explanation for altered β-adrenergic sensitivity in the elderly. *N Engl J Med* 1984;**310**:815.

Greenblatt DJ, Sellers EM, Shader RI: Drug disposition in old age. *N Engl J Med* 1982;**306**:1081.

Jarvik L (editor): *Clinical Pharmacology and the Aged Patient.* Raven, 1981.

Kohn RR: *Principles of Mammalian Aging.* Prentice-Hall, 1978.

Pagliaro LA, Pagliaro AM (editors): *Pharmacologic Aspects of Aging.* Mosby, 1983.

Ritschel WA: Pharmacokinetics in the aged. Chap 10, pp 219–256, in: *Pharmacologic Aspects of Aging.* Pagliaro LA, Pagliaro AM (editors). Mosby, 1983.

Roberts J, Steinberg GM (editors): Effects of aging on adrenergic receptors. (Symposium.) *Fed Proc* 1986;**45**:40.

Roe DA: *Drugs and Nutrition in the Geriatric Patient.* Churchill Livingstone, 1984.

Rowe JW: Health care of the elderly. *N Engl J Med* 1985; **312**:827.

Rowe JW, Besdine RW: Approach to the elderly patient: Physiologic and clinical considerations. Chap 1, pp 3–11, in: *Drug Treatment in the Elderly*. Vestal RE (editor). ADIS Health Science Press, 1984.

Salzman C: Geriatric psychopharmacology. *Annu Rev Med* 1985;**36**:217.

Schmucker DL: Age-related changes in drug disposition. *Pharmacol Rev* 1979:**30**:445.

Schmucker DL: Aging and drug disposition: An update. *Pharmacol Rev* 1985;**37**:133.

Vestal RE (editor): *Drug Treatment in the Elderly*. ADIS Health Science Press, 1984.

Vestal RE: Wood AJJ, Shand DG: Reduced β-adrenoceptor sensitivity in the elderly. *Clin Pharmacol Ther* 1979;**26**:181.

65

Dermatologic Pharmacology

Dirk B. Robertson, MD, & Howard I. Maibach, MD

The skin offers a number of special problems and opportunities to the therapist. Topical therapy is especially appropriate for diseases of the skin, although some dermatologic diseases respond as well or better to drugs administered systemically.

The general pharmacokinetic principles governing the use of drugs applied to the skin are the same as those involved in other routes of drug administration (Chapters 1 and 3). However, human skin, though often depicted as a simple 3-layered structure, is a complex series of diffusion barriers. Quantitation of the flux of drugs and drug vehicles through these barriers is the basis of pharmacokinetic analysis of dermatologic therapy; techniques for making such measurements are rapidly increasing in number and sensitivity.

Major variables that determine pharmacologic response to drugs applied to the skin include the following:

(1) Regional variation in drug penetration: For example, the scrotum, face, axilla, and scalp are far more permeable than the forearm and may require less drug for equivalent effect.

(2) Concentration gradient: Increasing the concentration gradient increases the mass of drug transferred per unit time, just as in the case of diffusion across other barriers (Chapter 1). Thus, resistance to topical corticosteroids can sometimes be overcome by use of higher concentrations of drug.

(3) Dosing schedule: Because of its physical properties, the skin acts as a reservoir for many drugs. As a result, the "local half-life" may be long enough to permit once-daily application of drugs with short systemic half-lives. For example, once-daily application of corticosteroids appears to be just as effective as multiple applications in many situations.

(4) Vehicles and occlusion: An appropriate vehicle maximizes the ability of the drug to penetrate the outer layers of the skin. In addition, through their physical properties (moistening or drying effects), vehicles may themselves have important therapeutic effects.

Occlusion (application of a plastic wrap to hold the drug and its vehicle in close contact with the skin) is extremely effective in maximizing absorption of many drugs.

DERMATOLOGIC VEHICLES

Topical medications usually consist of active ingredients incorporated in a vehicle that facilitates cutaneous application. Important considerations in selection of a vehicle include the solubility of the active agent in the vehicle; the rate of release of the agent from the vehicle; the ability of the vehicle to hydrate the stratum corneum, thus enhancing penetration; the stability of the therapeutic agent in the vehicle; and interactions, chemical and physical, of the vehicle, stratum corneum, and active agent. Vehicles have traditionally been considered pharmacologically inert; however, owing to their unique physical properties, many are therapeutically beneficial themselves.

Depending upon the vehicle, dermatologic formulations may be classified as tinctures, wet dressings, lotions, gels, aerosols, powders, pastes, creams, and ointments. The ability of the vehicle to retard evaporation from the surface of the skin increases in this series, being least in tinctures and wet dressings and greatest in ointments. In general, acute inflammation with oozing, vesiculation, and crusting is best treated with drying preparations such as tinctures, wet dressings, and lotions, while chronic inflammation with xerosis, scaling, and lichenification is best treated with more lubricating preparations such as creams and ointments. Tinctures, lotions, gels, and aerosols are convenient for application to the scalp and hairy areas. Emulsified vanishing type creams may be used in intertriginous areas without causing maceration.

Emulsifying agents are used to provide homogeneous, stable preparations when mixtures of immiscible liquids such as oil-in-water creams are compounded. Examples include alkyl sulfates (sodium lauryl sulfate), glyceryl monostearate, polyoxyethylene sorbitan monostearate and monooleate (polysorbate 80), and polyethylene glycols (Carbowax). These emulsifying agents are commonly found in lotions, creams, and ointments containing oily constituents and water. Some patients develop irritation from these agents. Substituting a preparation that does not contain them or using one containing a lower concentration may resolve the problem. Other additives widely used in dermatologic preparations include cetyl palmitate and related esters, which improve the consistency and appearance of creams; stearic acid and stearyl alcohol, which act as lubricants, emollients, and antifoaming agents; and methylcellulose and gum tragacanth, which are inert compounds used as suspending agents in pastes and ointments. The methyl and propyl esters of *p*-aminobenzoic acid (methylparaben and propylparaben) frequently are added as preservatives.

ANTIBACTERIAL AGENTS

TOPICAL ANTIBACTERIAL PREPARATIONS

Topical antibacterial agents may be useful in preventing infections in clean wounds, in the early treatment of infected dermatoses and wounds, in reducing colonization of the nares by staphylococci, in axillary deodorization, and in the management of acne vulgaris. The efficacy of antibiotics in these topical applications is not uniform. The general pharmacology of the antimicrobial drugs is discussed in Chapters 42–54.

Numerous topical anti-infectives contain corticosteroids in addition to antibiotics. There is no convincing evidence that topical corticosteroids inhibit the antibacterial effect of antibiotics when the 2 are incorporated in the same preparation. In the treatment of secondarily infected dermatoses, which are usually colonized with streptococci, staphylococci, or both, combination therapy may prove superior to corticosteroid therapy alone. Antibiotic-corticosteroid combinations may be useful in treating diaper dermatitis, otitis externa, and impetiginized eczema.

The selection of a particular antibiotic depends of course upon the diagnosis and, whenever possible, in vitro culture and sensitivity studies of clinical samples. The pathogens isolated from most infected dermatoses are group A beta-hemolytic streptococci, *Staphylococcus aureus,* or both. The pathogens present in surgical wounds will be those resident in the environment. Information about regional epidemiologic data and the prevailing patterns of drug resistance is therefore important in selecting a therapeutic agent. Prepackaged topical antibacterial preparations that contain multiple antibiotics are available in fixed dosages well above the therapeutic threshold. These formulations offer the advantages of efficacy in mixed infections, broader coverage for infections due to undetermined pathogens, and delayed microbial resistance to any single component antibiotic.

BACITRACIN & GRAMICIDIN

Bacitracin and gramicidin are polypeptide antibiotics, active against gram-positive organisms such as streptococci, pneumococci, and staphylococci. In addition, most anaerobic cocci, neisseriae, tetanus bacilli, and diphtheria bacilli are sensitive. Bacitracin is compounded in an ointment base alone or in combination with neomycin, polymyxin B, or both. The use of bacitracin in the anterior nares temporarily decreases colonization by pathogenic staphylococci. Microbial resistance may develop following prolonged use. Bacitracin-induced contact urticaria syndrome occurs rarely. Allergic contact dermatitis occurs more frequently. Bacitracin is poorly absorbed through the skin, so systemic toxicity is rare.

Gramicidin is available only for topical use, in combination with other antibiotics such as neomycin, polymyxin, bacitracin, and nystatin. Systemic toxicity limits this drug to topical use. The incidence of sensitization following topical application is exceedingly low in therapeutic concentrations.

POLYMYXIN B SULFATE

Polymyxin B is a polypeptide antibiotic effective against gram-negative organisms, including *Pseudomonas aeruginosa, Escherichia coli, Enterobacter,* and *Klebsiella.* Most strains of *Proteus* and *Serratia* are resistant, as are all gram-positive organisms. Topical preparations may be compounded in either a solution or ointment base. Numerous prepackaged antibiotic combinations containing polymyxin B are available. Detectable serum concentrations are difficult to achieve from topical application, but the total daily dose applied to denuded skin or open wounds should not exceed 200 mg in order to reduce the likelihood of neurotoxicity and nephrotoxicity. Hypersensitivity to topically applied polymyxin B sulfate is uncommon.

NEOMYCIN & GENTAMICIN

Neomycin and gentamicin are aminoglycoside antibiotics active against gram-negative organisms, including *E coli, Proteus, Klebsiella,* and *Enterobacter.* Gentamicin generally shows greater activity against *P aeruginosa* than neomycin. Gentamicin is also more active against staphylococci and group A betahemolytic streptococci. Widespread topical use of gentamicin, especially in a hospital environment, should be avoided to slow the appearance of gentamicin-resistant organisms.

Neomycin is available in numerous topical formulations, both alone and in combination with polymyxin, bacitracin, and other antibiotics. It is also available as a sterile powder for topical use. Gentamicin is available as an ointment or cream.

Topical application of neomycin rarely results in detectable serum concentrations. However, in the case of gentamicin, serum concentrations of 1–18 μg/mL are possible if the drug is applied in a water-miscible preparation to large areas of denuded skin, as in burned patients. Both drugs are water-soluble and are excreted primarily in the urine. Renal failure may permit the accumulation of these antibiotics, with possible nephrotoxicity, neurotoxicity, and ototoxicity.

Neomycin frequently causes sensitization, particularly if applied to eczematous dermatoses or if compounded in an ointment vehicle. When sensitization occurs, cross-sensitivity to streptomycin, kanamycin, paromomycin, and gentamicin is possible.

TOPICAL ANTIBIOTICS IN ACNE

Several parenteral antibiotics that have traditionally been used in the treatment of acne vulgaris have been shown to be effective when applied topically. Currently, 3 antibiotics are so utilized: clindamycin phosphate, erythromycin base, and tetracycline hydrochloride. The effectiveness of topical therapy is less than that achieved by systemic administration of the same antibiotic. Therefore, topical therapy is generally effective only in mild to moderate cases of inflammatory acne.

Clindamycin

Clindamycin has in vitro activity against *Propionibacterium (Corynebacterium) acnes;* this has been postulated as the mechanism of its beneficial effect in acne therapy. Approximately 10% of an applied dose is absorbed, and rare cases of bloody diarrhea and pseudomembranous colitis have been reported following topical application. The hydroalcoholic vehicle may cause drying and irritation of the skin, with complaints of burning and stinging. Allergic contact dermatitis is uncommon.

Erythromycin

In topical preparations, the base of erythromycin rather than a salt is used to facilitate penetration. Although the mechanism of action of topical erythromycin in inflammatory acne vulgaris is unknown, it is presumed to be due to its inhibitory effects on *P acnes.* One of the possible complications of topical therapy is the development of antibiotic-resistant strains of organisms, including staphylococci. If this occurs in association with a clinical infection, topical erythromycin should be discontinued and appropriate systemic antibiotic therapy started. Adverse local reactions may include a burning sensation at the time of application and drying and irritation of the skin. Allergic hypersensitivity appears to be uncommon.

Tetracycline

Two topical tetracycline antibiotics are currently available for topical treatment of acne vulgaris: (1) tetracycline hydrochloride in a hydroalcoholic base containing *n*-decyl methyl sulfoxide and (2) meclocycline sulfosalicylate in a cream base. The pharmacology of the tetracycline antibiotics is presented in Chapter 44. Serum levels of tetracycline obtained from continued twice-daily topical use of hydroalcoholic preparations are 0.1 μg/mL or less, and no demonstrable absorption has been reported following extensive twice-daily topical application of the meclocycline sulfosalicylate preparation over 4 weeks.

The beneficial effect of these preparations on acne vulgaris has been attributed to their inhibitory action on *P acnes.* Their use is associated with temporary yellow staining of the skin, which is most noticeable in fair-skinned individuals. Although photosensitivity has not been a problem, this hazard should be considered when using these potentially phototoxic antibiotics. As with all tetracycline derivatives, these agents should not be used in patients who are pregnant or have a history of significant renal or hepatic dysfunction.

ANTIFUNGAL AGENTS

The treatment of superficial fungal infections caused by dermatophytic fungi may be accomplished (1) with topical antifungal agents, eg, clotrimazole, miconazole, econazole, tolnaftate, and haloprogin; or (2) with orally administered agents, eg, griseofulvin and ketoconazole. Superficial infections caused by *Candida* sp may be treated with topical applications of clotrimazole, miconazole, econazole, nystatin, or amphotericin B. Chronic generalized mucocutaneous candidiasis is responsive to long-term therapy with oral ketoconazole.

TOPICAL ANTIFUNGAL PREPARATIONS

CLOTRIMAZOLE, MICONAZOLE, & ECONAZOLE

The imidazoles, such as clotrimazole, miconazole, and econazole, have a wide range of activity against dermatophytes *(Epidermophyton, Microsporum,* and *Trichophyton)* and yeasts, including *Candida albicans* and *Pityrosporon orbiculare,* the cause of tinea versicolor (see Chapter 48). These agents are chemically related to ketoconazole, whose structure is shown on p 556.

Miconazole (Monistat) is available for topical application as a cream or as a lotion, and as vaginal cream or suppositories for use in vulvovaginal candidiasis. An injectable form for intravenous administration in the treatment of potentially fatal systemic fungal infections is also available. Clotrimazole (Lotrimin, Mycelex) is available for topical application to the skin as a cream or as a lotion, and as vaginal cream and tablets for use in vulvovaginal candidiasis. Econazole (Spectazole) is available as a cream for topical application. Topical antifungal-corticosteroid fixed combinations have recently been introduced on the basis of providing more rapid symptomatic improvement than an antifungal agent alone. Clotrimazole-betamethasone cream is one such example.

Twice-daily application to the affected area will generally result in clearing of superficial dermatophyte infections in 2–3 weeks, although the medication should be continued until eradication of the organism is confirmed. Paronychial and intertriginous candidiasis can be treated effectively by any of these agents when applied 3–4 times daily.

Adverse local reactions to clotrimazole, miconazole, and econazole may include stinging, pruritus, erythema, and local irritation. Allergic contact dermatitis appears to be uncommon.

CICLOPIROX OLAMINE

Ciclopirox olamine is a synthetic broad-spectrum antimycotic agent with inhibitory activity against dermatophytes, *Candida* species, and *P orbiculare*. This agent appears to inhibit the uptake of precursors of macromolecular synthesis; the site of action is probably the cell membrane.

Ciclopirox olamine

Pharmacokinetic studies indicate that 1–2% of the dose is absorbed when applied as a solution on the back under an occlusive dressing. Ciclopirox olamine is available as a 1% cream (Loprox) for the topical treatment of dermatomycosis, candidiasis, and tinea versicolor. The incidence of adverse reactions has been low. Pruritus and worsening of clinical disease have been reported. The potential for delayed allergic contact hypersensitivity appears small.

TOLNAFTATE

Tolnaftate is a synthetic antifungal compound that is effective topically against dermatophyte infections caused by *Epidermophyton*, *Microsporum*, and *Trichophyton*. It is also active against *P orbiculare* but not against *Candida*.

Tolnaftate

Tolnaftate (Aftate, Tinactin) is available as a cream, solution, powder, or powder aerosol for application twice daily to infected areas. Recurrences following cessation of therapy are common, and infections of the palms, soles, and nails are usually unresponsive to tolnaftate alone. The powder or powder aerosol may be used chronically following initial treatment in patients susceptible to tinea infections. Tolnaftate is generally well tolerated and rarely causes irritation or allergic contact sensitization.

HALOPROGIN

Haloprogin is a synthetic halogenated phenolic ether, active against *Epidermophyton*, *Microsporum*, and *Trichophyton* as well as *P orbiculare*. Although this compound does exhibit in vitro activity against *Candida*, its use is generally restricted to the treatment of dermatophyte infections and tinea versicolor.

Haloprogin

Haloprogin (Halotex) is available as cream or solution. There is only slight penetration of intact skin, and systemic toxicity following topical application has not been observed. The small amounts of drug that are absorbed are converted to trichlorophenol, which is excreted predominantly in the urine. Twice-daily application to the affected area usually results in clearing in 2–3 weeks. Infections of the palms, soles, and nails are generally resistant to topical therapy. Adverse reactions include local irritation, burning sensations, vesiculation, increased maceration, and exacerbation of the preexisting lesion. Contact with the eyes must be avoided. Allergic contact hypersensitivity is uncommon.

NYSTATIN & AMPHOTERICIN B

Nystatin and amphotericin B are useful in the topical therapy of *C albicans* infections but ineffective against dermatophytes. Nystatin is limited to topical treatment of cutaneous and mucosal *Candida* infections because of its narrow spectrum and negligible absorption from the gastrointestinal tract following oral administration. Amphotericin B has a broader antifungal spectrum and is used intravenously in the treatment of many systemic mycoses and to a lesser extent in the treatment of cutaneous *Candida* infections.

The recommended dosage for topical preparations of nystatin in treating paronychial and intertriginous candidiasis is application 2 or 3 times a day. Oral candidiasis (thrush) is treated by holding 5 mL (infants,

2 mL) of nystatin oral suspension in the mouth for several minutes 4 times daily before swallowing. An alternative therapy for thrush is to retain a vaginal tablet in the mouth until dissolved 4 times daily. Recurrent or recalcitrant perianal, vaginal, vulvar, and diaper area candidiasis may respond to oral nystatin, 0.5–1 million units in adults (100,000 units in children) 4 times daily in addition to local therapy. Vulvovaginal candidiasis may be treated by insertion of 1 vaginal tablet twice daily for 14 days, then nightly for an additional 14–21 days.

Amphotericin B (Fungizone) is available for topical use in cream, ointment, and lotion form. The recommended dosage in the treatment of paronychial and intertriginous candidiasis is application 2–4 times daily to the affected area.

Adverse side effects associated with oral administration of nystatin include mild nausea, diarrhea, and occasional vomiting. Topical application is nonirritating, and allergic contact hypersensitivity is exceedingly uncommon. Topical amphotericin B is well tolerated and only occasionally locally irritating. Hypersensitivity is exceedingly rare. The drug may cause a temporary yellow staining of the skin, especially when the cream vehicle is used.

ORAL ANTIFUNGAL AGENTS

GRISEOFULVIN

Griseofulvin is effective orally against dermatophyte infections caused by *Epidermophyton, Microsporum,* and *Trichophyton* (Chapter 48). It is ineffective against *Candida* and *P orbiculare*.

Griseofulvin's antifungal activity has been attributed to inhibition of hyphal cell wall synthesis, effects on nucleic acid synthesis, and inhibition of mitosis. Griseofulvin interferes with microtubules of the mitotic spindle and with cytoplasmic microtubules. The destruction of cytoplasmic microtubules may result in impaired processing of newly synthesized cell wall constituents at the growing tips of hyphae. Griseofulvin is active only against growing cells.

Following the oral administration of 1 g of micronized griseofulvin, peak serum levels of 1.5–2 μg/mL are obtained in 4–8 hours. The drug can be detected in the stratum corneum 4–8 hours following oral administration, with the highest concentration in the outermost layers and the lowest in the base. Reduction of particle size greatly enhances absorption. Ultramicronized griseofulvin achieves bioequivalent plasma levels with half the dose of micronized drug. In addition, solubilizing griseofulvin in polyethylene glycol enhances absorption even further. Micronized griseofulvin is available as 250-mg and 500-mg tablets, and ultramicronized drug is available as 125-mg, 165-mg, and 330-mg tablets and as 250-mg capsules.

The usual adult dose of the micronized ("micro-size") form of the drug is 500 mg daily in single or divided doses with meals; occasionally, 1 g/d is indicated in the treatment of recalcitrant infections. The pediatric dose is 10 mg/kg of body weight daily in single or divided doses with meals. An oral suspension is available for use in children.

Griseofulvin is most effective in treating tinea infections of the scalp and glabrous (nonhairy) skin. In general, infections of the scalp respond to treatment in 4–6 weeks, and infections of glabrous skin will respond in 3–4 weeks. Dermatophyte infections of the nails respond only to prolonged administration of griseofulvin. Fingernails may respond to 6 months of therapy, whereas toenails are quite recalcitrant to treatment and may require 8–18 months of therapy; relapse almost invariably occurs.

Adverse side effects seen with griseofulvin therapy include headaches, nausea, vomiting, diarrhea, photosensitivity, peripheral neuritis, and occasionally mental confusion. Griseofulvin is derived from a *Penicillium* mold, and cross-sensitivity with penicillin may occur. It is contraindicated in patients with porphyria or hepatic failure or those who have had hypersensitivity reactions to it in the past. Its safety in pregnant patients has not been established. Leukopenia and proteinuria have occasionally been reported, and in patients undergoing prolonged therapy, routine evaluation of hepatic, renal, and hematopoietic systems may be desirable. Coumarin anticoagulant activity may be altered by griseofulvin, and anticoagulant dosage may require adjustment.

KETOCONAZOLE

Ketoconazole is a water-soluble synthetic anti-fungal imidazole derivative active against many fungi and yeasts, including dermatophytes, *Candida, P orbiculare,* and numerous dimorphic fungi responsible for systemic mycoses.

As explained in Chapter 48, imidazole derivatives, including ketoconazole, act by affecting the permeability of the cell membrane of sensitive cells through alterations of the biosynthesis of lipids, especially sterols, in the fungal cell.

Ketoconazole (Nizoral) is the first imidazole derivative available for oral treatment of systemic mycoses. Patients with chronic mucocutaneous candidiasis respond well to a once-daily dose of 200 mg of ketoconazole, with a median clearing time of 16 weeks. Most patients require long-term maintenance therapy. Variable results have been reported in treatment of chromomycosis.

Ketoconazole has been shown to be quite effective in the therapy of cutaneous infections caused by *Epidermophyton, Microsporum,* and *Trichophyton* species. Infections of the glabrous skin often respond within 2–3 weeks to a once-daily oral dose of 200 mg. Palmar-plantar skin is slower to respond, often taking 4–6 weeks at a dosage of 200 mg twice daily. Infections of the hair and nails may take even longer before resolving with low cure rates noted for tinea capitis. Tinea versicolor is very responsive to short courses (2 weeks) of a once-daily dose of 200 mg.

Nausea or pruritus has been noted in approximately 3% of patients taking ketoconazole. More significant side effects include gynecomastia, elevations of hepatic enzyme levels, and hepatitis. Caution is advised when using ketoconazole in patients with a history of hepatitis, and hepatic failure should be considered a relative contraindication to its use.

ANTIVIRAL AGENTS

ACYCLOVIR

Acyclovir is a synthetic guanine analog with inhibitory activity against members of the herpesvirus family, including herpes simplex types 1 and 2. As explained in Chapter 49, acyclovir is phosphorylated preferentially by herpes simplex virus–coded thymidine kinase and, following further phosphorylation, the resultant acyclovir triphosphate interferes with herpesvirus DNA polymerase and viral DNA replication. Indications and usage of parenteral acyclovir in the treatment of cutaneous infections are discussed in Chapter 49.

Topical acyclovir (Zovirax) is available as a 5% ointment for application to primary cutaneous herpes simplex infections and to limited mucocutaneous herpes simplex virus infections in immunocompromised patients. In primary infections, the use of topical acyclovir shortens the duration of viral shedding and may decrease healing time. In localized, limited mucocutaneous infections in immunocompromised patients, its use may be associated with a decrease in the duration of viral shedding. There is no evidence that the topical use of acyclovir is of any benefit in the treatment of recurrent disease in nonimmunocompromised patients. Indiscriminate use of acyclovir may result in the selection of resistant strains of herpes simplex virus, which are deficient in viral-coded thymidine kinase. This should be considered when contemplating the use of topical acyclovir in other than nonimmunocompromised patients with primary herpes simplex infection.

Adverse local reactions to acyclovir may include pruritus and mild pain with transient stinging or burning.

ECTOPARASITICIDES

LINDANE
(Hexachlorocyclohexane)

The gamma isomer of hexachlorocyclohexane was commonly called gamma benzene hexachloride,

which was a misnomer, since no benzene ring is present in this compound. Lindane is an effective pediculicide and scabicide.

Percutaneous absorption studies using a solution of lindane in acetone have shown that almost 10% of a dose applied to the forearm is absorbed, to be subsequently excreted in the urine over a 5-day period. Serum levels following the application of a commercial lindane lotion reach maximum at 6 hours and decline thereafter with a half-life of 24 hours. After absorption, lindane is concentrated in fatty tissues, including the brain.

Lindane (Kwell, Scabene) is available as a shampoo, lotion, or cream. For pediculosis capitis or pubis, 30 mL of shampoo is worked into a lather and left on the scalp or genital area for 5 minutes and then rinsed off. If living lice are present 1 week after treatment, reapplication may be required. Recent concerns about the toxicity of lindane have altered treatment guidelines for its use in scabies; the current recommendation calls for a single application to the entire body from the neck down, left on for 8–12 hours, and then washed off. Patients should be re-treated only if active mites can be demonstrated, and never within 1 week of initial treatment.

Much controversy exists about the possible systemic toxicities of topically applied lindane used for medical purposes. Concerns about neurotoxicity and hematotoxicity have resulted in warnings that lindane should be used with caution in infants, children, and pregnant women. The current USA package insert recommends that it not be used as an antiscabetic in premature infants and in patients with known seizure disorders. The risk of adverse systemic reactions to lindane appears to be minimal when it is used properly and according to directions in adult patients. However, local irritation may occur, and contact with the eyes and mucous membranes should be avoided.

CROTAMITON

Crotamiton, N-ethyl-*o*-crotonotoluidide, is a scabicide with some antipruritic properties. Its mechanism of action is not known, and studies on percutaneous absorption have not been performed.

Crotamiton (Eurax) is available as cream or lotion. Suggested guidelines for scabies treatment call for 2 applications to the entire body from the chin down at 24-hour intervals, with a cleansing bath 48 hours after the last application. Crotamiton is an effective agent that can be used as an alternative to lindane. Allergic contact hypersensitivity and primary irritation may

Crotamiton

occur, necessitating discontinuation of therapy. Application to acutely inflamed skin or to the eyes or mucous membranes should be avoided.

BENZYL BENZOATE

Benzyl benzoate is effective as a pediculicide and scabicide. It has generally been supplanted by lindane. The mechanism of action of benzyl benzoate is unknown. Although it appears to be relatively nontoxic after topical application, there are no studies of its toxic potential in the treatment of scabies.

SULFUR

Sulfur has a long history of use as a scabicide. Although it is nonirritating, it has an unpleasant odor, is staining, and is disagreeable to use. It has been replaced by more aesthetic and effective scabicides in recent years, but it remains a possible alternative drug for use in infants and pregnant women. The usual formulation is 5% precipitated sulfur in petrolatum.

MALATHION

Malathion is an organophosphate cholinesterase inhibitor (Chapter 6) which is an effective pediculicide and is indicated for the treatment of pediculosis capitis. In vitro studies have shown malathion to be both lousicidal and ovicidal at a concentration of 0.5%.

Malathion (Prioderm) is available as an alcohol-based 0.5% lotion. For pediculosis capitis, one application of 30 mL is applied to dry hair and scalp and allowed to remain for 8–12 hours before shampooing. Patients should be re-treated only if active lice can be demonstrated 7–10 days after initial treatment. Approximately 8% of an applied dose in an acetone vehicle is percutaneously absorbed. Although animal studies have not shown malathion to be carcinogenic, mutagenicity has not been determined, and caution is therefore advised with use in pregnant women, nursing mothers, and infants. This formulation is a weak primary irritant and is unlikely to cause allergic contact hypersensitivity.

PYRETHRINS & PIPERONYL BUTOXIDE

Combinations of pyrethrins and piperonyl butoxide are available as topical pediculicides. Pyrethrins are neurotoxic to *Pediculus capitis, Pediculus corporis,* and *Pthirus pubis.* The combination of pyrethrins with piperonyl butoxide appears to be synergistically lousicidal.

These agents are available over the counter (RID, A-200 Pyrinate), and it is recommended that they be applied undiluted to affected areas for 10 minutes and then washed off with warm water and soap. Second applications may be necessary, but consecutive applications should be separated by at least 24 hours.

AGENTS AFFECTING PIGMENTATION

HYDROQUINONE & MONOBENZONE

Hydroquinone and monobenzone, the monobenzyl ether of hydroquinone, are used to *reduce hyperpigmentation* of the skin. Topical hydroquinone usually results in temporary lightening, whereas monobenzone causes irreversible depigmentation.

Hydroquinone   Monobenzone

The mechanism of action of these compounds appears to involve inhibition of the enzyme tyrosinase, thus interfering with the biosynthesis of melanin. In addition, monobenzone may be toxic to melanocytes, resulting in permanent depigmentation. Some percutaneous absorption of these compounds takes place, because monobenzone may cause hypopigmentation at sites distant from the area of application.

Hydroquinone may be useful in treating melasma, lentigines, and ephelides but is of minimal benefit in treating postinflammatory hyperpigmentation, particularly when the melanin is no longer confined to the epidermis but has dropped down into the dermis. Most lesions treated with hydroquinone will respond with only a temporary lightening; when the medication is discontinued, the lesions return to their original color. Patients should be encouraged to use an opaque sunscreen to block the melanogenic long wavelengths of ultraviolet light. Hydroquinone is usually applied twice daily to the area to be lightened.

Monobenzone is used only when permanent irreversible depigmentation is desired, ie, in patients with disseminated vitiligo who have a few remaining areas of normal pigmentation. It is applied to the area to be depigmented twice daily until all pigmentation has resolved. As noted above, monobenzone has been reported to cause depigmentation at sites distant from the treatment area, and this should be explained to any patient in whom only local depigmentation is desired.

Both hydroquinone and monobenzone may cause local irritation. Allergic sensitization to these compounds does occur, and it is advisable to do a patch test on a small area of the body prior to use on the face. Contact of the drug with the eyes must be avoided. An unusual ochronosislike syndrome of hyperpigmentation has been reported in patients using hydroquinone cream in areas of intense sunlight exposure.

TRIOXSALEN & METHOXSALEN

Trioxsalen and methoxsalen are members of the naturally occurring tricyclic furocoumarins used for centuries in India for the *repigmentation* of depigmented macules of vitiligo. With the recent development of high-intensity long-wave ultraviolet fluorescent lamps, photochemotherapy with oral methoxsalen for psoriasis and with oral trioxsalen for vitiligo has been under intensive investigation.

Trioxsalen

Methoxsalen

Psoralens must be photoactivated by long-wavelength ultraviolet light in the range of 320–400 nm (UVA) to produce a beneficial effect. Psoralens intercalate with DNA and, with subsequent UVA irradiation, cyclobutane adducts are formed with pyrimidine bases. Both monofunctional and bifunctional adducts may be formed, the latter causing interstrand crosslinks. These DNA photoproducts may inhibit DNA synthesis.

In the treatment of vitiligo, 10 mg of trioxsalen (Trisoralen) is given orally 2 hours prior to measured periods of ultraviolet exposure, either from sunlight or an artificial light source. Methoxsalen (Oxsoralen) may be used in the treatment of vitiligo in a dosage of 20 mg orally 2 hours prior to light exposure. Topical methoxsalen may be used to treat small vitiliginous lesions, but extreme caution is necessary to prevent severe erythema and blistering. Dilution of the 1% lotion to a concentration of 1:1000 or 1:10,000 is helpful to avoid excessive reactions. The use of oral and topical methoxsalen in the treatment of psoriasis is still investigational. Any UVA light source used for photochemotherapy should be calibrated regularly to prevent excessive exposure.

In the treatment of psoriasis, 0.5 mg/kg of methoxsalen is given 2 hours prior to measured doses of UVA exposure. Initial UVA doses (in joules/cm^2) are determined by the patient's skin characteristics for sunburning and tanning. During the clearing phase of therapy, UVA exposure is given 2–3 times per week, with adjustments in UVA dosage if necessary. After clearing has occurred, the patient is maintained in remission with periodic treatments.

The major long-term risks of psoralen photochemotherapy are cataracts and skin cancer. Therefore, when oral psoralens are given, patients should wear UVA-opaque sunglasses and avoid exposure to sunlight from the time of ingestion, during their light treatment, and through the remaining hours of daylight on treatment days. The psoralens are contraindicated in persons under 12 years of age and in those who have received ionizing radiation or have porphyria, discoid or systemic lupus erythematosus, or xeroderma pigmentosum. Acute side effects include erythema, pruritus, severe burns from excessive exposure, and nausea from orally administered psoralens. In view of the delayed erythema caused by psoralens and UVA, treatments should never be given less than 48 hours apart.

SUNSCREENS

Topical medications useful in protecting against sunlight contain either chemical compounds that absorb ultraviolet light, called **sunscreens;** or opaque materials such as titanium dioxide that reflect light, called **sunshades.** The 2 classes of chemical compounds most commonly used in sunscreens are *p*-aminobenzoic acid (PABA) and its derivatives and the benzophenones.

p-Aminobenzoic acid

Most sunscreen preparations are designed to absorb ultraviolet light in "B" ultraviolet wavelength range from 280 to 320 nm, which is the range responsible for most of the erythema and tanning associated with sun exposure. Chronic exposure to light in this range induces aging of the skin and photocarcinogenesis. Para-aminobenzoic acid and its esters are the most effective available absorbers in the B region. Para-aminobenzoic acid in 55–70% alcohol is the most efficient agent, while padimate A (pentyl *p*-dimethylaminobenzoate), padimate O (2-ethylhexyldimethyl-*p*-aminobenzoate), and glyceryl *p*-aminobenzoate are somewhat less efficient but often utilized for their other qualities. Para-aminobenzoic acid may photooxidize to produce a yellow stain on light-colored fabrics, while the *p*-aminobenzoic acid esters do not stain as easily.

The benzophenones include oxybenzone, dioxybenzone, and sulisobenzone. These compounds provide a broader spectrum of absorption from 250 to 360 nm, but their effectiveness in the UVB erythema range is less than that of *p*-aminobenzoic acid. Several of the newer ultraprotective sunscreens contain a combination of *p*-aminobenzoic acid, its esters, and a benzophenone.

The protection factor (PF) of a given sunscreen is a measure of its effectiveness in absorbing erythrogenic ultraviolet light. It is determined by measuring the minimal erythema dose (MED) with and without the sunscreen in a group of normal people. The ratio of the minimal erythema dose with sunscreen to the minimal erythema dose without sunscreen is the protection factor. If the protection factor value is determined in field tests using sunlight rather than an artificial light source, it may be called the sun protection factor (SPF). Fair-skinned individuals who sunburn easily are advised to use a product with a high protection factor of 10–15; those with darker skins may use a sunscreen with a lower protection factor of 6–8.

Sunscreens should be applied 1 hour before sun exposure, and reapplication is advised after swimming or profuse sweating. Some recently introduced products have greater resistance to removal, thereby reducing the need for reapplication. Tingling and stinging sometimes occur with application of *p*-aminobenzoic acid preparations. Allergic contact and photocontact sensitization can occur with *p*-aminobenzoic acid, its esters, and benzophenones. Immediate contact sensitivity with resulting urticaria has been reported with the benzophenones.

ACNE PREPARATIONS

RETINOIC ACID

Retinoic acid, also known as tretinoin or *trans*-retinoic acid, is the acid form of vitamin A. It is an effective topical treatment for acne vulgaris. Several analogs of vitamin A, eg, 13-*cis*-retinoic acid (isotretinoin), have recently been shown to be effective in various dermatologic diseases when given *orally*. Vitamin A alcohol is the physiologic form of vitamin A. The topical therapeutic agent, retinoic acid, is formed by the oxidation of the alcohol group, with all 4 double bonds in the side chain in the *trans* configuration as shown.

Retinoic acid is insoluble in water but soluble in many organic solvents. It is susceptible to oxidation and ester formation, particularly when exposed to light. Topically applied retinoic acid remains chiefly in the epidermis, with less than 10% absorption into the circulation. The small quantities of retinoic acid absorbed following topical application are metabolized by the liver and excreted in bile and urine.

Retinoic acid has several effects on epithelial tissues. It stabilizes lysosomes, increases ribonucleic acid polymerase activity, increases prostaglandin E_2, cAMP, and cGMP levels, and increases the incorporation of thymidine into DNA. Its action in acne has been attributed to decreased cohesion between epidermal cells and increased epidermal cell turnover. This is thought to result in the expulsion of open comedones and the transformation of closed comedones into open ones.

Topical retinoic acid (Retin-A) is applied initially in a concentration sufficient to induce slight erythema with mild peeling. The concentration or frequency of application may be decreased if too much irritation is produced. Topical retinoic acid should be applied to dry skin only, and care should be taken to avoid contact with the corners of the nose, eyes, mouth, and mucous membranes. During the first 4–6 weeks of therapy, comedones not previously evident may appear and give the impression that the acne has been aggravated by the retinoic acid. However, with continued therapy, the lesions will clear, and in 8–12 weeks optimal clinical improvement should occur.

The most common adverse side effects of topical retinoic acid are the erythema and dryness that occur in the first few weeks of use, but these can be expected to resolve with continued therapy. Animal studies suggest that tretinoin may increase the tumorigenic potential of ultraviolet radiation. In light of this, patients using retinoic acid should be advised to avoid or minimize sun exposure and use a protective sunscreen. Allergic contact dermatitis to topical retinoic acid is rare.

ISOTRETINOIN

Isotretinoin (Accutane) is the first orally administered synthetic retinoid available in the USA, where its use is currently restricted to cystic acne. The precise mechanism of action of isotretinoin in cystic acne is not known, although it appears to act by inhibiting sebaceous gland size and function. The drug is well absorbed, extensively bound to plasma albumin, and has an elimination half-life of 10–20 hours.

Retinoic acid

Isotretinoin

Most cystic acne patients respond to 1–2 mg/kg, given in 2 divided doses daily for 4–5 months. If severe cystic acne persists following this initial treatment, after a period of 2 months, a second course of therapy may be initiated. Common adverse effects resemble hypervitaminosis A and include dryness and itching of the skin and mucous membranes. Less common side effects are headache, corneal opacities, pseudotumor cerebri, inflammatory bowel disease, anorexia, alopecia, and muscle and joint pains. These effects are all reversible on discontinuation of therapy. Skeletal hyperostosis has been observed in patients receiving isotretinoin with premature closure of epiphyses noted in children treated with this medication. Lipid abnormalities (triglycerides, HDL) are frequent; their clinical relevance is unknown at present. Teratogenicity has been observed in patients taking isotretinoin; therefore, women of childbearing potential *must* use an effective form of contraception for at least 1 month before, throughout isotretinoin therapy, and for one or more menstrual cycles following discontinuation of treatment. It is additionally recommended that a pregnancy test be obtained within 2 weeks before starting therapy in these patients.

ETRETINATE

Etretinate (Tigason) is an aromatic retinoid, not yet available in the USA, that is quite effective in the treatment of psoriasis, especially pustular forms. It is given orally at a dosage of 1–5 mg/kg/d, starting with 0.5 mg/kg/d in patients with erythrodermic psoriasis. Chronic dosing studies reveal a slow terminal elimination phase of several months' duration. Adverse effects attributable to etretinate therapy are similar to those seen with isotretinoin and resemble hypervitaminosis A. Lipid abnormalities are not frequently seen with etretinate; however, transient liver enzyme elevations have been reported. Etretinate is more teratogenic than isotretinoin in the animal species studied to date, which is of special concern in view of its prolonged elimination time after chronic administration.

BENZOYL PEROXIDE

Benzoyl peroxide is an effective topical agent in the treatment of acne vulgaris. It penetrates the stratum corneum or follicular openings unchanged and is converted metabolically to benzoic acid within the epidermis and dermis. Less than 5% of an applied dose is absorbed from the skin in an 8-hour period.

Benzoyl peroxide

It has been postulated that the mechanism of action of benzoyl peroxide in acne is related to its antimicrobial activity against *P acnes* and to its peeling and comedolytic effects.

To decrease the possibility of irritation, application should be limited to a low concentration (2.5%) once daily for the first week of therapy and increased in frequency and strength if the preparation is well tolerated.

Benzoyl peroxide is a potent contact sensitizer in experimental studies, and this adverse effect may occur in up to 1% of acne patients. Care should be taken to avoid contact with the eyes and mucous membranes. Benzoyl peroxide is an oxidant and may rarely cause bleaching of the hair or colored fabrics.

ANTI-INFLAMMATORY AGENTS

TOPICAL CORTICOSTEROIDS

The remarkable efficacy of topical corticosteroids in the treatment of inflammatory dermatoses was noted soon after the introduction of hydrocortisone in 1952. Subsequently, numerous analogs have been developed that offer extensive choices of potencies, concentrations, and vehicles. The therapeutic effectiveness of topical corticosteroids is based primarily on their anti-inflammatory activity. Definitive explanations of the effects of corticosteroids on endogenous mediators of inflammation such as histamine, kinins, lysosomal enzymes, and prostaglandins await further experimental clarification. The antimitotic effects of corticosteroids on human epidermis may account for an additional mechanism of action in psoriasis and other dermatologic diseases associated with increased cell turnover. The general pharmacology of these endocrine agents is discussed in Chapter 38.

The original topical glucocorticosteroid was hydrocortisone, the natural glucocorticosteroid of the adrenal cortex (Fig 65–1). Prednisolone and methylprednisolone are active to the same extent as hydrocortisone. The 9α-fluoro derivatives of hydrocortisone were active topically, but their salt-retaining properties made them undesirable even for topical use. The 9α-fluorinated steroids dexamethasone and betamethasone subsequently developed did not have any advantage over hydrocortisone. However, triamcinolone and fluocinolone, the acetonide derivatives of the fluorinated steroids, have a distinct advantage in topical therapy. Similarly betamethasone is not very active topically, but attaching a 5-carbon valerate chain to the 17-hydroxyl position results in a compound over 300 times as active as hydrocortisone for topical use. Fluocinonide is the 21-acetate derivative of fluocinolone acetonide; the addition of the 21-acetate enchances the topical activity about 5-fold. Fluorination of the steroid is not required for high

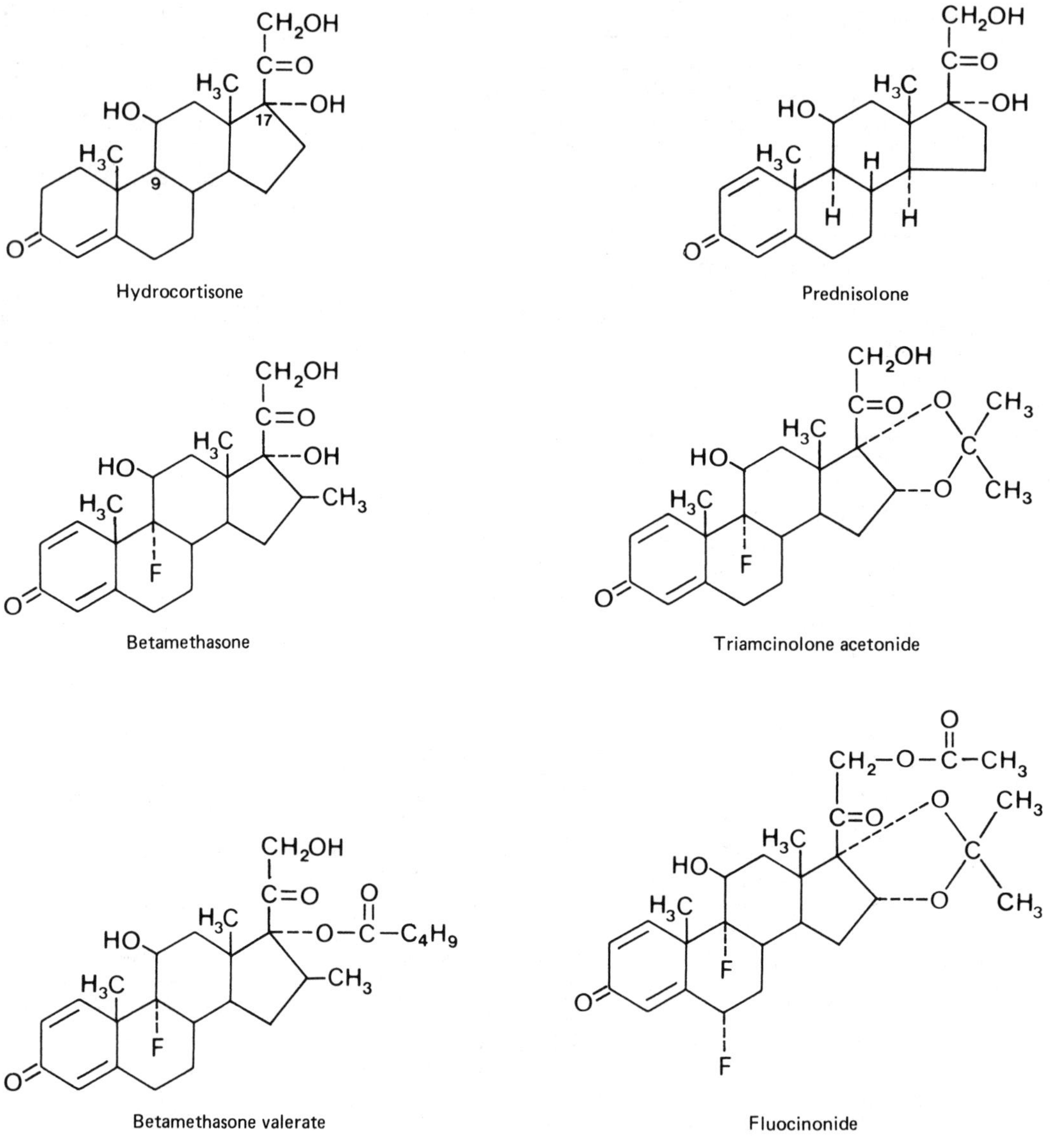

Figure 65-1. Chemical structures of several glucocorticoids.

potency; hydrocortisone valerate and butyrate have activity similar to that of triamcinolone acetonide.

Corticosteroids are only minimally absorbed following application to normal skin, eg, approximately 1% of a dose of hydrocortisone solution applied to the ventral forearm is absorbed. The newer analogs may not owe their increased efficacy to enhanced penetration. Those corticosteroids for which published data exist are absorbed to no greater—and perhaps to a lesser—degree than hydrocortisone. However, occlusion with an impermeable film, such as plastic wrap, is an effective method of enhancing penetration, yielding a 10-fold increase in absorption for all these agents. There is a marked regional anatomic variation in corticosteroid penetration. Compared to the absorption from the forearm, hydrocortisone is absorbed 0.14 times as well through the plantar foot arch, 0.83

times as well through the palm, 3.5 times as well through the scalp, 6 times as well through the forehead, 9 times as well through vulvar skin, and 42 times as well through scrotal skin. Penetration is increased severalfold in the inflamed skin of atopic dermatitis; and in severe exfoliative diseases, such as erythrodermic psoriasis, there appears to be little barrier to penetration.

Experimental studies on the percutaneous absorption of hydrocortisone fail to reveal a significant increase in absorption when applied on a repetitive basis compared to a single dose, and a single daily application may be effective in most conditions. Ointment bases tend to give better activity to the corticosteroid than do cream or lotion vehicles. Novel vehicles, including gels, may not retain their optimal drug delivery qualities if they are diluted, even with the same base. Increasing the concentration of a corticosteroid increases the penetration but not to the same degree. For example, approximately 1% of a 0.25% hydrocortisone solution is absorbed from the forearm. A 10-fold increase in concentration causes a 4-fold increase in absorption.

Table 65–1 groups topical corticosteroid formulation according to approximate relative efficacy. Table 65–2 lists major dermatologic diseases in order of their responsiveness to these drugs. In the first group of dis-

Table 65–1. Relative efficacy of some topical corticosteroids in various formulations.

Lowest efficacy	
0.25–2.5%	Hydrocortisone
0.25%	Methylprednisolone acetate (Medrol)
0.04%	Dexamethasone* (Hexadrol)
0.1%	Dexamethasone* (Decaderm)
1.0%	Methylprednisolone acetate (Medrol)
0.5%	Prednisolone (Meti-Derm)
0.2%	Betamethasone* (Celestone)
Low efficacy	
0.01%	Fluocinolone acetonide* (Fluonid, Synalar)
0.01%	Betamethasone valerate* (Valisone)
0.025%	Fluorometholone* (Oxylone)
0.025%	Triamcinolone acetonide* (Aristocort, Kenalog, Triacet)
0.1%	Clocortolone pivalate* (Cloderm)
0.03%	Flumethasone pivalate* (Locorten)
Intermediate efficacy	
0.2%	Hydrocortisone valerate (Westcort)
0.1%	Hydrocortisone butyrate (Locoid)
0.025%	Betamethasone benzoate* (Benisone, Flurobate, Uticort)
0.025%	Flurandrenolide* (Cordran)
0.1%	Betamethasone valerate* (Valisone)
0.05%	Desonide (Tridesilon)
0.025%	Halcinonide* (Halog)
0.05%	Desoximetasone* (Topicort L.P.)
0.05%	Flurandrenolide* (Cordran)
0.1%	Triamcinolone acetonide*
0.025%	Fluocinolone acetonide*
High efficacy	
0.05%	Betamethasone dipropionate* (Diprosone, Diprolene)
0.1%	Amcinonide* (Cyclocort)
0.25%	Desoximetasone* (Topicort)
0.5%	Triamcinolone acetonide*
0.2%	Fluocinolone acetonide* (Synalar-HP)
0.05%	Diflorasone diacetate* (Florone, Maxiflor)
0.1%	Halcinonide* (Halog)
0.05%	Fluocinonide* (Lidex, Topsyn)

*Fluorinated steroids.

Table 65–2. Dermatologic disorders responsive to topical corticosteroids ranked in order of sensitivity.

Very responsive
Atopic dermatitis
Seborrheic dermatitis
Lichen simplex chronicus
Pruritus ani
Later phase of allergic contact dermatitis
Later phase of irritant dermatitis
Nummular eczematous dermatitis
Stasis dermatitis
Psoriasis, especially of genitalia and face

Less responsive
Discoid lupus erythematosus
Psoriasis of palms and soles
Necrobiosis lipoidica diabeticorum
Sarcoidosis
Lichen striatus
Pemphigus
Familial benign pemphigus
Vitiligo
Granuloma annulare

Least responsive: intralesional injection required
Keloids
Hypertrophic scars
Hypertrophic lichen planus
Alopecia areata
Acne cysts
Prurigo nodularis
Chondrodermatitis nodularis helicus

eases, low- to medium-efficacy corticosteroid preparations often produce clinical remission. In the second group, it is often necessary to use high-efficacy preparations, occlusion therapy, or both. Once a remission has been achieved, every effort should be made to maintain the patient with a low-efficacy corticosteroid.

The limited penetration of topical corticosteroids can be overcome in certain clinical circumstances by the intralesional injection of relatively insoluble corticosteroids, eg, triamcinolone acetonide, triamcinolone diacetate, triamcinolone hexacetonide, and betamethasone acetate-phosphate. When these agents are injected into the lesion, measurable amounts remain in place and are gradually released for 3–4 weeks. This form of therapy is often effective for the lesions listed in Table 65–2 that are generally unresponsive to topical corticosteroids. The dosage of the triamcinolone salts should be limited to 1 mg per treatment site, ie, 0.1 mL of 10 mg/mL suspension, to decrease the incidence of local atrophy (see below).

Adverse Effects

All absorbable topical corticosteroids possess the potential to suppress the pituitary-adrenal axis (Chapter 38). Although most patients with pituitary-adrenal axis suppression demonstrate only a laboratory test abnormality, cases of severely impaired stress response can occur. Iatrogenic Cushing's syndrome may occur as a result of protracted use of topical corticosteroids in large quantities. Applying potent corticosteroids to extensive areas of the body for prolonged periods, with or without occlusion, increases the likelihood of systemic side effects. Fewer of these factors are required to produce adverse systemic effects in children, and growth retardation is of particular concern in the pediatric age group.

Adverse local effects of topical corticosteroids include the following: atrophy, which may present as depressed, shiny, often wrinkled "cigarette paper"–appearing skin with prominent telangiectases and a tendency to develop purpura and ecchymosis; steroid rosacea, with persistent erythema, telangiectatic vessels, pustules, and papules in central facial distribution; perioral dermatitis, steroid acne, alterations of cutaneous infections, hypopigmentation, hypertrichosis, and increased intraocular pressure; and allergic contact dermatitis, which may be confirmed by patch testing with high concentrations of corticosteroids, ie, 1% in petrolatum, because topical corticosteroids are not irritating. Topical corticosteroids are contraindicated in individuals who demonstrate hypersensitivity to them.

TAR COMPOUNDS

Coal tar preparations have been used in dermatologic practice since the late 19th century, chiefly in the treatment of psoriasis. Coal tar is the principal byproduct of the destructive distillation of bituminous coal and an exceedingly complex mixture, containing about 10,000 compounds. These include naphthalene, phenanthrene, fluoranthrene, benzene, xylene, toluene, phenol, cresols, other aromatic compounds, pyridine bases, ammonia, and peroxides. Chiefly because of the complexity of coal tar and the difficulties of isolating topically active fractions, analyses of the rates of absorption, blood levels, and excretion of specific compounds have been inadequate. Dermatologically useful tar compounds are also derived from the destructive distillation of shale rock, yielding ichthammol, and the heartwood of *Juniperus oxycedrus,* yielding juniper tar. Coal tar is available in many over-the-counter preparations in the form of bath additives, shampoos, and hydroalcoholic base gels. Coal tar may also be compounded in accordance with *United States Pharmacopeia, National Formulary,* or other formulations in concentrations ranging from 2 to 10%.

Liquor carbonis detergens (LCD) is a coal tar solution prepared by extracting coal tar with alcohol and an emulsifying agent, such as polysorbate 80. This solution contains 20 g of coal tar per 100 mL and may be compounded in concentrations of 2–10% in creams, ointments, or shampoos.

Tar preparations are used mainly in the treatment of psoriasis, dermatitis, and lichen simplex chronicus. The phenolic constituents endow these compounds with antipruritic properties, making them particularly valuable in the treatment of chronic lichenified dermatitis. Acute dermatitis with vesiculation and oozing

may be irritated by even weak tar preparations, which should be avoided. However, in the subacute and chronic stages of dermatitis and psoriasis, these preparations are quite useful and offer an alternative to the use of topical corticosteroids.

The most common adverse reaction to coal tar compounds is an irritant folliculitis, necessitating discontinuation of therapy to the affected areas for a period of 3–5 days. Phototoxicity and allergic contact dermatitis may also occur. Tar preparations should be avoided in patients who have previously exhibited sensitivity to them. Care should be exercised when using tar compounds in patients with erythrodermal or generalized pustular psoriasis, because of the risk of total body exfoliation.

KERATOLYTIC & DESTRUCTIVE AGENTS

SALICYLIC ACID

Salicylic acid was chemically synthesized in 1860 and has been extensively used in dermatologic therapy as a keratolytic agent. It is a white powder quite soluble in alcohol but only slightly soluble in water.

Salicylic acid

Salicylic acid is absorbed percutaneously and distributed in the extracellular space, with maximum plasma levels occurring 6–12 hours after application. Since 50–80% of salicylate is bound to albumin, transiently increased serum levels of free salicylates are found in patients with hypoalbuminemia. The urinary metabolites of topically applied salicylic acid include salicyluric acid and acyl and phenolic glucuronides of salicylic acid; only 6% of the total recovered is unchanged salicylic acid. About 95% of a single dose of salicylate is excreted in the urine within 24 hours after its absorption.

The mechanism by which salicylic acid produces its keratolytic and other therapeutic effects is poorly understood. The drug may solubilize cell surface proteins that keep the stratum corneum intact, thereby resulting in desquamation of keratotic debris. Salicylic acid is keratolytic in concentrations of 3–6%. In concentrations greater than 6%, it can be destructive to tissues.

Salicylism and death have occurred following topical application. In an adult, 1 g of a topically applied

6% salicylic acid preparation will raise the serum salicylate level not more than 0.5 mg/dL of plasma; the threshold for toxicity is 30–50 mg/dL. Higher serum levels are possible in children, who are therefore at a greater risk to develop salicylism. In cases of severe intoxication, hemodialysis is the treatment of choice (see p 746). It is advisable to limit both the total amount of salicylic acid applied and the frequency of application. Urticarial, anaphylactic, and erythema multiforme reactions may occur in patients allergic to salicylates. Topical use may be associated with local irritation, acute inflammation, and even ulceration with the use of high concentrations of salicylic acid. Particular care must be exercised when using the drug on the extremities of diabetics or patients with peripheral vascular disease.

PROPYLENE GLYCOL

Propylene glycol is extensively used in topical preparations because it is an excellent vehicle for organic compounds. Propylene glycol has recently been used alone as a keratolytic agent in 40–70% concentrations, with plastic occlusion, or in gel with 6% salicylic acid.

$$CH_3-CH-CH_2$$
$$\quad\;\; |\quad\;\; |$$
$$\quad\;\; OH\;\; OH$$

Propylene glycol

Only minimal amounts of a topically applied dose are absorbed through normal stratum corneum. Percutaneously absorbed propylene glycol is oxidized by the liver to lactic acid and pyruvic acid, with subsequent utilization in general body metabolism. Approximately 12–45% of the absorbed agent is excreted unchanged in the urine. Propylene glycol is an effective keratolytic agent for the removal of hyperkeratotic debris. This keratolytic effect is attributed to reversible and irreversible changes in epidermal structure proteins. Propylene glycol increases the solubility of proteins in water and also denatures proteins, with the maximum effect seen in a concentration range of 61–77%. The addition of salicylic acid to propylene glycol may augment the keratolytic effect of propylene glycol by lowering the pH of the preparation, thus enhancing subsequent protein denaturation.

Propylene glycol is also an effective humectant and increases the water content of the stratum corneum. The hygroscopic characteristics of the agent may help it to develop an osmotic gradient through the stratum corneum, thereby increasing hydration of the outermost layers by drawing water out from the inner layers of the skin.

Propylene glycol is used under polyethylene occlusion or with 6% salicylic acid for the treament of ichthyosis, palmar and plantar keratodermas, psoriasis, pityriasis rubra pilaris, keratosis pilaris, and hypertrophic lichen planus.

In concentrations greater than 10%, propylene glycol may act as an irritant in some patients; those with eczematous dermatitis may be more sensitive. Allergic contact dermatitis occurs with propylene glycol, and at present a 4% aqueous propylene glycol solution is recommended for the purpose of patch testing.

UREA

Urea in a compatible cream vehicle or ointment base has a softening and moisturizing effect on the stratum corneum. It has the ability to make creams and lotions feel less greasy, and this has been utilized in dermatologic preparations to decrease the oily feel of a preparation that otherwise might feel unpleasant. It is a white crystalline powder with a slight ammonia odor when moist.

$$H_2N-\overset{\displaystyle O}{\overset{\displaystyle \|}{C}}-NH_2$$

Urea

Urea is absorbed percutaneously, although the precise amount absorbed is not well documented. It is distributed predominantly in the extracellular space and excreted in urine. Urea is a natural product of metabolism, and systemic toxicities with topical application do not occur.

Urea allegedly increases the water content of the stratum corneum, presumably as a result of the hygroscopic characteristics of this naturally occurring molecule. Urea is also keratolytic. The mechanism of action appears to involve alterations in prekeratin and keratin, leading to increased solubilization. In addition, urea may break hydrogen bonds that keep the stratum corneum intact.

As a humectant, urea is used in concentrations of 2–20% in creams and lotions. As a keratolytic agent, it is used in 20% concentration in diseases such as ichthyosis vulgaris, hyperkeratosis of palms and soles, xerosis, and keratosis pilaris. Concentrations of 30–50% in ointment base applied to the nail plate under occlusion have been useful in softening the nail prior to avulsion. Concentrations of 10–20% applied to the diaper area, groin, or areas of eczematous dermatitis may be associated with an unpleasant stinging sensation that may necessitate discontinuation of the preparation.

PODOPHYLLUM RESIN

Podophyllum resin, an alcoholic extract of *Podophyllum peltatum,* commonly known as mandrake root or May apple, is used in the treatment of condyloma acuminatum and other verrucae. It is a mixture of podophyllotoin, alpha and beta peltatin, desoxypodophyllotoxin, dehydropodophyllotoxin, and other compounds. It is soluble in alcohol, ether, chloroform, and compound tincture of benzoin.

Podophyllotoxin

Percutaneous absorption of podophyllum resin occurs, particularly in intertriginous areas and from applications to large moist condylomas. It is soluble in lipids and therefore is distributed widely throughout the body, including the central nervous system.

The major use of podophyllum resin is in the treatment of condyloma acuminatum. Podophyllotoxin and its derivatives are active cytotoxic agents with specific affinity for the microtubule protein of the mitotic spindle. Normal assembly of the spindle is prevented, and epidermal mitoses are arrested in metaphase. A 25% concentration of podophyllum resin in compound tincture of benzoin is recommended for the treatment of condyloma acuminatum. Application should be restricted to wart tissue only, to limit the total amount of medication used and to prevent severe erosive changes in adjacent tissue. In treating cases of large extensive condylomas, it is advisable to limit application to sections of the affected area to minimize systemic absorption. The patient is instructed to wash off the preparation 2–3 hours after the initial application, since the irritant reaction is variable. Depending on the individual patient's reaction, this period can be extended to 6–8 hours on subsequent applications. If 3–5 applications have not resulted in significant resolution, other methods of treatment should be considered.

Toxic symptoms associated with excessively large applications include nausea, vomiting, alterations in sensorium, muscle weakness, neuropathy with diminished tendon reflexes, coma, and even death. Local irritation is common, and inadvertent contact with the eye may cause severe conjunctivitis. Use during pregnancy is contraindicated in view of possible cytotoxic effects on the fetus.

CANTHARIDIN

Cantharidin is the active irritant isolated from cantharides, or dried blister beetles—*Lytta (Cantharis) vesicatoria,* also known as Russian fly or Spanish fly. The ability of insects of the *Cantharis* type to produce vesicles and bullae on human skin led to the investigation of possible therapeutic uses of the vesicant can-

tharidin in dermatology. The major clinical use is in the treatment of molluscum contagiosum and verruca vulgaris, particularly periungual warts.

Cantharidin

The amount of cantharidin absorbed following cutaneous application is unknown. It is excreted by the kidney, and in cases of oral ingestion of significant amounts, marked irritation of the entire urinary tract has resulted, with pain, urinary urgency, and priapism.

Cantharidin acts on mitochondrial oxidative enzymes, resulting in decreased ATP levels. This leads to changes in the epidermal cell membranes, acantholysis, and blister formation. This effect is entirely intraepidermal, and no scarring ensues.

The main use of cantharidin is in the treatment of verruca vulgaris. Periungual warts are treated by applying this mixture to the wart surface, allowing it to dry, and occluding it with a nonporous plastic tape. A blister will form that will resolve in 7–14 days, at which time the area is debrided and any remaining wart is re-treated. Several applications may be required to effect a cure. Plantar warts are treated by paring and then applying several layers of cantharidin. An occlusive plastic tape is then applied. The resulting blister is removed in 10–14 days, and any residual wart is re-treated. Molluscum contagiosum will often respond to a single application without occlusion. Painless application and lack of residual scarring make cantharidin ideally suited for treatment of children.

A ring of warts may develop at the periphery of a cantharidin-treated wart as a result of intraepidermal inoculation. These may be re-treated with cantharidin or by an alternative method. Systemic toxic effects have not been observed with topical therapy, although ingestion of as little as 10 mg has resulted in abdominal pain, nausea, vomiting, and shock.

FLUOROURACIL

Fluorouracil is a fluorinated pyrimidine antimetabolite that resembles uracil, with a fluorine atom substituted for the 5-methyl group. Its systemic pharmacology is described in Chapter 58. Fluorouracil is used topically for the treatment of multiple actinic keratoses and intralesionally for keratoacanthomas.

The pharmacokinetics of intralesional therapy have not been determined. Approximately 6% of a topically applied dose is absorbed—an amount insufficient to produce adverse systemic effects. Most of the absorbed drug is metabolized and excreted as carbon

Fluorouracil

Table 65–3. Miscellaneous oral medications used in dermatology.

Drug or Group	Conditions	
Antihistamines	Pruritus (any cause)	See also Chapter 15.
Antimalarials	Lupus erythematosus, photosensitization	See also Chapter 34.
Antimetabolites	Psoriasis, pemphigus, pemphigoid	See also Chapter 58.
Dapsone	Dermatitis herpetiformis, erythema elevatum diutinum, pemphigus, pemphigoid, bullous lupus erythematosus	See also Chapter 46.
Corticosteroids	Pemphigus, pemphigoid, lupus erythematosus, allergic contact dermatoses, and certain other dermatoses	See also Chapter 38.

dioxide, urea, and α-fluoro-β-alanine. A small percentage is eliminated unchanged in the urine. Fluorouracil inhibits thymidylate synthetase activity, interfering with the synthesis of deoxyribonucleic acid and to a lesser extent ribonucleic acid. These effects are most marked in atypical, rapidly proliferating cells.

The response to treatment begins with erythema and progresses through vesiculation, erosion, superficial ulceration, necrosis, and finally reepithelialization. Fluorouracil should be continued until the inflammatory reaction reaches the ulceration and necrosis stage, usually in 3–4 weeks, at which time treatment should be terminated. The healing process may continue for 1–2 months after therapy is discontinued. Local adverse reactions may include pain, pruritus, a burning sensation, tenderness, and residual postinflammatory hyperpigmentation. Excessive exposure to sunlight during treatment may increase the intensity of the reaction and should be avoided. Allergic contact dermatitis to fluorouracil has been reported, and its use is contraindicated in patients with known hypersensitivity. Intralesional injections of keratoacanthomas with a 5% aqueous solution of fluorouracil have recently been advocated. Weekly injections of 25–50 mg are given until 70–80% involution of the lesion is

noted. If the lesion does not involute after 5 injections, excisional surgery is performed. Local reactions include erythema, inflammation, and subsequent necrosis of the tumor. Systemic adverse effects have not been observed and are not anticipated in view of the comparatively small amounts of fluorouracil administered on a weekly basis.

MISCELLANEOUS ORAL MEDICATIONS

A number of drugs used primarily for other conditions also find use as oral therapeutic agents for dermatologic conditions. A few of these are listed in Table 65–3.

REFERENCES

General

Bronaugh R, Maibach HI: *Percutaneous Penetration: Principles and Practices.* Marcel Dekker, 1985.

Wester RC, Maibach HI: Cutaneous pharmacokinetics: Ten steps to percutaneous absorption. *Drugs Metab Rev* 1983;**14:**169.

Antibacterial Drugs

Eady EA, Holland KT, Cunliffe WJ: Topical antibiotics in acne therapy. *J Am Acad Dermatol* 1981;**5:**455.

Leyden JJ et al: Topical antibiotics and topical antimicrobial agents in acne therapy. *Acta Derm Venereol [Suppl] (Stockh)* 1980;**89:**75.

Meleney FL, Johnson BA: Bacitracin. *Am J Med* 1949;**7:**794.

Milstone EM, McDonald AJ, Scholhamer CF: Pseudomembranous colitis after topical application of clindamycin. *Arch Dermatol* 1981;**117:**154.

Newton BA: The properties and mode of action of the polymyxins. *Bacteriol Rev* 1965;**20:**14.

Rasmussen JE: Topical antibiotics. *J Dermatol Surg* 1976; **2:**69.

Wachs GN, Maibach HI: Cooperative double blind trial of an antibiotic corticoid combination in impetiginized atopic dermatitis. *Br J Dermatol* 1976;**95:**323.

Antifungal Drugs

Borgers M: Mechanism of action of antifungal drugs, with special reference to the imidazole derivatives. *Rev Infect Dis* 1980;**2:**520.

Codish SD, Tobias JS, Monaco AP: Systemic mycotic infections—Part 1. *Hosp Med* (June) 1978;**14:**6.

Graybill JR et al: Ketoconazole treatment of chronic mucocutaneous candidiasis. *Arch Dermatol* 1980;**116:**1137.

Heel RC et al: Econazole: A review of its antifungal activity and therapeutic efficacy. *Drugs* 1978;**16:**177.

Hermann HW: Clinical efficacy studies of haloprogin, a new topical antimicrobial agent. *Arch Dermatol* 1972;**106:**839.

Jones HE: Ketaconazole. *Arch Dermatol* 1982;**118:**217.

Jones HE, Simpson JG, Artis WW: Oral ketoconazole: An effective and safe treatment for dermatophytosis. *Arch Dermatol* 1981;**117:**129.

Katz R, Cahn B: Haloprogin therapy for dermatophyte infections. *Arch Dermatol* 1972;**106:**837.

Knight AG: The activity of various griseofulvin preparations and the appearance of oral griseofulvin in the stratum corneum. *Br J Dermatol* 1974;**91:**49.

Robinson HM Jr, Raskin J: Tolnaftate, a potent topical antifungal agent. *Arch Dermatol* 1965;**94:**372.

Sakurai K et al: Mode of action of 6-cyclohexyl-1-hydroxy-4-

methyl-2(1H)-pyridone ethanolamine salt (ciclopirox olamine). *Chemotherapy* 1978;**25**:68.

Sawyer PR et al: Miconazole: A review of its antifungal activity and therapeutic efficacy. *Drugs* 1975;**9**:406.

Shah VP, Epstein Wl, Riegelman S: Role of sweat in accumulation of orally administered griseofulvin in skin. *J Clin Invest* 1974;**53**:1673.

Stritzler C: Cutaneous candidiasis treated with topical amphotericin B. *Arch Dermatol* 1966;**93**:101.

Urcuyo FG, Zaias N: The successful treatment of pityriasis versicolor by systemic ketoconazole. *J Am Acad Dermatol* 1982;**6**:24.

Weber K, Wehland J, Herzog W: Griseofulvin interacts with microtubules both in vivo and in vitro. *J Mol Biol* 1976;**102**:817.

Weinstein MJ, Oden EM, Moxx E: Antifungal properties of tolnaftate in vitro and in vivo. *Antimicrob Agents Chemother* 1964;**4**:595.

Zalias N, Battistini F: Superficial mycoses: Treatment with a new broad spectrum antifungal agent: 1% clotrimazole solution. *Arch Dermatol* 1977;**113**:307.

Antiviral Agents

Corey L et al: A trial of topical acyclovir in genital herpes simplex virus infection. *N Engl J Med* 1982;**306**:1313.

Douglas JM et al: A double-blind study of oral acyclovir for suppression of recurrences of genital herpes simplex virus infection. *N Engl J Med* 1984;**310**:1551.

Mertz GJ et al: Double-blind placebo-controlled trial of oral acyclovir in first episode genital herpes simplex virus infection. *JAMA* 1984;**252**:1147.

Pagano JS: Acyclovir comes of age. *J Am Acad Dermatol* 1982;**6**:396.

Ectoparasiticides

Cubela V, Yawalkar SJ: Clinical experience with crotamiton cream and lotion in the treatment of infants with scabies. *Br J Clin Pract* 1978;**32**:229.

Konstantinou D, Stanoeva L, Yawalkar SJ: Crotamiton cream and lotion in the treatment of infants and young children with scabies. *J Int Med Res* 1979;**7**:443.

Orkin M et al (editors): *Scabies and Pediculosis.* Marcel Dekker, New York, 1985.

Rasmussen JE: The problem of lindane. *J Am Acad Dermatol* 1981;**5**:507.

Schacter B: Treatment of scabies and pediculosis with lindane preparation: An evaluation. *J Am Acad Dermatol* 1981;**5**:517.

Agents Affecting Pigmentation

Engasser PG, Maibach HI: Cosmetics and dermatology: Bleaching creams. *J Am Acad Dermatol* 1981;**5**:143.

Epstein JH et al: Current status of oral PUVA therapy for psoriasis. *J Am Acad Dermatol* 1979;**1**:106.

Kaidbey KH, Kligman AM: An appraisal of the efficacy and substantivity of the new high-potency sunscreens. *J Am Acad Dermatol* 1981;**4**:566.

Mosher DB, Parrish JA, Fitzpatrick TB: Monobenzylether of hydroquinone: A retrospective study of treatment of 18 vitiligo patients and a review of the literature. *Br J Dermatol* 1977;**97**:669.

Pathak MA, Kramer DM, Fitzpatrick TB: Photobiology and photochemistry of furocoumarins (psoralens). In: *Sunlight and Man: Normal and Abnormal Photobiologic Responses.* Tokyo Univ Press, 1974.

Sayre RM et al: Performance of six sunscreen formulations on human skin. *Arch Dermatol* 1979;**115**:46.

Acne Preparations

Ehmann CW, Voorhees JJ: International studies of the efficacy of etretinate in the treatment of psoriasis. *J Am Acad Dermatol* 1982;**6**:692.

Heel RC et al: Vitamin A acid: A review of its pharmacological properties and therapeutic use in the topical treatment of acne vulgaris. *Drugs* 1977;**14**:401.

Isotretinoin. *Med Lett Drugs Ther* (Sept 3) 1982;**24**:79.

Nacht S et al: Benzoyl peroxide: Percutaneous penetration and metabolic disposition. *J Am Acad Dermatol* 1981;**4**:31.

Peck GL et al: Isotretinoin versus placebo in the treatment of cystic acne. *J Am Acad Dermatol* 1982;**6**:735.

Plewig G, Kligman AM: *Acne Morphogenesis and Treatment.* Springer-Verlag, 1975.

Thomas JR, Doyle MB: The therapeutic uses of topical vitamin A acid. *J Am Acad Dermatol* 1981;**4**:505.

Anti-inflammatory Agents

Grupper C: The chemistry, pharmacology and use of tar in the treatment of psoriasis. In: *Psoriasis: Proceedings of the International Symposium, Stanford University.* Farber E, Cos AJ (editors). Stanford Univ Press, 1971.

Maibach HI, Stoughton RB: Topical corticosteroids. Chap 13, p 174, in: *Steroid Therapy.* Arzanoff DL (editor). Saunders, 1975.

Miller JA, Munro DD: Topical corticosteroids: Clinical pharmacology and therapeutic use. *Drugs* 1980;**19**:119.

Robertson DB, Maibach HI: Topical corticosteroids: A review. *Int J Dermatol* 1982;**21**:59.

Keratolytic & Destructive Agents

Ashton H, Frenk E, Stevenson CJ: Urea as a topical agent. *Br J Dermatol* 1971;**84**:194.

Chamberlain MJ, Reynolds AL, Yeoman WB: Toxic effects of podophyllum applications in pregnancy. *Br Med J* 1972;**3**:391.

Epstein WL, Kligman AM: Treatment of warts with cantharidin. *Arch Dermatol* 1958;**77**:508.

Fine JD, Arndt KA: *Propylene Glycol: A Review.* Excerpta Medica, 1980.

Geotte DK: Topical chemotherapy with 5-fluorouracil. *J Am Acad Dermatol* 1981;**4**:633.

Geotte DK, Odom RB: Successful treatment of keratoacanthoma with intralesional fluorouracil. *J Am Acad Dermatol* 1980;**2**:212.

Goldsmith LA, Baden HP: Propylene glycol with occlusion for treatment of ichthyosis. *JAMA* 1972;**220**:579.

Roenigk H, Maibach HI (editors): *Psoriasis.* Marcel Dekker, 1985.

Taylor JR, Halprin KM: Percutaneous absorption of salicylic acid. *Arch Dermatol* 1975;**111**:740.

Ward J et al: Fatal systemic poisoning following podophyllin treatment of condyloma acuminata. *South Med J* 1954;**47**:1204.

Dermatotoxicology

Maibach H (editor): *Dermatotoxicology,* 2nd ed. Hemisphere Press, 1985.

Drugs Used in Gastrointestinal Diseases

66

David F. Altman, MD

Many drugs discussed elsewhere in this book have applications in the treatment of gastrointestinal diseases. Antimuscarinic drugs inhibit the food-stimulated secretion of gastric acid and also affect intestinal smooth muscle; these drugs are useful in some forms of functional bowel disease. Muscarinic agonists stimulate smooth muscle and are used to promote gastrointestinal motility. Some phenothiazines have excellent antiemetic properties, and narcotic analgesics and some of their derivatives are useful antidiarrheal medications by virtue of their ability to inhibit intestinal motility.

Several other groups of medications are used almost exclusively in gastrointestinal disease; these are grouped and discussed according to their therapeutic uses below.

DRUGS USED IN PEPTIC ULCER DISEASE

The pathogenesis of peptic ulcer disease is not completely understood. It is clear that gastric acid and a peptic ulcer. However, factors relating to mucosal pepsin secretion are necessary for the development of resistance to acid and pepsin are also important, particularly in gastric ulcer disease. Currently, drugs are available that have some effect on each of these factors.

ANTACIDS

Gastric antacids are weak bases that react with gastric hydrochloric acid to form a salt and water. Their usefulness in peptic ulcer disease thus lies in their ability to reduce gastric acidity and, since pepsin is inactive in solutions above pH 4, to reduce peptic activity.

Most antacids in current use are combinations of aluminum, magnesium, and calcium salts (Table 66–1). The differences among antacids relate to the rapidity of their reaction with gastric acid, their neutralizing capacity, their gastrointestinal side effects, and their systemic complications. Price to the consumer varies widely.

Sodium bicarbonate, the active ingredient in baking soda, is highly soluble and reacts almost instantaneously with hydrochloric acid:

$$NaHCO_3 + HCl \rightarrow NaCl + H_2O + CO_2$$

However, this compound is highly soluble and is absorbed rapidly from the gut. Thus, it may promote

Table 66–1. Representative liquid antacids.

Proprietary Preparation	Ingredients	Acid-Neutralizing Capacity (meq/mL)	Volume Containing 140 meq (mg/5 mL)	Sodium Content (mg/5 mL)	Cost of High-Dose Regimen*
Maalox T.C.	Aluminum hydroxide, magnesium hydroxide	4.2	33	1.2	$ 46.58
Titralac	Calcium carbonate	4.2	33	11.0	40.99
Delcid	Aluminum hydroxide, magnesium hydroxide	4.1	34	1.5	45.72
Mylanta-II	Aluminum hydroxide, magnesium hydroxide, simethicone	3.6	39	1.1	58.39
Gelusil-II	Aluminum hydroxide, magnesium hydroxide, simethicone	3.0	47	1.3	60.52
Ripan	Magaldrate	2.7	50	0.7	60.93
Maalox Plus	Aluminum hydroxide, magnesium hydroxide, simethicone	2.3	61	2.5	71.28
ALternaGEL	Aluminum hydroxide	2.4	60	2.0	89.44
Amphojel	Aluminum hydroxide	1.4	100	7.0	168.53

*Cost to the pharmacist of 1 month's treatment with high-dose regimen (see text) based on manufacturers' listings in *Drug Topics Red Book* 1982.

systemic alkalosis and fluid retention and is not recommended for long-term use.

Calcium carbonate reacts more slowly than sodium bicarbonate but is very effective in neutralizing gastric acid:

$$CaCO_3 + 2HCl \rightarrow CaCl_2 + H_2O + CO_2$$

However, approximately 10% of the calcium chloride produced is absorbed, with the potential side effects of hypercalcemia, milk-alkali syndrome, and acid rebound. This antacid is therefore not recommended for long-term use.

Aluminum hydroxide reacts with hydrochloric acid in similar fashion:

$$Al(OH)_3 + 3HCl \rightarrow AlCl_3 + 3H_2O$$

However, there is wide variability in the solubility of various aluminum hydroxide preparations and therefore wide variations in the rate of acid neutralization. The aluminum chloride formed is generally insoluble and often causes constipation. It also binds certain drugs (eg, tetracycline) and phosphate, preventing their absorption. This effect on phosphate absorption is used to therapeutic advantage in patients with chronic renal failure and bone diseases.

Magnesium hydroxide (milk of magnesia) reacts with acid almost as promptly as does sodium hydroxide:

$$Mg(OH)_2 + 2HCl \rightarrow MgCl_2 + 2H_2O$$

Unlike sodium hydroxide, however, the relative insolubility of magnesium hydroxide slows its emptying from the stomach, thus prolonging its neutralizing effect. Magnesium salts produced are poorly absorbed and are responsible for the well-known cathartic effect of this compound. A small amount of magnesium is absorbed, but this is of clinical significance only when renal insufficiency impairs its urinary excretion.

Clinical Use of Antacids

After a meal, gastric acid is produced at a rate of about 45 meq/h. A single dose of 156 meq of antacid given 1 hour after a meal effectively neutralizes gastric acid for 2 hours. A second dose given 3 hours after eating maintains the effect for over 4 hours after the meal. The dose-response relationship of antacids is variable, depending on the gastric secretory capacity (some individuals are "hypersecretors," some "hyposecretors") and the rate at which the antacid is emptied from the stomach.

In addition, as implied by the discussion of the individual antacid compounds, antacids vary widely in their potency. The relative amounts of the various compounds and their reactivity will not be clear on the product label. However, commercially available antacids vary as much as 7-fold in vitro acid-neutralizing capacity.

Antacids can be effective in promoting healing of duodenal ulcers. Their benefit in gastric ulcers is less clear. In the best controlled trial of duodenal ulcer therapy, 140 meq of antacid given 1 and 3 hours after each meal and at bedtime accelerated the healing of duodenal ulcers, although pain relief was not much better than that seen with placebo. Different doses of antacid are required to achieve this degree of neutralizing capacity, depending on the commercial product used (Table 66–1). Tablet antacids are generally weak in their neutralizing capacity, and a large number of tablets would be required for this high-dose regimen. They are not recommended for the treatment of active peptic ulcer. The efficacy of lower doses of liquid antacids has not been demonstrated.

Thus, an optimum antacid regimen for peptic ulcer disease—one that would maximally neutralize gastric acid throughout a 24-hour period—would use 140 meq of a liquid antacid given 1 and 3 hours after meals and at bedtime. The actual volume of antacid given should be adjusted to provide 140 meq of acid-neutralizing effect. A final important factor in such a regimen is palatability. Patients will often state a preference for one antacid over another.

Adverse reactions to antacids often include a change in bowel habits. As has been mentioned, magnesium salts often have a cathartic effect, and aluminum hydroxide may be constipating. These problems can be managed by either combining or alternating compounds with these effects. Other potential problems with antacids relate to cation absorption (sodium, magnesium, aluminum, calcium) and systemic alkalosis. Fortunately, these become clinical problems only in patients with renal impairment. In large doses, the sodium content of some antacids may become an important factor in patients with congestive heart failure.

Antacids have long been a mainstay of therapy for gastroesophageal reflux. However, they appear to have little impact on the natural history of the disease. Antacid in combination with alginic acid (Gaviscon) does lead to reduced acid reflux and symptomatic improvement.

Antacids have been used for pain relief from esophagitis, gastric ulcer, and duodenal ulcer. However, placebo-controlled trials have shown no effect of a single "effective" antacid dose for pain relief in any of these conditions.

H₂ RECEPTOR ANTAGONISTS

Since their introduction in the mid 1970s, these compounds have gained wide acceptance. The 2 major drugs in use are **cimetidine** and **ranitidine** (Chapter 15). These agents are capable of over 90% reduction in basal, food-stimulated, and nocturnal secretion of gastric acid after a single dose. Many trials have demonstrated their effectiveness in promoting the healing of duodenal and gastric ulcers and preventing their recurrence. They are important in the medical management of Zollinger-Ellison syndrome and gastric hypersecretory states seen in systemic mastocytosis.

The usual adult dose of cimetidine is 300 mg 4 times daily with meals and at bedtime, although 400 mg twice daily might be equally effective. The drug can be given intravenously at the same dose. Occasionally, larger doses are necessary—up to 2400 mg per 24 hours—particularly in patients with Zollinger-Ellison syndrome. The dose should be reduced in patients with renal insufficiency, in whom the drug's half-life is prolonged. A dose of 400 mg at bedtime prevents ulcer recurrence. However, giving up cigarettes may be more important than medications in preventing recurrence in smokers.

Although both H_2 receptor antagonists have been generally well tolerated with few side effects reported, several adverse reactions have occurred with cimetidine, for which there has been longer experience. Confusional states have been seen particularly in older patients. Antiandrogenic properties have been blamed for the occasional gynecomastia and male sexual dysfunction seen. Rare cases of leukopenia are reported. Cimetidine also delays hepatic microsomal metabolism of some drugs, such as warfarin, theophylline, diazepam, and phenytoin.

Ranitidine, a substituted alkylfuran, is on a milligram basis 5–10 times more potent than cimetidine and appears to have a slightly longer duration of effect. The usual adult dose is 150 mg twice daily. Preliminary reports indicate fewer adverse effects and drug interactions with ranitidine than with cimetidine, but clinical experience is limited.

Although combinations of H_2 receptor antagonists and antacids are widely prescribed, there is little rationale for this practice. High-dose antacids reduce bioavailability of both cimetidine and ranitidine. However, higher 24-hour intragastric pH has been reported in patients receiving the combination of antacids and H_2 receptor antagonists.

MUCOSAL PROTECTIVE AGENTS

Sucralfate

Sucralfate (Carafate), or aluminum sucrose sulfate, is a sulfated disaccharide recently developed for use in peptic ulcer disease.

R: $SO_3 [Al_2 (OH)_5] \cdot 16H_2O$

Sucralfate

Its mechanism of action is thought to involve selective binding to necrotic ulcer tissue, where it may act as a barrier to acid, pepsin, and bile. In addition, sucralfate may directly absorb bile salts. The drug has been shown to be effective in the healing of duodenal ulcers. It is not absorbed systemically, and few side effects have been reported. The dosage is 1 g 4 times daily on an empty stomach (at least 1 hour before meals). It also requires an acid pH to be activated and so should not be administered simultaneously with antacids or an H_2 receptor antagonist.

Colloidal Bismuth Compounds

These compounds also appear to work by selective binding to an ulcer and by coating it to protect the ulcer from acid and pepsin. **Tripotassium dicitrato bismuthate (De-Nol)** has been extensively tested in Europe and shown to be superior to placebo in the healing of both duodenal and gastric ulcers. Side effects have been minimal, and the encephalopathy reported with long-term use of other bismuth compounds has not been noted.

Carbenoxolone

This synthetic derivative of glycyrrhizic acid (an agent extracted from licorice) has been shown to be effective in healing both gastric and duodenal ulcers. The mechanism of action of carbenoxolone is not clear but is thought to involve an increase in the production, secretion, and viscosity of intestinal mucus. Although its ulcer-healing properties are evident, the drug has a major aldosteronelike side effect, so that hypertension, fluid retention, and hypokalemia have limited its clinical usefulness. The concurrent administration of spironolactone controls the fluid retention but also abolishes the ulcer-healing effect; thiazides prevent sodium retention without abolishing the beneficial effect in peptic disease.

Carbenoxolone, although widely used in Europe, is investigational in the USA.

Prostaglandins

These derivatives of arachidonic acid are discussed in detail in Chapter 17. Certain prostaglandins, especially prostaglandin E_2, are produced by the gastric mucosa and are thought to have a major role in gastric cytoprotection. When administered orally, methyl analogs of prostaglandin E_2 have been shown to be effective in healing not only peptic ulcers but also gastric lesions produced in experimental animals by the administration of aspirin and indomethacin. The mechanism of cytoprotection by prostaglandin E_2 is not known but may be related to stimulation of gastric secretion of mucus. The clinical usefulness of prostaglandins is limited by the diarrhea they induce. Newer prostaglandin derivatives without this effect are being developed; none of those presently available are approved for use in peptic disease.

OTHER AGENTS

Cholinoceptor antagonists (discussed in greater detail in Chapter 7) are now most useful as adjuncts to H_2 receptor antagonists, especially in those patients refractory to treatment with the latter or those with nocturnal pain. **Pirenzapine,** an antimuscarinic agent with activity apparently specific to gastric receptors, is under investigation and may prove more useful in ulcer therapy.

Tricyclic antidepressants (discussed in Chapter 28) also may promote the healing of peptic ulcers, but their precise mechanism of action (H_2 receptor blockade, antimuscarinic, or both) is not clear, and careful clinical trials have not been done (see Ries reference).

Omeprazole is a substituted benzimidazole that is a potent inhibitor of the gastric proton pump hydrogen-potassium ATPase. A single daily dose inhibits essentially 100% of gastric acid secretion. Although the drug is still under investigation, the development of gastric carcinoid tumors in experimental animals receiving it has raised questions about the potential adverse effects of long-term acid suppression.

DRUGS PROMOTING GASTROINTESTINAL MOTILITY

Cholinergic mechanisms are responsible for modulating motor phenomena in the gut; thus it is not surprising that cholinomimetic agents such as **bethanechol** are effective in promoting gastrointestinal motility.

Metoclopramide (Reglan), recently promoted as a gut stimulant, also has cholinomimetic properties, apparently sensitizing intestinal smooth muscle to the action of acetylcholine rather than acting directly on acetylcholine receptors. In addition, the drug is a potent dopamine antagonist, particularly at central dopamine receptors.

Metoclopramide
(methoxychloroprocainamide)

These properties contribute to the stimulant effects of metoclopramide in the gastrointestinal tract. The drug acts to hasten esophageal clearance, raise lower esophageal sphincter pressure, accelerate gastric emptying, and shorten small bowel transit time. The central dopamine antagonist effect is principally responsible for its antiemetic properties.

Clinical applications follow these effects. Metoclopramide is useful for facilitating small bowel intubation. In addition, in patients with gastric motor failure—particularly diabetic gastroparesis but possibly also after vagotomy and in other disorders of gastric emptying—metoclopramide can produce significant symptomatic relief. In patients with chronic gastroesophageal reflux disease, metoclopramide has

been effective in decreasing the incidence of heartburn, although long-term effects are uncertain. Finally, the drug is an effective antiemetic, particularly useful in association with cancer chemotherapy and in emergency surgery or labor and delivery to prevent aspiration of gastric contents.

Metoclopramide is rapidly absorbed, with peak concentrations after a single oral dose seen in 40–120 minutes. Its plasma half-life is about 4 hours, and the drug is excreted mainly by the kidneys. The usual dose is 10 mg 4 times daily with meals and at bedtime. Larger doses, up to 1–2 mg/kg, have been used in conjunction with cancer chemotherapy. A dose of 20 mg given by slow intravenous infusion is used for small bowel intubation.

The most common side effects of metoclopramide are somnolence, nervousness, and dystonic reactions. Parkinsonism and tardive dyskinesia have also been reported. The drug also causes increased pituitary prolactin release, and galactorrhea and menstrual disorders have been reported.

PANCREATIC ENZYME REPLACEMENT PRODUCTS

Steatorrhea occurs in pancreatic insufficiency when lipase output is reduced below 10% of normal. It is estimated that in the postprandial period, approximately 100,000 units of lipase are delivered to the intestinal lumen per hour. Thus, the goal of pancreatic enzyme replacement should be to deliver at least 10,000 units per hour. However, because of inactivation of the enzyme below pH 4, only about 8% of the ingested lipase activity reaches the distal duodenum.

Different pancreatic enzyme preparations vary markedly in enzyme activity. Manufacturers' listings of enzyme content may not always match a well-standardized in vitro laboratory assay. Two major types of preparation in use are pancreatin, an alcoholic extract of hog pancreas, and pancrelipase, a lipase-enriched hog pancreas preparation. The enzyme content of several pancreatic enzyme preparations as measured by in vitro assay is given in Table 66-2. As indicated in the table, variation in enzyme content can be partly compensated for by increases in dosage; the in vivo response—measured as reduction in stool fat and nitrogen—can be appreciable.

Various dosage schedules have been recommended for pancreatic enzyme replacement, but there appears to be little difference between giving the medication with meals and giving it every 2 hours through the day. Because individual dosage requirements vary, it is essential that the result of therapy—the daily stool fat excretion—be monitored and the number of capsules or tablets increased until a therapeutic effect is seen. Supplementing the regimen with cimetidine enhances the effectiveness of the enzymes, presumably by decreasing the destruction of enzyme activity by gastric acid.

Because the enzyme preparations have a high

Table 66–2. Enzyme activities in some pancreatic enzyme replacement products.
(nd = data not available.)

Proprietary Preparation	Amount (Units per Tablet or Capsule)			Number of Tablets or Capsules per Meal	Percentage Reduction in Feces	
	Lipase	Trypsin	Amylase		Fat	Nitrogen
Ilozyme*	3600	3444	329,600	3	48	nd
Cotazyme*	2014	1797	499,200	5	nd	35
Pancrease*	2005	nd	nd	3	73	40
Viokase†	1636	1828	277,333	6	49	40
Phazyme	210	620	15,800	nd	nd	nd

*Generic pancrelipase.
†Generic pancreatin.

purine content, uric acid renal stones may be seen as a side effect. Also, the lactose in the pills may be sufficient to cause symptoms in lactose-intolerant patients. Finally, pancreatic enzyme replacement is expensive, costing up to $1500 per year for adequate therapy.

LAXATIVES

Laxatives of various types are widely prescribed and more widely purchased without prescription, indicating a cultural preoccupation with "regularity." Laxatives are best classified by their mechanism of action as irritants or stimulants, bulking agents, and stool softeners.

IRRITANT OR STIMULANT LAXATIVES

Castor oil is hydrolyzed in the upper small intestine to ricinoleic acid, a local irritant that increases intestinal motility. The onset of action is prompt and continues until the compound is excreted via the colon.

Cascara, senna, and **aloes** contain emodin alkaloids that are liberated after absorption from the intestine and are excreted into the colon, where peristalsis is stimulated. Thus, their onset of activity is delayed for 6–8 hours. Chronic stimulation of the colon is thought to lead to chronic colonic distention and perpetuation of the perceived need for laxatives.

Phenolphthalein and **bisacodyl,** which are chemically similar, are also potent colonic stimulants. Their action may be prolonged by an enterohepatic circulation.

BULK LAXATIVES

Hydrophilic colloids, prepared from the indigestible parts of fruits, vegetables, and seeds, form gels within the large intestine, distending the intestine and thereby stimulating its peristaltic activity. Agar, psyllium seed, and methylcellulose all act in this manner as well. Bran and other forms of vegetable fiber have the same effect.

Saline cathartics such as magnesium citrate and magnesium hydroxide also distend the bowel and stimulate its contractions. These nonabsorbable salts hold water in the intestine by osmotic force and cause distention.

STOOL SOFTENERS

Agents that become emulsified with stool serve to soften it and make passage easier. Examples are **mineral oil, glycerin suppositories,** and detergents such as **dioctyl sodium sulfosuccinate (docusate).**

ANTIDIARRHEAL DRUGS

The 2 most widely used prescription drugs for diarrhea are **diphenoxylate** (with atropine), a weak analog of meperidine, and **loperamide,** which is chemically related to haloperidol. Their mechanism of action on the gut is similar to that of the opioids (Chapter 29). Loperamide may not cross the blood-brain barrier and thus may cause less sedation and be less addicting than diphenoxylate. Neither drug should be used in patients with severe ulcerative colitis, since toxic megacolon may be precipitated. It has been suggested that these drugs may prolong the duration of diarrhea in patients with *Shigella* or *Salmonella* infection.

Adsorbents such as **kaolin** and **pectin** are also widely used. Their action is through their ability to adsorb compounds from solution, presumably binding potential intestinal toxins. Overall, however, they are much less effective than the drugs mentioned above.

DRUGS USED FOR THE DISSOLUTION OF GALLSTONES

Cholesterol is solubilized in aqueous bile by the combined effect of bile acids and lecithin, which, together with cholesterol, form the mixed micelle. When cholesterol is secreted in bile in relative excess to lecithin and bile acids, cholesterol crystals precipitate and may coalesce into cholesterol gallstones. Patients with cholesterol gallstones have a diminished total body bile acid pool, and consequently their bile is saturated with cholesterol. Subsequently, it has been found that oral administration of the recently approved drug **chenodeoxycholic acid (Chenix;** chenodiol), a primary bile acid, can reduce the concentration of cholesterol in bile; the mechanism is incompletely understood. Chronic therapy with chenodiol is capable of causing gallstone dissolution in some patients.

The usefulness of chenodiol in the medical treatment of gallstones was elucidated by the National Cooperative Gallstone Study, the results of which were published in 1981. In this study, patients were assigned to either a "high-dose" (750 mg/d), "low-dose" (350 mg/d), or placebo group. Over a 2-year period of high-dose therapy, only 13.5% of patients had complete dissolution of stones. Dissolution was more successful in thin people and those with small or floating stones. Diarrhea occurred in 41% of patients receiving the high dose of chenodiol. It was pointed out later that few of the patients in the high-dose group received the recommended dose of 15 mg/kg, but such a dose would presumably cause even more severe diarrhea.

Ursodeoxycholic acid, the 7β epimer of chenodiol, may be a more potent desaturating agent for cholesterol in bile. It has also been reported to cause fewer side effects. It is investigational.

The role of medical therapy in the treatment of gallstones remains to be defined. Gallstone dissolution by the oral administration of bile acids is only useful for cholesterol gallstones. Radiopaque stones are rarely if ever cholesterol stones; however, fewer than 75% of radiolucent stones are cholesterol stones. In addition, this therapy is successful only in patients with functioning gallbladders. Several studies have shown a high recurrence rate for stones after treatment was stopped, presumably committing patients to lifelong therapy. These factors, together with the relatively low incidence of complete dissolution and the potentially high incidence of side effects, suggest that surgery will remain the favored therapeutic approach except in highly selected patients.

Monooctanoin (glyceryl-1-monooctanoate, Moctanin) is a newly approved agent that is infused into the common bile duct through a catheter or T tube to dissolve retained bile duct stones. Stones may be completely dissolved or sufficiently reduced in size to facilitate their subsequent removal.

DRUGS USED IN THE TREATMENT OF CHRONIC INFLAMMATORY BOWEL DISEASE

The principal drugs used in the treatment of chronic inflammatory bowel disease (ulcerative colitis, Crohn's disease) are corticosteroids and other immunosuppressive agents, which are discussed elsewhere, and **sulfasalazine.** Sulfasalazine was introduced in the 1940s for the treatment of rheumatoid arthritis. It has subsequently been shown to be effective in ulcerative colitis, Crohn's colitis, and less so in Crohn's disease of the small intestine. In ulcerative colitis, it is more effective in maintaining than in obtaining clinical remission.

Sulfasalazine

Sulfasalazine combines sulfapyridine with 5-aminosalicylic acid linked by an azo bond. The drug is poorly absorbed from the intestine, and the azo linkage is broken down by the bacterial flora in the colon. Most evidence suggests that the nonabsorbed salicylate moiety is the most active part of the drug. The mechanism of action of sulfasalazine is unknown. Recent studies have suggested either a cytoprotective role, perhaps by inhibition of breakdown of prostaglandin $F_{2\alpha}$, or a suppressant effect on immune function.

The usual therapeutic dose of sulfasalazine is 3–4 g daily in divided doses. Smaller doses, usually 2 g/d, are needed to maintain remission in ulcerative colitis. Dose-related side effects such as malaise, nausea, abdominal discomfort, or headache occur in up to 20% of patients given 4 g/d. Some of these effects may be avoided by beginning at a lower dose and slowly increasing to the desired dosage level or by using enteric-coated or liquid suspension preparations. The inhibition of folic acid absorption by sulfasalazine has been reported, so that supplemental folate should be administered. Finally, as with other sulfonamides, serum sickness–like reactions and severe bone marrow suppression have occasionally been seen.

Azodisalicylate, a diazotized form of 5-aminosalicylic acid currently under investigation, may provide a new means of delivering the active moiety of sulfasalazine to the distal bowel while avoiding the latter's side effects, most of which are attributable to the sulfapyridine.

DRUGS USED IN THERAPY OF PORTAL-SYSTEMIC ENCEPHALOPATHY

The broad-spectrum, nonabsorbable antibiotic neomycin (Chapter 45) has been combined with dietary restriction of protein for the treatment of portal-systemic encephalopathy. **Lactulose (Cephulac),** a synthetic disaccharide (galactose-fructose) that is not absorbed, is also effective in this condition.

The mechanism of action of lactulose is unclear. It is apparently degraded by intestinal bacteria to lactic acid, acetic acid, and other organic acids. It is thought that this may facilitate the "trapping" of ammonium ion or other putative central nervous system toxins in the intestinal tract. Modification of the normal intestinal flora by lactulose has been suggested as another mechanism of action, but this has not been demonstrated with certainty.

Lactulose is available as a syrup and is given in doses of 15–30 mL 4 times daily or until the patient has 4 or 5 soft bowel movements daily. The drug is well tolerated and may be given in combination with neomycin, although this combination has no clear advantage over lactulose alone. Lactulose may also be administered as an enema.

REFERENCES

Peptic Ulcer Disease

Drake D, Hollander D: Neutralizing capacity and cost effectiveness of antacids. *Ann Intern Med* 1981;**94:**215.

Graham DY, Patterson DJ: Double-blind comparison of liquid antacid and placebo in the treatment of symptomatic reflux esophagitis. *Dig Dis Sci* 1983;**28:**559.

Grossman MI et al: Peptic ulcer: New therapies, new diseases. *Ann Intern Med* 1981;**95:**609.

Peterson WL et al: Healing of duodenal ulcer with an antacid regimen. *N Engl J Med* 1977;**297:**341.

Ries RK, Gilbert DA, Katon W: Tricyclic antidepressant therapy for peptic ulcer disease. *Arch Intern Med* 1984;**144:**566.

Sachs G: Pump blockers and ulcer disease. (Editorial.) *N Engl J Med* 1984;**310:**785.

Sontag S et al: Cimetidine, cigarette smoking and recurrence of duodenal ulcer. *N Engl J Med* 1984;**311:**689.

Gastrointestinal Motility

Albibi R, McCallum RW: Metoclopramide: Pharmacology and clinical application. *Ann Intern Med* 1983;**98:**86.

Schulze-Delrieu K: Drug therapy: Metoclopramide. *N Engl J Med* 1981;**305:**28.

Pancreatic Insufficiency

DiMagno EP et al: Fate of orally ingested enzymes in pancreatic insufficiency: Comparison of two dosage schedules. *N Engl J Med* 1977;**296:**1318.

Graham DY: Enzyme replacement therapy of exocrine pancreatic insufficiency in man: Relation between in vitro enzyme activities and in vivo potency in commercial pancreatic extracts. *N Engl J Med* 1977;**296:**1314.

Laxatives

Binder HJ, Donowitz M: A new look at laxative action. *Gastroenterology* 1975;**69:**1001.

Gallstone Therapy

Danziger RG et al: Dissolution of cholesterol gallstones by chenodeoxycholic acid. *N Engl J Med* 1972;**286:**1.

Schoenfield LJ et al: Chenodiol (chenodeoxycholic acid) for dissolution of gallstones: The National Cooperative Gallstone Study. *Ann Intern Med* 1981;**95:**257.

Thistle JL, Hofmann AF: Efficacy and specificity of chenodeoxycholic acid therapy for dissolving gallstones. *N Engl J Med* 1973;**289:**655.

Tint GS et al: Ursodeoxycholic acid: A safe and effective agent for dissolving cholesterol gallstones. *Ann Intern Med* 1982;**97:**351.

Inflammatory Bowel Disease

Goldman P, Peppercorn MA: Sulfasalazine. *N Engl J Med* 1975;**293:**20.

Klotz U et al: Therapeutic efficacy of sulfasalazine and its metabolites in patients with ulcerative colitis and Crohn's disease. *N Engl J Med* 1980;**303:**1499.

Portal-Systemic Encephalopathy

Conn HO, Lieberthal MM: *The Hepatic Coma Syndromes and Lactulose.* Williams & Wilkins, 1978.

67

Clinical Interpretation of Drug Concentrations

Nicholas H.G. Holford, MB, ChB, MSc, MRCP (UK), FRACP

Improvements in drug analysis methods during the past 15 years have greatly increased the number of drugs that can be measured in body fluids, and the development of pharmacokinetics has defined the use of such measurements in therapeutics. The rationale for making such measurements lies in the fact that for many therapeutic situations, drug concentration *in the blood* determines the clinical response; variations in clinical response, eg, treatment failure, often result from variations in drug concentration that are predictable from pharmacokinetic considerations.

PHARMACOKINETICS & PHARMACODYNAMICS

The basic principles outlined in Chapters 1–3 can be applied to the interpretation of clinical drug concentration measurements on the basis of 3 major pharmacokinetic variables: absorption, clearance, and volume of distribution; and 2 pharmacodynamic variables: maximum effect attainable in the target tissue and the sensitivity of the tissue to the drug.

Pharmacokinetic Concepts

A. Absorption: The amount of drug that enters the body depends on the patient's compliance with the prescribed regimen and on the rate and extent of transfer from the site of administration to the blood.

Overdosage and underdosage—both aspects of failure of compliance—can frequently be detected by concentration measurements when gross deviations from expected values are obtained. If compliance is found to be adequate, malabsorption abnormalities in the small bowel may be the cause of abnormally low concentrations. Variations in the extent of bioavailability are rarely caused by irregularities in the manufacture of the particular drug formulation. More commonly, variations in bioavailability are seen with drugs such as propranolol that undergo extensive metabolism during absorption.

B. Clearance: Clearance reflects the ability of the body to eliminate drug—by metabolism (eg, in the liver) or by excretion of unchanged drug (eg, by the kidneys). It is defined as the factor that relates the average plasma concentration to the maintenance dose (see equation [2], below). For dose calculations the units of clearance are conveniently expressed as liters per hour (L/h). For example, the clearance of creatinine is 6 L/h in a person with normal renal function.

Abnormal clearance may be anticipated when there is major impairment of the function of the heart, kidney, or liver. The extent of the abnormality will depend upon the predominant route of elimination as well as the extent of functional loss. Creatinine clearance is a useful quantitative indicator of renal function. Drug clearance may be a useful indicator of the functional consequences of heart or liver failure, with greater precision than clinical findings or other laboratory tests. For example, when renal function is changing rapidly, estimation of the clearance of aminoglycoside antibiotics may be a more accurate indicator of glomerular filtration than serum creatinine.

C. Volume of Distribution: The apparent volume of distribution depends on the extent of drug penetration and binding to tissues. The smallest possible value for a drug injected into the blood is the plasma volume. Very large volumes may result if there is extensive tissue binding; eg, digoxin has an apparent volume of distribution of about 500 L per 70 kg.

The volume of distribution may be overestimated in obese patients if based on total body weight and the drug does not enter fatty tissues well, as is the case with digoxin. In contrast, abnormal accumulation of fluid—edema, ascites, pleural effusion—can markedly increase the volume of distribution of drugs such as tobramycin that are hydrophilic and have small volumes of distribution (10–20 L/70 kg).

Table 3–1 (pp 24–25) gives typical values of drug absorption, clearance, and volume of distribution in healthy adults.

Pharmacodynamic Concepts

A. Maximum Effect: All pharmacologic responses must have a maximum effect (E_{max}). No matter how high the drug concentration goes, a point will be reached beyond which no further increment in response is achieved.

If increasing the dose does not lead to a further clinical response, it is possible that the maximum effect has been reached. This can be verified by demonstrating that an increase in dose results in increased drug concentration without further drug effect. Recognition of maximum effect is helpful in avoiding ineffectual increases of dose with the attendant risk of toxicity.

B. Sensitivity: The sensitivity of the target organ to drug concentration is reflected by the concentration required to produce 50% of maximum effect. This concentration, known as the EC50, can be used to define the potency of one drug with respect to another.

Failure of response that is due to diminished sensitivity to the drug can be detected by measuring drug concentrations that are usually associated with therapeutic response in a patient who is not getting better. This may be a result of abnormal physiology—eg, hyperkalemia diminishes responsiveness to digoxin; or drug antagonism—eg, calcium channel blockers impair the inotropic response to digoxin. Increased sensitivity to the drug is usually signaled by exaggerated responses to small or moderate doses. The pharmacodynamic nature of this sensitivity can be confirmed by drug concentrations that are low in relation to the observed effect.

THE TARGET CONCENTRATION STRATEGY

Recognition of the essential role of concentration in linking pharmacokinetics and pharmacodynamics has led to the target concentration strategy. Pharmacodynamic principles can be used to predict the concentration required to achieve a particular degree of therapeutic effect. This "target concentration" can then be achieved by using pharmacokinetic principles to arrive at a suitable dosing regimen.

CLEARANCE

Clearance is the single most important factor determining drug concentrations. The interpretation of drug concentrations depends upon a clear understanding of 3 factors that may influence clearance. These are the dose, blood flow, and the intrinsic function of the liver or kidneys. Each of these factors should be considered when interpreting clearance estimated from a drug concentration measurement. It must also be recognized that changes in protein binding may mislead the unwary to believe there is a change in clearance when in fact drug elimination is not altered.

Most drug elimination pathways will become saturated if the dose is high enough. The relation between dose rate and average steady-state concentration (C_{ss}) is shown in Fig 67–1 and is expressed mathematically in equation (1):

$$\text{Dose rate} = \frac{EC}{K_m + C_{ss}} \times C_{ss} \qquad \ldots (1)$$

This equation is similar to the Michaelis-Menten statement of enzyme kinetics. The maximum elimination capacity (EC) corresponds to V_{max} of the Michaelis-Menten equation, and K_m is the concentration at which the rate of elimination is 50% of EC. It is important to note that in the nonlinear region (the right-hand side of Fig 67–1), the increase in steady-state concentration is much faster than the increase in dose rate. If dose rate exceeds elimination capacity, steady state cannot be achieved: the concentration will keep on rising as long as dosing continues. This kind of capacity-limited elimination becomes important

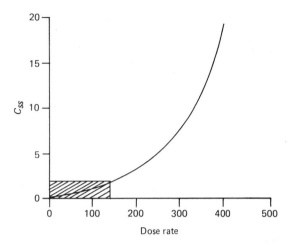

Figure 67–1. The relationship between dose rate and steady-state concentration (C_{ss}). Drugs with linear elimination occupy the shaded area. Drugs with nonlinear elimination encompass the whole curve. The units of dose rate and C_{ss} are arbitrary but are typical of phenytoin (EC = 500 mg/d, K_m = 5 mg/L).

when steady-state concentration is greater than K_m. It is an example of nonlinear pharmacokinetics caused by concentration-dependent clearance. This pattern of drug elimination is important for 3 drugs in common clinical use: propranolol, phenytoin, and aspirin.

Fortunately, the target concentration for most drugs used in clinical practice is usually less than their K_m, and steady-state concentration is always proportionate to the dose rate (shaded area in Fig 67–1). This is the region of linear pharmacokinetics. One major pathway of elimination, glomerular filtration, is never capacity-limited, and drugs excreted only by this route will have linear pharmacokinetics. Equation (1) reduces to a simpler form when steady-state concentration is much less than K_m:

$$\text{Dose rate} = \text{Clearance} \times C_{ss} \qquad \ldots (2)$$

This equation is often used to estimate total body clearance.

Blood Flow & Clearance

Drug elimination from liver and kidney may be dependent upon blood flow if blood clearance is similar to organ blood flow—about 90 L/h for the liver and 70 L/h for the kidneys (Table 1–3). Clearance of drugs such as lidocaine, morphine, and verapamil approaches hepatic blood flow, and they are said to have a high extraction ratio. Excretion of drugs with high extraction ratios is largely dependent upon blood flow to the eliminating organ.

Intrinsic Clearance

The functional ability of the liver to metabolize a drug or the kidney to filter or secrete a drug (the intrinsic clearance) will influence clearance independently of blood flow. In heart failure the clearance of theophylline is halved not because of reduced blood flow (theophylline extraction ratio is less than 5%) but because the congested liver is less capable of drug metabolism. A high extraction ratio drug such as lidocaine will have even greater impairment of clearance because of reductions in both intrinsic clearance and blood flow.

Clearance & Protein Binding

Many drugs are avidly bound by plasma proteins. This is not detected in clinical drug concentration determinations, because bound and unbound drug are measured together by most routine analytical methods. Clearance of drugs with high extraction ratios is unaffected by changes in protein binding, because these drugs are stripped completely from plasma proteins. Clearance of drugs with low extraction ratios, however, will appear to be inversely proportionate to the degree of drug-protein binding. This is because the elimination mechanism (filtration, secretion, or metabolism) is available only to unbound drug. Clearance of unbound drug is unaffected by protein binding changes, but total drug concentration will vary with the extent of binding. Clearance estimated from total drug concentration will therefore appear to vary with changes in protein binding. (See Chapter 3, Part I, for more detailed discussion.)

Factors Affecting Protein Binding

A. Albumin Concentration: Drugs such as phenytoin, salicylates, and disopyramide are extensively bound to plasma albumin. Albumin levels are low in many disease states, resulting in lower total drug concentrations.

B. Orosomucoid Concentration: Orosomucoid (α_1-acid glycoprotein) is an important protein binding site for drugs such as quinidine, lidocaine, and propranolol. It is increased in acute inflammatory disorders and causes major changes in total plasma concentration of these drugs even though drug elimination is unchanged.

C. Drug Concentration: The binding of drugs to plasma proteins is capacity-limited. Therapeutic concentrations of salicylates, disopyramide, and prednisolone show concentration-dependent protein binding. Because unbound drug concentration is determined by clearance—which is not altered, in the case of these low-extraction-ratio drugs, by protein binding—increases in dose will cause proportionate changes in the pharmacodynamically important unbound concentration, but total drug concentration will increase less rapidly because protein binding approaches saturation at higher concentrations.

THE VALUE OF DRUG CONCENTRATION MEASUREMENTS

A single drug concentration measurement typically costs about 20 times as much as a common laboratory test such as serum sodium or blood glucose. This is because the procedures are technically demanding and are performed in relatively small numbers. However, the information generated by a drug concentration measurement is potentially of more value than that provided by a serum sodium or blood glucose determination, because the amount of drug intake is often known more precisely than sodium or glucose intake, and drug distribution and elimination mechanisms are often simple and well understood. A single drug concentration measurement may often be relied upon to predict the consequences of dosing changes for days or even weeks.

Assessment of dosing regimen compliance and drug identification in suspected poisoning or overdose are sometimes possible only by measuring drug concentrations in the blood. Estimation of clearance and volume of distribution, prediction of future drug concentrations, rational design of dosing regimens, and assessment of functional impairment due to disease are also greatly facilitated by appropriate drug concentration measurements.

INTERPRETATION OF DRUG CONCENTRATION REPORTS

Dosing History

An accurate dosing history is essential to obtain maximum value from a drug concentration measurement. In fact, if the dosing history is unknown or incomplete, a drug concentration measurement loses all predictive value.

Timing

Quantitative interpretation of drug concentrations relies upon appropriately timed blood samples and accurate recording of time of collection. Blood samples should be drawn at a time (specified below) that provides maximum pharmacokinetic information about the patient.

Expected Concentration

The information to be gained from a drug concentration measurement must be interpreted in light of its expected value. The expected value is calculated from the dosing history, the condition of the patient, and the timing of the blood samples. Comparison of the expected value with the drug concentration measurement permits rational adjustment of future dosing.

TIMING OF DRUG CONCENTRATION MEASUREMENTS

Absorption

Information about the rate and extent of drug absorption in a particular patient is rarely of great clinical importance. Absorption usually occurs during the first 2 hours after a drug dose but varies according to food intake, posture, and activity. Therefore, it is important to avoid drawing blood until absorption is complete (about 2 hours after an oral dose). Attempts to measure peak concentrations early after oral dosing are usually unsuccessful and compromise the validity of the measurement, because one cannot be certain whether absorption is complete.

Clearance

The commonest pharmacokinetic indication for concentration measurements is to estimate clearance. Individual variations in clearance are much greater than variations in absorption or volume of distribution and are the single most important factor in successful pursuit of the target concentration strategy. Because the average steady-state concentration is most commonly used to predict drug effect (Table 3–1), the required dosing rate can be easily calculated from equation (2) above if clearance is known.

Conversely, clearance is readily estimated from the dosing rate and steady-state concentration. Blood samples should be appropriately timed to estimate steady-state concentration. Provided steady state has been reached (at least 3 half-lives of constant dosing), a sample obtained near the midpoint of the dosing interval will usually be close to steady-state concentration.

Volume of Distribution

Estimation of volume of distribution is sometimes feasible, especially if more than one measurement is available or if the drug is given intravenously. However, it is seldom important in individual cases to revise the expected value for volume of distribution. Plasma concentrations can be used to estimate volume of distribution when measured at the start of dosing, before extensive elimination has occurred (equation [1], Chapter 3, Part I), or—in combination with predosing (trough) concentration—immediately after a dose when input is complete (equations [9] and [10], Chapter 3, Part I).

THE INFLUENCE OF DOSING INTERVAL & HALF-LIFE ON OPTIMAL SAMPLING TIMES

Dosing Interval Much Longer Than Half-Life

Drugs given at intervals that are much longer than one half-life (eg, tobramycin, penicillin, prednisolone) are almost completely eliminated by the time the next dose is given (Fig 67–2). The timing of the blood sample is crucial to its interpretation. For example, tobramycin concentrations measured soon after the dose has been given reflect the volume of distribution and are little affected by clearance. Just before the next dose, however, the concentration is affected by both volume and clearance. Small errors in knowledge of the sample time can produce large errors in revising volume or clearance estimates. It is usually advisable to draw 2 samples, one just before the dose and another after the dose has been given, so that both volume and clearance can be accurately determined.

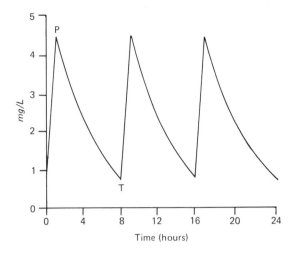

Figure 67–2. Time course of drug concentration in plasma for a drug when dosing interval is greater than half-life. A typical plasma concentration time curve is shown for tobramycin (half-life 2.2 hours) given every 8 hours by infusion over 1 hour. Ideal sampling times are at the end of the infusion (P, peak) and just before the next dose (T, trough).

Dosing Interval About Equal to Half-Life

The great majority of drugs are given about once every half-life (Fig 67–3). This is because many have half-lives between 4 and 8 hours and traditionally are given 3 or 4 times a day. The typical peak-to-trough drug concentration ratio is 2:1 when the dosing interval equals the half-life. A sample drawn in the middle of the dosing interval will be a good estimate of steady-state concentration if more than 3 half-lives have elapsed since starting regular dosing.

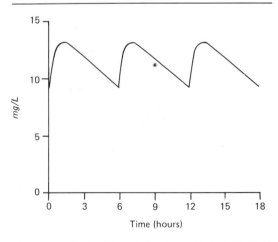

Figure 67–3. Dosing interval about equal to half-life. Typical plasma concentration time curve for theophylline (half-life 9 hours) given every 6 hours by mouth. Ideal sampling time is at the midpoint of the dosing interval (*).

Dosing Interval Much Less Than Half-Life

Some drugs with small clearance (eg, phenobarbital) or large volumes of distribution (eg, digoxin) have half-lives longer than a day. To encourage patient compliance, they are usually given once a day; the peak-to-trough variation is therefore usually quite small (Fig 67–4). For example, phenobarbital has a half-life of 5 days, and trough concentrations at steady state are only 10% lower than the peak. Blood samples drawn within a few hours after the first dose will accurately reflect the volume of distribution, and at steady state a sample drawn at any time will closely estimate steady-state concentration and allow clearance to be calculated.

FREQUENCY OF DRUG CONCENTRATION MEASUREMENTS

It is often valuable to obtain a drug concentration measurement on admission to hospital. This has 2 purposes: First, if the measurement is made rapidly, it can indicate whether a loading dose is required to supplement concentrations achieved by outpatient dosing or, conversely, whether maintenance dosing should be reduced or stopped if the concentration is too high. Second, the actual measurement compared with the expected concentration provides an estimate of outpatient compliance.

Hospital admissions are frequently associated with rapid, erratic dosing adjustments. If an accurate dosing history is kept, a second measurement made 2 or 3 half-lives after admission may provide essential information for future dosing adjustment. A constant dosing regimen should be established as soon as possible in order to achieve and maintain the target concentration. Further measurements should be considered if

the clinical state of the patient, especially clearance, is changing, eg, in heart failure. Measurements taken at intervals less than one half-life apart are of little value. At least 3 half-lives should be allowed to elapse after establishing a constant dosing regimen to obtain the most information about clearance.

OTHER BIOLOGIC FLUIDS

Therapeutic drug concentrations are most commonly measured in serum, plasma, or blood. The choice among these 3 is usually dictated by analytical requirements, and there is no pharmacokinetic or pharmacodynamic reason to prefer one over the other.

Saliva has been used instead of blood in order to avoid venipuncture. Unfortunately, salivary concentrations are influenced by factors such as saliva flow rate and pH that are not readily controlled and that result in an unacceptable variability in the ratio of concentration in saliva to concentration in blood. Reliable salivary concentrations usually impose more inconvenience on the patient than blood sampling and have found little favor except in pediatric practice.

Cerebrospinal fluid drug concentration measurements are sometimes useful for monitoring penetration of this compartment by antibiotics during treatment of intrathecal infections. However, their use for this purpose is semiquantitative and can give only rough guidance for future dosing. Concentrations of methotrexate in cerebrospinal fluid have been related to central nervous system toxicity and may be used in predicting when the target concentration for stopping leucovorin rescue therapy will be reached.

THE IMPORTANCE OF KNOWING THE EXPECTED VALUE

Interpretation of drug concentrations and their application to therapeutics hinges on knowing the expected values for the pharmacokinetic parameters of absorption, volume, and clearance and the pharmacodynamic parameters of maximum effect and sensitivity.

Pharmacokinetic parameters can be used to predict the drug concentration in a blood sample. Comparison of the measured concentration with the predicted one can then be used to decide if compliance was good, if the sample was drawn at the indicated time, if an error was made by the laboratory in measuring or reporting the result, or if revision of the expected pharmacokinetic parameters is required.

If pharmacokinetic revision is performed, deviations from the expected values for volume or clearance should be critically examined for reasonableness in direction and magnitude. For example, if tobramycin is administered to an emaciated patient, the expected tobramycin clearance using a prediction of creatinine production rate based on body weight (see equation [3], below) is likely to be too high because the actual

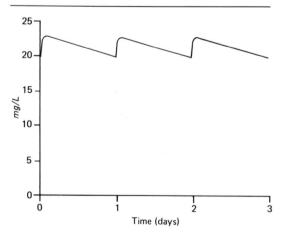

Figure 67–4. Dosing interval much less than half-life. A typical plasma concentration time curve is shown for phenobarbital (half-life 110 hours) given every 24 hours by mouth. Ideal sampling time is anywhere in the dosing interval.

creatinine production rate (per unit of body weight) will be lower as a result of muscle wasting.

Pharmacodynamic parameters can be used to predict whether a symptom or sign is drug-related. For example, a patient taking phenytoin who has a posterior fossa tumor may have nystagmus because of the drug or because of the tumor. Phenytoin-induced nystagmus usually does not appear until blood concentrations exceed 15 mg/L; a low phenytoin level may be used to identify the tumor as the more likely cause. However, withdrawal of phenytoin altogether may be required to resolve the issue, because the patient may have an unusually high sensitivity to this effect.

If a patient continues to have seizures and if repeated measurements after increasing doses have confirmed that concentrations are increasing and higher than those usually required, it should be assumed that the maximum effect has been achieved and another agent should be added or substituted.

Caution should be exercised in using drug concentrations in diagnosis. The inherent individual variability in pharmacodynamics should be recognized and weighed with other clinical features before a decision is made.

INITIAL PREDICTION OF INDIVIDUAL PHARMACOKINETICS

Typical values for absorption, clearance, and volume of distribution for many drugs measured by clinical laboratories are presented in Table 3–1. However, these values must sometimes be adjusted to reflect the clinical status of the patient.

Absorption

Quantitative adjustment of absorption parameters is rarely required. Patients with small bowel malabsorption can be expected to have reduced absorption. Digoxin bioavailability may be impaired in some patients by bacterial metabolism in the gut; this is difficult to identify in advance but may account for a marked increase in bioavailability that sometimes occurs when antibiotics are given.

Clearance

Drugs cleared by the renal route often require adjustment of clearance in proportion to renal function. This can be conveniently estimated from the creatinine clearance, determined from a single blood sample.

$$\begin{aligned} \text{Creatinine} \\ \text{clearance} \\ \text{(L/h)} \end{aligned} = \frac{160 - \text{Age (years)}}{22 \times \text{Serum creatinine (mg/dL)}} \\ \times \frac{\text{Weight (kg)}}{70} \\ (\times\ 0.9\ \text{if female}) \qquad \ldots (3)$$

The predicted clearance in women is 90% of the calculated value, because they have a smaller muscle

mass per kilogram and it is muscle mass that determines creatinine production. Because of the difficulty of obtaining complete urine collections, creatinine clearance calculated in this way is at least as reliable as estimates of production rate based on urine collection. Ideal body weight should be used for obese patients, and correction should be made for muscle wasting in severely ill patients.

The clearance of drugs excreted only by glomerular filtration is expected to be the same as the estimated creatinine clearance. If tubular secretion or reabsorption is important, renal clearance of the drug can often be estimated from creatinine clearance, eg, renal clearance of procainamide is about 3 times that of creatinine clearance.

Liver failure will impair drug clearance, but there are few reliable estimates of the quantitative effect. The presence of liver disease (eg, acute viral hepatitis, alcoholic cirrhosis) does not usually change drug elimination until liver dysfunction is severe enough to produce signs of neurologic impairment.

Volume of Distribution

Volume of distribution is commonly calculated from total body weight. If a patient is obese, drugs that do not readily penetrate fat (eg, tobramycin and digoxin) should have their volumes calculated from ideal body weight as shown below:

$$\begin{aligned} \text{Ideal body weight (kg)} &= 52 + 1.9\ \text{kg/in over 5 feet} \\ &\quad \text{(men)} \\ &= 49 + 1.7\ \text{kg/in over 5 feet} \\ &\quad \text{(women)} \qquad \ldots (4) \end{aligned}$$

Patients with edema, ascites, or pleural effusions offer a larger volume of distribution to the aminoglycoside antibiotics (eg, tobramycin) than is predicted by total body weight. In such patients, the total weight should be corrected as follows: Subtract an estimate of the weight of the excess fluid accumulation. Use the resultant "normal" body weight to calculate the normal volume of distribution. Finally, this normal volume should be increased by 1 L for each estimated kilogram of excess fluid. This correction is important because of the relatively small volumes of distribution of these water-soluble drugs.

Half-Life

Once the volume of distribution and clearance are known, the expected half-life can be calculated as follows:

$$\text{Half-life} = \frac{0.7 \times \text{Volume}}{\text{Clearance}} \qquad \ldots (5)$$

It is important to understand that volume of distribution and clearance are quite independent. A change in volume will not influence clearance, nor will a change in clearance alter volume. The half-life of a drug is determined by these 2 independent factors: volume of distribution, reflecting body size and composition; and clearance, reflecting organ size and function (mainly liver and kidney).

Time to Steady State

A practical guide to the time it will take for drug concentrations to reach steady state can be obtained by multiplying the half-life by 4. This is very close to the time it will take to reach 90% of the steady-state value.

Elimination Capacity

Drugs with capacity-limited elimination are difficult to study in patients with disease. As a consequence, little quantitative information is available to guide adjustment of elimination capacity estimates in a particular individual. Enzyme induction, eg, by anticonvulsants, may raise the elimination capacity substantially in some patients.

Percent Unbound in Plasma

Changes in protein binding may be caused by alterations in plasma protein concentration (albumin, orosomucoid), affinity to plasma proteins (phenytoin affinity is decreased in renal failure), or drug displacement interactions (valproic acid increases unbound phenytoin by half, from 10% to 15%).

Bioavailability & Drug Formulation

The bioavailability of intravenous doses, by definition, is always 100%. Care must be taken to adjust doses for the actual amount of active drug when the dose is given as a complex or salt. For example, theophylline is always given intravenously as aminophylline, a complex containing 80% theophylline.

REVISING PHARMACOKINETIC PARAMETERS USING MEASURED CONCENTRATIONS

The commonsense approach to the interpretation of drug concentrations compares predictions of pharmacokinetic parameters and expected concentrations to measured values. For example, if a patient is taking 0.25 mg of digoxin a day, a physician may expect (from application of equation [2]) the digoxin concentration to be about 1 ng/mL. This is based on the assumptions of typical bioavailability of 65% and total clearance of about 7 L/h. If the patient has heart failure, the concentration is expected to be about 1.5 ng/mL (expected clearance of 4.5 L/h). Suppose that the concentration actually measured is 2 ng/mL. Common sense would suggest halving the daily dose to achieve a target concentration of 1 ng/mL. This approach has used a revised clearance of 3.5 L/h (using equation [2], p 789).

This technique will often be misleading if steady state has not been reached. For example, if a loading dose of 1 mg of digoxin is given intravenously and the concentration is measured before a second dose hours later, it may be 1 ng/mL. However, this measurement says little about clearance and should not be used to determine the required maintenance dose. At least a week of regular dosing (3–4 half-lives) must elapse before the implicit method will be reliable. Failure to compare the expected concentration with the measured value in patients taking digoxin and quinidine explains why the major pharmacokinetic interaction between these 2 drugs went unnoticed for over 10 years, yet the doubling of steady-state concentrations by the action of quinidine on digoxin clearance can be detected in almost every patient taking this drug combination.

INTERPRETATION OF DRUG CONCENTRATIONS— COMMON SITUATIONS

Theophylline

A. On Admission: Blood should be drawn immediately before and 15–30 minutes after an intravenous loading dose. The change in concentration may be used with the size of the loading dose to determine the volume of distribution. If the target concentration has not been reached, the amount of additional theophylline required to get there can be calculated from the second blood level and the volume of distribution.

It is important to compare the estimate of volume obtained in this way with the expected value (0.5 L/kg). Blood levels obtained too soon after a loading dose will not permit normal drug distribution to the tissues, and the estimated volume will be too small compared with the expected value.

The level measured before the loading dose can be helpful in assessing compliance and the patient's clearance. Levels higher than expected based upon the dosing history and a clearance of 2.8 L/h per 70 kg should lead to caution in the maintenance dose that is to be prescribed. Most frequently the measured admission blood level will be lower than expected because of poor compliance. This information is valuable later for confronting the patient and emphasizing the need for regular use of theophylline if it is to be of any value in preventing hospital admissions. In this situation an average clearance should be assumed to predict the required maintenance dose. A low admission blood level should not be used to justify a higher than average maintenance dose. If this is done, high concentrations and toxicity such as vomiting will be frequent.

B. At the End of Intravenous Treatment: Blood drawn just before the end of a maintenance intravenous infusion of theophylline can be used to obtain an accurate estimate of clearance. This can then be used to predict the oral maintenance dose required to achieve the therapeutic target concentration. An abnormally low clearance is an additional factor favoring a contribution of heart failure to dyspnea in the older patient with airway obstruction.

At least 30 hours of constant rate infusion should elapse before accepting the measured level as a steady-state value. This time will be proportionately longer if the calculated clearance is lower than average.

Digoxin

The pharmacokinetic interpretation of digoxin concentrations is usually straightforward. Most patients will have been taking the drug for a long time. If the level is less than 1 ng/mL and is close to the value predicted from the patient's expected clearance, then it is unlikely that digoxin is of any therapeutic benefit at the current dose. On the other hand if the level is lower than predicted, a failure of compliance should be strongly considered and patient education may add some worthwhile improvement.

Tobramycin

Rational use of aminoglycoside drug concentrations requires that blood be drawn at least 30 minutes after the end of the infusion of the first dose and 2 or 3 half-lives later (usually just before the second dose)

(Fig 67–2). It may often take 24 hours before the results are known; therefore the earlier samples are taken in a course of treatment, the sooner dose adjustments can be made to reflect individual differences in volume and clearance.

Interpretation of the postinfusion concentration must be done with care. The volume of distribution may be roughly estimated from the dose divided by the concentration taken after the first dose. If the concentration appears to be too high (over 10 mg/L) but the volume is much smaller than the average 0.25 L/kg, then it is probable that the sample was drawn too soon after the infusion was stopped, when a significant fraction of the dose had yet to be distributed. It is important not to reduce the dose in these circumstances because the patient will be undertreated. Blood samples should be obtained again with the postinfusion sample drawn at a later time. The difference between the pre- and postinfusion levels can be used with the dose to check the apparent volume of distribution.

REFERENCES

Azarnoff DL: Use of pharmacokinetic principles in therapy. (Editorial.) *N Engl J Med* 1973;**289**:635.

Benet LZ: Effect of route of administration and distribution on drug action. *J Pharmacokinet Biopharm* 1978;**6**:559.

Bjornsson TD: Use of serum creatinine concentrations to determine renal function. *Clin Pharmacokinet* 1979;**4**:200.

Burton ME, Vasko MR, Brater DC: Comparison of drug dosing methods. *Clin Pharmacokinet* 1985;**10**:1.

Holford NHG: Theophylline: Designing the optimum dosing regimen. *Hosp Ther* 1985;**2**:21.

Holford NHG, Sheiner LB: Understanding the dose-effect relationship. *Clin Pharmacokinet* 1981;**6**:429.

Levy R, Shand D (editors): Clinical implications of drug-protein binding. *Clin Pharmacokinet* 1984;**9(Suppl)**:1.

Sokolow M, Edgar AL: Blood quinidine concentrations as a guide to the treatment of cardiac arrhythmias. *Circulation* 1950;**1**:576.

Whiting B et al: Clinical pharmacokinetics: A comprehensive system for therapeutic drug monitoring and prescribing. *Br Med J* 1984;**288**:541.

Winter ME: *Basic Clinical Pharmacokinetics*. Applied Therapeutics, 1980.

Zito RA, Reid PR: Lidocaine kinetics predicted by indocyanine green clearance. *N Engl J Med* 1978;**298**:1160.

68 Therapeutic & Toxic Potential of Over-the-Counter Agents

Mary Anne Koda-Kimble, PharmD

In the United States, drugs are divided by law into 2 classes: those restricted to sale by prescription only and those for which directions for safe use by the public can be written. The latter category constitutes the nonprescription or over-the-counter (OTC) drugs. The American public spends approximately $7.4 billion annually on an estimated 300,000 OTC products to medicate themselves for self-diagnosed ailments ranging from warts to psoriasis. These 300,000 products represent about 700 active ingredients in various forms and combinations. It is thus apparent that many are no more than "me too" products advertised to the public in ways that suggest that there are significant differences between them. For example, the current (seventh) edition of *Handbook of Nonprescription Drugs* lists 82 different internal analgesic products almost all of which contain aspirin, acetaminophen, salicylamide, phenacetin, or a combination of these agents as their primary ingredients. They are made different from one another by the addition of questionable ingredients such as caffeine or antihistamines; by brand names chosen to suggest a specific use ("feminine pain," "nighttime pain," "arthritis"); or by their special dosage form (enteric-coated tablets, liquids, sustained-release products, powders, seltzers). There is a price attached to all of these gimmicks, and in most cases a less expensive generic product can be equally effective. It is probably safe to assume that the public is generally overwhelmed and confused by the wide array of products presented and will probably use those that are most heavily advertised.

Since 1972, the Food and Drug Administration has been engaged in a methodical review of OTC ingredients for both safety and efficacy. There have been 2 major outcomes of this review: (1) ingredients designated as ineffective or unsafe for their claimed therapeutic use are being eliminated from OTC product formulations (eg, antimuscarinic agents have been eliminated from OTC sleep aids); and (2) agents previously available by prescription only have been made available for OTC use because they were judged by the review panel to be generally safe and effective for consumer use without medical supervision (eg, topical hydrocortisone 0.5%, diphenhydramine, ibuprofen). Some OTC ingredients previously available in low doses only are now available in higher concentrations. Table 68–1 lists some prescription drugs that have been recommended for OTC use. Although no final

regulations have been issued on any of these recommendations, the FDA's position has been to allow manufacturers to incorporate these ingredients into their OTC formulations upon publication of the review panel's preliminary report unless it (the FDA) finds compelling reason to dissent.

There are 3 reasons why it is critical for the clinician to be familiar with this class of products. First, many of the ingredients contained in these products are effective in treating common ailments, and it is important to be able to help the patient select a safe, effective product. (See Table 68–2.) Second, many of the active ingredients contained in OTC drugs may worsen existing medical conditions or interact with prescription medications. (See Appendix I, Drug Interactions.) Finally, the misuse or abuse of OTC products may actually produce significant medical complications. A general awareness of these products and their formulation will enable clinicians to more fully appreciate the potential for OTC drug-related problems in their patients.

Table 68–2 lists examples of OTC products that may be used effectively to treat medical problems commonly encountered in ambulatory patients. The selection of one ingredient over another may be important in patients with certain medical problems or in patients taking certain prescription medications. These are discussed in detail in other chapters. The recommendations listed in Table 68–2 are based upon the efficacy of the ingredients and on the principles set forth in the following paragraphs:

(1) Select the product that is simplest in formulation with regard to ingredients and dosage form. In general, single-ingredient products are preferred. Although some combination products contain effective doses of all ingredients, others contain therapeutic doses of some ingredients and subtherapeutic doses of others. Furthermore, there may be differing durations of action among the ingredients, and there is always a possibility that the clinician or patient will be unaware of the presence of certain active ingredients in the product. Aspirin, for example, is present in many cough and cold preparations; a patient unaware of this may take separate doses of analgesic in addition to that contained in the cold preparation.

(2) Select a product that contains a therapeutically effective dose.

(3) Select a product that lists its ingredients and

Table 68–1. Ingredients that have been recommended by over-the-counter (OTC) review panel
to be switched from prescription to OTC status.

Ingredient and Dosage	Indication	Single-Ingredient Product Examples
Systemic		
Brompheniramine 4 mg every 4–6 hours	Antihistamine	Dimetane Extentabs
Chlorpheniramine 4 mg every 4–6 hours	Antihistamine	Chlor-Trimeton
Diphenhydramine hydrochloride 25–50 mg every 4–6 hours	Antihistamine Antitussive Sleep aid	Benadryl Benylin Syrup Sominex 2, Sleep-Eze 3
Doxylamine 7.5–12.5 mg every 4–6 hours	Antihistamine	None
Dyclonine hydrochloride 0.05–0.10%	Oral local anesthetic, analgesic	None
Fluoride (various salts) Sodium 0.05% rinse Stannous 0.1% rinse Acidulated phosphate 0.02% rinse	Dental caries prophylactic	None
Methoxyphenamine hydrochloride 100 mg every 4–6 hours	Bronchodilator*	None
Promethazine hydrochloride 6.25–12.5 mg every 8–12 hours	Antihistamine*	None
Pseudoephedrine hydrochloride and sulfate 60 mg every 4–6 hours	Nasal decongestaqnt	D-Feda, Sudafed
Pyrantel pamoate 11 mg/kg as single dose	Anthelmintic (pinworms)	None
Topical		
Ephedrine sulfate 2–25%	Hemorrhoidal vasoconstrictor	None
Epinephrine hydrochloride 100–200 μg aqueous solution 4 times daily	Hemorrhoidal vasoconstrictor	None
Haloprogin 1%	Antifungal (anticandidal*)	None
Hydrocortisone (base and various salts) 0.5–1%	Anti-inflammatory (antifungal*) Dandruff (seborrheic dermatitis) Antipruritic, anti-inflammatory	None Aeroseb-HC CaldeCort, Cortaid, Lanacort
Miconazole nitrate 2%	Antifungal (anticandidal*)	None
Nystatin 100,000 units/g	Anticandidal*	None
Oxymetazoline hydrochloride 0.1%	Nasal decongestant	Afrin, Duration, Neo-Synephrine 12 Hour
Phenylephrine hydrochloride 0.5 mg aqueous solution 4 times daily	Hemorrhoidal vasoconstrictor	None
Xylometazoline 0.1%	Nasal decongestant	Dristan Long Lasting Nasal Mlst, Neo-Synephrine II Long Acting,Sine-Off Once-A-Day, Sinex Long-Acting Decongestant Nasal Spray

*Despite review panel recommendation, the FDA has dissented from OTC use for this application at this time.

their amounts. The label of a product should always be read carefully, since ingredients may be changed without public notification or change in brand name.

(4) Recommend a generic product if one is available.

(5) Be wary of "gimmicks" or advertising claims that claim specific superiority over similar products.

(6) For children, the dose, dosage form, and palatability of the product will be prime considerations.

Certain ingredients in OTC products should be avoided or used with caution in selected patients because they may exacerbate existing medical problems or interact with prescription medications the patient is

Table 68–2. Ingredients of known efficacy for selected over-the-counter (OTC) classes.

OTC Category	Ingredient and Dosage	Product Examples	Comments
Allergy preparations	Chlorpheniramine 4 mg every 4–6 hours; 12 mg every 12 hours	Chlor-Trimeton (4 mg/tablet or 10 mL syrup), Long Acting Chlor-trimetron* (8 mg/tablet), Teldrin Time-Released Capsules* (8 mg and 12 mg/capsule).	Antihistamines alone relieve most symptoms associated with allergic rhinitis or hay fever. Chlorpheniramine and brompheniramine cause less drowsiness than diphenhydramine, metha-pyriline, pyrilamine, doxylamine, and phento-loxamine. Occasionally, symptoms unrelieved by the antihistamine respond to the addition of a sympathomimetic.
	Brompheniramine 4 mg every 4–6 hours; 12 mg every 12 hours	Symptom 3 (4 mg/10 mL), Dimetane Extentab* (12 mg).	
	Diphenhydramine* 25–50 mg every 4–6 hours	Benadryl (25 mg/capsule; 12.5 mg/5 mL elixir).	
	Chlorpheniramine (4 mg) with pseudoephedrine (60 mg)	Chlor-Trimeton Decongestant (per tablet), Novafed A Syrup (per 10 mL), Sudafed Plus.	
	Chlorpheniramine (4 mg) with phenylpropanolamine (37.5 mg)	Novahistine, elixir and tablets (per 10 mL or 2 tablets); Tria-minicin Allergy (per tablet).	
	Triprolidine HCl* (2.5 mg) with pseudophendrine (60 mg)	Actifed.	
Analgesics and antipyretics	Aspirin 300–600 mg every 4–6 hours	Generic, Bayer Aspirin (325 mg/tablet).	There are numerous product modifications, in-cluding the addition of antacid, caffeine, and methapyriline; enteric-coated tablets and selt-zers; long-acting or extra-strength formula-tions; and various mixtures of analgesics. None have any substantial advantage over a single-ingredient product. Acetaminophen lacks anti-inflammatory activity but is available as a liquid; this dosage form is used primarily for infants and children who cannot chew or swallow tablets. Aspirin should be used cau-tiously in certain individuals (see text). Avoid products that contain phenacetin, eg, A.S.A. compound, Bromo-Seltzer, A.P.C. Capsules. Extra-strength formulations contain 400–600 mg of active ingredient.
	Acetaminophen 300–600 mg every 4–6 hours	Generic, Datril, Tylenol (325 mg/tablet—various strengths available).	
	Ibuprofen* 200–400 mg every 4–6 hours	Advil, Nuprin (200 mg/tablet).	
Antacids	Magnesium hydroxide and aluminum hydroxide combi-nations	Gelusil, Gelusil II, Maalox No. 1, Maalox No. 2, Mylanta, Mylanta II, Wingel.	Combinations of magnesium and aluminum hydroxide are less likely to cause constipation or diarrhea and offer high neutralizing capac-ity. The "II" formulations are approximately twice as potent on a mL/mL basis. The prod-ucts listed are liquid products with a low sodium content.
Antitussives	Codeine 10–20 mg every 4–6 hours (with guaifenesin)	Cheracol, Robitussin A-C (both contain 2 mg/mL).	In doses required for cough suppression, the addictive liability associated with codeine is low. Codeine is a Schedule V narcotic, and its OTC sale is restricted in some states. The efficacy of expectorants, which are included in almost all antitussives, is questionable. Guai-fenesin has the least potential for toxicity. Watch for hidden ingredients in these products.
	Dextromethorphan 10–20 mg every 4 hours or 30 mg every 6 hours (with guaifenesin)	Cheracol D (2 mg/mL), 2/G-DM (3 mg/mL), Novahistine Cough Formula (5 mg/mL), Pertussin 8-Hour Cough Formula (1.5 mg/mL), Robitussin-DM (3 mg/mL).	
Decongestants	Topical Oxymetazoline	Afrin.	Topical sympathomimetics are effective in the acute management of rhinorrhea associated with common colds and allergies. Long-acting agents (oxymetazoline and xylometazoline) are generally preferred, although phenyleph-rine is equally effective. Oral decongestants have a prolonged duration of action but may cause more systemic effects. Pseudoephedrine has the least CNS stimulatory effect. Phenyl-propanolamine is also effective. Phenyl-ephrine is unpredictably absorbed.
	Xylometazoline	Dristan Long Lasting Nasal Mlst, Neo-Synephrine II, Sinex-L.A., Sinutab Nasal Spray.	
	Phenylephrine	Allerest, Coricidin Nasal Spray, Neo-Synephrine, NTZ.	
	Oral Pseudoephedrine 60 mg every 4 hours or 120 mg every 12 hours	Novafed (30 mg/5 mL), Sudafed (30 mg/tablet or 5 mL), Sudafed SA (120 mg/capsule).	

Table 68–2 (cont'd). Ingredients of known efficacy for selected over-the-counter (OTC) classes.

OTC Category	Ingredient and Dosage	Product Examples	Comments
Decongestants (cont'd)	Oral (cont'd) Phenylpropanolamine 25 mg every 4 hours	No single-ingredient product available.	
Laxatives	Bulk formers	Metamucil, Serutan.	The safest laxatives for chronic use include the bulk formers and stool softeners. Saline laxatives and stimulants may be used acutely but not chronically (see text).
	Stool softeners—docusate sodium	Generic, Colace, Coloctyl, Doxinate.	
	Saline laxatives	Phillips' Milk of Magnesia.	
Sleep aids	Diphenhydramine 25–50 mg at bedtime	Sominex 2, Sleep-Eze 3 (25 mg/tablet or capsule); Sleepinal (50 mg).	Diphenhydramine, an antihistamine with well-documented CNS depressant effects, is now available over the counter for sedative use.

*Previously available by prescription only. Now available over the counter.

taking. Many of the more potent OTC ingredients are "hidden" in products where their presence would not ordinarily be expected (Table 68–3). This lack of awareness of the ingredients present in OTC products and the belief by many physicians that OTC products are "ineffective and harmless" may cause diagnostic confusion and perhaps interfere with therapy.

For example, innumerable OTC products, including cough and cold preparations, decongestants, and appetite control products, contain sympathomimetics. These agents should be avoided or used cautiously in insulin-dependent diabetics and patients with hypertension, angina, or hyperthyroidism. Aspirin should be avoided by individuals with active peptic ulcer disease, certain platelet disorders, or patients taking oral anticoagulants.

Finally, overuse or misuse of OTC products may induce significant medical problems. A prime example is rebound congestion from the regular use of nasal sprays for more than 3–4 days. The improper and chronic use of some antacids (eg, aluminum hydroxide) may cause constipation and even impaction in elderly people as well as hypophosphatemia. Laxative abuse (chiefly by older people) can result in abdominal cramping and fluid and electrolyte disturbances. Insomnia, nervousness, and restlessness can result from the use of sympathomimetics or caffeine hidden in many OTC products (Table 68–3). The chronic systemic use of some analgesics containing large amounts of caffeine may produce rebound headaches, and

long-term use of analgesics, especially those containing phenacetin, has been associated with interstitial nephritis. Acute ingestion of large amounts of aspirin or acetaminophen by adults or children causes serious toxicity. Antihistamines may cause sedation or drowsiness, especially when taken concurrently with sedative-hypnotics, tranquilizers, alcohol, or other central nervous system depressants. Finally, antihistamines, local anesthetics, antibiotics, antibacterial agents, counterirritants, *p*-aminobenzoic acid (PABA), preservatives, and deodorants contained in a myriad of OTC topical and vaginal products may induce allergic reactions.

There are 3 major drug information sources for OTC products. *Handbook of Nonprescription Drugs* is the most comprehensive resource for OTC medications; it evaluates ingredients contained in major OTC drug classes and lists the ingredients included in many OTC products. *Physicians' Desk Reference for Nonprescription Drugs,* a compendium of manufacturers' information regarding OTC products, is somewhat incomplete with regard to the number of products included and the consistency of information provided. *The Medicine Show,* a consumer guide to the use of OTC products, critically evaluates these products and discusses their rational use. It is well written and factually correct. Any clinician who seeks more specific information regarding OTC products should find these references useful.

Table 68–3. Hidden ingredients in over-the-counter (OTC) products.

Hidden Drug or Drug Class	OTC Class Containing Drug	Product Examples
Alcohol	Cough syrups/cold preparations.	Breacol (10%), Cotussis (20%), Formula 44D (20%), Halls (22%), Novahistine DMX (10%), NyQuil Nighttime Colds Medicine (25%), Pertussin 8-Hour Cough Formula (9.5%), Prunicodeine (25%), Romilar III (20%), Romilar CF (20%), Tussar SF (12%).
	Mouthwashes.	Astring-O-Sol (65%), Cepacol Mouthwash/Gargle (14%), Listerine Antiseptic (75%), Scope (19%).
Antihistamines	Analgesics.	Allerest Headache Strength Tablets, Excedrin PM, Percogesic, Sinarest Tablets.
	Asthma products.	Bronitin, Primatene M.
	Cold/allergy products.	Many. Alka-Seltzer Plus, Allerest, Chlor-Trimeton, Contac, Coricidin, Co-Tylenol, Dristan, Novahistine, NyQuil, Sinarest, Sine-Off, Sinutab, Super Anahist, Triaminic, Triaminicin, 4-Way Cold Tablets.
	Dermatologic preparations.	Pyribenzamine Cream or Ointment.
	Menstrual products.	Cardui, Pamprin, Sunril.
	Motion sickness products, antiemetics.	Bonine, Dramamine, Marezine.
	Sleep aids.	Compoz Tablets, Nervine, Nyutol, Sleep-Eze, Sominex.
	Topical decongestants.	Dristan, Sinex.
Antimuscarinic agents	Antidiarrheals.	Donnagel, Donnagel-PG.
	Cold/allergy preparations.	Sinulin Tablets.
	Hemorrhoidal products.	Tanicaine Rectal Ointment or Suppositories, Wyanoids Hemorrhoidal Suppositories.
Aspirin and other salicylates	Analgesics.	Many. Alka-Seltzer, Anacin, Aspergum, Cope, Ecotrin, Excedrin, Fizrin Powder, Measurin, Persistin, Stanback Tablets and Powder, Vanquish.
	Antidiarrheals.	Pepto-Bismol (bismuth subsalicylate).
	Cold/allergy preparations.	Alka-Seltzer Plus, Congespirin, Coricidin, Dristan Tablets, Sine-Off, Triaminicin, 4-Way Cold Tablets.
	Menstrual products.	Diurex (potassium salicylate), Midol.
	Sleep aids.	Quiet World Tablets, Tranquil Capsules (sodium salicylate).
Caffeine	Analgesics.	Anacin, Bromo-Seltzer, Cope, Excedrin, Stanback Tablets and Powder, Vanquish.
	Cold/allergy products.	Coryban D, Dristan, Super Anahist, Triaminicin.
	Menstrual/diuretic products.	Aqua-Ban, Midol, Tri-Aqua.
	Stimulants.	Awake, NoDoz, Vivarin.
	Weight control products.	Anorexin Capsules, Spantrol Capsules.
Estrogens	Hair creams.	Le Kair.
Local anesthetics (usually benzocaine)	Antitussives.	Formula 44 Cough Disc, Silexin Cough Tablets, Vicks Cough Silencer Tablets.
	Dermatologic preparations.	Americaine First Aid Spray or Ointment, Dermoplast, Nupercainal Cream or Ointment, Medi-Quick, Solarcaine, Unguentine Spray, Unguentine Plus.
	Hermorrhoidal products.	Americaine, Anusol Ointment, Lanacane Medicated Creme, Nupercainal Cream or Ointment, Tronolane Anesthetic Hemorrhoidal Cream.
	Lozenges.	Cepacol Troches, Hold, Spec-T Sore Throat Products, Trokettes, Vicks Throat Lozenges.
	Toothache, cold sore, and teething products.	Baby OraJel, Benzodent, Numzident, Orabase with Benzocaine, OraJel teething lotion, toothache drops.
	Weight loss products.	Diet Trim Tablets, Slim Line Candy and Gum, Spantrol.
Sodium (mg/tablet or mg/5 mL or as stated)	Analgesics.	Alka-Seltzer Effervescent Pain Reliever and Antacid (521), Bromo-Seltzer (717), Fizrin Powder (673), sodium salicylate (50 mg/300 mg).
	Antacids.	Alka-Seltzer Effervescent Antacid (276), Amphojel Liquid (7), A.M.T. (7), BisoDol (157), Rolaids (53), Soda Mint (89).

Table 68–3 (cont'd). Hidden ingredients in over-the-counter (OTC) products.

Hidden Drug or Drug Class	OTC Class Containing Drug	Product Examples
Sodium (mg/tablet or mg/5 mL or as stated) (cont'd)	Cough syrups.	Coryban D (31), Cerose (38), Dristan (59), Pertussin 8-Hour Cough Formula (24), Formula 44 (68), Vicks Cough Syrup (54).
	Laxatives.	Instant Mix Metamucil (250 mg/packet), Fleets Enema (5000 mg, of which 250–300 mg is absorbed), Phospho-Soda (55), Sal Hepatica (1000).
Sympathomimetics	Analgesics.	Allerest Headache Strength Tablets, Sinarest Tablets, Sine-Aid Sinus Headache Tablets.
	Asthma products.	Bronkaid, Bronkotabs, Primatene, Tedral.
	Cold/allergy preparations.	Many. Alka-Seltzer Plus, Allerest, Chlor-Trimeton Decongestant, Contac, Coricidin 'D' Decongestant Tablets, Co-Tylenol, Dristan, Novafed, Novahistine Sinus Tablets, NyQuil, Sinarest, Sine-Aid, Sine-Off, Sinutab, Sudafed, Super Anahist, Triaminicin, 4-Way Cold Tablets.
	Cough syrups.	Cerose DM, Formula 44D, Robitussin-PE, Triaminic Expectorant, Triaminicol, and many others.
	Hemorrhoidal products.	A-Caine, Epinephricaine Rectal Ointment, HTO Stainless Manzan Hemorrhoidal Tissue Ointment, Pazo Hemorrhoid Ointment, Wyanoids Ointment.
	Lozenges.	Spec-T Sore Throat/Decongestant, Sucrets Cold Decongestant Formula.
	Menstrual products.	Femcaps, Fluidex-Plus with Diadax.
	Topical decongestants.	Many. Afrin, Benzedrex, Neo-Synephrine Hydrochloride, NTZ, Privine Sinex, Vicks Inhaler.
	Weight control products.	Appedrine Tablets, Dexatrim Capsules, Dietac Diet Aid Capsules or Tablets, Prolamine Capsules.

REFERENCES

Estrogens in cosmetics. *Med Lett Drugs Ther* (June 21) 1985; **27**:54.

The Medicine Show, 5th ed. Editors of Consumer Reports Books, 1980.

Penna RP et al (editors): *Handbook of Nonprescription Drugs,* 7th ed. American Pharmaceutical Association, 1982.

Physicians' Desk Reference for Nonprescription Drugs, 2nd ed. Medical Economics, 1986.

Widger HN: *Widger's Guide to Over-the-Counter Products.* JP Tarcher, 1979.

69 Prescription Writing

Paul W. Lofholm, PharmD

THE PRESCRIPTION

A prescription is a physician's order to prepare or dispense a specific treatment—usually medication—for an individual patient. The physician's decision to prescribe a drug assumes that the patient has been evaluated and a diagnosis arrived at and that it is rational to prescribe drugs. Much of this book is devoted to discussions of the pharmacologic principles of drug action used to select the drug of choice. This chapter deals with the techniques of prescription writing once the therapeutic agent is selected and the legal, economic, and social factors involved in that process.

While a prescription can be written on any piece of paper (as long as all of the legal elements are present), it usually takes a particular form. A typical printed prescription form for outpatients is shown in Fig 69–1.

In the hospital setting, drugs are prescribed on a particular page of the patient's hospital chart called the physician's order sheet. Such a prescription order is known as a **chart order,** and the contents of that prescription are specified by the medical staff rules. The patient's name is typed or written on the form; therefore, the orders consist of the name and strength of the medication, the dose, the route and frequency of administration, the date, other pertinent information, and the signature of the prescriber. Often the duration of therapy or the number of doses is not specified; therefore, medications are continued until the prescriber discontinues the order or until it is terminated as a matter of policy routine.

A typical chart order might be as follows:

6/14/84 (1) Ampicillin 500 mg IV q6h × 5 days
(2) ASA 0.6 g per rectum q4h prn temp over 101

(Signed) John B. Doe, M.D.

Thus, the elements of the hospital chart order are equivalent to the central elements (8–11) of the outpatient prescription.

Whether in the hospital or in an office practice setting, the implications of each element of the prescription should be understood.

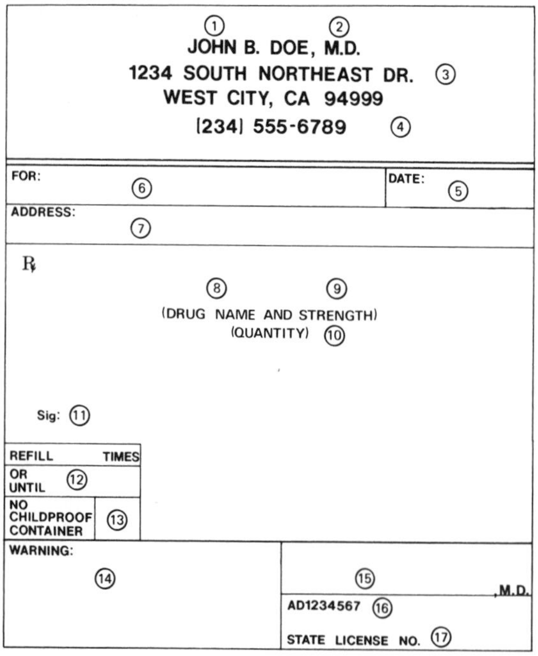
① ②
JOHN B. DOE, M.D.
1234 SOUTH NORTHEAST DR. ③
WEST CITY, CA 94999
(234) 555-6789 ④

FOR: ⑥ DATE: ⑤
ADDRESS: ⑦

℞
⑧ ⑨
(DRUG NAME AND STRENGTH)
(QUANTITY) ⑩

Sig: ⑪

REFILL TIMES
OR UNTIL ⑫
NO CHILDPROOF CONTAINER ⑬
WARNING: ⑭

⑮ M.D.
AD1234567 ⑯
STATE LICENSE NO. ⑰

Figure 69–1. Common form of outpatient prescription. Circled numbers are explained in the text.

Elements of the Prescription

The first 4 elements of the outpatient prescription establish the identity of the prescriber: name, license classification (ie, professional degree), address, and office telephone number. Before dispensing a prescription, the pharmacist must establish the prescriber's bona fides and should be able to contact the prescriber by telephone should any question arise. Element ⑤ is the date the prescription was written. It should be near the top of the prescription form or at the beginning (left margin) of the order. Since the order has legal significance and usually has some temporal relationship to the date of the patient-physician interview, a pharmacist should refuse to fill a prescription without verification by telephone if too much time has elapsed since its writing.

Elements ⑥ and ⑦ identify the patient by name and address. The patient's name and full address should be clearly spelled out.

The body of the prescription contains the elements ⑧ to ⑪ that specify the medication, the quantity to be dispensed, the dose, and complete directions for use. When writing the drug name (element ⑧), either the brand name (proprietary name) or generic name (non-proprietary name) may be used. Reasons for using one or the other are discussed below. The strength of the medication (element ⑨) should be written in metric units. However, the prescriber should be familiar with both systems now in use: apothecary and metric. For practical purposes, the following approximate conversions are useful:

1 grain (gr) = 0.065 grams (g), often rounded to 60 milligrams (mg)
15 gr = 1 g
1 ounce (oz) = 30 milliliters (mL)
1 teaspoonful (tsp) = 5 mL
1 tablespoonful (tbsp) = 15 mL
1 quart (qt) = 1000 mL
20 drops (gtt) = 1 mL
2.2 pounds (lb) = 1 kilogram (kg)
1 minim = 1 drop

The strength of a solution is usually expressed as the quantity of solute in sufficient solvent to make 100 mL; for instance, 20% potassium chloride solution is 20 grams per deciliter (g/dL).

The quantity of medication prescribed should reflect the anticipated length of therapy, the cost, the need for continued contact with the clinic or physician, the potential for abuse, and the potential for toxicity or overdose. Consideration should be given also to the standard sizes in which the product is available and whether this is the initial prescription of the drug or a repeat prescription or refill. If 10 days of therapy are required to effectively cure a streptococcal infection, an appropriate quantity for the full course should be prescribed. Birth control pills are often prescribed for 1 year or until the next examination is due; however, some patients may not be able to afford a year's supply at one time; therefore, a 3-month supply might be ordered, with refill instructions to renew 3 times or for 1 year (element ⑫). Finally, when first prescribing medications that are to be used for the treatment of a chronic disease, the initial quantity should be small, with refills for larger quantities. The purpose of beginning treatment with a small quantity of drug is to reduce the cost if the patient cannot tolerate the drug. Once it is determined that tolerance is not a problem, a larger quantity purchased less frequently is usually less expensive.

The directions for use (element ⑪) must be drug-specific and patient-specific. The simpler the directions, the better; and the fewer the number of doses (and drugs) per day, the better. Patient noncompliance (failure to adhere to the drug regimen) is a major cause of treatment failure. To help patients remember to take their medications, prescribers often give an instruction that medications be taken at or around mealtimes and at bedtime. However, it is important to inquire about the patient's eating habits and other life-style patterns, since many patients do not eat 3 regularly spaced meals a day, especially if they are sick or dieting.

The instructions on how and when to take medi-cations, the duration of therapy, and the purpose of the medication must be explained to each patient by the physician and by the pharmacist. Furthermore, the drug name, the purpose for which it is given, and the duration of therapy should be written on each label so that the drug may be identified easily in case of overdose. An instruction to "take as directed" may save the time it takes to write the orders out but often leads to noncompliance, patient confusion, and medication error. The directions for use must be clear and concise to avoid toxicity and to obtain the greatest benefits from therapy.

Patient education has been of concern to the FDA and professional groups and has resulted in several experimental programs. The United States Pharmacopeial Convention (USP) annually publishes a 2-volume work entitled *USP DI* ("dispensing information"). The first volume contains information for the professional (prescriber) and the second consists of short informational notes prepared for patients' use in understanding the drugs they are given. Over 300 medications are covered in the current (1986) edition. Information about *USP DI* may be obtained from the USP Drug Information Division, 12601 Twinbrook Parkway, Rockville, MD 20852.

A program sponsored by the American Medical Association has the potential for similar usefulness to patients. Patient medication instruction (PMI) sheets are being prepared that provide patient information about individual drugs or classes of drugs. The content of the PMI sheet is very similar to that of the *USP DI* note for the same drug. The PMI sheets will be distributed by prescribers at their discretion directly to patients.

Although directions for use are no longer written in Latin, many Latin apothecary abbreviations (and some others included below) are still in use. Knowledge of these abbreviations is essential for the dispensing pharmacist and often useful for the prescriber. Abbreviations still commonly used are listed in Table 69–1.

Elements ⑫ to ⑭ of the prescription include refill information, waiver of the requirement for childproof containers, and additional labeling instructions (eg, name of drug on label, "may cause drowsiness," "do not drink alcohol"). Most pharmacists now put the name of the medication on the label unless directed otherwise by the prescriber (some medications have the name of the drug stamped or imprinted on the tablet or capsule). Pharmacists should place the expiratory date for the drug on the label. If the patient or prescriber does not request waiver of childproof containers, the pharmacist or dispenser must place the medication in such a container. Pharmacists may not refill a prescription medication without authorization from the prescriber. Prescribers may grant authorization to renew prescriptions at the time of writing the prescription or over the telephone. Finally, the prescriber may request that special warning notices be placed on the label by the pharmacist.

Elements ⑮ to ⑰ are the prescriber's signature and other identification data.

Table 69–1. Common abbreviations.

Dose
dr, teaspoonful
g or **gm,** gram
gr, grain
gtt, drops
mcg, μ**g,** microgram
mg, milligram
Route
ad, right ear
as, left ear
au, each ear
od, right eye
os, left eye
ou, each eye
po, by mouth
supp, suppository
vag, vaginally
Frequency
ac, before meals
ad lib, freely at pleasure
bid, twice a day
h, hour
hs, at bedtime
pc, at meals
prn, as needed
q, every
qd, every day
qid, four times a day
qod, every other day
stat, at once, immediately
tid, three times a day
ut dict, as directed
Miscellaneous
a̅a̅, of each
cap, capsule
c̅, with
n.r., no refill
qs ad, add a sufficient amount to make
rep, repeat, refill
s̅, without
s̅s̅, one-half
sig, directions for use
tab, tablet

LEGAL FACTORS (USA)

The United States government recognizes 2 classes of drugs: (1) over-the-counter (OTC) drugs and (2) those that require a prescription from a licensed prescriber (legend drugs). OTC drugs are those that can be safely self-administered by the layman for self-limiting conditions and for which appropriate labels can be written for lay comprehension. Half of all drug doses consumed by the American public are OTC drugs.

Prescription drugs are controlled by the US Food and Drug Administration. They are identified by the federal legend statement: "Caution: Federal law prohibits dispensing without a prescription." This statement, as well as the package insert, is part of the packaging requirements for all prescription drugs. The package insert is the official brochure setting forth the indications, contraindications, warnings, and dosing for the drug.

The prescriber controls who may obtain prescription drugs by writing and signing a prescription order. The pharmacist may purchase these drugs, but they may only be dispensed on the order of a legally qualified prescriber. The patient may legally possess these drugs only when the drug vial or container has the pharmacist's label properly affixed to it. Thus, a "prescription" is actually 3 things: the physician's order, the written order to which the pharmacist refers when dispensing, and the patient's medication vial with a label affixed.

While the federal government controls the drugs and their labeling and distribution, the individual states control who may prescribe drugs through their licensing boards, ie, the Board of Medical Examiners. Physicians, dentists, veterinarians, and podiatrists acting within the scope of their practice are licensed to prescribe drugs. These prescribers must pass examinations, pay fees, and—in the case of some states and some professions—meet other requirements for relicensure such as continuing education. If these requirements are met, the prescriber is licensed to order dispensing of drugs.

The federal government and the states further impose special restrictions on drugs with a potential for abuse. Drugs with abuse potential include opiates, hallucinogens, stimulants, and depressants (Chapter 30). Special requirements must be met when these drugs are to be prescribed. The Controlled Drug Act requires prescribers and dispensers to register with the Drug Enforcement Agency (DEA), pay a fee, receive a personal registration number, and keep records of all controlled drugs prescribed or dispensed. The registration period is for 1 year. Every time a controlled drug is prescribed, a valid DEA number must appear on the prescription blank. Controlled drugs are classified according to their potential for abuse as shown in Table 69–2.

Prescriptions for substances with a high potential

Table 69–2. Classification of controlled substances. (See inside front cover for examples.)

	Potential for Abuse	Other
Class I	High	No accepted medical use; lack of accepted safety as drug.
Class II	High	Current accepted medical use. Abuse may lead to psychologic or physical dependence.
Class III	Less than I or II	Current accepted medical use. Moderate or low potential for physical dependence and high potential for psychologic dependence.
Class IV	Less than III	Current accepted medical use. Limited potential for dependence.
Class V	Less than IV	Current accepted medical use. Limited dependence possible.

for abuse (class II) cannot be refilled. Prescriptions for class III, IV, and V drugs can be refilled, but there is a 5-refill maximum, and in no case may the prescription be refilled after 6 months from the date of writing. Class II drug prescriptions may not be transmitted over the telephone, and some states require a special state-issued prescription blank. These restrictive prescribing laws are intended to limit the amount of drugs of abuse that are made available to the public.

Labeled & Unlabeled Uses of Drugs

In the USA, the FDA approves a drug only for the specific uses proposed and documented by the manufacturer when it approves a New Drug Application (NDA; see Chapter 4). These approved (labeled) uses or indications are set forth in the package insert that accompanies the drug. For a variety of reasons, these labeled indications may not include all the conditions in which the drug might be useful. Therefore, a clinician may wish to prescribe the agent for some other, unapproved (unlabeled) clinical condition, often on the basis of adequate or even compelling scientific evidence. Federal laws governing FDA regulations and drug use place no restrictions on such unapproved use.* Even if the patient suffers injury from the drug, its use for an unlabeled purpose does not in itself constitute "malpractice." However, the courts may consider the package insert labeling as a complete listing of the indications for which the drug is considered safe unless the clinician can show (from the literature, etc) that his or her use of the agent is considered reasonable by his peers.

SOCIOECONOMIC FACTORS

Generic Prescribing

Prescribing by generic name offers the pharmacist flexibility in selecting the particular drug product to fill the order and the patient a potential savings if there is price competition. The brand name of a popular diuretic is, eg, Esidrix by Ciba. The generic (public, nonproprietary) name of the same chemical substance adopted by United States Adopted Names (USAN) and approved by the Food and Drug Administration (FDA) is hydrochlorothiazide. All hydrochlorothiazide drug products in the USA meet the pharmaceutical standards expressed in *United States Pharmacopeia* (USP). However, there are many manufacturers, and prices vary as much as 2-fold. For other drugs, the difference in cost between the trade name

product and generic products varies from less than 2-fold to more than 10-fold.

In some states and in many hospitals, pharmacists have the option of supplying a generically equivalent drug product even if a proprietary name has been specified in the order. In office practice, drug product selection laws enable the pharmacist to make that selection, and in many hospitals the pharmacy and therapeutics committee through its drug formulary policies establish the dispensing practices of the pharmacist. If the physician wants a particular brand of drug product dispensed, handwritten instruction to "dispense as written" or words of similar meaning are required. Unfortunately, it is not certain that generic prescribing or substitution results in lower total prescription costs (see Krawelski reference, below). Some government-subsidized health care programs require that pharmacists dispense the cheapest generically equivalent product in the inventory. However, the principles of drug product selection by pharmacists do not permit substituting one therapeutic agent for another; ie, dispensing trichlormethiazide for hydrochlorothiazide would not be permitted without the prescriber's permission even though the 2 drugs may be considered pharmacodynamically equivalent.

It should not be assumed that all generic drug products are as satisfactory as trade name products, though most generics are satisfactory. Bioavailability—the effective absorption of the drug product—varies between manufacturers and sometimes between different lots of a drug produced by the same manufacturer. In the case of drugs with a low therapeutic index, poor solubility, or a high ratio of inert ingredients to active drug content, a specific manufacturer's product might well give more consistent results. In the case of life-threatening diseases, the advantages of generic substitution are probably outweighed by the clinical urgency so that the prescription should be filled as written.

Other Cost Factors

The private pharmacist bases his or her charges on the cost of the drug plus a fee for providing a professional service. Each time a prescription is dispensed, there is a fee. The prescriber controls the frequency of filling prescriptions by authorizing refills and specifying the quantity to be dispensed. Thus, the prescriber can save the patient money by prescribing standard sizes (so that drugs do not have to be repackaged) and, when chronic treatment is involved, by ordering the largest quantity consistent with safety and expense. Thus, optimal prescribing often involves consultation between the prescriber and the pharmacist.

---

*"Once a product has been approved for marketing, a physician may prescribe it for uses or in treatment regimens or patient populations that are not included in the approved labeling. Such 'unapproved' or, more precisely, 'unlabeled' uses may be appropriate and rational in certain circumstances, and may, in fact, reflect approaches to drug therapy that have been extensively reported in medical literature." (*FDA Drug Bull* 1982;**12**:4.)

REFERENCES

Business and Professions Code, Chap 9, Div 2, Pharmacy Law. Department of Consumer Affairs, Sacramento, Calif, 1985.

Final Report: Task Force on Prescription Drugs. Department of Health, Education, and Welfare, 1969.

Hoover JE: *Dispensing of Medication*, 8th ed. Mack Publishing Co., 1976.

Hoover JE: *Remington's Pharmaceutical Sciences*, 16th ed. Mack Publishing Co., 1980.

Jerome JB, Sagan P: The USAN nomenclature system. *JAMA* 1975;**232**:294.

Kickoff for AMA's new PMI program. (Medical News.) *JAMA* 1982;**248**:1031.

Krawelski JE, Pitt L, Dowd B: The effects of competition on prescription-drug-product substitution. *N Engl J Med* 1983; **309**:213.

United States Pharmacopeial Convention: *1986 USP DI*. Vol 1: *Advice for the Health Care Provider;* Vol 2: *Advice for the Patient*, 6th ed. United States Pharmacopeial Convention, Inc., 1986.

Use of approved drugs for unlabeled indications. *FDA Drug Bull* 1982;**12**:4.

Some Aspects of Veterinary Pharmacology

70

J. Desmond Baggot, MVM, MRCVS, PhD, DSc

The range of species in which drugs are used and studied is what distinguishes veterinary from human pharmacology. While the mechanism of action of a drug is often the same in humans and other mammalian species, the intensity and duration of the effects produced can vary widely. This implies that species variations in the response produced by a fixed dose of drug can be attributed to differences either in pharmacokinetic processes (absorption, distribution, and elimination) or in the pharmacodynamic sensitivity of tissue receptor sites. Since it has been found that dosage appropriate for the species can offset differences in the intensity of the response produced by a number of drugs, it is generally assumed that the range of therapeutic plasma concentrations in animals is the same as in humans. For example, the plasma concentration of pentobarbital at which dogs and goats awaken from anesthesia induced by an intravenous dose (25 mg/kg) of the drug is the same, but the duration of anesthesia and rate of decline in plasma concentrations vary between the species (Fig 70–1). Studies on thiopental, digoxin, theophylline, and aspirin

(analgesic effect) provide further support for this assumption. Premedication with acetylpromazine appears to lengthen the duration of thiopental anesthesia in dogs, but it does not change the plasma thiopental concentration at which the dogs awaken from anesthesia (20 μg/mL) or alter the rate of elimination (half-life and body clearance) of the drug.

In other orders of animals (eg, birds, amphibians, fish), these differences may be even more extreme. For example, the average half-life of amikacin in gopher snakes is about 72 hours compared with 1.0, 1.7, and 2.3 hours in dogs, horses, and humans, respectively. However, there are few pharmacokinetic data available for nonmammalian species, and this chapter will emphasize the usual sport and companion species (dog, cat, horse) and farm animals (cow, goat, sheep, pig).

Species Variations in Drug Response

Variation among species in response to a drug can generally be minimized by using a dosage level of the drug appropriate for the species of animal (Table

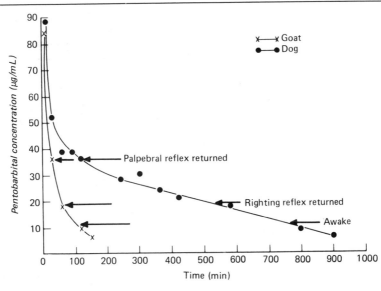

Figure 70–1. Pentobarbital concentrations in plasma of dogs and goats following intravenous administration of an anesthetic dose (25 mg/kg). Arrows indicate the plasma drug concentrations and related times at which reflexes returned. (Modified and reproduced, with permission, from Baggot JD: *Principles of Drug Disposition in Domestic Animals.* Saunders, 1977.)

70–1). In the case of aspirin, the dosage *level* that will produce an analgesic effect is the same (10 mg/kg) for dogs and cats, but the dosage *interval* is much longer for cats. This dosage regimen aims at maintaining plasma salicylate concentrations within the range of 25–100 μg/mL. A similar situation applies to oral maintenance dosage with chloramphenicol in that the drug can be administered at the same dosage level (25 mg/kg) to dogs and cats, but a longer interval between successive doses is required in cats. The slower elimination of these and other drugs for which glucuronide conjugation is a major metabolic pathway can be attributed to the relative deficiency in glucuronyl transferase activity in the cat. Acetaminophen toxicity is often encountered in cats, because glucuronide conjugation occurs slowly and N-hydroxylation leads to a toxic metabolite (Chapter 3). Intoxication can be treated, as in humans, with acetylcysteine. Traditionally, morphine is known to cause "maniacal" excitement in cats. However, when administered in a dosage appropriate for the relief of intense visceral pain, morphine produces similar sedative and analgesic effects in dogs and cats. Whether the 10-fold difference in dosage level reflects a species difference in accessibility of morphine to its site of central nervous system action or a difference in sensitivity of opiate receptors between dogs and cats is not known. Premedication with a phenothiazine tranquilizer can prevent the excitement induced by morphine in cats, an effect that might be attributed to blockade of central dopamine receptors. Meperidine (5 mg/kg intramuscularly) does not cause a dose-related species variation in response. Xylazine, a nonnarcotic sedative analgesic, has been found clinically to be the most useful drug for alleviating moderate pain in ruminant animals (ie, cattle, sheep, and goats). Based on a comparison of dosage levels required to produce equivalent analgesic effects, the ruminant species appear to be 10 times more sensitive to the drug than are the nonruminant species (ie, horses, dogs, and cats). At relatively low doses (0.66 mg/kg intramuscularly or subcutaneously) for the species, xylazine is a reliable central emetic in cats. A single parenteral dose (0.1 mg/kg) of apomorphine, which causes marked excitement in cats, is the most effective emetic agent in dogs. The varying susceptibility of different species to neuromuscular blockade with succinylcholine can be attributed to variations in activity of plasma pseudocholinesterase, the enzyme that hydrolyzes and thereby inactivates the drug.

ABSORPTION, DISTRIBUTION, & ELIMINATION

Comparative Aspects of Gastrointestinal Absorption

Dietary habit serves as a useful basis for grouping the species of domestic animals when comparing the systemic availability of a drug preparation given orally. The carnivorous species (dogs and cats), like the omnivorous pig, are monogastric animals. The absorption process in these species is thought to resemble that in humans, in that drugs are absorbed by passive nonionic diffusion, mainly in the upper small intestine. Presystemic elimination (first-pass effect; Fig 3–2) will decrease the systemic availability of a drug following oral administration (Table 70–2). This can be attributed to metabolism or degradation in the gut lumen, metabolism in the gut epithelium occurring during absorption, or metabolism in the liver preceding entry of drug into the systemic circulation. This can contribute to variations between dogs and cats in the fraction of an oral dose that is available systemically. The variation between these species is small,

Table 70–1. Some examples of species variations in drug dosage.

Drug and Route	Species	Dose
Aspirin (oral)	Dog	10 mg/kg at 8-hour intervals
	Cat	10 mg/kg at 24-hour intervals
Chloramphenicol palmitate (oral)	Dog	25 mg/kg at 8-hour intervals
	Cat	25 mg/kg at 12-hour intervals
Morphine sulfate (IM, single dose)	Dog	1 mg/kg
	Cat	0.1 mg/kg
Xylazine hydrochloride (IM, single dose)	Dog	2 mg/kg
	Cat	2 mg/kg
	Horse	2 mg/kg
	Ruminant	0.2 mg/kg
Succinylcholine chloride (IV, single dose)	Dog	0.3 mg/kg
	Cat	1 mg/kg
	Horse	0.1 mg/kg
	Ruminant	0.02 mg/kg

Table 70–2. Some drugs that undergo presystemic elimination in the dog when given by the oral route.

Drug	Dose	Systemic Availability (percent)	Site of Metabolism
Lidocaine	10 mg/kg	15	Liver
Salicylamide	30 mg/kg	22	Gut wall and liver
Aspirin	250 mg (total)	45	Gut wall and liver
Levodopa	25 mg/kg	44	Gut lumen or gut wall (or both)
Sulfadimethoxine	55 mg/kg	50	Liver
Flunitrazepam	2 mg/kg	0	Gut wall and liver
Propranolol	80 mg (total)	2–17	Liver

however, compared with the difference between carnivorous species and the herbivorous animals.

The herbivorous species are composed of the horse and the ruminant species (cattle, sheep, and goats). The horse, unlike the ruminant species, is a monogastric animal. Horses are selective grazing animals that feed continuously, and their nutritional status depends on microbial digestion of polysaccharides, a process that takes place in the colon. (Guinea pigs similarly depend on microbial digestion in the cecum.) Disturbance of the colonic microflora, resulting from either a disease condition or the action of an antimicrobial agent, can seriously threaten the life of the horse. In a study of the bioavailability of various oral preparations of phenylbutazone, it was shown that feeding had a considerable influence on both the shape of the plasma concentration–time curve and the area under the curve. Administration of phenylbutazone, either as a paste formulation before feeding or as the powder in a small bran mash, provided a peak plasma concentration of the drug at 2–3 hours after dosing and almost complete absorption. However, when the drug was administered after feeding, absorption was greatly delayed and variable in extent. The toxic potential associated with phenylbutazone therapy may not be as high in the horse as in humans, since chronic therapy (exceeding 5 days) is not recommended for horses, and metabolism of both the parent drug and oxyphenbutazone takes place quite rapidly. At therapeutic dosage (4.4 mg/kg), the half-life of phenylbutazone in the horse is 6 hours, compared with up to 72 hours in humans. Thus, bioavailability studies carried out in humans or dogs cannot be used to predict the rate and extent of absorption of drugs from the gastrointestinal tract of the horse.

A unique feature of digestive physiology in the ruminant animal is that fermentation takes place continuously in the reticulorumen. The contents of the voluminous forestomach vary from fluid to semisolid in consistency, and the pH is normally maintained within the range 5.5–6.5. Although the organ is lined with stratified squamous epithelium, the nonionized form of weak organic acids and bases passively diffuses through the mucosa. When a drug is given orally to a ruminant animal, it enters a large volume of ruminal contents that have an acidic reaction produced by microbial fermentation processes. The ruminal microflora can inactivate drugs by hydrolytic or reductive reactions. Chronic oral dosage with a "broad-spectrum" antimicrobial agent (such as a tetracycline or sulfonamide) can suppress activity of ruminal microflora, thereby interfering with carbohydrate digestion, which is an essential function of the forestomach. The dosage regimen for aspirin in cows (100 mg/kg, administered at 12-hour intervals) can be expected to maintain plasma salicylate concentrations in the range of 40–60 μg/mL. Slow absorption from the rumen rather than the half-life of salicylate, which is less than an hour, is the basis for the 12-hour dosage interval.

Thus, the considerable differences in anatomic arrangement and digestive physiology between carnivorous and herbivorous species and, among the latter, between the horse and ruminant animals make it unrealistic to extrapolate information on absorption of orally administered drugs from one type of species to another.

Absorption Through the Skin

Many drugs are used for their effects on the skin and are applied topically (Chapter 65). If they do not penetrate the stratum corneum, they are ineffective (unless given for control of external parasites). On the other hand, if they are absorbed too rapidly into the circulation, they may produce systemic toxicity. Because of the very different anatomy of the skin in different species, the rate of absorption of drugs may vary over a 30-fold range (Table 70–3).

Drug Distribution

The drug distribution pattern, by which is meant the amount of drug that enters each organ and tissue, is determined by physiologic factors and certain physicochemical properties of the drug. These factors include blood flow to tissues, the mass of various organs and tissues, the ability of the drug to pass through cellular membranes, and drug binding to plasma proteins and extravascular tissue components. In general, patterns of blood flow—on a flow per unit of organ weight basis—are similar for most of the mammals. However, the relative size of some organs varies markedly, especially between ruminant and nonruminant species. Differences in body composition may largely acount for species variations in the distribution pattern of drugs. For example, the gastrointestinal tract and its contents constitute 4.6% of body weight in dogs and 20.3% in goats. Skeletal muscle mass varies much less: 54% in dogs and 46% in goats. Since drug passage across membranes takes place primarily by passive diffusion, lipid solubility and degree of ionization are the major physicochemical properties that determine distribution of weak organic electrolytes (Chapter 1). Definitive information on the distribution of a drug can be obtained only by measuring levels of

Table 70–3. Rate of absorption of an organophosphate cholinesterase inhibitor through the excised skin of the dorsal thorax.[*]

Species	Rate (μg/cm^2/min)
Pig	0.3
Dog	2.7
Monkey	4.2
Goat	4.4
Cat	4.4
Guinea pig	6
Rabbit	9.3
Rat	9.3

[*]Modified and reproduced, with permission, from Baggot JD: *Principles of Drug Disposition in Domestic Animals.* Saunders, 1977.

the drug in the various organs and tissues of the body (such as kidney, liver, heart, skeletal muscle, and fat).

In animals produced for meat, drugs that are used to prevent parasitism or to accelerate growth must be withdrawn from the diet before slaughter to minimize the drug residues in the meat that is sold. Definitive information of the type described above must be obtained in such tissues to confirm predictions of appropriate withdrawal times for each drug. Therefore, the drug residue profile should be determined in the edible tissues of the food-producing animals, especially cattle, sheep, pigs, and—of recent concern—fish.

Plasma Protein Binding

Although species variations in extent of binding occur, these variations are small and generally not of clinical significance. It is only for drugs that have extensive (> 80%) protein binding that species variations may assume importance, since extensive binding restricts distribution and may affect (either hinder or facilitate) elimination depending on the mechanism of elimination.

The extent of binding depends upon both the affinity of the protein (usually albumin) for the drug and the protein concentration in plasma. A decrease in either apparent affinity (which can occur in uremia or result from competition between extensively bound acidic drugs for albumin binding sites) or in plasma albumin concentration (chronic liver disease) can cause an increase in the percentage of free (unbound) drug in the plasma (Chapter 3). Consequently, more drug is available for extravascular distribution, which may give increased concentrations at the site of action, and for elimination by passive transfer (diffusion, glomerular filtration). The significance of decreased protein binding can be seen in perspective by considering the fraction of drug in the body that is in the plasma. Decreased binding is likely to assume clinical significance (by increasing pharmacologic response) only with drugs that bind extensively (> 80%) and have relatively small volumes of distribution (such as phenytoin, warfarin). The anticoagulant effect of warfarin may be enhanced when the drug is used concurrently with phenylbutazone, as in the treatment of navicular disease in horses.

Passage of Antimicrobial Agents Into Milk

It has been shown that only the lipid-soluble nonionized fraction of an organic electrolyte that is free (unbound) in the plasma diffuses into milk. In normal lactating cows, weak acids produce ratios of milk ultrafiltrate concentration to plasma ultrafiltrate concentration that are less than or equal to unity; organic bases, excluding aminoglycoside antibiotics (which are polar), attain concentration ratios greater than 1 (Table 70–4). There is close agreement between equilibrium concentration ratios obtained experimentally and those calculated theoretically by either of the following forms of the Henderson-Hasselbalch equation:

For an acid,

Table 70–4. Passage of antimicrobial agents from the systemic circulation into milk.*

Drug	pK_a	Milk pH	Concentration Ratio (Milk Ultrafiltrate:Plasma Ultrafiltrate)*	
			Theoretical	Experimental
Organic acids				
Ampicillin	2.7, 7.2	6.8	0.26	0.24–0.30
Benzylpenicillin (G)	2.7	6.8	0.25	0.13–0.26
Cephaloridine	3.4	6.8	0.25	0.24–0.28
Cloxacillin	2.7	6.8	0.25	0.25–0.30
Sulfadimethoxine	6.1	6.6	0.20	0.23
Sulfamethazine	7.4	6.6	0.58	0.59
Organic bases				
Erythromycin	8.8	6.8	3.9	8.7
Kanamycin	(7.8)	6.8	3.1	0.60–0.80
Lincomycin	7.6	6.8	2.83	2.50–3.60
Trimethoprim	7.6	6.5–6.8	2.8–5.3	2.90–4.90
Tylosin	7.1	6.8	2.0	3.5
Amphoteric				
Oxytetracycline		6.5–6.8		0.75

*It is important to know the dosing regimen, since an equilibrium state will not be established by a single administration of the drug.

$$R_{milk/plasma} = \frac{1 + 10^{(pH_m - pK_a)}}{1 + 10^{(pH_p - pK_a)}} \quad \ldots (1)$$

or, for a base,

$$R_{milk/plasma} = \frac{1 + 10^{(pK_a - pH_m)}}{1 + 10^{(pK_a - pH_p)}} \quad \ldots (2)$$

where pH_m and pH_p are the pH reactions of milk and plasma, respectively, and pK_a is the negative logarithm of the acidic ionization (or dissociation) constant of the drug. It can be concluded that the mammary gland epithelium behaves as a lipid barrier separating blood of pH 7.4 from milk, which has a lower pH value (normal pH range of cow's milk is 6.5–6.8). The general validity of these equations enables one to make predictions on milk withholding periods based on the bioavailability and disposition kinetics of the drug in the target species of animal. The milk:plasma concentration ratio of an antimicrobial agent reflects its capacity to penetrate cellular barriers in general and may be useful in predicting accessibility to infection sites. (However, because of the difference in pH between milk and plasma, "trapping" of ionized bases in milk exaggerates the penetrative capacity of bases; the reverse effect results in underestimates of penetration of the lipid barrier by acidic drugs.) Lipophilic antimicrobial agents attain high milk:plasma concentration ratios and are far more likely to reach relatively inaccessible infection foci than antibiotics that are polar.

Equation (1) or (2) can be used to predict passage of an organic acid or base, respectively, from the systemic circulation into other fluids (eg, aqueous humor, saliva, synovial fluid, cerebrospinal fluid), taking into account the pH reaction of the fluid and the pK_a value for the drug (Tables 70–4 and 1–1). There are significant species differences in the pH of certain fluids. For example, the usual pH of human saliva is acidic (pH 6.4); the pH of horse saliva is 7.4; and the saliva of cattle is alkaline (pH 8.4).

Elimination Processes

A. Metabolism: As in humans, the majority of drugs administered to animals are eliminated by a combination of hepatic metabolism and renal excretion processes. The liver is the principal organ for metabolism of drugs; the hepatic microsomal enzyme systems mediate a variety of oxidative reactions and glucuronide conjugation. Other tissues, including plasma, kidney, lung, and intestinal mucosa, as well as gut microflora, can contribute to the metabolism of a drug. The major metabolic pathways can be predicted for many compounds based on the functional groups present in the molecule. While oxidative, reductive, and hydrolytic reactions are present in all species, certain synthetic reactions are either defective or absent in some species (Table 70–5). The cat synthesizes glucuronide conjugates slowly, because it is deficient in glucuronyl transferase. Like the cat, the human infant and neonatal animals of different species synthesize glucuronide conjugates of drugs such as salicylates and acetaminophen at a slow rate. Sulfate conjugation appears to be deficient in the pig and has been attributed to limited availability of sulfate for conjugation. The deficiency in this synthetic pathway does not appear to delay elimination of drugs in the pig, probably because glucuronide conjugates, an alternative pathway, are rapidly synthesized. Studies showing the complete absence of the N^4-acetylated derivative of sulfonamide compounds in the urine of dogs have led researchers to conclude that dogs are unable to acetylate aromatic amino groups. However, the inability to acetylate this type of amino group does not hinder elimination of these drugs in dogs.

The importance of alternative metabolic pathways is well demonstrated by the metabolism of lidocaine (Table 70–6). Although the amount of metabolism by any single pathway varied among species by up to 100-fold, the total urinary excretion (53.8–85%) varied by less than 2-fold.

Table 70–5. Species with a defective metabolic pathway.

Species	Metabolic Reaction	Functional Group(s)	Type of Defect
Cat	Glucuronide synthesis	–OH, –COOH –NH₂, =NH, –SH	Slow rate
Dog	Acetylation	Aromatic –NH₂	Absent
Pig	Sulfate conjugation	Aromatic –OH, aromatic –NH₂	Low extent

Table 70–6. Species variations in the metabolism of lidocaine.*

Compound	Percentage of Dose Recovered in Urine			
	Rat	Guinea Pig	Dog	Human
Lidocaine	0.2	0.5	2	2.8
Monoethylglycinexylidide	0.7	14.9	2.3	3.7
Glycinexylidide	2.1	3.3	12.6	2.3
3-Hydroxylidocaine	31.2	0.5	6.7	1.1
3-Hydroxymonoethylglycine-xylidide	36.9	2	3.1	0.3
2,6-Xylidine	1.5	16.2	1.6	1
4-Hydroxy-2,6-dimethylaniline	12.4	16.4	35.2	72.6
Total	85.0	53.8	63.5	83.8

*Reproduced, with permission, from Baggot JD: *Principles of Drug Disposition in Domestic Animals.* Saunders, 1977.

B. Renal Excretion: The fraction of the systemically available dose that is excreted unchanged in the urine is a quantitative measure of the contribution of renal excretion to overall drug elimination. From the fraction excreted unchanged one can estimate the effect of an alteration of urinary pH on the rate of drug elimination. It is only when a substantial fraction of the dose is excreted unchanged that a change in urinary pH will significantly alter the rate of elimination (usually expressed as half-life) of a drug. Comparison of the 24-hour cumulative urinary excretion of a number of lipid-soluble drug substances in different species has indicated that the herbivorous species excrete a smaller fraction of the dose unchanged in the urine than the carnivorous species. Trimethoprim is a good example: Less than 5% of a dose is excreted unchanged in ruminant species (cows, goats), while in the dog 20% is excreted unchanged, and in humans 47% is unchanged. This suggests that herbivorous species (or their gastrointestinal microflora) metabolize trimethoprim more extensively than other species. In the case of lipid-soluble drugs, the rate of metabolism to less lipid-soluble metabolites usually determines the duration of pharmacologic effect. As a result, species differences in the rate of metabolism of these drugs most often underlie variations in the duration of pharmacologic effect following the administration of a fixed dose. In general, humans metabolize drugs less efficiently than do the domestic animals, herbivorous species in particular.

Renal excretion is the principal process of elimination for drugs that are predominantly ionized at physiologic pH and for compounds (such as drug metabolites) with limited lipid solubility. The renal handling of drugs and metabolites is complex and, depending on the physicochemical properties of the compound, the following mechanisms may be involved: (1) glomerular filtration of molecules that are free (unbound) in the plasma; (2) carrier-mediated excretion of certain polar organic compounds by the proximal tubular cells; and (3) pH-dependent passive reabsorption of the nonionized lipid-soluble moiety of weak organic electrolytes (acids or bases).

Extensive binding to plasma proteins limits the availability of a drug for glomerular filtration but does not hinder proximal tubular excretion. This is reflected in the similar rates of elimination of cloxacillin and ampicillin in a single species of animal. These 2 semisynthetic penicillins, which are excreted by the same renal mechanisms, have the same half-life (1.2 hours in cows, 1.3 hours in humans), although cloxacillin is 80% and ampicillin only 20% bound to plasma albumin.

There appears to be a species difference, though unlikely to be of clinical importance, in the rate of elimination of some drugs that are removed from the body by renal excretion. The carnivorous species eliminate most drugs that are excreted unchanged by glomerular filtration somewhat more rapidly than the herbivorous species. This may be attributed to the higher rate of glomerular filtration. Creatinine clearance, for example, is 1.46 mL/min/kg in horses and 1.68 in cows, but 4.3 in dogs and even higher in cats.

The usual urinary reaction of carnivorous animals is acidic (pH 5.5–7), while that of herbivorous species is alkaline (pH 7–8). In any species, however, urinary pH is dependent mainly on dietary habit. In the human, the urinary reaction is generally acidic, but it can vary over a wide range of pH (5–7.5). Suckling and milkfed animals generally excrete an acid urine even if when mature they characteristically excrete alkaline urine. Since the pH of plasma is maintained within a narrow range (7.3–7.5), a large pH gradient may exist between plasma and urine. This influences the extent of reabsorption of weak organic electrolytes with pK_a values in the range of urinary pH (5–8) and thereby the rate of their elimination.

C. Biliary Excretion: Certain drugs (eg, nafcillin, tetracyclines), iopanoic acid, and glucuronide conjugates of a variety of compounds, which include lipophilic drugs (chloramphenicol, morphine) and endogenous steroidal substances, are excreted by the liver into bile. Most of the compounds excreted in bile are polar, and most have molecular weights about 300. Species variations in the extent of biliary excretion are likely to occur only with compounds of molecular weight between 300 and 500. The species may be grouped together as "good" (rats, dogs, chickens), "moderate" (cats, sheep), and "poor" (guinea pigs, rabbits, rhesus monkeys, and probably humans) biliary excretors. Compounds excreted in the bile enter the small intestine and, depending on their lipid solubility, some (such as the tetracyclines) may be reabsorbed. Glucuronide conjugates may be hydrolyzed by β-glucuronidase, which is present in the intestinal microorganisms, and the liberated compound can then be reabsorbed. This cycle, consisting of biliary excretion followed by reabsorption from the intestine, is known as the "enterohepatic circulation" of a drug. When a significant fraction of the dose undergoes enterohepatic circulation, elimination of the compound is delayed. Biliary excretion is an important mechanism of elimination for organic anions and cations that are too polar to be reabsorbed from the intestine.

SOME APPLICATIONS OF PHARMACOKINETICS IN VETERINARY MEDICINE

An optimal dosage regimen can be defined as one that will maintain plasma concentrations of the drug within the therapeutic range for the duration of therapy. The use of pharmacokinetics in the design and evaluation of drug dosage forms provides an approach to the rational choice and optimal dosage of a drug. Kinetic parameters derived from single-dose studies can be used to predict the steady-state plasma concentrations that multiple dosing schedules will produce. The utility of pharmacokinetics in clinical pharmacology rests largely on the premise that the therapeutic range of plasma concentrations can be defined for a drug.

Comparative pharmacokinetic studies provide a technique for elucidating differences in absorption and disposition processes that may underlie the species variations in response to fixed dosage of a drug. These studies provide a basis for the selection of a test species from which pharmacokinetic information can be extrapolated for application in humans.

The prediction of preslaughter withdrawal times for drug preparations developed for use in the food-producing animals represents an application of pharmacokinetics in the field of **drug residues.** This application depends on selection of the appropriate compartmental model and validity of the assumption that the decline in plasma concentrations parallels the rate of removal of the drug from edible tissues (skeletal muscle, heart, liver, kidney). An important requirement of the experimental design in drug residue studies is that the pharmacokinetic behavior of the drug be determined at both ends of the range of recommended dosage levels. A disproportionate increase in tissue residue levels of drug with increase in dose is evidence that the drug shows nonlinear pharmacokinetic behavior. It is important to stress that insight into the drug residue "profile" can only be obtained by linking fixed-dose pharmacokinetic studies of blood levels with measurement of the amount of drug in selected tissues of the target species of animal. This approach has an economic aspect in that it leads to a considerable reduction in the total number of animals required for study.

The Disposition Curve

Disposition is the term used to describe the simultaneous effects of distribution and elimination—ie, the processes that occur subsequent to the absorption of a drug. The disposition curve, usually plotted on semilogarithmic paper, describes graphically the plasma concentration profile of a drug following the intravenous injection of a single dose (Fig 70–2). For most drugs, in veterinary as in human pharmacokinet-

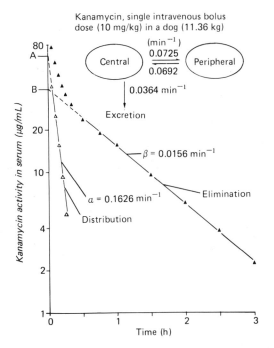

Kanamycin, single intravenous bolus
dose (10 mg/kg) in a dog (11.36 kg)

Figure 70–2. Analysis of the disposition kinetics of kanamycin in a dog given a single intravenous dose (10 mg/kg) of kanamycin sulfate. The elimination phase is represented by a least squares linear regression line, based on measured activity of kanamycin in serum samples (▲) between 0.5 and 3 hours after drug administration. The regression line that represents distribution phase is based on calculated data points (△). Note the much smaller value of β compared to α. Inset is a schematic representation of the 2-compartment open model; values of the individual rate constants (microconstants) associated with the model are given. (Modified and reproduced, with permission, from Baggot JD: *Principles of Drug Disposition in Domestic Animals.* Saunders, 1977.)

ics, the curve can be fitted to a sum of exponential terms:

$$C_p = \sum_{i=1}^{n} A_i e^{-k_i t} \qquad \ldots (3)$$

where C_p is the plasma drug concentration at time t after the administration of a single intravenous dose and A_i and k_i represent a series of "hybrid" coefficients and exponents, respectively, that can be related to intrinsic rate constants of corresponding compartmental pharmacokinetic models. For most drugs, 2 or 3 exponential terms are sufficient to describe the equation that will fit the experimental data points. This implies that the pharmacokinetic behavior of such drugs can be interpreted in terms of a 2- or 3-compartment open model (Fig 70–2).

The completeness of the disposition curve depends not only on the frequency and duration of blood sampling but also on the sensitivity of the analytic procedure used to measure concentrations of the drug in plasma. Incomplete determination of the curve can lead to error in values of the experimental constants which, in turn, will affect accuracy of all pharmacokinetic terms and the predictions based on these terms. The most common error is overestimation of the terminal exponent (β), due either to sampling for too short a period of time or using an analytic procedure that is not sensitive enough to measure concentrations of the drug in plasma during the "true" elimination phase of disposition. A significant consequence of this error is that the steady-state plasma concentration produced by multiple-dose therapy will differ from that predicted. Likewise, predicted tissue drug residues and pre-slaughter withdrawal times will be in error. Species comparisons in the rate of drug elimination, based on half-life, may be invalid. It follows that complete determination of the disposition curve is of paramount importance both in predicting optimal dosage and as a basis for comparing the disposition kinetics of a drug in different species.

Pharmacokinetic Parameters

The elimination phase of drug disposition may be characterized by 2 parameters, namely, half-life ($t_{1/2}$) and apparent volume of distribution (V_d). The half-life of a drug expresses the time required for the plasma concentration—as well as the amount of drug in the body—to decrease by one-half through the process of elimination. It is dependent upon the clearance and volume of distribution:

$$t_{1/2} = \frac{0.693 \times V_d}{Cl} \qquad \ldots (4)$$

The half-life values of most therapeutic agents are independent of the dose administered, since their overall elimination obeys first-order kinetics. First-order (exponential) elimination implies that a constant fraction of the amount of drug in the body is eliminated in each equal interval of time.

There is considerable variation among the species of domestic animals in the half-lives of drugs that are eliminated by hepatic metabolism (Table 70–7). As noted above, herbivorous species appear to metabolize most lipid-soluble drugs far more rapidly than carnivorous species. However, there are many exceptions to this trend, and the half-life of a drug that undergoes extensive metabolism should not be extrapolated from one species to another. Based on the relative rates of glomerular filtration, it can be predicted that the half-lives of drugs that are eliminated entirely by this renal excretion mechanism (such as the aminoglycoside antibiotics) will be somewhat shorter in dogs and cats than in horses and the ruminant species. This difference in half-life is unrelated to diet and urinary pH reaction.

Selection of a dosing interval should always take into account the half-life and the range of therapeutic plasma concentrations, if these are known for the species in question. Extrapolation from one species to another may result in completely ineffective therapy. For example, the range of therapeutic plasma concentra-

Table 70–7. Species variations in elimination half-lives (hours) of drugs that undergo hepatic metabolism.

Drug	Ruminant Species	Horse	Dog	Cat	Human
Pentobarbital	0.8	1.5	4.5	4.9	22.3
Thiopental	3.3		8.5		11.5
Ketamine	1	0.7	1	1.1	2.5
Amphetamine	0.6	1.4	4.5*	6.5*	10–15*
Salicylate	0.8	1	8.6	35	4–8[†]
Phenylbutazone	43	3–6[†]	2.5–6[†]		72[†]
Trimethoprim	0.8	3.2	3		10.6
Sulfadimethoxine	9	11	13.2	10.2	40
Chloramphenicol	4.2	0.9	4.2	5.1	2.7
Theophylline		15.2	5.7	7.8	9
Antipyrine	3.1	2.8	3.2		12.7

*Half-life can be markedly influenced by urinary pH.
[†]Half-life is dose-dependent.

tions for an anticonvulsant drug may be the same in humans and dogs, but the half-life of most anticonvulsants is considerably shorter in dogs (Table 70–8). Short half-life makes dosing of many potentially effective anticonvulsant drugs impractical for therapeutic use in dogs.

The apparent volume of distribution provides an estimate of the *extent* of distribution but does not reveal the distribution *pattern* of a drug. As noted in Chapter 1, distribution volumes are not directly related to physiologic compartments, and it is incorrect to make inferences about the distribution pattern of a drug based on its volume of distribution. The most notable species differences in volume of distribution have been found between monogastric (dogs and cats) and ruminant (cattle, sheep, goats) animals, particularly for lipid-soluble organic bases. Following parenteral administration to ruminants, these drugs passively diffuse from the systemic circulation into ruminal liquor (pH 5.5–6.5), where they become "trapped" by ion-

Table 70–8. Therapeutic plasma concentrations and half-lives of anticonvulsant drugs in humans and dogs.

Drug	Therapeutic Range of Plasma Concentrations (μg/mL)	Average Half-Life (hours)	
		Human	Dog
Phenobarbital*	10–25	86	41
Primidone	10–25	8	2
Phenytoin[†]	10–20	24	6
Sodium valproate	40–100	16	2.5
Carbamazepine*	3–12	24	1.5
Diazepam	0.6–?	24–36	8
Clonazepam	0.01–0.08	40	

*Chronic medication induces hepatic microsomal oxidative activity.
[†]Half-life is dose-dependent.

ization. This process is part of the normal distribution pattern for lipid-soluble drugs. Because of the very large volume of ruminal liquor, a large fraction of an administered dose may be distributed to this area. The colon, by acting similarly as a reservoir, can contribute to the apparent volume of distribution of lipid-soluble drugs in horses.

Body clearance is based on the concept of the body acting as a drug-eliminating system and represents the sum of individual clearances of a drug by the organs of elimination (liver and kidneys). It can be calculated by dividing the systemically available dose of drug by the area under the plasma concentration–time curve. For comparisons between species, clearance is best expressed as mL/min/kg. In Table 70–9, the half-life, apparent volume of distribution, and body clearance of some drugs are compared in the horse and the dog. A knowledge of the body clearance of a drug ($Cl_{systemic}$) is essential for determining the dosing rate (ie, the dose per unit time) that would be required to produce a given average steady-state concentration ($C_{p,ss_{avg}}$) of the drug:

$$\frac{F \times Dose}{Dosing\ interval} = C_{p,ss_{avg}} \times Cl_{systemic} \quad \ldots (5)$$

where F is the fraction of the dose that enters the systemic circulation intact (compare p 30, Chapter 3). For example, to produce a sustained bronchodilator effect with theophylline, the average steady-state plasma concentration should be maintained at 10 μg/mL. The clearance of theophylline in the horse and cat is 40 mL/h/kg, which is similar to the average clearance in man (41 mL/h/kg). The clearance in dogs is much higher, approximately 100 mL/h/kg. The desired steady-state plasma concentration can be achieved by administering aminophylline orally at a dosing rate appropriate for the species of animal, which is 10 mg/kg at 8-hour intervals to dogs and 5 mg/kg at 12-hour intervals to horses or cats.

DOSAGE REGIMENS

The therapeutic effectiveness of a drug product can be greatly influenced by the dosage regimen, which includes route of administration, size of dose, and interval between successive doses. Both the dosage regimen and the duration of therapy depend on the therapeutic objectives, and in veterinary medicine the species of animal is an additional consideration.

Drug Administration

Antimicrobial agents and anthelmintics are the 2 most widely used classes of drugs in veterinary medicine. Anthelmintic drugs are used primarily to suppress internal parasite burdens to a tolerable level. The administration of an anthelmintic to a large number of animals, such as a herd of cattle or flock of sheep, could be considered an example of mass medication and is similar to mass public health treatment

Table 70–9. Comparison of some pharmacokinetic parameters for selected drugs in the horse and dog.*

Drug	Half-Life (hours)		Volume of Distribution (mL/kg)		Clearance (mL/min/kg)	
	Horse	Dog	Horse	Dog	Horse	Dog
Hepatic metabolism						
Theophylline	14.8	5.7	856	824	0.67	1.67
Amphetamine	1.4	4.5	2610	2670	21.8	6.85
Ketamine	0.7	1	1625	2492	26.8	28.8
Xylazine	0.8	0.5	2456	2517	34	58.1
Hepatic metabolism and renal excretion						
Salicylate	1	8.7	180	189	2.1	0.25
Sulfadimethoxine	11.1	13.2	211	410	0.22	0.36
Renal excretion						
Penicillin G	0.4	0.5	163	156	4.8	3.6
Kanamycin	1.8	0.9	228	255	1.5	3.2
Digoxin	23.1	28	4890	9460	2.44	3.94

*Drugs are divided into groups based on the principal process of elimination. For individual references, write to the author of this chapter.

programs in human medicine. Selection of the anthelmintic drug as well as the time of the year and the frequency at which animals are medicated depend on the class of helminth parasite, the species of animal to be dosed, and the overall cost of the medication program.

Antimicrobial Therapy

While some antimicrobial agents (such as tylosin and monensin) are used as feed additives in food-producing animals, treatment of bacterial infections is the more important indication for administration of antimicrobial agents. In the management of an ill animal in which bacterial infection is either present or strongly suspected, the initial question should be whether or not an antimicrobial agent is indicated. If the answer is yes, selection of the most useful agent requires that the following factors be taken into account: the susceptibility of the infecting organism, the nature (pH reaction) and location of the infection focus, the disposition of potentially effective antimicrobial agents in the species of animal affected, and the antimicrobial preparations that are available as pharmaceutical products. Additional considerations in the selection of an antimicrobial preparation for administration to an animal patient include the convenience afforded by the dosage regimen (which relates to the dosage form and its route and frequency of administration) and the cost of such treatment. The latter may be relative to the "value" placed on the animal. In the food-producing animals, the residue potential and withdrawal times (milk and preslaughter) must be considered in the selection of an antimicrobial preparation and its route of administration.

Samples on which bacterial sensitivity tests can be performed must be collected before initiating antimicrobial therapy. It is particularly desirable to have the bacterial susceptibility pattern supported by minimum inhibitory concentration (MIC) values when infections are caused by *Staphylococcus aureus* and members of the Enterobacteriaceae family.

Long-Acting Parenteral Preparations

In farm animals, the administration of multiple doses of a drug at short intervals is impractical; a prolonged-release parenteral preparation is often the most convenient dosage form. Commonly used examples include procaine penicillin G (buffered aqueous suspension or in oil containing aluminum monostearate) and oxytetracycline base in 2-pyrrolidone. A single dose (25,000 units/kg) of procaine penicillin G (in buffered aqueous suspension) injected either intramuscularly or subcutaneously, can maintain effective levels of penicillin G for 24 hours in most species, although the half-life of penicillin G is less than an hour. While oxytetracycline base in 2-pyrrolidone should not be administered to horses, this preparation is approved for intramuscular administration to cattle, in which a single dose (20 mg/kg) will maintain effective serum concentrations of oxytetracycline for 48 hours. It is important that the formulation of parenteral (including prolonged-release) preparations be such that their intramuscular injection does not cause tissue damage and persistence of residual levels at the site of injection. The tissue-damaging effect of various drugs (oxytetracycline, neomycin, erythromycin, tylosin, sulfonamides, trimethoprim, lidocaine, diazepam, and digoxin) and some vehicles was reviewed by Rasmussen (see references).

It is well known that formulation can affect the bioavailability of a drug from various dosage forms and thereby influence therapeutic effectiveness. When comparing the bioavailability of a drug from different parenteral preparations, the location of the intramuscular (or subcutaneous) injection site should be the same or at least comparable.

The serum concentration–time curves obtained in different species given amoxicillin aqueous suspension (10%) by intramuscular injection appear to vary in a systematic way (Fig 70–3). The trend shown is that the smaller animals (piglets, dogs, and cats) gave an early high peak that was followed by a rapid decline in amoxicillin concentration, while the larger animals (calves and horses) produced a lower and relatively constant concentration of antibiotic in the serum. It is not known whether other drugs show this pattern.

THE NEONATAL PERIOD

The neonatal period is that time span from birth to 1 month of age. During this period, many, if not most, of the unexpected responses shown to the "usual" dosage level of drugs can be attributed to differences in drug disposition between neonatal and adult animals of the same species. Alteration in the pattern of distribution may be related to the difference in the relative volumes of the body fluid compartments coupled with the lower extent of plasma protein binding in the neonatal animal. Both total body water and the extracellular fluid volume, expressed as a percentage of body weight, are higher during the neonatal period (Chapter 63). There are marked deficiencies in some of the prominent processes of elimination (hepatic microsomal metabolic pathways and renal excretion mechanisms) in neonatal animals, particularly during the first 5 days of life. These differences in disposition are likely to alter the intensity and duration of the pharmacologic effects produced by a drug. While the effect may be either greater or less depending on the

drug, its duration will invariably be prolonged when microsomal-mediated metabolism or renal excretion is the principal process by which the drug is eliminated. Theoretically, a modification of the dosing rate (ie, the dose per unit time) could compensate for the anticipated alteration in response. In practice, however, it is exceedingly difficult to predict the dosage adjustment that may be required, since the rate of development of the elimination processes is not only variable but is also species-dependent. Absorption and disposition processes are most "unusual" in the first 24 hours after birth.

Neonatal Absorption

Orally administered absorbable antimicrobial agents are well absorbed in the neonatal animal, and, at least during the first week of life, their systemic availability may even be higher than in the adult animal. For example, the systemic availability of amoxicillin administered orally as a 5% suspension of the trihydrate is 30–50% in 5- to 10-day-old foals compared with 5–15% in adult horses. Since the rumen takes 8–12 weeks to develop and become functional, the bioavailability profile of drugs administered orally to neonatal calves is similar to that obtained in monogastric species. Chloramphenicol, for example, administered as an oral solution, is well absorbed in neonatal calves, and oral dosage (25 mg/kg at 12-hour intervals) will maintain therapeutically effective plasma concentrations of the antibiotic. In older calves, oral administration of chloramphenicol fails to produce effective plasma concentrations ($> 5 \mu g/mL$), since the antibiotic is inactivated in the rumen by a reductive reaction. It is interesting that the oral dosage regimen for chloramphenicol in neonatal calves is the same as that used in adult cats. The effectiveness of the 12-hour dosage interval relates to the relatively slow synthesis of the glucuronide conjugate of chloramphenicol. The half-life of chloramphenicol, which is 14 hours in 1-day-old calves, decreases to 7.5 hours in calves 7 days of age and at 10–12 weeks is only slightly longer than in adult cows (4.2 hours). This decrease is caused partly by increased drug "trapping" in the developing rumen and partly by development of metabolic capacity.

Neonatal Metabolic Pathways

The rate of development of hepatic microsomal oxidative reactions during the neonatal period may vary with the species of animal. It has been shown that piglets require 4–6 weeks for the cytochrome P-450–dependent, mixed function oxidase system to develop activity similar to that in the adult pig. In a study of the disposition kinetics of antipyrine in the cow, it was found that the half-life of antipyrine in calves 6 weeks of age (7.3 ± 1.8 hours, n = 5) was one-fourth of that in the 1-day-old calf but approximately twice as long as in adult cows. These changes in the half-life directly reflected changes in antipyrine clearance. Such results clearly show that this metabolic pathway is not fully developed in calves even at 6

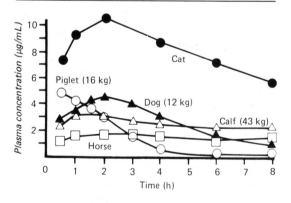

Figure 70–3. Effect of species and weight on bioavailability. Amoxicillin aqueous suspension (10%) was administered by intramuscular injection to all species at the same dosage level (7 mg/kg) except cats (10–12 mg/kg). (Modified and reproduced, with permission, from Marshall AB, Palmer GH: Injection sites and drug bioavailability. Page 59 in: *Trends in Veterinary Pharmacology and Toxicology.* Van Miert ASJPAM, Frens J, van der Kreek FW [editors]. Elsevier, 1980.)

weeks of age. The half-life of trimethoprim is 40 minutes in adult goats and 4–5 times longer in newborn kids. A period of 40–50 days after birth is required for the half-life of trimethoprim to decrease to the value found in the adult goat.

Neonatal Renal Excretion

Renal function, calculated from clearances of inulin and *p*-aminohippuric acid (which are indicative of glomerular filtration rate and effective renal plasma flow, respectively), is low in neonatal animals of most species, including the human. Both glomerular filtration and proximal tubular secretion are depressed. Although neonatal renal capacity may be "immature" relative to that of the adult, it adequately serves its normal function. However, when young animals are treated with drugs, the combined effect of slow hepatic microsomal metabolism (oxidation and glucuronide conjugation) and inefficient renal excretion mechanisms can decrease considerably the removal of lipid-soluble agents and their metabolites from the body. A possible exception is the neonatal calf, which, unlike neonatal animals of other species, appears to have well-developed glomerular filtration, at least after the first day of life.

DISEASE STATES

The presence of a disease state can alter the disposition kinetics of a drug. It has been shown that peni-

Table 70–10. Disposition kinetics of imidocarb (4 mg/kg) in normal dogs and dogs with *Escherichia coli* endotoxemia or *Trypanosoma evansi* infection.

Pharmacokinetic Parameter	Normal	E coli Endotoxemia	T evansi Infection
$t_{1/2}$ (min)	207 ± 45	198 ± 38	266 ± 73
Cl (mL/min · kg)	1.47 ± 0.38	0.89 ± 0.33	2.21 ± 0.49
V_d (mL/kg)	390 ± 92	188 ± 61	722 ± 202

cillin G distributes more widely in febrile than in normal animals. Increased penetration of the blood-brain barrier may contribute to effectiveness of penicillin in the treatment of some meningeal infections when the drug is administered during the acute febrile stage of the disease. Even though infectious diseases have in common the presence of fever, the nature of the altered disposition varies with the pathophysiology of the disease condition. In a study of the disposition kinetics of the antiprotozoal drug imidocarb in disease-induced and control dogs, it was found that corresponding changes occurred in the volume of distribution and the body (systemic) clearance of the drug, so that the half-life of imidocarb remained unchanged (Table 70–10). Thus half-life alone is not a reliable pharmacokinetic parameter on which to base the decision as to whether the disposition of a drug is altered in the presence of a disease state.

REFERENCES

Baggot JD: Distribution of antimicrobial agents in normal and diseased animals. *J Am Vet Med Assoc* 1980;**176**:1085.

Baggot JD: *Principles of Drug Disposition in Domestic Animals*. Saunders, 1977.

Baggot JD, Short CR: Drug disposition in the neonatal animal, with particular reference to the foal. *Equine Vet J* 1984;**16**:364.

Dalton RG: Renal function in neonatal calves: Inulin, thiosulphate and para-aminohippuric acid clearance. *Br Vet J* 1968;**124**:498.

Elliot DL et al: Pet-associated illness. *N Engl J Med* 1985;**313**:985.

Greenblatt DJ: Predicting steady state serum concentrations of drugs. *Annu Rev Pharmacol Toxicol* 1979;**19**:347.

Marshall AB, Palmer GH: Injection sites and drug bioavailability. In: *Trends in Veterinary Pharmacology and Toxicology*. Van Miert ASJPAM, Frens J, van der Kreek FW (editors). Elsevier, 1980.

Nouws JFM et al: Comparative plasma ampicillin levels and bioavailability of five parenteral ampicillin formulations in ruminant calves. *Vet Q* 1982;**4**:62.

Pope DG, Baggot JD: The basis for selection of the dosage form. In: *Formulation of Veterinary Dosage Forms*. Blodinger J (editor). Marcel Dekker, 1983.

Rasmussen F: Tissue damage at the injection site after intramuscular injection of drugs in food-producing animals. In: *Trends in Veterinary Pharmacology and Toxicology*. Van Miert ASJPAM, Frens J, van der Kreek FW (editors). Elsevier, 1980.

Reiche R, Mulling M, Frey H-H: Pharmacokinetics of chloramphenicol in calves during the first weeks of life. *J Vet Pharmacol Ther* 1980;**3**:95.

Riviere JE: Calculation of dosage regimens of antimicrobial drugs in animals with renal and hepatic dysfunction. *J Am Vet Med Assoc* 1984;**185**:1094.

Short CR, Davis LE: Perinatal development of drug-metabolizing enzyme activity in swine. *J Pharmacol Exp Ther* 1970;**174**:185.

Williams RT: Species variations in drug biotransformations. In: *Fundamentals of Drug Metabolism and Drug Disposition*. LaDu BN, Mandel HG, Way EL (editors). Williams & Wilkins, 1971.

Appendix I:
Important Drug Interactions

Philip D. Hansten, PharmD

MECHANISMS OF DRUG INTERACTIONS

One of the factors that can alter the response to drugs is the concurrent administration of other drugs. There are several mechanisms by which drugs may interact, but most can be categorized as pharmacokinetic (absorption, distribution, metabolism, excretion), pharmacodynamic, or combined toxicity. Knowledge of the mechanism by which a given drug interaction occurs is often clinically useful, since the mechanism may influence both the time course and the methods of circumventing the interaction. Some important drug interactions occur as a result of 2 or more mechanisms.

Pharmacokinetic Mechanisms

The gastrointestinal **absorption** of drugs may be affected by concurrent use of other agents that (1) have a large surface area upon which the drug can be adsorbed, (2) bind or chelate, or (3) alter gastrointestinal motility. One must distinguish between effects on adsorption *rate* and effects on *extent* of absorption. A reduction in only the absorption rate of a drug is seldom clinically important, whereas a reduction in the extent of absorption will be clinically important if it results in subtherapeutic serum levels of the drug.

The mechanisms by which drug interactions alter drug **distribution** include (1) competition for plasma protein binding and (2) displacement from tissue binding sites. Although competition for plasma protein binding can increase the free concentration (and thus the effect) of the displaced drug in plasma, the increase tends to be temporary owing to a compensatory increase in drug disposition. The importance of protein binding displacement has probably been overemphasized; only a few drugs are known to manifest clinically important interactions by this mechanism (eg, oral anticoagulants, sulfonylureas, hypoglycemics). Displacement from tissue binding sites would tend to increase the blood concentration of the displaced drug. Such a mechanism is partially responsible for the elevation of serum digoxin concentration by concurrent quinidine therapy.

The **metabolism** of drugs can be stimulated or inhibited by concurrent therapy. Induction (stimulation) of hepatic microsomal drug-metabolizing enzymes can be produced by drugs such as barbiturates, carbamazepine, glutethimide, phenytoin, primidone, and rifampin. Enzyme induction does not take place quickly; maximal effects usually occur after 7–10 days and require an equal or longer time to dissipate after the enzyme inducer is stopped. Drugs that may inhibit hepatic microsomal metabolism of other drugs include allopurinol, chloramphenicol, cimetidine, disulfiram, isoniazid, metronidazole, phenylbutazone, propoxyphene, and sulfonamides. Inhibition of metabolism generally takes place more quickly than enzyme induction and may begin as soon as sufficient hepatic concentration of the inhibitor is achieved. However, if the half-life of the affected drug is long, it may take a week or more to reach a new steady-state serum level.

The renal **excretion** of active drug can also be affected by concurrent drug therapy. The renal excretion of certain drugs that are weak acids or weak bases may be influenced by other drugs that affect urinary pH. This is due to changes in ionization of the drug, thus altering its lipid solubility and therefore its ability to be absorbed back into the blood from the kidney tubule. For some drugs, active secretion into the renal tubules is an important elimination pathway. This process may be affected by concurrent drug therapy, thus altering serum drug levels and pharmacologic response.

Pharmacodynamic Mechanisms

When drugs with similar pharmacologic effects are administered concurrently, an additive or synergistic response is usually seen. The 2 drugs may or may not act on the same receptor to produce such effects. Conversely, drugs with opposing pharmacologic effects may reduce the response to one or both drugs. Pharmacodynamic drug interactions are relatively common in clinical practice, but adverse effects can be minimized if the interactions are anticipated and appropriate countermeasures taken.

Combined Toxicity

The combined use of 2 or more drugs, each of which has toxic effects on the same organ, can greatly increase the likelihood of organ damage. For example, concurrent administration of 2 nephrotoxic drugs can produce kidney damage even though the dose of either drug alone may have been insufficient to produce toxicity. Furthermore, some drugs can enhance the organ toxicity of another drug even though the enhancing drug has no intrinsic toxic effect on that organ.

PREDICTABILITY OF DRUG INTERACTIONS

The designations listed below will be used here to *estimate* the predictability of the drug interactions. These estimates are intended to indicate simply whether or not the interaction will occur and do not always mean that the interaction is likely to produce an adverse effect. Whether the interaction produces an adverse effect or not depends upon (1) the presence or absence of factors that predispose to the adverse effects of the drug interaction (diseases, organ function, dose of drugs, etc) and (2) *awareness* on the part of the prescriber, so that appropriate monitoring can be ordered or preventive measures taken.

HP Highly predictable. Interaction occurs in almost all patients receiving the interacting combination.

P Predictable. Interaction occurs in most patients receiving the combination.

NP Not predictable. Interaction occurs only in some patients receiving the combination.

NE Not established. Insufficient data available on which to base estimate of predictability.

ALCOHOL

Properties Promoting Drug Interaction
(1) Chronic alcoholism results in enzyme induction.

(2) Acute alcohol intoxication tends to inhibit drug metabolism (whether person is alcoholic or not).

(3) Severe alcohol-induced hepatic dysfunction may inhibit ability to metabolize drugs.

(4) Disulfiramlike reaction in the presence of certain drugs.

(5) Additive central nervous system depression with other central nervous system depressants.

Clinically Documented Interactions
Acetaminophen: [NE] Increased formation of hepatotoxic metabolites.

Anticoagulants, oral: [NE] Increased hypoprothrombinemic effect with acute alcohol intoxication.

Central nervous system depressants: [HP] Additive or synergistic central nervous system depression.

Insulin: [NE] Acute alcohol intake may increase hypoglycemic effect (especially in fasting patients).

Drugs that may produce a disulfiramlike reaction:
Cephalosporins: [NP] Disulfiramlike reactions noted with cefamandole, cefoperazone, and moxalactam.

Chloral hydrate: [NP] Mechanism not established.

Disulfiram: [HP] Inhibits aldehyde dehydrogenase.

Metronidazole: [NP] Mechanism not established.

Sulfonylureas: [NE] Chlorpropamide is most likely to produce a disulfiramlike reaction; acute alcohol intake may increase hypoglycemic effect (especially in fasting patients).

ALLOPURINOL

Properties Promoting Drug Interaction
Inhibits hepatic drug-metabolizing enzymes.

Clinically Documented Interactions
Anticoagulants, oral: [NP] Increased hypoprothrombinemic effect.

Azathioprine: [P] Decreased azathioprine detoxification resulting in increased azathioprine toxicity.

Mercaptopurine: [P] Decreased mercaptopurine metabolism resulting in increased mercaptopurine toxicity.

ANTACIDS

Properties Promoting Drug Interaction
(1) Antacids may adsorb drugs in gastrointestinal tract, thus reducing absorption.

(2) Antacids tend to speed gastric emptying, thus delivering drugs to absorbing sites in the intestine more quickly.

(3) Some antacids (eg, magnesium hydroxide + aluminum hydroxide) alkalinize the urine somewhat, thus altering excretion of drugs sensitive to urinary pH.

Clinically Documented Interactions
Digoxin: [NP] Reduced gastrointestinal absorption of digoxin.

Iron: [P] Reduced gastrointestinal absorption of iron with some antacids.

Salicylates: [P] Increased renal clearance of salicylates due to increase urine pH; occurs only with large doses of salicylates.

Sodium polystyrene sulfonate: [NE] Binds antacid cation in gut, resulting in metabolic alkalosis.

Tetracyclines: [HP] Reduced gastrointestinal absorption of tetracyclines.

ANTICHOLINERGICS: SEE ANTIMUSCARINICS

ANTICOAGULANTS, ORAL

Properties Promoting Drug Interaction
(1) Metabolism inducible.

(2) Susceptible to inhibition of metabolism.

(3) Highly bound to plasma proteins.

(4) Anticoagulant response altered by drugs that affect clotting factor synthesis or catabolism.

Clinically Documented Interactions

Drugs that may increase anticoagulant effect:

Amiodarone: [P] Mechanism not established.

Anabolic steroids: [P] Alter clotting factor disposition?

Chloramphenicol: [NE] Inhibits dicumarol metabolism (possibly also warfarin).

Cimetidine: [HP] Inhibits anticoagulant metabolism.

Clofibrate: [P] Mechanism not established.

Danazol: [NE] Impaired synthesis of clotting factors?

Dextrothyroxine: [P] Enhances clotting factor catabolism?

Disulfiram: [P] Inhibits anticoagulant metabolism.

Metronidazole: [P] Inhibits anticoagulant metabolism.

Miconazole: [NE] Mechanism not established.

Phenylbutazone: [HP] Inhibits anticoagulant metabolism.

Quinidine: [NP] Additive hypoprothrombinemia.

Salicylates: [HP] Platelet inhibition; [P] Large doses have hypoprothrombinemic effect.

Sulfinpyrazone: [NE] Mechanism not established.

Sulindac: [NP] Mechanism not established.

Sulfonamides: [NE] Inhibit anticoagulant metabolism; displace protein binding.

Thyroid hormones: [P] Enhance clotting factor catabolism.

Trimethoprim-sulfamethoxazole: [P] Inhibits anticoagulant metabolism; displaces from protein binding.

See also Alcohol; Allopurinol.

Drugs that may decrease anticoagulant effect:

Barbiturates: [P] Enzyme induction.

Carbamazepine: [P] Enzyme induction.

Cholestyramine: [P] Reduces absorption of anticoagulant.

Glutethimide: [P] Enzyme induction.

Primidone: [P] Enzyme induction.

Rifampin: [P] Enzyme induction.

Effects of anticoagulants on other drugs:

Hypoglycemics, oral: [P] Dicumarol inhibits hepatic metabolism of tolbutamide and chlorpropamide.

Phenytoin: [P] Dicumarol inhibits metabolism of phenytoin.

ANTIDEPRESSANTS, TRICYCLIC

Properties Promoting Drug Interaction

(1) Inhibition of amine uptake into postganglionic adrenergic neuron.

(2) Antimuscarinic effects may be additive with other antimuscarinic drugs.

(3) Metabolism inducible.

Clinically Documented Interactions

Barbiturates: [P] Increased antidepressant metabolism.

Cimetidine: [P] Inhibits antidepressant metabolism.

Clonidine: [P] Reduced antihypertensive effect; mechanism unknown.

Guanadrel: [P] Reduced uptake of guanadrel into sites of action.

Guanethidine: [P] Reduced uptake of guanethidine into sites of action.

Sympathomimetics: [P] Enhanced pressor response to norepinephrine, epinephrine, and phenylephrine.

ANTIMUSCARINICS

Properties Promoting Drug Interaction

(1) Decreased gastrointestinal motility. This may increase bioavailability of poorly soluble drugs and reduce bioavailability of drugs degraded in gut.

(2) Combined use of more than one antimuscarinic increases likelihood of antimuscarinic adverse effects.

Clinically Documented Interactions

Levodopa: [P] Increased degradation of levodopa in gut; serum levodopa levels lowered.

Combined antimuscarinics: [P] Antimuscarinic adverse effects (eg, paralytic ileus, urinary retention, blurred vision).

BARBITURATES

Properties Promoting Drug Interaction

(1) Induction of hepatic microsomal drug-metabolizing enzymes.

(2) Additive central nervous system depression with other central nervous system depressants.

Clinically Documented Interactions

Beta-adrenoceptor blockers: [P] Increased beta blocker metabolism.

Central nervous system depressants: [HP] Additive central nervous system depression.

Corticosteroids: [P] Increased corticosteroid metabolism.

Doxycycline: [P] Increased doxycycline metabolism.

Estrogens: [P] Increased estrogen metabolism.

Phenothiazines: [P] Increased phenothiazine metabolism.

Quinidine: [P] Increased quinidine metabolism.

Valproic acid: [P] Decreased phenobarbital metabolism.

See also Anticoagulants, Oral; Antidepressants, Tricyclic.

BETA-ADRENOCEPTOR BLOCKERS

Properties Promoting Drug Interaction

(1) Beta blockade (especially with nonspecific agents such as propranolol) alters response to sympathomimetics with beta-agonist activity (eg, epinephrine).

(2) Beta blockers that undergo extensive first-pass metabolism may be affected by drugs capable of altering this process.

(3) Beta blockers may reduce hepatic blood flow.

Clinically Documented Interactions

Drugs that may increase beta blocker effect:

Chlorpromazine: [P] Reduces metabolism of propranolol.

Cimetidine: [P] Reduces metabolism of propranolol; additive bradycardia.

Furosemide: [P] Reduces metabolism of propranolol.

Hydralazine: [P] Reduces metabolism of propranolol.

Drugs that may decrease beta blocker effect:

Enzyme inducers: [P] Barbiturates, phenytoin and rifampin may enhance beta blocker metabolism; other enzyme inducers may produce similar effects.

Nonsteroidal anti-inflammatory drugs: [P] Indomethacin reduces antihypertensive response; other prostaglandin inhibitors probably also interact.

Effects of beta blockers on other drugs:

Clonidine: [NE] Hypertensive reaction if clonidine is withdrawn while patient is taking propranolol.

Insulin: [P] Inhibition of glucose recovery from hypoglycemia; inhibition of symptoms of hypoglycemia (except sweating); increased blood pressure during hypoglycemia.

Lidocaine: [NE] Reduced plasma clearance of intravenous lidocaine; increased plasma lidocaine levels.

Prazosin: [P] Increased hypotensive response to first dose of prazosin.

Sympathomimetics: [P] Enhanced pressor response to epinephrine (and possibly other sympathomimetics); this is more likely to occur with nonspecific beta blockers.

BILE ACID–BINDING RESINS
(Cholestyramine, Colestipol)

Properties Promoting Drug Interaction

(1) Resins may bind with orally administered drugs in gastrointestinal tract.

(2) Resins may bind in gastrointestinal tract with drugs that undergo enterohepatic circulation, even if the latter are given parenterally.

Clinically Documented Interactions

Acetaminophen: [NE] Reduced gastrointestinal absorption of acetaminophen.

Digitalis glycosides: [NE] Reduced gastrointestinal absorption of digitoxin (possibly also digoxin).

Thiazide diuretics: [P] Reduced gastrointestinal absorption of thiazides.

Thyroid hormones: [P] Reduced thyroid absorption.

See also Anticoagulants, Oral.

CARBAMAZEPINE

Properties Promoting Drug Interaction

(1) Induction of hepatic microsomal drug-metabolizing enzymes.

(2) Susceptible to inhibition of metabolism.

Clinically Documented Interactions

Doxycycline: [P] Increased doxycycline metabolism.

Erythromycin: [NE] Decreased carbamazepine metabolism.

Estrogens: [P] Increased estrogen metabolism.

Isoniazid: [P] Decreased carbamazepine metabolism.

Propoxyphene: [HP] Decreased carbamazepine metabolism.

Troleandomycin: [P] Decreased carbamazepine metabolism.

See also Anticoagulants, Oral.

CHLORAMPHENICOL

Properties Promoting Drug Interaction

Inhibits hepatic drug-metabolizing enzymes.

Clinically Documented Interactions

Sulfonylurea hypoglycemics: [P] Inhibited sulfonylurea metabolism.

Phenytoin: [P] Inhibited phenytoin metabolism.

See also Anticoagulants, Oral.

CIMETIDINE

Properties Promoting Drug Interaction

(1) Inhibits hepatic microsomal drug-metabolizing enzymes. (Ranitidine does not appear to do so.)

(2) May reduce hepatic blood flow, thus reducing first-pass metabolism of highly extracted drugs. (However, the significance of this mechanism is not established.)

(3) May increase bone marrow suppression caused by other drugs.

Clinically Documented Interactions

Benzodiazepines: [P] Inhibits metabolism of alprazolam, chlordiazepoxide, diazepam, halazepam, prazepam, and clorazepate but not oxazepam, lorazepam, or temazepam.

Carmustine: [NE] Increased bone marrow suppression.

Ketoconazole: [NE] Decreased gastrointestinal absorption of ketoconazole due to increased pH in gut.

Lidocaine: [P] Inhibits metabolism of lidocaine; increased serum lidocaine.

Phenytoin: [NE] Inhibits phenytoin metabolism; increased serum phenytoin.

Procainamide: [P] Decreased renal excretion of procainamide; increased serum procainamide levels.

Quinidine: [P] Decreased metabolism of quinidine; increased serum quinidine levels.

Theophylline: [P] Inhibits theophylline metabolism; increased plasma theophylline.

See also Anticoagulants, Oral; Antidepressants, Tricyclic; Beta-Adrenoceptor Blockers.

DIGITALIS GLYCOSIDES

Properties Promoting Drug Interaction

(1) Digoxin susceptible to inhibition of gastrointestinal absorption.

(2) Digitalis toxicity may be increased by drug-induced electrolyte imbalance (eg, hypokalemia).

(3) Digitoxin metabolism inducible.

(4) Renal excretion of digoxin susceptible to inhibition.

Clinically Documented Interactions

Drugs that may increase digitalis effect:

Amiodarone: [P] Increased plasma digoxin concentrations by unknown mechanisms.

Diltiazem: [P] Increased plasma digoxin (usually 20–30%) due to reduced renal and nonrenal clearance.

Erythromycin: [NP] Increased gastrointestinal absorption of digoxin in certain patients.

Potassium-depleting drugs: [P] Increased likelihood of digitalis toxicity.

Quinidine: [HP] Reduced renal digoxin excretion; displacement of digoxin from tissue binding sites; digitoxin may also be affected.

Spironolactone: [NE] Reduced renal digoxin excretion and interference with some serum digoxin assays.

Verapamil: [P] Increased serum digoxin levels.

Drugs that may decrease digitalis effect:

Kaolin-pectin: [P] Reduced gastrointestinal digoxin absorption.

Penicillamine: [NE] Decreased serum digoxin.

Sulfasalazine: [NE] Reduced gastrointestinal digoxin absorption.

See also Antacids; Bile Acid–Binding Resins.

DISULFIRAM

Properties Promoting Drug Interaction

(1) Inhibits hepatic microsomal drug-metabolizing enzymes.

(2) Inhibits aldehyde dehydrogenase.

Clinically Documented Interactions

Benzodiazepines: [P] Inhibits metabolism of chlordiazepoxide and diazepam but not lorazepam and oxazepam.

Metronidazole: [NE] Confusion and psychoses reported in patients on this combination; mechanism unknown.

Phenytoin: [P] Inhibits phenytoin metabolism.

See also Alcohol; Anticoagulants, Oral.

ESTROGENS

Properties Promoting Drug Interaction

(1) Metabolism inducible.

(2) Enterohepatic circulation of estrogen may be interrupted by alteration in bowel flora (eg, due to antibiotics).

Clinically Documented Interactions

Ampicillin: [NP] Interruption of enterohepatic circulation of estrogen; possible reduction in oral contraceptive efficacy.

Corticosteroids: [P] Increased corticosteroid effect; mechanism not established.

Diazepam: [NE] Reduced diazepam metabolism.

Griseofulvin: [NE] Possible inhibition of oral contraceptive efficacy; mechanism unknown.

Phenytoin: [NP] Increased estrogen metabolism; possible reduction in oral contraceptive efficacy.

Rifampin: [NP] Increased estrogen metabolism; possible reduction in oral contraceptive efficacy.

See also Barbiturates; Carbamazepine.

LEVODOPA

Properties Promoting Drug Interaction

(1) Levodopa degraded in gut prior to reaching sites of absorption. Agents that alter gastrointestinal motility may alter degree of intraluminal degradation.

(2) Antiparkinsonism effect of levodopa susceptible to inhibition by other drugs.

Clinically Documented Interactions

Clonidine: [NE] Inhibits antiparkinsonism effect.

Monoamine oxidase inhibitors: [P] Hypertensive reaction (carbidopa prevents the interaction).

Papaverine: [NE] Inhibits antiparkinsonism effect.

Phenothiazines: [P] Inhibits antiparkinsonism effect.

Phenytoin: [NE] Inhibits antiparkinsonism effect.

Pyridoxine: [P] Inhibits antiparkinsonism effect (carbidopa prevents the interaction).

See also Antimuscarinics.

LITHIUM

Properties Promoting Drug Interaction

(1) Renal lithium excretion sensitive to changes in

sodium balance. (Sodium depletion tends to cause lithium retention.)

(2) Susceptible to drugs enhancing central nervous system lithium toxicity.

Clinically Documented Interactions

Diurectics (sodium-depleting): [P] Reduced renal excretion of lithium; furosemide may be less likely to produce this effect than thiazide diuretics.

Haloperidol: [NP] Occasional cases of neurotoxicity in manic patients, especially with large doses of one or both drugs.

Methyldopa: [NE] Increased likelihood of central nervous system lithium toxicity.

Nonsteroidal anti-inflammatory drugs (NSAIDs): [NE] Indomethacin reduces renal lithium excretion; possibly other NSAIDs do the same.

MONOAMINE OXIDASE INHIBITORS (MAOI)

Properties Promoting Drug Interaction

(1) Increase norepinephrine stored in adrenergic neuron. Displacement of these stores by other drugs may produce acute hypertensive response.

(2) MAOI have intrinsic hypoglycemic activity.

Clinically Documented Interactions

Antidiabetic agents: [P] Additive hypoglycemic effect.

Guanethidine: [P] Reversal of the hypotensive action of guanethidine.

Narcotic analgesics: [NP] Some patients develop hypertension, rigidity, excitation; meperidine may be more likely to interact than morphine.

Phenylephrine: [P] Hypertensive episode, since phenylephrine is metabolized by monoamine oxidase.

Sympathomimetics (Indirect-Acting): [HP] Hypertensive episode due to release of stored norepinephrine.

See also Levodopa.

NONSTEROIDAL ANTI-INFLAMMATORY DRUGS (NSAIDs)

Properties Promoting Drug Interaction

(1) Prostaglandin inhibition may result in reduced renal sodium excretion, impaired resistance to hypertensive stimuli, and reduced renal lithium excretion.

(2) Most NSAIDs inhibit platelet function; may increase likelihood of bleeding due to other drugs that impair hemostasis.

(3) Most NSAIDs are highly bound to plasma proteins.

(4) Phenylbutazone may inhibit hepatic microsomal drug metabolism (also seems to act as enzyme inducer in some cases).

(5) Phenylbutazone may alter renal excretion of some drugs.

Clinically Documented Interactions

Captopril: [P] Reduced antihypertensive response to captopril.

Furosemide: [P] Reduced diuretic, natriuretic, and antihypertensive response to furosemide with indomethacin (possibly also other NSAIDs).

Phenytoin: [P] Reduced hepatic phenytoin metabolism.

Thiazides: [P] Reduced antihypertensive response to thiazides.

Triamterene: [NE] Reduced renal function noted with triamterene plus indomethacin in both healthy subjects and patients.

See also Anticoagulants, Oral; Beta-Adrenoceptor Blockers; Lithium.

PHENYTOIN

Properties Promoting Drug Interaction

(1) Induces hepatic microsomal drug metabolism.

(2) Susceptible to inhibition of metabolism.

Clinically Documented Interactions

Drugs whose metabolism is stimulated by phenytoin:

Corticosteroids: [P] Reduced serum corticosteroid levels.

Doxycycline: [P] Reduced serum doxycycline levels.

Methadone: [P] Reduced serum methadone levels; withdrawal symptoms.

Quinidine: [P] Reduced serum quinidine levels.

Theophylline: [NE] Reduced serum theophylline levels.

Verapamil: [NE] Increased verapamil metabolism; reduced verapamil effect.

See also Estrogens.

Drugs that inhibit phenytoin metabolism:

Chloramphenicol: [P] Increased serum phenytoin.

Isoniazid: [NP] Increased serum phenytoin; problem primarily with slow acetylators of isoniazid.

See also Disulfiram; Phenylbutazone.

POTASSIUM-SPARING DIURETICS (Amiloride, Spironolactone, Triamterene)

Properties Promoting Drug Interaction

(1) Additive effects with other agents increasing serum potassium concentration.

(2) May alter renal excretion of substances other than potassium (eg, digoxin, hydrogen ions).

Clinically Documented Interactions

Captopril: [NE] Additive hyperkalemic effect.

Potassium supplements: [P] Additive hyperkalemic effect; especially a problem in presence of renal impairment.

See also Digitalis Glycosides; Nonsteroidal Antiinflammatory Drugs.

PROBENECID

Properties Promoting Drug Interaction

(1) Interference with renal excretion of drugs that undergo active tubular secretion, especially weak acids.

(2) Inhibition of glucuronide conjugation of other drugs.

Clinically Documented Interactions

Clofibrate: [P] Reduced glucuronide conjugation of clofibric acid.

Methotrexate: [P] Reduced renal methotrexate excretion.

Penicillin: [P] Reduced renal penicillin excretion.

Salicylates: [P] Reduced uricosuric effect of probenecid (interaction unlikely with less than 1.5 g of salicylate daily).

QUINIDINE

Properties Promoting Drug Interaction

(1) Metabolism inducible.

(2) Renal excretion susceptible to changes in urine pH.

Clinically Documented Interactions

Acetazolamide: [P] Reduced renal quinidine excretion due to increased urinary pH; elevated serum quinidine.

Amiodarone: [NE] Increased serum quinidine levels; mechanism not established.

Rifampin: [P] Enhanced hepatic quinidine metabolism.

See also Anticoagulants, Oral; Barbiturates; Cimetidine; Digitalis Glycosides; Phenytoin.

RIFAMPIN

Properties Promoting Drug Interaction

Induction of hepatic microsomal drug-metabolizing enzymes.

Clinically Documented Interactions

Corticosteroids: [P] Increased corticosteroid hepatic metabolism; reduced corticosteroid effect.

Sulfonylurea hypoglycemics: [P] Increased hepatic metabolism of tolbutamide and probably other sulfonylureas metabolized by the liver (including chlorpropamide).

Verapamil: [NE] Increased verapamil metabolism; reduced verapamil effect.

See also Anticoagulants, Oral; Beta-Adrenoceptor Blockers; Estrogens.

SALICYLATES

Properties Promoting Drug Interaction

(1) Interference with renal excretion of drugs that undergo active tubular secretion.

(2) Salicylate renal excretion dependent on urinary pH when large doses of salicylate used.

(3) Salicylates may displace drugs from plasma protein binding sites.

(4) Aspirin (but not other salicylates) interferes with platelet function.

(5) Large doses of salicylates have intrinsic hypoglycemic activity.

Clinically Documented Interactions

Carbonic anhydrase inhibitors: [NE] Increased salicylate toxicity due to decreased blood pH.

Heparin: [NE] Increased bleeding tendency with aspirin, but probably not with other salicylates.

Methotrexate: [P] Reduced renal methotrexate clearance; increased methotrexate toxicity.

Sulfinpyrazone: [HP] Reduced uricosuric effect of sulfinpyrazone (interaction unlikely with less than 1.5 g of salicylate daily).

See also Antacids; Anticoagulants, Oral; Probenecid.

THEOPHYLLINE

Properties Promoting Drug Interaction

(1) Susceptible to inhibition of hepatic metabolism.

(2) Metabolism inducible.

Clinically Documented Interactions

Erythromycin: [P] Inhibition of hepatic theophylline metabolism.

Smoking: [HP] Enhanced hepatic theophylline metabolism.

Troleandomycin: [P] Inhibition of hepatic theophylline metabolism.

See also Cimetidine.

REFERENCES

Cluff LE, Petrie JC: *Clinical Effects of Interaction Between Drugs*. Excerpta Medica, 1974.

Hansten PD: *Drug Interactions*, 5th ed. Lea & Febiger, 1985.

Hansten PD: *Drug Interactions Newsletter*. Applied Therapeutics. [Monthly.]

Hartshorn EA: *Drug Interactions Update*. American Society of Hospital Pharmacists. [Yearly.]

Mangini RJ (editor): *Drug Interaction Facts*. Lippincott. [Quarterly.]

Rizack MA (editor): *The Medical Letter Handbook of Adverse Interactions*. The Medical Letter, 1985.

Smith NT, Miller RD, Corbascio AN: *Drug Interactions in Anesthesia*. Lea & Febiger, 1981.

Stockley I: *Drug Interactions*. Blackwell, 1981.

Appendix II:
Drug Effects on Laboratory Tests

Philip D. Hansten, PharmD, & Lisa A. Lybecker, PharmD

THE EFFECTS OF DRUGS ON COMMON CLINICAL LABORATORY PROCEDURES (Table 1)

With the increasing number of available drugs and the increasing number and complexity of tests performed by the clinical laboratory, drug-induced interference with test results is occurring with greater frequency. Table 1 has been prepared to assist clinicians and laboratory personnel in identifying such drug effects. In an effort to keep the information clinically relevant, no information from animal studies and limited information from in vitro studies have been included.

Although an effort has been made to cover each area thoroughly, it is inevitable that a listing of this type will be incomplete. The reader may wish to add to the chart on the basis of personal reading and experience.

Types of Drug Interference

Alterations in clinical laboratory results caused by drugs may be grouped into 2 general categories:

A. Effects Due to Pharmacologic or Toxic Properties of Drugs: Here, a true change is produced in the level of the variable being measured. In Table 1, changes of this nature are designated as increase (+) or decrease (−). The magnitude of the change depends upon a variety of factors such as dosage of drug, duration of administration, condition of patient, etc.

B. Effects Due to Interference With the Testing Procedure: In this case, the drug or its metabolite becomes a contaminant that may alter the value obtained or interfere with the measurement. This type of interference is indicated in Table 1 as increase (●) or decrease (○). It should be noted that drugs may affect one method of performing a given laboratory procedure and have no effect on another. For this reason, the specific testing method affected has been specified whenever possible.

Arrangement of Table 1

Table 1 lists the drugs that may affect the results of the laboratory tests indicated at the top. Tests less commonly influenced by drug administration are included in the column headed Other Tests.

All drugs are listed alphabetically by generic name, with common trade names and other names in parentheses. Some general drug classifications have been used. If a drug falls into one of the categories listed below, it should be sought under that general classification.

Aluminum antacids
Aminoglycosides
Anabolic steroids
Barbiturates
Calcium antacids
Cephalosporins
Contrast media, iodine-containing
Corticosteroids
Digitalis glycosides
Estrogens
Gold salts
Inorganic iodides
Iron, oral
Mercurial diuretics
Monoamine oxidase inhibitors
Oral contraceptives
Phenothiazines
Progestogens
Salicylates
Sulfonamides
Tetracyclines
Thiazide diuretics
Tricyclic antidepressants

Acetaminophen:

Overdose may produce liver damage with hyperbilirubinemia.

Hypoglycemia has been reported with large doses. False decreases have also been reported (glucose oxidase-peroxidase method), as well as false-positive readings (Yellow Spring Instrument glucose analyzer).

May cause false increases in urinary 5-HIAA (screening methods using nitrosonaphthol reagent).

Possible false increase for metanephrine determination by Shoup and Kissenger methods (liquid chromatography with electrochemical determination).

An acetaminophen metabolite may give false-positive screening for phenylalanine by chromatographic analysis.

Alcohol, ethyl:

Acute intoxication may produce myopathy, with elevation of serum aldolase, CPK, and SGOT.

Acute intoxication may enhance hypoprothrombinemic effect of oral anticoagulants.

The diuresis produced results in a lighter urine.

Attacks of acute intermittent porphyria may be precipitated by ethanol.

Allopurinol:

May enhance hypoprothrombinemic effect of oral anticoagulants.

Aminoglycosides:

Oral aminoglycosides may decrease serum cholesterol.

False increase in urine protein (Ponceau Red method); true proteinuria may also occur.

Oral aminoglycosides may reduce urinary urobilinogen.

Oral aminoglycosides may decrease blood ammonia in patients with hepatic disease.

Gentamicin has been associated with decreased serum magnesium.

Oral aminoglycosides may decrease urinary estrogen excretion.

Aminosalicylic acid:

Reportedly may produce acute pancreatitis, with elevated serum amylase.

May cause reddening of the urine if toilet bowl recently cleaned by hypochlorite bleach.

Will produce yellow color with Ehrlich's reagent test for porphobilinogen or urobilinogen.

Ampicillin:

Intramuscular ampicillin may result in increased serum CPK levels.

Anabolic steroids:

May decrease blood glucose in diabetic patients.

May enhance hypoprothrombinemic effect of oral anticoagulants.

Norethandrolone (Nilevar) may elevate SGOT.

Testosterone treatment increases urinary excretion of 17-ketosteroids, whereas methyltestosterone does not appear in the urine.

Ascorbic acid:

Large doses may produce false increase in serum bilirubin (SMA 12/60).

May produce false elevations in uric acid determinations (except enzymatic methods).

Large doses may produce false positives by copper reduction methods (eg, Clinitest), and false negatives by glucose oxidase methods (eg, Clinistix, Tes-Tape).

May interfere with the determination of urinary 17-hydroxycorticosteroids by a modification of the Reddy, Jenkins, Thorn procedure (*Metabolism* 1952;**1**:511 and 1954;**3**:489).

Azathioprine:

Pancreatitis has been reported following azathioprine administration.

May decrease serum uric acid in patients with gout.

Barbiturates:

Serum amylase may be decreased in barbiturate poisoning.

Enzyme induction by barbiturates may reduce serum bilirubin; rare instances of liver injury may increase serum bilirubin.

Prolonged use of barbiturates as anticonvulsants has resulted in osteomalacia with elevated serum alkaline phosphatase.

May inhibit hypoprothrombinemic effect of oral anticoagulants.

Attacks of acute intermittent porphyria may be precipitated by barbiturates.

Bromsulphalein (BSP):

May interfere with alkaline phosphatase determinations.

May produce false-positive tests for acetone by reacting with sodium nitroprusside (as found in some reagent strips).

Caffeine:

Coffee reportedly may result in spurious elevations in serum uric acid as done by an adaptation of the method of Bittner (*Am J Clin Pathol* 1963;**40**:423).

Calcium antacids:

Large doses of calcium carbonate may produce hypercalcemia.

Table 1. Effects of drugs on common laboratory tests.

Legend:

+ = Increase (pharmacologic or toxic effect)
- = Decrease (pharmacologic or toxic effect)
N = See notes (below)
● = Increase (test interference)
○ = Decrease (test interference)
★ = Present or positive

	BLOOD, SERUM, OR PLASMA													URINE										OTHER TESTS
Drug	Amylase	Bilirubin	Cholesterol	Coombs (Direct)	CPK	Glucose	Thyroxine	Phosphatase, Alk.	Potassium	Prothrombin Time	SGOT and SGPT	Urea Nitrogen	Uric Acid	Color	Catecholamines	Glucose (Cu Reduction)	5-HIAA	Ketones	Porphyrins	Protein	Steroids	Urobilinogen	VMA	Other Tests
Acetaminophen	N	N		★		N					+				N	●	N			●				Blood and urine phenylalanine (N)
Acetazolamide (Diamox)		+				-		-				+	+	+						●		+		Blood ammonia +
Acetohexamide (Dymelor)						-	-	+					-				-							
Alcohol, ethyl	+	-	N		N	-		+		+	+	-	+	N	+	N	-		N					Serum aldolase (N); plasma cortisol +; serum lactate +
Allopurinol (Zyloprim)	+	+						+			+		-											
Aluminum antacids								+																Serum phosphate –
Aminocaproic acid (Amicar)					+				+															
Aminoglycosides		N						+	+		+	+		N					N	N		N		Blood ammonia (N); serum magnesium (N); urine estriol (N)
Aminosalicylic acid (PAS)	N	-	-				-	-	+		+			N		●			N					
Amphotericin B (Fungizone)	+	+			+			-	-			+				●				★				
Ampicillin				★	N																			Urine estriol –
Anabolic steroids		+	-			+	-			N	N	N				N					N			
Ascorbic acid	N	N										N	N		N	N				N				
Asparaginase (Elspar)	+	+	-			+		+	+	+	+	N												Blood ammonia +; serum albumin –
Azathioprine (Imuran)	N	+					-	+		+	+	N												
Barbiturates	N	N				N	N	N	N	+	+					N			N	○				Metyrapone response –; serum calcium –; GGT* +; thyroxine –
Bumetanide (Bumex)	+							-	-		+	+	+		+									Serum calcium –
Caffeine			+			+						N											●	
Calcium antacids								+																Serum calcium (N)
Captopril (Capoten)		+	+	★				+												★				Serum albumin –
Carbamazepine (Tegretol)	N	N				N	N	+		+										N				Serum sodium –; serum calcium –

*GGT: Gamma glutamyl transpeptidase.

Carbamazepine:
Jaundice has occurred; incidence must await further trials.
May inhibit hypoprothrombinemic effect of oral anticoagulants.
May produce false-positive Zimmermann reaction for 17-ketosteroids and 17-hydroxycorticosteroids.

Carbenicillin:
Intramuscular administration may result in increased serum CPK levels.

Cephalosporins:
Larger doses may adversely affect renal function, with elevation of the BUN.
Cephalosporins (excluding moxalactam) may form an interfering color in copper reduction methods for urinary glucose, but the effect is usually minor.
Large doses of cephalothin may produce false increases in urinary 17-ketosteroids (Zimmermann reaction).
Cefoxitin and cephalothin (very rarely) may cause positive interference in determining creatinine with methods involving the Jaffe alkaline picrate reaction.

Chloral hydrate:
May transiently increase the hypoprothrombinemic response to oral anticoagulants.
Large doses reportedly may cause false elevation of BUN (nesslerization method).
Attacks of acute intermittent porphyria may be precipitated.
May interfere with fluorimetric test for urine catecholamines.
May interfere with the determination of urinary 17-hydroxycorticosteroids by a modification of the Reddy, Jenkins, Thorn procedure (*Metabolism* 1952;**1**:511 and 1954;**3**:489).

Chloramphenicol:
May see false increases in urea nitrogen (nesslerization method) or false decreases (Berthelot method).

Chloroquine:
May color urine rusty yellow or brown.
May be a precipitating factor in porphyria.

Chlorpropamide:
Serum cholesterol may increase owing to cholestasis or decrease owing to reduced synthesis.
May be a precipitating factor in porphyria.
May cause hyponatremia due to syndrome of inappropriate antidiuretic hormone secretion.

Chlorthalidone:
Has produced pancreatitis, with resultant increase in serum amylase.
Excessive use has produced hypokalemic myopathy with elevated CPK.

Chlorzoxazone:
May color urine orange or purplish-red.

Cholestyramine:
Has produced hyperchloremic acidosis in children.
Absorption of orally administered thyroid hormones is decreased if cholestyramine is given within several hours.

Cimetidine:
May enhance hypoprothrombinemic effect of oral anticoagulants.
Phenol in intravenous cimetidine may turn urine green.

Clindamycin:
Intramuscular administration of clindamycin appears to increase serum CPK levels in a majority of patients.

Clofibrate:
Glucose tolerance tends to improve in diabetics receiving clofibrate.
May enhance the hypoprothrombinemic effect of oral anticoagulants.

Clonidine:
Chronic therapy reduces urine catecholamines, but abrupt withdrawal may increase them.

Codeine:
May elevate serum amylase, but less potent than other opiates (eg, morphine) in this regard.
May produce elevated transaminase levels in certain patients.

Colchicine:
Reported to have an unpredictable antithyroid effect.

Table 1 (cont'd). Effects of drugs on common laboratory tests.

Legend:
+ = Increase (pharmacologic or toxic effect)
- = Decrease (pharmacologic or toxic effect)
N = See notes (below)
● = Increase (test interference)
○ = Decrease (test interference)
★ = Present or positive

Drug	Amylase	Bilirubin	Cholesterol	Coombs (Direct)	CPK	Glucose	Thyroxine	Phosphatase, Alk.	Potassium	Prothrombin Time	SGOT and SGPT	Urea Nitrogen	Uric Acid	Color	Catecholamines	Glucose (Cu Reduction)	5-HIAA	Ketones	Porphyrins	Protein	Steroids	Urobilinogen	VMA	OTHER TESTS
Carbenicillin (Geopen, Pyopen)					N				-															Bleeding time +
Cephalosporins				★						+	+	N			N	N				★	N			Serum creatinine (N)
Chloral hydrate (Noctec)								+		+		N			N	●			N		N			
Chloramphenicol (Chloromycetin)		+										N				●						-		
Chlordiazepoxide (Librium)		+						+		+	+								+					
Chloroquine (Aralen)														N					N					Serum sodium (N)
Chlorpropamide (Diabinese)		+	N	★		-		+		+	+								N					Serum calcium +; blood ammonia +
Chlorthalidone (Hygroton)					N	+		-					+											
Chlorzoxazone (Paraflex)		+																						
Cholestyramine (Cuemid)			-				N		+	+				N										Serum chloride (N)
Cimetidine (Tagamet)											N			N										Serum creatinine +; serum prolactin +
Cisplatin (Platinol)									-	N		+	+											Serum magnesium -; serum calcium -
Clindamycin (Cleocin)					N																			
Clofibrate (Atromid-S)			-		+	N	-	-		+	+		-											Serum aldolase +
Clonidine (Catapres)															N								-	Plasma growth hormone +
Cloxacillin (Tegopen)											+													
Codeine	N										+													Lipase +
Colchicine			-				N																	
Colistin (Coly-Mycin)	N	N						-				+								★				
Contrast media, iodine-containing	N												-											
Corticosteroids	N	+											N		N	N				N	N			Urine estriol -; serum calcium -
Cyclophosphamide (Cytoxan)										+						+				N	N			Serum cholinesterase -

Contrast media, iodine-containing:
Cholangiography may result in transient elevations of serum amylase.
Cholecystographic media can result in increased serum bilirubin.
May see false decreases in urinary metanephrines (Crout modification of Pisano method).
Sodium diatrizoate (Hypaque) may form a black color in copper reduction tests for glucose.
Iodoalphionic acid (Priodax), iopanoic acid (Telepaque), and sodium diatrizoate (Hypaque) may give false positives with sulfosalicylic acid and nitric acid, but not with heat and acetic acid.
May decrease values for 17-ketogenic steroids (Rutherford-Nelson method).

Corticosteroids:
Have produced pancreatitis, with resultant increase in serum amylase.
May increase the requirement for coumarin anticoagulants.
Corticosteroids are weak uricosurics but may produce severe hyperuricemia in patients with acute leukemia.
Potent corticosteroids decrease urinary 17-ketosteroid and 17-hydroxycorticosteroid excretion.

Cyclophosphamide:
Rapid lysis of tumor cells in patients with lymphomas or leukemias may result in hyperkalemia.

Cyproheptadine:
Although depression of fasting blood glucose has been reported, subsequent studies have not confirmed this.

Danazol:
Decreases high-density lipoprotein cholesterol level.
Concentrations of total thyroxine and cortisol may be decreased and the percentage of free thyroxine and cortisol increased.

Dapsone:
Occasional hepatotoxicity with elevated bilirubin, alkaline phosphatase, and transaminases.
Occasional reports of hypoalbuminemia.

Dextrothyroxine:
Enhances hypoprothrombinemic effect of oral anticoagulants.

Digitalis glycosides:
Intramuscular digoxin may increase serum CPK.

Disopyramide:
Occasional hepatotoxicity with elevated serum bilirubin, alkaline phosphatase, and transaminases.
Fasting hypoglycemia may occur, especially in elderly.

Disulfiram:
Inhibits decrease in serum cholesterol that normally occurs when alcoholics abstain.
Enhances hypoprothrombinemic effect of oral anticoagulants.

Epinephrine:
Epinephrine and related agents used in asthma by inhalation may increase urinary catecholamines and urinary VMA.

Erythromycin:
The estolate salt may produce cholestatic hepatitis with elevated bilirubin levels.
May cause false increase of transaminases done by colorimetric methods. The estolate salt may produce true increases in transaminase owing to hepatic toxicity.
May produce false elevation in fluorimetric determinations for urinary catecholamines.

Estrogens:
Oral contraceptives have been associated with pancreatitis and elevated serum amylase.
Cholesterol usually unchanged or decreased in postmenopausal women. Massive elevation of cholesterol and triglyceride occasionally reported.
May increase cortisol-binding proteins, resulting in moderate decrease in urinary 17-ketosteroids and 17-hydroxycorticosteroids.

Ethacrynic acid:
Has been implicated in the production of pancreatitis, with resultant increase in serum amylase.
Both hypoglycemia (in uremic patients) and hyperglycemia (in diabetics) have been reported.
May cause uricosuria if given intravenously and urate retention if given orally.
May slightly decrease urinary cortisol excretion.

Table 1 (cont'd). Effects of drugs on common laboratory tests.

+ = Increase (pharmacologic or toxic effect)
− = Decrease (pharmacologic or toxic effect)
N = See notes (below)

● = Increase (test interference)
○ = Decrease (test interference)
★ = Present or positive

Drug	Amylase	Bilirubin	Cholesterol	Coombs (Direct)	CPK	Glucose	Thyroxine	Phosphatase, Alk.	Potassium	Prothrombin Time	SGOT and SGPT	Urea Nitrogen	Uric Acid	Color	Catecholamines	Glucose (Cu Reduction)	5-HIAA	Ketones	Porphyrins	Protein	Steroids	Urobilinogen	VMA	Other Tests
Cyproheptadine (Periactin)	+																							
Danazol (Danocrine)		N	N				N	+	+	+	+													GGT*; prolactin −; cortisol (N)
Dapsone (Avlusulfon)		N						N		N	N									+				Serum albumin (N)
Dextrothyroxine (Choloxin)			−			+	+			N						+								
Diazoxide (Hyperstat)						+							+			+								
Digitalis glycosides					N																			Serum estrogen +
Disopyramide (Norpace)		N				N		N		N	N													
Disulfiram (Antabuse)		+	N				+	+	N	+	+				−								−	
Epinephrine		N				+		+				+			N								N	
Erythromycin		N					+	+	N	N	N				N									
Estrogens	N	+	N			+	+	+		+	+					+					N			Serum ceruloplasmin +; serum iron +; plasma cortisol +
Ethacrynic acid (Edecrin)	N					N			−			N	N								N			
Ethambutol (Myambutol)										+	+		+											
Ethchlorvynol (Placidyl)								+	N	N	+													
Ethinamate (Valmid)										N											N			
Ethionamide (Trecator-SC)		+					−	+		+	+													
Furazolidone (Furoxone)														N										
Furosemide (Lasix)	N					+	+	+	−			+	+											Blood ammonia +; serum calcium −
Glucagon						+			N															Serum calcium −
Glucose infusions						+			−			−				N								Blood ammonia (N)
Glutethimide (Doriden)								N	N			−									●			Serum calcium (N)
Glyceryl guaiacolate (Robitussin)																	●						N	

*GGT: Gamma glutamyl transpeptidase.

Ethchlorvynol:
May depress the anticoagulant activity of the coumarin anticoagulants.

Ethinamate:
May markedly increase the absorption in 17-ketosteroid determinations (modified Zimmermann reaction).

Furazolidone:
May color urine brown.

Furosemide:
Has precipitated pancreatitis, with resultant increase in serum amylase. (Also, small increases in serum amylase occur regularly.)

Glucagon:
May enhance response to oral anticoagulants.

Glucose:
Intravenous glucose may produce glycosuria in some patients.
Some studies have shown that a large glucose load may increase blood ammonia in patients with cirrhosis and portasystemic shunts; however, further studies have indicated that this effect is small.

Glutethimide:
Long-term use occasionally results in osteomalacia, with elevated alkaline phosphatase and reduced serum calcium.
May enhance metabolism of coumarin anticoagulants.

Glyceryl guaiacolate:
May cause a color change during screening methods for VMA, but final measurement apparently is not affected.

Gold:
Gold-induced nephrotic syndrome of colitis may lower serum albumin, globulins, or both.

Griseofulvin:
May depress anticoagulant activity of coumarin anticoagulants.
May precipitate acute attack in patients with porphyria.

Guanethidine:
Has antidiabetic activity and may decrease insulin requirements.

Heparin:
In acquired hemolytic anemia, heparin may cause the direct Coombs test to become negative.
Reportedly may increase blood glucose; confirmation is needed.
Free thyroxine may be falsely low (Amerlex method) or falsely high (Liquisol method).
Hyperkalemia in predisposed patients, due to heparin-induced decrease in aldosterone synthesis.
May decrease urinary 5-HIAA excretion in patients with carcinoid syndrome.

Hydralazine:
Occasional hepatotoxicity with elevated bilirubin, alkaline phosphatase, and transaminase.

Indomethacin:
Has produced pancreatitis, with resultant increase in serum amylase.
Hyperkalemia has occurred in some patients, and in others the hypokalemia of Bartter's syndrome has improved.

Inorganic iodides:
Occasionally produce thyrotoxicosis with elevated serum thyroxine.
May interfere with the determination of urinary 17-hydroxycorticosteroids by a modification of the Reddy, Jenkins, Thorn procedure (*Metabolism* 1952;1:511 and 1954;3:489).

Insulin:
Insulin-induced hypoglycemia results in release of epinephrine, thus increasing urinary excretion.

Iron, oral:
Administration of ferrous sulfate and ferrous fumarate has resulted in false-positive benzidine tests for occult blood in the stools.
May interfere with serum calcium (EDTA titration method).

Isoniazid:
Both true glycosuria and false-positive copper reduction tests have been reported.
Acetonuria may occur with isoniazid intoxication.
Although isoniazid is reported to increase blood ammonia, some studies have failed to confirm this.
Isoniazid intoxication may increase serum lactate.

Table 1 (cont'd). Effects of drugs on common laboratory tests.

Legend:
+ = Increase (pharmacologic or toxic effect)
− = Decrease (pharmacologic or toxic effect)
N = See notes (below)
● = Increase (test interference)
○ = Decrease (test interference)
★ = Present or positive

Drug	BLOOD, SERUM, OR PLASMA													URINE										OTHER TESTS
	Amylase	Bilirubin	Cholesterol	Coombs (Direct)	CPK	Glucose	Thyroxine	Phosphatase, Alk.	Potassium	Prothrombin Time	SGOT and SGPT	Urea Nitrogen	Uric Acid	Color	Catecholamines	Glucose (Cu Reduction)	5-HIAA	Ketones	Porphyrins	Protein	Steroids	Urobilinogen	VMA	
Gold salts		+																		★				Serum proteins (N)
Griseofulvin (Fulvicin, Grifulvin)								+			+									★				
Guanethidine (Ismelin)						N						+			−								−	
Heparin			−			N			+	+	+													
Hydralazine (Apresoline)		N		★				+		N	N					●			N					
Imipramine (Tofranil)		+	+					+															−	
Indomethacin (Indocin)	N	+		★				+	−	+	+	+					−							Serum calcium −
Insulin						−			−															
Iodides, inorganic							N								N									Stool blood (N); serum calcium (N)
Iron, oral		+																						Blood ammonia (N); blood lactate (N)
Isoniazid (INH)		+		★		+		+			+					N		N						
Isotretinoin (Accutane)											+													Serum triglycerides +
Levodopa (L-dopa)	N	N		★									N	N		N	−	N					N	
Levothyroxine (Synthroid)					N		N			N														
Lidocaine						+	−																	
Lithium carbonate						+				N	N													
Mefenamic acid (Ponstel)				N						N										★			N	Urine bilirubin ●
Meperidine (Demerol)		+																		★				
Mephenesin (Sinan, Tolserol)																	●						N	
Meprobamate (Equanil, Miltown)		+						+		N											N		N	Metyrapone response −

Levodopa:
May produce false increase in serum bilirubin (SMA 12/60).
May produce false increases for serum uric acid by colorimetric methods but not when uricase is used. True increases also reported.
Urine may darken on standing.
Both false-positive Clinitest and false-negative glucose oxidase reactions may occur, especially with large doses.
May interfere with ferric chloride tests for urine ketones, Ketostix, and possibly Acetest.
Small increase in urinary VMA excretion, but VMA measured by Pisano method may be falsely decreased.

Levothyroxine:
Serum thyroxine levels increased to normal or above normal in adequately treated patients.
Increasing thyroid hormone activity enhances anticoagulant effect of coumarins.

Lidocaine:
Intramuscular lidocaine may increase serum CPK.

Lithium carbonate:
Preliminary studies indicate that urinary VMA excretion may be somewhat increased.

Mefenamic acid:
Autoimmune hemolytic anemia may occur after prolonged therapy.
May increase response to oral anticoagulants.

Meperidine:
May elevate transaminase levels in certain patients.

Mephenesin:
May cause color changes during screening methods for VMA, but final measurement apparently is not affected.

Meprobamate:
May increase the absorbance in measurements for 17-ketosteroids (Zimmermann reaction).
May inhibit antiprothrombinemic effect of warfarin.

Mercurial diuretics:
Meralluride (Mercuhydrin) may produce false negatives for urinary glucose as measured by glucose oxidase methods (eg, Clinistix, Tes-Tape).

Methenamine:
Produces false elevation in urinary 17-hydroxycorticosteroids by method of Reddy (*Metabolism* 1954;**3**:489).
May interfere with tests for urinary urobilinogen.

Methicillin:
Intrathecal administration may result in false-positive CF protein using Du-Pont method (trichloroacetic acid method).

Methocarbamol:
Parenteral preparations may contain polyethylene glycol, which may increase urea retention in patients with renal impairment.
Urine may darken on standing.
May produce false increases in urinary VMA by screening method of Gitlow but not in quantitative procedure of Sunderman.

Methotrexate:
Nephropathy with elevated urea nitrogen has been reported.
Hyperuricemia may occur owing to rapid lysis of tumor cells.

Methyldopa:
May produce sialadenitis with increased amylase.
Urine may darken on standing.
Does not appreciably affect VMA determinations.

Methylene blue:
Colors the urine blue.

Metronidazole:
Enhances hypoprothrombinemic effect of oral anticoagulants.
May cause darkening of urine.

Miconazole:
May enhance hypoprothrombinemic effect of oral anticoagulants.
May cause false increases in urine protein (turbimetric method).

Monoamine oxidase inhibitors:
Although MAO inhibitors have been reported to reduce blood ammonia, some of these agents have produced hepatotoxicity and thus could be dangerous in patients with impaired liver function.
Nialamide may decrease the response to metyrapone.
Phenelzine (Nardil) may decrease serum cholinesterase levels.

Table 1 (cont'd). Effects of drugs on common laboratory tests.

Legend:
- + = Increase (pharmacologic or toxic effect)
- − = Decrease (pharmacologic or toxic effect)
- N = See notes (below)
- ● = Increase (test interference)
- ○ = Decrease (test interference)
- ★ = Present or positive

Drug	Amylase	Bilirubin	Cholesterol	Coombs (Direct)	CPK	Glucose	Thyroxine	Phosphatase, Alk.	Potassium	Prothrombin Time	SGOT and SGPT	Urea Nitrogen	Uric Acid	Color	Catecholamines	Glucose (Cu Reduction)	5-HIAA	Ketones	Porphyrins	Protein	Steroids	Urobilinogen	VMA	Other Tests
Mercurial diuretics													+			N								
Methenamine (Mandelamine, Uritone)		+													●		○				N	N		Urine estriol ○
Methicillin (Dimocillin, Staphcillin)												+					●						N	Cerebrospinal fluid protein (N)
Methocarbamol (Robaxin)												N		N						★			N	
Methotrexate	N							+			+	N	N											
Methyldopa (Aldomet)	N	+		★				+			+	+		N	●		−						N	
Methylene blue														N										
Metronidazole (Flagyl)									N	N				N						N				Serum triglycerides +
Miconazole (Monistat i.v.)			+			−			N	N							−	N	N				−	
Monoamine oxidase inhibitors (MAOI)																								Blood ammonia (N); metyrapone response (N); serum cholinesterase (N)
Morphine	+										N				●	●				N				
Nafcillin (Unipen)											+													
Nalidixic acid (NegGram)		+	−			N					+	+				●					N			Serum lactate +
Nicotinic acid (large doses)		+				+		+			+	+			●	N								
Nitrofurantoin (Furadantin)		N						N			+			N										
Nitroglycerin															+								+	
Novobiocin (Albamycin)		N																						
Oral contraceptives	N	+	N				+	+		N	+	N							N	N	N			Metyrapone response −; serum cortisol +; serum calcium (N); serum phosphate (N); serum prolactin +
Oxacillin (Prostaphlin)																				N				
Pargyline (Eutonyl)						−											−						−	
Penicillamine (Cuprimine)							−				+									★				
Penicillin G				★					N							●				N	N			

Morphine:
May elevate transaminase levels in certain patients.
Attacks of acute intermittent porphyria may be precipitated.

Nafcillin:
Large doses may produce false positives for urine protein (sulfosalicylic acid method) and interfere with the interpretation of the trichloroacetic acid method.

Nalidixic acid:
Large doses or overdoses may produce false elevations in blood glucose (Somogyi-Nelson procedure).
May cause false elevation of urinary 17-ketosteroids (Zimmermann reaction).

Nicotinic acid:
May impair glucose tolerance, resulting in glycosuria.

Nitrofurantoin:
Cholestatic jaundice occasionally occurs following nitrofurantoin.
May cause false decrease in alkaline phosphatase or a true increase owing to hepatitis.
May tint urine brown.

Novobiocin:
May produce jaundice with an increase in unconjugated but not conjugated bilirubin in plasma; also, a yellow pigment may occur in the plasma that interferes with icterus index and bilirubin determinations.

Oral contraceptives:
Hyperlipidemic patients have developed pancreatitis following initiation of oral contraceptive use.
Oral contraceptives have been reported to elevate serum cholesterol.
A decrease in the hypoprothrombinemic effect of oral anticoagulants may occur.
May affect the handling of porphyrins by the liver; urinary coproporphyrin excretion may be increased.
The estrogenic component may increase cortisol-binding proteins, resulting in a moderate decrease in urinary 17-ketosteroids and 17-hydroxycorticosteroids.
May cause hypocalcemia and hypophosphatemia, resulting in secondary hyperparathyroidism.

Oxacillin:
High doses in infants may cause azotemia and proteinuria.

Penicillin G:
Massive intravenous doses of penicillin G sodium may produce hypokalemia. Penicillin G potassium can produce hyperkalemia.
Massive doses may yield false-positive results for proteinuria when turbidity measures are used (eg, heat and acetic acid, sulfosalicylic acid).
Intravenous doses may produce false elevations of 17-ketogenic steroids (Norymberski method) and a less marked increase in 17-ketosteroid determinations (Zimmermann reaction).

Pentamidine:
Isolated reports of acute pancreatitis with elevated serum amylase.
Tends to produce hypoglycemia but rarely may produce hyperglycemia.

Pentazocine:
Causes sphincter of Oddi spasm, indicating that elevations of serum amylase may occur.

Phenazopyridine:
May color urine orange to orange-red.
May produce interfering colors for urine ketones by Ketostix or Gerhardt ferric chloride method.
May produce falsely high readings in the assay of porphyrins by spectrophotofluorimetry.
May interfere with Ames reagent strips for urine protein as well as the nitric acid ring test.
May yield a pink to red color in Ehrlich's test for urobilinogen.

Phenothiazines:
Intramuscular chlorpromazine may result in increased CPK levels.
Chlorprothixene may result in significant uricosuria.
May color urine pink to red or red-brown.
Chlorpromazine may result in high apparent values for urine metanephrines (Pisano method).
May interfere with diacetic acid determinations.
May cause false increases in 17-ketosteroids (Zimmermann reaction).
Chlorpromazine may produce moderate decreases in urinary VMA excretion.

Table 1 (cont'd). Effects of drugs on common laboratory tests.

+ = Increase (pharmacologic or toxic effect)
− = Decrease (pharmacologic or toxic effect)
N = See notes (below)
● = Increase (test interference)
○ = Decrease (test interference)
★ = Present or positive

	BLOOD, SERUM, OR PLASMA													URINE										OTHER TESTS
	Amylase	Bilirubin	Cholesterol	Coombs (Direct)	CPK	Glucose	Thyroxine	Phosphatase, Alk.	Potassium	Prothrombin Time	SGOT and SGPT	Urea Nitrogen	Uric Acid	Color	Catecholamines	Glucose (Cu Reduction)	5-HIAA	Ketones	Porphyrins	Protein	Steroids	Urobilinogen	VMA	
Pentamidine	N					N						+												
Pentazocine (Talwin)	N																							
Phenazopyridine (Pyridium)		+	+					+						N				N	N	N	N	N		Urine bilirubin ●
Phenothiazines		+	+		N	+	+	+			+	+	N	N	N		○	N	N	N	N	●	N	Metyrapone response −; serum albumin −
Phenylbutazone (Butazolidin)	N	N	+					+	−		+	+	N											
Phenytoin (Dilantin)		N	+			+	−	+			+													Metyrapone response −; serum calcium −
Polymyxin B (Aerosporin)												+								★				
Primaquine																								
Probenecid (Benemid)		+						+		+	+		−			●					N			
Procainamide (Pronestyl)		+						+			+								N		N	N		
Procaine													+						N		N	N		
Progestogens							+						+											
Propoxyphene (Darvon)		+				N		+		+	+			N	N						N			
Propranolol (Inderal)		N				−	N			N	+	+												
Propylthiouracil		+					−		+	+	+													
Pyrazinamide (PZA)		+						+	N	N	+		+								N			
Quinacrine (Atabrine)		+						+			+		+	N										
Quinethazone (Hydromox)						+							+											
Quinidine		+		★			−	+	+	+	+				●		N				N			
Reserpine							−							N	N		N				N		N	
Riboflavin														N	●									
Rifampin (Rifadin, Rimactane)	+	+		★				+		N	+	N		N										

Phenylbutazone:

May occasionally produce hepatitis with hyperbilirubinemia.

Parotitis, with resultant elevation of serum amylase, is a rare complication of phenylbutazone therapy.

Markedly enhances hypoprothrombinemic effect of oral anticoagulants.

Phenylbutazone is a weak uricosuric.

Phenytoin:

Serum bilirubin tends to be low (owing to phenytoin-induced enzyme induction), but hepatotoxicity with jaundice occasionally occurs.

Slightly decreases excretion of 17-ketosteroids and 17-hydroxycorticosteroids.

Probenecid:

May decrease urinary 17-ketosteroid excretion.

Procaine:

May react with Ehrlich's reagent in test for porphyrins or urobilinogen.

Propoxyphene:

Has produced hypoglycemia in a patient with impaired renal function.

Preliminary evidence indicates that propoxyphene may cause false decreases in urinary 17-hydroxycorticosteroids (Porter-Silber) and 17-ketosteroids (Zimmermann reaction).

Propranolol:

False increases in serum bilirubin (by SMA 12/60) in uremic patients taking propranolol.

Total and free thyroxine levels may be increased by doses of 160 mg or greater, while serum triiodothyronine levels tend to decrease.

False decrease in urine metanephrines (Pisano method).

Pyrazinamide:

May decrease plasma prothrombin levels owing to its hepatotoxicity.

Urinary 17-ketosteroids may be decreased, followed by a return to normal.

Quinacrine:

May color the urine yellow.

Quinidine:

May interfere with the determination of urinary 17-hydroxycorticosteroids by a modification of the Reddy, Jenkins, Thorn procedure.

Reserpine:

May cause slight initial increase in excretion of 5-HIAA.

May cause slight increase in absorbance in 17-hydroxycorticosteroid measurements (modified Glenn-Nelson technique).

Chronic administration decreases urinary catecholamine and VMA excretion; however, increases in both may be seen during the first day or 2 of therapy.

Riboflavin:

Large doses may produce yellow discoloration in urine.

Rifampin:

Inhibits hypoprothrombinemic effect of oral anticoagulants.

May produce acute renal failure with elevated urea nitrogen.

May produce red-orange color in urine.

Salicylates:

Salicylism has resulted in pancreatitis, with resultant increase in serum amylase.

Large doses may decrease serum cholesterol.

Salicylate overdose may increase serum CPK.

The salicylates have variable effects on blood glucose; a hypoglycemic action may be seen (especially in diabetics), and both hyperglycemia and hypoglycemia have occurred from salicylate intoxication.

Large doses (eg, 3–5 g/d) can cause uricosuria; smaller doses result in urate retention.

Aspirin may interfere with fluorescence methods for urinary 5-HIAA.

May produce an interfering color in ferric chloride test for acetoacetic acid.

False increases with various methods for urinary VMA, but false *decreases* may occur with Pisano method.

Sulfonamides:

Reports have appeared describing pancreatitis, with elevated serum amylase, following sulfasalazine and sulfamethizole.

Jaundice has been produced, owing to both acute hemolytic anemia and hepatotoxicity.

Some sulfonamides enhance the hypoprothrombinemic effect of oral anticoagulants.

May color urine rusty yellow or brownish.

May react with Ehrlich's reagent in test for porphyrins or urobilinogen. May also precipitate an attack of acute intermittent porphyria.

Sulfisoxazole may lead to false-positive results for proteinuria by turbidity and by heat and acid methods; also, many sulfonamides may result in crystalluria with true proteinuria.

Table 1 (cont'd). Effects of drugs on common laboratory tests.

+ = Increase (pharmacologic or toxic effect)
− = Decrease (pharmacologic or toxic effect)
N = See notes (below)
● = Increase (test interference)
○ = Decrease (test interference)
★ = Present or positive

Drug	Amylase	Bilirubin	Cholesterol	Coombs (Direct)	CPK	Glucose	Thyroxine	Phosphatase, Alk.	Potassium	Prothrombin Time	SGOT and SGPT	Urea Nitrogen	Uric Acid	Color	Catecholamines	Glucose (Cu Reduction)	5-HIAA	Ketones	Porphyrins	Protein	Steroids	Urobilinogen	VMA	Other Tests
Salicylates	N	+	N		N	N	−	+	−	+	+		N		−	●	N	N		★			N	Urine estriol −
Spironolactone (Aldactone)									+			+									●			Plasma cortisol ●
Succinylcholine (Anectine)									+			+												
Sulfinpyrazone (Anturane)													−											
Sulfonamides	N	N	+				−	+		N	+					●			N	N		N		
Sulindac (Clinoril)	N	N	N			N		N		N	N			N	●	●				N				
Tetracyclines	N		N			N		+		N	+	+				N						−		Serum lipase (N)
Thiabendazole (Mintezol)											+						−							
Thiazide diuretics	+		+			+		−	−		+	+	+			N					N			Blood ammonia +; serum calcium +; serum sodium (N); serum magnesium −
Thyroglobulin (Proloid)			−				N																	
Thyroid, desiccated			−			+	N			N														
Tolazamide (Tolinase)		+				−		+			+				N				N					
Tolbutamide (Orinase)		+				−	−	+			+				N					N				
Tolmetin (Tolectin)																				N				
Triamterene (Dyrenium)						+		+			+	+	+	N										
Tricyclic antidepressants		+				N				N	+	+		N	N								−	Serum prolactin (N)
Triiodothyronine (Cytomel)			−				−																	
Trimethadione (Tridione)											+	+								★				
Valproic acid (Depakene)	N	+				+		+			+													Blood ammonia +
Verapamil						N									N									Serum prolactin +
Vitamin A		N						N		N	N													Serum calcium (N)

Sulindac:
Isolated cases of pancreatitis, with elevated serum amylase.
Isolated cases of liver function abnormalities (eg, increased serum bilirubin, alkaline phosphatase, transaminases).
Isolated cases of proteinuria have occurred.

Tetracyclines:
Prolonged high doses have resulted in pancreatitis in certain patients, with elevations in serum amylase and lipase.
Oral chlortetracycline may reduce serum cholesterol.
Oxytetracycline has produced hypoglycemic effects in diabetics but apparently not in normal subjects.
Intravenous tetracycline may decrease plasma prothrombin activity; also, tetracyclines may reduce the vitamin K–producing bacteria in the gut.
Parenteral forms containing ascorbic acid may cause false negatives in urinary glucose by glucose oxidase methods (eg, Clinistix, Tes-Tape).

Thiabendazole:
Hyperglycemia may occur (incidence is low).

Thiazide diuretics:
May cause hyperglycemia and glycosuria in patients predisposed to diabetes.
May cause slight decrease in urinary cortisol excretion.
Has been associated with hyponatremia due to syndrome of inappropriate antidiuretic hormone secretion.

Thyroglobulin; desiccated thyroid:
Effects on serum thyroxine should be consistent with metabolic effects.
Increasing thyroid hormone activity increases anticoagulant effect of coumarins.

Tolbutamide:
A metabolite may cause false-positive tests for proteinuria when turbidity procedures are used (eg, heat and acetic acid, sulfosalicylic acid).

Tolmetin:
False-positive reactions for urinary protein with sulfosalicylic acid method due to precipitation of the decarboxylic acid metabolite.

Triamterene:
May produce a pale blue fluorescence in the urine.
False increases in urinary metanephrines (Sandhu and Freed method).

Tricyclic antidepressants:
Both increases and decreases in serum glucose have been noted.
False-positive interference in urinary metanephrine determination (Pisano method by imipramine).
Amoxapine may increase prolactin levels; women usually experience a greater response than men.

Triiodothyronine:
Increasing thyroid hormone activity increases hypoprothrombinemic effect of coumarins.

Troleandomycin (triacetyloleandomycin):
May cause false elevations of 17-ketosteroids (Drekter) and 17-hydroxycorticosteroids (Porter-Silber).

Valproic acid:
Isolated cases of pancreatitis with increased serum amylase.

Verapamil:
May improve glucose tolerance in patients with non–insulin-dependent diabetes.

Vitamin A:
Intoxication may produce hepatotoxicity with increased bilirubin, alkaline phosphatase, and transaminase.
Intoxication may produce hypercalcemia.

CONVERSION TABLES

Fahrenheit/Celsius Temperature Conversion
($°F = 9/5°C + 32; °C = 5/9[°F - 32]$)

°F	°C	°F	°C
90	= 32.2	100	= 37.8
91	= 32.8	101	= 38.3
92	= 33.3	102	= 38.9
93	= 33.9	103	= 39.4
94	= 34.4	104	= 40.0
95	= 35.0	105	= 40.6
96	= 35.6	106	= 41.1
97	= 36.1	107	= 41.7
98	= 36.7	108	= 42.2
99	= 37.2	109	= 42.8

Milliequivalent Conversion Factors

meq/L of:	Divide mg/dL or vol% by:
Calcium	2.0
Chloride (from Cl)	3.5
(from NaCl)	5.85
CO_2 combining power	2.222
Magnesium	1.2
Phosphorus	3.1 (mmol)
Potassium	3.9
Sodium	2.3

Metric System Prefixes
(Small Measurement)

In accordance with the decision of several scientific societies to employ a universal system of metric nomenclature, the following prefixes have become standard in many medical tests and journals.

k	kilo-	10^3
c	centi-	10^{-2}
m	milli-	10^{-3}
μ	micro-	10^{-6}
n	nano- (formerly millimicro, mμ)	10^{-9}
p	pico- (formerly micromicro, μμ)	10^{-12}
f	femto-	10^{-15}
a	atto-	10^{-18}

Household Equivalents (Approximate)

1 tsp = 6 mL
1 tbsp = 15 mL
1 oz (eg, medicine glass) = 30 mL
1 cup = 8 fluid oz = 240 mL
1 quart = 946 mL

Apothecary Equivalents

Metric			Approximate Apothecary Equivalents		Metric			Approximate Apothecary Equivalents	
30	g	...	1	oz	20	mg	...	1/3	gr
6	g	...	90	gr	15	mg	...	1/4	gr
5	g	...	75	gr	12	mg	...	1/5	gr
4	g	...	60	gr	10	mg	...	1/6	gr
3	g	...	45	gr	8	mg	...	1/8	gr
2	g	...	30	gr	6	mg	...	1/10	gr
1.5	g	...	22	gr	5	mg	...	1/12	gr
1	g	...	15	gr	4	mg	...	1/15	gr
0.75	g	...	12	gr	3	mg	...	1/20	gr
0.6	g	...	10	gr	2	mg	...	1/30	gr
0.5	g	...	7 ½	gr	1.5	mg	...	1/40	gr
0.4	g	...	6	gr	1.2	mg	...	1/50	gr
0.3	g	...	5	gr	1	mg	...	1/60	gr
0.25	g	...	4	gr	0.8	mg	...	1/80	gr
0.2	g	...	3	gr	0.6	mg	...	1/100	gr
0.15	g	...	2 ½	gr	0.5	mg	...	1/120	gr
0.12	g	...	2	gr	0.4	mg	...	1/150	gr
0.1	g	...	1 ½	gr	0.3	mg	...	1/200	gr
75	mg	...	1 ¼	gr	0.25	mg	...	1/250	gr
60	mg	...	1	gr	0.2	mg	...	1/300	gr
50	mg	...	¾	gr	0.15	mg	...	1/400	gr
40	mg	...	⅔	gr	0.12	mg	...	1/500	gr
30	mg	...	½	gr	0.1	mg	...	1/600	gr
25	mg	...	⅜	gr					

Pounds to Kilograms
(1 kg = 2.2 lb; 1 lb = 0.45 kg)

lb	kg	lb	kg	lb	kg	lb	kg	lb	kg
5	2.3	50	22.7	95	43.1	140	63.5	185	83.9
10	4.5	55	25.0	100	45.4	145	65.8	190	86.2
15	6.8	60	27.2	105	47.6	150	68.0	195	88.5
20	9.1	65	29.5	110	49.9	155	70.3	200	90.7
25	11.3	70	31.7	115	52.2	160	72.6	205	93.0
30	13.6	75	34.0	120	54.4	165	74.8	210	95.3
35	15.9	80	36.3	125	56.7	170	77.1	215	97.5
40	18.1	85	38.6	130	58.9	175	79.4	220	99.8
45	20.4	90	40.8	135	61.2	180	81.6		

Feet and Inches to Centimeters
(1 cm = 0.39 in; 1 in = 2.54 cm)

ft	in	cm	ft	in	cm	ft	in	cm	ft	in	cm	ft	in	cm
0	6	15.2	2	4	71.1	3	4	101.6	4	4	132.0	5	4	162.6
1	0	30.5	2	5	73.6	3	5	104.1	4	5	134.6	5	5	165.1
1	6	45.7	2	6	76.1	3	6	106.6	4	6	137.1	5	6	167.6
1	7	48.3	2	7	78.7	3	7	109.2	4	7	139.6	5	7	170.2
1	8	50.8	2	8	81.2	3	8	111.7	4	8	142.2	5	8	172.7
1	9	53.3	2	9	83.8	3	9	114.2	4	9	144.7	5	9	175.3
1	10	55.9	2	10	86.3	3	10	116.8	4	10	147.3	5	10	177.8
1	11	58.4	2	11	88.8	3	11	119.3	4	11	149.8	5	11	180.3
2	0	61.0	3	0	91.4	4	0	121.9	5	0	152.4	6	0	182.9
2	1	63.5	3	1	93.9	4	1	124.4	5	1	154.9	6	1	185.4
2	2	66.0	3	2	96.4	4	2	127.0	5	2	157.5	6	2	188.0
2	3	68.6	3	3	99.0	4	3	129.5	5	3	160.0	6	3	190.5

Desirable Weights (Pounds)

Men (Age 25 and Over)				Women (Age 25 and Over)*			
Height* Feet Inches	**Small Frame**	**Medium Frame**	**Large Frame**	**Height**[†] Feet Inches	**Small Frame**	**Medium Frame**	**Large Frame**
5 2	112–120	118–129	126–141	4 10	92– 98	96–107	104–119
5 3	115–123	121–133	129–144	4 11	94–101	98–110	106–122
5 4	118–126	124–136	132–148	5 0	96–104	101–113	109–125
5 5	121–129	127–139	135–152	5 1	99–107	104–116	112–128
5 6	124–133	130–143	138–156	5 2	102–110	107–119	115–131
5 7	128–137	134–147	142–161	5 3	105–113	110–122	118–134
5 8	132–141	138–152	147–166	5 4	108–116	113–126	121–138
5 9	136–145	142–156	151–170	5 5	111–119	116–130	125–142
5 10	140–150	146–160	155–174	5 6	114–123	120–135	129–146
5 11	144–154	150–165	159–179	5 7	118–127	124–139	133–150
6 0	148–158	154–170	164–184	5 8	121–131	128–143	137–154
6 1	152–162	158–175	168–189	5 9	126–135	132–147	141–158
6 2	156–167	162–180	173–194	5 10	130–140	136–151	145–163
6 3	160–171	167–185	178–199	5 11	134–144	140–155	149–168
6 4	164–175	172–190	182–204	6 0	138–148	144–159	153–173

*With shoes with 1-inch heels.

*For women between 18 and 25, subtract 1 lb for each year under 25.
[†]With shoes with 2-inch heels.

This table was derived primarily from data on the Build and Blood Pressure Study, 1959, Society of Actuaries. A useful discussion is presented in Seltzer CC, Mayer J: How representative are the weights of insured men and women? *JAMA* 1967;**201**:221.

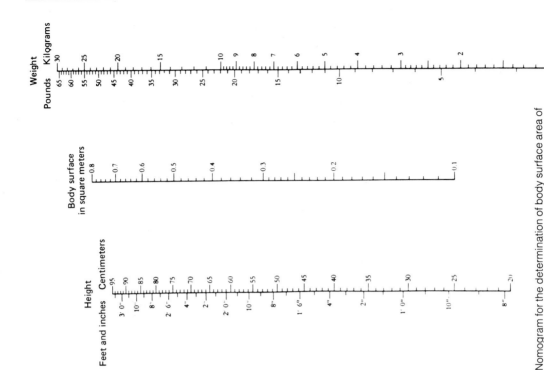

Nomogram for the determination of body surface area of children. (Reproduced, with permission, from Du Bois: *Basal Metabolism in Health and Disease.* Lea & Febiger, 1936.)

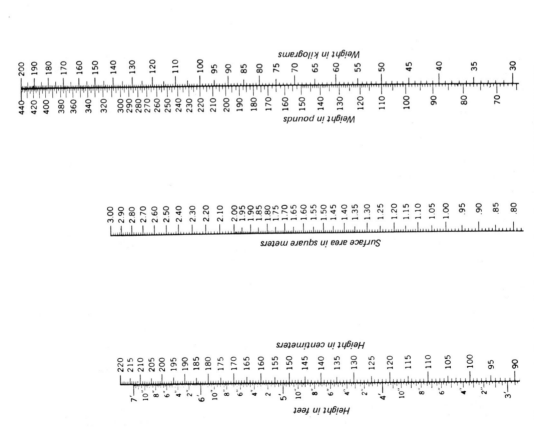

Nomogram for the determination of body surface area of children and adults. (Reproduced, with permission, from Boothby and Sandiford: *Boston MSJ* 1921;**184**:337.) [Revised 1979.]

Appendix III:
Trade Names/Generic Names

Note to Reader: In this text we have attempted to identify every drug by its "USAN" (United States Adopted Names) designation.* This name is also considered the generic name of the drug in the USA. Because some drugs are marketed under a multiplicity of trade names, not all of which are listed in the Index, we provide this Appendix. The list that follows gives the generic names of the drugs whose trade (or other) names are listed alphabetically (in capital letters). The impossible task of including all trade names is not attempted. The purpose of the list is to help the reader who knows a drug only by its trade or alternative name identify it by its current generic name.

A-200 PYRINATE: Pyrethrins, piperonyl butoxide
ABBOKINASE: Urokinase
ACCUTANE: Isotretinoin
ACETONYL: Aspirin
ACETOSPAN: Triamcinolone acetonide
ACHROMYCIN: Tetracycline hydrochloride
ACHROSTATIN V: Nystatin, tetracycline hydrochloride (combination product)
ACILLIN: Ampicillin
ACTAMER: Bithionol
ACTHAR: Corticotropin (injection)
ACTIDIL: Triprolidine hydrochloride
ACTI-DIONE: Cycloheximide
ACTIFED: Pseudoephedrine hydrochloride, triprolidine hydrochloride (combination product)
ACTRAPID: Insulin
ADALAT: Nifedipine
ADANON HYDROCHLORIDE: Methadone hydrochloride
ADAPIN: Doxepin hydrochloride
ADEMOL: Flumethiazide
ADRENALIN: Epinephrine
ADRIAMYCIN: Doxorubicin hydrochloride
ADROYD: Oxymetholone
ADRUCIL: Fluorouracil
ADVIL: Ibuprofen
AEROSPORIN: Polymyxin B sulfate
AFRIN: Oxymetazoline hydrochloride
AFTATE: Tolnaftate
AGRIBON: Sulfadimethoxine
AKINETON: Biperiden
ALBAMYCIN: Novobiocin
ALBON: Sulfadimethoxine
ALCAINE: Proparacaine hydrochloride
ALCOPAR: Bephenium hydroxynaphthoate

ALCOPARA: Bephenium hydroxynaphthoate
ALDACTAZIDE: Hydrochlorothiazide, spironolactone (combination product)
ALDACTONE: Spironolactone
ALDOCLOR: Chlorothiazide, methyldopa (combination product)
ALDOCORTIN: Aldosterone
ALDOMET: Methyldopa
ALDORIL: Hydrochlorothiazide, methyldopa (combination product)
ALERMINE: Chlorpheniramine maleate
ALIDASE: Hyaluronidase (injection)
ALKERAN: Melphalan
ALLEREST: Chlorpheniramine maleate, phenylpropanolamine hydrochloride (combination product)
ALLOFERIN: Alcuronium chloride
ALMOCARPINE: Pilocarpine hydrochloride
ALPHADROL: Fluprednisolone
ALPHA-RUVITE: Hydroxocobalamin
ALTAFUR: Furaltadone
ALTHOSE HYDROCHLORIDE: Methadone hydrochloride
ALUPENT: Metaproterenol sulfate
ALYSINE: Sodium salicylate
AMBILHAR: Niridazole
AMBODRYL HYDROCHLORIDE: Bromodiphenhydramine hydrochloride
AMCILL: Ampicillin
AMEN: Medroxyprogesterone acetate
AMERICAINE: Benzocaine
AMICAR: Aminocaproic acid
AMIFUR: Nitrofurazone
AMIKIN: Amikacin sulfate
AMINODUR: Aminophylline

*Names are listed in *USAN and the USP Dictionary of Drug Names* (1986 edition, United States Pharamacopeial Convention, Inc., 12601 Twinbrook Parkway, Rockville, MD 20852) and other sources. Many of the names are no longer current, either because the product itself has been discontinued or because the firm has discontinued production and no longer markets the drug under that name. Such items are listed for identification of drugs in the older literature, in patients' health records, in pharmacists' prescription files, etc.

AMITID: Amitriptyline hydrochloride
AMOXIL: Amoxicillin
AMPYROX: Methscopolamine bromide
AMSTAT: Tranexamic acid
AMYTAL: Amobarbital
ANADROL: Oxymetholone
ANALONE: Nandrolone decanoate
ANAPROX: Naproxen sodium
ANAREL: Guanadrel sulfate
ANAVAR: Oxandrolone
ANCEF: Cefazolin sodium
ANDROGYN LA: Testosterone enanthate
ANDRUSOL: Testosterone
ANECTINE: Succinylcholine chloride
ANHYDRON: Cyclothiazide
ANSPOR: Cephradine
ANTABUSE: Disulfiram
ANTEMAL: Pyrimethamine-sulfadoxine
ANTEPAR: Piperazine citrate
ANTHECOLE: Piperazine
ANTHIPHEN: Dichlorophen
ANTIMINTH: Pyrantel pamoate
ANTIVERT: Meclizine hydrochloride
ANTRENYL BROMIDE: Oxyphenonium bromide
ANTRYPOL: Suramin
ANTURANE: Sulfinpyrazone
APRESOLINE HYDROCHLORIDE: Hydralazine
    hydrochloride
APTINE: Alprenolol hydrochloride
AQUADIOL: Estradiol
AQUAMEPHYTON: Phytonadione
AQUATAG: Benzthiazide
AQUATENSEN: Methylclothiazide
ARALEN HYDROCHLORIDE: Chloroquine hy-
    drochloride (injection)
ARAMINE: Metaraminol bitartrate
ARFONAD: Trimethaphan camsylate
ARISTOCORT: Triamcinolone
ARPEZINE: Piperazine
ARQUEL: Meclofenamic acid
ARTANE: Trihexyphenidyl hydrochloride
ASELLACRIN: Somatropin
ASENDIN: Amoxapine
ASMATANE MIST: Epinephrine bitartrate
ASMINYL: Dyphylline
ASTIBAN: Stibocaptate
ATABRINE HYDROCHLORIDE: Quinacrine hy-
    drochloride
ATARAX: Hydroxyzine hydrochloride
ATHROMBIN-K: Warfarin potassium
ATIVAN: Lorazepam
ATROMID-S: Clofibrate
ATROVENT: Ipratropium bromide
AUGMENTIN: Amoxicillin and potassium clavuli-
    nate
AUTOPLEX: Activated factor IX complex
AVENTYL HYDROCHLORIDE: Nortriptyline hy-
    drochloride
AVLOCLOR: Chloroquine diphosphate
AVLOSULFON: Dapsone
AYGESTIN: Norethindrone acetate

AZAPEN: Methicillin sodium
AZLIN: Azlocillin
AZOLID: Phenylbutazone
AZULFIDINE: Sulfasalazine

BACTOCILL: Oxacillin sodium
BACTRIM: Trimethoprim-sulfamethoxazole (com-
    bination product)
BAL: Dimercaprol
BALUSIL: Chloroguanide
BANOCIDE: Diethylcarbamazine citrate
BANTHINE: Methantheline bromide
BASOQUIN: Amodiaquine dihydrochloride
BAYER 205: Suramin
BAYER 2502: Nifurtimox
BECLOVENT: Beclomethasone
BELGANYL: Suramin
BENACINE: Diphenhydramine hydrochloride, sco-
    polamine hydrobromide (combination product)
BENADRYL: Diphenhydramine hydrochloride
BENDECTIN: Doxylamine succinate, pyridoxine
    hydrochloride (combination product)
BENDOPA: Levodopa
BENEMID: Probenecid
BENISONE: Betamethasone benzoate
BENTYL: Dicyclomine hydrochloride
BENURON: Bendroflumethiazide
BENZEDREX: Propylhexedrine
BENZEDRINE: Amphetamine
BEROTEC: Fenoterol
BERUBIGEN: Cyanocobalamin
BETAGAN: Levobunolol
BETAPAR: Meprednisone
BETAPRED: Meprednisone
BETOPTIC: Butaxolol
BEZALIP: Bezafibrate
BICILLIN: Penicillin G benzathine
BiCNU: Carmustine
BILARCIL: Metrifonate
BILTRICIDE: Praziquantel
BISTRIUM BROMIDE: Hexamethonium bromide
BITIN: Bithionol
BLENOXANE: Bleomycin sulfate
BLEPHAMIDE LIQUIFILM: Prednisolone acetate,
    sulfacetamide sodium (combination product)
BLOCADREN: Timolol maleate
BONINE: Meclizine hydrochloride
BREOKINASE: Urokinase
BRETHINE: Terbutaline sulfate
BRETYLOL: Bretylium tosylate
BREVICON: Ethinyl estradiol, norethindrone (com-
    bination product)
BREVITAL SODIUM: Methohexital sodium
    (injection)
BRICANYL: Terbutaline sulfate
BROMSULPHALEIN: Sulfobromophthalein
    sodium
BRONKOMETER: Isoetharine
BRONKOSOL: Isoetharine
BUMEX: Bumetanide
BUPRENEX: Buprenorphine hydrochloride

BUTAZOLIDIN: Phenylbutazone

CAFERGOT: Caffeine, ergotamine tartrate (combination product)
CALAN: Verapamil hydrochloride
CALCIMAR: Calcitonin
CALCIPARINE: Calcium heparin
CAMOLAR HYDROCHLORIDE: Cycloguanil embonate
CAMOQUIN HYDROCHLORIDE: Amodiaquine hydrochloride
CANTIL: Mepenzolate bromide
CAPASTAT: Capreomycin
CAPOTEN: Captopril
CARAFATE: Sucralfate
CARBOCAINE: Mepivacaine hydrochloride
CARDIDIGIN: Digitoxin
CARDILATE: Erythrityl tetranitrate
CARDIZEM: Diltiazem hydrochloride
CARDRASE: Ethoxzolamide
CARICIDE: Diethylcarbamazine citrate
CATAPRES: Clonidine hydrochloride
CECLOR: Cefaclor
CEDUR: Bezafibrate
CEFADYL: Cephapirin sodium
CEFIZOX: Ceftizoxime sodium
CELBENIN: Methicillin sodium
CELESTONE: Betamethasone
CELONTIN: Methsuximide
CENERIDE: Praziquantel
CENTRAX: Prazepam
CEPHULAC: Lactulose
CERUBIDINE: Daunorubicin
CERVILAXIN: Relaxin
CESAMET: Nabilone
CESOL: Praziquantel
CHENIX: Chenodeoxycholic acid
CHLORIDIN: Pyrimethamine
CHLOROGUANIL: Chloroguanide
CHLOROMYCETIN: Chloramphenicol
CHLOROPTIC: Chloramphenicol
CHLOR-TRIMETON: Chlorpheniramine maleate
CHOLEDYL: Oxtriphylline
CHOLOXIN: Dextrothyroxine sodium
CHRONOGYN: Danazol
CHRONULAC: Lactulose
CHYMODIACTIN: Chymopapain
CIKLOCHIN: Cycloquine
CIN-QUIN: Quinidine sulfate
CIRCANOL: Ergoloid mesylates
CITANEST: Prilocaine hydrochloride
CLEOCIN: Clindamycin
CLINORIL: Sulindac
CLISTIN: Carbinoxamine maleate
CLODERM: Clocortolone pivalate
CLOMID: Clomiphene citrate
CLONOPIN: Clonazepam
CLOXAPEN: Cloxacillin sodium
CODROXOMIN: Hydroxocobalamin
COGENTIN: Benztropine mesylate
COGESTIN: Benztropine

COLESTID: Colestipol hydrochloride
COLY-MYCIN M: Colistimethate sodium
COMBANTRIN: Pyrantel pamoate
COMPAZINE: Prochlorperazine
CORDARONE: Amiodarone
CORDRAN: Flurandrenolide
CORGARD: Nadolol
CORT-DOME: Hydrocortisone
CORTEF: Hydrocortisone
CORTISPORIN: Bacitracin zinc, gramicidin, hydrocortisone (combination product)
CORTONE ACETATE: Cortisone acetate
CORTRIL: Hydrocortisone
CORTROSYN: Cosyntropin
CORVATON: Molsidomine
COSMEGEN: Dactinomycin
COTINAZIN: Isoniazid
COUMADIN: Warfarin sodium
CRASNITIN: Asparaginase
CRESCORMON: Somatropin
CRYSTODIGIN: Digitoxin
CRYSTOIDS: Hexylresorcinol
CUEMID: Cholestyramine
CUPRID: Trientine
CUPRIMINE: Penicillamine
CYCLOCORT: Amcinonide
CYCLOGYL: Cyclopentolate hydrochloride
CYCLOPAR: Tetracycline hydrochloride
CYCLO-PROSTIN: Epoprostenol
CYFOS: Ifosfamide
CYSTICID: Praziquantel
CYTADREN: Aminoglutethimide
CYTELLIN: Phytosterols (mixed)
CYTOMEL: Liothyronine
CYTOMINE: Liothyronine
CYTOSAR-U: Cytarabine
CYTOXAN: Cyclophosphamide

DALMANE: Flurazepam hydrochloride
DANOCRINE: Danazol
DANTRIUM: Dantrolene sodium
DAQUIN: Chlorazanil hydrochloride
DARANIDE: Dichlorphenamide
DARAPRAM: Pyrimethamine
DARAPRIM: Pyrimethamine
DARBID: Isopropamide iodide
DARICON: Oxyphencyclimine hydrochloride
DARVON: Propoxyphene hydrochloride
DATRIL: Acetaminophen
DAXOLIN: Loxapine succinate
DBI: Phenformin hydrochloride
DDAVP: Desmopressin acetate
DECADERM: Dexamethasone
DECADRON: Dexamethasone
DECAPRYN: Doxylamine
DECARIS: Levamisole
DECHOLIN: Dehydrocholic acid
DECLINAX: Debrisoquin sulfate
DECLOMYCIN: Demeclocycline hydrochloride
DELALUTIN: Hydroxyprogesterone caproate
DELATESTRYL: Testosterone enanthate

DELESTREC: Estradiol undecylate
DELESTROGEN: Estradiol valerate
DELTA-CORTEF: Prednisolone
DELTA-DOME: Prednisone
DELTALIN: Ergocalciferol
DELTASONE: Prednisone
DELTOIN: Methetoin
DEMEROL: Meperidine hydrochloride
DEMSER: Metyrosine
DEMULEN: Ethinyl estradiol, ethynodiol diacetate (combination product)
DENDRID: Idoxuridine
DE-NOL: Tripotassium dicitrato bismuthate
DEPAKENE: Valproic acid
DEPAKOTE: Divalproex sodium
DEPEN: Penicillamine
DEPINAR: Cyanocobalamin
DEPO-MEDROL: Methylprednisolone acetate
DEPO-PROVERA: Medroxyprogesterone acetate
DEPOVIRIN: Testosterone cypionate
DESFERAL: Deferoxamine mesylate
DESOXYN: Methamphetamine hydrochloride
DESYREL: Trazodone hydrochloride
DEXEDRINE: Dextroamphetamine
DIABETA: Glyburide
DIABINESE: Chlorpropamide
DIAMOX: Acetazolamide
DIAPID: Lypressin
DIBENZYLINE: Phenoxybenzamine hydrochloride
DICLOXIN: Dicloxacillin sodium
DICODID: Hydrocodone bitartrate
DIDRATE: Hydrocodone bitartrate
DIDREX: Benzphetamine hydrochloride
DIGISIDIN: Digitoxin
DIGITALINE NATIVELLE: Digitoxin
DIGUANYL: Chloroguanide
DILANTIN: Phenytoin
DILAUDID HYDROCHLORIDE: Hydromorphone hydrochloride
DIMETANE: Brompheniramine maleate
DIMOCILLIN: Methicillin
DINACRIN: Isoniazid
DIOGYN: Estradiol
DIPRIVAN: Disoprofol
DIPROLENE: Betamethasone dipropionate
DIPROSONE: Betamethasone dipropionate
DISCASE: Chymopapain
DISIPAL: Orphenadrine
DISOMER: Dexbrompheniramine
DISPERMIN: Piperazine
DIUCARDIN: Hydroflumethiazide
DIULO: Metolazone
DIUPRES: Chlorothiazide, reserpine (combination product)
DIURIL: Chlorothiazide
DOBUTREX: Dobutamine hydrochloride
DOLOBID: Diflunisal
DOLOPHINE: Methadone
DONNATAL: Atropine sulfate, hyoscyamine sulfate, phenobarbital, scopolamine hydrobromide (combination product)

DOPASTAT: Dopamine
DORIDEN: Glutethimide
DORSACAINE: Benoxinate hydrochloride
DRAMAMINE: Dimenhydrinate
DRINUPAL: Chloroguanide
DROCODE: Dihydrocodeine
DURABOLIN: Nandrolone phenpropionate
DURACILLIN: Penicillin G procaine (sterile)
DURANEST: Etidocaine
DURAQUIN: Quinidine gluconate
DYAZIDE: Hydrochlorothiazide, triamterene (combination product)
DYMELOR: Acetohexamide
DYRENIUM: Triamterene

ECODIDE: Echothiophate iodide
EDECRIN: Ethacrynic acid
EFUDEX: Fluorouracil
ELANTAN: Isosorbide mononitrate
ELAVIL: Amitriptyline hydrochloride
ELDISINE: Vindesine sulfate
ELECTROCORTIN: Aldosterone
ELIXICON: Theophylline
ELIXOPHYLLIN: Theophylline
ELKOSIN: Sulfisomidine
ELSPAR: Asparaginase
EMBEQUIN: Iodoquinol
EMCYT: Estramustine phosphate sodium
E-MYCIN: Erythromycin
ENDURON: Methyclothiazide
ENKADE: Encainide hydrochloride
ENOVID: Mestranol, norethynodrel (combination product)
ENTACYL: Piperazine
ENTERO-VIOFORM: Clioquinol
ENZEON: Chymotrypsin
ENZODASE: Hyaluronidase (injection)
EPITRATE: Epinephrine bitartrate
EQUA: Aspartame
EQUAGESIC: Aspirin, ethoheptazine citrate, meprobamate (combination product)
EQUAL: Aspartame
EQUANIL: Meprobamate
ERBAPRELINA: Pyrimethamine
ERGOMAR: Ergotamine tartrate
ERGOSTAT: Ergotamine tartrate
ERGOTRATE MALEATE: Ergonovine maleate
ERYTHROCIN: Erythromycin
ESIDRIX: Hydrochlorothiazide
ESKACILLIN: Penicillin G procaine (sterile)
ESTINYL: Ethinyl estradiol
ESTRACE: Estradiol
ESTRAGUARD: Dienestrol
ESTROVIS: Quinestrol
ETHAMIDE: Ethoxzolamide
ETHNOR: Levamisole
ETHRANE: Enflurane
ETRENOL: Hycanthone methanesulfonate
EURAX: Crotamiton
EUTHROID: Liotrix
EUTONYL: Pargyline hydrochloride

EVIPAL: Hexobarbital
EXNA: Benzthiazide

FACTREL: Gonadorelin hydrochloride
FALCIDAR: Pyrimethamine-sulfadoxine
FANSIDAR: Pyrimethamine-sulfadoxine
FASIGYN: Tinidazole
FEDRAZIL: Chlorcyclizine hydrochloride, pseudoephedrine hydrochloride (combination product)
FEIBA: Factor XIII inhibitor bypassing activity
FELDENE: Piroxicam
FEMINONE: Ethinyl estradiol
FILARABITS: Diethylcarbamazine citrate
FLAGYL: Metronidazole
FLAVOQUINE: Amodiaquine dihydrochloride
FLAXEDIL: Gallamine triethiodide
FLOLAN: Epoprostenol
FLORINEF: Fludrocortisone
FLORONE: Diflorasone diacetate
FLOROPRYL: Isoflurophate
FLUONID: Fluocinolone acetonide
FLUOROMAR: Fluroxene
FLUROBATE: Betamethasone benzoate
FOLVITE: Folic acid
FORANE: Isoflurane
FORHISTAL: Dimethindene
FORTRAL: Pentazocine
FULVICIN: Griseofulvin
FUNGIZONE: Amphotericin B
FURACIN: Nitrofurazone
FURADANTIN: Nitrofurantoin
FURAMIDE: Diloxanide furoate
FUROXONE: Furazolidone

GAMENE: Gamma benzene hexachloride
GAMMACORTEN: Dexamethasone
GAMMAR: Globulin, immune
GAMULIN: Globulin, immune
GANTRISIN: Sulfisoxazole
GEMONIL: Metharbital
GEOPEN: Carbenicillin disodium
GERMANIN: Suramin
GLIBENESE: Glipizide
GLUCOTROL: Glipizide
GLUTRIL: Glibornuride
GLYCOBARB: Glycopyrrolate
GRIFULVIN V: Griseofulvin
GUANATOL: Chloroguanide
GYNE-LOTRIMIN: Clotrimazole
GYNERGEN: Ergotamine tartrate

HALCION: Triazolam
HALDOL: Haloperidol
HALDRONE: Paramethasone acetate
HALOCHIN: Cycloquine
HALODRIN: Ethinyl estradiol, fluoxymesterone (combination product)
HALOG: Halcinonide
HALOTESTIN: Fluoxymesterone
HALOTEX: Haloprogin

HERBESSER: Diltiazem
HETRAZAN: Diethylcarbamazine citrate
HEXADROL: Dexamethasone
HISTALOG: Betazole hydrochloride
HISTIONEX: Phenyltoloxamine
HOLOCAINE HYDROCHLORIDE: Phenacaine hydrochloride
HUMATIN: Paromomycin sulfate
HUMORSOL: Demecarium bromide
HUMULIN: Human insulin
HYCODAN: Hydrocodone
HYDELTRA: Prednisolone
HYDERGINE: Ergoloid mesylates
HYDREA: Hydroxyurea
HYDRODIURIL: Hydrochlorothiazide
HYDROMOX: Quinethazone
HYDROPRES: Hydrochlorothiazide, reserpine (combination product)
HYGROTON: Chlorthalidone
HYKINONE: Menadione sodium bisulfite
HYKOLEX: Dehydrocholic acid
HYLOREL: Guanadrel sulfate
HYOSOL: Scopolamine hydrobromide
HYPERSTAT: Diazoxide

IFEX: Ifosfamide
ILOTYCIN: Erythromycin
IMFERON: Iron dextran (injection)
IMODIUM: Loperamide
IMURAN: Azathioprine
INDERAL: Propranolol hydrochloride
INDERIDE: Hydrochlorothiazide, propranolol hydrochloride (combination product)
INDOCIN: Indomethacin
INHISTON: Pheniramine
INNOVAR: Droperidol, fentanyl citrate (combination product)
INOCOR: Amrinone
INSULATARD: Semisynthetic human insulin
INTAL: Cromolyn sodium
INTROPIN: Dopamine hydrochloride
INVERSINE: Mecamylamine hydrochloride
ISMELIN: Guanethidine monosulfate
ISOCAINE: Mepivacaine
ISOPTIN: Verapamil hydrochloride
ISORDIL: Isosorbide dinitrate
ISUPREL HYDROCHLORIDE: Isoproterenol hydrochloride
IVADANTIN: Nitrofurantoin sodium

KAON: Potassium gluconate
KAYQUINONE: Menadione
KEFLEX: Cephalexin
KEFLIN: Cephalothin sodium
KEFLORIDIN: Cephaloridine
KEFORAL: Cephalexin
KEFZOL: Cefazolin sodium
KEMADRIN: Procyclidine
KENACORT: Triamcinolone
KENALOG: Triamcinolone acetonide
KETALAR: Ketamine hydrochloride

KETASET: Ketamine hydrochloride
KETRAX: Levamisole
KEVADON: Thalidomide
KITNOS: Etofamide
KONYNE: Factor IX complex
KWELL: Lindane

LAMPIT: Nifurtimox
LANODOXIN: Iodoquinol
LANOXIN: Digoxin
LARODOPA: Levodopa
LASIX: Furosemide
LEPADINA: Chloroguanide
LEUKERAN: Chlorambucil
LEVO-DROMORAN: Levorphanol tartrate
LEVOPA: Levodopa
LEVOPHED: Norepinephrine bitartrate
LEVOPROME: Methotrimeprazine
LEVOTHROID: Levothyroxine sodium
LIBRAX: Chlordiazepoxide hydrochloride, clidinium bromide (combination product)
LIBRIUM: Chlordiazepoxide hydrochloride
LIDANAR: Mesoridazine
LIDEX: Fluocinonide
LIDONE: Molindone
LINCOCIN: Lincomycin
LIORESAL: Baclofen
LIPANTHYL: Fenofibrate
LIPO-HEPIN: Heparin sodium
LIQUAEMIN SODIUM: Heparin sodium
LIQUAMAR: Phenprocoumon
LIQUAPEN: Penicillin G potassium
LITHANE: Lithium carbonate
LITHONATE: Lithium carbonate
LITHOTABS: Lithium carbonate
LOCOID: Hydrocortisone butyrate
LOCORTEN: Flumethasone pivalate
LODOSYN: Carbidopa
LOESTRIN: Ethinyl estradiol, norethindrone (combination product)
LOMIDINE: Pentamidine
LOMOTIL: Atropine sulfate, diphenoxylate hydrochloride (combination product)
LONITEN: Minoxidil
LO/OVRAL: Ethinyl estradiol, norgestrel (combination product)
LOPID: Gemfibrozil
LOPRESSOR: Metoprolol tartrate
LOPROX: Ciclopirox olamine
LORELCO: Probucol
LORFAN: Levallorphan tartrate
LORIDINE: Cephaloridine
LORINAL: Chloral hydrate
LOROTHIDOL: Bithionol
LOTRIMIN: Clotrimazole
LOXITANE: Loxapine
LOZOL: Indapamide
LUDIOMIL: Maprotiline
LUMINAL: Phenobarbital
LUPRON: Leuprolide
LYNORAL: Ethinyl estradiol

LYSODREN: Mitotane

MADRIBON: Sulfadimethoxine
MAKAROL: Diethylstilbestrol
MALOCIDE: Pyrimethamine
MANDELAMINE: Methenamine mandelate
MANSIL: Oxamniquine
MARCAINE: Bupivacaine hydrochloride
MARCOUMAR: Phenprocoumon
MARCUMAR: Phenprocoumon
MAREZINE: Cyclizine
MARINOL: Dronabinol
MARPLAN: Isocarboxazid
MATULANE: Procarbazine hydrochloride
MAXIDEX: Dexamethasone
MAXIFLOR: Diflorasone diacetate
MEBADIN: Oral dehydroemetine resinate
MEBARAL: Mephobarbital
MEBINOL: Clefamide
MECLOMEN: Meclofenamate sodium
MEDROL: Methylprednisolone acetate
MEFOXIN: Cefoxitin
MEGACE: Megestrol acetate
MELLARIL: Thioridazine
MELOXINE: Methoxsalen
MELTROL-50: Phenformin
MEPACRINE: Quinacrine
MEPADIN: Meperidine hydrochloride
MEPHYTON: Phytonadione
MERCODINONE: Hydrocodone bitartrate
MERITAL: Nomifensine
MESANTOIN: Mephenytoin
MESTINON: Pyridostigmine bromide
METAHYDRIN: Trichlormethiazide
METANDREN: Methyltestosterone
METAPREL: Metaproterenol sulfate
METATENSIN: Reserpine, trichlormethiazide (combination product)
METHADOSE: Methadone hydrochloride
METHERGINE: Methylergonovine maleate
METHIPOX: Pyrimethamine-sulfadoxine
METHORATE: Dextromethorphan hydrobromide
METICORTEN: Prednisone
METI-DERM: Prednisolone
METOPIRONE: Metyrapone
METUBINE: Dimethyltubocurarine
METYCAINE HYDROCHLORIDE: Piperocaine hydrochloride
MEXITIL: Mexiletine
MEZLIN: Mezlocillin
MICATIN: Miconazole
MICREST: Diethylstilbestrol
MICRONASE: Glyburide
MICRONOR: Norethindrone
MIDAMOR: Amiloride hydrochloride
MILONTIN: Phensuximide
MILTOWN: Meprobamate
MINIDIAB: Glipizide
MINIHIST: Pyrilamine maleate
MINIPRESS: Prazosin hydrochloride
MINOCIN: Minocycline hydrochloride

MINOCYN: Minocycline
MINODIAB: Glipizide
MINTEZOL: Thiabendazole
MIOSTAT: Carbachol
MITHRACIN: Mithramycin
MITOCIN-C: Mitomycin
MITOMYCIN C: Mitomycin
MOBAN: Molindone
MOCTANIN: Monooctanoin
MODICON: Ethinyl estradiol, norethindrone (combination product)
MODURETIC: Amiloride
MOGADON: Nitrazepam
MONISTAT IV: Miconazole
MONOTARD: Human insulin
MOTRIN: Ibuprofen
MOXAM: Moxalactam disodium
MUCOMYST: Acetylcysteine
MURCIL: Chlordiazepoxide hydrochloride
MUSTARGEN: Mechlorethamine hydrochloride
MUTAMYCIN: Mitomycin
MYAMBUTOL: Ethambutol hydrochloride
MYCELEX: Clotrimazole
MYCOSTATIN: Nystatin
MYDRIACYL: Tropicamide
MYLERAN: Busulfan
MYOCHRYSINE: Gold sodium thiomalate
MYSOLINE: Primidone
MYTELASE: Ambenonium

NALFON: Fenoprofen calcium
NALLINE: Nalorphine hydrochloride
NALUTRON: Progesterone
NAPHURIDE: Suramin
NAPROSYN: Naproxen
NAQUA: Trichlormethiazide
NARCAN: Naloxone hydrochloride
NARDIL: Phenelzine sulfate
NATURETIN: Bendroflumethiazide
NAVANE: Thiothixene
NEBCIN: Tobramycin sulfate (injection)
NEBS: Acetaminophen
NEGGRAM: Nalidixic acid
NEMBUTAL: Pentobarbital
NEO-ANTERGAN: Pyrilamine
NEOBIOTIC: Neomycin sulfate
NEOCAINE: Procaine hydrochloride
NEO-CORTEF: Hydrocortisone acetate, neomycin sulfate (combination product)
NEOPHYL: Dyphylline
NEOSPORIN: Neomycin sulfate, polymyxin B sulfate (combination product)
NEO-SYNEPHRINE: Phenylephrine
NEPTAZANE: Methazolamide
NESACAINE: Chloroprocaine hydrochloride
NETROMYCIN: Netilmicin sulfate
NEUTRAPEN: Penicillinase
NICLOCIDE: Niclosamide
NICONYL: Isoniazid
NIDATON: Isoniazid
NIGRIN: Streptonigrin

NILSTAT: Nystatin
NIOFORM: Clioquinol
NIPRIDE: Sodium nitroprusside
NISENTIL: Alphaprodine
NITRODISC: Nitroglycerin (tablets)
NITRONG: Nitroglycerin (tablets)
NITROPRESS: Sodium nitroprusside
NITROSPAN: Nitroglycerin (tablets)
NITROSTAT: Nitroglycerin (tablets)
NIVAQUINE: Chloroquine sulfate
NIZORAL: Ketoconazole
NOBESE: Phenylpropanolamine hydrochloride
NOCTEC: Chloral hydrate
NOLUDAR: Methyprylon
NOLVADEX: Tamoxifen citrate
NORCURON: Vecuronium
NORDETTE: Ethinyl estradiol, norgestrel (combination product)
NORFLEX: Orphenadrine citrate
NORINYL: Ethinyl estradiol, norethindrone (combination product)
NORINYL: Mestranol, norethindrone (combination product)
NORISODRINE SULFATE: Isoproterenol sulfate
NORLESTRIN: Ethinyl estradiol, norethindrone acetate (combination product)
NORLUTATE: Norethindrone acetate
NORLUTIN: Norethindrone
NORMODYNE: Labetalol
NORPACE: Disopyramide phosphate
NORPRAMIN: Desipramine hydrochloride
NOR-QD: Norethindrone
NOTEZINE: Diethylcarbamazine citrate
NOVAFED: Pseudoephedrine hydrochloride
NOVAHISTINE: Chlorpheniramine maleate, phenylephrine hydrochloride (combination product)
NOVANTRONE: Mitoxantrone
NOVOCAIN: Procaine
NOVOLIN L: Human insulin
NOVOLIN N: Human insulin
NOVOLIN R: Human insulin
NUBAIN: Nalbuphine hydrochloride
NUMORPHAN: Oxymorphone hydrochloride
NUPERCAINAL: Dibucaine
NUPERCAINE HYDROCHLORIDE: Dibucaine hydrochloride
NUPRIN: Ibuprofen
NUTRASWEET: Aspartame
NYDRAZID: Isoniazid

OBEDRIN-LA: Methamphetamine hydrochloride
OCUSERT: Pilocarpine
OGEN: Estropipate
OMNIPEN: Ampicillin
ONCOVIN: Vincristine sulfate
OPTIMIL: Methaqualone hydrochloride
ORACON: Dimethisterone, ethinyl estradiol (combination product)
ORAFLEX: Benoxaprofen
ORAGRAFIN: Ipodate

ORA-LUTIN: Ethisterone
ORA-TESTRYL: Fluoxymesterone
ORATROL: Dichlorphenamide
ORAVIRON: Methyltestosterone
ORENZYME: Chymotrypsin
ORETIC: Hydrochlorothiazide
ORETON: Testosterone
ORGATRAX: Hydroxyzine hydrochloride
ORINASE: Tolbutamide
ORTHO-NOVUM: Ethinyl estradiol, norethindrone
(combination product)
ORTHO-NOVUM: Mestranol, norethindrone (combination product)
OVCON: Ethinyl estradiol, norethindrone (combination product)
OVOCYLIN: Estradiol
OVRAL: Ethinyl estradiol, norgestrel (combination product)
OVRETTE: Norgestrel
OVULEN: Mestranol, ethynodiol diacetate (combination product)
OXLOPAR: Oxytetracycline hydrochloride
OXSORALEN: Methoxsalen
OXURASIN: Piperazine
OXYLONE: Fluorometholone
OXYZIN: Piperazine

PAGITANE: Cycrimine
PALUDRINE: Chloroguanide
PALUSIL: Chloroguanide
PAMELOR: Nortriptyline hydrochloride
PAMINE BROMIDE: Methscopolamine bromide
PANMYCIN: Tetracycline
PANTERIC: Pancreatin
PANWARFIN: Warfarin sodium
PARACORT: Prednisone
PARACORTOL: Prednisolone
PARAFLEX: Chlorzoxazone
PAREDRINE: Hydroxyamphetamine hydrobromide
PARENCILLIN: Penicillin G procaine (sterile)
PARFURAN: Nitrofurantoin
PARLODEL: Bromocriptine mesylate
PARNATE: Tranylcypromine sulfate
PAROIDIN: Parathyroid (injection)
PARSIDOL: Ethopropazine
PATHILON: Tridihexethyl chloride
PATHOCIL: Dicloxacillin sodium
PAVABID: Papaverine hydrochloride
PAVULON: Pancuronium bromide
PEDIAMYCIN: Erythromycin ethylsuccinate
PEGANONE: Ethotoin
PEMOPHYLLIN: Theophylline sodium glycinate
PEN A/N: Ampicillin sodium
PENAPAR VK: Penicillin V potassium
PENISEM: Penicillin G potassium
PENTAM 300: Pentamidine isethionate
PENTHRANE: Methoxyflurane
PENTOSTAM: Sodium stibogluconate
PENTOTHAL SODIUM: Thiopental sodium
PENTRITOL: Pentaerythritol tetranitrate
PEN-VEE K: Penicillin V potassium

PEPTAVLON: Pentagastrin
PERAZIL: Chlorcyclizine
PERCODAN: Aspirin, oxycodone hydrochloride
(combination product)
PERCOGESIC WITH CODEINE: Acetaminophen,
codeine phosphate (combination product)
PERCORTEN ACETATE: Desoxycorticosterone
acetate
PERGONAL: Menotropins
PERIACTIN: Cyproheptadine hydrochloride
PERIN: Piperazine
PERITRATE: Pentaerythritol tetranitrate
PERMAPEN: Penicillin G benzathine
PERMITIL: Fluphenazine hydrochloride
PERSANTINE: Dipyridamole
PERTOFRANE: Desipramine hydrochloride
PETHIDINE HYDROCHLORIDE: Meperidine hydrochloride
PHENAPHEN: Acetaminophen
PHENERGAN: Promethazine hydrochloride
PHENOXENE: Chlorphenoxamine
PHENURONE: Phenacemide
PHOSPHOLINE IODIDE: Echothiophate iodide
PHYLLOCONTIN: Aminophylline
PIPANOL: Trihexyphenidyl hydrochloride
PIPERAT: Piperazine
PIPIZAN: Piperazine
PITOCIN: Oxytocin (injection)
PITRESSIN: Vasopressin
PLACIDYL: Ethchlorvynol
PLAQUENIL: Hydroxychloroquine
PLASIN: Chloroguanide
PLATINOL: Cisplatin
POLARAMINE: Dexchlorpheniramine
POLYCILLIN: Ampicillin
POLYMOX: Amoxicillin
POLYSPORIN: Bacitracin zinc, polymyxin B sulfate
(combination product)
PONSTAN: Mefenamic acid
PONSTEL: Mefenamic acid
PONTOCAINE: Tetracaine
POVAN: Pyrvinium pamoate
PRANONE: Ethisterone
PRANTAL: Diphemanil
PRANTURON: Gonadotropin, chorionic
PRED FORTE: Prednisolone
PRED MILD: Prednisolone
PREDNE-DOME: Prednisolone
PREGNYL: Gonadotropin, chorionic
PREGOVA: Menotropins
PRELUDIN: Phenmetrazine hydrochloride
PREMARIN: Estrogens, conjugated
PREPCORT: Hydrocortisone
PRESAMINE: Imipramine hydrochloride
PRE-SATE: Chlorphentermine hydrochloride
PRESSONEX: Metaraminol bitartrate
PRESSOROL: Metaraminol bitartrate
PRIMAXIN: Imipenem and cilastatin
PRINCIPEN: Ampicillin
PRIODERM: Malathion
PRIPSEN: Piperazine

PRISCOLINE HYDROCHLORIDE: Tolazoline hydrochloride
PRIVINE HYDROCHLORIDE: Naphazoline hydrochloride
PROAQUA: Benzthiazide
PRO-BANTHINE: Propantheline bromide
PROCAN: Procainamide hydrochloride
PROCARDIA: Nifedipine
PROCETOFEN: Fenofibrate
PRO-CORT: Hydrocortisone
PROCTOCORT: Hydrocortisone
PRODROXAN: Ethisterone
PROGESTAB: Ethisterone
PROGESTEROL: Progesterone
PROGESTORAL: Ethisterone
PROGLYCEM: Diazoxide
PROGUANIDE: Chloroguanide
PROGYNON: Estradiol
PROKETAZINE: Carphenazine
PROLIXIN: Fluphenazine hydrochloride
PROLOID: Thyroglobulin
PROLOPRIM: Trimethoprim
PROLUTON: Progesterone
PRONESTYL: Procainamide hydrochloride
PROPADRINE: Phenylpropanolamine hydrochloride
PROPLEX: Factor IX complex
PROPOQUIN: Amopyroquin
PROSTAPHLIN: Oxacillin sodium
PROSTIGMIN: Neostigmine bromide
PROSTIGMIN: Neostigmine methylsulfate
PROSTIN VR PEDIATRIC: Alprostadil
PROTEF: Hydrocortisone acetate, neomycin sulfate (combination product)
PROTOPAM CHLORIDE: Pralidoxime chloride
PROTROPIN: Somatrem
PROVENTIL: Albuterol
PROVERA: Medroxyprogesterone acetate
PROVIGAN: Promethazine hydrochloride
PSP-IV: Prednisolone sodium phosphate
PURINETHOL: Mercaptopurine
PURODIGIN, CRYSTALLINE: Digitoxin
PYMAFED: Pyrilamine maleate
PYOPEN: Carbenicillin disodium
PYRATHYN: Methapyrilene hydrochloride
PYRIBENZAMINE: Tripelennamine
PYRIDIUM: Phenazopyridine

QUAALUDE: Methaqualone
QUANTREL: Pyrantel with oxantel pamoate
QUARZAN: Clidinium
QUELICIN: Succinylcholine chloride
QUESTRAN: Cholestyramine resin
QUIDE: Piperacetazine
QUINADOME: Iodoquinol
QUINAGLUTE: Quinidine gluconate
QUINAMIN: Quinine sulfate
QUINE: Quinine sulfate
QUINICARDINE: Quinidine sulfate
QUINIDEX: Quinidine sulfate
QUINITE: Quinine sulfate

RAU-SED: Reserpine
RAUZIDE: Bendroflumethiazide, *Rauwolfia serpentina* (combination product)
REDISOL: Cyanocobalamin
REGITINE: Phentolamine
REGLAN: Metoclopramide hydrochloride
REGONOL: Pyridostigmine bromide
REGROTON: Chlorthalidone, reserpine (combination product)
RELEASIN: Relaxin
RELEFACT-TRH: Protirelin
REMSED: Promethazine hydrochloride
RENAFUR: Nifuradene
RENESE: Polythiazide
RESERPOID: Reserpine
RESOCHIN: Chloroquine diphosphate
RESPAIRE: Acetylcysteine
RESTORIL: Temazepam
RETET: Tetracycline hydrochloride
RETIN-A: Tretinoin
RhoGAM: Rh_o (D) immune globulin
RID: Pyrethrins, piperonyl butoxide
RIDAURA: Auranofin
RIFADIN: Rifampin
RIMACTANE: Rifampin
RIMIFON: Isoniazid
RITALIN HYDROCHLORIDE: Methylphenidate hydrochloride
ROBAXIN: Methocarbamol
ROBINUL: Glycopyrrolate
ROBITUSSIN: Glyceryl guaiacolate
ROHYPNOL: Flunitrazepam
ROMILAR: Dextromethorphan hydrobromide
RONDOMYCIN: Methacycline hydrochloride
RONIACOL: Nicotinyl alcohol
RUFEN: Ibuprofen

SALISBURYSTIN: Pentamustine
SALURON: Hydroflumethiazide
SALUTENSIN: Hydroflumethiazide, reserpine (combination product)
SANDIMMUNE: Cyclosporine
SANDRIL: Reserpine
SANSERT: Methysergide maleate
SARENIN: Saralasin acetate
SAVORQUIN: Iodoquinol
SCABENE: Lindane
SEBAQUIN: Iodoquinol
SECONAL: Secobarbital
SEMIKON: Methapyrilene
SEMOXYDRINE: Methamphetamine
SENSORCAINE: Bupivacaine hydrochloride
SEPTRA: Trimethoprim-sulfamethoxazole (combination product)
SERAX: Oxazepam
SERENIUM: Ethoxazene hydrochloride
SERENTIL: Mesoridazine
SERNYLAN: Phencyclidine hydrochloride
SEROMYCIN: Cycloserine
SERPASIL: Reserpine
SERPILOID: Reserpine

SINEMET: Carbidopa, levodopa (combination product)
SINEQUAN: Doxepin hydrochloride
SKELAXIN: Metaxolone
SLO-BID: Theophylline
SLO-PHYLLIN: Theophylline
SODIUM VERSENATE: Edetate disodium
SOLASKIL: Levamisole
SOLFOTON: Phenobarbital
SOLGANAL: Aurothioglucose
SOLU-CORTEF: Hydrocortisone
SOLU-MEDROL: Methylprednisolone
SOLU-PREDALONE: Prednisolone
SOMOPHYLLIN: Aminophylline
SOPOR: Methaqualone
SORBITRATE: Isosorbide dinitrate
SORQUAD: Isosorbide dinitrate
SPARINE: Promazine hydrochloride
SPECTAZOLE: Econazole
SPONTIN: Ristocetin
STADOL: Butorphanol
STAPHCILLIN: Methicillin sodium
STECLIN: Tetracycline hydrochloride
STELAZINE: Trifluoperazine hydrochloride
STENTAL: Phenobarbital
STERANE: Prednisolone
STILBETIN: Diethylstilbestrol
STREPTASE: Streptokinase
STRYCIN: Streptomycin sulfate (sterile)
SUBLIMAZE: Fentanyl citrate
SUCOSTRIN CHLORIDE: Succinylcholine chloride
SULFACTOL: Sodium thiosulfate
SULFALAR: Sulfisoxazole
SULFAMYLON: Mafenide
SULFATRYL: Trisulfapyrimidines (oral suspension)
SULFIZIN: Sulfisoxazole
SULFONSOL: Trisulfapyrimidines (oral suspension)
SULFOSE: Trisulfapyrimidines (oral suspension)
SULTRIN: Sulfabenzamide, sulfacetamide, sulfathiazole (combination product)
SUMOX: Amoxicillin
SUMYCIN: Tetracycline hydrochloride
SUPEN: Ampicillin
SUPRARENIN: Epinephrine bitartrate
SURITAL: Thiamylal sodium (injection)
SURMONTIL: Trimipramine
SUSADRIN: Nitroglycerin (tablets)
SUS-PHRINE: Epinephrine
SUX-CERT: Succinylcholine chloride
SYMMETREL: Amantadine hydrochloride
SYNALAR: Fluocinolone acetonide
SYNANDRETS: Methyltestosterone
SYNANDROL: Testosterone propionate
SYNCILLIN: Phenethicillin potassium
SYNEMOL: Fluocinolone acetonide
SYNERONE: Testosterone propionate
SYNESTROL: Dienestrol
SYNGESTERONE: Progesterone

SYNGESTRETS: Progesterone
SYNGESTROTABS: Ethisterone
SYNKAYVITE: Menadiol sodium diphosphate
SYNTHROID: Levothyroxine sodium
SYNTOCINON: Oxytocin (injection)
SYTOBEX: Cyanocobalamin

TACE: Chlorotrianisene
TAGAMET: Cimetidine
TALWIN: Pentazocine
TAMBOCOR: Flecainide acetate
TANDEARIL: Oxyphenbutazone
TAO: Troleandomycin
TAPAR: Acetaminophen
TAPAZOLE: Methimazole
TARACTAN: Chlorprothixene
TASK: Dichlorvos
TEDRAL: Ephedrine hydrochloride, phenobarbital, theophylline (combination product)
TEGISON: Etretinate
TEGOPEN: Cloxacillin sodium
TEGRETOL: Carbamazepine
TELDRIN: Chlorpheniramine maleate
TELOPAR: Oxantel pamoate
TEMARIL: Trimeprazine tartrate
TEMGESIC: Buprenorphine
TEMPRA: Acetaminophen
TENORMIN: Atenolol
TENSILON: Edrophonium chloride
TERFONYL: Trisulfapyrimidines (oral suspension)
TERRA-CORTRIL: Hydrocortisone acetate, oxytetracycline hydrochloride (combination product)
TERRAMYCIN: Oxytetracycline
TERRASTATIN: Nystatin, oxytetracycline (combination product)
TESTATE: Testosterone enanthate
TESTORA: Methyltestosterone
TESTOSTROVAL: Testosterone enanthate
TESTRED: Methyltestosterone
TETRACYN: Tetracycline
TETRAMINE: Oxytetracycline hydrochloride
THEACITIN: Theophylline sodium acetate
THEELIN: Estrone
THEELOL: Estriol
THENYLENE HYDROCHLORIDE: Methapyrilene hydrochloride
THEOCALCIN: Theobromine calcium salicylate
THEOCIN: Theophylline sodium acetate
THEO-DUR: Theophylline
THEOLAIR: Theophylline
THEOPHYL: Theophylline
THEPHORIN: Phenindamine tartrate
THIOSULFIL: Sulfamethizole
THIURETIC: Hydrochlorothiazide
THORAZINE: Chlorpromazine
THYLOGEN MALEATE: Pyrilamine maleate
THYLOQUINONE: Menadione
THYPINONE: Protirelin
THYRACTIN: Thyroglobulin

THYRAR: Thyroid
THYROLAR: Liotrix
THYROPROTEIN: Thyroglobulin
THYTROPAR: Thyrotropin
TICAR: Ticarcillin disodium
TIGASON: Etretinate
TIMOLATE: Timolol maleate
TIMOPTIC: Timolol maleate
TIMOPTOL: Timolol maleate
TINACTIN: Tolnaftate
TINDAL: Acetophenazine maleate
T-IONATE-PA: Testosterone cypionate
TIRIAN: Chloroguanide
TISIN: Isoniazid
TOBREX: Tobramycin
TOFRANIL: Imipramine hydrochloride
TOLECTIN: Tolmetin sodium
TOLINASE: Tolazamide
TOLSEROL: Mephenesin
TONOCARD: Tocainide
TOPAZONE: Furazolidone
TOPICORT: Desoximetasone
TOPICYCLINE: Tetracycline hydrochloride
TOPILAN: Chloroprednisone acetate
TOPSYN: Fluocinonide
TORECAN: Thiethylperazine
TOTACILLIN: Ampicillin
TRACRIUM: Atracurium
TRAL: Hexocyclium
TRAMACIN: Triamcinolone acetonide
TRAMISOL (as hydrochloride): Levamisole hydrochloride
TRANDATE: Labetalol hydrochloride
TRANMEP: Meprobamate
TRANXENE: Clorazepate dipotassium
TRASYLOL: Aprotinin
TRECATOR-SC: Ethionamide
TREMIN: Trihexyphenidyl hydrochloride
TREST: Methixene
TRIACET: Triamcinolone acetonide
TRIAZURE: Azaribine
TRICOFURON: Furazolidone, nifuroxime (combination product)
TRIDESILON: Desonide
TRIDIONE: Trimethadione
TRILAFON: Perphenazine
TRIMETON: Pheniramine
TRIMOX (as trihydrate): Amoxicillin
TRIMPEX: Trimethoprim
TRIND: Chlorpheniramine maleate, phenylpropanolamine hydrochloride (combination product)
TRI-NORINYL: Ethinyl estradiol, norethindrone (combination product)
TRIPERIDOL: Trifluperidol
TRIPHASIL: Ethinyl estradiol, norgestrel (combination product)
TRIPTIL: Protriptyline hydrochloride
TRISEM: Trisulfapyrimidines (oral suspension)
TRISORALEN: Trioxsalen
TROBICIN: Spectinomycin hydrochloride

TROCINATE: Thiphenamil
TRONOLANE: Pramoxine hydrochloride
TRONOTHANE HYDROCHLORIDE: Pramoxine hydrochloride
TROSINONE: Ethisterone
TRUOZINE: Trisulfapyrimidines (oral suspension)
TUBARINE: Tubocurarine chloride
TUINAL: Amobarbital sodium, secobarbital sodium (combination product)
TYLAN: Tylosin
TYLENOL: Acetaminophen
TYLOSTERONE: Diethylstilbestrol, methyltestosterone (combination product)
TYLOX: Acetaminophen, oxycodone hydrochloride (combination product)
TYMTRAN: Cyclophosphamide
TYVID: Isoniazid

U-GENCIN: Gentamicin sulfate
ULCERBAN: Sucralfate
ULTANDREN: Fluoxymesterone
ULTRACEF: Cefadroxil
ULTRASUL: Sulfamethizole
UNAKALM: Ketazolam
UNIDIGIN: Digitoxin
UNIPEN: Nafcillin sodium
UNIPRES: Hydralazine hydrochloride, hydrochlorothiazide, reserpine (combination product)
UNISOM: Doxylamine succinate
URECHOLINE: Bethanechol chloride
URITONE: Methenamine
UROPEN: Hetacillin potassium
UTERACON: Oxytocin (injection)
UTICILLIN VK: Penicillin V potassium
UTICORT: Betamethasone benzoate
UTIMOX: Amoxicillin

VAGESTROL: Diethylstilbestrol
VALADOL: Acetaminophen
VALISONE: Betamethasone valerate
VALIUM: Diazepam
VALMID: Ethinamate
VALPIN 50: Anisotropine
VANACTANE: Viomycin
VANCERIL: Beclomethasone dipropionate
VANCOCIN HYDROCHLORIDE: Vancomycin hydrochloride
VANDID: Ethamivan
VANSIL: Oxamniquine
VAPO-ISO: Isoproterenol hydrochloride
VARDAX: Sulmazole
VASOCON: Naphazoline hydrochloride
VASOCON-A: Antazoline phosphate, naphazoline hydrochloride (combination product)
VASOTEC: Enalapril
VASOXYL: Methoxamine hydrochloride
VATENSOL: Guanoclor sulfate
V-CILLIN: Penicillin V
VECTRIN: Minocycline hydrochloride
VEETIDS: Penicillin V potassium

VELBAN: Vinblastine sulfate
VELOSEF: Cephradine
VELOSULIN: Semisynthetic human insulin
VENTOLIN: Albuterol sulfate
VEPESID: Etoposide
VERMAGO: Piperazine
VERMIDOL: Piperazine
VERMOX: Mebendazole
VEROXIL: Piperazine
VERSAPEN: Hetacillin
VERSENATE: Ethylenediamine-tetraacetic acid
VERSENE CA: Edetate calcium disodium
VERSTRAN: Prazepam
VESPRIN: Triflupromazine hydrochloride
VETALAR: Ketamine hydrochloride
VIBRAMYCIN: Doxycycline
VINISIL: Povidone
VIOCIN SULFATE: Viomycin sulfate (sterile)
VIOFORM: Clioquinol
VIRA-A: Vidarabine
VIRAZOLE: Ribavirin
VIROPTIC: Trifluridine
VISKEN: Pindolol
VISTARIL: Hydroxyzine
VISTRAX: Hydroxyzine hydrochloride, oxyphency-
    climine hydrochloride (combination product)
VI-TWEL: Cyanocobalamin
VIVACTIL: Protriptyline hydrochloride
VONTIL: Thioproperazine mesylate
VONTROL: Diphenidol

WELFERON: Interferon
WELLBUTRIN: Bupropion hydrochloride
WESTCORT CREAM: Hydrocortisone valerate
WINSTROL: Stanozolol
WINTOMYLON: Nalidixic acid

WYACORT: Methylprednisolone
WYAMINE SULFATE: Mephentermine sulfate
WYAMYCIN E: Erythromycin ethylsuccinate
WYAMYCIN S: Erythromycin stearate
WYCILLIN: Penicillin G procaine (sterile)
WYGESIC: Acetaminophen, propoxyphene hy-
    drochloride (combination product)
WYMOX: Amoxicillin
WYNESTRON: Estrone
WYTENSIN: Guanabenz acetate

XANAX: Alprazolam
XYLOCAINE: Lidocaine

YODOXIN: Iodoquinol
YOMESAN: Niclosamide
YUTOPAR: Ritodrine hydrochloride

ZACTANE: Ethoheptazine citrate
ZACTIRIN: Aspirin, ethoheptazine citrate (combi-
    nation product)
ZANOSAR: Streptozocin
ZARONTIN: Ethosuximide
ZAROXOLYN: Metolazone
ZENTAL: Albendazole
ZEPHIRAN: Benzalkonium chloride
ZIDE: Hydrochlorothiazide
ZIRADRYL: Diphenhydramine hydrochloride, zinc
    oxide (combination product)
ZOLYSE: Chymotrypsin
ZOMAX: Zomepirac sodium
ZOVIRAX: Acyclovir
ZYLOPRIM: Allopurinol

Index

The indexers have tried to emphasize major discussions of drugs and drug groups, so that drugs mentioned in passing or in minor applications may not be listed. Disease names are indexed also, however, so that it should be possible to locate every mention of a drug the reader is interested in. Trade names of combination remedies are indexed without generic components in most cases, but the components are listed on the page cited. The reader should consult the Trade Names/Generic Names Appendix as a means of quick reference to identify generic names when only the trade name is known. British readers should note that only American generic and trade names are indexed, but the indexers feel that the differences are either trivial (phenobarbit*al,* -barbit*one*) or both rare and well known (meperidine, pethidine).

Analgesic(s) (cont'd)
  nonopioid, **408–409**
  opioid,
    and antagonists, **336–349**
    basic pharmacology of, **336–344**
    clinical pharmacology of, 344
    OTC
      hidden ingredients in, 800
      ingredients of, 798
Analgesic sedatives, as cytochrome
    P-450 inhibitor, 40
Anaphylaxis
  mechanisms of, 714
  sympathomimetic drugs in, 93
Anaprox (naproxen), 401
Ancylostoma duodenale
  albendazole for, 642
  drugs for, 642
  tetrachloroethylene for, 660
Androgen replacement therapy, 480
  preparations for, 480
Androgenic hormones, for breast can-
    cer, 694
Androgens, 478
  for breast cancer, 694
  for cancer chemotherapy, 687, 688
    dosages and toxicities of, 682
  preparations available, 479
  suppression of, 481
Androstanolone, 479
Anectine (succinylcholine), 296, 841
Anemia(s), **362–371**
  and alcohol abuse, 257
  androgens for, 480
  aplastic, and chloramphenicol, 528
  folic acid for, 365
  pernicious, 370
  vitamin B_{12} for, 365
Anesthesia
  local, H_1 antagonists in, 189
  and neuromuscular blocking drugs,
    301
  opioid analgesics for, 286, 345
  sedative-hypnotics in, 248
  signs and stages of, 280
  surgical, stage of, 280
  general, **279–288**
    basic pharmacology of, **279–283**
    clinical pharmacology of, **284–288**
    sites of action of, 235
    types of, 279
  inhaled, **284–286**
  intravenous, **286–287**
  local, **289–294**
    and autonomic transmission, 60
    basic pharmacology of, **289–292**
    clinical pharmacology of, **293–294**
  in OTC products, 800
"Angel dust," abuse of, 357
Angina
  classic, 134
  of effort, 134
    nitrate effects in, 128
  mixed, 135
  Prinzmetal's, 199
  treatment of, nitrate and nitrite drugs
    for, 129
  unstable, 135
    nitrate effects in, 129
  variant, 134
    diagnosis of, ergonovine in, 199
    nitrate effects in, 129

Angina pectoris
  drugs used in, clinical pharmacology
    of, **134–136**
  general management of, 136
  treatment of, **125–137**
Angioplasty, transluminal coronary,
    135
Angiostrongylus cantonensis, drugs for,
    642
Angiotensin, **201–205,** 421
  analogs of, 204
  biosynthesis of, 201
  inhibitors of, **120–121**
  for hypertension, 107
Angiotensin I, 202
Angiotensin II
  actions of, 203
  and angiotensinogen production, 202
  and autonomic transmission, 60
  metabolism of, 204
  and renin secretion, 202
  structure of, 204
Angiotensin receptors, 203
Angiotensin-converting enzyme, 201
Angiotensinogen, 202
Anhydron (cyclothiazide), 176
Aniline
  phase I biotransformation reactions
    in, 40
  phase II biotransformation reactions
    in, 40
Animal(s)
  absorption, distribution, and elimina-
    tion in, **808–812**
  antimicrobial drug therapy in, 815
  breast milk of, antimicrobial agents
    in, 810
  defective metabolic pathway in, 811
  and disease states, drug kinetics in,
    817
  disposition curve in, 812
  dosage regimens in, 814
  drug absorption through skin in, 809
  drug administration in, 814
  drug residues in, 812
  elimination half-lives in, 814
  neonatal, **816**
    absorption in, 816
    metabolic pathways in, 816
    renal excretion in, 817
  parenteral preparations in, long-act-
    ing, 815
  pharmacokinetics in, 812, 813
  plasma protein binding in, 810
Animal proteins, hypersensitivity to,
    599
Anion gap acidosis, drug-induced, 742
Anion inhibitors, 442
Anion overdose, loop agents for, 174
Anisotropine, dosage of, 79
Anorexin Capsules, 800
ANP (atrial natriuretic peptide), 208
Ansamycin, 545
Antabuse (disulfiram), 833
Antacids, 781
  aluminum, and laboratory tests, 829
  and antimicrobials, 584
  calcium, and laboratory tests, 829
  OTC
    hidden ingredients in, 800
    ingredients of, 798, 800

Antacids (cont'd)
  interactions with other drugs, 820
  liquid, 781
  and tetracyclines, 530
Antagonism, drug
  mechanisms of, 15
  physiologic, 16
Antagonist(s)
  for adrenoceptors, selectivity of, 96
  chemical, 16
  competitive, 11
  defined, 9
  irreversible, 11
  opioid, 349
Antazoline, 189
Antepar (piperazine), 654
Anterior pituitary hormones, **423–433**
Anthelmintic drugs, **641–664**
Anthiphen (dichlorophen), 644
Anthracyclines, for cancer chemother-
    apy, 678
Anthrax
  drugs for, 575
  vaccine for, 598
Antiadrenoceptor actions, of H_1 antago-
    nists, 189
Antiandrogens, 481
Antiarrhythmic drugs
  and aging, 760
  basic pharmacology of, **155–166**
  and cardiac sodium channel, interac-
    tion of, 158
  clinical pharmacology of, **166–167**
  membrane actions of, 159
  and neuromuscular blocking drugs,
    302
  properties of, 160
Antiarrhythmic therapy, principles of,
    166
Antibacterial agents. *See also specific*
    drugs and classes of drugs.
  topical, **765–766**
Antibiotics. *See also specific drugs and*
    classes of drugs.
  for amebiasis, 635
  for cancer chemotherapy, 668,
    678–682
  for neuromuscular blocking drugs,
    302
  topical, in acne, 766
Antibodies
  antilymphocyte, 710
    clinical use of, 712
  as immunosuppressive agents, 709
Antibody-immunoglobulin, structural
    characteristics of, 706
Anticancer drugs
  cell cycle relationships of, 668
  investigational, 686
  miscellaneous, **684**
    dosages and toxicities of, 685
Anticholinergic drugs. *See* Antimus-
    carinic drugs.
Anticholinesterases
  poisoning due to, 745
  sites of action of, 235
Anticholinoceptor actions, of H_1 antag-
    onists, 189
Anticoagulants
  and alcohol, 820
  and allopurinol, 820

Fluphenazine, 320
  dosages of, 320
  pK$_a$ of, 2
  structure of, 316
  for tics, 313
Fluprednisolone, 453
Flurandrenolide, efficacy of, 775
Flurazepam, 244
  biodispositional properties of, 246
  chemical structure of, 242
  dosage of, 251
  hepatic clearance of, effects of age
    on, 757
  pharmacokinetics of, 244
Flurobate (betamethasone benzoate),
    775
Fluorocarbons, as drugs of abuse, 360
Fluoroxene, as cytochrome P-450 in-
    hibitor, 40
Flutamide, 481
FMN, 38
Folacin, structure of, 366
Folic acid
  in anemia, 365
  deficiency of, 370
  structure of, 367, 675
Follicle-stimulating hormone, 421, **430**
Follicular development and regression,
    during normal menstrual cycle,
    461
Food and Drug Administration, 48
Food, Drug, and Cosmetic Act (1938),
    48
Formaldehyde, as antimicrobial, 602
Formic acid blood levels, in methanol
    intoxication, 260
Formula 44 Cough Disc, 800
Formula 44D, 800
4-Way Cold Tablets, 800
Foxglove, toxic syndromes of, 742
Framycetin, 536
Francisella tularensis, drugs for, 575
"Free base," 355
FSH, 421, **430**
Ftorafur, 676, 686
  structure of, 676
5-FU (fluorouracil), 676
FUDR, 676
Full agonists, 13
Fulvicin (griseofulvin), 835
Fungi, drugs for, **554–558,** 576
  topical, **766–768**
Fungizone (amphotericin B), 635, 768
Furacin (nitrofurazone), 605
Furadantin (nitrofurantoin), 605
Furamide (diloxanide furoate), 628,
    632
Furosemide, pharmacokinetic parame-
    ters of, 24
Furazolidone, 569
  and laboratory tests, 833
Furosemide, 172
  and beta-adrenoceptor blockers, 822
  for chronic heart failure, 147
  for hypertension, 108
  and laboratory tests, 833
  and NSAIDs, 824
  pK$_a$ of, 2
  structure of, 172
Furoxone (furazolidone), 833
Fusobacterium, drugs for, 575

**GABA (gamma-aminobutyric acid),
  236, 238, 245**
  CNS pharmacology of, 238
GABA-benzodiazepine-chloride channel
    receptor complex, proposed model
    of, 247
GABA-modulin, 246
Gallamine, 296
  autonomic effects of, 301
  structure of, 297
Gallstones, dissolution of, 785
Gametocides, 618
Gamma benzene hexachloride, 769
Gamma globulin, 559, 590
  clinical use of, in immunosuppres-
    sion, 712
Gamma-aminobutyric acid (GABA),
    236, 245
Ganglion-blocking drugs
  as antihypertensive agents, 112
  pharmacology of, **81–83**
Gardnerella vaginalis, metronidazole
    for, 638
Gasoline
  as drug of abuse, 360
  toxic syndromes of, 741
Gastric acid secretion, testing of, 187
Gastric lavage, in poisoning, 744
Gastric ulcer, cimetidine for, 192
Gastrointestinal absorption, in animals,
    808
Gastrointestinal disease, eicosanoids in,
    220
Gastrointestinal motility, drugs promot-
    ing, 784
Gastrointestinal tract
  and alcohol abuse, 256
  and aspirin, 399
  and bromocriptine, 310
  carcinomas of, 696
  and chloramphenicol, 527
  and cholinergic stimulants, 66, 67
  and cholinesterase inhibitors, 71, 72
  diseases of, drugs used in, **781–787**
  disorders of
    antimuscarinic agents for, 78, 79
    due to oral contraceptives, 475
  in drug excretion, 5
  and emetine and dehydroemetine,
    631
  and erythromycins, 566
  and ganglion-blocking drugs, 82
  and lead, 732
  and levodopa, 308
  and methylxanthines, 226
  and morphine, 343
  and serotonin, 194
  smooth muscle of
    and eicosanoids, 217
    and histamine, 186
    and sympathomimetic drugs, 88
    and tetracyclines, 530
    and thyroid hormones, 440
Gating mechanism, 152
Gaviscon, 782
Gelusil, 798
Gelusil-II, 781, 798
Gemfibrozil
  for hyperlipidemias, 391
  for hyperlipoproteinemias, 387
  structure of, 392

Gemonil (metharbital), 268
Gene-active hormones, 418
General anesthetics, **279–288**
  basic pharmacology of, **279–284**
  clinical pharmacology of, **284–287**
  types of, 279
Generalized seizures
  defined, 275
  drugs for, 276
Generic prescribing, 805
Genitourinary tract
  and antimuscarinic agents, 78, 79
  and cholinergic stimulants, 67
  and ganglion-blocking drugs, 82
  and morphine, 343
  and sympathomimetic drugs, 88, 93
Gentamicin, 512, **537,**
  absorption of, in neonate, 751
  in microbial infections, 576, 577
  pharmacokinetic parameters of, 24
  in renal failure, 581
  structure of, 534
  topical, 765
  for urinary tract infections, 571
Gentisic acid, structure of, 398
Geopen (carbenicillin), 831
Geriatric pharmacology, **756–763**
  practical aspects of, 762
Germanin (suramin), 637, 659
GH, 416, 419, **425**
Giardia lamblia, purine metabolism in,
    612
Giardiasis
  metronidazole for, 637
  treatment of, 638
GIH, 425
Gilles de la Tourette's syndrome, 306,
    313
  antipsychotics for, 319
Gingivitis, metronidazole for, 638
Glabrous skin, tinea infections of, 768
Glanders, drugs for, 575
Glandular kallikreins, 205
Glaucoma
  beta-blocking drugs for, 102
  carbonic anhydrase inhibitors for,
    171
  cholinesterase inhibitors for, 69, 71
  and levodopa, 309
  sympathomimetic drugs in, 93
Glibenclamide (glyburide), 493
  structure and dosage of, 492
Glicentin, 495
Glipizide, structure and dosage of, 492
Glipizide (Glucotrol), 492, 493
Glomerular filtration, in drug excretion,
    5
Glomerulopathy, minimal change, and
    lithium, 325
Glucagon, 421, **494–496**
  amino acid sequence of, 494
  and laboratory tests, 833
Glucocorticoids, 418, **449–457**
  as antirheumatics, 407
  and bone mineral homeostasis, 500
  in hypercalcemia, 503
  in immunosuppression, 707
  intermediate-acting, 453
  long-acting, 453
  metabolism of, 41
  short-acting, 453

Lange Medical Publications titles are available at all medical bookstores within the USA. If you wish to order directly from the publisher, please complete and mail the attached postage-paid card. Where applicable, availability is indicated in parentheses.

1. **Current Medical Diagnosis & Treatment 1986,** Krupp et al (A0025-5) **$29.50**

2. **Current Pediatric Diagnosis & Treatment, 9th ed.,** Kempe et al (A1414-0) **$29.00** (9/86)

3. **Current Obstetric & Gynecologic Diagnosis & Treatment, 6th ed.,** Benson (A1412-4) **$28.00** (11/86)

4. **Current Emergency Diagnosis & Treatment, 2nd.,** Mills et al (A0027) **$28.00**

5. **Current Surgical Diagnosis & Treatment, 7th ed.,** Way (A0019) **$31.50**

6. **Basic & Clinical Pharmacology, 3rd ed.,** Katzung (A0553-6) **$28.00** (9/86)

7. **Pharmacology: A Review,** Katzung & Trevor (A0031) **$13.00**

8. **Review of General Psychiatry,** Goldman (A0030) **$24.00**

9. **Basic & Clinical Endocrinology, 2nd ed.,** Greenspan & Forsham (A0547-8) **$27.00** (9/86)

10. **Basic & Clinical Immunology, 6th ed.,** Stites et al (A0548-6) **$27.50** (11/86)

11. **Harper's Review of Biochemistry, 20th ed.,** Martin et al (A0003) **$24.50**

12. **Biochemistry: A Synopsis,** Colby (A0033) **$13.00**

13. **Basic Histology, 5th ed.,** Junqueira et al (A0570-0) **$21.50**

14. **Review of Medical Physiology, 12th ed.,** Ganong (A0013) **$22.50**

15. **Physiology: A Study Guide,** Ganong (A0032) **$12.00**

16. **Review of Medical Microbiology, 17th ed.,** Jawetz et al (A8432-5) **$20.00** (9/86)

17. **Correlative Neuroanatomy & Functional Neurology, 19th ed.,** Chusid (A0001) **$19.50**

18. **General Urology, 11th ed.,** Smith (A0009) **$24.00**

19. **General Ophthalmology, 11th ed.,** Vaughan & Asbury (A3108-6) **$22.00**

20. **Principles of Clinical Electrocardiography, 12th ed.,** Goldman (A0008) **$19.00**

21. **Clinical Cardiology, 4th ed.,** Sokolow & McIlroy (A0023) **$26.50** (6/86)

22. **Electrocardiography: Essentials of Interpretation,** Goldschlager & Goldman (A0029) **$13.00**

23. **Physician's Handbook, 21st ed.,** Krupp et al (A0002) **$16.50**

24. **Handbook of Pediatrics, 15th ed.,** Silver et al (A3635-8) **$16.50** (10/86)

25. **Handbook of Poisoning, 12th ed.,** Dreisbach & Robertson (A3643-2) **$16.50** (12/86)

26. **Handbook of Obstetrics & Gynecology, 9th ed.,** Benson (A3627-5) **$16.50** (11/86)

ORDER CARD

Please send me the following books. If I wish, I may return the book(s) within 30 days and receive a full credit/refund.

1. Krupp (A0025-5) $29.50
2. Kempe (A1414-0) $29.00
3. Benson (A1412-4) $28.00
4. Mills (A0027-1) $28.00
5. Way (A0019-8) $31.50
6. Katzung (A0553-6) $28.00
7. Katzung (A0031-3) $13.00
8. Goldman (A0030-5) $24.00
9. Greenspan (A0547-8) $27.00

10. Stites (A0548-6) $27.50
11. Martin (A0003-2) $24.50
12. Colby (A0033-9) $13.00
13. Junqueira (A0570-0) $21.50
14. Ganong (A0013-1) $22.50
15. Ganong (A0032-1) $12.00
16. Jawetz (A8432-5) $20.00
17. Chusid (A0001-6) $19.50
18. Smith (A0009-9) $24.00

19. Vaughan (A3108-6) $22.00
20. Goldman (A0008-1) $19.00
21. Sokolow (A0023-0) $26.50
22. Goldschlager (A0029-7) $13.00
23. Krupp (A0002-4) $16.50
24. Silver (A3635-8) $16.50
25. Dreisbach (A3643-2) $16.50
26. Benson (A3627-5) $16.50

☐ Payment enclosed, including handling charge.
☐ Charge to my   ☐ VISA   ☐ Mastercard

Name _____

Address _____

City/State/Zip _____

Signature _____

Affiliation _____

Card Number _____

Expiration Date _____

Amount $ _____
State Tax $ _____
Handling $ _____
TOTAL $ _____

Mail and make check payable to:

Appleton-Century-Crofts
25 Van Zant St.
E. Norwalk, CT 06855

Prices are subject to change without notice. Prices advertised are applicable in the U.S., its territories and possessions only. For orders outside the U.S. and Canada contact: Prentice-Hall Intl., Englewood Cliffs, NJ 07632. In Canada, contact: Prentice-Hall Canada, Scarborough, Ontario, M1P 2J7.

BUSINESS REPLY MAIL
FIRST CLASS PERMIT NO. 150 E. NORWALK, CT

POSTAGE WILL BE PAID BY ADDRESSEE

NO POSTAGE
NECESSARY
IF MAILED
IN THE
UNITED STATES

APPLETON-CENTURY-CROFTS
LANGE MEDICAL PUBLICATIONS

DEPARTMENT B
25 VAN ZANT STREET
EAST NORWALK, CT 06855

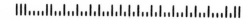